The Great Ormond Street Hospital

Manual of Children and Young People's Nursing Practices

The Great Ormond Street Hospital

Manual of Children and Young People's Nursing Practices

Second Edition

Edited by

Elizabeth Anne Bruce

MSc, BSc (hons), RN (Child), RN (Adult)
Clinical Nurse Specialist, Pain Control Service, and Project Lead,
Nursing Great Ormond Street Hospital for Children NHS Foundation Trust
London, UK

Janet Williss

MSc, BSc, RN (Child), RN (Adult), ONC Cert
Formerly Deputy Chief Nurse
Great Ormond Street Hospital for Children NHS Foundation Trust
London, UK

Faith Gibson

PhD, MSc, RN (Child), RN (Adult), ONC cert, Cert Ed, RNT, FRCN, FAAN
Professor of Child Health and Cancer Care, University of Surrey
Director of Research, Nursing and Allied Health
Great Ormond Street Hospital for Children NHS Foundation Trust
London, UK

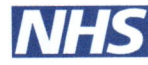

Great Ormond Street Hospital for Children
NHS Foundation Trust

WILEY Blackwell

This edition first published 2023
© 2023 John Wiley & Sons Ltd

Edition History
© 2012 Great Ormond Street Hospital for Children NHS Foundation Trust. Published 2012 by Blackwell Publishing Ltd.

All rights reserved. No part of this publication may be reproduced, stored in a retrieval system, or transmitted, in any form or by any means, electronic, mechanical, photocopying, recording or otherwise, except as permitted by law. Advice on how to obtain permission to reuse material from this title is available at http://www.wiley.com/go/permissions.

The right of Elizabeth Anne Bruce, Janet Williss, and Faith Gibson to be identified as the authors of the editorial material in this work has been asserted in accordance with law.

Registered Offices
John Wiley & Sons, Inc., 111 River Street, Hoboken, NJ 07030, USA
John Wiley & Sons Ltd, The Atrium, Southern Gate, Chichester, West Sussex, PO19 8SQ, UK

For details of our global editorial offices, customer services, and more information about Wiley products visit us at www.wiley.com.

Wiley also publishes its books in a variety of electronic formats and by print-on-demand. Some content that appears in standard print versions of this book may not be available in other formats.

Trademarks: Wiley and the Wiley logo are trademarks or registered trademarks of John Wiley & Sons, Inc. and/or its affiliates in the United States and other countries and may not be used without written permission. All other trademarks are the property of their respective owners. John Wiley & Sons, Inc. is not associated with any product or vendor mentioned in this book.

Limit of Liability/Disclaimer of Warranty
The contents of this work are intended to further general scientific research, understanding, and discussion only and are not intended and should not be relied upon as recommending or promoting scientific method, diagnosis, or treatment by physicians for any particular patient. In view of ongoing research, equipment modifications, changes in governmental regulations, and the constant flow of information relating to the use of medicines, equipment, and devices, the reader is urged to review and evaluate the information provided in the package insert or instructions for each medicine, equipment, or device for, among other things, any changes in the instructions or indication of usage and for added warnings and precautions. While the publisher and authors have used their best efforts in preparing this work, they make no representations or warranties with respect to the accuracy or completeness of the contents of this work and specifically disclaim all warranties, including without limitation any implied warranties of merchantability or fitness for a particular purpose. No warranty may be created or extended by sales representatives, written sales materials or promotional statements for this work. The fact that an organization, website, or product is referred to in this work as a citation and/or potential source of further information does not mean that the publisher and authors endorse the information or services the organization, website, or product may provide or recommendations it may make. This work is sold with the understanding that the publisher is not engaged in rendering professional services. The advice and strategies contained herein may not be suitable for your situation. You should consult with a specialist where appropriate. Further, readers should be aware that websites listed in this work may have changed or disappeared between when this work was written and when it is read. Neither the publisher nor authors shall be liable for any loss of profit or any other commercial damages, including but not limited to special, incidental, consequential, or other damages.

Library of Congress Cataloging-in-Publication Data

Names: Bruce, Elizabeth Anne, editor. | Williss, Janet, editor. |
  Gibson, Faith, editor.
Title: The Great Ormond Street Hospital manual of children and young
  people's nursing practices / edited by Elizabeth Anne Bruce, Janet Williss, Faith Gibson.
Other titles: Great Ormond Street Hospital manual of children's nursing
  practices | Manual of children and young people's nursing practice
Description: 2nd edition. | Hoboken, NJ : Wiley-Blackwell, 2023. | Preceded
  by The Great Ormond Street Hospital manual of children's nursing
  practices / edited by Susan Macqueen, Elizabeth Anne Bruce, Faith
  Gibson. 2012. | Includes bibliographical references and index.
Identifiers: LCCN 2020021837 (print) | LCCN 2020021838 (ebook) | ISBN
  9781118898222 (paperback) | ISBN 9781119099710 (adobe pdf) | ISBN
  9781119099703 (epub)
Subjects: MESH: Great Ormond Street Hospital for Children NHS Foundation
  Trust. | Pediatric Nursing–methods | Evidence-Based Nursing | Infant |
  Child | Adolescent
Classification: LCC RJ245 (print) | LCC RJ245 (ebook) | NLM WY 159 |
  DDC 618.92/00231–dc23
LC record available at https://lccn.loc.gov/2020021837
LC ebook record available at https://lccn.loc.gov/2020021838

Cover Design: Wiley
Cover Image: Courtesy of The Great Ormond Street Hospital Children's Charity

Set in 9/10pt Rockwell by Straive, Pondicherry, India
Printed and bound by CPI Group (UK) Ltd, Croydon, CR0 4YY

Contents

Foreword — xiii
Editorial panel — xiv
List of contributors — xv
Introduction — xx

1 Assessment — 1
Sue Chapman, Eileen Brennan, and Lindy May

Introduction — 2
Section 1: General principles — 2
Section 2: Present illness — 4
Section 3: Past history — 4
Section 4: Family history — 5
Section 5: Vital signs and baseline measurements — 6
Section 6: Assessment of body systems — 19
References — 25

Procedure guidelines
1.1 General principles of assessment — 2
1.2 Present illness — 4
1.3 Past history — 4
1.4 Family history — 5
1.5 Monitoring plan and early warning score — 6
1.6 Measuring temperature — 6
1.7 Measuring heart rate — 7
1.8 Measuring respiratory rate — 8
1.9 Measuring blood pressure — 8
1.10 Measuring oxygen saturation — 14
1.11 Growth assessment — 14
1.12 Measuring height — 15
1.13 Measuring weight — 16
1.14 Measuring head circumference — 18
1.15 Assessing the respiratory and cardiovascular systems — 19
1.16 Assessing the neurological system — 20
1.17 Assessing nutrition — 22
1.18 Assessing elimination and sexual development — 22
1.19 Assessing skin and hygiene — 23
1.20 Assessing mobility — 24
1.21 Assessing development — 25
1.22 Other relevant information — 25

2 Allergy and anaphylaxis — 29
Róisín Fitzsimons

Introduction — 30
Allergy and the immune response — 30
Diagnosis and management of allergy — 30
Management of anaphylaxis — 32
Food allergy — 34
Respiratory allergy — 37
Allergens in the healthcare setting — 39
Conclusion — 41
References — 41

3 Biopsies — 43
Zoe Wilks, Eileen Brennan, Nikki Bennett-Rees, Alex M. Barnacle, Kishore Minhas, and Anne-Marie Kao

Introduction — 44
Liver biopsy — 44
Punch skin biopsy — 49
Renal biopsy — 54
Bone marrow aspirate and trephine — 57
References — 59

Procedure guidelines
3.1 Preoperative preparation (liver biopsy) — 46
3.2 Perioperative procedure (liver biopsy) — 47
3.3 Postoperative care (liver biopsy) — 48
3.4 Punch skin biopsy — 50
3.5 Preparation of the CYP (skin biopsy) — 50
3.6 Preparation of equipment (skin biopsy) — 51
3.7 Punch skin biopsy procedure — 51
3.8 Postprocedural care (skin biopsy) — 53
3.9 Preoperative procedure (renal biopsy) — 55
3.10 Postoperative procedure (renal biopsy) — 56
3.11 Preparation of equipment and environment (aspiration/trephine) — 57
3.12 Preparation of CYP and family (aspiration/trephine) — 57
3.13 Aspiration/trephine procedure — 58
3.14 Postprocedure care (aspiration/trephine) — 58

4 Administration of blood components and products — 61
Kate Khair, Lisa Baldry, and Rachel Moss

Introduction — 62
An overview of blood transfusion — 62
Administration of blood components — 66
Coagulation factors — 70
Conclusion — 71
References — 71

Procedure guidelines
4.1 Preparation – CYP and family (transfusion) — 63
4.2 Preparation – prescription (transfusion) — 63
4.3 Preparation – transfusion — 63
4.4 Infuse component – identity check and administration — 65
4.5 Infuse product – observations, recordings and traceability — 65
4.6 Reaction management (transfusion) — 66
4.7 Infuse component (albumin) — 67
4.8 Observations and recordings (albumin) — 67
4.9 Preparation – CYP and family (immunoglobulin) — 68
4.10 Preparation – prescription (immunoglobulin) — 68
4.11 Preparation – equipment for intravenous or subcutaneous infusion of immunoglobulin — 68

Contents

4.12	Procedure – intravenous infusion (immunoglobulin)	69
4.13	Procedure – subcutaneous infusion (immunoglobulin)	69
4.14	Reaction management (immunoglobulin)	70
4.15	Completing the infusion (immunoglobulin)	70

5 Bowel care — 73
Helen Johnson and June Rogers

Introduction	74
Diarrhoea	74
Constipation	74
Laxatives	75
Preparation for investigations or surgery	76
Treatment of faecal soiling/incontinence	76
Products to help with the management of faecal incontinence/soiling	76
Factors to note	84
Stoma pouch selection	85
References	85

Procedure guidelines

5.1	Administering a rectal suppository	78
5.2	Administering an enema	79
5.3	Rectal washout on an infant	80
5.4	Anal irrigation	80
5.5	Antegrade colonic enema (ACE washout)	81
5.6	Stoma siting	82
5.7	Changing a pouch	83

6 Burns and scalds — 87
Brian McGowan and Sally Robertson

Introduction	88
Common causes of burns in CYPs	88
Overview of anatomy of the skin	88
Classification of burns	89
First aid following a burn	89
Assessment	90
Fluid resuscitation for major burns	90
Wound healing	91
Wound care	92
Choice of dressing	94
Nutrition	94
Psychological care following a burn	94
References	96

Procedure guidelines

6.1	First aid following a burn	89
6.2	Assessment of a burn	90
6.3	Dressing changes	92
6.4	Referral to the community children's nursing team	94
6.5	Ongoing care of the child	95
6.6	Health promotion and education following a burn	95

7 Complementary and alternative medicine (CAM) — 99
Jenni Hallman

Introduction and definitions	100
A brief history of CAM and surrounding legislation	100
The five most commonly used CAM	101
Disclosure of CAM to healthcare practitioners	102
Massage therapy	102
A practical example of a massage therapy service	103
Case studies	109
Conclusion	110
References	110

Procedure guideline

7.1	Massage	103

8 Administration of systemic anti-cancer treatment (SACT) — 113
Emily Baker, Nicky Farrell, Bhumik Patel, Cindy Sparkes, and Julie Bayliss

Introduction	114
Legislation and recommendations	114
Consent	114
Safe handling	114
Reconstitution and preparation of chemotherapeutic agents	114
Personal protective equipment (PPE)	115
Work practices	115
Safe administration of SACT	115
Routes of administration	116
References	122

Procedure guideline

8.1	Administration of SACT via the intravenous route	118
8.2	Administration of SACT via the oral route	121
8.3	Extravasation (Adapted from EONS 2012)	121

9 Early recognition and management of the seriously ill child — 123
Denise Welsby and Liesje Andre

Introduction	124
Prevention: The 'chain of prevention'	124
Early recognition of the seriously ill child	124
Rapid assessment using the A-E assessment tool	125
'Just in case'/'just in time' training and situational awareness	127
AVPU (neurological observations)	127
Supporting the CYP using the structured A-E assessment tool	127
References	130

10 Fluid balance — 133
Eileen Brennan, John Courtney, and Josephine Jim

Introduction	134
Maintenance of fluid requirements	134
Fluid balance in the ill CYP	134
Renal replacement therapy (RRT)	134
Vascular access	136
Haemofiltration (HF)	136
Haemodialysis (HD)	136
Dialysis fluid for HD	137
Haemofiltration	139
Peritoneal dialysis (PD)	139
Types of PD	139
Preparing the CYP for dialysis access	141
References	154
Further reading	155

Procedure guidelines

10.1	Fluid input/output	141
10.2	Preparation of the CYP and family for HD/HF	142
10.3	Inserting a catheter (HD/HF)	142
10.4	Preparing the equipment (HF)	143
10.5	Preparation for HF	144
10.6	Starting CRRT	144
10.7	Monitoring and maintaining CRRT	146
10.8	Discontinuing CRRT	147
10.9	Commencing HD	149
10.10	Discontinuing HD	150
10.11	Preparation (PD)	150
10.12	Preparation for surgery (PD)	151
10.13	Starting PD for AKI	151
10.14	Care of the CYP on PD	153
10.15	Special considerations (PD)	153
10.16	Discontinuing PD	154

11 Personal hygiene and pressure ulcer prevention — 157
Sarah Kipps, Rachel Allaway, and Sarah Carmichael

Introduction	158
Bathing	158
Toileting	159
Nappy and incontinence pad care	161
Nail care	165
Oral hygiene	165
Oral assessment	166
Eye care	169
Ear care	170
Pressure ulcer prevention and management	171
Management of pressure ulcers	176
Conclusion	177
References	197

Procedure guidelines
11.1	Assessment for bathing	178
11.2	Baby bathing	178
11.3	Topping and tailing	180
11.4	Washing and bathing the CYP	180
11.5	Bed bathing	181
11.6	Bathing the CYP with special needs	182
11.7	Assessment of toileting needs	182
11.8	Toileting the CYP	183
11.9	Assessing nappy rashes	185
11.10	Routine nappy care	185
11.11	Nail assessment	187
11.12	Nail care	187
11.13	Oral assessment	188
11.14	Oral hygiene tools	189
11.15	Performing oral care	191
11.16	Oral health promotion	192
11.17	Oral care during compromised health	192
11.18	Eye care	194
11.19	Administration of eye drops	195
11.20	Insertion of contact lenses	196
11.21	Removal of soft contact lenses	196
11.22	Removal of gas permeable contact lenses and all contact lenses	196
11.23	Care of contact lenses	196
11.24	Administration of ear drops	197

12 Immunisation — 201
Helen Bedford

Introduction	202
Routine immunisation schedule for CYPs in the UK	202
Special risk groups	203
Immunity	203
Types of vaccine	204
General considerations	204
Specific diseases and the vaccines	206
Vaccines not in general use in UK	213
Storage and administration of vaccines	213
Ensuring good uptake	213
Vaccine safety scares	214
Immunisation of healthcare workers	214
Conclusion	215
References	215
Further reading	216

Procedure guideline
12.1	Administration of vaccines	205

13 Infection prevention and control — 217
Barbara Brekle

Introduction	218
Financial burden of healthcare associated infections	218
The health and social care act 2008: Code of practice on the prevention and control of infections and related guidance	218
Antibiotic resistance and antimicrobial stewardship	219
The chain of infection	219
Standard precautions	221
Isolation nursing	239
Management of exposure to blood and body fluids	240
Reporting of injuries, diseases and dangerous occurrences regulations	242
Decontamination of equipment and the environment	243
References	245
Further reading	247

Procedure guidelines
13.1	Hand decontamination techniques	233
13.2	Hand drying techniques	234
13.3	Inoculation with blood or body fluids	242
13.4	Dealing with spillage of blood or other body fluids	243

14 Intravenous and intra-arterial access and infusions — 249
Anne Ho, Hannah Barron, and Lorna O'Rourke

Introduction	250
Aseptic nontouch technique (ANTT®) for intravenous therapy	250
Visual infusion phlebitis (VIP)	260
Types of central venous access devices (CVADs)	268
CVAD dressings	269
Common CVAD complications	280
Safety aspects for staff and families	287
Neonatal longlines (PICCs); nursing management	294
Arterial lines	298
References	306
Further reading	309

Procedure guidelines
14.1	ANTT® for intravenous therapy	251
14.2	General principles: cannulation	255
14.3	Planning and preparation for peripheral venous cannulation	256
14.4	Peripheral venous cannulation	256
14.5	Cannula dressing	259
14.6	Flushing the peripheral venous cannula	261
14.7	Administration of a bolus medication via a peripheral cannula	262
14.8	Administration of an infused medication via a peripheral cannula	263
14.9	Blood sampling from a peripheral cannula	265
14.10	Removal of a peripheral cannula	267
14.11	CVAD: CVAD dressing	271
14.12	CVAD: changing the needle-free access device	272
14.13	Accessing CVADs: flushing	272
14.14	Accessing CVADs: administration of a medication bolus	273
14.15	Accessing CVADs: administration of a medication infusion via a syringe pump	274
14.16	Accessing CVADs: administration of a medication infusion via a volumetric pump	275
14.17	Accessing an implanted port	277
14.18	De-Accessing an implanted port	279
14.19	Assessing a CVAD for occlusions	283
14.20	Instillation of alteplase into a CVAD	284
14.21	Immediate care of a PICC or Hickman® with a fracture, hole, or split	287
14.22	Action required with a pulled-out PICC or Hickman®	287

14.23	Repair of a single lumen Groshong® NXT ClearVue® PICC	288
14.24	Repair of a Broviac® or Hickman®	290
14.25	Removal of a noncuffed PICC stitched in situ	293
14.26	Neonatal longline dressing change	296
14.27	Neonatal longlines: nursing care (general)	297
14.28	Removal of neonatal longlines	298
14.29	Intra-arterial lines: preparation of child and family	298
14.30	Insertion of an intra-arterial line	299
14.31	Preparation: system setup (inter-arterial infusion)	301
14.32	Maintenance: calibration	301
14.33	Maintenance: maintaining patency	302
14.34	Maintenance: observations	302
14.35	Blood sampling (arterial)	303
14.36	Troubleshooting: dampened trace	304
14.37	Troubleshooting: abnormal readings	305
14.38	Troubleshooting: puncture site bleeding	305
14.39	Troubleshooting: circulation compromise	305
14.40	Troubleshooting: no waveform	305
14.41	Removal of arterial cannula	306

15 Investigations — 313
Barbara Brekle, Annabel Linger, Di Robertshaw, and Melanie Hiorns

Introduction	314
Collection of microbiological specimens	314
Ward-based investigations	331
Radiological investigations	346
References	353

Procedure guidelines

15.1	Taking a blood culture	315
15.2	Capillary blood sampling	317
15.3	Collecting a sample of chest drain fluid	320
15.4	Collecting fungal samples	321
15.5	Collecting gastric samples	321
15.6	Collecting a nasopharyngeal aspirate	322
15.7	Collecting sputum samples	322
15.8	Collecting a stool (faecal) specimen	323
15.9	Taking a cough swab	323
15.10	Taking an ear swab	324
15.11	Taking an eye swab	324
15.12	Collecting nose swabs	325
15.13	Taking an oral fluid (saliva) swab	325
15.14	Collecting pernasal swabs	326
15.15	Taking skin (screening) swabs	326
15.16	Taking throat swabs	326
15.17	Taking a vulval swab for the investigation of simple vaginal discharge	327
15.18	Taking a wound swab	328
15.19	Collecting a urine specimen	328
15.20	Collecting vesicular fluid	330
15.21	Blood glucose monitoring	332
15.22	Three-lead continuous ECG monitoring	335
15.23	Performing a 12-lead ECG	337
15.24	Measuring glomerular filtration rate	339
15.25	Care of the CYP during a radiological investigation	347

16 Learning (intellectual) disabilities — 357
Jim Blair

Introduction	358
Principles underpinning practice	358
Families as allies	358
What is a learning (intellectual) disability?	358
The need for change in services and practice	359
Challenges health professionals face when working with people with learning (intellectual) disabilities	359
See the person and understand behaviour that challenges	359
Diagnostic overshadowing	360
Positive behaviour support reducing the use of restrictive practices	361
Becoming an adult: All change	361
Making decisions: Consent to treatment	361
Health needs and the transition	362
Getting care right in practice	362
Reasonable care adjustments	362
Hospital passport	362
Protocols to improve care outcomes	362
The learning (intellectual) disability protocol for preparation for theatre and recovery	364
Getting communication right	364
Pictures say more than words	364
Books beyond words	364
Tips to getting it right	364
Conclusion	365
Useful websites	365
References	365

17 Administration of medicines — 367
Jacqueline Robinson-Rouse, Mandy Matthews, Emily Baker, and Bhumik Patel

Section 1: General principles	368
Introduction	368
Child development considerations	370
Checking the medicine prescription	370
Drug calculations	370
Section 2: Routes of administration	371
Oral	371
Enteral via a tube or device	372
Buccal	372
Sublingual	373
Intranasal	374
Inhalation	374
Rectal	375
Intradermal (ID), subcutaneous (SC), and intramuscular (IM)	376
Intradermal	377
Subcutaneous	377
Intramuscular	378
Intravenous	380
Intraosseous	380
Intrathecal	380
Epidural	381
Transdermal (skin patches)	381
References	402

Procedure guidelines

17.1	Oral medication administration	384
17.2	Enteral tube administration	384
17.3	Buccal and sublingual administration	386
17.4	Intranasal administration	387
17.5	Inhalation administration	388
17.6	Rectal administration	390
17.7	Preparation of medication for injections using an aseptic nontouch technique	392
17.8	Intradermal (ID) administration	393
17.9	Subcutaneous (SC) administration	394
17.10	Intramuscular (IM) administration	396
17.11	Intraosseous administration	398
17.12	Intrathecal administration	398
17.13	Skin patch administration	402

18 Mental health — 405
Sharon Philips and Caroline Grindrod

What is mental health?	406
How common are mental health difficulties?	406
Somatoform disorders and medically unexplained symptoms	407
Anxiety disorders	407
Psychosis	408
Eating disorders	408
References	413

Procedure guideline

18.1	Managing meal times	412

19 Moving and handling — 415
Kathleen Owen and Janet Brooks

Introduction	416
Why Is the legislation important?	416
Moving and handling risk assessment	416
Musculoskeletal health and wellbeing	417
Education and training	418
Documentation	421
Equipment	421
References	425

20 Neonatal care — 427
Heather Parsons, Marie-Anne Kelly, Monika Sedlbauer, and Jane Burgering

Introduction	428
Neonatal thermoregulation	428
Developmental care	433
Vitamin K administration	435
Umbilical cord care	436
Newborn blood spot screening	438
Phototherapy – neonatal jaundice	443
Neonatal fluid management	444
References	449

Procedure guidelines

20.1	Preparation for umbilical care	437
20.2	Care of the umbilicus if soiled or sticky	437
20.3	Newborn blood spot screening	439
20.4	When to undertake newborn blood spot screening	439
20.5	Collecting the blood spot sample	440

21 Neurological care — 453
Nicola Barnes, Sophie Boella, Lindy May, Ainsley Moven, and Jody O'Connor

Introduction	454
Section 1: Neurological observations	454
Types of painful stimuli	462
Section 2: Seizures	463
Physiology of seizures	464
Care of the CYP with Seizures	465
Classification of seizures	468
Section 3: External ventricular drainage	470
References	479

Procedure guidelines

21.1	Neurological observations	454
21.2	Nursing management of the CYP during seizures	466
21.3	Introduction to external ventricular drainage	471
21.4	Inform the CYP and family	472
21.5	Neurological assessment	473
21.6	Drain management: positioning of drain	473
21.7	Drain management: drainage	474
21.8	Drain management: connecting or changing the system	475
21.9	Drain management: patency of drain: repairing a catheter	476
21.10	Drain management: patency of drain: unblocking of catheter	476
21.11	Drain management: fluid and electrolyte balance	477
21.12	Accessing the drain: CSF sampling	477
21.13	Accessing the drain: giving intrathecal drugs	478
21.14	Exit site care	478
21.15	Removal of the drain	479

22 Nutrition and feeding — 481
Vanessa Shaw and Sarah Kipps

Introduction	482
Nutritional requirements	482
Nutrition from preterm to adolescence	483
Breastfeeding	488
Enteral feeding	489
Parenteral nutrition	490
References	515

Procedure guidelines

22.1	Adding fortifier to EBM on the ward	496
22.2	Inserting and managing the nasogastric tube	498
22.3	Inserting and managing the nasojejunal tube	501
22.4	Management where both a gastric and a jejunal tube are inserted	503
22.5	Administration of enteral feeds	507
22.6	Monitoring CYPs on enteral feeds	509
22.7	Delivery of PN in the hospital setting	510
22.8	Sham feeding	513

23 Orthopaedic care — 519
Nathan Askew, Edel Broomfield, Penny Howard, Carole Irwin, Deborah Jackson, and Nicola Wilson

Introduction	520
Traction	520
Skeletal pin site care	520
Neurovascular observations	520
Care of a plaster cast	520
Removal of plaster casts	520
Use of crutches	521
Orthopaedic traction	521
Care of a CYP in traction	521
Gallows traction	521
Modified gallows traction/abduction traction/hoop traction	527
Skin traction	527
Slings and springs suspension	528
Spinal traction	528
References	539
Further reading	540

Procedure guidelines

23.1	How to perform neurovascular observations	524
23.2	Management of acute compartment syndrome	526
23.3	Handling a newly applied plaster cast	526
23.4	Preparation and equipment (cutting a plaster)	527
23.5	Splitting a cast	529
23.6	How to window a cast	529
23.7	Reinforcing a cast	529
23.8	Removing a cast	530
23.9	Performing basic care needs (CYP in a cast)	531
23.10	Assessment (walking aid)	532
23.11	Checking safety of crutches	533
23.12	Education of CYP and carers (crutches)	533

Contents

23.13	Management of traction	536
23.14	Applying skin traction	537
23.15	Nursing care of the CYP in traction	538
23.16	Nursing care of the CYP receiving spinal traction	539

24 Pain management — 541
Elizabeth Anne Bruce

Introduction	542
General principles of pain management	542
Pain assessment	545
Administration of entonox	550
Epidural analgesia	555
Patient and nurse controlled analgesia (PCA/NCA)	565
Prevention and management of opioid-related complications	566
Sucrose	571
References	573
Further reading	575

Procedure guidelines

24.1	Pain assessment on admission	547
24.2	Pain assessment using a self-report tool	548
24.3	CYP assessment for use of entonox	551
24.4	Preparation for entonox use	552
24.5	Administration of entonox	553
24.6	Managing side-effects of entonox	554
24.7	After use	555
24.8	Storage	555
24.9	Transfer of the CYP following epidural insertion	557
24.10	Nursing care of an epidural (general)	557
24.11	Nursing care of an epidural (observations)	558
24.12	Epidural related complications	561
24.13	Technical problems	563
24.14	Discontinuing the epidural	564
24.15	Preparation for PCA/NCA use	566
24.16	Setting up a PCA/NCA infusion	567
24.17	Technical problems (PCA/NCA)	568
24.18	Care of the CYP receiving PCA/NCA	568
24.19	Prevention and management of opioid-related complications	569
24.20	Sucrose administration	572

25 Palliative care — 577
June Hemsley

Introduction	578
Assessment of symptoms	579
Pain in palliative care: PCA and proxy PCA	580
Nausea and vomiting	580
Constipation and diarrhoea	581
Dyspnoea	581
Hydration and nutrition	582
Haemorrhage	582
Agitation	582
Seizures	582
Signs of impending death	583
Conclusion	584
References	591
Further reading	593

Procedure guidelines

25.1	Assessment of symptoms	584
25.2	Care of patient receiving PCA/PPCA for palliative care	585
25.3	Assessment and management of nausea and vomiting	586
25.4	Assessment and management of constipation and diarrhoea	586
25.5	Management of dyspnoea	587
25.6	Management of hydration and nutrition	588
25.7	Management of haemorrhage	589
25.8	Management of agitation	590
25.9	Management of seizures	591
25.10	Recognising signs of impending death	591

26 Perioperative care — 595
Ciara McMullin, Anthony Baker, Claire Cook, Yvonne Hambley, and Melissa Silva

Introduction	596
Preoperative preparation	596
Intra operative care	597
Recovery	597
References	617
Further reading	619

Procedure guidelines

26.1	Pre-admission	598
26.2	Admission to hospital	598
26.3	Immediately prior to theatre	600
26.4	Care in the anaesthetic room	601
26.5	Care in the operating theatre	602
26.6	Care in recovery	609

27 Play as a therapeutic tool — 621
Jennifer Dyer, Janet Holmes, Denise Cochrane, and Nigel Mills

Introduction	622
The development of play in hospital	622
Normal play for development	622
Types of play	623
Functions of play	623
Development of play	623
The importance of play for children in hospital	623
The functions of play in hospital	623
Siblings	624
The health play specialist (HPS)	624
HPS training	624
The play worker (PW)	625
Preparation for surgery and procedures	625
Aims of play preparation	625
Preadmission programmes	626
Preparation session	626
Postprocedural play	627
The reluctant CYP	627
Adolescents	627
Children and young people with additional needs or a learning disability (LD)	627
Distraction techniques	628
Distraction Tools and Resources	630
Relaxation	630
Guided imagery	631
Therapeutic play	631
Desensitisation	632
Arts in health	633
References	633
Further reading	634
Useful websites	634

Procedure guideline

27.1	Using distraction during a painful/frightening procedure	629

28 Poisoning and overdose — 635
Robert Cole

Nonaccidental ingestion and self-harm	636
Health promotion strategies	637
Common ingestions	637
Initial management following poisoning or overdose	639
Care of the parent/carer	640
Treatment of ingested poisons	640
Gastric lavage	640
References	644

Procedure guidelines
28.1 Patient consent and preparation — 642
28.2 Preparation of equipment (gastric lavage) — 642
28.3 Procedure (gastric lavage) — 642
28.4 Postprocedure (gastric lavage) — 643

29 Respiratory care — 645
Elizabeth Leonard, Charlotte Donovan, Emma Shkurka, Joanne Cooke, Heather Hatter, Maura O'Callaghan, Vicky Robinson, Catherine Spreckley, Ana Marote, Harriet Clark, and Jade Rand

Introduction — 646
Airway suction — 646
Nasopharyngeal airway — 649
Oxygen therapy — 657
Chest drain management — 663
Noninvasive ventilation (NIV) — 672
Long-term ventilation (LTV) — 676
References — 680

Procedure guidelines
29.1 Suction: training, assessment and preparation — 647
29.2 Performing suction — 648
29.3 Preparation for a NPA — 651
29.4 Inserting the NPA — 654
29.5 Observations post NPA insertion — 656
29.6 Ongoing care of an NPA and discharge planning — 656
29.7 Education, assessment, and preparation for oxygen administration — 660
29.8 Administration of oxygen therapy — 660
29.9 Continuous assessment of the CYP receiving oxygen therapy — 661
29.10 Discharge planning for the CYP on long-term oxygen — 662
29.11 Preparation for insertion of a chest drain — 665
29.12 Postprocedure care of a chest drain — 665
29.13 Specific chest drain observations — 666
29.14 Ongoing chest drain care and prevention of complications — 669
29.15 Changing a chest drain chamber — 670
29.16 Removal of a chest drain — 670
29.17 Preparation for NIV — 673
29.18 NIV mask placement and care — 673
29.19 NIV humidification and oxygen — 674
29.20 NIV safety, tolerance, and compliance — 675
29.21 Ongoing care of NIV — 675
29.22 Assessment for LTV and transitional care — 676
29.23 Management of a CYP on LTV — 676
29.24 Leaving the clinical area with LTV — 677
29.25 Discharge planning for a CYP with LTV — 678
29.26 The management of acute illness in a CYP with a tracheostomy at home — 680

30 Resuscitation — 683
Denise Welsby

Introduction — 684
Early warning scoring (EWS) — 684
Aetiology of cardiorespiratory arrest — 684
Airway management — 684
Recovery position — 689
Circulation management — 693
Basic life support — 696
Choking — 701
Cardiopulmonary arrest management — 704
Defibrillation — 707
Resuscitation team — 710
Ethical considerations — 710
References — 711

Procedure guidelines
30.1 Head positioning (airway management) — 687
30.2 Pharyngeal airways — 688
30.3 Placing a child in a recovery position — 690
30.4 Self-inflating bag mask valve ventilation — 691
30.5 Preparation for insertion of an IO cannula — 694
30.6 Procedure for a manually inserted cannula — 695
30.7 Procedure for an EZ-IO inserted cannula — 695
30.8 Using the IO cannula — 696
30.9 Basic life support (BLS) provision — 697
30.10 Management of the choking infant/child — 702
30.11 Management of nonshockable rhythms (asystole and PEA) — 704
30.12 Management of shockable rhythms (ventricular fibrillation and pulseless ventricular tachycardia) — 705
30.13 Manual defibrillation with self-adhesive pads — 707

31 Safeguarding children and young people — 713
Janice Baker and Danya Glaser

Introduction — 714
Safeguarding: An individual and corporate responsibility — 714
Background — 714
Defining child maltreatment — 714
The effects of abuse and neglect — 716
Intra-familial risk factors — 716
Extra-familial risk factors — 719
The legal framework — 719
Improving child protection and safeguarding practice — 719
Professional responsibilities — 724
Procedures where there are concerns or suspicions about fabricated or induced illness (FII) — 725
Pre-discharge planning procedure — 725
Referral to children's social care — 725
Looked after children (LAC) — 726
Conclusion — 726
References — 726

32 Tracheostomy care and management — 729
Joanne Cooke

Introduction — 730
Care of the CYP with a tracheostomy — 730
Ongoing care and management: TRACHE care bundle — 735
Tracheostomy tube changes (planned) — 745
Tracheostomy tubes for CYPs — 746
Discharge planning — 749
Decannulation — 749
References — 750
Further reading — 751

Procedure guidelines
32.1 Preparation of the bed space for a new tracheostomy — 731
32.2 Care and assessment of potential complications of a new tracheostomy — 733
32.3 Other tracheostomy care needs — 735
32.4 Tape changes (cotton) — 737
32.5 Tracheostomy resuscitation — 742
32.6 Suctioning a tracheostomy tube — 743
32.7 Tube changes — 746
32.8 Preparation for discharge — 749

33 Urinary catheter care — 753
Donna Wyan

Introduction — 754
Types of catheters — 754
Risk factors — 754
References — 767

Procedure guidelines

33.1 Catheter insertion: preparation — 756
33.2 Urethral catheter insertion — 757
33.3 Catheter care: general — 759
33.4 Catheter care: entry site — 761
33.5 Emptying a catheter drainage bag — 762
33.6 Maintaining catheter drainage — 763
33.7 Flushing suprapubic, urethral or mitrofanoff catheters — 763
33.8 Removal of suprapubic and urethral catheters — 765
33.9 Discharge planning — 766

34 Drug withdrawal: prevention and management — 769
Rebecca Saul

Introduction — 770
Definitions — 770
Incidence of withdrawal — 770
Mechanisms of tolerance — 770
Overall aims of withdrawal management — 770
Prevention of withdrawal symptoms — 771
Assessment of the symptoms of withdrawal — 771
Management of withdrawal of opioid and benzodiazepine therapy — 771
Pharmacological weaning management — 772
References — 777

Procedure guidelines

34.1 Prevention of opioid or benzodiazepine withdrawal symptoms — 772
34.2 Assessment of opioid and benzodiazepine withdrawal — 773
34.3 Taking a patient history — 773
34.4 Creating a weaning plan — 774
34.5 Conversion from intravenous to oral medication — 775
34.6 Clonidine — 776
34.7 Non-pharmacological management — 776

35 When a child or young person dies — 779
Rachel Cooke

Introduction — 780
Communication and responsibilities following a death of a CYP — 780
Legal aspects: Certification, notification, and registration — 780
Personal care of the CYP (previously known as last offices) — 787
Moving the CYP to the mortuary and aftercare — 788
Post-mortem — 792
Bereavement — 792
Self-care and debrief — 792
References — 794
Further reading — 794

Procedure guidelines

35.1 Communication and responsibilities — 783
35.2 Legal aspects: certification, registration, post-mortem, and organ and tissue donation — 785
35.3 Personal care of a CYP (previously known as last offices) — 788
35.4 Moving a CYP to the mortuary and aftercare — 790

Index — 795

Foreword

It is my great pleasure to be asked to write the Foreword to the second edition of the *Great Ormond Street Hospital Manual of Children and Young People's Nursing Practices*.

The Hospital for Sick Children opened in 1852 with just 10 beds. Since then, and throughout its 171-year history, Great Ormond Street Children's Hospital (GOSH) has remained a hospital dedicated to the care of children and young people and has established a reputation for being at the leading edge of care, education, and research, both nationally and internationally.

Healthcare for children across the world continues to develop as advancements in medical science, technology, and pharmacology lead to innovation and treatment breakthroughs, making the impossible possible. Children and young people with rare and complex conditions come from across the United Kingdom and the rest of the world to access our highly specialised services. Excellence in nursing is fundamental to what we can offer and plays a key role in the delivery of high standards of care and practice that we constantly strive to influence and achieve, working in collaboration with the children and young people themselves and their families. Now, more so than ever before, nurses play such a pivotal role in improvements in patient care and experience by championing developments in digital technology, making access to care and treatment easier and equitable.

Florence Nightingale once stated 'it is the real test of a nurse whether she can nurse a sick infant' (Nightingale 1859, p. 116). This manual is an inspiring body of work, contributed to by many, which showcases the profession of children's nursing, of which we are extremely proud. It supports the delivery of evidence-based practice across a wide variety of topics, updated original guidance, as well as introducing new aspects of practice, and is essential reading for *all* nurses and other healthcare professionals involved in caring for children and young people across acute, community, and primary care settings.

Reference

Nightingale F 1859 (1952) *Notes on Nursing: What it Is, and What It Is Not.* London, UK, Harrison.

Tracy Luckett
Chief Nurse
Great Ormond Street Hospital for Children NHS Foundation Trust

Editorial Panel

Nathan Askew MSc Adv P, BSc (Hons), Dip HE Nursing (Child)
Formerly Lead Nurse and Advanced Practitioner, Surgery
Great Ormond Street Hospital for Children NHS
Foundation Trust
London, UK

Julie Bayliss RN (Adult), RN (Child), BSc, MSc, ANP, NMP
Consultant Nurse, Paediatric Palliative Care
Great Ormond Street Hospital for Children NHS
Foundation Trust
London, UK

Elizabeth Anne Bruce MSc, BSc (Hons), RN (Adult), RN (Child)
Clinical Nurse Specialist, Pain Control Service
Great Ormond Street Hospital for Children NHS
Foundation Trust
London, UK

John Courtney RN (Adult), RN (Child), MA, PgDip, ENB415
Formerly Assistant Chief Nurse
Great Ormond Street Hospital for Children NHS
Foundation Trust
London, UK

Faith Gibson PhD, MSc, RN (Child), RN (Adult), ONC cert, Cert Ed, RNT, FRCN, FAAN
Professor of Child Health and Cancer Care
University of Surrey
Guildford, UK
Director of Nursing and Allied Health Research
Great Ormond Street Hospital for Children NHS
Foundation Trust
London, UK

Anna Gregorowski RN (Child), BSc Nursing, MSc
Formerly Nurse Consultant in Adolescent Health
Great Ormond Street Hospital for Children NHS
Foundation Trust
London, UK

Kate Khair RN (Adult), RN (Child), MSc, MCGI, PhD
Formerly Clinical Academic Careers Fellow
Centre for Outcomes Research and Experience in Children's Health Illness and Disability (ORCHID)
Great Ormond Street Hospital for Children NHS
Foundation Trust
London, UK

Elizabeth Leonard RN (Adult), RN (Child), BA (Hons), MSc
Head of Education (Operational)
Great Ormond Street Hospital for Children NHS
Foundation Trust
London, UK

Lindy May RN (Adult), RN (Child), MSc (Neuroscience), Diploma in Counselling, PhD
Formerly Nurse Consultant, Neurosurgery
Great Ormond Street Hospital for Children NHS
Foundation Trust
London, UK

Liz Smith RN (Adult), RN (Child), Advanced Diploma and MSc in Child Development
Lead Advanced Nurse Practitioner and ECMO Coordinator, Cardiorespiratory Services
Great Ormond Street Hospital for Children NHS
Foundation Trust
London, UK

Mark Whiting PhD, MSc, BSc Nursing, RN (Child)
Consultant Nurse, Children's Specialist Services, Hertfordshire Community NHS Trust and WellChild Professor of Community Children's Nursing
University of Hertfordshire
Hatfield, UK

Janet Williss MSc, BSc, RN (Child), RN (Adult), ONC Cert
Formerly Deputy Chief Nurse
Great Ormond Street Hospital for Children NHS
Foundation Trust
London, UK

List of Contributors

Rachel Allaway BSc (Hons), Children's Nursing,
Clinical Nurse Specialist, Tissue Viability,
Great Ormond Street Hospital for Children NHS
Foundation Trust, London, UK
(Chapter 11)

Liesje Andre RN (Adult), RN (Child), PGCME,
Formerly Lead Nurse, Resuscitation,
Great Ormond Street Hospital for Children NHS
Foundation Trust, London, UK
(Chapter 9)

Nathan Askew MSc Adv P, BSc (Hons), DipHE Nursing (Child),
Formerly Lead Nurse and Advanced Practitioner, Surgery,
Great Ormond Street Hospital for Children NHS
Foundation Trust, London, UK
(Chapter 23, Editor)

Anthony Baker
Formerly Practice Educator, Theatres,
Great Ormond Street Hospital for Children NHS
Foundation Trust,
(Chapter 26)

Emily Baker DipHE Nursing Child Branch,
BSc (Hons) Children's Cancer Nursing, MA
Practice Education,
Senior Clinical Research Nurse Haematology/Oncology,
Great Ormond Street Hospital for Children NHS
Foundation Trust, London, UK
(Chapters 8, 17)

Janice Baker SCPHN-HV RM RN (Adult),
Formerly Head of Safeguarding and Named Nurse,
Great Ormond Street Hospital for Children NHS
Foundation Trust, London, UK
(Chapter 31)

Lisa Baldry FIBMS,
Formerly Chief Biomedical Scientist,
Great Ormond Street Hospital for Children NHS
Foundation Trust, London, UK
(Chapter 4)

Dr. Alex M. Barnacle BM, MRCP, FRCR,
Consultant Interventional Radiologist,
Great Ormond Street Hospital for Children NHS
Foundation Trust, London, UK
(Chapter 3)

Nicola Barnes RN (Child), MSc Paediatric Advanced Practice,
Advanced Nurse Practitioner for Epilepsy Surgery,
Great Ormond Street Hospital for Children NHS
Foundation Trust, London, UK
(Chapter 21)

Hannah Barron RN (Child),
Senior Staff Nurse, PICU,
Great Ormond Street Hospital for Children NHS
Foundation Trust, London, UK
(Chapter 14)

Julie Bayliss RN (Adult), RN (Child), BSc, MSc, ANP, NMP,
Consultant Nurse, Paediatric Palliative Care
Great Ormond Street Hospital for Children NHS
Foundation Trust, London, UK
(Chapter 8, Editor)

Helen Bedford RN (Adult), RHV, PhD, MSc (Nursing Studies), BSc
Nursing (Hons), FFPH, FRCPCH,
Professor of Children's Health, UCL,
Great Ormond Street Hospital for Children NHS
Foundation Trust, London, UK
(Chapter 12)

Nikki Bennett-Rees RN (Child), RN (Adult), Diploma Advanced
Nursing,
Formerly Clinical Nurse Specialist, Bone Marrow Transplant,
Great Ormond Street Hospital for Children NHS
Foundation Trust, London, UK
(Chapter 3)

Jim Blair RNLD, CNLD, DipSW, MA, BSc, BA, MSDipHE, PGDipHE,
Formerly Consultant Nurse, Intellectual (Learning) Disabilities,
Great Ormond Street Hospital for Children NHS
Foundation Trust, London, UK
Associate Professor Learning Disabilities, Kingston University and
St. George's University of London, London, UK
(Chapter 16)

Sophie Boella RN (Child),
Neurology Nurse,
Great Ormond Street Hospital for Children NHS
Foundation Trust, London, UK
RNLD, CNLD, DipSW, MA, BSc, BA, MSDipHE, PGDipHE,
(Chapter 21)

Barbara Brekle RN (Child), BSc (Hons),
Deputy Lead Nurse, Infection Prevention and Control,
Great Ormond Street Hospital for Children NHS
Foundation Trust, London, UK
(Chapters 13, 15)

Eileen Brennan RN (Adult), RN (Child), MSc,
Formerly Nurse Consultant in Paediatric Nephrology,
Great Ormond Street Hospital for Children NHS
Foundation Trust, London, UK
(Chapters 1, 3, 10)

Janet Brooks
Back Care Advisor,
Great Ormond Street Hospital for Children NHS
Foundation Trust, London, UK
(Chapter 19)

List of Contributors

Edel Broomfield RN (Child), DipHE, BSC, MSc,
Lead Spinal Advanced Nurse Practitioner,
Great Ormond Street Hospital for Children NHS
Foundation Trust, London, UK
(Chapter 23)

Elizabeth Anne Bruce MSc, BSc (Hons), RN (Adult),
RN (Child),
Clinical Nurse Specialist, Pain Control Service,
Great Ormond Street Hospital for Children NHS
Foundation Trust, London, UK
(Chapter 24, Editor)

Jane Burgering
Formerly Practice Educator, NICU,
Great Ormond Street Hospital for Children NHS
Foundation Trust, London, UK
(Chapter 20)

Sarah Carmichael BSc (Hons), Children's Nursing,
Formerly Clinical Nurse Specialist, Tissue Viability,
Great Ormond Street Hospital for Children NHS
Foundation Trust, London, UK
(Chapter 11)

Sue Chapman RN (Adult), RN (Child),
AdvDip Child Development, MSc PCCN (Advanced Practice),
PhD Child Health,
Formerly Clinical Site Director,
Great Ormond Street Hospital for Children NHS
Foundation Trust, London, UK
(Chapter 1)

Harriet Clark RN (Child) BSc (Hons) Children's Nursing,
Practice Educator,
Great Ormond Street Hospital for Children NHS
Foundation Trust, London, UK
(Chapter 29)

Denise Cochrane
Play Specialist Team Leader,
Great Ormond Street Hospital for Children NHS
Foundation Trust, London, UK
(Chapter 27)

Robert Cole RN (Adult), RN (Child), MA Ed, PGDip Ed; BSc
(Hons) with ENB Higher Award; ENB 199; ENB 998;
ENB A53, APLS Instructor,
Head of Nursing for Children and Young People,
University Hospital Lewisham, Lewisham & Greenwich NHS Trust,
London, UK
(Chapter 28)

Claire Cook
Formerly Team Leader for Spinal Surgery,
Great Ormond Street Hospital for Children NHS
Foundation Trust, London, UK
(Chapter 26)

Joanne Cooke TD, MSc, BSc (Hons), RN (Adult),
RN (Child), NT,
Advanced Nurse Practitioner, ENT/Tracheostomies,
Great Ormond Street Hospital for Children NHS
Foundation Trust, London, UK
(Chapters 29, 32)

Rachel Cooke RN (Child),
Bereavement Services Manager,
Great Ormond Street Hospital for Children NHS
Foundation Trust, London, UK
(Chapter 35)

John Courtney MA, PgDip, RN (Adult), RN (Child),
Formerly Assistant Chief Nurse,
Great Ormond Street Hospital for Children NHS
Foundation Trust, London, UK
(Chapter 10, Editor)

Charlotte Donovan BSc (Hons) Physiotherapy,
Paediatric Physiotherapist, PICU and NICU,
Great Ormond Street Hospital for Children NHS
Foundation Trust, London, UK
(Chapter 29)

Jennifer Dyer
Senior Play Specialist Team Leader,
Great Ormond Street Hospital for Children NHS
Foundation Trust, London, UK
(Chapter 27)

Nicky Farrell RN (Adult), RN (Child), BSc (Hons) Nursing,
DipHE Child Health, ENB 998, ENB 240,
Macmillan Clinical Nurse Specialist, Neuro-Oncology-
Endocrinology,
Great Ormond Street Hospital for Children NHS
Foundation Trust, London, UK
(Chapter 8)

Róisín Fitzsimons RN (Adult), RN (Child), DipHE,
BSc (Hons), MSc (Allergy), RNC, MCGI, PhD,
Formerly Consultant Nurse, Children's Allergy Service,
Guy's & St Thomas' NHS Foundation Trust, London, UK
(Chapter 2)

Dr. Danya Glaser MBBS, DCH, FRCPsych, Hon FRCPCH,
Honorary Child and Adolescent Psychiatrist,
Great Ormond Street Hospital for Children NHS
Foundation Trust, London, UK
(Chapter 31)

Caroline Grindrod
Formerly CNS, Eating Disorders Team, Adolescent
Mental Health Unit,
Great Ormond Street Hospital for Children NHS
Foundation Trust, London, UK
(Chapter 18)

Jenni Hallman RN (Adult), RN (Child), BSc (Hons) Children's
Oncology Nursing,
Formerly Oncology Complementary Therapy Nurse Specialist,
Great Ormond Street Hospital for Children NHS
Foundation Trust, London, UK
(Chapter 7)

Yvonne Hambley RN (Adult), DipHE Child Health,
Sister, Recovery,
Great Ormond Street Hospital for Children NHS Foundation Trust,
London, UK
(Chapter 26)

Heather Hatter RN (Adult), RN (Child), Bsc (Hons), Dip Nursing,
Formerly Practice Educator, Respiratory Medicine,
Great Ormond Street Hospital for Children NHS Foundation Trust, London, UK
(Chapter 29)

June Hemsley RN, BSc, MSc (Child), NMP
Advanced Nurse Practitioner,
Louis Dundas Centre for Oncology Outreach and Palliative Care,
Great Ormond Street Hospital for Children NHS Foundation Trust, London, UK
(Chapter 25)

Melanie Hiorns FRCR, FRCP
Clinical Director International and Private Patients,
and Consultant Radiologist,
Great Ormond Street Hospital for Children NHS Foundation Trust, London, UK
(Chapter 15)

Anne Ho RN (Child), BSc
Central venous Access CNS,
Great Ormond Street Hospital for Children NHS Foundation Trust, London, UK
(Chapter 14)

Janet Holmes BSc (Hons), NNEB, HPSET,
Senior Health Play Specialist,
Great Ormond Street Hospital for Children NHS Foundation Trust, London, UK
(Chapter 27)

Penny Howard RN (Adult), RN (Child),
Clinical Nurse Specialist, Orthopaedics,
Great Ormond Street Hospital for Children NHS Foundation Trust, London, UK
(Chapter 23)

Carole Irwin BSc (Hons), ENB 219, PGCE,
Formerly Clinical Project Manager,
Great Ormond Street Hospital for Children NHS Foundation Trust, London, UK
(Chapter 23)

Deborah Jackson BSc (Hons) in Physio, MSc in Advanced Physiotherapy, MCSP, SRP,
Clinical Specialist Physiotherapist,
Great Ormond Street Hospital for Children NHS Foundation Trust, London, UK
(Chapter 23)

Josephine Jim RN (Child), BSc,
Sister, PICU,
Great Ormond Street Hospital for Children NHS Foundation Trust, London, UK
(Chapter 10)

Helen Johnson RN (Adult), RN (Child), ENB 216, BSc (Hons),
Formerly Clinical Nurse Specialist Stoma Care,
Great Ormond Street Hospital for Children NHS Foundation Trust, London, UK
(Chapter 5)

Anne-Marie Kao
Formerly Nurse Practitioner, Dermatology,
Great Ormond Street Hospital for Children NHS Foundation Trust, London, UK
(Chapter 3)

Marie-Anne Kelly RN (Child), ENB 405
Formerly Neonatal Clinical Nurse Specialist,
Great Ormond Street Hospital for Children NHS Foundation Trust, London, UK
(Chapter 20)

Kate Khair RN (Adult), RN (Child), MSc, MCGI, PhD,
Formerly Clinical Academic Careers Fellow, Centre for Outcomes Research and Experience in Children's Health Illness and Disability (ORCHID),
Great Ormond Street Hospital for Children NHS Foundation Trust, London, UK
(Chapter 4, Editor)

Sarah Kipps
Formerly Practice Educator, Nursing Quality,
Great Ormond Street Hospital for Children NHS Foundation Trust, London, UK
(Chapters 11, 22)

Elizabeth Leonard RN (Adult), RN (Child), BA (Hons), MSc,
Head of Education (Operational),
Great Ormond Street Hospital for Children NHS Foundation Trust, London, UK
(Chapter 29, Editor)

Annabel Linger RN (Child), Dip HEd Nursing Sciences, BSc (Hons) Child Health Nursing, ENB 405, ENB 998,
Sister, NICU,
Great Ormond Street Hospital for Children NHS Foundation Trust, London, UK
(Chapter 15)

Ana Marote
Formerly Ward Sister, Respiratory,
Great Ormond Street Hospital for Children NHS Foundation Trust, London, UK
(Chapter 29)

Mandy Matthews RN (Adult), RN (Child), PGDip in Learning and Teaching for Professional Practice,
Formerly Head of International Practice Development,
Great Ormond Street Hospital for Children NHS Foundation Trust, London, UK
(Chapter 17)

Lindy May RN (Adult), RN (Child), MSc (Neuroscience), Diploma in Counselling, PhD,
Formerly Nurse Consultant, Neurosurgery,
Great Ormond Street Hospital for Children,
NHS Foundation Trust, London, UK
(Chapters 1, 21, Editor)

Brian McGowan RN (Child), MSc, SFHEA,
Lecturer in Higher Education Practice,
Ulster University, Belfast, UK
(Chapter 6)

List of Contributors

Ciara McMullin BSc Hons (Paeds), DipN (Adult),
Head of Nursing and Patient Experience,
Great Ormond Street Hospital for Children NHS
Foundation Trust, London, UK
(Chapter 26)

Nigel Mills
Formerly Adolescent Nurse Specialist,
Great Ormond Street Hospital for Children NHS
Foundation Trust, London, UK
(Chapter 27)

Dr. Kishore Minhas MBCHB, MSc, FRCR,
Consultant Interventional Radiologist,
Great Ormond Street Hospital for Children NHS
Foundation Trust, London, UK
(Chapter 3)

Rachel Moss RN (Adult),
Senior Transfusion Practitioner,
Great Ormond Street Hospital for Children NHS
Foundation Trust, London, UK
(Chapter 4)

Ainsley Moven RN (Child), PgDip,
Nurse Practitioner, Neurosurgery,
Great Ormond Street Hospital for Children NHS
Foundation Trust, London, UK
(Chapter 21)

Maura O'Callaghan RN (Adult), RN (Child), ANP,
Lead Nurse, ECMO/VAD,
Cardiorespiratory Unit,
Great Ormond Street Hospital for Children NHS
Foundation Trust, London, UK
(Chapter 29)

Jody O'Connor RN (Child), DipHE, BSc (hons) Neuroscience,
MSc ANP,
Advanced Nurse Practitioner, Neurosurgery,
Great Ormond Street Hospital for Children NHS
Foundation Trust, London, UK
(Chapter 21)

Lorna O'Rourke RN (Adult), RN (Child), BSc (Hons),
Ward Sister, NICU,
Great Ormond Street Hospital for Children NHS
Foundation Trust, London, UK
(Chapter 14)

Kathleen Owen
Formerly Back Care Advisor and Moving and
Handling Trainer,
Great Ormond Street Hospital for Children NHS
Foundation Trust, London, UK
(Chapter 19)

Heather Parsons RN (Child), BSc (Hons) Neonatal Nursing,
Practice Educator, NICU,
Great Ormond Street Hospital for Children NHS
Foundation Trust, London, UK
(Chapter 20)

Bhumik Patel MPharm, MSc, PGCert,
Senior Specialist Pharmacist in Paediatric Palliative Care,
Great Ormond Street Hospital for Children NHS
Foundation Trust, London, UK
(Chapters 8, 17)

Sharon Philips
Formerly Ward Sister, Adolescent Mental Health Unit,
Great Ormond Street Hospital for Children NHS
Foundation Trust, London, UK
(Chapter 18)

Jade Rand RN(Child) BSc (Hons) Children's
Nursing, PG Cert Practice Education,
Practice Educator, Respiratory,
Great Ormond Street Hospital for Children NHS
Foundation Trust, London, UK
(Chapter 29)

Di Robertshaw RN (Adult), RN (Child), RNT, BSc (Hons)
Child Health, DipN (Paediatrics), DipNE,
Practice Educator, Cardiac,
Great Ormond Street Hospital for Children NHS
Foundation Trust, London, UK
(Chapter 15)

Sally Robertson MA, Pg. Cert, BA, RN Child Dip,
Head of Education,
Great Ormond Street Hospital for Children NHS
Foundation Trust, London, UK
(Chapter 6)

Vicky Robinson DipHe and BSc (Hons) Children's Nursing,
RN (Child),
CNS Non-invasive ventilation,
Great Ormond Street Hospital for Children NHS
Foundation Trust, London, UK
(Chapter 29)

Jacqueline Robinson-Rouse RN (Child),
BSc (Hon), MSc,
Formerly Lead Nurse, Nursing Workforce,
Great Ormond Street Hospital for Children NHS
Foundation Trust, London, UK
(Chapter 17)

June Rogers RN (Adult), RN (Child), BSc (Hons), MSc,
Children's Bladder and Bowel Nurse Specialist,
Bladder & Bowel UK, Manchester, UK
(Chapter 5)

Rebecca Saul RN (Child), RN (Adult), MSc,
Clinical Nurse Specialist Paediatric Pain,
Great Ormond Street Hospital for Children NHS
Foundation Trust, London, UK
(Chapter 34)

Monika Sedlbauer MSc Adv Paed N,
Formerly Practice Educator, NICU,
Great Ormond Street Hospital for Children NHS
Foundation Trust, London, UK
(Chapter 20)

List of Contributors

Vanessa Shaw MBE, MA, PGDip Dietetics, RD, FBDA,
Honorary Associate Professor of Paediatric Dietetics,
Plymouth University,
Honorary Senior Lecturer,
UCL Great Ormond Street Institute, London, UK
(Chapter 22)

Emma Shkurka BSc (Hons) Physiotherapy, MRes Clinical Practice,
Paediatric Critical Care Physiotherapist,
NIHR Clinical Doctoral Research Fellow,
Great Ormond Street Hospital for Children NHS
Foundation Trust, London, UK
(Chapter 29)

Melissa Silva BSc (nursing), MSc (Nursing Education),
Formerly Practice Educator,
Great Ormond Street Hospital for Children NHS
Foundation Trust, London, UK
(Chapter 26)

Cindy Sparkes RN (Child), MSc, PGCE,
Lead Educator, Haematology and Oncology,
Great Ormond Street Hospital for Children
NHS Foundation Trust, London, UK
(Chapter 8)

Catherine Spreckley RN (Child), BSc (Hons), PGCE, PGDip
Formerly Practice Educator, Respiratory,
Great Ormond Street Hospital for Children NHS
Foundation Trust, London, UK
(Chapter 29)

Denise Welsby RN (Adult),
EPALs Subcommittee faculty member, instructor and course director, Resuscitation Council UK,
Head of Resuscitation Services,
Great Ormond Street Hospital for Children NHS
Foundation Trust, London, UK
(Chapters 9, 30)

Zoe Wilks RN (Adult), RN (Child), BSc (Hons) Child Health,
Adv Dip Ch Dev,
Formerly Modern Matron,
Great Ormond Street Hospital for Children NHS
Foundation Trust, London, UK
(Chapter 3)

Nicola Wilson MNurSci, PGCert Ed, DTN
Lead Practice Educator,
Great Ormond Street Hospital for Children NHS
Foundation Trust, London, UK
(Chapter 23)

Donna Wyan DipHE (Child), BSc (Hons), Independent Prescriber,
Urology Nurse Practitioner,
Great Ormond Street Hospital for Children NHS
Foundation Trust, London, UK
(Chapter 33)

Introduction

We made a decision to write this introduction last. We wanted to set the scene for what was to follow and therefore needed to know what followed before we put finger to keyboard. Our intention here is to highlight a number of principles that should underpin all clinical care given in community and hospital settings, all of which are the cornerstone of the content of chapters in this textbook. The guidelines contained herein are not intended to replace individual assessment and personalised treatment and care of the child or young person (CYP) and their carers/family. Instead, our intention in presenting this information is to bring to nurses and other healthcare professionals delivering healthcare to CYPs the latest evidence that underpins clinical care; the *how to* and *why* of many of the clinical procedures undertaken. The first principle that guides us in our work regards individualised care.

Individualised care

The mission for Great Ormond Street Hospital for Children NHS Foundation Trust (GOSH) is to put the 'child first and always' (GOSH 2020). This continues to underpin the work of every person employed at the hospital. To deliver on this mission, each CYP needs to be seen as a 'whole' being in the context of their family, carers, school, friends, and local community. This perspective should involve an understanding that, as CYPs grow up and develop, their needs will change. Knowledge of child development, family structures, communication patterns and the wider social networks CYPs live within is important for us to understand how we approach care delivery. Using a family systems approach to nursing is not new, but we, and the practitioners who have contributed to this textbook, would recommend its use to ensure that the focus is on the care of the whole family (Hemphill and Dearmun 2010). We would also suggest having in place an ideal care delivery model (Pordes et al. 2019) that includes the creation of proactive plans based on the goals of the family and CYP, where multidisciplinary, shared decision-making is facilitated and recorded, and a professional such as a key worker familiar with the CYP and family is involved to address comprehensive needs (Ogourtsova et al. 2018).

CYPs also have rights as human beings and need special care and attention (United Nations International Children's Emergency Fund [UNICEF] 1989). This Convention was the first legally binding international instrument to incorporate the full range of human rights for CYPs; civil, cultural, economic, political, and social rights. Each CYP has the right:

- For survival – to be given food and water and opportunities for healthy growth.
- To develop to the fullest – to achieve and enjoy through education.
- To protection from harmful influences, abuse, and exploitation – to stay safe.
- To participate fully in family, cultural, and social life – to make a positive contribution and achieve economic well-being.

Now, 30 years since it was ratified (https://www.unicef.org/child-rights-convention), readers are encouraged to take a few minutes to watch some of the more recent videos that show what CYPs are doing to use their rights; see, for example, https://www.youtube.com/watch?v=y4udqAY2Bqc and https://www.youtube.com/watch?v=DtzlxpDRiMk.

Our role in healthcare is to ensure that CYPs reach their fullest potential, and thus limit whenever we can the short- and long-term effects that result from health changes. Most CYPs will experience the healthcare system in some way during their life; for example, vaccinations, school health checks, dental checks, sexual health, maternity services, or, if they become unwell, a visit to their local doctor or a hospital referral. It is important that within each of these different contexts the CYP is seen as an individual within the family. Throughout this textbook there are many examples of approaches to ensure this aim will be achieved in your approaches to care.

Family-centred care

Our second principle is the need to fully understand the methods of a family-centred approach to care. This takes the notion of individualised care further, with family-centred care (FCC) viewed as a central tenet of CYPs' nursing (Coleman 2002). An FCC model is widely used in the care of CYPs in hospital. This encompasses the holistic psychosocial-economic need to always see CYPs within a family concept. Hutchfield (1999) analysed the concepts of FCC and found that partnership with parents, parent participation, and care by parent were the most common systems applied in practice. These systems were meant to help clarify for parents their caring roles, and make explicit how professionals and parents would work together. 'The social construct of family-centred care has been refined again and again and within this construct parents have moved from a passive presence to being allowed to take on a more active role in their child's care in hospital' (Coleman 2002, p. 9).

More recently, O'Connor et al. (2019) undertook a concept analysis of FCC and concluded that the concept continues to evolve. Attributes included parental participation in care, the development of respectful and trusting partnerships and information sharing, with all family members as care recipients. O'Connor et al. (2019) reaffirm that the effectiveness of family-centred care has not been measured sufficiently and argue that although nurses can support the principles of it, very few can really define it and say what works best in different situations; empirical evidence continues to be absent. Despite this lack of evidence and lack of a single definition of FCC, we would strongly support the application of an FCC approach to care, in which nurses work within family structures to care for CYPs effectively and support family members in their roles, whether they be nursing or family roles; where parents are able to negotiate with health staff to determine what this participation will involve and negotiate new roles for themselves in sharing the care of their sick CYP. Parents should be involved in the

Table I.1 Relevant legislation and policies.

Policy	URL
The Human Rights Act 1998	https://www.equalityhumanrights.com/en/human-rights/human-rights-act
The Children Act 2004 – The legal framework for England and Wales	www.legislation.gov.uk/ukpga/2004/31/contents
Protection of Vulnerable Groups (Scotland) Act 2007	www.legislation.gov.uk/asp/2007/14/contents
Protection of Children (Scotland) Act 2003	www.legislation.gov.uk/asp/2003/5/contents
Children (Northern Ireland) Order 1995	www.legislation.gov.uk/nisi/1995/755/contents/made
Safeguarding Vulnerable Groups (Northern Ireland) Order 2007	www.legislation.gov.uk/nisi/2007/1351/contents
Children and Young Persons Act 2008	www.legislation.gov.uk/ukpga/2008/23/pdfs/ukpga_20080023_en.pdf
The Children's Plan (Department for Children, Schools and Families 2007)	https://assets.publishing.service.gov.uk/government/uploads/system/uploads/attachment_data/file/325111/2007-childrens-plan.pdf
Children and Families Act 2014	www.legislation.gov.uk/ukpga/2014/6/contents/enacted
Children and Social Work Act 2017	www.legislation.gov.uk/ukpga/2017/16/contents/enacted
Healthy Children: Transforming Child Health Information (NHS England 2016)	https://www.england.nhs.uk/wp-content/uploads/2016/11/healthy-children-transforming-child-health-info.pdf
Working Together to Safeguard Children (HM Government 2018)	https://assets.publishing.service.gov.uk/government/uploads/system/uploads/attachment_data/file/779401/Working_Together_to_Safeguard-Children.pdf
Protecting Children from Trafficking and Modern Slavery (National Society for the Prevention of Cruelty to Children (NSPCC) 2021)	https://learning.nspcc.org.uk/child-abuse-and-neglect/child-trafficking-and-modern-slavery
The Children Act 1989 Guidance and Regulations (Department for Education (DfE) 2021)	https://assets.publishing.service.gov.uk/government/uploads/system/uploads/attachment_data/file/441643/Children_Act_Guidance_2015.pdf
Female Genital Mutilation Act 2003	www.legislation.gov.uk/ukpga/2003/31/contents

decision-making process. We recommend the family-centred practice continuum described by Coleman et al. (2003) to practitioners; this will help you help parents/carers decide on the degree in which they may be active participants in their child's care, including planning, delivery, and management. As suggested by Al-Motlaq et al. (2019), guidance documented in this textbook reflects the philosophy of FCC and its major components.

Making reasonable adjustments to care

Under the Equality Act (2010), health services must consider the needs of people with disabilities in the way they organise their buildings, policies, and services. These are called 'reasonable adjustments' and reflect the fact that some people with disabilities may have particular needs that standard services do not adequately meet. This could relate to, for instance, people with learning and/or physical disabilities. Making reasonable adjustments for CYPs in our care is our third principle. In the context of this textbook, this relates to the need for tailored information and advice to be offered in formats and languages that people can understand; for extra time to be offered to people who have particular communication needs or difficulty understanding what is being said; and ensuring that CYPs and their families are fully prepared for a clinical procedure by listening to what their individual needs might be.

We know that developmentally appropriate and individually tailored preparatory information has a positive effect on CYP's experiences of clinical procedures (Bray et al. 2019a). We also know that there is an added complexity when working with CYPs who have a learning disability, whereby 'individually tailoring' may well require additional preparatory time. Added to this, we are well aware of the range of practices that fall within the term *physical holding*, used to facilitate a clinical procedure being completed (Bray et al. 2018). There is a need for more evidence on how clinical practice guidelines inform professional practice and CYP's views of how their opinions and choices should be sought and attended to in the process of a procedure being completed. But in the meantime, we recommend an initial assessment, working closely with parents/carers in order to understand fully a CYP's needs; this might well reveal social communication difficulties associated with autism, or the presence of challenging behaviour (Absoud et al. 2019). Bray et al. (2019b) have highlighted that during a clinical procedure there are many factors that can 'tip' the balance toward a CYP's expressed wishes being undermined and their feelings of being held against their will. An initial assessment can anticipate the presence of these factors. The need to balance different agendas, rights, and priorities within the momentum that can build during a clinical procedure requires professionals to feel equipped to enact a 'clinical pause': an opportunity to establish a balanced approach that acknowledges the CYP's agency within healthcare procedures. Initial assessment and clinical pause are two approaches that inform and enable a nurse's ability to make a reasonable adjustment.

Legislation and policy relevant to care

Our fourth principle stresses the need for clinical professionals working with CYPs to be conversant with legislation and general guidance for the welfare of CYPs. There is a complex legal framework relevant to the provision of care and treatment to CYPs, and this may vary across the four countries in the UK as well as across international boundaries. Added to this, the development of human rights law has contributed to the increasing recognition of the need to give greater weight to the views of CYPs as they develop their understanding and ability to make their own decisions. However, there are occasions when the adults with the responsibility for the care and treatment of young people have to make decisions and take actions on their behalf to ensure their well-being. Therefore, knowledge regarding the various legal frameworks will always be timely, and it falls to the professional to keep this up to date. Access to computers at unit/ward level makes this task much easier than it ever was, with access to professional databases and PubMed. In addition, organisations such as the Care Quality Commission (CQC 2022) produce lists of legislation that may be relevant to health and social care. In Table I.1 we draw the reader's attention to some of the legislation and policies relevant in the UK today and include websites where up-to-date information can be found.

Code of conduct that underpins care

Our fifth principle is the need to be conversant with the Nursing and Midwifery Council (NMC) code of conduct. Nurses and other healthcare staff must act as advocates for the CYP when necessary (NMC 2018). The people in your care must be able to trust you with their health and well-being. The Code is shaped around four statements, which state that good nurses will:

1 Prioritise people
2 Practise effectively
3 Preserve safety
4 Promote professionalism and trust

As a professional, you are personally accountable for actions and omissions in your practice and you must always be able to justify your decisions. The Code should be considered alongside the NMC's rules, standards, guidance, and advice, available from www.nmc-uk.org. The NMC web site is kept up to date and should be able to guide you in aspects of the code and guidance; your role as a practitioner is to keep up to date with this.

Delivering culturally sensitive care

As nurses, we need to be confident in our role to deliver culturally sensitive care to families; this is our sixth principle. Family ethnicity includes race, culture, religion, and nationality, which impact on a family or person's identity and how they are seen by others. Health is shaped by many different factors such as lifestyle, material wealth, educational attainment, job security, housing conditions, psychosocial stress, discrimination, and the health services. We know that health inequalities exist within different ethnic minority groups and represent the cumulative effect of these factors over the course of life; they can be passed on from one generation to the next through maternal influences on baby and child development. Initiatives aimed at reducing poverty, social exclusion, and difficulty in accessing health services have the potential to tackle the root causes of health inequalities. Some community initiatives aiming to reduce health inequalities and social exclusion by targeting deprived areas are Health Action Zones (www.haznet.org.uk), Neighbourhood Renewal (www.neighbourhood.statistics.org.uk), the New Deal for Communities (www.communities.gov.uk), Sure Start (http://www.early-years.org/surestart/), and more. Recently, the Spearhead Area initiatives (National Audit Office 2010; Barr et al. 2017). An understanding of such schemes can help nurses to be aware of support networks available to the families in our care.

The concept of 'culture' is not homogeneous and one should avoid using generalisations in explaining families' beliefs or behaviours. One should differentiate between the rules of a culture, which governs how one *should* think and behave, and how people actually behave in real life. Generalisations can be dangerous as they often lead to misunderstandings, prejudices, and discrimination. There may be conflict within a family that holds certain beliefs when their CYP has been influenced by different outside social forces. Cultural background has an important influence on many aspects of a CYP's life, including their beliefs, behaviours, perceptions, emotions, language, religion, rituals, family structure, diet, dress, body image, and concepts of space and time. It also plays a part in attitudes to illness, pain, and other misfortunes (Helman 2007). It is important to interpret behaviour or beliefs within its particular context, which is made up of historical, economic, social, political, and geographical elements. This may, for example, have an influence on CYPs or parents who are nonadherent with their medical/nursing care and are seen as 'difficult.'

In most cultures, boys and girls are socialised in different ways and this varies throughout the world. For example, men may play a more predominate part in public life in some cultures, but the 'grandmother' of the family (who is seen as being wiser) may be the decision maker on the way the CYP is brought up. Artificial changes of the body, such as body piercing, tattooing, or artificial fattening are often deemed as notions of beauty in some cultures. Extreme cases such as female circumcision or female genital mutilation (FGM) and severe obesity will affect health and well-being and should be dealt with accordingly. For more information on FGM, which is illegal in the UK see Chapter 31: Safeguarding Children and Young People. Different religious beliefs may include ritual immersions, fasts, food taboos, circumcision, communal feasts, and mass pilgrimages. Some of these may be associated with health concerns such as malnutrition with food taboos, where cultural beliefs and practices misalign with best practices in healthcare (Aghajari et al. 2019). The challenge relates to providing culturally competent care and effectively communicating with families from diverse cultural and ethnic backgrounds who have different health beliefs, practices, values, and languages (Tavallali et al. 2017).

Healthcare professionals should not assume that everyone knows how his or her body works. Many people see it as a 'plumbing system' or machine, and believe that body parts and cavities are connected by pipes (Helman 2007). It is important to ensure that families and CYPs understand their particular health problem and that this is communicated by both oral and written information in their native language, using props that might best help us explain what is happening. An interpreting service should be available to families and CYPs whose first language is not English. Healthcare workers must be sensitive to the world that CYPs and their families live in and ensure that cultural differences or even different views on health are taken into consideration, recorded where necessary, and communicated appropriately to the clinical team.

Consent and involving CYPs in decisions about their care

Throughout this text-book there is an emphasis on ensuring CYPs are communicated with directly and wherever possible are involved in all decisions about their healthcare. We know from many different sources that CYPs want to be involved in the discussions and decisions that affect their health (Royal College of Paediatrics and Child Health, [RCPCH] (2017). In addition, the UN Convention on the Rights of the Child outlines the legal requirements for engaging and involving CYPs in the strategic influence of their healthcare. Article 12 recommends that:

> Children have the right to give their opinions freely on issues that affect them. Adults should listen and take children seriously (UNICEF 1989).

Involving CYPs in decisions about their healthcare can help their understanding of the disease and treatment, reduce their fears, and help them feel more prepared and to cope better. Although there is minimal evidence about what approaches work best for involving CYPs in decision making, we are supportive of communication practices that assist CYPs in this decision-making process (Boland et al. 2019).

In all the relevant sections of this textbook the authors have provided supporting literature on the issue of consent relevant to clinical procedures. We thought this an important seventh principle, and

Introduction

want to highlight in particular the guidance that should be fully understood by all nurses delivering healthcare to CYPs, see for example the recommendations from the Care Quality Commission (CQC 2019). There are a number of documents we want to recommend in this section and list them here. All are based on English law: Healthcare practitioners must follow professional and local guidelines and ensure they are kept up to date, as further legal developments may occur and the law may differ in other countries.

General Medical Council (2018a): *Protecting Children and Young People*	https://www.gmc-uk.org/ethical-guidance/ethical-guidance-for-doctors/protecting-children-and-young-people
General Medical Council (2018b): *0–18 Years: Guidance for All Doctors*	https://www.gmc-uk.org/ethical-guidance/ethical-guidance-for-doctors/0-18-years
Wilacy and Tidy (2021): *Consent to Treatment in Children*	https://patient.info/doctor/consent-to-treatment-in-children-mental-capacity-and-mental-health-legislation
British Medical Association (2021): *Children and Young People Ethics Toolkit*	https://www.bma.org.uk/advice-and-support/ethics/children-and-young-people/children-and-young-people-ethics-toolkit
RCPCH (2012): *Pre-procedure Pregnancy Checking*	www.rcpch.ac.uk/sites/default/files/Guidance.pdf

All the above guidance should be read in conjunction with the Human Tissue Act (2004) and the Mental Capacity Act (2005). They should be read in conjunction with the issues highlighted in each section of this textbook. We would also refer you to sources on YouTube; in particular, look for accounts of CYPs talking about what this process is like – see, for example, https://www.youtube.com/watch?v=837PKaIAk24.

Restrictive physical interventions and clinical holding

NHS Trusts are committed to providing the best-quality care from a compassionate, caring, and competent workforce. As we have discussed, this is best achieved by working in partnership with CYPs and their families to obtain their consent for procedures. However, there are times when the CYP may need to be held still or 'restrained', with or without their explicit consent or that of their parents/carers, so that care can be delivered safely and effectively. This can raise many complex legal, ethical, and practical issues. Clinical holding refers to immobilisation, which may be by splinting or by using limited force. It may be a method of helping CYPs, with their or their parent/carer's permission, to manage a painful procedure quickly and effectively. 'Clinical holding has been distinguished from restrictive physical intervention by the degree of force used, the intention of the hold, and the agreement of the child' (Royal College of Nursing (RCN) 2019).

As just discussed, valid consent should be sought for all forms of healthcare and is particularly important if the CYP must be held still or 'restrained'. This section provides guidance to all staff regarding the use of restrictive physical interventions (formerly known as restraint) and clinical holding of CYPs. It is designed to be read in conjunction with other local and national policies and guidelines. Recent government guidelines focus primarily on restraint in social, educational and community settings (HM Government 2019) and there is currently no precise government guidance on the use of restrictive physical interventions, restraint or clinical holding of CYPs in hospital. The following documents have been incorporated into the principles that underpin this policy and may provide additional information to guide good practice:

- The Children Act 1989
- Human Rights Act 1998
- The United Nations Convention on the Rights of the Child (1989)
- Positive and Proactive Care: Reducing the Need for Restrictive Interventions (DH 2014)
- The Mental Health Act (1983)
- Restrictive Physical Interventions and Therapeutic Clinical Holding of Children and Young People: Guidance for Nursing Staff (RCN 2019)

Individual practitioners remain accountable for protecting the rights and the best interests of their patients while maintaining the standards of practice set out by their own professional body (Nursing and Midwifery Council 2015, updated 2018).

Principles of good practice

- Restrictive physical intervention or clinical holding should be used as the last resort and not the first line of intervention (RCN 2019).
- There should be openness about who decides what is in the CYP's best interest. Where possible, these decisions should be made with the full agreement and involvement of the CYP and their parent or carer (RCN 2019).
- Staff should not be deterred from normal social contact; however, they should try to ensure that a CYP does not misinterpret any physical contact. Developmental age and gender should be considerations in deciding the level of appropriate physical contact.
- Staff should ascertain the significance of physical contact through discussion with the CYP, family, professionals, and previous carers. If the CYP is not comfortable with physical contact, this should be recorded and considered throughout their stay; however, this would not necessarily mean physical contact would be withheld if considered necessary. Cultural factors will be significant in determining what is considered to be acceptable in terms of physical contact.
- Clinical holding and restrictive physical intervention should be employed to achieve outcomes that reflect the best interests of the CYP (i.e. to deliver safe and effective care) and/or others affected by their behaviour (i.e. to prevent the CYP from causing injury to him- or herself or others).
- Serious consideration must be given to the appropriateness of applying to the High Court if there are indications that physical force or unusual restraint needs to be used in order to give treatment, even if the parents/carers consent.
- Clinical holding or restrictive physical intervention should not arouse sexual feelings or expectations (RCN 2019) and should cease if the CYP gives any indication of this.
- Where a member of staff feels it would be inappropriate to respond to a CYP seeking physical contact, the reasons for denying such contact should be explained.
- There should be sufficient staff available who are trained and confident in safe and appropriate techniques and alternatives to restrictive physical intervention and clinical holding of CYPs.
- Staff working within mental health units and services should receive specialist and regular updates to maintain skills as appropriate. These staff can act as a resource within the Trust, should specialist techniques be required.
- There is guidance for parents to read, please see https://www.gosh.nhs.uk/conditions-and-treatments/procedures-and-treatments/therapeutic-holding/.

Prevention

- Staff should communicate with CYPs in a way that maximises and promotes their understanding of their illness and treatment. Time

Introduction

- spent talking and explaining procedures to them and their family may avoid the need for clinical holding or restrictive physical intervention altogether.
- Clinical holding and restrictive physical intervention should be used only if other preventive strategies such as dialogue, diversion, and distraction techniques have been unsuccessful. Clinical staff should be trained and competent in these preventive strategies and in clinical holding and restrictive physical intervention of CYPs for clinical procedures.
- Clinical staff working in 'high-risk' specialist areas (e.g. mental health units) may need additional training in de-escalation techniques.

Specific advice regarding infants and young children

- When young children are being cared for in hospital, it will not usually seem practicable to seek consent from their parents/carers for every routine intervention such as blood or urine tests or X-rays that may require a degree of restraint. However, it should be remembered that, by law, such consent is required. Therefore, discussion of the procedures with the child and their parent/carer should take place in advance to obtain their consent.
- If the child or their parents/carers specify that they wish to be asked before certain procedures are initiated, this must happen, unless the delay involved in contacting them would put the child's health at risk.

Clinical holding for planned procedures

- For planned procedures (e.g., to pass a nasogastric tube or to take blood), consent should be sought in accordance with local policy. If staff will have to hold the CYP to carry out the procedure, the person giving consent should be made aware of this and their consent sought. Consent may be verbal and sought in advance of the procedure (i.e. on admission).
- The involvement of parents/carers may reduce the level of clinical holding needed. Consideration should be given to full parental involvement in the examination and/or treatment, as this may significantly reduce the CYP's anxiety. Staff should recognise that the procedure may be as stressful and distressing for the parent/carer as for the CYP and should ensure that appropriate support is available.
- Gentle protective containment of the CYP with bolsters, pads, and light straps to gain and maintain the correct positioning for diagnostic imaging, or to protect the restless CYP from self-injury, is acceptable. Parents/carers may gently restrain their own child (e.g. to limit movement during cannulation).
- Staff should, if at all possible, have an established relationship with the CYP and should clearly explain what they are doing and why.

Clinical holding in emergency situations

- If consent has not been sought and it is necessary to hold a CYP to perform an emergency or urgent intervention, there should be careful consideration of whether the procedure is really necessary, and whether delaying the procedure to contact the parents/carers would put the CYP's health at risk. Wherever possible, the procedure should be delayed until consent has been obtained (RCN 2019).
- If immediate initiation of the procedure is deemed to be in the CYP's best interests, every effort should be made to gain their cooperation.

Restrictive physical intervention (restraint)

- Restrictive physical intervention is permissible in circumstances where staff are attempting to (i) avert an immediate danger or injury to the CYP or another individual, or (ii) avoid immediate damage to property, where any other course of action would be likely to fail.
- Staff should take steps in advance to avoid the need for restrictive physical intervention, such as through dialogue and diversion, and the CYP should be warned verbally that physical restraint will be used unless they desist.
- Restrictive physical intervention is distinguished from clinical holding by the degree of force required. At all times, the degree of force used must be reasonable and proportionate to both the behaviour of the individual to be controlled and the nature of the harm they may cause. These judgements must be made at the time, taking account of all the circumstances, including any known history of other events requiring restraint.
- The minimum necessary force should be used.
- The techniques deployed should be those for which staff are trained and familiar with, and are able to use safely. The team leader should be clearly identified and should ensure that all staff are aware of their individual roles during the period of restraint.
- Restrictive physical intervention should avert danger by preventing or deflecting a CYP's action or by removing a physical object. Averting harm by causing or threatening hurt, pain, or distress is unacceptable (except in wholly exceptional circumstances such as self-defence).
- Restrictive physical intervention should not be used purely to force adherence with staff instruction when there is no immediate risk to people or property.
- Every effort should be made to secure the presence of other staff before applying restraint. The number of staff needed will vary with the situation. If possible, a member of staff of the same sex as the CYP should be present.
- Restrictive physical intervention should be disengaged by degrees as the CYP calms down in response to physical contact. As soon as it is safe, restraint should be gradually relaxed to allow the CYP to regain self-control.
- Debriefing of the CYP and everyone involved should take place as soon after the incident as possible (RCN 2019).
- The senior nurse and the CYP's parents/carers must be made aware of all incidents requiring a restrictive physical intervention and the CYP's doctor should be informed of incidents lasting more than 30 minutes.
- All incidents should be fully documented and the Trust's local procedures for reporting incidents should be followed.

Documentation

- All staff involved must keep detailed and accurate records of each occasion where a CYP is held or 'restrained'.
- An incident report form must be completed and reported in accordance with local policies whenever restrictive physical intervention is used.

Communication and handover to improve quality of care

Communication, and the ability to communicate complex information to CYPs and family members, features in all our stated principles so far. We encourage practitioners to learn effective communication strategies to ensure CYPs and their parents/carers have the information they need in the appropriate format (Matthews 2010). In principle number 9, we want to turn to the importance of communication between professionals. Nurses have always had a 'ritual' for handing over patient information from one another when changing shifts but the quality and accuracy of the information has often been called into question. One of the greatest sources of frustration for CYPs and their families is the lack of integration and communication between different services within an organisation or between organisations.

Handover is the system by which the responsibility for immediate and ongoing care is transferred between healthcare professionals. CYPs and their families expect and should have a designated consultant and nurse to coordinate the multidisciplinary team. However, at times (e.g. at night, during weekends, or during an emergency admission), the responsibility for care must pass from one team or consultant to another (Royal College of Physicians 2011). Poor handover between doctors, nurses, and multidisciplinary teams is a common cause of error in hospitals and a major preventable cause of patient harm. It can lead to inefficiencies, repetitions, delayed decisions, repeated investigations, incorrect diagnoses, incorrect treatment, and poor communication with the patient. Some hospitals do not even have a handover protocol in place (Royal College of Physicians 2011). The handover should be written or recorded and each professional involved in the CYP's care should have access to it at all times. There is no reason why CYPs or their parents should not listen to their own handover unless this is felt to be medically inappropriate.

Communication during verbal handover should also be standardised to improve accuracy and safety. A communication tool developed by the US Navy and adapted for healthcare (Hohenhaus et al. 2006) has been further adapted by clinical teams at GOSH. A 'D' (decisions) has been added to the acronym SBAR (situation, background, assessment, recommendation) to 'round off' each conversation and improve clarity (SBARD). Over one third of wards at GOSH have improved the efficiency and effectiveness of their handover using the SBARD communication tool. On average, wards using SBARD have reduced the length of time spent in handover by 30–50% – that is 10–20 minutes twice each day. Nurses who now use SBARD also report that their handovers feel safer and more effective, as everyone involved focuses on patient care needs for the next shift and beyond, rather than reviewing what has happened in the past. This method is also being used to communicate the needs of the deteriorating CYP. Although yet to be formally evaluated within the context of CYPs' healthcare, we are recommending its use to readers of this textbook, and refer you to studies that have looked at the quality of handover (Ruhomauly et al. 2019).

Of further assistance in our approach to communication between professionals is the increasing use of electronic patient records and the introduction of a paperless NHS (Parliamentary Office of Science and Technology 2016). The increased use of electronic patient records in the NHS means that up-to-date information about patients is readily available to a range of health professionals who are treating and caring for those patients (Griffith 2019); assisting in more effective communication between professionals.

The nine principles outlined here briefly are, we suggest, important to all the chapters that follow. Delivering safe care, managing procedures effectively, and working with all family members sensitively are important to ensure that we as nurses can be confident of delivering high quality care. Nurses have a central role in helping CYPs and their family members to manage the demands of clinical procedures as part of a unique illness experience. Even when the procedure has been undertaken many times before and we are caring for 'expert patients,' our attention to individualised patient assessment will enable us to work effectively alongside family members. The latest research and evidence for procedures must underpin all our approaches to care. Nurses have a responsibility to provide the highest standard of care; to do that they must keep up to date. The chapters that follow facilitate this level of knowledge and practice, and point readers to places where they can continue to stay current. We conclude by reminding nurses of their responsibilities, and would encourage use of journals such as *Evidence-Based Nursing* and *Worldviews on Evidence-Based Nursing*, alongside speciality journals and National Institute for Health and Care Excellence (NICE) Evidence search tools for authoritative evidence for healthcare.

References

Absoud, M., Wake, H., Ziriat, M., and Hassiotis, A. (2019). Managing challenging behaviour in children with possible learning disability. *BMJ* 365: l663. https://doi.org/10.1136/bmj.l1663.

Aghajari, P., Valizadeh, L., Zamanzadeh, V. et al. (2019). Cultural sensitivity in paediatric nursing care: a concept analysis using the hybrid method. *Scandinavian Journal of Caring Sciences* 33: 609–620.

Al-Motlaq, M.A., Carter, B., Neill, S. et al. (2019). Toward developing consensus on family centred care: an international descriptive study and discussion. *Journal of Child Health Care* 23 (3): 458–467.

Barr, B., Higgerson, J., and Whitehead, M. (2017). Investigating the impact of the English health inequalities strategy: time trend analysis. *BMJ* 358: j3310. https://doi.org/10.1136/bmj.j3310.

Boland, L., Graham, I.D., Legare, F. et al. (2019). Barriers and facilitators of pediatric shared decision-making: a systematic review. *Implementation Science* 14: 7. https://doi.org/10.1186/s13012-018-0851-5.

Bray, L., Carter, B., Ford, K. et al. (2018). Holding children for procedures: an international survey of health professionals. *Journal of Child Health Care* 22 (2): 205–215.

Bray, L., Appleton, V., and Sharpe, A. (2019a). The information needs of children having clinical procedures: will it hurt? Will I feel scared? What can I do to stay calm? *Child: Care, Health and Development* 45: 737–743.

Bray, L., Ford, K., Dickinson, A. et al. (2019b). A qualitative study of health professionals' views on the holding of children for clinical procedures: constructing a balanced approach. *Journal of Child Health Care* 23 (1): 160–171.

British Medical Association (2021). *Children and young people ethics toolkit*. https://www.bma.org.uk/advice-and-support/ethics/children-and-young-people/children-and-young-people-ethics-toolkit (accessed 03 February 2023).

Care Quality Commission (CQC) (2022). Regulations for service providers and managers: related legislation. www.cqc.org.uk/guidance-providers/regulations-enforcement/regulations-service-providers-managers-relevant (accessed 03 February 2023).

CQC (2019) Brief guide: capacity and competence to consent in under 18s. https://www.cqc.org.uk/sites/default/files/Brief_guide_Capacity_and_consent_in_under_18s%20v3.pdf (accessed 29 March 2022).

Children (Northern Ireland) Order (1995). www.legislation.gov.uk/nisi/1995/755/contents/made (accessed 03 February 2023).

The Children Act (1989). London, HMSO.

The Children Act (2004). www.legislation.gov.uk/ukpga/2004/31/notes/division/2/2/1/2 (accessed 03 February 2023).

Children and Families Act (2014). www.legislation.gov.uk/ukpga/2014/6/contents/enacted (accessed 03 February 2023).

Children and Social Work Act (2017). www.legislation.gov.uk/ukpga/2017/16/contents/enacted (accessed 03 February 2023).

Children and Young Persons Act (2008). www.legislation.gov.uk/ukpga/2008/23/pdfs/ukpga_20080023_en.pdf (accessed 03 February 2023).

Coleman, V. (2002). The evolving concept of family-centred care. In: *Family-Centred Care: Concept, Theory and Practice* (eds. L. Smith, V. Coleman and M. Bradshaw), 3–18. Hampshire: Palgrave.

Coleman, V., Smith, L., and Bradshaw, M. (2003). Enhancing consumer participation using the practice continuum tool for family-centred care. *Paediatric Nursing* 15 (8): 28–31.

Department for Children, Schools and Families (2007). The children's plan. https://assets.publishing.service.gov.uk/government/uploads/system/uploads/attachment_data/file/325111/2007-childrens-plan.pdf (accessed 03 February 2023).

Department for Education (DfE) (2015). The Children Act 1989 guidance and regulations. https://assets.publishing.service.gov.uk/government/uploads/system/uploads/attachment_data/file/1000549/The_Children_Act_1989_guidance_and_regulations_Volume_2_care_planning__placement_and_case_review.pdf (accessed 03 February 2023).

DH (2014). Positive and Proactive Care: reducing the need for restrictive interventions. https://www.gov.uk/government/publications/positive-and-proactive-care-reducing-restrictive-interventions (accessed 3 February 2023).

Equality Act (2010). p2, c2, s20. www.legislation.gov.uk/ukpga/2010/15/contents (accessed 03 February 2023).

General Medical Council (2018a). Protecting children and young people: the responsibilities of all doctors. https://www.gmc-uk.org/ethical-guidance/ethical-guidance-for-doctors/protecting-children-and-young-people (accessed 03 February 2023).

General Medical Council (2018b). 0–18 years: Guidance for all doctors. https://www.gmc-uk.org/ethical-guidance/ethical-guidance-for-doctors/0-18-years (accessed 03 February 2023).

Great Ormond Street Hospital for Children NHS Foundation Trust (GOSH) (2020). About us: Who we are. https://www.gosh.nhs.uk/about-us/who-we-are/ (accessed 03 February 2023).

Griffith, R. (2019). Electronic records, confidentiality and data security: the nurses responsibility. *British Journal of Nursing* 28 (5): 313–314.

Introduction

Helman, C. (2007). *Culture, Health and Illness*, 5e. London: Hodder Arnold Publications.

Hemphill, A.L. and Dearmun, A.K. (2010). Working with children and families. In: *A Textbook of Children's and Young People's Nursing* (eds. A. Glasper and J. Richardson), 17–29. Churchill Livingstone Elsevier.

HM Government (2018). Working together to safeguard children. https://www.gov.uk/government/publications/working-together-to-safeguard-children–2 (accessed 03 February 2023).

HM Government (2019). Reducing the need for restraint and restrictive intervention. https://www.gov.uk/government/publications/reducing-the-need-for-restraint-and-restrictive-intervention (accessed 03 February 2023).

Hohenhaus, S., Powell, S., and Hohenhaus, J.T. (2006). Enhancing patient safety during hands-off: standardized communication and teamwork using the SBAR method. *American Journal of Nursing* 106 (8): 72A–72B.

Human Rights Act (1998). London, HMSO. https://www.equalityhumanrights.com/en/human-rights/human-rights-act (accessed 03 February 2023).

Human Tissue Act (2004). www.hta.gov.uk/policies/human-tissue-act-2004 (accessed 03 February 2023).

Hutchfield, K. (1999). Family-centred care: a concept analysis. *Journal of Advanced Nursing* 29 (5): 1178–1187.

Matthews, J. (2010). Communicating with children and their families. In: *A Textbook of Children's and Young People's Nursing* (eds. A. Glasper and J. Richardson), 121–136. Churchill Livingstone Elsevier.

Mental Capacity Act (2005). www.legislation.gov.uk/ukpga/2005/9/contents (accessed 03 February 2023).

Mental Health Act (1983). *Code of Practice, Department of Health and Welsh Office*. London: The Stationery Office.

National Audit Office (2010). Tackling inequalities in life expectancy in areas with the worst health and deprivation. www.nao.org.uk/wp-content/uploads/2010/07/1011186.pdf (accessed 03 February 2023).

National Service Framework for Children, Young People and Maternity Services (2007). https://webarchive.nationalarchives.gov.uk/+/www.dh.gov.uk/en/Publicationsandstatistics/Publications/PublicationsPolicyAndGuidance/Browsable/DH_4094329 (accessed 03 February 2023).

National Society for the Prevention of Cruelty to Children (2021). https://learning.nspcc.org.uk/child-abuse-and-neglect/child-trafficking-and-modern-slavery (accessed 03 February 2023).

NHS England (2016). Healthy children: transforming child health information. https://www.england.nhs.uk/wp-content/uploads/2016/11/healthy-children-transforming-child-health-info.pdf (accessed 03 February 2023).

Nursing and Midwifery Council (2015, updated 2018). *The Code: Professional standards of practice and behaviour for nurses, midwives and nursing associates*. London: NMC. https://www.nmc.org.uk/standards/code/ (accessed 03 February 2023).

Nursing and Midwifery Council (NMC) (2018). The code: Professional standards of practice and behaviour for nurses, midwives and nursing associates. www.nmc.org.uk/standards/code (accessed 03 February 2023).

O'Connor, S., Brenner, M., and Coyne, I. (2019). Family-centred care of children and young people in the acute hospital setting: a concept analysis. *Journal of Clinical Nursing*. https://doi.org/10.1111/jocn.14913.

Ogourtsova, T., O'Donnell, M., and Majnemer, A. (2018). Coach, care coordinator, navigator or keyworker? *Review of Emergent Terms in Childhood Disability. Physical & Occupational Therapy in Pediatrics*. https://doi.org/10.1080/01942638.2018.1521891.

Parliamentary Office of Science and Technology (2016). Electronic health records. https://post.parliament.uk/research-briefings/post-pn-0519 (accessed 03 February 2023).

Pordes, E., Gordon, J., Sanders, L.M., and Cohen, E. (2019). Models of care delivery for children with medical complexity. *Pediatrics* 141 (sz93): e2 0171284.

Protection of Children (Scotland) Act (2003). www.legislation.gov.uk/asp/2003/5/contents (accessed 03 February 2023).

Protection of Vulnerable Groups (Scotland) Act (2007). www.legislation.gov.uk/asp/2007/14/contents (accessed 03 February 2023).

Royal College of Nursing (2019). Restrictive physical interventions and the clinical holding of children and young people: Guidance for nursing staff. https://www.rcn.org.uk/professional-development/publications/pub-007746 (accessed 03 February 2023).

Royal College of Paediatrics and Child Health (RCPCH) (2012). *Preprocedure pregnancy checking: guidance for clinicians*. www.rcpch.ac.uk/sites/default/files/Guidance.pdf (accessed 03 February 2023).

Royal College of Physicians (2011). Acute Care Toolkit 1 – Handover. www.rcplondon.ac.uk/guidelines-policy/acute-care-toolkit-1-handover (accessed 03 February 2023).

Royal College of Paediatrics and Child Health (2017). Involving children and young people in specialised commissioning. https://www.rcpch.ac.uk/resources/involving-children-young-people-specialised-commissioning (accessed 30 Jan 2023).

Ruhomauly, Z., Betts, K., Coupe, K.J. et al. (2019). Improving the quality of handover: implanting SBAR. *Future Healthcare Journal* 6 (2): 1, s54–67.

Tavallali, A.G., Jirwe, M., and Kabir, Z.N. (2017). Cross-cultural encounters in paediatric care: minority ethnic parents' experiences. *Scandinavian Journal of Caring Sciences* 31: 54–62.

United Nations International Children's Emergency Fund (UNICEF) (1989). United Nations Convention on the Rights of the Child. UNICEF. London. https://www.unicef.org/child-rights-convention (accessed 03 February 2023).

Wilacy, H. and Tidy, C. (2021). *Consent to treatment in children: mental capacity and mental health legislation*. https://patient.info/doctor/consent-to-treatment-in-children-mental-capacity-and-mental-health-legislation (accessed 03 February 2023).

Chapter 1

Assessment

Sue Chapman[1], Eileen Brennan[2], and Lindy May[3]

[1]RN (Adult), RN (Child), AdvDip Child Development, MSc Paediatric Critical Care Nursing (Advanced Practice), PhD Child Health; Clinical Site Director; Great Ormond Street Hospital, London, UK

[2]RN (Adult), RN (Child), MSc; Nurse Consultant in Paediatric Nephrology; GOSH

[3]RN (Adult), RN (Child), MSc (Neuroscience), Diploma in Counselling, PhD; Formerly Nurse Consultant, Neurosurgery; GOSH

Chapter contents

Introduction	2
Section 1: General principles	2
Section 2: Present illness	4
Section 3: Past history	4
Section 4: Family history	5
Section 5: Vital signs and baseline measurements	6
Section 6: Assessment of body systems	19
References	25

Procedure guidelines

1.1 General principles of assessment	2	
1.2 Present illness	4	
1.3 Past history	4	
1.4 Family history	5	
1.5 Monitoring plan and early warning score	6	
1.6 Measuring temperature	6	
1.7 Measuring heart rate	7	
1.8 Measuring respiratory rate	8	
1.9 Measuring blood pressure	8	
1.10 Measuring oxygen saturation	14	
1.11 Growth assessment	14	
1.12 Measuring height	15	
1.13 Measuring weight	16	
1.14 Measuring head circumference	18	
1.15 Assessing the respiratory and cardiovascular systems	19	
1.16 Assessing the neurological system	20	
1.17 Assessing nutrition	22	
1.18 Assessing elimination and sexual development	22	
1.19 Assessing skin and hygiene	23	
1.20 Assessing mobility	24	
1.21 Assessing development	25	
1.22 Other relevant information	25	

The Great Ormond Street Hospital Manual of Children and Young People's Nursing Practices, Second Edition. Edited by Elizabeth Anne Bruce, Janet Williss, and Faith Gibson.
© 2023 John Wiley & Sons Ltd. Published 2023 by John Wiley & Sons Ltd.

Introduction

Assessment forms the first part of any nursing activity and is the first step in delivering nursing care. Without a comprehensive assessment of the child or young person (CYP) and family's needs, care cannot be planned, delivered, or evaluated effectively (Broom 2007). For most CYPs and their families, the nursing assessment is often the first contact that they have with the nursing team and it is important that this is seen as a positive, helpful, and informative process (Moorey 2010a).

Each CYP and member of their family should be approached as an individual. Much about the CYP's illness or problem can be discovered through observing them at play, or interacting with their family, without the nurse needing to touch or examine them.

To aid ease of use, this chapter is organised into six distinct sections.

Section 1: General Principles: This section outlines the general principles that should run throughout the assessment process, and which should support the nurse's assessment of the CYP.

Section 2: Present Illness: Issues surrounding the CYP's present illness are then explored and this includes examining the current issues that have brought the CYP into the healthcare setting.

Section 3: Past History: For many CYPs, their current problems may be related to previous illnesses and/or injuries, so this forms an important part of the assessment process.

Section 4: Family History: Likewise, many conditions may be hereditary or have a tendency to run in families, so the health history of other family members may provide important information on actual or potential health problems for the CYP.

Section 5: Vital Signs and Baseline Measurements: The measuring of vital signs is a core essential skill for all healthcare practitioners working with infants and CYPs (RCN 2017). It provides valuable information about the CYP's state of health and can identify signs of illness, disease, or deterioration, allowing early intervention and treatment. Standards for assessing, measuring, and monitoring vital signs in infants and CYPs have been described (RCN 2017). Vital signs are also a core component of a paediatric track and trigger or early warning system. These systems can assist staff in recognising CYPs 'at risk' of deterioration (Chapman et al. 2016) and form part of the safe system framework for those at risk of deterioration recommended by the Royal College of Paediatrics and Child Health (RCPCH 2018). Other routine measurements, such as height and weight, provide essential information about the CYP's growth and development, which is especially important in cases of chronic illness.

Section 6: Review of Body Systems: The subsequent physical examination is separated into nine 'systems' based on the approach used throughout the 'admission assessment' documentation currently in use at Great Ormond Street Hospital. The information gained thus far should be utilised to guide the nurse on the structure and depth of the physical examination of each system. The process is not designed to be fragmented, but to encourage the nurse to structure the examination around the CYP and family's individual needs, while providing a comprehensive healthcare assessment. Not every system will need to be examined to the same depth, but if actual or potential problems are identified within a certain system, special attention should be paid to examining that area in detail. The 'systems review' section is designed to be read in conjunction with other relevant chapters of this book.

Finally, assessment is an ongoing, dynamic process. Although this chapter provides a structured approach to performing a full nursing assessment, it is not designed to be prescriptive and the nurse should remain responsive to the CYP and family's needs at all times. Assessment of the CYP is also addressed in many other chapters in this book, including but not limited to Chapter 9: Early Recognition and Management of the Seriously Ill Child; Chapter 21: Neurological Care (neurological observations); Chapter 23: Orthopaedic Care (neurovascular observations); and Chapter 24: Pain Management (pain assessment).

Section 1: General principles

Procedure guideline 1.1 General principles of assessment

Statement	Rationale
1 Before undertaking the assessment, the nurse should consider the CYP's age, gender, culture, and religious beliefs, as well as their physical and developmental needs.	1 These factors should influence how the nurse approaches the assessment process.
2 Throughout the assessment process the nurse should refer any serious concerns about any aspect of the CYP's well-being to a senior nursing or medical colleague.	2 To ensure that if help is immediately required, it is sought quickly and from the appropriate source.
3 The nurse should be familiar with the parent-held child health record (commonly known as the 'red book'), previous healthcare records, and referral letter if appropriate.	3 To guide the assessment process, avoid unnecessary repetition, and highlight priorities for assessment.

Procedure guideline 1.1 General principles of assessment *(continued)*

Statement	Rationale
4 Establish who has parental responsibility (PR) for the CYP.	4 Only a person with PR can consent to any form of care or treatment (including the assessment process) of a CYP under 16 years of age (unless they are considered competent to consent for themselves). Fathers do not automatically acquire PR and either parent can have this revoked by the Court.
5 Establish a rapport with the CYP and family by: • Introducing yourself by name and role. • Establishing what they would like to be called. • Being welcoming in a warm, friendly fashion. • Maintaining good eye contact throughout the assessment process.	5 To reduce any anxiety they may have and promote effective assessment (Moorey 2010a).
6 Ensure all explanations are described in language appropriate for the CYP's age and development (Moorey 2010b), taking into account any learning and/or physical disabilities (Thurgate 2006).	6 To ensure understanding.
7 Use jargon-free, nontechnical terms throughout the assessment process. If jargon is unavoidable, ensure this is clearly explained and documented.	7 To ensure understanding.
8 Explain to the CYP and family the purpose and format of the assessment process (Moorey 2010b).	8 To reduce any anxiety that they may have. Cooperation and open communication is more likely if they understand what is happening and why.
9 Select the environment where the assessment is to be conducted. Ensure it is warm and private and if possible is decorated in an age-appropriate manner (Engel 2006).	9 To promote comfort for the CYP and maintain confidentiality. The needs of an adolescent are different to those of an infant.
10 When recording the health assessment, use the CYP and family's own words wherever possible.	10 To ensure accuracy of information.
11 Encourage the CYP and family to ask questions and voice any concerns.	11 To ensure effective communication and reduce anxiety. Parents/carers' concerns about their child may provide an important clue about the CYP's overall condition (Moorey 2010a).
12 Establish the CYP and family's first language. If it is not spoken English, do they need an interpreter or signer to be present? Are there any other language needs, such as British Sign Language or Makaton?	12 Effective communication is essential to the assessment process.
13 Use a mixture of open and closed questions.	13 Open questions elicit broader, more general information. Closed questions can be used to gain more specific information and clarify information.
14 Clarify your understanding of the issues by reflecting back the CYP and family's statements, such as 'when you said that you had a headache in your tummy, did you mean that your tummy was hurting?'	14 To ensure correct interpretation of the information provided.
15 a) If equipment is used to measure or assess the CYP it should be appropriate for their needs and staff should be trained in its use. b) Equipment must be checked, calibrated, and cleaned prior to use in accordance with manufacturer's guidelines and local policies (RCN 2017).	15 a) To ensure appropriate assessment and accurate measurement. b) To prevent cross-infection.
16 All assessments and measurements should be documented as soon as possible after they have been recorded. All entries should be signed and dated, and a note made of any action taken as a result of the assessment.	16 To facilitate inter-professional communication and accurately record the CYP's progress.

Section 2: Present illness

Procedure guideline 1.2 Present illness

Statement	Rationale
1 Find out what the CYP and family's reason for attending the hospital or clinic is.	1 This will provide important information about their perception of their needs and healthcare problems.
2 Ascertain what they consider to be the main health problem or need.	2 The needs of the CYP and family may not be the same as those perceived by the healthcare workers. This will also help the nurse to structure the assessment process.
3 Ask the CYP and family to describe the symptoms of the illness or problem in their own words.	3 To structure the assessment process and ensure effective assessment and communication.
4 a) If they have symptoms of pain, what words or sounds does the CYP use to describe their pain? b) Establish with the CYP and family the exact location, duration, and frequency of the pain. Does anything trigger the pain to start? What helps to relieve the pain (including over-the-counter medicines used)? c) Severity may be assessed using pain assessment tools appropriate for the CYP's age.	4 a) To ensure effective communication and assessment of pain. b) Establishing factors that aggravate or relieve the pain may help with the diagnosis and the planning of nursing care. c) Pain assessment tools will help to more accurately monitor the CYP's pain and response to treatment. For further information, see Chapter 24: Pain Management.
5 Does the CYP have any known infections?	5 If so, they may need to be isolated to prevent the spread of infection. For further information, see Chapter 13: Infection Prevention and Control.

Section 3: Past history

Procedure guideline 1.3 Past history

Principle	Rationale
1 Taking details of the CYP's past history and illnesses is an important part of the assessment process.	1 The CYP's past history may offer important information about their current healthcare issues (Miller and Hinton 2014).
2 CYPs who are experiencing developmental or neurological problems and all those under two years of age should have their prenatal, birth, and neonatal history assessed (Engel 2006).	2 The prenatal, birth, and neonatal history is especially important for these CYPs as developmental and neurological problems may be related to their prenatal and birth history (Sables-Baus and Robinson 2011).
3 The prenatal history should include details about maternal health, any infections or medications taken, abnormal maternal bleeding, weight gain, and the duration of and any other difficulties encountered during the pregnancy (Sables-Baus and Robinson 2011).	3 To provide a comprehensive assessment.
4 The birth history should include the duration of labour, type of delivery, and any maternal complications.	4 To provide a comprehensive assessment.
5 The neonatal history should include weight and condition at birth, as well as details of any admission to special care or neonatal intensive care. Any other complications or difficulties, such as respiratory distress, jaundice, or feeding problems should also be noted. The results of an infant's Guthrie test should be established.	5 To provide a comprehensive assessment.
6 Has the CYP been in hospital before? If so, when was this and what was wrong with them? More detailed information may be found within the CYP's healthcare records.	6 The current illness may be related to previous illness or past surgery.
7 How has the CYP responded to previous illnesses, procedures, and hospitalisations?	7 A CYP who is chronically ill or who has been in hospital numerous times may need different support from one who has never been in hospital before. Identification of procedures that are known to distress the CYP (such as venepuncture) enables practitioners to adopt strategies to lessen the distress.

Procedure guideline 1.3 Past history *(continued)*

Principle	Rationale
8. a) What medicines is the CYP currently taking? Note the dosage and frequency of all medications, including 'over-the-counter' medicines. b) Establish the CYP and parent/carer's understanding of the drugs and the reasons for their use.	8. a) To allow a review of the current medications and ensure that the current regimen is continued. b) The assessment also provides an opportunity for education surrounding their medications.
9. Is the CYP allergic to anything? If so, what are the medicines or products that they are allergic to? a) What type of reaction did they have to the medicine/product? Who told you that it was an allergic reaction? b) Has the CYP taken this or similar drugs/products after this reaction occurred? If yes, did they experience similar problems?	9. Failure to document a serious allergy places the CYP at risk of anaphylaxis if the medicine/product is subsequently given. The CYP and family may mistake a medication's side effects for an allergy (e.g. gastrointestinal (GI) disturbance during antibiotic therapy). Misdiagnosing a reaction can lead to the CYP being deprived of effective treatment.
10. Has the CYP had any of the common communicable diseases such as chickenpox, mumps, or measles? Have they been in recent contact with anyone else who has these illnesses?	10. It is important to establish if they have acquired immunity to any of these common illnesses, as well as establishing that they are not currently an infection risk to other children.
11. Has the CYP been immunised? If so, take details of which vaccinations they have received and when. Check this against the current recommended immunisation schedule. a) Make a note of any vaccinations they have not received and the reason why.	11. They may be at risk of illness if they have not received their vaccinations. The assessment may also provide an opportunity for education and health promotion. For further information see Chapter 12: Immunisations.

Section 4: Family history

Procedure guideline 1.4 Family history

Principle	Rationale
1. What is the family composition? Who lives at home with the CYP? Do they have siblings? If so, what are their names and ages?	1. To develop an understanding of the CYP as an individual and member of a family.
2. Are the parents/carers employed? If so, what are their occupations? If both parents work, who cares for the CYP?	2. Parental occupation can have an impact on the health and well-being of the CYP and family. Financial difficulties may adversely affect the health and well-being of the family and the individual.
3. Where do the CYP and family live? Do they own their own house or rent? How long have they lived at that address?	3. Problems with housing can have a significant effect on the CYP's physical, emotional, and psychological well-being (Harker 2006). Hospitalisation that is a significant distance from the family home may affect the ability of other family members to visit and lead to isolation and stress.
4. Ask about the health of the parents, grandparents, and siblings. Do they have any current health concerns or have they suffered from serious illness in the past?	4. The health of the CYP's family may give clues to the nature of the CYP's illness (Miller and Hinton 2014). Inherited diseases such as cystic fibrosis, congenital heart disease may be identified through examination of the family history.
5. Does the CYP attend school? Which one? Overall, how are they progressing? Are there any problems that the parents/carers or CYP are aware of?	5. Problems at school may negatively impact on health (Oberklaid 2014). Problems may be related to current health problems (e.g. difficulties with hearing or eyesight may affect the ability to learn) or can be the cause of health problems (e.g. bullying at school may lead to anxiety, causing behavioural problems, weight loss, sleeping difficulties, etc. (Wolke et al. 2014).
6. Does the family see any other medical or allied health professionals on a regular basis?	6. Other professionals may provide important information about the CYP and family. Communication and liaison with other healthcare teams is equally important.
7. Do the CYP and/or family have any other concerns regarding the CYP's general health and social needs?	7. To enable them to voice concerns about issues that may not have been covered within the assessment.

Section 5: Vital signs and baseline measurements

Procedure guideline 1.5 Monitoring plan and early warning score

Statement	Rationale
1 All CYPs admitted to hospital should have a documented monitoring plan (RCN 2011).	1 To facilitate communication among the multiprofessional team members.
2 The monitoring plan should be reviewed at least daily by the multiprofessional team.	2 To ensure the plan is appropriate for the CYP's needs.
3 All CYPs should also be assessed using a Paediatric Early Warning System or similar tool (RCN 2017).	3 To detect early signs of deterioration and ensure appropriate escalation to a senior healthcare worker if needed (Chapman et al. 2010). See Chapter 9: Early Recognition and Management of the Seriously Ill Child.

Procedure guideline 1.6 Measuring temperature

Statement	Rationale
1 Core temperature varies in childhood and is dependent on a number of factors including age, environmental factors, and illness.	1 It is important to assess temperature against age appropriate values, taking into account environmental factors and current state of health.
2 Peripheral temperature monitoring is useful for CYPs where there are concerns about fluid balance status or peripheral perfusion.	2 A significant difference between the core and peripheral temperature may indicate poor perfusion to the skin from dehydration or shock (Advanced Life Support Group 2011 (ALSG) 2016).
3 a) All CYPs should have a temperature recorded on admission (RCN 2017). b) The ongoing frequency of temperature monitoring should reflect the CYP's clinical condition.	3 a) To establish a baseline. b) To provide individualised care.
4 a) If the temperature reading falls outside the normal range, measurements should be taken more frequently until the temperature normalises. b) Fever in children under 5 years should be assessed using the National Institute for Health and Clinical Excellence (NICE) guidelines (NICE 2019).	4 a) To assess temperature instability and severity, to monitor disease progression and to monitor temperature control techniques. b) Infection is the leading cause of death in children under the age of 5 years. Therefore fever must be assessed using a systematic approach (NICE 2019).
5 a) The site and equipment selected for temperature measurement should take into account the CYP's age, local policy guidance and the preferences of the CYP and family (RCN 2011; Sund-Levander and Grodzinsky 2013). b) The manufacturer's instructions and local guidelines for the selected temperature measurement device should be followed. c) Infants under the age of 4 weeks should have their temperature measured with an electronic thermometer in the axilla (NICE 2019). d) Infants and children from 4 weeks to 5 years should have their temperature measured with an electronic/chemical dot thermometer in the axilla or an infra-red tympanic thermometer (NICE 2019; RCN 2017). e) The rectal route is not recommended unless other routes and methods are impossible or impractical (RCN 2017).	5 a) To ensure safety and improve adherence. b) Individual devices vary in the time needed to ensure accurate measurement, cleaning, and calibration requirements. e) There is a risk of bowel perforation, discomfort, and distress to the CYP due to the invasive nature of this route (El-Radhi 2013).
6 *Axillary temperature measurement:* a) It may be helpful to place younger children on their parent's/carer's lap. b) Measurements via this route may be inaccurate in the early stages of a fever (El-Radhi 2014).	6 a) To ensure safety and improve adherence. b) Peripheral vasoconstriction may cool the skin and sweating may cause the skin temperature to be lower than the core temperature, resulting in inaccurate readings (El-Radhi 2014).

Procedure guideline 1.6 Measuring temperature (continued)

Statement	Rationale
7 Oral temperature measurement: a) Ensure the CYP is sitting or lying. b) Do not measure the temperature via this route if the CYP has had a hot or cold drink in the previous 20 minutes. c) Avoid this route if the CYP is uncooperative, comatose, tachypnoeic, seizure-prone, or had recent oral surgery (El-Radhi 2013).	7 a–b) To prevent inaccurate readings. c) To prevent complications.
8 Tympanic temperature measurement: a) Ensure the CYP is sitting or lying. b) Perform an ear tug: For children under 1 year, pull the ear straight back. For CYPs aged 1 to adult, pull the ear up and back. c) While tugging the ear, fit the probe snugly into the ear canal (with a firm seal around the external auditory meatus), orientating the tip toward the tympanic membrane. d) Avoid using tympanic thermometer measurements in children under three years of age (El-Radhi 2014). It may also be difficult in children with very small external ear canals. e) Do not use this route if the CYP has acute otitis media, sinusitis, or had recent surgery to the ear.	8 b) To straighten the ear canal in order to allow a clear view of the eardrum. c) To allow the sensor to measure the heat from the eardrum and not the sides of the ear canal. d) They may be inaccurate in children under 3 years of age (El-Radhi 2014). e) To avoid causing damage to the eardrum.
9 Rectal temperature measurement: a) If the rectal route must be used, younger infants may be placed in the supine position with knees flexed toward the abdomen. b) For older CYPs, place prone or lying on their side. c) Do not use if the CYP has had anal or rectal surgery, chemotherapy, or has diarrhoea or rectal irritation (Engel 2006).	9 a) To ensure safety and improve adherence. b) To ensure safety and improve adherence. c) To prevent secondary complications.
10 Assess the temperature against age-appropriate values. a) The measurement should be documented according to local policy and the method and device from which the temperature was recorded should be noted.	10 Normal temperature varies slightly with age. a) To ensure accuracy, consistency, and comparability.

Procedure guideline 1.7 Measuring heart rate

Statement	Rationale
1 In older CYPs, heart rate can be assessed by palpating the radial artery (Rawlings-Anderson and Hunter 2008; RCN 2011). In infants and children under 2 years of age, auscultation of the apical beat with a stethoscope is recommended (Howlin and Brenner 2010; RCN 2017).	1 To provide an accurate record. The pulse is difficult to palpate in younger children (Howlin and Brenner 2010).
2 If the CYP is crying or very distressed, wait until they are calmer (Engel 2006).	2 Crying and distress may increase the pulse rate.
3 Count the pulse for a full minute (Howlin and Brenner 2010). Electronic data should be cross-checked by auscultation or palpation of the pulse (RCN 2017).	3 To ensure an accurate reading, as the pulse may be irregular (Rawlings-Anderson and Hunter 2008; RCN 2011).
4 If using palpation, assess if the pulse is regular and of normal volume.	4 An irregular pulse may indicate cardiac abnormalities. A bounding pulse may indicate patent ductus arteriosus or aortic regurgitation, while a thready, weak pulse may indicate sepsis, severe dehydration, congestive heart failure, or aortic stenosis (Howlin and Brenner 2010).
5 Assess the heart rate against age-appropriate values (Bonafide et al. 2013; Fleming et al. 2011; Rawlings-Anderson and Hunter 2008) taking into account factors such as exercise, fever, anxiety, and stress (Howlin and Brenner 2010; Nijman et al. 2012). Document the heart rate on the appropriate chart, noting the CYP's activity at the time.	5 To identify if the values are abnormal and ensure accuracy, consistency, and comparability.

Procedure guideline 1.8 Measuring respiratory rate

Statement	Rationale
1 Avoid letting the CYP know that respirations are being counted.	1 Self-consciousness may alter the respiratory rate and depth.
2 If the CYP is crying or very distressed, you may have to wait until they are calmer.	2 To gain an accurate recording, as crying and distress may increase the respiratory rate (Aylott 2006).
3 In infants and young children, place a hand just below the child's xiphoid process. Observation alone is adequate in the older CYP.	3 To assess the infant/CYP's breathing.
4 a) Count the breaths for 1 full minute. b) Observe the rate, rhythm, depth, and effort.	4 a) To ensure an accurate reading as the respirations of infants and young CYP may be irregular (RCN 2011). b) Respirations should be regular, of normal depth and normal effort. Deep sighing respirations (Kussmaul breathing) may indicate acidosis or poisoning.
5 a) Assess respiratory rate against age-appropriate values, taking into account factors such as exercise, fever, anxiety, and stress (Howlin and Brenner 2010; Nijman et al. 2012). b) Document the respiratory rate on the appropriate chart.	5 a) Normal respiratory rate varies with age (Bonafide et al. 2013; Fleming et al. 2011). Rapid respiratory rates (tachypnoea) may indicate fever, anxiety, pain, or respiratory distress. Low respiratory rates (bradypnoea) may indicate overdosage with opiates. Bradypnoea following a period of respiratory distress may indicate exhaustion. This is a clinical emergency and appropriate action must be taken (ALSG 2016). b) To ensure accuracy, consistency, and comparability.

Procedure guideline 1.9 Measuring blood pressure

Statement	Rationale
1 The CYP should be calm, relaxed, and stress free, in a warm environment, with tight or restrictive clothing removed from the limb identified for measurement.	1 To minimise the effect of extraneous influences which may temporarily alter the blood pressure (BP) (Perloff et al. 1993). Anxiety and distress may cause the BP to be artificially high.
2 The CYP should be in a seated position with the measurement taken on the right arm.	2 The right arm is generally the preferred arm for blood pressure measurement for consistency and comparison with international reference tables. International reference tables for BP centiles are based on manual readings measured on arms only. A diagnosis of high BP can be made only on arm BP measurements. Treatment for hypertension should never be started without first establishing an arm BP.
3 a) Position the CYP in a seated position for 3–5 minutes with their feet on the ground and their legs uncrossed (Beevers et al. 2001a; Foster-Fitzpatrick et al. 1999). b) The arm should be well supported, horizontal, and positioned at the level of mid-sternum. c) Leg BP should only be measured in exceptional circumstances. If the BP has to be measured on the leg the infant/CYP should be lying flat on the bed for 5 minutes.	a) BP can be significantly increased if the legs are crossed (Foster-Fitzpatrick et al. 1999). If the CYP is lying down, the BP may read slightly lower due to peripheral amplification of the pulse pressure (Lurbe et al. 2009; Beevers et al. 2001a). b) If the CYP's arm is below or above the level of the heart, the BP can be overestimated or underestimated by 10 mmHg respectively (Perloff et al. 1993). c) BP measurement in legs should never be used as a diagnostic measurement of hypertension because of the artefactual abnormalities found in leg measurements.
4 Choose the correct blood pressure cuff, ensuring: The inflatable part of the cuff (the bladder) is long enough to encircle at least 90% and preferably 100% of the upper arm circumference (Figure 1.1).	4 To ensure an accurate recording (Howlin and Brenner 2010; Lurbe et al. 2009; Vyse 1987).

Procedure guideline 1.9 Measuring blood pressure (continued)

Statement	Rationale
The width of the bladder should ideally be the full length from under the arm axilla to the olecranon (elbow) or the largest cuff that can fit onto the upper arm and still allow auscultation of the brachial artery. If these criteria cannot both be met, the largest cuff available for the arm should be used (Beevers et al. 2001a).	
Apply the correct cuff ensuring that: a) It fits firmly and is well secured (Perloff et al. 1993). b) The centre of the cuff bladder (usually labelled artery) is placed over the brachial artery. c) The tubing from the cuff is not crossing the auscultatory area. d) There is no IV cannula or infusion on the limb.	b) Too narrow a cuff will yield a reading that is falsely high. Too wide a cuff, if not correctly fitted, may result in a lower reading (Howlin and Brenner 2010). d) To reduce the risk of tissue damage and extravasation.
5 *For measurements using automated devices only:* a) Set the correct patient size (neonate/ paediatric/ adult) on the monitor. b) Set the monitor for a single measurement or automatic measurement as required. c) Start the measurement procedure following the manufacturer's instructions. d) Keep the arm still during measurement. e) Ensure that the cuff is not wrapped too tightly around the limb if the BP is to be measured continuously (Rationale 47). f) Continue to point 11.	5 a) If the monitor inflation settings are too high this may cause considerable discomfort to the CYP and cause increased BP due to pain. d) Movement artefact is often responsible for falsely high readings or an inability for the monitor to register a reading, but this is not always the case. In this situation a manual BP should be taken.
If the oscillometric device inflates and deflates repeatedly without displaying the BP, this can indicate the BP is either too low or high for the automated monitor to register (Lurbe et al. 2009). If this occurs, a manual BP should be measured (see Figure 1.1).	
6. *For manual measurements using stethoscope or Doppler:* a) Position the manometer • Vertically at eye level. • Not more than 1 m from the observer (Perloff et al. 1993). b) Ensure you are comfortably positioned and able to inflate and deflate the cuff gradually with ease before proceeding (Perloff et al. 1993). c) For measurements using the stethoscope continue to point 8.	6 a) To prevent observer error (Beevers et al. 2001b). b) To prevent injury to staff and ensure the procedure is performed accurately on the first attempt, preventing unnecessary repeating of the procedure and reduce the risk of further distressing the CYP (Perloff et al. 1993).
7 *For measurements using the Doppler only:* a) Place the Doppler over the position of maximal pulsation of the brachial artery in the arm or radial pulse in the wrist and pump up the cuff. b) When the pulse sound disappears, this is the estimated systolic BP. c) Now deflate the cuff.	7 a) Prevents underestimation of systolic pressure by misreading the Korotkoff sound; this will ensure that the auscultatory gap is not missed (Perloff et al. 1993) b) A doppler cannot identify the diastolic BP because it detects only the acoustic waves moving toward the transducer.
8 *For measurements using stethoscope palpation or Doppler:* a) Gently place the stethoscope Doppler/fingers gently over artery to feel/hear the CYP's pulse b) Inflate the bladder rapidly and steadily to a pressure of 30mmHg above the previously estimated systolic BP (McAlister and Straus 2001). c) Reduce the cuff pressure at 2–3mmHg per second.	8 a) Pressing too firmly on the artery could occlude it, affecting the accuracy and reproducibility of the measurement (Perloff et al. 1993). b) A slow inflation can cause venous congestion and increases the likelihood of an inaccurate measurement. c) A rapid deflation can result in recording errors (Nolan and Nolan 1993). NB: Using the Accoson Greenlight device reduces this risk as it displays a green light when the reduction of pressure is at the recommended speed (Graves et al. 2004).
9 a) Listen for repetitive, clear tapping sounds. When first heard for two consecutive beats, the first consecutive beat indicates the systolic BP (McAlister and Straus 2001). b) Mentally note this value to the nearest 2mmHg (Beevers et al. 2001b). c) For measurement using the Doppler, continue to point 11.	9 a) This is Korotkoff phase 1 sound, which identifies the systolic blood pressure (Howlin and Brenner 2010; McAlister and Straus 2001).

(continued)

Procedure guideline 1.9 Measuring blood pressure *(continued)*

Statement	Rationale
10 *For measurements using stethoscope only:* a) Continue to reduce the cuff pressure at 2–3 mmHg per second. b) The point at which repetitive sounds disappear (Phase 5) is the diastolic BP (Beevers et al. 2001b; McAlister and Straus 2001) c) Mentally note this value to the nearest 2 mmHg (Beevers et al. 2001b). d) If Korotkoff sounds can be heard to 0 mmHg, repeat the measurement after at least 1 minute's rest with less pressure on the stethoscope. e) If the Korotkoff sounds persist, identify the diastolic pressure at the point where the sound becomes muffled (Howlin and Brenner 2010; McAlister and Straus 2001). f) Document that Korotkoff phase 4 sound (K4) has been used.	10 b) This is Korotkoff phase 5 sound (K5), which identifies the diastolic blood pressure (Howlin and Brenner 2010; McAlister and Straus 2001) d) The sounds persist in some CYPs. e) This is Korotkoff phase 4 sound (K4) (Howlin and Brenner 2010; McAlister and Straus 2001)
11 Continue to completely deflate the cuff rapidly (McAlister and Straus 2001).	11 To prevent discomfort.
12 a) Document the BP using arrows with the tips pointing up for the systolic BP (∧) and pointing down (∨) for the diastolic value. The tip of the arrow should indicate the value. b) Note the CYP's position, limb used, cuff size, and method of measurement. c) Document if they were anxious, restless, or distressed during the procedure.	12 a) For consistency and accuracy of documentation. b) There are many factors that can cause a spuriously high reading, which may lead to unnecessary instigation and inappropriate treatment (Beevers et al. 2001b).
13 a) Assess the significance of the measurement by reference to local guidelines or recognised reference ranges. b) If the BP readings are above the expected level for gender, age, and height and the CYP is calm and not in any discomfort during the BP measurement, it should be re-measured three times, leaving at least 1 minute between readings. c) Make sure the cuff bladder size is correct and continue to monitor. If the readings obtained are consistently high a 4-limb BP should be measured. If the problem continues a manual BP is recommended using a Doppler for infants and small children and a stethoscope for older CYPs (Figure 1.1). d) If the BP measurement is consistently high and there are no other contributing factors, a measurement should be performed on both arms and legs (Beevers et al. 2001a; Perloff et al. 1993) and the arm with the highest reading, which should then be used regularly (McAlister and Straus 2001). e) Report significant differences in limb recordings to a medical practitioner.	13 a) There are no automated monometers that have been validated for use in hypertensive CYPs (Lunn et al. 2009). b) Automated devices tend to under-read at low BP and over-read at very high BP, and this may be clinically significant, especially for children/young people with hypertension. c) The pressure differences between arms can be >10 mmHg in some hypertensive CYPs (McAlister and Straus 2001). d) A high reading on the right arm BP and a low reading on the leg BP can be a sign of coarctation of the aorta, which can be confirmed by bilateral weak femoral pulses and echocardiogram. e) To ensure prompt action if required.
14 a) If repeated measurements are required, where possible the same limb, cuff size, position, and method should be used. b) If the CYP's BP is to be monitored continually, make sure the cuff is not wrapped too tightly around the limb. c) Remove and reapply the BP cuff hourly, observing the colour, warmth, and sensitivity of the limb.	14 a), b) To ensure consistent and reproducible measurements (National High Blood Pressure Education Program Working Group on High Blood Pressure in Children and Adolescents 2004). c) Frequent repeated measurement can cause purpura, ischaemia, and neuropathy.
15 a) If the reading is difficult to ascertain (common in small, unsettled children) stop, take a rest, and retry when the CYP is settled. b) If it is necessary to repeat the recording, the cuff should be allowed to fully deflate, and a minute elapse before the next measurement is attempted (Ramsay et al. 1999). c) The CYP should be fully settled before the measurement is attempted. Consider distraction therapy or referral to a play specialist if the CYP is particularly anxious. For further information, see Chapter 27: Play as a Therapeutic Tool. For definitions of blood pressure categories see Figure 1.3. For BP centile chart see Figure 1.4.	15 a) To obtain an accurate reading. BP readings will be elevated in unsettled CYPs. b) To prevent venous congestion, resulting in an inaccurate BP (Nolan and Nolan 1993). c) To prevent falsely high readings due to distress.

Chapter 1 Assessment

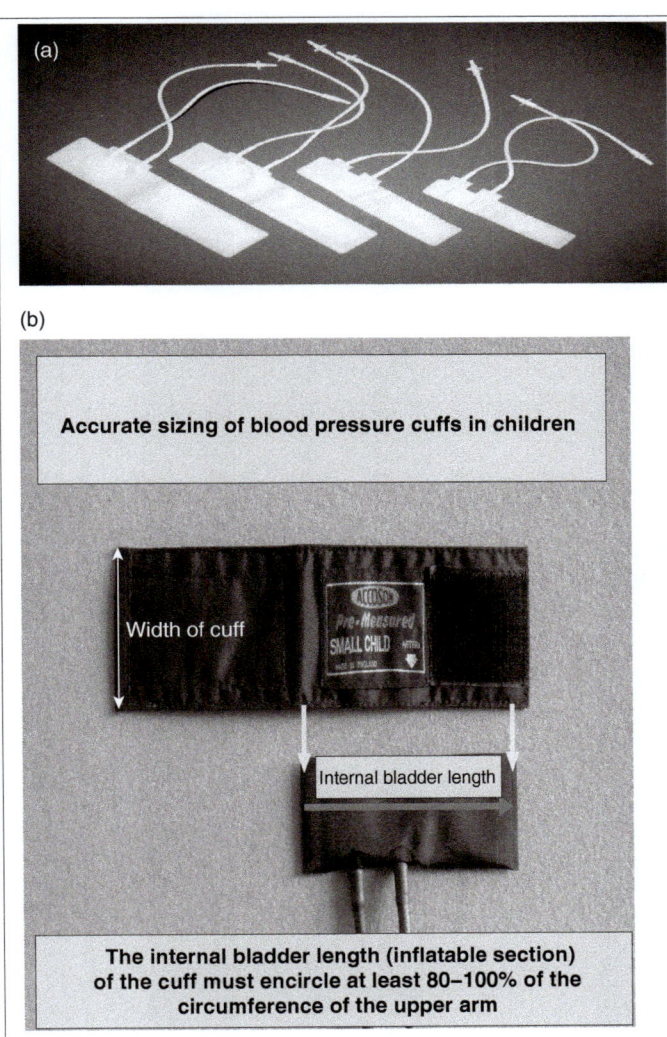

Figure 1.1 Blood pressure cuffs. (a) Integrated bladder; (b) cuff with internal bladder.

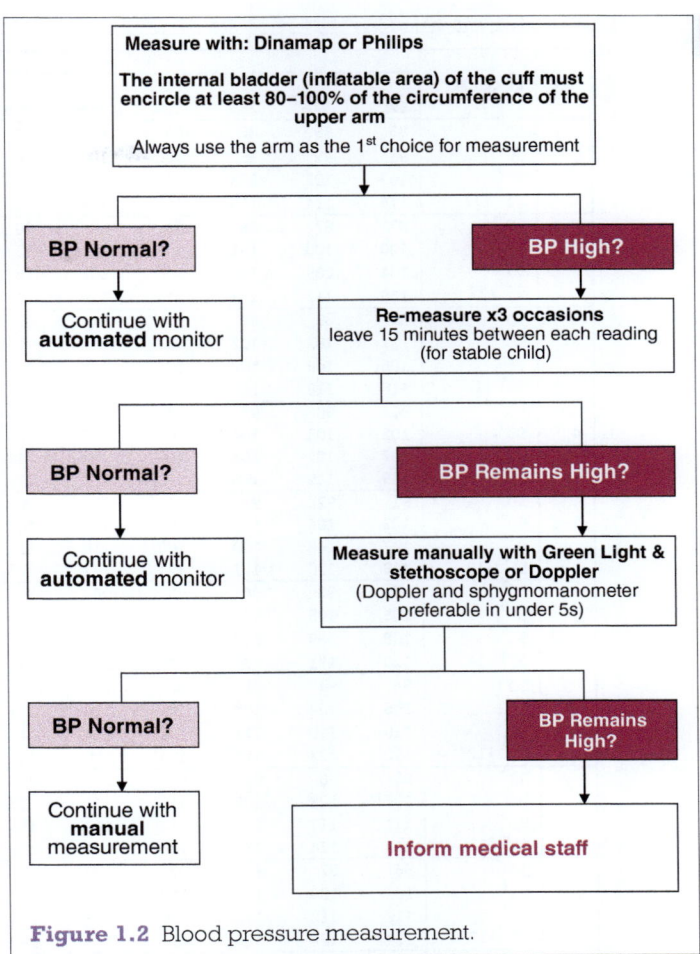

Figure 1.2 Blood pressure measurement.

Categories	For Children Aged 1–<13 y	For Children Aged ≥13 y
Normal BP	<90th percentile	<120/<80 mm Hg
Elevated BP	≥90th percentile to <95th percentile or 120/80 mm Hg to <95th percentile (whichever is lower)	120/<80 to 129/<80 mm Hg
Stage 1 Hypertension	≥95th percentile to <95th percentile + 12 mmHg, or 130/80 to 139/89 mm Hg (whichever is lower)	130/80 to 139/89 mm Hg
Stage 2 Hypertension	≥95th percentile + 12 mm Hg, or ≥140/90 mm Hg (whichever is lower)	≥140/90 mm Hg

Figure 1.3 Updated Definitions of blood pressure Categories and Stages. *Source:* Flynn et al. (2017).

Age	BP centile	Boys - Height Centile												
		SBP							DBP					
		5%	10%	25%	50%	75%	90%	95%	5%	10%	25%	50%	75%	90%	95%
1	50th	85	85	86	87	88	88	40	40	40	41	41	42	42
	90th	98	99	99	100	100	101	101	52	52	53	53	54	54	54
	95th	102	102	103	103	104	105	105	54	54	55	55	56	57	57
	95th +12	114	114	115	115	116	117	117	66	66	67	67	68	69	69
2	50th	87	87	88	89	89	90	91	43	43	44	44	45	46	46
	90th	100	100	101	102	103	103	104	55	55	56	56	57	58	58
	95th	104	105	105	106	107	107	108	57	58	58	59	60	61	61
	95th +12	116	117	117	118	119	119	120	69	70	70	71	72	73	73
3	50th	88	89	89	90	91	92	92	45	46	46	47	48	49	49
	90th	101	102	102	103	104	105	105	58	58	59	59	60	61	61
	95th	106	106	107	107	108	109	109	60	61	61	62	63	64	64
	95th +12	118	118	119	119	120	121	121	72	73	73	74	75	76	76
4	50th	90	90	91	92	93	94	94	48	49	49	50	51	52	52
	90th	102	103	104	105	105	106	107	60	61	62	62	63	64	64
	95th	107	107	108	108	109	110	110	63	64	65	66	67	67	68
	95th +12	119	119	120	120	121	122	122	75	76	77	78	79	79	80
5	50th	91	92	93	94	95	96	96	51	51	52	53	54	55	55
	90th	103	104	105	106	107	108	108	63	64	65	65	66	67	67
	95th	107	108	109	109	110	111	112	66	67	68	69	70	70	71
	95th +12	119	120	121	121	122	123	124	78	79	80	81	82	82	83
6	50th	93	93	94	95	96	97	98	54	54	55	56	57	57	58
	90th	105	105	106	107	109	110	110	66	66	67	68	68	69	69
	95th	108	109	110	111	112	113	114	69	70	70	71	72	72	73
	95th +12	120	121	122	123	124	125	126	81	82	82	838	84	84	85
7	50th	94	94	95	97	98	98	99	56	56	57	58	58	59	59
	90th	106	107	108	109	110	111	111	68	68	69	70	70	71	71
	95th	110	110	111	112	114	115	116	71	71	727	73	73	74	74
	95th +12	122	122	123	124	126	127	128	83	83	84	85	85	86	86
8	50th	95	96	97	98	99	99	100	57	57	58	59	59	60	60
	90th	107	108	109	110	111	112	112	69	70	70	71	72	72	73
	95th	111	112	112	114	115	116	117	72	73	73	74	75	75	75
	95th +12	123	124	124	126	127	128	129	84	85	85	86	87	87	87
9	50th	96	97	98	99	100	101	101	57	58	59	60	61	62	62
	90th	107	108	109	110	111	112	113	70	71	72	73	74	74	74
	95th	112	112	113	115	116	118	119	74	74	75	76	76	77	77
	95th +12	124	124	125	127	128	130	131	86	86	87	88	88	89	89
10	50th	97	98	99	100	101	102	103	59	60	61	62	63	63	64
	90th	108	109	11	112	113	115	116	72	73	74	74	75	75	76
	95th	112	113	114	116	118	120	121	76	76	77	77	78	78	78
	95th +12	124	125	126	128	130	132	133	88	88	89	89	90	90	90
11	50th	99	99	101	102	103	104	106	61	61	62	63	63	63	63
	90th	110	111	112	114	116	117	118	74	74	75	75	75	76	76
	95th	114	114	116	118	120	123	124	77	78	78	78	78	78	78
	95th +12	126	126	128	130	132	135	136	89	90	90	90	90	90	90
12	50th	101	101	102	104	106	108	109	61	62	63	63	63	63	63
	90th	113	114	115	117	119	121	122	75	75	75	75	75	76	76
	95th	116	117	118	121	124	126	128	78	78	78	78	78	79	79
	95th +12	128	129	130	133	136	138	140	90	90	90	90	90	91	91
13	50th	103	104	105	108	110	111	112	61	60	61	62	63	64	65
	90th	115	116	118	12	124	126	126	74	74	74	75	76	77	77
	95th	119	120	122	125	128	130	131	78	78	78	78	80	81	81
	95th +12	131	132	134	137	140	142	143	90	90	90	90	92	93	93
14	50th	105	106	109	111	112	113	113	60	60	62	64	65	66	67
	90th	119	120	123	126	127	128	129	74	74	75	77	78	79	80
	95th	123	125	127	130	132	133	134	77	78	79	81	82	83	84
	95th +12	135	137	139	142	144	145	146	89	90	91	93	94	95	96
15	50th	108	110	112	113	114	114	114	61	62	64	65	66	67	68
	90th	123	124	126	128	129	130	130	75	76	78	79	80	81	81
	95th	127	129	131	132	134	135	135	78	79	81	83	84	85	85
	95th +12	139	141	143	144	146	147	147	90	91	93	95	96	97	97
16	50th	111	112	114	115	115	116	116	63	64	66	67	68	69	69
	90th	126	127	128	129	131	131	132	77	78	79	80	81	82	82
	95th	130	131	133	134	135	136	137	80	81	83	84	85	86	86
	95th +12	142	143	145	146	147	148	149	92	93	95	96	97	98	98
17	50th	114	115	116	117	117	118	118	65	66	67	68	69	70	70
	90th	128	129	130	131	132	133	134	78	79	80	81	82	82	83
	95th	132	133	134	135	137	138	138	81	82	84	85	86	86	87
	95th +12	144	145	146	147	149	150	150	93	94	96	97	98	98	99

Figure 1.4 Blood pressure levels for boys and girls by age and height percentiles. *Source:* Flynn et al. (2017).

Chapter 1 Assessment

Age	BP centile	Girls - Height Centile												
		SBP							DBP					
		5%	10%	25%	50%	75%	90%	95%	5%	10%	25%	50%	75%	90%	95%
1	50th	84	85	86	86	87	88	88	41	42	42	43	44	45	46
	90th	98	99	99	100	101	102	102	54	55	55	56	57	58	58
	95th	101	102	102	103	104	105	105	59	59	60	60	61	62	62
	95th +12	113	114	114	115	116	117	117	71	71	72	72	73	74	74
2	50th	87	87	88	89	90	91	91	45	46	47	48	49	50	51
	90th	101	101	102	103	104	105	106	58	58	59	60	61	62	62
	95th	104	105	106	106	107	108	109	62	63	63	64	65	66	66
	95th +12	116	117	118	118	119	120	121	74	75	75	76	77	78	78
3	50th	88	89	89	90	91	92	93	48	48	49	50	51	53	53
	90th	102	103	104	104	105	106	107	60	61	61	62	63	64	65
	95th	106	106	107	108	109	110	110	64	65	65	66	67	68	69
	95th +12	118	118	119	120	121	122	122	76	77	77	78	79	80	81
4	50th	89	90	91	92	93	94	94	50	51	51	53	54	55	55
	90th	103	104	105	106	107	108	108	62	63	64	65	66	67	67
	95th	107	108	109	109	110	111	112	66	67	68	69	70	70	71
	95th +12	119	120	121	121	122	123	124	78	79	80	81	82	82	83
5	50th	90	91	92	93	94	95	96	52	52	53	55	56	57	57
	90th	104	105	106	107	108	109	110	64	65	66	67	68	69	70
	95th	108	109	109	110	111	112	113	68	69	70	71	72	73	73
	95th +12	120	121	121	122	123	124	125	80	81	82	83	84	85	85
6	50th	92	92	93	94	96	97	97	54	54	55	56	57	58	59
	90th	105	106	107	108	109	110	111	67	67	68	69	70	71	71
	95th	109	109	110	111	112	113	114	70	71	72	72	73	74	74
	95th +12	121	121	122	123	124	125	126	82	83	84	84	85	86	86
7	50th	92	93	94	95	97	98	99	55	55	56	57	58	59	60
	90th	106	106	107	109	110	111	112	68	68	69	70	71	72	72
	95th	109	110	111	112	113	114	115	72	72	73	73	74	74	75
	95th +12	121	122	123	124	125	126	127	84	84	85	85	86	86	87
8	50th	93	94	95	97	98	99	100	56	56	57	59	60	61	61
	90th	107	107	108	110	111	112	113	69	70	71	72	72	73	73
	95th	110	111	112	113	115	116	117	72	73	74	74	75	75	75
	95th +12	122	123	124	125	127	128	129	84	85	86	86	87	87	87
9	50th	95	95	97	98	99	100	101	57	58	59	60	60	61	61
	90th	108	108	109	111	112	113	114	71	71	72	73	73	73	73
	95th	112	112	113	114	116	117	117	74	74	75	75	75	75	75
	95th +12	124	124	125	126	128	129	130	86	86	87	87	87	87	87
10	50th	96	97	98	99	101	102	103	58	59	59	60	61	61	62
	90th	109	110	111	112	113	115	116	72	73	73	73	73	73	73
	95th	113	114	114	116	117	119	120	75	75	76	76	76	76	76
	95th +12	125	126	126	128	129	131	132	87	87	88	88	88	88	88
11	50th	98	99	101	102	104	105	106	60	60	60	61	62	63	64
	90th	111	112	113	114	116	118	120	74	74	74	74	74	75	75
	95th	115	116	117	118	120	123	124	76	77	77	77	77	77	77
	95th +12	127	128	129	130	132	135	136	88	89	89	89	89	89	89
12	50th	102	102	104	105	107	108	108	61	61	61	62	64	65	65
	90th	114	115	116	118	120	122	122	75	75	75	75	76	76	76
	95th	118	119	120	122	124	125	126	78	78	78	78	79	79	79
	95th +12	130	131	132	134	136	137	138	90	90	90	90	91	91	91
13	50th	104	105	106	107	108	108	109	62	62	63	64	65	65	66
	90th	116	117	119	121	122	123	123	75	75	75	76	76	76	76
	95th	121	122	123	124	126	126	127	79	79	79	79	80	80	81
	95th +12	133	134	135	136	138	138	139	91	91	91	91	92	92	93
14	50th	105	106	107	108	109	109	109	63	63	64	65	66	66	66
	90th	118	118	120	122	123	123	123	76	76	76	76	77	77	77
	95th	123	123	124	125	126	127	127	80	80	80	80	81	81	82
	95th +12	135	135	136	137	138	139	139	92	92	92	92	93	93	94
15	50th	105	106	107	108	109	109	109	64	64	64	65	66	67	67
	90th	118	119	121	122	123	123	124	76	76	76	77	77	78	78
	95th	124	124	125	126	127	127	128	80	80	80	81	82	82	82
	95th +12	136	136	137	138	139	139	140	92	92	92	93	94	94	94
16	50th	106	107	108	109	109	110	110	64	64	65	66	66	67	67
	90th	119	120	122	123	124	124	124	76	76	76	77	78	78	78
	95th	124	125	125	127	127	128	128	80	80	80	81	82	82	82
	95th +12	136	137	137	139	139	140	140	92	92	92	93	94	94	94
17	50th	107	108	109	110	110	110	111	64	64	65	66	66	66	67
	90th	120	121	123	124	124	125	125	76	76	77	77	78	78	78
	95th	125	125	126	127	128	128	128	80	80	80	81	82	82	82
	95th +12	137	137	138	139	140	140	140	92	92	92	93	94	94	94

Figure 1.4 *(continued)*

Procedure guideline 1.10 Measuring oxygen saturation

Statement	Rationale
1 Pulse oximetry provides a measure of arterial blood oxygen saturation. It does NOT assess the level of tissue oxygenation or the adequacy of ventilation. Carbon dioxide levels may be high despite normal oxygen saturation levels.	1 Pulse oximetry forms only one part of respiratory status assessment. It is important to remember that serious respiratory complications may still be present despite normal oxygen saturation levels.
2 Select the site to apply the probe. Potential sites include fingers, toes, earlobes, and the bridge of the nose (Higgins 2005). The site with the best pulsatile flow should be selected initially and reviewed. The most appropriate probe for the site selected should be used.	2 Site selection is an important factor in the quality of the reading.
3 Apply the probe and operate the equipment according to the manufacturer's instructions.	3 To ensure safe practice.
4 Assess pulse detection by comparing the signal with the CYP's pulse.	4 To assess the reliability of the recording.
5 Set appropriate alarm parameters in light of the CYP's current condition.	5 To detect deterioration at an early stage.
6 Rotate the probe site regularly.	6 To prevent skin damage.
7 Record the oxygen saturation levels, alongside concurrent oxygen therapy and other clinically significant findings such as respiratory effort, consciousness level, and position.	7 To ensure that recordings are clinically relevant.
8 Pulse oximetry may not be accurate in the following circumstances: • High ambient light levels (fluorescent and xenon lights) • Nail varnish present (Hakverdioğlu et al. 2014) • Motion artefact • Reduced pulse volume • Hypotension • Low cardiac output • Vasoconstriction • Hypothermia • Presence of other haemoglobins: carboxyhaemoglobin (carbon monoxide poisoning), and methaemoglobin (congenital or acquired) • Surgical and imaging dyes: methylene blue, indocyanine green, and indigo carmine cause falsely low readings. However pulse oximetry is NOT affected by anaemia, jaundice, or skin pigmentation (Resuscitation Council [UK] 2011).	8 Pulse oximetry should be used with caution in these circumstances, and alternative means of assessing oxygenation should be used (e.g. blood gas analysis).

Procedure guideline 1.11 Growth assessment

Statement	Rationale
1 Growth assessment encompasses height, weight, and head circumference.	1 All three measurements are needed to provide a comprehensive assessment of the CYP.
2 Assessment of growth is vital and provides a sensitive guide to: • health, • development, • nutritional status, • the response to treatment. (Hall 2000).	2 A healthy, adequately nourished, and emotionally secure CYP grows at an optimal rate (Stanhope et al. 1994). A slow rate of growth could suggest a pathological disorder requiring diagnosis and possible treatment, e.g. malabsorption, an eating disorder, hypertension, psychosocial problems, craniopharyngioma (Sherwood et al. 1986; Skuse 1989). CYPs with disabilities may be particularly at risk (Lionti et al. 2013).
3 While single measurements provide an indication of expected "normal values", serial measurements are more useful.	3 Serial measurements allow progress to be tracked over time and the relationship between the three measurements to be assessed (Schilg and Hulse 1997).

Procedure guideline 1.12 Measuring height

Statement	Rationale
1 All CYPs in hospital should have their height measured and plotted on a centile chart every three months.	1 Hospitalised CYPs are at nutritional risk. Serial measurements allow for a more accurate assessment of growth rate.
2 The appropriate equipment to measure the height of the CYP should be selected. This is dependent on the CYP's age and developmental and physical ability.	2 To obtain an accurate measurement and maintain the safety of the CYP and staff.
3 Infants and children under two years of age and those who are unable to stand (or find standing difficult) should be measured using a length board or mat (RCPCH 2021). Children and young people over 2 years should be measured using a rigid upright measure with a T piece or a stadiometer (RCPCH 2021).	3 To ensure accuracy and avoid inconsistencies in measurement.
4 A CYP who has one leg shorter than the other should be measured standing on the longest leg.	4 To ensure accuracy and avoid inconsistencies in measurement.
5 In some forms of short stature, body proportions may also be clinically relevant, e.g. achondroplasia, or after spinal irradiation. The most useful body proportion is the relationship between trunk length and leg length. This is obtained by measuring a sitting height and subtracting this from the total height. CYPs who need to be measured lying down should have their crown–rump length measured, i.e. head to bottom. This measurement is then subtracted from their total length.	5 To ensure accuracy and avoid inconsistencies in measurement.
6 Remove shoes or other footwear before measurement. Infants should have nappies removed.	6 To ensure accuracy and avoid inconsistencies in measurement.
7 When measuring a CYP who is standing, they must be positioned with: • feet together and flat on the ground • heels touching the back plate of the measuring instrument • legs must be straight • buttocks against the backboard • scapula, wherever possible, against the backboard • arms loosely at their side.	7 To ensure an accurate measurement. Poor positioning results in inaccurate measurement.
8 When measuring a CYP in the supine position, two people are required: a) Place the measuring board on a firm surface and lay the CYP on the board. b) One person should ensure the head is held in contact with the headboard. c) The other person should position the CYP with: • feet together and flat against the foot board • heels touching the back plate of the measuring instrument • legs straight and in alignment with the body • buttocks against the backboard • scapula, wherever possible, against the backboard. d) The ankles should be held to ensure this position is maintained and firm pressure may need to be applied to keep the legs in position. e) The CYP should be completely aligned and flat on the board.	8 To ensure stability of the measuring device and obtain an accurate measurement. To ensure that the head and body are in complete alignment.
9 When measuring a CYP who is standing, they must be positioned with: (a) feet together and flat on the ground (b) heels touching the back plate of the measuring instrument (c) legs must be straight (d) buttocks against the backboard (e) scapula, wherever possible, against the backboard (f) arms loosely at their side.	9 Poor positioning may result in inaccurate measurement.
10 In both measurement methods, the CYP's head should be positioned with the lower margins of the orbit in the same horizontal plane as the external auditory meatus, i.e. the corner of the eyes horizontal to the middle of the ear (see Figure 1.5) (Lynch-Caris et al. 2008).	10 This position is referred to as the Frankfort plane and ensures accuracy of measurement (Horan et al. 2014; RCPCH 2021).

(continued)

Procedure guideline 1.12 Measuring height *(continued)*

Statement	Rationale
11 The measuring instrument should then be read (ensuring it is at eye level for the standing method) when the CYP has fully exhaled. Record the measurement to the last complete millimetre (Himes 2009).	11 To ensure accuracy and avoid inconsistencies in measurement.
12 It is good practice to take three measurements and use the average (RCPCH 2021).	12 To ensure accuracy and avoid inconsistencies in measurement.
13 For documentation see final section of Procedure guideline 1.14	
14 Any abnormality or deviation from the expected centile should be reported to the CYP's doctor.	14 To facilitate appropriate management.

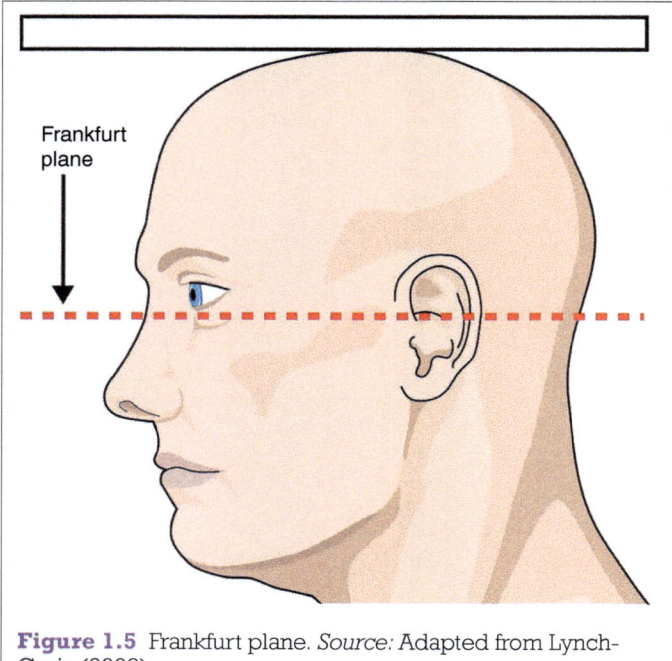

Figure 1.5 Frankfurt plane. *Source:* Adapted from Lynch-Caris (2008).

Procedure guideline 1.13 Measuring weight

Statement	Rationale
1 CYPs should be weighed on admission and at least weekly thereafter.	1 To establish a baseline for future assessment and to monitor growth. Hospitalised CYPs and those with disabilities are at nutritional risk (Joosten and Hulst 2008; Lionti et al. 2013).
a) Infants should be weighed in the first week as part of the assessment of feeding and thereafter as needed (RCPCH 2021). If there is professional concern or if parents wish, babies can be weighed at 6–8 weeks, 12 and 16 weeks (RCPCH 2021). Thereafter babies should usually be weighed at 12–13 months at the time of routine immunisations.	a) To identify problems early to allow monitoring and intervention if needed.
b) Infants and CYP should be weighed more frequently if there is concern about their health and well-being. However in general, babies should be weighed no more than: • once a month from 2 weeks to 6 months of age • once every two months from 6 to 12 months of age • once every three months over the age of 1 year (RCPCH 2021).	b) Infant weights measured too closely together can be misleading (RCPCH 2021).
2 Children under two years of age should be weighed naked. CYPs over 2 years of age should be weighed in minimal clothing or vest and pants (RCPCH 2012). Nappies, shoes and slippers should be removed and ensure no dolls or teddies held before measurement (RCPCH 2021).	2 To ensure accuracy and avoid inconsistencies in measurement.

Procedure guideline 1.13 Measuring weight *(continued)*

Statement	Rationale
3 If clothing has not been removed or the CYP is weighed with additional equipment, such as a splint or cast, this must be recorded in the CYP's healthcare records.	3 To maintain an accurate record.
4 Class III clinical electronic sales in metric settings should be used (RCPCH 2021). The appropriate type of scales should be selected dependent on the CYP's age and developmental and physical ability. If the CYP is very sick or unable to sit unaided, the CYP should be supported by a carer and weighed together on the scales. The carer should then be weighed alone and their weight subtracted from the combined weight of the CYP and carer.	4 To obtain an accurate measurement and maintain the safety of the CYP and staff.
5 The CYP must be completely on the scales and their weight fully borne.	5 To ensure an accurate measurement.
6 Record the figure shown on the scales to the last complete gram for infants under 4 kg and to the last 100 g for older CYPs above 4 kg.	6 Rounding up the measurement will produce an inaccurate measurement.
7 Help to re-dress the CYP.	7 To maintain comfort and dignity.
8 For documentation see final section of Procedure guideline 1.14	
9 Interpreting results: The centile describes the percentage of the population expected to be below that line. Half of all children should be between 25–75th centile. a) Infant measurements need to be interpreted in relation to length, growth potential and any earlier measurements of the baby (RCPCH 2021). b) For infants, if there is significant weight loss, or weight is still below birth weight at 2 weeks of age, the % weight loss must be calculated. Weight loss = difference between current weight and birth weight Percentage weight loss = weight loss ÷ birth weight × 100%. c) Babies do not all grow at the same rate, so a baby's weight often does not follow a particular centile line, especially in the first year. For infants, some weight loss in the first weeks of life is common, but 80% of infants will have regained this by 2 weeks of age. A weight loss of 10% or more at any stage should be escalated to the treating paediatrician. d) For infants, acute illness may lead to sudden weight loss and a weight centile fall, but this should return to its normal centile within two to three weeks (RCPCH 2021). e) A sustained drop through two or more weight centile spaces is unusual and should trigger a fuller assessment including measuring length/height (RCPCH 2021).	9 a) To ensure measurements are interpreted accurately. To provide individualised care. b) To ensure weight loss is calculated accurately. c) Recovery of birth weight by 2 weeks suggests that feeding is effective, and that the child is well (RCPCH 2021). Fewer than 5% of babies lose more than 10% of their weight at any stage, and only 1 in 50 are 10% or more lighter than birth weight at 2 weeks (RCPCH 2021). d) Fewer than 2% of infants have sustained weight loss and this may indicate underlying health or social issues (RCPCH 2021). e) To identify problems early to allow monitoring and intervention if needed..
10 For CYPs, abnormality or deviation from the expected centile should trigger a fuller assessment and be reported to the paediatrician. Weight loss of more than 10%, or a weight below 0.4th centile needs careful assessment (RCPCH 2021). a) If the weight is above the 99.6th centile, calculate body mass index (BMI) (RCPCH 2021). Calculating Body Mass Index: BMI uses height and weight to calculate if the weight is healthy. A child whose weight is average for their height will have a BMI between the 25th and 75th centiles, whatever their height centile. BMI above the 91st centile suggests that the child is overweight; a child above the 98th centile is very overweight (clinically obese) (RCPCH 2021). BMI below the 2nd centile is unusual and may reflect under-nutrition (RCPCH 2021).	10 To identify problems early to allow monitoring and intervention if needed. a) BMI allows better interpretation of weight. Weight above the 99.6th centile may indicate obesity and needs to be interpreted taking account of the CYPs height.

Procedure guideline 1.14 Measuring head circumference

Statement	Rationale
1 Head circumference should be measured: a) Around birth, but ideally not within the first 24 hours. b) At the 8 week check and at any time after that if there are any worries about the child's head growth or development (RCPCH 2021).	1 a) To identify problems early to allow monitoring and intervention if needed. b) Measurements taken in the first 24-hours are unreliable as the head will have been subjected to moulding (RCPCH 2021)
2 Any CYP with a known or suspected neurological or craniofacial abnormality will need their head circumference recorded more frequently.	2 To monitor the CYP's condition. An increase in the volume of cerebrospinal fluid (CSF) can result in an increase in head circumference.

Preparation:

Statement	Rationale
3 Inform the family, and CYP if age appropriate, of the following: • that a measurement of head circumference measurement is required • the reason for the measurement • what it entails • the likely duration of the procedure	3 To obtain informed consent, reduce anxiety, and aid compliance.
4 Remove hats, bonnets, hair clips and plats and braids wherever possible.	4 To allow for accurate measurement.

Measurement technique:

Statement	Rationale
1 Use a disposable paper or plastic tape measure.	1 To minimise the risk of cross-infection.
2 Measure the circumference at the point where the head circumference is widest. Take three measurements and use the average (RCPCH 2021).	2 To ensure consistent and accurate measurement.
3 Head circumference centile measurements should track within one centile space.	3 The head circumference centile may show some variation over time, but fewer than 1% of infants drop or rise through more than 2 centile spaces after the first few weeks (RCPCH 2021).
4 Report any fall or rise through 2 or more centile spaces (RCPCH 2021).	4 Very rapid head growth with upward centile crossing can be a sign of hydrocephalus or other problems. Slowing of head growth, with a fall down the centiles may also be a sign of underlying problems of brain or skull growth and development.

Documentation of height, weight and head circumference:

Statement	Rationale
1 Record the CYP's height, weight and head circumference in their healthcare records as appropriate. Documentation should include the date and time of the measurement as well as the name of the person who performed the procedure.	1 To maintain accurate and consistent documentation.
2 The CYP's weight should be plotted on a standardised growth chart, such as the UK-WHO growth chart (RCPCH 2021).	2 To compare the growth against evidence-based data (Wright et al. 2013).
3 The correct chart should be chosen dependant on the child's age and for infants, gestation.	3 To ensure measurements are interpreted accurately.
4 Use a calendar or date wheel to calculate age. Age should be calculated in weeks for the first 6–12 months and calendar months thereafter. Count forward from the date of birth using the day of birth (RCPCH 2021).	4 Age errors are common (RCPCH 2021).
5 Record measurements and date in ink Plot data points in pencil. Use a dot and do not join up	5 Plotting errors are common and may need to be adjusted.
6 A child is on a centile if within 1/4 space of the line or between the two centiles if not. A centile space is the distance between two centile lines (RCPCH 2021).	
7 Escalate any concerns about the CYP's height, weight and/or head circumference to the appropriate clinician.	7 These may indicate underlying problems of growth and development which need further investigation.

Section 6: Assessment of body systems

Procedure guideline 1.15 Assessing the respiratory and cardiovascular systems

Statement	Rationale
1 Observe and note the CYP's activity level. Are they: a) Calm and behaving appropriately? b) Restless or agitated? c) Listless and drowsy?	1 This is a valuable indicator of their overall state of health. b) Agitation and restlessness may indicate shock or hypoxia. c) Drowsiness and listlessness may indicate serious problems such as late shock or a neurological problem (ALSG 2016)
2 Observe their body posture.	2 A CYP may alter their body position to alleviate symptoms: A CYP with severe airway obstruction or respiratory distress may sit upright in a 'tripod' position to ease their breathing (ALSG 2016). 'Squatting' may indicate a diagnosis of Tetralogy of Fallot (Massoure et al. 2014).
3 Note their general colour. Is this normal for the CYP?	3 Skin colour varies between and within different ethnic groups. Parents/carers will generally have noticed if the CYP's colour has altered from the baseline. Skin colour may indicate underlying disease problems. Pallor (especially when combined with drowsiness and fever in infants) may indicate serious problems such as shock or hypoxia (Hewson et al. 2000). A yellow tinge (jaundice) may indicate liver problems.
4 Observe for peripheral and central cyanosis (blue/purple discolouration). Check the colour of the CYP's tongue.	4 Peripheral cyanosis may be due to vasoconstriction and can be a healthy response to a cold environment. Central cyanosis is a blue or purple discolouration of the tongue and indicates severe hypoxaemia, polycythaemia, or cardiac or pulmonary disease (Shobi et al. 2012).
5 Observe the CYP for mottling and oedema. Look at the hands and nails for colour, shape and condition.	5 Pallor and mottling may indicate heart disease or shock. Oedema may be present in congestive heart failure or renal failure (Howlin and Brenner 2010). Finger clubbing is due to chronic hypoxia and may indicate a chronic heart or lung condition (Howlin and Brenner 2010; Tully et al. 2012). Splinter haemorrhages (small red or black lines in the fingernail beds) may be present in infective endocarditis (Tully et al. 2012).
6 Look at the shape of the CYP's chest. Are there any deformities of the chest wall?	6 Prominence of the sternum and costal cartilages may indicate respiratory or cardiac problems. In older CYPs, a round chest is often indicative of a chronic lung disorder.
7 Does the chest move symmetrically on breathing?	7 In health, the chest should move symmetrically. Decreased movement on one side may indicate pneumonia, pneumothorax, or inhalation of a foreign body.
8 Are there signs of recession (in-drawing of the chest wall)? If so, where is it located and how marked is it (mild, moderate or severe)?	8 Recession is more commonly seen in younger children as their ribs and chest wall are more compliant (Aylott 2006). Recession generally indicates increased work of breathing and respiratory distress (Aylott 2006). The degree of recession generally correlates to the severity of the condition. Severe recession, especially in older CYPs and if accompanied by other signs of respiratory distress, is a sign of severe illness and should be referred to a doctor immediately (ALSG 2016; Carter and Laird 2005; Hewson et al. 2000).
9 Are there visible pulsations or scars? Where are they located?	9 Visible pulsation may be present in health, especially in thin CYPs (Howlin and Brenner 2010). Bulging of the left chest or obvious lifting of the chest wall during contraction (a heave) may indicate left ventricular enlargement or other cardiac problems (Howlin and Brenner 2010). Scars may indicate previous surgery for respiratory or cardiac problems.

(continued)

Procedure guideline 1.15 Assessing the respiratory and cardiovascular systems *(continued)*

Statement	Rationale
10. Does the CYP make any noises when they are breathing? If so, what do they sound like and when do they occur (on inspiration, expiration or both)?	10. Stridor (a high-pitched sound that is generally worse on inspiration) indicates severe upper airway obstruction and may be due to infection (such as croup or epiglottis), post-traumatic injury, neoplasia, or developmental problems such as subglottic haemangioma or laryngomalacia (Carter and Laird 2005; Sasidaran et al. 2011). Wheeziness may indicate asthma, an acute respiratory tract infection or foreign body inhalation. Grunting is a sign of severe respiratory distress (ALSG 2016; Aylott 2006).
11. Are there any problems with the CYP's ears, nose, and throat?	11. Ear, nose, and throat problems are common in CYPs and although most are relatively minor, some may require immediate assessment and treatment (Carter and Laird 2005).
12. Does the CYP have a cough? a) If so, what does it sound like and when does it occur? b) Is the cough productive? If so, describe the nature of the expectorant.	12. a) A severe barking cough, especially with stridor, may indicate croup (Sasidaran et al. 2011). A paroxysmal prolonged bout of coughing (sometimes ending in a sharp intake of breath) may indicate pertussis (whooping cough). b) A productive cough is rare in CYPs and may indicate cystic fibrosis.
13. Do the CYP and/or family have any other concerns regarding the CYP's respiratory or cardiovascular needs?	13. To allow the CYP and family to voice concerns about any issues that may not have been covered within the assessment.

Procedure guideline 1.16 Assessing the neurological system

Statement	Rationale
1. Ask the parent/carer the age at which the CYP first rolled over, sat unaided, crawled, walked, spoke their first words, spoke their first sentence, and dressed without help (Engel 2006). Assess these against developmental guidelines.	1. A through history of the CYP's development is important in order to plan nursing care appropriate for their developmental age. The assessment can also identify neurological and developmental abnormalities.
2. Check the CYP's head circumference against age-appropriate values.	2. A large head (especially within the frontal area) may indicate hydrocephalus. A small head (microcephaly) may be linked to abnormality during the prenatal period (maternal infection, drug use), chromosomal abnormality, or perinatal trauma.
3. a) Observe the CYP for any abnormal movement. Do they move all their limbs? Do they have a normal gait? Are there any areas of flaccidity or spasticity? b) Does the CYP and/or parent/carer identify any problems with movement?	3. a) Abnormal limb movement may be seen while observing the CYP at play and may result from neurological problems or local injury to a limb. b) Parents/carers and CYPs may have concerns that require further investigation.
4. If indicated, assess the CYP's motor responses. Assess the CYP's limb movement and power (Table 1.1) (Dawes et al. 2007). Assess each limb separately and compare right and left to identify any differences. b) Ask the CYP to hop, skip, and walk heel-to-toe to assess balance and gross motor skills.	4. In-depth assessment of the motor system is only required if there is a suspicion of neurological problems. b) Inability or difficulty to perform any of these may indicate cerebellar dysfunction (Cox 2008).
5. If indicated, assess the CYP's cranial nerves (Table 1.2) (Sables-Baus and Robinson 2011).	5. Testing of the cranial nerves will identify any abnormalities and establish a baseline for further assessment.
6. If indicated, assess the CYP's pupil responses and Glasgow Coma Score (see Chapter 21: Neurological Care)	6. To establish a baseline.
7. Do the CYP and/or family have any other concerns regarding the CYP's neurological needs?	7. To allow the CYP and family to voice concerns about issues that may not have been covered within the assessment.

Table 1.1 Observation of limb movement

Observation	Result	Method
Normal power	The patient will be able to push against resistance with no difficulty.	To determine whether the patient has normal power, or mild or severe weakness. Each limb is assessed and recorded separately. Arms: while holding the wrist ask the patient to pull you toward him or her and then push you away. Legs: holding the top of the ankle ask the patient to lift his or her leg off the bed then holding the back of the ankle ask the patient to pull the leg toward him or her.
Miid weakness	The patient will be able to push against resistance but will be easily overcome.	
Severe weakness	The patient will be able to move his or her limbs independently but will be unable to move against resistance.	
Spastic flexion	The patient's limbs will flex in response to painful stimuli. Arms, wrists and possibly the thumb will bend inwards. Legs will pull upwards.	To determine a response of spastic flexion or extension, apply central painful stimuli. If no response is elicited use peripheral painful stimulus.
Extension	The patient's limbs will extend in response to painful stimuli. Elbows, wrists and fingers will straighten stiffly down the side of the body. Legs will stiffen and feet will point downwards.	
No response	There is no motor response despite central and peripheral painful stimuli.	

Source: Adapted from Woodward (1997).

Table 1.2 Testing cranial nerve function of a child

Cranial nerve	Name	Type and when to test	How to test	Abnormal
Cranial nerve I	Olfactory	Test those with head trauma and abnormal mental status	With child's eyes closed occlude one nostril and present an aromatic substance that is non-noxious	
Cranial nerve II	Optic nerve	Papilledema with increased intracranial pressure; optic atrophy	Using the ophthalmoscope to examine the ocular fundus to determine the colour, size, and shape of the optic disc.	
Cranial nerves III, IV, VI	Oculomotor, trochlear, and abducens nerves	Motor function, sensory function, and corneal reflex	Check pupils for size, regularity and equality and consensual light reaction and accommodation. Nysstagmus is a back-and-forth oscillation of the eyes.	Increasing intracranial pressure causes a sudden, unilateral, dilated, and nonreactive pupil. Nystagmus occurs with disease of the vestibular system, cerebellum, or brain stem
Cranial nerve V	Trigeminal nerve	Muscles of mastication, sensory function and corneal reflex	Palpate the temporal and masseter muscles as the person clenches the teeth. Lightly touch a cotton wisp to forehead, cheeks and chin. Place wisp of cotton on the cornea, coming in from the side.	
Cranial nerve VII	Facial nerve	Motor and sensory function	Note mobility and facial symmetry as person responds to request to: smile, frown, close eyes tightly, lift eyebrows, show teeth.	Muscle weakness is shown by flattening of the nasolabial fold, drooping of one side of the face, lower eyelid sagging. These may indicate central nervous system lesions and peripheral nervous system lesions.
Cranial nerve VIII	Acoustic (vestibulocochlear) nerve		Ability to hear normal conversation, by whispered voice, and by Weber and Rinne tuning fork.	

(continued)

Table 1.2 Testing cranial nerve function of a child *(continued)*

Cranial nerve	Name	Type and when to test	How to test	Abnormal
Cranial nerve IX and X	Glossopharyngeal and vagus nerves	Motor and sensory function	Depress tongue with tongue blade and note pharyngeal movement as the person says "ahhh"; the uvula and soft palate should rise in the midline and tonsillar pillars should move medially.	Absence or asymmetry of soft palate, uvula deviates to side, or asymmetry of tonsillar pillar movements indicate an abnormal finding.
Cranial nerve XI	Spinal accessory nerve		Check for symmetry of sternomastoid and trapezius muscles by asking the person to turn head and shrug shoulders against resistance.	Atrophy or muscle weakness or paralysis indicate abnormal findings.
Cranial nerve XII	Hypoglossal nerve		Inspect tongue. No wasting or tremors should be present. Note the forward thrust in the midline as the person protrudes the tongue.	Atrophy or fasciculations or tongue deviates to side with lesions of hypoglossal nerve.

This information was published in Jarvis (2008).

Procedure guideline 1.17 Assessing nutrition

Statement	Rationale
1 Measure the CYP's weight and height and check these against age-appropriate values, growth charts, and previous records. Use of a nutrition screening tool may highlight CYPs at risk (Gerasimidis et al. 2010; White et al. 2014).	1 To establish if the CYP is growing and developing normally. CYPs in hospital are particularly at risk of malnutrition (Aurangzeb et al. 2012).
2 Is the CYP gaining weight and growing? Are the parents/carers concerned about any aspect of development?	2 Parents/carers are generally the first people to detect poor nutrition or weight gain. Failure to thrive may indicate a number of chronic conditions such as gastro-oesophageal reflux, cardiac, respiratory, liver and renal disease, malignancy, and endocrine and metabolic disorders (Joosten and Hulst 2008).
3 What is the CYP's normal feeding regimen? Do they need help with eating or drinking? Do they use a knife and fork or their fingers to feed themselves? Do they drink from a cup/beaker/bottle?	3 Continuing the CYP's normal regimen will help to decrease anxiety and stress.
4 For infants, are they breast- or bottle-fed and if so, which milk do the parents/carers use?	4 To maintain the current feeding regimen.
5 What are the CYP's likes and dislikes? Are there any foods to which the CYP is allergic or cannot tolerate?	5 To establish the CYP's current regimen and aid the planning of nursing care.
6 Does the CYP require a special diet or food supplements?	6 Wherever possible, these should be continued while the CYP is in hospital.
7 Does the CYP require any additional nutritional support such as overnight feeding or total parenteral nutrition?	7 To establish the CYP's current regimen and aid the planning of nursing care.
8 Is the CYP seeing any other professional, such as a dietician or nurse specialist?	8 To ensure effective communication between professionals, which may offer additional information about the CYP.
9 Do the CYP and/or family have any other concerns regarding the CYP's nutritional needs?	9 To allow the CYP and family to voice concerns about issues that may not have been covered within the assessment.

Procedure guideline 1.18 Assessing elimination and sexual development

Statement	Rationale
1 What is the CYP's normal toilet regimen? Can they use the toilet unaided? For younger children, are they potty trained?	1 To plan the CYP's individual care and maintain the CYP and family's normal routine wherever possible.
2 What is the colour and consistency of the CYP's urine? Does it have an odour? Does it hurt when they pass urine?	2 Dark, concentrated urine may indicate dehydration. Cloudy and/or smelly urine may indicate infection. Red or brown urine suggests haematuria.

Procedure guideline 1.18 Assessing elimination and sexual development *(continued)*

Statement	Rationale
3 What is the colour and consistency of the CYP's faeces? Do they have an odour? Does it hurt when they defecate	3 Black stools may indicate melaena from gastrointestinal bleeding. Grey- or clay-coloured stools in a CYP with persistent jaundice may indicate biliary atresia (Davenport 2012). Pale, loose, bulky, offensive stools may indicate coeliac disease (Tran 2014). Liquid or watery green stools may indicate diarrhoea due to infection, inflammation, chemotherapy, or laxative use. Ribbon-like stools may indicate Hirschsprung's disease (Engel 2006).
4 Is the CYP constipated? Do they need aperients, such as laxatives, suppositories or enemas? If so, how often are they required?	4 To maintain current therapy and promote normal bowel actions. Recurrent constipation may indicate more serious gastrointestinal issues (Nurko and Zimmerman 2014).
5 Is there any abnormal discharge from the genital area?	5 Abnormal discharge may result from the presence of a foreign body or infection. Sexually transmitted diseases may result from consensual sex or sexual abuse.
6 In older boys, have they reached puberty? If so, at what age did this occur?	6 Puberty in boys usually starts between 11 and 14 years and is considered delayed if there are no signs by age 14 years (Villanueva and Argente 2014).
7 In older girls, have they developed secondary sexual characteristics (breasts, pubic hair)? If so, at what age did this occur?	7 Breast development before 8 years of age may be normal, but needs further assessment. Puberty in girls is considered delayed if there are no signs by age 13 years (Villanueva and Argente 2014).
8 In older females, have they started menstruating? Are there any problems such as heavy or frequent bleeding or pain? What was the date of their last period?	8 Menstruation problems are a common concern for adolescent females (Bennett and Gray 2014). The possibility that the young person could be pregnant should be examined. CYPs may not declare this in front of their parents/carers.
9 For older children and adolescents, are they sexually active (remembering that they may not disclose this if their parents/carers are present)? If so, are they practising safe sex and using contraception?	9 Adolescents may be sexually active and not disclose this to their parents/carers. The health assessment may be an appropriate opportunity for health promotion and discussion about sexual health.
10 Do the CYP and/or family have any other concerns regarding the CYP's elimination needs or sexual development?	10 To allow the CYP and family to voice concerns about issues that may not have been covered within the assessment.

Procedure guideline 1.19 Assessing skin and hygiene

Statement	Rationale
1 Observe the general colour and pigmentation of the skin.	1 Overall skin colour varies between individuals and across ethnic groups. A yellow discolouration may indicate jaundice or liver disease; redness may indicate inflammation or bruising, and paleness may indicate anaemia, or shock.
2 Observe the general condition of the CYP's hair. What is the texture and colour? Is it normally distributed?	2 To establish a baseline for future assessment.
3 Observe the general condition of the CYP's nails. What are their shape and colour?	3 To establish a baseline and identify any problems (Piraccini and Starace 2014).
4 Observe the general condition of the CYP's mouth. Ask about their normal dental routine. When did they last visit the dentist?	4 To establish a baseline for future assessment.
5 Is there any abnormal odour?	5 This may indicate a fungal infection or poor personal hygiene.
6 Are there any abnormal areas of skin? If so, describe their location and appearance.	6 To establish a baseline for future assessment and help to plan nursing care.
7 Is there a rash? If so, describe the duration, site of onset, how it has developed, and if it has spread. Is it transient or persistent? Does it itch? Has the CYP started taking any medication recently?	7 When assessing a rash, it is important to take a thorough history (Watkins 2013). Allergic reactions, eczema, chickenpox (varicella zoster) and bacterial infections such as impetigo may be very pruritic (itchy). Acute urticaria presents with itchy, white or red, raised oedematous weals (hives) and may be triggered by an allergy. A maculopapular rash may indicate a drug reaction or infectious disease (Watkins 2013). Skin may be dried and cracked in eczema and needs regular moisturisation.

(continued)

Procedure guideline 1.19 Assessing skin and hygiene (continued)

Statement	Rationale
8 Does the rash blanch when pressure is applied?	8 Haemorrhagic rashes do not fade under pressure and may be associated with meningococcal septicaemia, acute leukaemia, or Henoch-Schonlein purpura (Nielsen et al. 2001). These are potentially life-threatening and more experienced advice should be sought immediately.
9 Is anyone else in the family affected?	9 Infestations (such as scabies) or infectious diseases may affect other CYPs or adults in the same household.
10 Does anyone else in the family have a history of skin disorders?	10 Diseases such as eczema or psoriasis can run in families.
11 What is the CYP's normal hygiene routine? Do they prefer a bath or shower? Are there any soaps or products they or their parents/carers would not use?	11 Maintaining the CYP's normal regimen will help to reduce anxiety and promote continuity. For further information see Chapter 11: Personal Hygiene and Pressure Ulcer Prevention.
12 Does the CYP need any assistance with hygiene needs?	12 To plan their nursing care.
13 Establish with the CYP and carer their level of involvement and participation in meeting their hygiene needs.	13 To plan their nursing care.
14 Are there any bruises? If so, where are they located, what is the size and colour, and how did they happen?	14 Bruises may frequently be found on the legs of toddlers as they learn to walk. Multiple bruises or unusual patterns/locations may be indicative of non-accidental injury and should be referred to a senior colleague for assessment. Suspicions of abuse should be documented and referred to the appropriate social worker. For further information see Chapter 31: Safeguarding Children and Young People.
15 Does the CYP have any wounds? If so, describe their reason, location, size, and appearance. Does the wound need any form of dressings? If so, describe when and how this is changed.	15 Wounds may indicate previous surgery or illness and may need regular reassessment and re-dressing.
16 Assess the CYP for potential or actual risk of pressure sores using a recognised tool.	16 To assess risk on admission and establish a baseline. For further information see Chapter 11: Personal Hygiene and Pressure Ulcer Prevention.
17 Do the CYP and/or family have any other concerns regarding the CYP's skin or hygiene needs?	17 To allow the CYP and family to voice concerns about issues that may not have been covered within the assessment.

Procedure guideline 1.20 Assessing mobility

Statement	Rationale
1 Ask the parent/carer the age at which the CYP first rolled over, sat unaided, crawled, walked, and dressed without help. Assess these against normal developmental criteria.	1 A thorough history of the CYP's development is important in order to plan nursing care appropriate for their developmental age. The assessment can also identify mobility and developmental abnormalities (Sharma 2011).
2 How does the CYP normally mobilise? How far can they walk independently?	2 To plan appropriate and individualised nursing care.
3 Observe the CYP for any abnormalities of movement and assess against 'age-appropriate' development.	3 Abnormal movement may result from neurological problems or local injury to the affected limb.
4 If the CYP can walk, observe the gait and note any abnormalities.	4 Infants and toddlers tend to walk bow-legged with a wide-based gait. Limping may indicate a variety of abnormalities including trauma, septic arthritis/osteomyelitis, transient synovitis, slipped femoral capital epiphysis, developmental hip dysplasia, irritable hip, scoliosis, or cerebral palsy (Perry et al. 2011).
5 Does the CYP need any mobility aids such as crutches or a wheelchair?	5 To plan appropriate and individualised nursing care.
6 Do the CYP and/or family have any other concerns regarding the CYP's development or mobility?	6 To allow the CYP and family to voice concerns about issues that may not have been covered within the assessment and provide valuable information during the assessment (Sharma 2011).

Procedure guideline 1.21 Assessing development

Statement	Rationale
1 How does the CYP address his parents/carers (e.g. Mummy, Daddy, Mamma, etc.)?	1 To ensure effective communication and promote the CYP's sense of security.
2 Does the CYP have any special toys or comforters? Have they brought them with them?	2 To promote the CYP's normal regimen and sense of security.
3 What is the CYP's normal daily routine? What time do they wake, eat meals, and go to sleep? a) How has the CYP reacted to their illness?	3 To plan the CYP's individual care and maintain the family's normal routine wherever possible. a) To plan individualised nursing care as CYPs react differently to illness.
4 Is the diagnosis and prognosis of the CYP's illness known to the CYP and/or family? What exactly do they understand about their current condition?	4 To maintain confidentiality and plan appropriate and individualised nursing care. To ensure adequate psychological and emotional support.
5 Does the CYP have any emotional, developmental, or mental health problems?	5 To plan appropriate and individualised nursing care and facilitate early diagnosis and intervention (Bellman et al. 2013).
6 Do the CYP and/or family have any other concerns regarding their emotional or psychological needs?	6 To allow the CYP and family to voice concerns about issues that may not have been covered within the assessment (Sharma 2011).

Procedure guideline 1.22 Other relevant information

Statement	Rationale
1 Do the family have a health visitor? If so, what is their name and contact details?	1 The health visitor may provide valuable information on the CYP's development and progress (Bellman et al. 2013).
2 Do the family see any other medical or allied health professionals on a regular basis?	2 Other professionals may provide important information about the CYP and family. Communication and liaison with other healthcare teams is equally important.
3 Does the CYP or family have any other specific needs or difficulties?	3 To plan appropriate and individualised nursing care. The CYP's parents/carers may also have specific health needs or disabilities that affect their ability to care for the CYP at home and/or in hospital.
4 Does the CYP have any problems with their hearing, speech, or eyesight? If so, what specifically are the problems and when was this last assessed?	4 In order to plan the CYP's nursing care and ensure effective communication.
5 Do the CYP and family have any other questions about any aspect of their care?	5 To ensure that all concerns have been addressed and all aspects of the CYP's care recorded.

References

Advanced Life Support Group (ALSG) (2016) (6th edition). *Advanced Paediatric Life Support*. Wiley-Blackwell.

Aurangzeb, B., Whitten, K.E., Harrison, B. et al. (2012). *Prevalence of malnutrition and risk of under-nutrition in hospitalized children*. Clinical Nutrition (Edinburgh, Scotland) 31 (1): 35–40.

Aylott, M. (2006). *Assessing the sick child: Part 2a, Respiratory assessment*. Paediatric Nursing 18 (9): 38–44.

Beevers, G., Lip, G.Y., and O'Brien, E. (2001a). *ABC of hypertension. Blood pressure measurement. Part I, Sphygmomanometry: factors common to all techniques*. British Medical Journal 322 (7292): 981–985.

Beevers, G., Lip, G.Y., and O'Brien, E. (2001b). *ABC of hypertension: Blood pressure measurement. Part II, Conventional sphygmomanometry: technique of auscultatory blood pressure measurement*. British Medical Journal 322 (7293): 1043–1047.

Bellman, M., Byrne, O., and Sege, R. (2013). *Developmental assessment of children*. British Medical Journal 346: e8687.

Bennett, A.R. and Gray, S.H. (2014). *What to do when she's bleeding through: the recognition, evaluation, and management of abnormal uterine bleeding in adolescents*. Current Opinion in Pediatrics 26 (4): 413–419.

Bonafide, C.P., Brady, P.W., Keren, R. et al. (2013). *Development of heart and respiratory rate percentile curves for hospitalized children*. Pediatrics 131 (4).

Broom, M. (2007). *Exploring the assessment process*. Paediatric Nursing 19 (4): 22–25.

Carter, S. and Laird, C. (2005). *10 assessment and care of ENT problems*. Emergency Medicine Journal 22 (2): 128–139.

Chapman, S.M., Grocott, M.P.W., and Franck, L.S. (2010). *Systematic review of paediatric alert criteria for identifying hospitalised children at risk of critical deterioration*. Intensive care medicine 36 (4): 600–611.

Chapman, S.M., Wray, J., Oulton, K., and Peters, M.J. (2016). *Systematic review of paediatric track and trigger systems*. Resuscitation. 109: 87–109.

Cox, B. (2008). *The principles of neurological assessment*. Practice Nurse 36 (7): 45–50.

Davenport, M. (2012). *Biliary atresia: clinical aspects*. Seminars in pediatric surgery 21 (3): 175–184.

Dawes, E., Lloyd, H., and Durham, L. (2007). *Monitoring and recording patients' neurological observations*. Nursing Standard 22 (10): 40–45.

El-Radhi, A.S. (2013). *Temperature measurement: the right thermometer and site*. British Journal of Nursing 22 (4): 208–211.

El-Radhi, A.S. (2014). *Determining fever in children: the search for an ideal thermometer*. British Journal of Nursing 23 (2): 91–94.

Engel, J.K. (2006). *Mosby's Pocket Guide to Pediatric Assessment*, 5e. Mosby.

Fleming, S., Thompson, M., Stevens, R. et al. (2011). *Normal ranges of heart rate and respiratory rate in children from birth to 18 years of age:*

a systematic review of observational studies. Lancet 377 (9770): 1011–1018.

Flynn, J.T., Kaelber, D.C., Baker-Smith, C.M. et al. (2017). *Clinical practice guideline for screening and management of high blood pressure in children and adolescents.* Pediatrics 140 (3): e20171904.

Foster-Fitzpatrick, L., Ortiz, A., Sibilano, H. et al. (1999). *The effects of crossed leg on blood pressure measurement.* Nursing Research 48 (2): 105–108.

Gerasimidis, K., Keane, O., Macleod, I. et al. (2010). *A four-stage evaluation of the Paediatric Yorkhill Malnutrition Score in a tertiary paediatric hospital and a district general hospital.* The British Journal of Nutrition 104 (5): 751–756.

Graves, J.W., Tibor, M., Murtagh, B. et al. (2004). *The Accoson Greenlight 300, the first non-automated mercury-free blood pressure measurement device to pass the International Protocol for blood pressure measuring devices in adults.* Blood Pressure Monitoring 9 (1): 13–17.

Hakverdioğlu, Y.G., Akin, K.E., and Dizer, B. (2014). *The effect of nail polish on pulse oximetry readings.* Intensive & Critical Care Nursing 30: 111–115. https://doi.org/10.1016/j.iccn.2013.08.003.

Hall, D.M. (2000). *Growth monitoring.* Archives of Disease in Childhood 82 (1): 10–15.

Harker, L. (2006). *Chance of a Lifetime: The Impact of Bad Housing on children's Lives.* Shelter UK.

Harris, S.R. (2013). *Congenital idiopathic microcephaly in an infant: congruence of head size with developmental motor delay.* Developmental Neurorehabilitation 16: 129–132.

Hewson, P., Poulakis, Z., Jarman, F. et al. (2000). *Clinical markers of serious illness in young infants: a multicentre follow-up study.* Journal of Paediatrics and Child Health 36 (3): 221–225.

Higgins, D. (2005). *Pulse oximetry.* Nursing Times 101 (6): 34–35.

Himes, J.H. (2009). *Challenges of accurately measuring and using BMI and other indicators of obesity in children.* Pediatrics 124 (Suppl 1): S3–S22.

Horan, M., Gibney, E., Molloy, E., and McAuliffe, F. (2014). *Methodologies to assess paediatric adiposity.* Irish Journal of Medical Science 184 (1): 53–68.

Howlin, F. and Brenner, M. (2010). *Cardiovascular assessment in children: assessing pulse and blood pressure.* Paediatric Nursing 22 (1): 25–35.

James, H.E., Perszyk, A.A., MacGregor, T.L., and Aldana, P.R. (2015). *The value of head circumference measurements after 36 months of age: a clinical report and review of practice patterns.* Journal of Neurosurgical Pediatrics 16 (2): 186–194. https://doi.org/10.3171/2014.12.PEDS14251.

Jarvis, C. (2008). *Physical Examination and Health Assessment,* 5e, 685. Elsevier.

Joosten, K.F.M. and Hulst, J.M. (2008). *Prevalence of malnutrition in pediatric hospital patients.* Current Opinion in Pediatrics 20 (5): 590–596.

Lionti, T., Reid, S.M., Reddihough, D. et al. (2013). *Monitoring height and weight: findings from a developmental paediatric service.* Journal of Paediatrics and Child Health 49 (12): 1063–1068.

Lunn, A., Blyton, D., and Watson, A.R. (2009). *Blood pressure measurement in children: declining standards?* Archives of Disease in Childhood 94 (12): 995.

Lurbe, E.C.R., Cruickshank, J.K., Dillon, M.J. et al. (2009). *Management of high blood pressure in children and adolescents: recommendations of the European Society of Hypertension.* Journal of Hypertension 27 (9): 1719–1742.

Lynch-Caris, T., Majeske, K.D., Brelin-Fornari, J., and Nashi, S. (2008). *Establishing reference values for cervical spine range of motion in pre-pubescent children.* Journal of Biomechanics 41 (12): 2714–2719.

Massoure, P.-L., Roche, N.C., and Czitrom, D. (2014). *Squatting.* Archives of Cardiovascular Diseases 107 (1): 67–68.

McAlister, F.A. and Straus, S.E. (2001). *Measurement of blood presssure: an evidence based review.* British Medical Journal 322: 908–911.

Miller, E.M. and Hinton, R.B. (2014). *A pediatric approach to family history of cardiovascular disease: diagnosis, risk assessment, and management.* Pediatric Clinics of North America 61 (1): 187–205.

Moorey, S. (2010a). *Unplanned hospital admission: supporting children, young people and their families.* Paediatric Nursing 22 (10): 20–23.

Moorey, S. (2010b). *Unplanned hospital admission: supporting children, young people and their families.* Paediatric Nursing 22 (10): 20–23.

National High Blood Pressure Education Program Working Group on High Blood Pressure in Children and Adolescents (2004). *The fourth report on the diagnosis, evaluation, and treatment of high blood pressure in children and adolescents.* Pediatrics 114 (2 Suppl 4th Report): 555–576.

National Institute for Health and Clinical Excellence (NICE) 2019. Fever in under 5s: assessment and initial management. NG143. https://www.nice.org.uk/guidance/ng143 (accessed 15 August 2022).

Nielsen, H.E., Andersen, E.A., Andersen, J. et al. (2001). *Diagnostic assessment of haemorrhagic rash and fever.* Archives of Disease in Childhood 85 (2): 160–165.

Nijman, R.G., Thompson, M., van Veen, M. et al. (2012). *Derivation and validation of age and temperature specific reference values and centile charts to predict lower respiratory tract infection in children with fever: prospective observational study.* BMJ 345: e4224.

Nolan, J. and Nolan, M. (1993). *Can nurses take an accurate blood pressure?* British Journal of Nursing 2 (14): 724–729.

Nurko, S. and Zimmerman, L.A. (2014). *Evaluation and treatment of constipation in children and adolescents.* American family physician 90 (2): 82–90.

Oberklaid, F. (2014). *Struggling at school – A practical approach to the child who is not coping.* Australian Family Physician 43 (4): 186–188.

Perloff, D., Grim, C., Flack, J. et al. (1993). *Human blood pressure determination by sphygmomanometry.* Circulation 88 (5): 2460–2470.

Perry, D.C., Harper, A.R., and Bruce, C.E. (2011). *A limping child.* British Medical Journal 342: d3565.

Piraccini, B.M. and Starace, M. (2014). *Nail disorders in infants and children.* Current Opinion in Pediatrics 26 (4): 440–445.

Ramsay, L.E., Williams, B., Johnston, G.D. et al. (1999). *British Hypertension Society guidelines for hypertension management 1999: summary.* British Medical Journal 319 (7210): 630–635.

Rawlings-Anderson, K. and Hunter, J. (2008). *Monitoring pulse rate.* Nursing Standard 22 (31): 41–43.

Resuscitation Council (UK) (2011). *European Paediatric Life Support,* Thirde. London: Resuscitation Council.

Royal College of Nursing (RCN) (2011). *Standards for Assessing, Measuring and Monitoring Vital Signs in Infants, Children and Young People,* 2e. Royal College of Nursing.

Royal College of Nursing (RCN) (2017). *Standards for Assessing, Measuring and Monitoring Vital Signs in Infants, Children and Young People,* 2e. Royal College of Nursing.

Royal College of Paediatrics and Child Health (RCPCH) (2021). Growth charts. https://www.rcpch.ac.uk/resources/growth-charts (accessed 4 April 2021).

Royal College of Paediatrics and Child Health (RCPCH) (2018). Safe system framework for children at risk of deterioration. https://www.rcpch.ac.uk/resources/safe-system-framework-children-risk-deterioration (accessed 15 August 2022).

Sables-Baus, S. and Robinson, M.V. (2011). *Pediatric neurologic exam.* International Emergency Nursing 19 (4): 199–205.

Sasidaran, K., Bansal, A., and Singhi, S. (2011). *Acute upper airway obstruction.* Indian Journal of Pediatrics 78 (10): 1256–1261.

Schilg, S. and Hulse, T. (1997). *Growth, Monitoring and Assessment in the Community: A Guide to Good Practice.* London: Child Growth Foundation.

Sharma, A. (2011). *Developmental examination: birth to 5 years.* Archives of Disease in Childhood. Education and Practice Edition 96 (5): 162–175.

Sherwood, M.C., Stanhope, R., Preece, M.A. et al. (1986). *Diabetes insipidus and occult intracranial tumours.* Archives of Disease in Childhood 61: 1222–1224.

Shobi, A., Tullu, M.S., Bhatia, S. et al. (2012). *An unusual cause of central cyanosis in a nine-year-old boy.* Journal of Postgraduate Medicine 58 (4): 314–317.

Skuse, D.H. (1989). *ABC of child abuse. Emotional abuse and delay in growth.* Bmj 299: 113–115.

Sniderman, A. (2010). *Abnormal head growth.* Pediatrics in Review 31: 382–384.

Stanhope, R., Wilks, Z., and Hamill, G. *Failure to grow: lack of food or lack of love?* Professional care of mother and child 4: 234–237.

Stoner, A. and Walker, J. (2006). *Growth assessment: how do we measure up?* Paediatric Nursing 18 (7): 26–28.

Sund-Levander, M. and Grodzinsky, E. (2013). *Assessment of Body Temperature Measurement Options.* British Journal of Nursing 22 (16): 942, 944–950.

Thurgate, C. (2006). *Living with disability: part 3 communication and care.* Nursing Children and Young People 18 (5): 40–44.

Tran, T.H. (2014). *Advances in pediatric celiac disease*. Pediatrics 26 (5): 589–589.

Tully, A.S., Trayes, K.P., and Studdiford, J.S. (2012). *Evaluation of nail abnormalities*. American Family Physician 85 (8): 779–787.

Villanueva, C. and Argente, J. (2014). *Pathology or Normal Variant: What Constitutes a Delay in Puberty?* Hormone Research in Paediatrics 82: 213–221.

Voss, L.D. (2000). *Standardised technique for height measurement*. Archives of Disease in Childhood 82: 14–15.

Vyse, T.J. (1987). *Sphygmomanometer bladder length and measurement of blood pressure in children*. Lancet 1 (8532): 561–562.

Watkins, J. (2013). *Looking at common rashes and adverse drug reactions*. British Journal of School Nursing 8 (4): 169–172.

White, M., Lawson, K., Ramsey, R. et al. (2014). *A simple nutrition screening tool for pediatric inpatients*. JPEN Journal of Parenteral and Enteral Nutrition. https://doi.org/10.1177/0148607114544321.

Wolke, D., Lereya, S.T., Fisher, H.L. et al. (2014). *Bullying in elementary school and psychotic experiences at 18 years: a longitudinal, population-based cohort study*. Psychological Medicine 44 (10): 2199–2211.

Woodward, S., 1997. Neurological observations: 3. Limb responses. Nursing Times, 93, 47, suppl 1-2.

Wright, C.M., Williams, A.F., and Cole, T.J. (2013). *Advances in growth chart design and use: the UK experience*. World Review of Nutrition and Dietetics 106: 66–74.

Chapter 2

Allergy and anaphylaxis

Róisín Fitzsimons

MSc (Allergy), BSc Hons, DipHE, RNC, formerly Consultant Nurse, Children's Allergy Service,
Guy's & St Thomas' NHS Foundation Trust, London, UK

Chapter contents

Introduction	30	Respiratory allergy	37
Allergy and the immune response	30	Allergens in the healthcare setting	39
Diagnosis and management of allergy	30	Conclusion	41
Management of anaphylaxis	32	References	41
Food allergy	34		

The Great Ormond Street Hospital Manual of Children and Young People's Nursing Practices, Second Edition. Edited by Elizabeth Anne Bruce, Janet Williss, and Faith Gibson.
© 2023 John Wiley & Sons Ltd. Published 2023 by John Wiley & Sons Ltd.

Introduction

Allergic conditions or hypersensitivity reactions are common and their prevalence is increasing. They cause a range of symptoms from mild reactions, such as rashes and sneezing, to severe, life-threatening reactions such as anaphylaxis. Food is the most common cause of allergic reactions, with most children and young people (CYPs) who have a food allergy showing sensitisation to specific foods by the age of 2 years. Other allergic diseases such as eczema, asthma, and allergic rhinitis are increasing in prevalence across the world. Approximately 40% of CYPs in the UK have a diagnosed condition, such as asthma, eczema, allergic rhinitis, or food allergy. With increasing awareness of allergic disease, many more parents/carers believe their child has an allergy. Unfortunately there is a need for greater knowledge regarding the management of allergic disease by healthcare workers in the UK and more adequate allergy care for CYPs. Consequences of the lack of understanding and provision include heightened anxiety, risk taking, inappropriate food exclusion with nutritional consequences and unnecessary omission of vaccination because of fear of an allergic reaction. National Institute for Health and Care Excellence (NICE) guidelines are now available for the diagnosis and assessment of food allergy in CYPs in primary care (NICE 2011b).

The range of allergic diseases is wide and it is outside the realm of this chapter to cover all of them; the following aspects will be explored:

1. Allergy and the immune response
2. Diagnosis and management of allergy
3. Management of anaphylaxis
4. Food allergy
5. Respiratory allergy
6. Allergens in the healthcare setting.

Further reading is recommended and a number of useful websites are suggested at the end of the chapter.

Table 2.1 The Gell-Coombs classification for allergic responses

Type I	Immunoglobin E (IgE)–mediated (immediate) hypersensitivity
Type II	Antibody-mediated hypersensitivity
Type III	Immune-complex interactions
Type IV	Cell-mediated (delayed) hypersensitivity

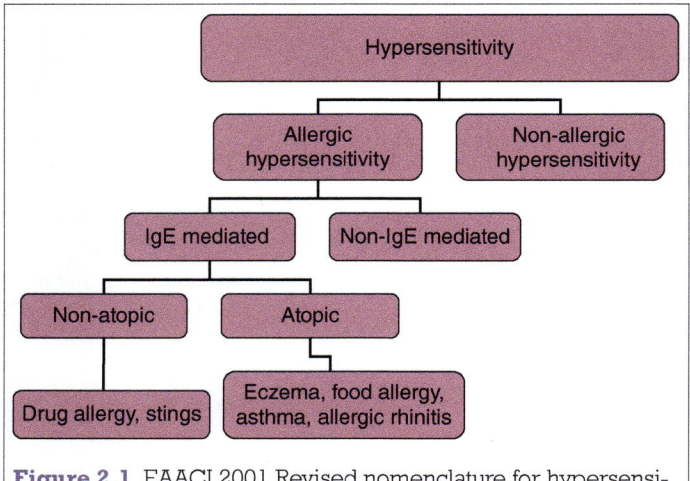

Figure 2.1 EAACI 2001 Revised nomenclature for hypersensitivity reactions (Johansson 2004).

Allergy and the immune response

The word "allergy" is derived from the Greek, meaning altered reactivity. The immune system is responsible for allergic responses and the Gell-Coombs classification for allergic responses was proposed in the 1960s and has been used widely for many years (Mirakian et al. 2009) (Table 2.1).

A revised nomenclature for allergy was devised by the European Academy of Allergy and Clinical Immunology (EAACI) taskforce in 2001 (Figure 2.1) (Johansson et al. 2001). This has helped to simplify and define 'allergic responses' to reactions as either IgE- or non-IgE-mediated, and it is more common now for clinicians to use this definition, which aids the diagnosis and management of reactions (Johansson et al. 2004).

Allergic reactions are inappropriate immune responses by an atopic individual to a protein within a substance, which is usually harmless. The production of immunoglobulin E (IgE) and subsequent allergic reactions are a response of the immune system to an allergen (antigen). The first part of this process is the uptake of the allergen by an antigen-presenting cell. The allergen passes through the body's barriers, such as the skin, nasal mucosa, respiratory or gastrointestinal tract, and is captured and internalised by an antigen-presenting cell, the most efficient of which are dendritic cells. The antigen is broken down by the dendritic cell and through a series of complex immune processes immunoglobulin E (IgE) is produced. IgE binds with high-affinity receptors known as FcεR1 on the outside of mast cells, an effector cell in the allergic response found in all tissues of the body. When IgE on the mast cell subsequently comes into contact with the specific allergen, it triggers the mast cell to degranulate and release its contents: histamine, tryptase, heparin, and leukocytes, mediators of an allergic response.

As histamine is released by mast cells it acts on surrounding blood vessels, causing them to dilate. This initial vasodilatation causes redness (erythema) in the skin, which occurs rapidly after the release of histamine. As the blood vessels dilate, their walls become permeable and plasma leaks out, causing swelling (oedema). Histamine also stimulates the nerves to cause further vasodilatation and the sensation of feeling itchy. The release of mediators also sends signals via cytokines to recruit the effector cells in the allergic response, T helper cells and eosinophils, which cause inflammation, the late phase of the allergic response, and can lead to a systemic reaction.

Atopy is the predisposition to produce IgE on encountering a potential allergen. How atopy manifests itself is known as allergic disease and can include: asthma, eczema, allergic rhinitis and conjunctivitis, food allergy, and, in severe cases, anaphylaxis. An atopic individual may have one or all of these conditions. A phenomenon known as 'the allergic march' has been recognised, where symptoms follow an atopic pattern. Many CYPs present as young babies with eczema, develop food allergies within the first few years of life, and then in their mid-childhood to teenage years, develop asthma and allergic rhinitis (Nissen et al. 2013).

Diagnosis and management of allergy

Diagnosis of allergy

Accurate history is the cornerstone of allergy diagnosis and should underpin a decision to perform testing. Diagnosis of allergy should begin with a careful allergy-focused history of symptoms and their relation to foods eaten, the home environment, pets, seasons of the year, and medication. Family history is important, as it gives an indication as to whether the CYP is at increased risk of being atopic. CYPs who have either one or both parents with an atopic disease are at increased risk of being atopic themselves. This may manifest as eczema or food allergy as a baby, or allergic rhinitis in adulthood, as the parent passes on a genetic predisposition to develop an allergic disease rather than a specific allergy itself; hence, a CYP whose parent has peanut allergy may not develop an allergy to peanuts themselves.

History alone is not enough to confirm allergy. Firm diagnosis requires confirmatory testing. Two common tests used to assess atopic CYPs are skin prick tests and specific IgE (SpIgE) testing (formerly known as RAST testing). Skin prick tests are simple and inexpensive to perform and they give immediate results.

Skin prick testing

Skin prick testing (SPT) introduces the allergen into the top layer of skin. If the CYP is allergic to the allergen a wheal and flare (hive) will appear at the site within 15–20 minutes. The skin is marked to identify each allergen, a small droplet of the allergen is placed on the skin, with at least 2 cm between each droplet, and the skin is pricked gently with a metal lancet at a 90° angle through the allergen, which is then carefully removed with tissue. To avoid contamination the CYP should remain as still as possible to prevent the droplets running into one another and a new lancet should be used for each allergen and care taken when wiping the droplets away. After 15 minutes, the wheal is measured in millimetres at the widest point and recorded. The size of the wheal relates to the likelihood of clinical allergy but not to severity of reaction. A negative (saline) and positive (histamine) control should be performed to ensure the CYP reacts appropriately and validates the test (Høst et al. 2003).

There is a small theoretical risk that a severe systemic reaction could occur when SPT is performed and therefore SPT should be carried out in a clinical area where facilities are available for resuscitation. The clinician performing SPT should ensure the CYP is well and if they have asthma, it is well controlled, and the CYP is neither requiring a bronchodilator nor is wheezy on the day of testing. There are some situations when SPT is not appropriate, for example, if the CYP has severe eczema, as a clear patch of skin may not be available and itching as a response to SPT may cause the CYP more discomfort. Some CYPs have a condition called dermatographism, where their skin marks quite easily and SPT may return false positive results to all allergens tested. If the CYP has taken an antihistamine or medicine containing a sedative (e.g. cough medicine), the SPT may give a false negative response, which could lead to an unsafe diagnosis. Proper use of positive and negative control tests ensures this is detected and thus prevented. Immediate diagnosis of an allergy with SPT enables patients to receive accurate information regarding allergen avoidance and a management plan detailing how to treat an allergic reaction at their clinic visit (see Figure 2.2).

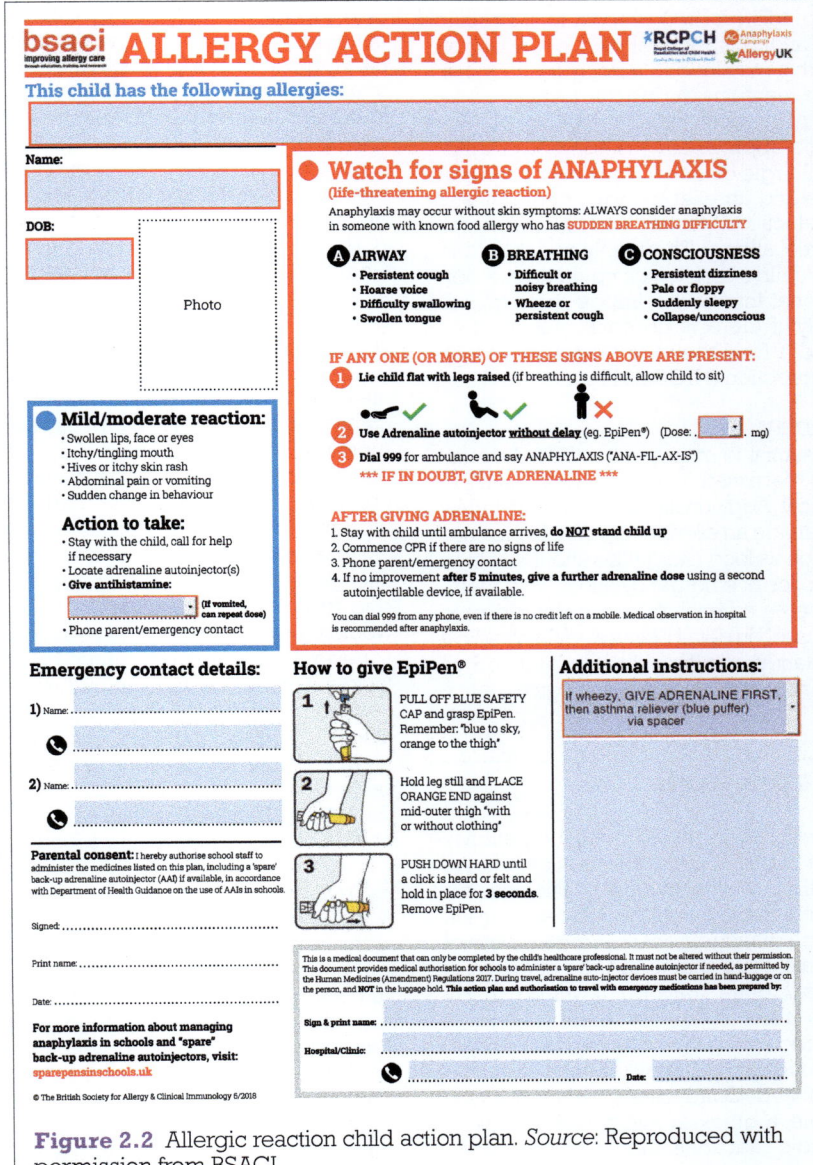

Figure 2.2 Allergic reaction child action plan. *Source*: Reproduced with permission from BSACI.

Table 2.2 A comparison of SPT and SpIgE testing

Test	Advantages	Disadvantages
Skin prick testing	• Convenient • Quick • Visual • Cheap • High sensitivity	• Must stop taking antihistamines at least 48 hours prior to testing • Close monitoring, oxygen, suction, and rescue medication required • May elicit false negative and positive results • Requires trained person
Specific IgE	• Patient does not have to stop taking antihistamines • No risk of systemic reaction	• Long wait for results • Expensive • Blood test can be distressing

Table 2.3 Children at increased risk of anaphylaxis (Muraro et al. 2007; NICE 2011a)

Absolute risk of anaphylaxis, i.e. should be prescribed an adrenaline auto-injector device	Relative risk of anaphylaxis
Coexistent asthma	Reacted to trace quantities of allergen, i.e. vapour or topical contact
Previous anaphylaxis to food, drug, or insect sting	Peanut or tree nut allergy
Food dependent exercised induced anaphylaxis (FDEIA)	Teenager with a food allergy
Idiopathic anaphylaxis	Living in a remote area, far from medical services

Specific IgE testing

SpIgE testing is not as instantaneous as SPT (see Table 2.2 for advantages and disadvantages of both), as blood must be taken from the patient and sent to a laboratory where it undergoes a process to measure the amount of IgE (in Ku/l) present to a specific allergen. The results may take a long time to return, depending on local laboratory facilities, and this may lead to a delay in diagnosis and risk of subsequent allergic reactions during this period.

The under-provision of allergy services within the UK may cause a delay for the CYP in receiving appropriate assessment, diagnosis, and management of their allergic disease. This delay may lead the family to turn to alternative and unreliable forms of diagnostic techniques, such as Vega (bioelectrical) testing and kinesiology, to confirm and treat any suspected allergy. The family may exclude foods unnecessarily from their child's diet, which could have a detrimental effect on their nutritional intake and impair their growth and development. Alternatively, if there is no confirmation of an allergy, the CYP may not avoid a food they are allergic to, which puts them at risk of an allergic reaction (NICE 2011b).

The management of allergy

Avoidance of the allergen is essential to ensuring the CYP does not have an allergic reaction; this is discussed in the sections relating to specific disease processes below. Additionally, the CYP and family should be given strategies to manage an allergic reaction. In the case of potentially severe allergies such as food allergy, this should include a written treatment plan, prescription of emergency and rescue medication, and training in how to use an adrenaline auto-injector device (AAI), if appropriate. This is discussed in detail below. Regular medical review and assessment is important, particularly during childhood, as the course of allergic conditions may change as the child grows.

Management of anaphylaxis

Anaphylaxis is an increasing problem in the UK, with food allergy being the most common cause in CYPs. While allergen avoidance is the mainstay of management, it is vital that when reactions occur they are quickly recognised and managed appropriately. If there are signs of anaphylaxis, first-line management is administration of intramuscular adrenaline—a safe drug that is rapidly effective in most cases, although a second dose may be required. Early administration of adrenaline is associated with better outcomes and where there is uncertainty regarding the severity of a reaction, it is best to err on the side of caution and administer the adrenaline (Royal College of Paediatrics and Child Health 2011; Muraro et al. 2007). In milder reactions, a quick-acting antihistamine is sufficient. CYPs at risk of allergic reactions should have an individualised treatment plan in place at school (see Figure 2.2). An accidental reaction should be used as an opportunity to consider how to reduce the chance of a repeat occurrence and ensure that there is an appropriate ongoing medical care plan in place.

Anaphylaxis is a serious systemic allergic reaction, rapid in onset, which may lead to death and differs from other allergic reactions due to its severity and the involvement of respiratory and/or cardiovascular symptoms. While hypotension and shock are more commonly seen as part of anaphylaxis in adults, it is respiratory features that are most commonly implicated in severe reactions in childhood (Muraro et al. 2007). The Resuscitation Council (2008), Royal College of Paediatrics and Child Health (2011) and National Institute for Health and Care Excellence (NICE) (2011a) all provide guidelines for the management of anaphylaxis (Figure 2.3).

The most common cause of allergic reactions in CYPs is food. Common allergens include milk and eggs (which are often outgrown), as well as peanuts, tree nuts, fish, and shellfish (which are seldom outgrown). Other, less common causes of anaphylaxis include insect stings, latex, and medications such as penicillin (see Table 2.3).

The fundamental principle of managing allergy is to avoid the allergen. Unfortunately, in severe food allergies, even small exposures (particularly by mouth) may cause severe reactions. However, most reactions to food are mild, self-limiting, and respond well to antihistamines such as chlorphenamine. Severe reactions are more common in CYPs who have had a history of severe reactions or who also have asthma. This is because those with poorly controlled asthma may already have inflamed and narrowed airways. If an allergic reaction were to occur, any additional airway narrowing due to the systemic release of allergic inflammatory mediators would cause respiratory distress and anaphylaxis.

Severity of a reaction cannot be predicted and may depend on factors such as the amount and state of the allergen ingested (e.g. cooked/uncooked), alcohol consumption, exercise, and intercurrent illness. Therefore, the EAACI taskforce for anaphylaxis in CYPs has identified criteria that assist clinicians in categorising those who may be at higher risk of anaphylaxis and should be prescribed an AAI device. This includes anyone who has had an anaphylaxis previously or who has both asthma and a food allergy (Muraro et al. 2010).

Adrenaline

Adrenaline, the optimal drug for treating an allergic reaction, increases vasoconstriction, reduces oedema, causes bronchodilation, and inhibits the release of inflammatory mediators, such as histamine and tryptase. In the event of a severe allergic reaction, the priority is to administer intramuscular adrenaline. Adrenaline is a safe drug which is rapidly effective, although a further dose may be required if there is no improvement in the symptoms and an ambulance has not arrived within five minutes of administration. Of individuals who have required a dose of adrenaline, 20% have required a further dose (Muraro et al. 2007; Noimark et al. 2012).

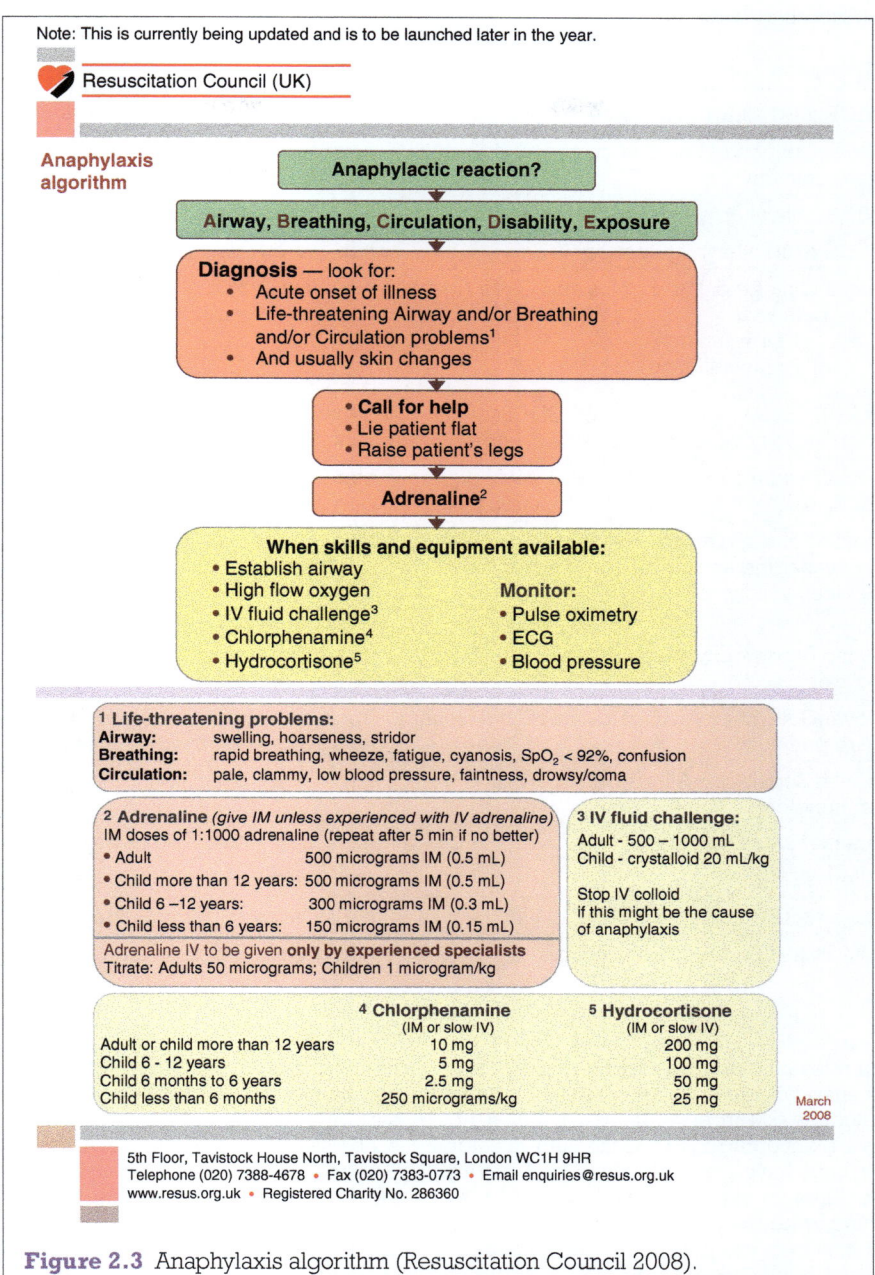

Figure 2.3 Anaphylaxis algorithm (Resuscitation Council 2008).

AAI devices (Epipen, Jext) are syringes and needles preloaded with adrenaline. Anyone who carries an AAI should have two with them at all times as they are single use only (Medicines and Healthcare products Regulatory Agency [MHRA] 2017). For CYPs, it is advisable they should be prescribed four devices; two to keep at home and two at school. Families should be encouraged to check and make a note of the expiry date of the AAI, as most last for approximately 12–18 months and should be renewed before they expire. Table 2.4 provides the doses of the different AAI devices available for three different weight banded groups of CYPs (BMJ Group 2022).

An individual with a diagnosed food allergy should have a formal emergency treatment plan in place, with which all carers should be familiar. The emergency plan is unique to each child, identifies what the individual is allergic to, and clearly outlines how to treat an allergic reaction should one occur (Ewan et al. 2016). Families are strongly advised to keep this emergency management plan with the emergency medications (antihistamines, AAI, and inhalers if the CYP is asthmatic), which should be available at all times. The British Society of Allergy and Clinical Immunology (BSACI) has developed management plans, which can be downloaded from their website (www.bsaci.org) and personalised (Figure 2.2).

Training regarding how and when to administer an AAI device should be provided at diagnosis, and should be re-iterated at

Table 2.4 Doses of adrenaline auto-injector devices (BMJ 2022)

Weight of child	Dose of adrenaline auto device
10–30 kg	Epipen junior 0.15 mg Jext 0.15 mg
>30 kg	Epipen 0.3 mg Jext 0.3 mg

Box 2.1 Useful Websites (Accessed 16 August 2022)

Topic	Resource	Link
Food allergy	NICE food allergy guidance	https://www.nice.org.uk/guidance/qs118
	Royal College of Paediatrics and Child Health care pathway	https://www.rcpch.ac.uk/resources/allergy-care-pathway-food-allergy
	NICE milk allergy in children guidance	https://cks.nice.org.uk/topics/cows-milk-allergy-in-children/
Drug allergy	NICE drug allergy guidance	https://www.nice.org.uk/guidance/cg183
	Royal College of Paediatrics and Child Health care pathways • Drug allergy • Latex allergy	https://www.rcpch.ac.uk/resources/allergy-care-pathway-drug-allergy https://www.rcpch.ac.uk/resources/allergy-care-pathway-latex-allergy
	British Society for Allergy and Clinical Immunology vaccine advice	https://www.bsaci.org/wp-content/uploads/2021/10/BSACI-vaccine-recommendations-for-children-2021-FINAL.pdf
Allergic reactions	British Society for Allergy and Clinical Immunology paediatric allergy action plans	https://www.bsaci.org/professional-resources/resources/paediatric-allergy-action-plans/
	Spare Pens in Schools a multiagency resource for managing anaphylaxis and adrenaline devices in schools	https://www.sparepensinschools.uk/
	Gov.uk Using emergency adrenaline auto injectors in schools	https://www.gov.uk/government/publications/using-emergency-adrenaline-auto-injectors-in-schools
	Royal College of Paediatrics and Child Health care pathway	https://www.rcpch.ac.uk/resources/allergy-care-pathway-anaphylaxis
General resources	British Society for Allergy and Clinical Immunology	https://www.bsaci.org/
	Anaphylaxis Campaign	https://www.anaphylaxis.org.uk/
	Allergy UK	https://www.allergyuk.org/
	Allergy Academy	https://www.allergyacademy.org/
	The British Dietetic Association	https://www.bda.uk.com/

subsequent meetings with relevant healthcare workers. Early use of adrenaline during an anaphylactic reaction results in rapid recovery and a better outcome (Ewan et al. 2016; MHRA 2017; Muraro et al. 2007). Carers are encouraged to use the auto-injector as soon as signs of anaphylaxis have been identified and before calling an ambulance. Features of an anaphylaxis manifest as increased work of breathing, wheeze, stridor, persistent cough, hoarse voice and the CYP may become pale, floppy, or unresponsive. Some young people and adults have described a 'feeling of impending doom'. Good advice for carers is that if they are unsure whether the reaction warrants use of an AAI, it is best to err on the side of caution and administer adrenaline immediately.

Following this, many CYP's emergency plans will advise carers to call for help and to give an antihistamine, if the CYP is able to swallow, to reduce symptoms of a pruritic urticarial rash. The CYP's salbutamol inhaler can be given via a spacer device, following administration of adrenaline, to act locally to reduce the symptoms of respiratory distress. Following an anaphylaxis and administration of the AAI, the CYP should be placed in a lying position (or sitting if the child has respiratory distress), legs elevated, and should avoid physical activity. If an ambulance has not arrived within five minutes of administration of adrenaline and they are still exhibiting signs of an anaphylaxis, a second AAI should be administered (MHRA 2017; Muraro et al. 2007).

In order to minimise the risk of accidental exposure to the food the CYP is allergic to, communication with schools and nurseries is vital. All carers involved in the care of the CYP with a food allergy should be aware of allergens they need to avoid, as well as their treatment plan. Emergency medication should be readily available, and all staff should be able to identify the CYP and be confident in identifying and managing an allergic reaction. School nurses or community nurses who have been trained to provide teaching and support to nurseries/schools regarding management of allergies in schools and administration of AAIs, should provide regular updates. Treatment plans should be written and agreed in partnership with the CYP and their carer, the school and healthcare professional supporting the school and family, and emergency medication should be available at all times (Department of Health [DH] 2014; Muraro et al. 2010). New legislation has come into effect that has led to the amendment of the Human Medicines Regulations, allowing schools to purchase their own adrenaline devices. This will enable schools to ensure they have spare AAI devices for use in an emergency (DH 2017). There are a number of online resources available to assist with the management of allergy and other long-term conditions in school; see Box 2.1.

Food allergy

Common food allergens in children include milk and egg (which are often outgrown) as well as peanuts, tree nuts, fish, and shellfish (which are seldom outgrown). Around 6–8% of children in the UK suffer from a food allergy and there has been an increase in peanut and tree nut allergies, with almost 1 in 50 children affected. Most British classrooms now contain at least one CYP with a food allergy. This has implications for families, carers, schools, and primary care (NICE 2011b).

Allergic reactions to food may present in a variety of ways, due to different underlying mechanisms. Food allergy falls under the umbrella of food hypersensitivity, and includes both IgE- and non-IgE-mediated food allergy. IgE-mediated allergic reactions to food often occur on the second or subsequent exposure to the allergen. Sensitisation (and subsequent allergy) may occur without ingestion of the allergen. It is now thought that cutaneous exposure to peanut, for example, may lead to sensitisation in atopic infants with eczema (Du Toit et al. 2015). In the past, delayed allergies were referred to as intolerances (e.g. cow's milk intolerance), which imply a nonimmune-mediated process. However, improved understanding means that while exact details of the underlying mechanisms are unclear, it is now recognised that there is an immunological basis involving T cells (Fox and Thompson 2007).

Most food allergies are diagnosed in the first few years of life, when new foods are introduced into the child's diet. Cow's milk is the most common food allergy in childhood, followed closely by hen's egg, soya, peanuts, tree nuts, fin fish, shell fish, sesame, and wheat, although these vary across the world. Most children who are cow's milk, hen's egg, wheat, or soya allergic, outgrow this by school age, whereas other allergies are less frequently outgrown.

Diagnosis

Any CYP who is believed to have a food allergy would benefit from being seen at a specialist children's allergy clinic, where medical history, examination and allergy testing can be performed. History is the cornerstone of accurate diagnosis of a food allergy and will guide the clinician as to which allergens should be tested for.

Timing of the allergic reaction is important in establishing if this was an IgE- or non-IgE-mediated allergic reaction, or indeed an allergic reaction at all. How long after the food was consumed did the CYP react? An IgE-mediated reaction typically occurs within 30 minutes of ingesting the food but can occur up to 2 hours after ingestion. This close relationship between ingestion and reaction aids the diagnosis of IgE-mediated allergies. Reproducibility of symptoms is also key to uncovering an allergic response; it is unlikely that a CYP would suddenly become allergic to a food if they have eaten it without adverse effect on numerous previous occasions (NICE 2011b).

Some CYPs can tolerate small amounts of the allergen, such as egg as a baked ingredient in cakes, but refuse plain egg. For some food allergens, the state of the allergen (cooked or raw) can affect the protein structure. In the case of egg, when it is heated up the protein is broken down and it becomes less allergenic, therefore it is common to tolerate small amounts of the allergen in a highly processed form but not tolerate it in a rawer form. Young children may not be able to vocalise that they are having an allergic reaction and may feel a strange sensation in their mouths, complaining their mouth feels 'itchy, spicy, or tickly'. These children may be deemed a 'fussy eater', therefore it should be ascertained, whether they can eat a whole portion of the suspected food, as refusal may be a sign of an allergic response, the local release of histamine in the mouth, causing a strange sensation.

Food allergies can be subtler, causing delayed symptoms often related to ongoing exposure to the food due to its inclusion in the diet (see Table 2.5). Delayed reactions are not so obvious and a CYP may continue to eat or be offered a particular food and suffer from persistent symptoms such as eczema or reflux, or they may start to refuse to eat the food. These delayed, or non-IgE-mediated allergies tend to be more of a problem in infancy and are most commonly due to milk, although soya, wheat, and egg are also common allergens implicated in non-IgE allergies.

Family and past medical history also help when establishing the CYP's allergic status. Babies who suffer from eczema are at risk of having food allergies. The more severe the eczema and the earlier in life that it begins, the more likely there is to be a food allergy. For example, a baby with severe eczema, unresponsive to moderate topical treatment, before three months of age may be suffering from and should be assessed for food allergies.

Testing

SPT and SpIgE are the only validated confirmatory tests used in the diagnosis of IgE-mediated food allergy. Measurement of the size of the SPT wheal or level of SpIgE in the blood helps to ascertain the likelihood of a CYP being allergic to a suspect food. It is a common misconception among parents/carers that the larger the size of the wheal or higher the level of SpIgE, the more severe an allergic reaction will be. This is not the case; there are no tests that can give an indication of the severity of an allergic reaction. For some common food allergens, validated studies have demonstrated that a wheal above a certain size or SpIgE above a certain level has a 95% predictive value that the CYP is clinically allergic, although results vary between populations (Table 2.6). The size of the SPT wheal or level of SpIgE may vary over time and may indicate when a CYP has outgrown their allergy. Therefore, children are reviewed and retested regularly to see if they have developed tolerance. This is helpful when deciding which children should have an oral food challenge (OFC) to explore the possibility they may be able to tolerate the allergen (Høst et al. 2003; Nowak-Wegzyrn et al. 2009; Roberts and Lack 2000).

Results of SPT and SpIgE tests must be treated with caution; an incorrect diagnosis may prove fatal if the CYP was still allergic to a food and they were to consume the allergen based on a false negative result. This highlights the importance of accurate history taking. If a CYP had a good history of reacting to a food but had a negative or low SPT or SpIgE result, they fall into a 'grey area' and the only safe way to know if food can be eaten is to perform an OFC in a supervised, safe clinical environment. Recent advances in allergy testing have led to the development of more sophisticated methods of testing, such as component resolved diagnostics and basophil activation test. These are still in the exploratory stage, but may one day become commonplace in clinical practice, replacing time-consuming and risky OFC (Santos et al. 2015).

Table 2.5 Presentation of IgE- and non-IgE-mediated allergic responses to food (NICE 2011b)

IgE-mediated allergic reactions	Non-IgE-mediated allergic reactions
Skin	Skin
• Urticaria	• Eczema
• Oedema	Gastrointestinal
• Itching	• Gastro-oesophageal reflux
Gastrointestinal	• Food protein induced enterocolitis syndrome
• Vomiting	• Enteropathy
• Diarrhoea	• Proctocolitis
Respiratory	• Failure to thrive
• Wheezing	• Constipation
• Anaphylaxis	
Circulatory	
• Anaphylaxis	
• Decreased blood pressure	

Table 2.6 95% specificity in predicting the outcome of food challenges (Sporik et al. 2000)

Allergen	Size of wheal in children > 2 years	Size of wheal in children < 2 years	Level of SpIgE in children > 2 years	Level of SpIgE in children < 2 years
Cow's milk	8 mm	6 mm	15 kU/l	5 kU/l
Hen's egg	7 mm	5 mm	7 kU/l	2 kU/l
Peanut	8 mm	4 mm	14 kU/l	14 kU/l

Table 2.7 Examples of food challenge doses (Guys and St Thomas' Oral Food Challenge Protocol, 0–6 years)

Dose	Cow's milk	Hen's egg
1	3 ml	0.7 g
2	9.1 ml	2.1 g
3	30 ml	6.8 g
4	136 ml	21 g

Oral food challenge (OFC)

The OFC is conducted as an inpatient procedure. It involves feeding the CYP the suspected allergen in increasing portions until the CYP has consumed 8–10 g of dried weight of protein of the allergen or an appropriate portion size of the allergen. The OFC must be performed on a children's ward, so that the CYP can be observed for any sign of an allergic reaction. All rescue medications should be close at hand, and the OFC must be supervised by a specialist nurse, who has skills and experience in the recognition and treatment of an allergic reaction. A resuscitation team and facilities for paediatric resuscitation and acute monitoring should be available in case of a severe anaphylaxis requiring advanced life support.

The OFC is the gold standard test as it can objectively demonstrate tolerance or allergy. An OFC entails the child consuming increasing amounts of the food over a period of approximately 2 hours, with 15–30 minutes between each dose. Table 2.7 shows examples of OFC doses. The allergen can be disguised in any vehicle that will facilitate the CYP eating the food. This can be anything from cow's milk mixed with soya milk, which the CYP may be familiar with drinking, to cod in jam sandwiches, to disguise the taste. As long as the vehicle is something the CYP has eaten before and is not allergic to, and it helps the CYP eat the challenge allergen, anything goes! (Nowak-Wegzyrn et al. 2009; Sampson et al. 2012).

If at any point during the OFC the CYP exhibits any sign of an allergic reaction, the OFC will be stopped immediately and the CYP will be treated for an allergic reaction according to its severity. They should be observed for a period of at least two hours once they have finished consuming the food, regardless of whether they tolerate the top dose or if the OFC is discontinued at an earlier portion because they have reacted (Nowak-Wegzyrn et al. 2009).

Preparation

There are a number of factors that need to be considered when performing an OFC. Preparation is essential to ensure the OFC is performed safely and runs smoothly. The family should be fully informed of the procedure before the appointment; this includes providing them with written information and discussing the procedure with them, either at an outpatient appointment or on the telephone before the OFC. This will help the family prepare the CYP for the OFC, which will hopefully ensure the day goes well. The family should also be aware that if the CYP has a negative OFC and consumes the required amount of allergen, they must incorporate the food into their diet at home at least twice a week to maintain tolerance (Du Toit et al. 2015). In addition to understanding the purpose and benefits of an OFC, it is important the family members are aware of the risks. As the purpose of an OFC is to diagnose allergy or tolerance to an allergen, there is a real risk the child may have an allergic reaction during the challenge. An essential part of explaining the procedure is to outline the possibility of an allergic reaction, including life-threatening anaphylaxis, steps that are taken to reduce the risk of an anaphylaxis occurring, and how a reaction will be treated, should one occur.

To ensure the safety of the OFC there are a number of measures that need to be taken. The CYP should be well on the day of the OFC and should have stopped taking antihistamines, which can mask the early signs of an allergic reaction. Long-acting antihistamines, such as cetirizine and loratidine, should be stopped five days before the OFC; short-acting antihistamines, such as chlorphenamine, should be stopped 48 hours before the OFC. The CYP should not have had a viral illness, exacerbation of asthma, eczema, or allergic rhinitis in the week preceding the OFC. If the CYP is unwell in any way they could have a more severe allergic reaction if they were to react to the allergen. If there are any exacerbations of atopic disease it is difficult to know if the CYP is reacting during the OFC; for example, if their eczema is very troublesome and they are itchy it is often difficult to gauge during the OFC if they are having a reaction or if this amount of itch is normal for them. Similarly, it is best to challenge someone with allergic rhinitis out of the pollen season, as it may be difficult for them to stop taking their antihistamines. Or if they develop rhinorrhea during the course of the OFC, it may cause confusion as to whether this is a response to the challenge allergen or part of their concurrent rhinitis.

Troubleshooting

The CYP and their family may be very anxious about the OFC as they are being exposed to something they are possibly allergic to and have previously been warned could prove life-threatening if accidentally consumed. The role of the nurse is to explain to the family why the OFC is being performed, build up their confidence, and gain their trust. The CYP may be anxious due to previous experience, so having the opportunity to speak to a specialist nurse or dietician before the OFC will help them to build their confidence to either continue with the OFC, or develop strategies to manage their allergy with confidence at home.

Some CYPs may get mid-way through the OFC and decide they no longer want to eat the food. This is a difficult situation because, if they have not consumed enough of the allergen, we cannot say with certainty they are not allergic. To give the CYP a diagnosis of allergy at this point could mean that they will continue to avoid a food to which they may not be allergic. This has a huge impact on the family's quality of life and may have implications on the child's nutritional requirements. Alternatively, if the CYP was allergic to the food and they were told they could consume it, this could have disastrous consequences, as they could have an allergic reaction on subsequent exposure at home. This is where bringing in food the CYP commonly eats, e.g. soya milk or a favourite sandwich filling, can help to disguise the challenge allergen. The skills of a play specialist, or rewards such as stickers may help to encourage the CYP to continue eating.

Often the CYP may report subjective symptoms of an allergic reaction, such as itchy throat or abdominal pain, or a younger child may become very quiet and withdrawn. These symptoms must be taken seriously as they may herald a more severe allergic reaction. However, many children are very anxious about consuming the challenge food and these symptoms may be due to fear rather than a genuine allergic reaction. This is a difficult situation to manage; it would be unwise to stop the challenge without a definitive diagnosis, yet you do not want to elicit an anaphylaxis. There are a number of approaches that may be utilised in this situation; in the first instance, preparing the CYP and gaining their trust, by explaining the procedure so they feel reassured, should help avoid this scenario. Distraction is very useful (e.g. engaging the CYP in an activity such as having a story read to them or playing a computer game) to see if the symptoms disappear. If the symptoms persist and the CYP cannot be distracted, a discussion with the family should then ensue, to make a decision as to whether or not to stop the OFC. If it is felt this is not an allergic response, the OFC should proceed with caution; it may be wise to repeat the previous dose and see if the symptoms persist. If the symptoms do persist or get worse, the OFC should be stopped and the allergy confirmed. If they do not persist the OFC will continue.

Following a negative OFC, where the CYP has tolerated the food, the allergen can be reintroduced into the child's diet. If the OFC was positive and the CYP reacted, the family should be advised to strictly avoid that allergen; at this point a dietician is essential either to guide reintroduction or to give assistance with avoidance strategies.

Unfortunately there are no reliable tests available for delayed non-IgE-mediated food allergies. A food exclusion diet of between six and eight weeks, under the guidance of a paediatric dietician and subsequent reintroduction of the suspected allergen is the recommended method to confirm a delayed allergy. The symptoms should disappear when the food is removed from the diet and return when the food is reintroduced (NICE 2011b).

Respiratory allergy

Increase in atopy is not limited to food allergy. It is estimated that 80% of asthma in CYPs is driven by aeroallergens and there is an increase in children presenting at a younger age with symptoms of allergic rhinitis. This disease now affects between 10% and 40% of CYPs across the world (Roberts et al. 2013). The link between asthma and allergic rhinitis is now much better understood. The nasal cavity is the beginning of the respiratory tract and the epithelium of the nasal mucosa has similarities to that of the lower airway. The nose acts as a gatekeeper, warming, humidifying, and filtering air before it passes through into the lungs. If the nasal passage becomes blocked and the nose cannot do its job, the child will begin to breathe through their mouth. Cold, dry air will pass into the respiratory tract and can cause bronchospasm. In addition, the air is not filtered, which allows small airborne particles to enter the lower airways, introducing infection and causing inflammation, which can lead to coughing, constriction of the airways, and symptoms of asthma (Roberts et al. 2013).

The inextricable link between asthma and allergic rhinitis is well established. In the 1990s an international group of clinicians got together to look at allergic rhinitis and its impact on asthma (ARIA). The group have produced guidelines and regular updates on the management of patients with allergic rhinitis and asthma. Upper airway symptoms of allergic rhinitis include rhinorrhea, sneezing, blocked nose, nose bleeds, headaches and ocular symptoms; red, watery, itchy eyes, which often become swollen and painful (Brożek et al. 2010).

Diagnosis

As with all allergic disease, diagnosis of a respiratory allergy begins with taking an accurate clinical history. History should include respiratory symptoms; whether these are persistent, time of year of onset, and how troublesome these symptoms are. This is important, as different aeroallergens are prevalent in the atmosphere at different times of year. For example, CYPs who notice exacerbation of asthma in the autumn months may well be sensitised to moulds such as Cladosporium, Alternaria, and Aspergillus, which are commonly found on decaying leaves, fruit and vegetables. CYPs who have symptoms of allergic rhinoconjunctivitis, such as runny nose, runny eyes, itchy nose, and sneezing during spring (February to April) are more likely to be sensitised to tree pollen, as this is in abundance in the atmosphere at these times. Those who have these symptoms later on in the year (May, June, and July) are likely to be grass pollen allergic, as this is the height of the grass pollen season. Others may have symptoms of allergic rhinitis all year round and these are caused by indoor aeroallergens such as house dust mite, cats and dogs (Roberts et al. 2013).

To fully assess the impact of the disease on an individual, severity must also be considered. The impact of respiratory allergy is often underestimated, but for CYPs who suffer with allergic rhinitis their quality of life is significantly affected. Those who are affected in the height of the pollen season report a huge impact on outdoor activities. They are unable to join in with their friends when playing sports, or enjoy trips to the park, and are woken frequently at night due to a runny or blocked nose, which causes them to be very tired during the day. In addition, CYPs with allergic rhinitis may take daily sedating antihistamines to combat the symptoms. These sedating antihistamines have an effect on their school lives, and they frequently underperform at school. Public exams are taken at the height of the grass pollen season when young people with allergic rhinitis are most affected, and they are more likely to perform better in their mock exams, which are held in the winter months, than exams that are held in the summertime, when compared with young people without allergic rhinitis (Roberts et al. 2013; Walker et al. 2007).

There are a number of presenting features of the CYP with allergic rhinitis: they may have dark circles under their eyes, due to vasodilation and inflammation in the blood vessels around the sinuses, which impinges on blood drainage (these are known as 'allergic shiners'). The CYP often has a nasal crease, which results from rubbing their nose frequently. This is often called the 'allergic salute' and a child may do this continuously during the consultation (Figure 2.4). They frequently mouth-breathe because their nose is blocked, and they are unable to breath adequately through their nose. This causes dry lips and some children may persistently lip-lick and develop a perioral rash (Roberts et al. 2013).

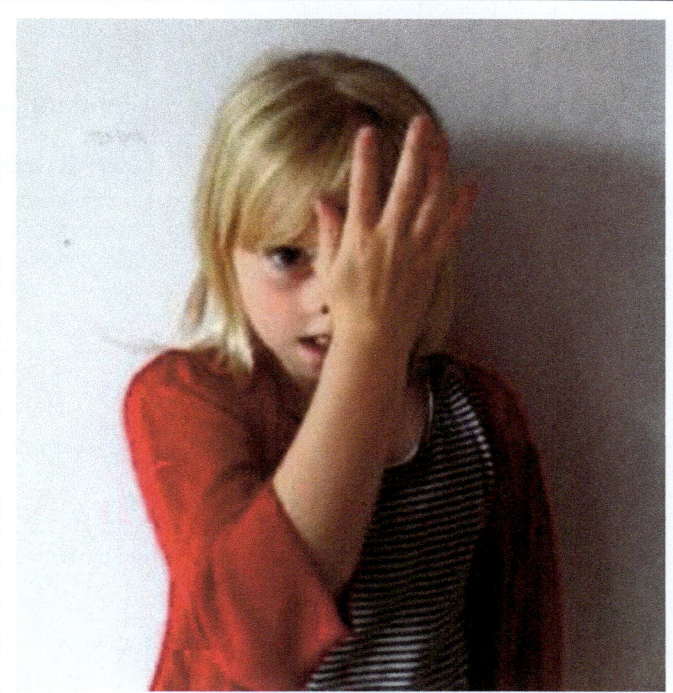

Figure 2.4 The 'allergic salute' in a child with allergic rhinitis.

The nasal mucosa of CYPs with allergic rhinitis often appears very red and inflamed, with visible inferior nasal turbinates and a clear, watery nasal discharge. This clinical picture and history is, therefore, suggestive of allergic rhinitis. The onset of symptoms and time of year when the CYP is affected can indicate to which aeroallergens they are likely to be sensitised. SPT to a panel of aeroallergens, as previously described, would confirm the suspected allergens driving the CYP's allergic rhinitis (Roberts et al. 2013).

Management

Avoidance of aeroallergens is hard to achieve, as they are found in abundance in the environment. Parents/carers may wish to try bed covers and mattress encasings and remove soft toys from the child's bed to reduce the exposure to house dust mite. However, these are costly and no proven benefit has been shown. The mainstay of management of persistent allergic rhinitis is pharmacotherapy (Roberts et al. 2013). When regular antihistamines are no longer having an effect, the first line treatment is an intranasal corticosteroid, which reduces the inflammation in the nasal mucosa. Correct administration technique is essential to ensure the nasal spray is effective (Figure 2.5). The CYP should sit or stand with their head bent forward, and the hand that is administering the nasal spray should be the opposite side to the nostril into which the nasal spray is administered. They must *not* sniff following administration, as this would cause the medication to be swallowed, rather than remaining on the area of inflammation (Scadding et al. 2008).

Pre-emptive administration of the intranasal corticosteroid should commence preseasonally, to ensure that there is minimal inflammation of the nasal mucosa before being exposed to the allergen. In addition, if the CYP continues to have symptoms of allergic rhinitis, a once-daily, nonsedating antihistamine should be administered regularly. A sedating antihistamine will only add to drowsiness and contribute to poor performance at school. In addition to the nasal spray and antihistamines, eye drops are useful for those who suffer from troublesome ocular symptoms. An advance in the treatment of allergic rhinitis is the addition of a leukotriene receptor antagonist (montelukast),

Nurses in Allergy

Standard Operating Procedure

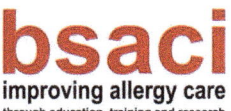

How to apply a nasal spray

- Always ensure hands are clean before applying a nasal spray
- Always ensure the spray device is working and primed
- Shake the bottle before use
- A spray can be applied either in the morning, or evening, or both

ACTION		RATIONALE
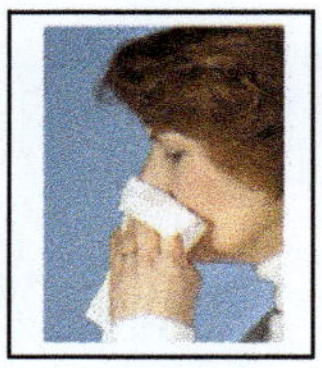 **Step 1.** Clear the nose	Gently blow the nose or nasal douche	This prepares the nasal area by removing mucus that otherwise would trap the medicated spray preventing it from reaching the nasal lining
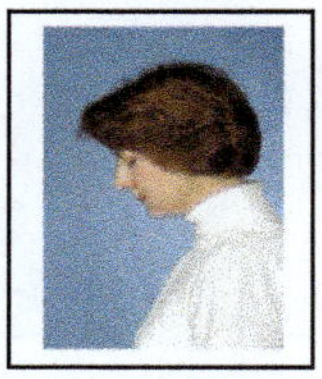 **Step 2.** Bend the head forward	Bring your chin to your chest	This position closes off the back of the throat and allows the spray to reach the correct area inside the nose
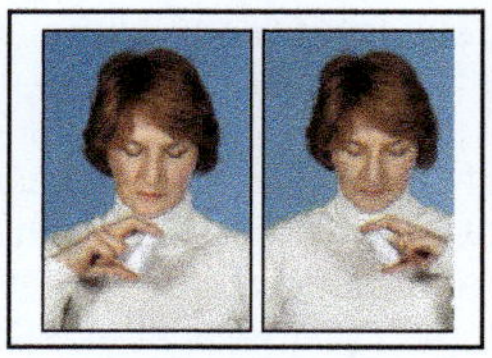 **Step 3.** Hold the spray in the opposite hand to the nostril in which you are about to apply the spray	How to hold and activate the spray will depend on the device being used. Follow manufacturer's instructions.	This ensures you aim the spray pointing it away from the septum, which has only a thin layer of membrane and can be easily damaged.
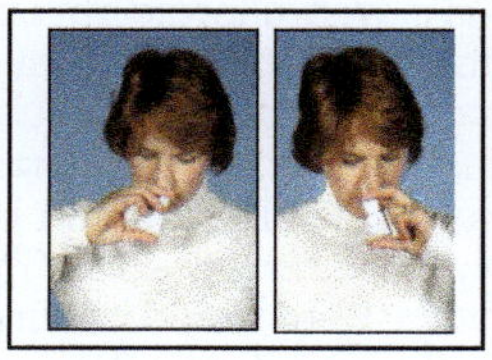 **Step 4.** Using the opposite hand to the nostril being treated, place the end of the spray bottle just inside the nostril aiming away from the septum, and pointing to the ear or eye.		This will ensure the spray is aimed toward the fleshy turbinates inside the nose.
Step 5. Activate the spray DO NOT sniff		Each spray will release a metered dose of the medication. Sniffing hard causes the medication to pass straight through the nasal cavity and be swallowed.
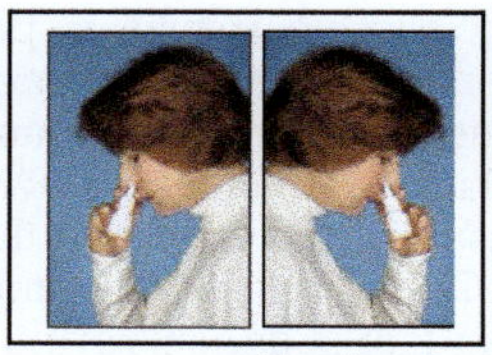 **Step 6.** Change hands and repeat this action in the other nostril		Using the opposite hand ensures that the spray bottle continues to be angled away from the septum.

Version 2
Production date: March 2017   Review Date: 2020   Page 2

Figure 2.5 Correct administration of an intranasal corticosteroid. *Source*: Used by kind permission of Janette Bartle and the BSACI Nurses Group (Nurses in Allergy Group 2017).

previously an add-on therapy for asthma, but the benefits of this drug for allergic rhinitis have been demonstrated (Brożek et al. 2017).

Despite maximal pharmacotherapy, some CYPs still have severe symptoms of allergic rhinitis and for these, specific immunotherapy may be considered. This is the administration of the allergen in small but increasing doses until maintenance dose has been reached. This can either be given sublingually or subcutaneously. Immunotherapy has been in existence for over 100 years; however, it went out of vogue in the UK during the 1980s and 1990s, due to a number of fatalities. It is much more widely used now, although only in specialised clinics where the clinicians have the knowledge and expertise to safely administer this treatment to a highly selected population. Immunotherapy is now widely used in children across the UK for the treatment of allergic rhinitis. There is evidence that treating the cause of allergic rhinitis with immunotherapy significantly reduces the risk of the development of asthma symptoms (Penagos et al. 2006; Radulovic et al. 2011; Roberts et al. 2013; Valovirta et al. 2017).

It is important to be aware of the association between allergic rhinitis and asthma. A blocked and inflamed nasal mucosa may be suggestive of lower airway inflammation. CYPs may be asymptomatic most of the year but develop symptoms during the pollen season. Therefore questioning and treatment should also include symptoms of asthma, such as nocturnal cough, wheeze and difficulty in breathing, or coughing following exertion (exercise, playing, laughing). Any reports of such symptoms must be investigated. A spirometry test is a reliable method of assessing lung function in CYPs who are symptomatic. It entails them blowing into a machine to measure the amount of air that can be expelled from the lungs in one second. A baseline reading is measured, following which salbutamol is administered and, 15–20 minutes later, a second test is performed. If the difference is more than 15% and there is a clinical history suggestive of lower airway inflammation, the CYP should be managed in accordance with the British Thoracic Society (2019) [updated] (2016) guidelines and followed up to monitor their progress.

Allergens in the healthcare setting

This section will focus on an area of allergy that causes concern for healthcare workers and can have implications for CYPs who may be allergic to certain medication or latex.

Drug allergy

While adverse reactions to drugs are a real concern, a large number of parents/carers believe their children have a drug allergy. Incorrect diagnosis of a drug allergy has far-reaching implications; if the CYP is allergic to a particular drug, subsequent exposure could cause an allergic reaction, potentially severe in nature and may be fatal. Therefore, if the CYP is allergic to a particular drug, they should be aware of the importance of informing all healthcare workers of this at every encounter. However, if the CYP is not allergic to the suspected drug and has not had any confirmatory testing, they may well avoid a particular drug unnecessarily and as a result, be treated with more expensive, less effective medication. Penicillin is commonly used to treat childhood infections and many parents/carers believe their children to be allergic to it. This is often based either on a family history of drug allergy or a rash that occurred at time of administration. Frequently a rash that develops at this time may be part of the infection process, rather than a response to the medication (Mirakian et al. 2015; NICE 2014).

Presentation

The drugs most commonly implicated in allergic reactions are beta-lactams, such as penicillin and cephalosporin. Nonsteroidal anti-inflammatory drugs (NSAIDs), insulin, anticonvulsants, and drugs used in anaesthesia, most commonly neuromuscular blocking agents (NMBAs) such as rocuronium and suxamethonium (Demoly et al. 2014; Kuyucu et al. 2014; NICE 2014). The Gell-Coombes classification of allergic response describes four types of responses to allergic reactions to drugs (Mirakian et al. 2009). Most commonly Type 1 IgE-mediated allergic reactions occur, usually caused by penicillin. The Type 4, non-IgE-mediated delayed hypersensitivity reactions are usually T-cell-mediated and are commonly driven by antibiotics, anticonvulsants, and NSAIDs (Mirakian et al. 2009).

Diagnosis

If the CYP is an inpatient at the time of a suspected adverse reaction the suspected drug should be stopped immediately and they should be treated appropriately. Antihistamines should be administered to reduce urticaria and puritus if the CYP exhibits symptoms of a mild allergic reaction. If the CYP experiences anaphylaxis, adrenaline should be administered as early as possible and local resuscitation guidelines for management of an anaphylaxis should be followed, after which the CYP should be referred to a specialist allergy service, where clinicians are experienced in the investigation of a suspected drug allergy in CYPs.

History is essential to establish accurate diagnosis, and this should include timing of administration of a drug and subsequent allergic reaction. If the CYP was an inpatient, their drug chart and notes are essential to help build up a clinical picture (NICE 2014, Mirakian et al. 2015). Included in the history should be any history of the CYP previously taking the drug and either reacting to it or tolerating it. If the suspected drugs were administered during anaesthesia it is essential that the anaesthesia records are forwarded to the allergy clinic and used as part of the diagnostic procedure. Parents/carers often take photos of rashes that have developed after taking a drug and these may be helpful to establish the type of reaction. A history of all drugs taken at the time of the reaction is essential, including any over-the-counter medications and homoeopathic remedies that may have been administered by carers (Ewan et al. 2009; Mirakian et al. 2015).

There are a number of risk factors that may predispose a CYP to be at increased risk of an allergic reaction to medication, including recurrent administration of the drug, either orally or topically. CYPs with chronic conditions such as cystic fibrosis may be at increased risk, due to prolonged use of antibiotics. Atopy is not a risk factor, but CYPs who are atopic may have a more severe reaction if they do react to a drug.

Testing

If a CYP is hospitalised at the time of an allergic reaction, blood should be taken immediately after the reaction to measure tryptase levels. Tryptase is released by mast cells at the time of an allergic reaction and is elevated in the blood up to 2 hours after the allergic reaction begins. It may remain elevated up to 7 hours after a reaction; hence blood should be taken again at 6 hours, then at 24 hours, to record the child's baseline level of tryptase, which will help in diagnosing an allergic reaction to a drug (NICE 2014).

SPT and intradermal testing (IDT) can be helpful in the diagnosis of drug allergy, particularly general anaesthesia. Neat concentrations of the drugs can cause an irritation reaction and therefore the drugs are diluted and SPT is performed as described earlier in the chapter. In the case of many drugs, such as NMBAs, other drugs used during general anaesthesia, insulins and drugs that are not available as oral preparations, the only definitive way to test for allergy or tolerance is IDT (Demoly et al. 2014; Ewan et al. 2009; Mirakian et al. 2009). IDT involves injecting a small amount of the drug (0.03 ml of the solution) into the top layer of the skin to raise a bleb of approximately 3 mm in diameter. After 15–20 minutes it can be measured to see if the size of the bleb has increased. SPT and IDT should be carried out by clinicians who are experienced in this procedure, as expertise is needed to interpret the results and differentiate a true positive result from an irritant reaction. A negative skin test should not automatically indicate tolerance to the drug, especially if the history is suggestive of an allergic reaction; hence, clinical expertise and judgement is essential.

Evidence has shown SPT and IDT is less helpful in children with suspected beta lactam (penicillin) allergy, where an oral provocation challenge is most reliable to confirm diagnosis or tolerance to the suspected drug (Mirakian et al. 2015). An oral drug challenge should be performed in an inpatient setting equipped to manage a severe allergic reaction. The suspected drug is administered to the CYP in increasing doses, starting with a 100th of the dose and increasing in four steps until a cumulative therapeutic dose has been administered. The doses are given in 30-minute intervals and the CYP is observed between doses. As with OFC, the CYP will be kept for 2 hours following the final administration of the dose. If the CYP reacts at any point the challenge will be stopped immediately and the reaction treated appropriately. If the CYP does not exhibit signs of an adverse reaction to the suspected drug, they will be discharged home on a course of that particular drug for three to five days. The duration of the course will depend on the history of onset of the suspected allergic reaction.

Management of drug allergy

If drug allergy has been diagnosed, management is strict avoidance of the allergen. The CYP and family should alert all healthcare workers of their allergic status. If the CYP is admitted to hospital, a red allergy name band should be worn and the allergy documented in their notes and on their prescription chart. They should be encouraged to wear an item that identifies that they have an allergy, such as a Medic Alert bracelet, which carries an internationally known symbol identifying the CYP and the drug to which they are allergic. A suitable alternative drug should be found so that they have a safe treatment option in the future. If there are no suitable alternatives and the CYP needs a particular drug that they are allergic to, desensitisation can be carried out so that they can use that drug. This is not a common procedure and should only be carried out under the guidance of an allergist, in a setting where full resuscitation facilities are available (Mirakian et al. 2015; NICE 2014).

Vaccination

Many parents/carers who have a child with a food allergy have concerns regarding immunisation of their child. This has come to the forefront in recent years with the drive to immunise increasing numbers of CYPs with swine flu and seasonal flu vaccines, not just those at high risk with conditions such as asthma. There have also been misplaced concerns about the MMR vaccine for those with an egg allergy. For more information see Chapter 12: Immunisation.

MMR Vaccine and egg allergy

A common misconception is that the MMR and some other vaccines contain egg and may cause an allergic reaction in those children allergic to egg. Alongside unfounded concerns relating to autism, these concerns were partly to blame for the dip in the immunisation rate for MMR in the UK in the late 1990s to less than 80%. A recent study has shown the uptake of vaccination in the egg allergic population has now increased to 90% (Fox et al. 2014) The BSACI has recently examined the suitability of MMR immunisation in egg allergic children (BSACI 2007). It was concluded that any hen's egg protein content is negligible, and is safe for use in CYPs who are allergic to hen's egg in the Primary Care setting (Clark et al. 2010). The only caution would be for those who have had anaphylaxis to a vaccine previously, and they should be referred to a specialist allergy or immunisation service. Vaccination should be postponed in CYPs who are unwell or who have poorly controlled asthma on the day scheduled for administration (Baxter 2003; Clark et al. 2010; Di Pietrantonj et al. 2021; Fox and Lack 2003; World Health Organization 2004).

Other vaccines and egg allergy

Anyone, irrespective of whether they have egg allergy, may be at risk of an allergic reaction to any vaccine, caused by one of the excipients, such as gelatine or neomycin contained in the vaccine. However, the concern of parents/carers who have a CYP with an egg allergy is not unfounded as some vaccines are grown on egg (Table 2.8). These children may be at higher risk of an allergic reaction when egg-containing vaccine is administered and should have the vaccine administered as a day case in hospital, where emergency medication and equipment is available.

Other allergies and vaccines

Severe allergic reactions or anaphylaxis to vaccines are extremely rare; however, there are many common, mild, vaccine-related adverse events or side effects. The World Health Organisation (WHO) (2004) acknowledges this and classifies adverse events following immunisations (AEFIs) according to four main categories, which are outlined below; examples given are not exhaustive and the Department of Health's *Green Book* provides further explanation of AEFIs (DH 2013):

1 Programme-related: This relates to incorrect practice of administering vaccines, including not allowing enough time between vaccinations, and incorrect reconstitution or administration of the vaccine.

Table 2.8 Vaccines grown on hens' eggs

Vaccines containing egg	Alternatives to egg-containing vaccine
Yellow fever vaccine	No vaccine alternative. A risk assessment should be performed. If the risk of the disease outweighs the risk of the vaccine and the vaccine should be given in a hospital setting. If not, the patient should check the area they are travelling to and if possible they should obtain an exemption certificate. However, they should be aware some countries will not allow travel without vaccination. Yellow fever vaccination can only be performed in a setting with a certificate to administer the vaccine, by staff with the appropriate knowledge and training.
Seasonal influenza vaccine	This vaccine is developed each year according to the strain of influenza. Studies have demonstrated the safety of the seasonal influenza nasal vaccine in children with egg allergy and is only contraindicated in children who have been admitted to intensive care following anaphylaxis to egg, these children should receive the vaccine in a hospital setting. Public Health England publishes advice each year in 'The Green Book' with regard to egg content of vaccines and the appropriate administration of the seasonal influenza vaccine and should be referred to when weighing up the risks and benefits of vaccination (DH 2020).
Rabies vaccine	Some Rabies vaccines are not grown on egg and are therefore suitable for CYPs with an egg allergy. If there is any uncertainty the CYP should be referred to a specialised high-risk vaccine service, where the vaccine can be administered.
Hepatitis A vaccines	One of the vaccines contains egg. An alternative should be given to egg allergic individuals.

2 Vaccine induced: These are events which are directly related to the administration of the vaccine, for example, redness and swelling at the site of administration, or a fever or rash following DTaP/HiB/IPV or MMR. These reactions are common and self-limiting; however, there have been reports of anaphylaxis following administration of vaccines and anyone administering a vaccine should remain vigilant.

3 Coincidental: Many CYPs develop a cold following administration of a vaccine, such as the influenza vaccine. This may have developed irrespective of the vaccination being administered, and commonly the influenza vaccine is administered in the winter months when cold viruses are prevalent.

4 Unknown: An adverse event which does not fit into any of the first three criteria.

AEFIs can be managed in a number of ways; in the first instance, preparation and managing parental/carers' expectations is essential. Vaccinations should be administered in settings equipped to provide resuscitation, by healthcare workers who are trained in administering vaccinations and managing emergency situations. The child's past medical history should be established, including previous responses to vaccination and any existing allergies. Carers should be advised that some events are normal after immunisation, such as fever within 48 hours following DTaP/HiB/IPV, and a rash or fever one week following the MMR vaccine.

Advice regarding management of fever and signs to observe for should be given.

An anaphylaxis commonly occurs within 30 minutes of exposure to the allergen and in the case of vaccines, other than previous anaphylaxis to a vaccine, there are no known predisposing factors that put CYPs at an increased risk of having an anaphylactic reaction to a vaccine. Any CYP who is suspected of having had an anaphylactic or allergic reaction to a vaccination, or who is at risk of one, should be referred to a specialist service within an allergy, immunology, or immunisation department for investigation if appropriate, and subsequent administration of vaccines in a hospital setting.

Latex allergy

Latex use is commonplace in industrialised societies, from tyres and dummies to surgical gloves and sundry medical products. Latex gloves were introduced for medical use more than 100 years ago. Other than three isolated incidents (two in Germany and one in the United States of America in 1927), there were no reports of systemic latex allergy until the late 1980s. It is now recognised that there is a risk associated with the wearing of latex gloves, particularly those with a powder lining.

Latex allergy affects an increasing number of the population and many healthcare providers have a latex-free policy. CYPs who undergo multiple surgical procedures have an increased risk of developing an allergy to latex, as numerous exposures perioperatively can lead to sensitization. Proteins in certain fruits (i.e. banana and avocado) cross-react with latex, and some CYPs who are allergic to these fruits may also be allergic to latex. Latex allergy should be suspected in CYPs who report an allergic reaction to balloons or sports equipment or who have had an allergic reaction in a healthcare setting, such as the dentist, when no other allergens are present. However, CYPs may also have come into contact with latex in the community, e.g. balloons or sports equipment, such as racquet handles. Therefore history should include questioning regarding tolerance of these items. If there is no reliable history of tolerance to latex and the CYP falls into a high-risk group, SPT or SpIgE testing could be performed. An equivocal result would warrant an inpatient challenge to latex (Cabañes et al. 2012; Wrangsjo et al. 2012).

Management of children and young people with a latex allergy

As with all allergens, avoidance is the mainstay of management to reduce the risk of allergic reaction. As there is an increased awareness of latex allergy, many trusts now have a latex-free policy, written in conjunction with the procurement department, to ensure products containing latex cannot be ordered, or it is brought to the requisitioner's attention that the product contains latex and an alternative is suggested. In addition, all CYPs who are allergic to latex need to be identified; for example, they should wear red 'allergy' wristbands, ensuring everyone caring for that CYP is aware of their allergy. In some instances, such as in theatre, where some products still contain latex, there are a number of measures that can be taken to minimise the child's risk of exposure. Where possible, latex products should be removed from the environment, the number of people in theatre at the time of the child's procedure should be kept to a minimum, and if possible a CYP with latex allergy should be first on the list for surgery (Wrangsjo et al. 2012). Not all dentists have moved to latex-free products, therefore parents/carers should be advised to tell all medical professionals if their child has a latex allergy and may like their child to wear a bracelet identifying their allergic status to all, just in case the CYP is ever in a position where they are unable to speak for themselves.

Any allergic reaction to latex should be treated in the same way as any other allergic reaction, and for an anaphylaxis, adrenaline should be administered at the earliest opportunity and help sought immediately. In a hospital setting, this would involve calling the resuscitation team; in the community, an ambulance should be called.

Conclusion

The incidence of atopy is increasing across the world and manifests in a variety of ways, from food allergy in the young child to asthma, allergic rhinitis in older CYPs, or drug allergy, which can affect CYPs regardless of their atopic status. Unfortunately the rapid increase in atopy is not mirrored by the provision of allergy services in the UK. However, with a better understanding and recognition of allergic presentations and the knowledge of how to treat and manage allergic disease, these CYPs are being referred to the appropriate specialists. In specialist clinics they can be managed in a safe way and receive the appropriate education and empowerment they need to manage their condition and achieve optimal quality of life.

References

Baxter, D.N. (2003). Measles immunization in children with a history of egg allergy. *Vaccine* 14 (2): 131–134.

BMJ Group, Pharmaceutical Society of Great Britain. & RCPCH Publications Ltd (2017). *British National Formulary for Children*. BMJ Publishing Group Ltd https://bnfc.nice.org.uk/ (accessed 16 August 2022).

British Society for Allergy and Clinical Immunology–Paediatric Allergy Group (BSACI) (2007). Recommendations for combined measles, mumps and rubella (MMR) vaccination in egg-allergic children. https://www.bsaci.org/wp-content/uploads/2021/10/BSACI-vaccine-recommendations-for-children-2021-FINAL.pdf (accessed 27 August 2022).

British Thoracic Society and Scottish Intercollegiate Guidelines Network (2019). British guidelines on the management of asthma. https://www.sign.ac.uk/media/1773/sign158-updated.pdf (accessed 16 August 2022).

Brożek, J.L., Bousquet, J., Agashi, I. et al. (2017). Allergic rhinitis and its impact on asthma (ARIA) guidelines - 2016 revision. 140(4): 950–958.

Cabañes, N., Igea, J.M., de la Hoz, B. et al. (2012). Latex allergy: position paper. *Journal of Investigational Allergology & Clinical Immunology* 22 (5): 313–330.

Clark, A.T., Skypala, I., Leech, S.C. et al. (2010). British Society for Allergy and Clinical Immunology guidelines for the management of egg allergy. *Clinical and Experimental Allergy* 40: 1116–1129.

Demoly, P., Adkinson, N.F., Brockow, K. et al. (2014). International consensus on drug allergy. *Allergy* 69: 420–437.

Department of Health (DH) (2013). Immunisation against infectious disease. https://www.gov.uk/government/collections/immunisationagainst-infectious-disease-the-green-book (accessed 16 August 2022).

Department of Health (DH) (2014). Supporting pupils with medical conditions at school. https://www.gov.uk/government/publications/supporting-pupils-at-school-with-medical-conditions--3 (accessed 16 August 2022).

Department of Health (DH) (2017). Guidance on the use of adrenaline auto-injectors in schools. https://www.gov.uk/government/publications/using-emergency-adrenaline-auto-injectors-in-schools (accessed 27 August 2022).

Di Pietrantonj, C., Rivetti, A., Marchione P., Debalini, M.G., Demicheli, V. (2021). Vaccines for measles, mumps, rubella, and varicella in children. https://www.cochranelibrary.com/cdsr/doi/10.1002/14651858.CD004407.pub5/full (accessed 27 August 2022).

Du Toit, G., Roberts, G., Sayre, P.H. et al. (2015). Randomized trial of peanut consumption in infants at risk for peanut allergy. *The New England Journal of Medicine* 372: 803–813. https://doi.org/10.1056/NEJMoa1414850.

Ewan, P.W., Dugué, P., Mirakian, R. et al. (2009). BSACI guidelines for the investigation of suspected anaphylaxis during general anaesthesia. *Clinical and Experimental Allergy* 40: 15–31.

Ewan, P.W., Brathwaite, N., Leech, S. et al. (2016). BSACI guideline: prescribing an adrenaline auto-injector. *Clinical & Experimental Allergy* 46: 1258–1280. https://onlinelibrary.wiley.com/doi/10.1111/cea.12788 (accessed 16 August 2022).

Fox, A. and Lack, G. (2003). Egg allergy and MMR vaccination. *British Journal of General Practice* 53: 801–802.

Fox, A.T. and Thompson, M. (2007). Adverse reactions to cows' milk. *Paediatrics and Child Health* 17 (7): 288–294.

Fox, A.T., Swan, K.E., Perkin, M. et al. (2014). The changing pattern of measles, mumps and rubella vaccine uptake in egg-allergic children. *Clinical & Experimental Allergy* 44: 999–1002.

Høst, A., Andrae, S., Charkin, S. et al. (2003). Allergy testing in children: why, who, when and how? *Allergy* 58 (7): 559–569.

Johansson, S.G.O., O'B Hourihane, J., Bousquet, J. et al. (2001). A revised nomenclature for allergy. An EAACI position statement from the EAACI nomenclature task force. *Allergy* 56: 813–824.

Johansson, S.G.O., Bieber, T., Dahl, R. et al. (2004). A revised nomenclature for allergy for global use: Report of the Nomenclature Review Committee of World Allergy Organization. *The Journal of Allergy and Clinical Immunology* 113: 832–836.

Kuyucu, S., Mori, F., Atanaskovic-Markovic, M. et al. (2014). Hypersensitivity reactions to non-betalactam antibiotics in children: An extensive review. *Pediatric Allergy and Immunology* 25: 534–543.

Medicines and Healthcare products Regulatory Agency (MHRA) (2017). Adrenaline auto-injectors: updated advice after European review. https://www.gov.uk/drug-safety-update/adrenaline-auto-injectors-updated-advice-after-european-review (accessed 16 August 2022).

Mirakian, R., Ewan, P.W., Durham, S.R. et al. (2009). BSACI guidelines for the management of drug allergy. *Clinical and Experimental Allergy* 39: 43–46.

Mirakian, R., Leech, S.C., Krishna, M.T. et al. (2015). Management of allergy to penicillins and other beta-lactams. *Clinical & Experimental Allergy* 45: 300–327.

Muraro, A., Roberts, G., Clark, A. et al. (2007). The management of anaphylaxis in childhood: position paper of EAACI. *Allergy* 62: 857–871.

Muraro, A., Clark, A., Beyer, K. et al. (2010). The management of the allergic child at school: EAACI/GA2LEN Task Force on the allergic child at school. *Allergy* 65: 681–689.

National Institute for Health and Care Excellence (NICE) (2011a). Anaphylaxis. Assessment to confirm an anaphylactic episode and the decision to refer after emergency treatment for a suspected anaphylactic episode CG134 London, National Institute for Health and Care Excellence. http://guidance.nice.org.uk/CG134 (accessed 16 August 2022).

National Institute for Health and Care Excellence (NICE) (2011b). Food allergy in under 19s: assessment and diagnosis. London: National Institute for Health and Clinical Excellence. www.nice.org.uk/guidance/CG116 (accessed 16 August 2022).

National Institute for Health and Care Excellence (NICE) (2014). Drug allergy: diagnosis and management of drug allergy in adults, children and young people CG183. London, National Institute for Health and Care Excellence. www.nice.org.uk/guidance/cg183 (accessed 16 August 2022).

Nissen, S.P., Kjær, H.F., Høst, A. et al. (2013). The natural course of sensitization and allergic diseases from childhood to adulthood. *Pediatric Allergy and Immunology* 24 (6): 549–555.

Noimark, L., Wales, J., Du Toit, G. et al. (2012). The use of adrenaline autoinjectors by children and teenagers. *Clinical and Experimental Allergy* 42: 284–292.

Nowak-Wegzyrn, A., Assaad, A., Bahana, S. et al. (2009). Work Group report: Oral food challenge testing. *The Journal of Allergy and Clinical Immunology* 123 (6): S365–S383.

Nurses in Allergy Group (2017). How to use a nasal spray. http://www.bsaci.org/Guidelines/SOPs (accessed 16 August 2022).

Penagos, M., Compalati, E., Tarantini, F. et al. (2006). Efficacy of sublingual immunotherapy in the treatment of allergic rhinitis in pediatric patients 3 to 18 years of age: a meta-analysis of randomized, placebo-controlled, double-blind trials. *Annals of Allergy, Asthma, and Immunology* 97: 141–148.

Radulovic, S., Wilson, D., Calderon, M., and Durham, S. (2011). Systematic reviews of sublingual immunotherapy (SLIT). *Allergy* 66: 740–752.

Resuscitation Council (UK) (2008). Emergency treatment of anaphylactic reactions. Guidelines for healthcare providers. http://www.resus.org.uk/pages/reaction.pdf (accessed 16 August 2022).

Roberts, G. and Lack, G. (2000). Food allergy-getting more out of your skin prick tests. *Clinical and Experimental Allergy* 30: 1495–1498.

Roberts, G., Xatzipsalti, M., Borrego, L.M. et al. (2013). Paediatric rhinitis: position paper of the European Academy of Allergy and Clinical Immunology. *Allergy* 68: 1102–1116.

Royal College of Paediatrics and Child Health (2011). Anaphylaxis care pathway www.rcpch.ac.uk/allergy/anaphylaxis (accessed 8 September 2017).

Sampson, H.A., van Wijk, R.G., Bindslev-Jensen, C. et al. (2012). PRACTALL consensus report: standardizing double-blind, placebo-controlled oral food challenges: American Academy of Allergy, Asthma & Immunology–European Academy of Allergy and Clinical Immunology. *The Journal of Allergy and Clinical Immunology* 130 (6): 1260–1274.

Santos, A.F., Du Toit, G., Douiri, A. et al. (2015). Distinct parameters of the basophil activation test reflect the severity and threshold of allergic reactions to peanut. *The Journal of Allergy and Clinical Immunology* 135 (1): 179–186.

Scadding, G.K., Durham, S.R., Mirakian, R. et al. (2008). BSACI guidelines for the management of allergic and non-allergic rhinitis. *Clinical and Experimental Allergy* 38: 19–42.

Sporik, R., Hill, D.J., and Hosking, C.S. (2000). Specificity of allergen skin testing in predicting positive open food challenges to milk, egg and peanut in children. *Clinical and Experimental Allergy* 30: 1540–1546.

Valovirta, E., Petersen, T.H., Piotrowska, T., Laursen, M.K., Andersen, J.S., Sørensen, H.F., and Klink, R., On behalf of the GAP investigators (2017). Results from the 5-year SQ grass sublingual immunotherapy tablet asthma prevention (GAP) trial in children with grass pollen allergy *The Journal of Allergy and Clinical Immunology* 141(2): 529–538.e13 https://www.jacionline.org/article/S0091-6749(17)31088-6/fulltext (accessed 16 August 2022).

Walker, S., Khan-Wasti, S., Fletcher, M. et al. (2007). Seasonal allergic rhinitis is associated with a detrimental effect on examination performance in United Kingdom teenagers: case-control study. *Journal of Allergy and Clinical Immunology* 120: 381–387.

World Health Organization (2004). Measles vaccines; WHO position paper. *Weekly Epidemiological Record* 14: 130–142.

Wrangsjo, K., Boman, A., Lid´en, C., and Meding, B. (2012). Primary prevention of latex allergy in health care–spectrum of strategies including the European glove standardization. *Contact Dermatitis* 66: 165–171.

Chapter 3

Biopsies

Zoe Wilks[1], Eileen Brennan[2], Nikki Bennett-Rees[3], Alex M. Barnacle[4], Kishore Minhas[5], and Anne-Marie Kao[6]

[1]BSc (Hons) Child Health, AdvDip Child Development, RN (Child), RN (Adult); Formerly Modern Matron, Great Ormond Street Hospital, London, UK

[2]RN (Child), RN (Adult), MSc; Nurse Consultant in Paediatric Nephrology, GOSH

[3]RN (Child), RN (Adult), Diploma Advanced Nursing; formerly Clinical Nurse Specialist, Bone Marrow Transplant, GOSH

[4]BM, MRCP, FRCR; Consultant Interventional Radiologist, GOSH

[5]MBCHB, MSc, FRCR; Consultant Interventional Radiologist, GOSH

[6]Formerly Nurse Practitioner, Dermatology, GOSH

Chapter contents

Introduction	44
Liver biopsy	44
Punch skin biopsy	49
Renal biopsy	54
Bone marrow aspirate and trephine	57
References	59

Procedure guidelines

3.1 Preoperative preparation (liver biopsy)	46
3.2 Perioperative procedure (liver biopsy)	47
3.3 Postoperative care (liver biopsy)	48
3.4 Punch skin biopsy	50
3.5 Preparation of the CYP (skin biopsy)	50
3.6 Preparation of equipment (skin biopsy)	51
3.7 Punch skin biopsy procedure	51
3.8 Postprocedural care (skin biopsy)	53
3.9 Preoperative procedure (renal biopsy)	55
3.10 Postoperative procedure (renal biopsy)	56
3.11 Preparation of equipment and environment (aspiration/trephine)	57
3.12 Preparation of CYP and family (aspiration/trephine)	57
3.13 Aspiration/trephine procedure	58
3.14 Postprocedure care (aspiration/trephine)	58

The Great Ormond Street Hospital Manual of Children and Young People's Nursing Practices, Second Edition. Edited by Elizabeth Anne Bruce, Janet Williss, and Faith Gibson.
© 2023 John Wiley & Sons Ltd. Published 2023 by John Wiley & Sons Ltd.

Introduction

This chapter includes guidelines on liver biopsy, punch skin biopsy, renal biopsy, and bone marrow aspirate and trephine (BMT). Care of the child or young person (CYP) undergoing general anaesthesia can be found in Chapter 26: Perioperative Care.

Liver biopsy

Introduction

The liver (Figures 3.1 and 3.2) is located in the upper right quadrant of the abdomen, just behind the lower portion of the ribs, which protect it from injury, and is the largest and most metabolically complex organ in the body. It carries out hundreds of different functions designed to maintain a favourable internal environment in the body (metabolic homeostasis), and helps to protect against infection. While there is an increasing role in the use of noninvasive tests for assessing liver disease, liver biopsy remains the gold standard for histopathological examination of the liver and is a valuable tool in the diagnosis, prognosis, and management of many paediatric liver diseases (Dezsofi et al. 2015). Liver biopsy is sometimes used in the investigation of CYPs with suspected liver disease, e.g. enlargement of liver and/or spleen, abnormal liver enzymes, an abnormal appearance of the liver on a scan, low blood sugar, raised blood ammonia, etc. The benefits and risks of a liver biopsy must be assessed carefully for each CYP and the results of other routine investigations taken into account.

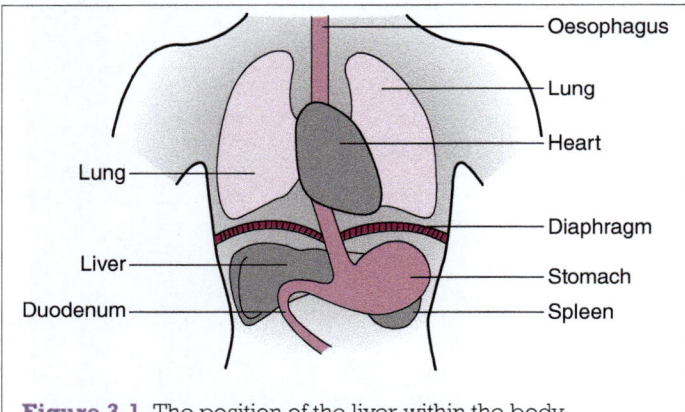

Figure 3.1 The position of the liver within the body.

Liver biopsy samples can be obtained by different methods, such as percutaneous core needle biopsy sampling, using a transjugular core needle approach, or by laparoscopic or open surgical techniques. Percutaneous core needle biopsy can be performed 'blind' or with contemporaneous ultrasound imaging, and the latter has shown to confer much greater success and safety (Siegel et al. 2005).

Ultrasound-guided percutaneous liver biopsy is associated with small but definite risks to the CYP, even in the most experienced hands, and therefore it should be performed only when the potential benefits of the test outweigh the risks. Knowing what the liver looks like (or how it functions biochemically, or whether it is the site of infection) under the microscope provides vital information that can lead to specific, effective treatment or define the likely disease outcome. This benefit should be continually re-evaluated as alternative diagnostic tests (e.g. DNA analysis) and new treatment options, such as new antiviral therapies in viral hepatitis and liver transplantation, become available.

In the majority of cases, percutaneous core needle sampling is the modality of choice, due to the relative technical ease of the procedure and its high diagnostic accuracy (Cohen et al. 1992; Franchi-Abella et al. 2014; Hoffer 2000; Lachaux et al. 1995; Litchtman et al. 1987; Nobili et al. 2003; Rivera-Sanfeliz et al. 2005).

Indications for liver biopsy

Liver biopsy (in combination with the CYP's clinical history, physical examination, data from imaging, and laboratory tests) is a powerful clinical tool for diagnosing, treating, and monitoring liver disease. At Great Ormond Street Hospital (GOSH), all liver biopsies are performed by the Interventional Radiology (IR) department, usually under general anaesthetic. Biopsies undertaken in a specialist paediatric IR facility is best practice, but is available only in a few centres across Europe. It is assumed that all CYP referred to IR for a liver biopsy will have had previous imaging of the liver and biliary tree to identify any anatomical abnormalities. This imaging will be reviewed by IR and discussed with the referring team prior to accepting the biopsy request. Indications for a liver biopsy include:

- Investigation of suspected diffuse liver disease, such as infective, autoimmune, cholestatic, and congenital forms of hepatitis, Langerhans' cell histiocytosis (LCH), metabolic liver disease such as Wilson's disease and glycogen-storage disorders, and some types of neuroblastoma (diffuse forms of stage 4 and stage 4S).
- Investigation of focal liver disease, such as mesenchymal hamartoma, teratoma, hepatoblastoma, rhabdoid tumour, sarcoma, non-Hodgkin lymphoma, hepatocellular carcinoma, and hepatic adenoma (Roebuck 2008).
- Diagnosis and work-up of congenital conditions such as biliary atresia.
- Management of liver transplant.
- Management of drug therapies that affect the liver parenchyma.

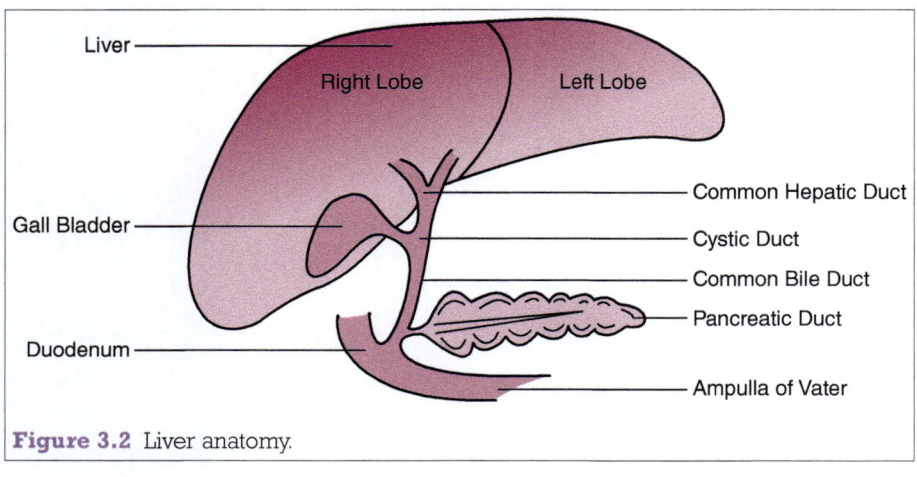

Figure 3.2 Liver anatomy.

Contraindications to liver biopsy

Contraindications to liver biopsy include:

- A CYP who is too unstable or critically unwell to undergo this procedure. There is an increased risk of mortality for an acutely sick CYP.
- Significant coagulopathy, significant thrombocytopenia (usually taken to be less than 80,000/mm^3). There is no published safe lower limit for platelet count, though studies usually consider levels below 50–100,000/mm^3 to be unsafe for a percutaneous approach (Franchi-Abella et al. 2014; Gonzalez-Vallina et al. 1993; Hatfield et al. 2008; Hoffer 2000; Lindor et al. 1996; Little et al. 1996; Nobili et al. 2003; Rivera-Sanfeliz et al. 2005; Schiemann et al. 2000; Sharma et al. 1982). Sharma et al. (1982) have shown that the risk of bleeding increases if the platelet count is below 60,000/mm^3. It makes sense that the risk of haemorrhage increases in the presence of abnormal clotting parameters (Lachaux et al. 1995), but it has also been noted that prebiopsy coagulation parameters were not predictive of subsequent complications. Importantly, operators should be wary of temporary correction of significant coagulopathies, as the abnormality may recur in the hours or days following the procedure, leading to delayed bleeding. In such circumstances, there should be a low threshold for considering a transjugular approach (Cohen et al. 1992; Franchi-Abella et al. 2014).
- Significant ascites. A small volume of ascites can probably be tolerated by most operators, particularly if the percutaneous biopsy track is to be plugged, though significant volumes of ascites should prompt consideration of a transjugular approach. Published studies vary in their definition of the volume of ascites, making interpretation of the data difficult. It may be that image-guided percutaneous procedures are less risky in cases of mild–moderate ascites than previously thought (Little et al. 1996).

Relative contraindications to liver biopsy include:

- Extra-hepatic biliary obstruction (Grant and Neuberger 1999).
- Acute cholangitis.

A CYP in whom any of these factors are present should be discussed with the IR team on a consultant-to-consultant basis, in order to decide whether the potential benefits of biopsy outweigh the risks; some of these factors may be only relative contraindications. In some cases, the transjugular biopsy route may be appropriate, as the risks of bleeding are greatly reduced using this technique.

Clotting abnormalities must be discussed with a consultant haematologist, and corrected, as far as possible, prior to the procedure.

CYPs on anticoagulant medication or a nonsteroidal should have their medication discussed with their clinical team and the haematology team prior to a decision to proceed with the biopsy.

A complete assessment is required to assess suitability of the CYP and the likelihood of complications.

Percutaneous liver biopsy should be avoided in specific patient categories as far as practicable:

- Soon after haematopoietic stem cell transplantation
- During sickle cell crises
- In cases of suspected haemophagocytic lymphohistiocytosis (Dezsofi et al. 2015).

Equipment for a percutaneous liver biopsy procedure

The following equipment is required:

- An ultrasound machine with a standard 13–6 MHz linear transducer. Occasionally a small parts 13–6 MHz linear probe is useful in infants.
- Coaxial core needle biopsy system. Semi-automated systems are available from various manufacturers (examples include Coaxial Temno: Allegiance Healthcare). Older series describe the use of aspiration needles, but more recent series have shown that automated devices are safe and accurate (Hoffer 2000; Rivera-Sanfeliz et al. 2005). There is no strong evidence to recommend a particular biopsy needle size; although the literature suggests that an 18G core needle sample is adequate for a diagnostic sample in the majority of cases (Hoffer 2000; Nobili et al. 2003). The Temno™ coaxial biopsy system currently used at GOSH allows for variation of the throw of the biopsy needle (1–2 cm). Ensuring adequate biopsy sample length increases the diagnostic yield (Short et al. 2013), and where permissible a 2 cm throw is used.
- The appropriate medium for the biopsy should be obtained from the relevant laboratory prior to the procedure to ensure optimal condition of the biopsy when it arrives in the laboratory for analysis. The medium is usually a very small amount of sterile normal saline in a sterile specimen pot. If saline is used, the sample must be transported immediately to the laboratory so that it can be processed correctly, e.g. some are fixed in formalin, some in glutaraldehyde, or frozen.
- Some investigations require that the liver is snap-frozen immediately and this will require solid carbon dioxide (cardice) or liquid nitrogen at the venue of the procedure.

The biopsy tract is routinely embolised with Gelfoam™, a haemostatic sponge which is able to absorb and hold many times its weight in blood within its interstices to promote haemostasis. The Gelfoam sponge pledgets can be deployed along the biopsy tract through the coaxial needle itself and no further puncture through the liver capsule is required. Biopsy tract embolization, particularly in children <10 kg, is shown to reduce the rate of adverse events (Lungren et al 2016).

Complications of liver biopsy

Paediatric studies suggest an overall complication rate for percutaneous biopsy of 0–6.83% (2.4–4.5% major complications) (Cohen et al. 1992; Gonzalez-Vallina et al. 1993; Lachaux et al. 1995; Nobili et al. 2003; Schiemann et al. 2000). Mortality rates are quoted at 0–0.6% (Cohen et al. 1992; Lachaux et al. 1995; Litchtman et al. 1987). The data is difficult to compare between series as authors vary in their definition of major and minor complications, and in the exclusion criteria they employ.

Major complications include intraperitoneal haemorrhage, biliary peritonitis, haemobilia, and injury to the duodenum, colon, or lung, and death. The risk of significant bleeding after an image-guided percutaneous liver biopsy, as measured by a decrease in haematocrit, is reported to be 1.2–2%. Lachaux et al. (1995), McGill et al. (1990) and Rivera-Sanfeliz et al. (2005) showed that the risk of significant bleeding is increased in malignant versus nonmalignant liver disease. Paediatric studies have shown that the risk of complications is greater in CYP with malignant disease, cirrhosis, or recent bone marrow transplant (Cohen et al. 1992; Lachaux et al. 1995). It may be that these CYP should always be considered for a transjugular biopsy approach.

Tumour seeding along the biopsy track remains a significant concern but, unlike in hepatocellular carcinoma in the adult population, it is rare in the commoner paediatric lesions such as hepatoblastoma. Minor complications include pain, subcapsular bleeding that does not require further intervention or a prolonged hospital stay, infection, minor bile leak or haemobilia, and arteriovenous fistula. With good operative technique, postoperative pain should be minimal and postoperative infection rare. Smaller risks include lack of an adequate sample (see earlier).

Following liver biopsy the CYP will return to the ward on a 'Liver Biopsy Postoperative Care Pathway'. This stipulates specialist one-to-one nursing with observations recorded every 15 minutes for the first two hours, every 30 minutes for the next two hours and hourly thereafter. At eight hours post biopsy the CYP should be reviewed by a senior member of the medical team to ensure

Procedure guideline 3.1 Preoperative preparation (liver biopsy)

Statement	Rationale
Percutaneous core needle biopsy technique	
1 Careful preparation prior to undertaking a liver biopsy is essential. Ideally, education should begin at an outpatient visit, prior to the biopsy. Explain the procedure in sufficient detail, with careful attention to anxiety and pain management issues. Explain the potential benefits and (at least to the parent/carer) the risks involved.	1 To provide information, minimise anxiety, maximize concordance, and ensure safety during and post procedure.
2 The CYP will usually be asked to complete a 6-hour fast. Some (those at risk of a low blood sugar) will require an intravenous infusion during this time.	2 To minimise the risk of postprocedure nausea and vomiting and aspiration of stomach contents.
3 In most instances, the biopsy procedure is undertaken on an inpatient basis, following the recommendations outlined below.	3 To maintain adequate hydration and electrolyte balance.
4 On the day before the biopsy, the clinical team reviews recent laboratory evaluation of prothrombin time activated, partial thromboplastin time, and complete blood count, including platelets.	4 To check the CYP's clotting status and to minimise the risk of haemorrhage.
5 Normal coagulation parameters and platelets >80,000 (sampled within the last month) are acceptable if the CYP's clinical condition is stable and they do not have cholestatic jaundice. If the CYP is unwell, the results should be from a sample collected within 24 hours of the biopsy. In an emergency situation the biopsy may proceed with fresh frozen plasma (FFP) cover to minimise the risk of haemorrhage, but this should be agreed by all parties prior to commencing the procedure. If there is abnormal coagulation or thrombocytopenia that cannot be corrected, a transjugular biopsy may be more appropriate.	5 To minimise the risk of haemorrhage.
6 Explain the procedure to the parents/carers and CYP as appropriate. The consent should include adequate understanding of the risks and benefits of the procedure, complications, postprocedural care, and home care.	6 To obtain informed and written consent (Department of Health (DH) 2001, 2009)
7 A premedication can be administered prior to attending theatre. This decision will be made by the anaesthetist in charge of the case. A play specialist may be able to assist in preparing the CYP for the procedure.	7 To make the experience less frightening or stressful.
8 An intravenous cannula may need to be inserted prior to the procedure.	8 To facilitate the anaesthetic induction and to manage fluid balance.
9 CYP with an underlying metabolic disorder or a history of hypoglycaemia should receive an intravenous infusion of glucose while fasting: 5% glucose 5–10 mg/kg/min 0.1–0.2 ml/kg/min 10% glucose 5–10 mg/kg/min 0.05–0.1 ml/kg/min	9 To prevent hypoglycaemia and minimise the risk of metabolic acidosis.
10 Record the CYP's blood glucose at 1–2 hourly intervals, depending on their underlying condition. The blood glucose should be maintained at 5–8 mmol/l. Medical staff should provide clear, written instructions of action to be taken in the event of hypoglycaemia during fasting.	10 To ensure the CYP's safety.

specialist nursing can be discontinued. Any rise in the Children's Early Warning Score (CEWS) should prompt immediate reporting to the clinical team. If internal bleeding is suspected the consultant in charge, the IR consultant, and a member of the surgical team should be consulted. Urgent imaging should be requested and this may prompt further interventions, including embolization or surgery. If the CYP remains well they can eat and drink two hours post-procedure, but should remain on bed rest for at least eight hours following liver biopsy.

Discharge planning

Recent literature suggests liver biopsies in children can be performed safely on an outpatient basis (Bolia et al. 2017), but at present all paediatric liver biopsies at GOSH are performed as inpatients. At discharge, the parents/carers should be supplied with a liver biopsy advice leaflet, if they do not already have one, so that they can be supported with advice when at home. They should be advised that the histology results are usually available no earlier than 2 days after the procedure being performed. This may be due

Chapter 3 Biopsies

Procedure guideline 3.2 Perioperative procedure (liver biopsy)

Statement	Rationale
1 Universal precautions and personal protective equipment (PPE) is standard practice within an intra-operative theatre environment.	1 To safeguard the practitioner and CYP.

Positioning

2 The CYP should be placed in a supine position.	2 To allow ultrasound examination of the abdomen.
3 Consider moving and handling risks when positioning and moving the CYP.	3 To ensure staff safety.

Procedure

4 A suitable biopsy site is identified by the radiologist, using ultrasound.	4 To ensure the safest approach to the liver parenchyma is used.
5 Prepare the field with alcohol-based solution (povidone–iodine) and place sterile drapes over the CYP.	5 To sterilise the operative field.
6 Administer local anaesthetic with 0.25% levobupivacaine 2.5 mg/ml in both superficial and deep planes. Lidocaine 1% buffered with sodium bicarbonate may be used for non-GA (general anaesthetic) cases, as it is less painful, but most children have this procedure performed under general anaesthetic.	6 To provide analgesia. Local anaesthetic minimises procedural pain. Levobupivacaine has a long duration of action and provides analgesia postoperatively.
7 A small nick in the skin is made with a surgical blade, usually using a subcostal approach, to allow introduction of the biopsy needle.	7 For ease of access.
8 The radiologist will then advance the coaxial biopsy needle through the skin and into the liver, under direct ultrasound guidance. While this is done, the anaesthetist usually ensures that the CYP is breath-holding, so that the passage of the needle through the liver capsule is accurate.	8 This allows the time spent in the liver to be kept to a minimum.
9 If the biopsy is nontargeted (for investigation of diffuse liver disease), the semi-automated inner needle of the coaxial system is fired twice, in slightly different areas of the liver, to ensure two good cores are obtained. This is done under real-time ultrasound guidance. The number of cores may vary depending on the clinical situation.	9 This technique allows collection of many cores with only one hole in the liver capsule.
10 In targeted biopsies (for focal liver lesions) the outer needle is usually advanced through normal liver parenchyma into the abnormal liver lesion and then the inner needle is used to sample from the area of abnormality; again, this is performed using real-time ultrasound guidance. The number of cores obtained may be as many as 15, so that the pathologist has enough tissue to ensure a diagnosis can be made.	
11 Once the biopsy samples have been taken, the inner needle of the system is removed and the track is filled with several plugs of a haemostatic substance such as gelatine foam sheets (Gel foam™, Pharmacia and Upjohn), as the outer needle is withdrawn.	11 The gelatine plugs minimise the risk of both tumour spill and bleeding (Smith et al. 1996). In one paediatric series, detectable bleeding occurred in three children (14%) despite biopsy track embolisation; two with focal disease and one with diffuse disease (Hoffer 2000). In another series, there was no statistical difference in complication rates between CYPs who did or did not undergo track embolisation (Hatfield et al. 2008).
12 The biopsy sample is obtained and placed in the correct medium, which is usually a very small amount of sterile normal saline in a sterile specimen container.	12 To ensure optimal condition of the biopsy arriving in the laboratory for analysis.
13 The biopsy site may be closed with a wound closure strip, e.g. Steri-strip and an adhesive dressing is then applied (Autio et al. 2002).	13 To close the wound and prevent infection.

(continued)

Procedure guideline 3.2 Perioperative procedure (liver biopsy) *(continued)*

Statement	Rationale
14 The CYP is then rolled onto the right side and postoperative instructions are given for them to remain in this position for 1 hour.	14 To help prevent bleeding or bile leakage: When the CYP is positioned on their right side, pressure is being applied to the liver to encourage haemostasis.
15 The practitioner undertaking the procedure must ensure that the sample is clearly labelled with the CYP's details, sample type, date and time, prior to sending it to the appropriate laboratory. A request form must accompany the sample and include accurate patient details and clear instructions for the analysis of the sample.	15 To ensure that the sample is analysed appropriately.
16 The operator performing the biopsy should record the procedure in the CYP's healthcare record, including: • How many passes were made. • Any medication administered. • Any apparent complications. • Specific postoperative care requirements.	16 To maintain an accurate record and documentation.

Procedure guideline 3.3 Postoperative care (liver biopsy)

Statement	Rationale
1 Measure and record vital signs: • Every 15 minutes for the first 2 hours • Every 30 minutes for 2 hours thereafter • Hourly thereafter until 8 hours post biopsy At 8 hours post biopsy, the CYP should be reviewed by a member of the clinical team (doctor) to ensure they are well enough to be discharged or to discontinue specialist nursing care, where appropriate (see discharge section). Any rise in pulse rate, fall in blood pressure, or respiratory distress should be reported immediately to the clinical team looking after the CYP. They will assess and determine the possible need for blood transfusion, clotting factors, platelets, etc. If significant bleeding is suspected they will need to inform the person who undertook the procedure and the consultant in overall charge of the CYP. A surgeon should be informed at this early stage. Urgent imaging, embolisation or surgery may be required.	1 To monitor CYP for complications, primarily haemorrhage, and to act promptly to restore circulating blood volume and stop bleeding.
2 Observe the actual site of the biopsy for any signs of bleeding, at the same time as vital signs are recorded, for the first 12-hour period after the procedure. An intravenous cannula must remain in situ for the 24-hour period post biopsy. **Note that most CYP who bleed post liver biopsy do so into the peritoneal cavity and therefore there is often no external sign of bleeding.**	2 Complications usually occur within the first 3 hours of liver biopsy as the blood pressure returns to normal parameters (Grant and Neuberger 1999).
3 **It is important to remember that a sick CYP may also deteriorate for reasons unrelated to the liver biopsy.** For example, a CYP with mitochondrial disease who appears slow to recover from anaesthesia may have an undetected severe hypoglycaemia.	3 Junior staff must inform a more senior nurse/doctor should this occur for advice/appropriate medical intervention.
4 Assess the need for analgesics postoperatively and administer as appropriate.	4 To relieve pain and help minimise the risk of complications.
5 The CYP may eat and drink two hours postprocedure, once awake and orientated.	5 To prevent aspiration and vomiting.

Chapter 3 Biopsies

Procedure guideline 3.3 Postoperative care (liver biopsy) *(continued)*

Statement	Rationale
6 They should remain on bed rest for eight hours postprocedure, but can be allowed brief toilet visits under the supervision of a nurse or responsible family member during this period, provided their vital signs are stable. The position in which the CYP should be nursed following liver biopsy is not significant. There is no consensus in the literature and no controlled trials have been carried out to assess the various possible positions. The child should be encouraged to adopt a position that is comfortable and reassuring (Grant and Neuberger 1999; Perraul et al. 1978). It can be difficult to ensure that children remain on bed rest for this period and creative thinking may need to be used. The family and play specialist could be involved in keeping the CYP occupied while on bed rest.	6 To minimise the risk of complications.
7 Ensure that the CYP has passed urine postanaesthetic.	7 To ensure they are not dehydrated or showing signs of urine retention.
8 Most CYP will remain in hospital for 24 hours post biopsy. Those who are otherwise well, with no clotting abnormalities, may be discharged 8 hours postprocedure, if the biopsy was performed early on the morning theatre list, but this decision must be discussed and agreed with all clinical teams prior to biopsy. **The CYP must then be reviewed by a senior doctor on the clinical team prior to discharge.** They should have a responsible person to stay with them on the first post biopsy night at home and should be able to return to hospital in a timely manner should the need arise.	8 To observe for late signs of complications.

to the complexity of the analysis being performed on the biopsy specimen. For microbiology and metabolic analysis, for example, these results will take longer. The family must also be made aware of how they will receive the results. Usually, results will be available at the next outpatient appointment for discussion with the CYP's consultant.

When the CYP goes home they can resume a degree of normal activity. There should be an interval of somewhere between 2 weeks and 3 months where they have restrictions and they may have to avoid contact sports and swimming for 6–8 weeks. This is to allow the internal organ to heal following the biopsy and to minimise the risk of internal haemorrhage postoperatively. Advice from the clinician relevant to the CYP's age and lifestyle is provided. However, parents/carers should prevent the CYP from indulging in rough-and-tumble play that might inadvertently cause trauma to the liver.

If a dressing and wound closure strip, e.g. Steri-strip, is in place it may be removed after three days or soaked off in the bath (Autio and Koozer 2002). If the skin looks red and inflamed and/or the CYP develops a pyrexia, parents/carers should seek medical advice from their GP. This may be due to infection and the CYP will need to visit their GP, who will contact the hospital for advice regarding whether they need to return to the hospital for blood test analysis and appropriate treatment.

It has been shown that delayed haemorrhage can occur up to 15 days after percutaneous liver biopsy in CYPs who develop a post biopsy coagulopathy. Parents/carers need to observe the CYP for signs of a high temperature, unexpected lethargy, and generally being unwell or irritable.

The occurrence of delayed haemorrhage is also documented after the reinstatement of warfarin therapy several days after percutaneous liver biopsy. The CYP's consultant must give the family clear advice regarding recommencing anticoagulant drugs (see Contraindications section earlier in this chapter).

Punch skin biopsy

Introduction

The skin is complex with an array of functions. It is the body's largest organ, protecting the deeper tissues and organs from mechanical damage, chemical damage, bacterial damage, ultraviolet radiation, and thermal damage. The skin aids in regulating body temperature, excretion of urea and uric acid, and synthesis of vitamin D (Marieb 2012). CYP can present with a wide range of skin anomalies, some of which can prove to be relatively normal, while others can be life threatening, making timely assessment and accurate diagnosis crucial. Many skin disorders can be diagnosed through direct observation and palpation but others may require referral to a dermatology specialist or expert. CYP with a persistent skin problem or an unusual presentation may be referred to a dermatologist for further investigations in order to achieve differential diagnosis prior to initiating a clinically effective treatment regime. This may involve a microscopic or histopathological examination of the area of skin involved, or additional radiological imaging. When a sample of the skin is required for the purpose of aiding an accurate diagnosis or further investigation, a minor surgical procedure is undertaken in order to obtain a biopsy sample.

There are various techniques that can be used to perform a skin biopsy such as a punch biopsy, shave biopsy, or surgical excision of part of a lesion (Nischal et al. 2008). A punch skin biopsy is considered the best technique to obtain diagnostic full-thickness skin specimens (Kupesic 2017). A circular blade is rotated into the skin through to the subcutaneous fat, obtaining a cylindrical specimen which is then histologically examined (Pickett 2011). Punch skin biopsies are useful in investigating neoplasms, pigmented lesions, and inflammatory lesions (Kupesic 2017). The procedure may be performed in a procedure room on the ward, outpatients or operating theatre. A punch skin biopsy should be undertaken only by a

Procedure guideline 3.4 Punch skin biopsy

Statement	Rationale
1. a) A local anaesthetic is used when carrying out the procedure. b) Oral sedation may also be required. c) An aseptic nontouch technique (ANTT) should be employed throughout the procedure.	1. a) To minimise pain, stress, and anxiety. b) In giving sedation the CYP is better able to tolerate the overall procedure. c) To minimise the risk of infection.
2. The site to be biopsied must be identified by the relevant multidisciplinary team. The preferred site is the axilla.	2. To aid the diagnosis for the CYP and family. To minimise visible scarring and provide a good cosmetic outcome.
3. Cytogenetics and chromosome specimens are sent via Biochemistry to a Cytogenetics department. Fibroblast culture specimens are sent to an Enzymology Laboratory.	
4. Universal precautions and personal protective equipment (PPE) must be adopted according to hospital policy.	4. To prevent contamination and safeguard the person performing the procedure.

Procedure guideline 3.5 Preparation of the CYP (skin biopsy)

Statement	Rationale
1. Obtain verbal and written consent from the CYP and family for the procedure (DH 2001; 2009; Nursing and Midwifery Council [NMC] 2015; Wellesley 2009) a) Allow enough time between giving information to the family and CYP and performing the procedure.	1. To ensure that informed consent is obtained and to allow the family to develop coping strategies. a) Too much or too little time and the CYP will become anxious. The better informed they are the better able they will be to develop coping strategies (Sclare and Waring 1995).
2. The CYP and family should be given Trust-specific information and directed to relevant websites, in particular direct to the GOSH website (https://www.gosh.nhs.uk/medical-information/procedures-and-treatments/skin-biopsy-punch-method).	2. To address any information requirements and to empower the CYP and family, alleviating any worries or concerns.
3. Inform the CYP and family of the following: • That a punch skin biopsy is necessary. • The reason for the biopsy. • What it entails. • The potential risks of a punch skin biopsy. • Whether there are any alternatives. • The duration of the procedure. • The expected cosmetic outcome. • What happens afterwards. • When to expect results.	3. To obtain informed written consent, minimise anxiety, empower the family, and promote concordance.
4. A play specialist and the named nurse should provide information according to the age and cognitive development of the CYP, in language they can understand: avoiding jargon and complex words (Duffin 2012). a) Discuss with the family, and CYP if appropriate, the method of distraction that will be used during the procedure. This will need to be appropriate for their age and level of cognitive development. For more information see Chapter 24: Play As a Therapeutic Tool. b) Identify with the parent/carer their role throughout the procedure, adopting the appropriate method of distraction to use during the procedure. The parent/carer may remain with their child if they wish to do so.	4. To prepare the CYP and family for the procedure. a) To distract and relax the CYP and divert their attention away from the invasive procedure (Langley 1999; Nilsson and Hallqvist 2013). b) To minimise anxiety and empower the family/carer.

Procedure guideline 3.6 Preparation of equipment (skin biopsy)

Statement	Rationale
1 Gather the following equipment:	2 To ensure a smooth and timely procedure with no unnecessary delays.
a) Clean dressing trolley or appropriate clean surface or tray.	a) To minimise the risk of infection
b) Skin Biopsy Pack (obtainable from a HSDU department), or a sterile dressing pack, containing sterile nonwoven swabs and a sterile towel.	b) Some literature suggests that fibres from cotton wool swabs shed and can become entwined in tissue and a focus for infection (Briggs 1996).
c) Alcohol based antiseptic cleaning solution, e.g. chlorhexidine gluconate 0.5%.	c) Active against a wide range of Gram-positive and negative organisms. Routine use of povidone–iodine solution should be avoided in small babies and children. Iodine absorption may cause hypothyroidism during a critical period of neurological development and stains the skin cells (Smerdely et al. 1989).
d) Local anaesthetic, e.g. lidocaine 1%. Lidocaine with adrenaline (epinephrine) is a powerful vasoconstrictor, therefore decreasing the bleeding in wounds. However, this may be contraindicated in areas of end artery flow, i.e. fingers and toes. This can cause palpitations and tremors, so is therefore used with caution.	
e) Disposable scalpel.	
f) Sterile gloves.	
g) Disposable plastic apron.	
h) Prescription chart.	
i) 2 ml syringe.	
j) Blue needle (23G).	
k) Orange needle (25G).	
l) Correctly labelled specimen pot containing the appropriate medium. This is decided by the type of investigation required.	
m) A sterile occlusive latex-free dressing, e.g. Cutiplast™ size 7.2 cm × 5 cm or Opsite™ size 6.5 cm × 5 cm.	m) A wound dressing serves several functions. It protects the wound from further insult, keeps the wound clean, and provides a moist environment that promotes healing (Autio et al 2002). It also minimises the risk of scarring. Choosing an appropriate dressing is difficult, especially with the wide and confusing range that is available for use today. For CYP, dressings must be easy to apply and remove; be able to withstand the rigors of children's activities; and be secure enough to prevent the child from interfering with the wound (Teare 1997).
n) Conforming bandage.	
o) Steri-strips.	
p) Tape.	
q) Disposable punch biopsy needle size 0.3 mm or 0.4 mm.	q) Any smaller and the sample will not be suitable for histopathological examination (Nischal et al. 2008)
r) Hypoallergenic dressing, e.g. Mepitel™.	r) To prevent further breakdown of fragile skin.

Procedure guideline 3.7 Punch skin biopsy procedure

Statement	Rationale
1 a) A topical local anaesthetic should be applied to the biopsy site prior to the procedure. Consult the CYP and family on the use of Ametop® cream.	1 a) To minimise pain during the procedure (Lawson et al. 1995, Tayeb et al. 2017).
b) Check for previous allergic reactions to the cream and use Emla® if necessary.	b) erythema is common with Ametop due to vasodilation.
c) If Emla™ is used, ensure that it remains in situ for the appropriate time. For more information see Chapter 24: Pain Management.	c) Emla™ is very slow acting.
2 The local anaesthetic used should be prescribed and checked according to the Administration of Medicines Policy.	2 To minimise risk.
3 While maintaining the dignity of the CYP, place them in a comfortable position, with the potential biopsy area exposed. Positioning will depend on the site of the skin biopsy. The position should be the most comfortable and reassuring for the CYP. Small children/infants can lie or sit on an adult's lap. Consider moving and handling risks issues and ensure a young child has their favourite cuddly toy or comforter with them throughout (RCN 2019; Robinson and Collier 1997).	3 To facilitate biopsy taking and to maintain safety, security and dignity. To minimise the stress to the CYP.

(continued)

Procedure guideline 3.7 Punch skin biopsy procedure *(continued)*

Statement	Rationale
4 Having performed a surgical ward hand wash and wearing the appropriate protective clothing, remove the local anaesthetic cream and wipe dry with a tissue or gauze. If able, confirm with the CYP whether the cream has caused numbness of the skin effectively. The biopsy area should be cleaned for 30 seconds with an alcohol based cleansing solution and allowed to dry for another 30 seconds (The Health Foundation (2015); Pratt et al. 2007; Royal College of Nursing (RCN) 2020).	4 To minimise the risk of infection and to prevent pain.
5 Check the CYP's name, date of birth, hospital number and allergies against their identification bracelet and the prescription chart.	5 To prevent a medication error.
6 The local anaesthetic should be prepared using an aseptic nontouch technique. Draw up in a 2 ml syringe with a blue needle (23G) and change to an orange needle (25G). a) Warn the CYP that they may feel a stinging or burning sensation with subcutaneous infiltration of the local anaesthetic. b) It should be injected subcutaneously using the 'spider technique'; lifting a skin fold to assure that the subcutaneous injection is accomplished. This forms a 'bleb' or small bump. c) Time must be allowed for the anaesthetic to take effect. Wait 2–3 minutes before proceeding.	6 To minimise the risk of infection. a) To prepare the CYP for the sensation. b) Less adipose tissue leads to greater risk of intra-muscular injection (King 2003; Winslow et al. 1997). c) To ensure maximum effectiveness of the anaesthetic.
7 To perform the procedure: a) Stretch the skin perpendicular to normal relaxation lines at time of biopsy. b) Introduce an appropriate sized disposable punch biopsy firmly at a perpendicular angle to the anaesthetised area of the skin surface. c) The sterile punch biopsy should be rotated through 45 degrees repeatedly with the cutting edge carrying the punch down onto the tissue and through to the subcutis. d) The guard on the sterile punch biopsy will prevent too deep a penetration into the skin. e) Withdraw the sterile biopsy punch needle while applying pressure on the puncture site with a nonwoven swab. This should release the skin specimen. f) If the sample is not released from the skin, use the plastic disposable forceps and disposable scalpel or sterile scissors to cut the sample. Apply minimum pressure with the forceps as a crush injury alters the histological appearance of the tissue sample. g) Specimens taken for rare metabolic disorders should be removed using a disposable scalpel blade. h) Place the specimen in the appropriate biopsy medium and ensure the container is correctly and clearly labelled. i) Apply continuous pressure to the biopsy site until bleeding stops. j) For immunocompromised CYPs, once bleeding has stopped apply some Fucidin® ointment to the site k) Apply wound closure strips in a 'star' pattern. l) Once haemostasis has been achieved, apply either: • A dry dressing, e.g. Cutiplast™ or Op-site™ or • a low-adherent dressing, e.g. Mepitel™, if the surrounding skin is fragile (White and Morris 2009). m) Dispose of used equipment and sharps according to local policy. Remove protective clothing and perform a clinical hand wash. n) Document the type of specimen the time, date and site where the biopsy was taken.	a) To immobilise the skin and increase the likelihood of gaining a more satisfactory cosmetic appearance. b) To facilitate effective biopsy taking. c) To ensure that the full thickness of the deeper dermis is obtained. d) To avoid damage to underlying tissue and to minimise pain and bleeding. f) To obtain sample and prevent damage to the fibroblasts and skin tissue. g) To ensure that the fibroblasts on the skin are not damaged. h) To prepare for laboratory analysis, to enable correct analysis and correctly identify the CYP. i) To achieve haemostasis. j) To minimise the risk of infection. k) To ensure the edges of the wound are drawn carefully together so as to promote effective healing and improve cosmetic outcome. Steri-strips work best on superficial low-tension wounds. They are inexpensive, and easy and painless to apply (Autio et al. 2002). l) To protect the site and minimise infection, To maintain comfort, prevent further irritation and provide a warm environment to promote healing m) To minimise the risk of an inoculation injury and cross-infection. n) To enable accurate analysis to take place.

Procedure guideline 3.7 Punch skin biopsy procedure (continued)

Statement	Rationale
o) Place the sample in a polythene specimen bag and send to the appropriate laboratory.	o) To minimise the risk of infection. Depending upon the medium used, there is also a risk of chemical injury to those handling the sample. To meet the Control of Substances Hazardous to Health Regulations (COSHH) and Health and Safety Regulations (Health and Safety Executive 2002).
p) Record the procedure in the CYP's healthcare records.	p) To maintain an accurate record (NMC 2015).
q) Time should be taken to give positive feedback to the CYP for tolerating the invasive procedure, and to the parent/carer for their valuable contribution.	q) To conclude the procedure with a positive outcome and to acknowledge the value of the involvement of parent/carer.

Procedure guideline 3.8 Postprocedural care (skin biopsy)

Statement	Rationale
1 Once the procedure has been completed the CYP may return to their bed or the playroom. a) Observe the biopsy dressing 10 minutes after completion of biopsy b) If sedation has been given, level of consciousness and vital signs must be monitored pre discharge.	1 To facilitate safety and comfort. a) To ensure bleeding has fully ceased before discharging the CYP. b) To ensure the CYP is awake and orientated prior to discharge.
2 Assess the CYP's need for analgesia. Oral analgesia may be required if the CYP experiences pain or discomfort. The analgesia must be prescribed and administered according to hospital Administration of Medicines Policy. Advise the family to give further analgesia at home if the child continues to experience discomfort	2 To relieve pain and to promote comfort.
3 The dressing should be observed intermittently within the first 24 hours for any signs of bleeding. The pressure dressing should be removed after this point. a) The CYP's doctor should be informed if bleeding is observed. b) Advise the parents to apply a pressure to the dressing site if bleeding reoccurs at home. The family/carer should be given clear instructions to contact the CYP's GP or other healthcare worker if a problem occurs.	3 To detect early signs of biopsy site complications as early detection prevents complications and poor wound healing (Tickle 2013).
4 A clean wound should be left untouched, leaving the exudates to nourish the natural healing process (Briggs 1996; Dealey 1994). a) The site should be left untouched and kept dry for 48 hours. b) The dressing may be removed after 48 hours. c) The Steri-strips may begin to fall off. Allow this to happen. If still intact they may be removed on the third day. Many CYP prefer to remove their own dressings by soaking them off in the bath or shower (Bale and Jones 1996). d) Once skin edges have sealed, bathing or showering is not likely to cause any further risk (Briggs 1997).	4 To minimise the risk of infection. CYP in good health have a vigorous healing reaction. Increased metabolism and good circulation contribute to increased rates of healing (Dealey 1994). a) Consider wound healing within the context of the CYP's disorder. c) To minimise the risk of scarring. d) To enable normal hygiene practices to resume.
5 Healing in immune-compromised CYP may be delayed because of reduced efficiency of the immune system. Secondary to this is a decreased resistance to infection, which in turn will delay healing (Butcher 2013).	
6 The CYP may be prescribed a prophylactic topical antibiotic. Those with an uncomplicated biopsy do not usually develop an infection. The first application is applied after haemostasis has occurred. a) The second application should be made 48 hours after the procedure when the dressing is removed.	6 To prevent infection. Use of adhesive tapes is also associated with decreased infection rates (Trott 1997). a) Antibiotics are often an overused prophylactic.
7 The topical antibiotics must be prescribed and given according to the Administration of Medicines Policy.	7 To maintain patient safety.

(continued)

Procedure guideline 3.8 Postprocedural care (skin biopsy) *(continued)*

Statement	Rationale
8 A written instruction sheet on the care of the biopsy site must be given to the main parent/carer on discharge. It should include education about the wound healing process, including a discussion of the return to normal activities. a) An outpatient appointment must be given to the family.	8 To educate the family, minimise the risk of infection, and promote healing of the biopsy site. a) To inform parents/carers of results and to recommend future action/treatment.
9 The CYP and family must be informed of the results of the procedure as soon as possible, although they should be advised that some biopsy results take 6–8 weeks depending on the nature of analysis of the biopsy. a) This discussion must be recorded in the CYP's healthcare records.	9 To keep the CYP and family informed. This may be due to time taken for the growing of skin cells. a) To provide an accurate record and documentation.

healthcare practitioner (HCP) who has been trained in this skill. Any training should acknowledge the physical act of the procedure, psychological aspects, and the sequence of events to ensure consistent and safe practice. Any HCPs who undertake this role should ensure that they work within their code of professional conduct and should be aware of developments in practice, research, and available products to ensure that their knowledge remains valid, up to date, and that their practice is safe and efficient (NMC 2015).

Prior to carrying out the biopsy, the exact area to be biopsied must be considered, as some conditions require affected and unaffected skin for diagnosis and therefore the biopsy is taken across the border of the lesion. Of equal importance is the age of the lesion, as a biopsy performed too early or too late may provide a false negative result (Nischal et al. 2008).

Renal biopsy

Introduction

A renal biopsy is undertaken to confirm a diagnosis or to monitor the effectiveness of a treatment regimen (Franke et al. 2014). It is a specialised, minimally invasive procedure with some significant and serious but rare complications, with an estimated incidence of less than 5% in the UK (Gupta et al. 2016). The procedure essentially involves the removal of a very small amount of kidney tissue (cortical and medullary) for microscopic analysis. There are several different techniques that can be used to obtain this tissue sample, including open, laparoscopic, and percutaneous (Fiorentino et al. 2016). The percutaneous method is the most commonly performed technique, unless the CYP has contraindications to this method. It is usually undertaken in theatre or interventional radiology with ultrasound guidance under either local or general anaesthesia, depending on the age and level of adherence of the CYP (Gupta et al. 2016).

A renal biopsy is usually performed by a specialist medical practitioner; however, an audit of practice in the UK by the British Association of Paediatric Nephrology (BAPN) identified that this was not always the case and highlighted a wide variation in techniques and preparation of CYP for a renal biopsy (Hussain et al. 2010). Following this publication the BAPN recommended guidance and the need for a standard protocol. The practice in the UK was then reaudited and published in 2016 (Gupta et al. 2016), showing improvements in preparation of CYP and a reduced in complication rate. The play specialist and nursing role in caring for a CYP undergoing a renal biopsy is very important and is principally to ensure appropriate preparation and safe recovery of the CYP (Gupta et al. 2016). There are several indications for a renal biopsy; a number of contraindications to the biopsy going ahead; and various complications that can occur after the biopsy has been performed, all of which it serves the nurse well to understand. A competent and knowledgeable nurse can fulfil a vital role within the specialist expert team, as that knowledge may enable early recognition of potential complications, and therefore swift investigation and correction. A specialist expert team is felt to be an important, if not fundamental, factor in the success and safety of the renal biopsy, and CYP should be referred to specialist centres if a renal biopsy is considered necessary (Rees et al. 2012).

Indications

Renal biopsies will be required for the following procedures:

- Persistent blood or protein in the urine.
- A history of glomerular nephritis.
- Acute kidney injury of uncertain aetiology.
- Rapid progressive renal failure of unknown aetiology.
- To confirm a diagnosis of systemic lupus erythematosus (SLE).
- To diagnose rejection post renal transplant.

Contraindications

To reduce the likelihood of complications there are a number of risk factors that need to be considered, and if possible corrected, prior to a kidney biopsy going ahead. These include uncontrolled hypertension, oedema, severe anaemia, and having a solitary kidney (Munoz et al. 2011). As bleeding is the most common and potentially serious complication of a biopsy (Gupta et al. 2016), severe anaemia should be corrected before the procedure as reducing the haemoglobin level further may be hazardous. Equally, CYP with hypertension are at greater risk of bleeding during the procedure (Munoz et al. 2011), so this condition should receive investigation and further management. To prevent the significant risk of bleeding, clotting screens (and bleeding times if the CYP has severe uraemia) should be checked and corrected if necessary prior to the procedure and any anticoagulation and antiplatelet therapy should be discussed with regard to the pre-emptive discontinuation of treatment. The CYP should have blood taken for group and save, in order that blood can be cross-matched if required or, if at high risk of bleeding, blood should be cross matched ready for use if necessary (Gupta et al. 2016).

A biopsy must always be preceded by an ultrasound of the kidneys to ensure that the CYP has two kidneys, in the usual position, to reduce any risk to their renal function (Gupta et al. 2016). In CYPs with transplanted kidneys, it is already known that there is only one functioning kidney, but the need for the biopsy outweighs the risks of the biopsy itself (Gupta et al. 2016). To reduce the risk of damaging the kidney the biopsy is performed under ultrasound guidance to ensure accurate localisation of the kidney (Franke et al. 2014).

Complications

As previously mentioned, bleeding is the most commonly seen complication after a biopsy; most often exhibited as haematuria, which is almost unavoidable as the kidney is such a vascular organ (Gupta et al. 2016). Microscopic haematuria is virtually always present and should not cause any anxiety, but macroscopic haematuria may occasionally be witnessed; both usually settle quickly with encouragement of fluids, which also has the benefit of reducing the risks of clots forming in the bladder. Persistent macroscopic haematuria may indicate bleeding at the site of the biopsy, possibly resulting in the need for a blood transfusion and very occasionally there may be a need for another operation or radiological procedure to stop the bleeding. Bed rest is generally thought to prevent the likelihood of haematomas and haematuria, although the optimal length of bed rest is heavily debated (Hussain et al. 2010).

Further complications that may occur include haematomas; small insignificant haematomas may never be noticed and are probably quite common, but there are a very small number of CYP who suffer from larger more noteworthy haematomas. These may cause significant loin pain and warrant further investigation. Minor discomfort and pain from insertion of the needle are also common after a biopsy over the site but usually easily controlled with mild analgesia such as paracetamol, but stronger pain relief may be required. Other potential, but rare, complications include peri-renal/retroperitoneal bleed, bleeding into the urinary tract and clots in the bladder, arterio-venous fistula and renal capsular tear (Franke et al. 2014). A nephrectomy may be required in extreme circumstances if the bleeding from a renal capsular tear is uncontrollable and all other procedures have failed. There is also a very small mortality risk, which, on examining the research, usually occurs only as a result of substantial haemorrhage, which is rare (Franke et al. 2014). The final potential problem, which requires a mention, is that of technical failure, where insignificant tissue is collected for analysis and a repeat biopsy is required). It is important the CYP and family understand all these potential risks before consenting to the procedure (Fiorentino et al. 2016).

Renal biopsy complications have been reported as uncommon after 6 hours and as a result, several units perform them as a day case (Hussain et al. 2003). If observations are normal, the biopsy site looks satisfactory, the CYP is pain free, tolerating food and drink, and has passed urine with no evidence of persistent macroscopic haematuria, they can be discharged. The CYP must also live within reasonable travelling distance of the hospital and on discharge it is important that the family fully understand all the potential complications. The CYP and family should be given written information before and after the procedure, which should specify include the following advice:

- Rest for a further 12–24 hours once discharged.
- Observe urine for signs of bleeding.
- Stay home from school for 2–3 days.
- Avoid strenuous exercise (for example bike riding and horse-riding) and contact sports for 4 weeks, as this provides time for maximum healing and minimises the likelihood of any further complications.

The CYP and family should have an outpatient clinic appointment booked, to receive the results when available, or be contacted sooner if there are other clinical concerns (Gupta et al. 2016).

Procedure guideline 3.9 Preoperative procedure (renal biopsy)

Statement	Rationale
1 Ensure that informed consent is gained and a consent form is completed. a. Ensure that the CYP has a correctly labelled name band in place.	1 To ensure the CYP and family are fully aware of any potential complications. a) To ensure that the correct CYP will receive the procedure.
2 A preoperative set of baseline observations should be performed, including: a) Temperature. b) Pulse rate. c) Respiratory rate. d) Blood pressure. e) Oxygen saturations.	2 To enable an accurate comparison to be made postoperatively. To assess for any contraindications (such as hypertension).
3 Ensure the following blood tests are performed: a) Full blood count. b) Urea and electrolytes (U&Es). c) Clotting screen. d) Group and save. e) Bleeding time if urea >40 mmol/l.	3 To ensure that the CYP is safely prepared for theatre.
4 The CYP may need to have any coagulation abnormalities corrected prior to procedure.	4 To reduce the risk of bleeding postoperatively.
5 Discuss anticoagulant or antiplatelet therapy with medical staff (usually discontinued for one week before and after the procedure).	5 To reduce the risk of bleeding postoperatively.
6 The CYP should be nil by mouth appropriately for the type of anaesthetic they will receive.	6 To ensure that the CYP is safely prepared for theatre.
7 Transplant patients may require hyper-hydration pre-procedure.	7 To avoid the risk of dehydration. This group are at increased risk of dehydration
8 A urinalysis ward dipstick should be performed before the CYP goes to theatre.	8 To assess the level of haematuria pretheatre (baseline), to enable an accurate comparison to be made postoperatively.
9 Ensure that an ultrasound is performed.	9 To ensure that the CYP has two kidneys to minimise the risk of subsequent renal failure if complications were to occur (unless they are a transplant patient where the benefits should outweigh the risks).
10 The CYP should receive age-appropriate preparation either by nursing staff or the play specialist (Price et al. 2000).	10 To reduce any anxiety.

Procedure guideline 3.10 Postoperative procedure (renal biopsy)

Statement	Rationale

1 Monitor the CYP's oxygen saturations on return, until stable. Record the CYP's:
a) Temperature.
b) Pulse rate.
c) Respiratory rate.
d) Blood pressure
   i ¼ hourly for 1 hour
   ii ½ hourly for 2 hours
   iii Hourly until discharge
Reduce or increase frequency of observations as condition dictates.
	1 To assess for complications such as respiratory distress, haemorrhage, pain, and infection.

2 Liberal fluids should be commenced post biopsy (unless the CYP is fluid restricted, in which case input should be closely monitored). IV fluids should be started if the CYP is unable to take fluids orally.	2 To promote good urine output in order to reduce and determine haematuria and the risk of clot formation.
3 Monitor the CYP's input and output.	3 To assess fluid status and kidney function.
4 Small urine samples from each void should be collected, labelled with time and date, and saved for duration of stay. a) These should be tested with a ward dipstick. b) Macroscopic haematuria and passing of clots should be reported to medical staff. Persistent bleeding may require postoperative bloods, an ultrasound, and overnight stay.	4 Microscopic haematuria is normal for 72 hours post biopsy, but should be decreasing throughout this period. a) To observe for diminishing haematuria. b) To ensure that any persistent bleeding can be treated promptly.
5 The biopsy site must be observed: • 1/4 hourly for 1 hour • 1/2 hourly for 2 hours • Hourly until discharge	5 To check for potential complications of a biopsy, which include bleeding, haematoma, and infection.
6 Keep the dressing dry and in place for 36–48 hours. a) Steri-strips will fall off.	6 To promote healing and reduce the risk of scarring.
7 a) The CYP's level of pain should be assessed when carrying out other observations and managed appropriately (for more information see Chapter 24: Pain Management). b) Any loin pain or excessive flank / abdominal pain should be reported.	7 a) To assess, manage, and treat pain appropriately. b) Site tenderness is normal post biopsy; excessive flank/abdominal pain may indicate haemorrhage; loin pain may indicate a large haematoma.
8 Commence diet when tolerating fluids. a) Assess the CYP for nausea and vomiting. Refer to medical practitioner for antiemetics as required.	8 To reintroduce normal feeding and maintain hydration. a) To minimise discomfort and dehydration.
9 The CYP should be kept on bed rest for four hours after the biopsy. a) Distressed toddlers may sit on carers' laps. b) A play specialist referral should be made.	9 To reduce the risk of haemorrhage, haematuria, and haematomas. a) To encourage them to stay on bed rest, and to reduce any distress and subsequent potential damage of any distress. b) To occupy the CYP while on bed rest.
10 The CYP should start to very gently mobilise prior to discharge.	10 To ensure they are safe to be discharged.
11 The CYP and family should receive a 'Kidney Biopsy – Information for Families' booklet (GOSH 2022).	11 To enable them to recognise complications more promptly.
12 The family should be aware that they should contact the ward if the CYP has blood in the urine or pain around site.	12 To ensure prompt treatment of any complications.
13 The CYP should be advised to avoid lifting, strenuous activity (e.g. bike riding, horse riding) and contact sports for 6 weeks.	13 Provides time for maximum healing and minimises the likelihood of any further complications (Rees et al. 2012).
14 The CYP's GP and Community Team should be informed that the CYP has had a biopsy.	14 To ensure that appropriate and fully informed assistance can be provided if required when the CYP is at home.
15 The school nurse should be informed that the CYP has had a biopsy.	15 To ensure that the school is aware that the CYP will be absent from school for 2–3 days and should not perform school sports for 6 weeks.

Bone marrow aspirate and trephine

Introduction
Healthy bone marrow is a complex tissue that is a fundamental requirement for normal living. The bone marrow contains stem cells for haemopoietic cells and stem cells that are precursors for nonhaemopoietic tissues, which are responsible for:

- Maintaining homeostasis
- Maintaining the body's defence system
- Transporting oxygen and carbon dioxide around the body.

A bone marrow aspiration is the removal of adequate amounts of bone marrow to confirm the diagnosis of a malfunctioning marrow. Furthermore, it can be repeated to monitor the CYP's response to treatment.

Bone marrow can be aspirated from a variety of sites that are rich in marrow. These sites are the sternum, tibia (in small infants only), and, the most usual site, the anterior and posterior iliac crests. Cells from the marrow are analysed for their characteristics such as shape, size, and number, and are used to aid diagnosis in CYP with haematological, oncological, immunological, metabolic, and infectious problems.

A bone marrow aspirate can be performed either under general anaesthetic, or more usually under local anaesthetic, and usually as a day case in the clinic setting.

Bone marrow trephine/biopsy is a procedure where a small core of both bone and marrow are removed. If this is required it is usually performed at the same time as an aspirate. A bone marrow trephine is used to establish further staging of a CYP's solid tumour by confirming the presence of metastatic disease.

Complications
Complications are extremely rare, the more common being:

1. Haemorrhage: This is most likely to occur in CYP who are thrombocytopenic, therefore, the platelet count must be checked before the following procedures:
    - A bone marrow aspirate; the platelet count must be greater than $10 \times 10^9/l$.
    - A bone marrow trephine; the platelet count must be greater than $30 \times 10^9/l$.
2. Bleeding/bruising: This can be avoided by applying pressure to the site and, if necessary, a pressure bandage.
3. Infection: If a pressure bandage or plaster has been applied, these must be removed by 24 hours post procedure, as leaving them on will expose the immune-compromised CYP to infection. The gentlest way to remove the dressing is to soak it off in a warm bath.

Procedure guideline 3.11 Preparation of equipment and environment (aspiration/trephine)

Statement	Rationale
1 To prepare the equipment and perform the aspiration/trephine, staff must perform a surgical hand wash and use an aseptic technique.	1 To minimise the risk of infection.
2 The following equipment should be prepared: • Alcohol-based antiseptic, e.g. chlorhexidene in alcohol • Sterile dressing pack • Sterile gloves • Selection of syringes – including 20 ml syringes and needles • Bone marrow aspiration needle • Bone marrow trephine needle (if required) • Microscope glass slides and container • Specimen bottles – plain and with heparin • Specimen pot with formalin for trephine, if required • Local anaesthetic, if required • Plaster	

Procedure guideline 3.12 Preparation of CYP and family (aspiration/trephine)

Statement	Rationale
1 Inform and prepare the CYP and family of the following: • Whether a bone marrow aspirate +/− trephine is required and why. • What the test involves. • The potential risks of the aspirate/trephine. • The approximate duration of the procedure.	1 To obtain informed consent, minimise anxiety, and promote concordance (DH 2009; Pinkerton et al. 1993).
2 Contact a play specialist or experienced nurse to work with the CYP.	2 To help prepare them for the procedure.
3 Ensure the appropriate hospital information leaflets are given to the family in a format which they can read.	3 To enable the family to have a full understanding of the procedure.
4 If a general anaesthetic is to be used, ensure a doctor obtains written consent.	4 To comply with hospital policy.
5 If an anaesthetic is to be used the CYP must be nil by mouth as per hospital policy.	5 To minimise the risk of aspiration of stomach contents while under anaesthesia.
6 Blood test results, i.e. full blood count +/− clotting, available prior to performing the procedure.	6 To reduce the risk of haemorrhage.

Procedure guideline 3.13 Aspiration/trephine procedure

Statement	Rationale
1 During the procedure under anaesthetic, monitor the CYP's: a) Oxygen saturations. b) Respiratory and pulse rate and pattern. c) Colour. d) Airway. e) Secretions. f) Consciousness level.	1 To monitor their cardiopulmonary systems. c-e) To determine the need for suction or atropine if excessive secretions. f) To observe if the CYP needs further anaesthetic.
2 During the procedure under local anaesthetic, the parents/carers may wish to remain with their child.	2 To offer comfort and support.
3 The local anaesthetic must be checked as prescribed. a) The doctor will administer the local anaesthetic into the prepared puncture site and must wait for it to take effect.	3 To comply with hospital policy. a) To ensure effectiveness of the anaesthetic.
4 Once the CYP is ready, position them with the side where the aspirate will be performed uppermost. This position must be maintained throughout the procedure, ensuring an adequate airway is maintained.	4 To facilitate effective aspiration. To maintain safety of the CYP.
5 The doctor performing the procedure will comply with universal precautions and clean the site of the aspiration with an alcohol-based antiseptic and allow the site to dry.	5 To minimise the risk of infection.
6 The marrow needle is inserted into the anaesthetised area and a 20 ml syringe is applied to the hub of the needle. If the marrow is hypercellular and difficult to aspirate, continue repeating the above procedure through the **same** skin puncture site until an adequate specimen is obtained.	6 To obtain an adequate sample for diagnosis.
7 Place the aspirate on the microscope slide and in the specimen pots.	7 To prepare sample for laboratory analysis.
8 Label slides and pots. Once dry, place the slides in the slide container.	8 To ensure slides have the correct CYP's details on them.
9 Withdraw the aspirate needle while applying pressure on the puncture site.	
10 Apply continuous pressure until the bleeding stops.	10 To minimise haematoma formation and pain.
11 Apply a dressing to the puncture site (i.e. plaster).	11 To minimise infection.
12 Dispose of used equipment as per hospital policy.	12 To comply with hospital policy.
13 Ensure specimens are sent to the appropriate laboratories.	13 To enable analysis to occur.
14 Record necessary information in appropriate healthcare records.	14 To ensure accurate data collection.

Procedure guideline 3.14 Postprocedure care (aspiration/trephine)

Statement	Rationale
1 Continue to monitor vital signs until the CYP is fully awake.	1 To ensure a safe recovery from anaesthetic.
2 Keep noise levels to a minimum while the CYP is regaining consciousness.	2 To minimise distress.
3 If the procedure was under general anaesthetic, ask the parents/carers to return once the CYP is rousable.	3 To minimise the distress for the CYP and anxiety for the parents/carers.
4 Ensure oxygen and suction are available by the CYP's bed, and are functioning.	4 To maintain a safe environment.
5 The CYP can return to their bed once rousable and may sleep in a semi-prone position. If awake they can be cared for in whichever position is most comfortable.	5 To maintain a clear airway.
6 Give prescribed analgesia if needed and repeat as often as necessary.	6 To minimise pain.
7 Resume oral fluids and diet once the CYP is fully awake.	7 To reintroduce normal feeding and maintain hydration. To minimise discomfort and dehydration.
8 Observe the puncture site for signs of bleeding. Contact the doctor if there are any problems.	8 To detect complications.
9 Inform the parents/carers: a) To repeat analgesia as prescribed. b) Their child may bathe/shower the following day. c) To remove the plaster/dressing within 24 hours.	9 a) To minimise pain. b) To continue normal hygiene practice. c) To minimise the risk of infection.
10 They will be informed of results as soon as possible.	10 To keep the family informed.

References

Autio, L., Koozer, K., and Olson (2002). *The four S's of wound management: staples, sutures, steri-strips and sticky stuff*. Holistic Nurse Practice 16 (2): 80–88.

Bale, S. and Jones, V. (1996). *Caring for children with wounds*. Journal of Wound Care 5 (4): 177–180.

Bolia, R., Matta, J., Malik, R., and Hardikar, W. (2017). *Outpatient Liver Biopsy in Children: Safety, Feasibility, and Economic Impact*. Journal of Pediatric Gastroenterology and Nutrition 65 (1): 86–88. https://journals.lww.com/jpgn/Fulltext/2017/07000/Outpatient_Liver_Biopsy_in_Children___Safety,19.aspx (accessed 05 September 2022).

Briggs, S.M. (1996). *The principles of a specific technique in wound care*. Professional Nurse 11 (12): 805–810.

Briggs, M. (1997). *The principles of a closed surgical wound care*. Journal of Wound Care 6 (6): 288–292.

Butcher, M. (2013). *Assessment, management and prevention of infected wounds*. Journal of Community Nursing 27 (4): 25–33.

Cohen, M.B., A-Kader, H.H., Lambers, D., and Heubi, J.E. (1992). *Complications of percutaneous liver biopsy in children*. Gastroenterology 102: 629–632.

Dealey, C. (1994). The care of wounds. Cambridge: Blackwell Science.

Department of Health (DH) (2001). Consent – what you have a right to expect: A guide for children and young people. https://ethics.grad.ucl.ac.uk/forms/DH_GuideForChildrenAndYoungPeople.pdf (accessed 05 September 2022).

The Health Foundation (2015). Infection prevention and control: lessons from acute care in England. http://www.health.org.uk/sites/default/files/InfectionPreventionAndControlLessonsFromAcuteCareInEngland.pdf (accessed 05 September 2022).

Department of Health (DH) (2009). Reference guide to consent for examination or treatment. https://assets.publishing.service.gov.uk/government/uploads/system/uploads/attachment_data/file/138296/dh_103653__1_.pdf (accessed 05 September 2022).

Dezsofi, A., Baumann, U., Dhawan, A. et al. (2015). *Liver biopsy in children: Position Paper of the ESPGHAN Hepatology Committee*. Journal of Pediatric Gastroenterology and Nutrition 60 (3): 408–420. https://journals.lww.com/jpgn/Fulltext/2015/03000/Liver_Biopsy_in_Children___Position_Paper_of_the.28.aspx (accessed 05 September 2022).

Duffin, C. (2012). *Not just fooling around: how play can help young patients overcome their fears*. Nursing Children and Young People 24 (10): 6–7s.

Fiorentino, M., Bolignano, D., Tesar, V. et al. (2016). *Renal Biopsy in 2015-from Epidemiology to Evidence-baseed Indications*. American Journal of Nephrology 43: 1–19. https://doi.org/10.1159/000444026.

Franchi-Abella, S., Cahill, A.M., Barnacle, A.M. et al. (2014). *Hepatobiliary intervention in children*. Cardiovascular and Interventional Radiology 37: 37–54.

Franke, M., Kramarczyk, A., Taylan, C. et al. (2014). *Ultrasound-guided percutaneous renal biopsy in 295 children and adolescents: role of ultrasound and analysis of complications*. PLoS One. https://doi.org/10.1371/journal.pone.0114737.

GOSH (2022). Kidney biopsy. https://www.gosh.nhs.uk/conditions-and-treatments/procedures-and-treatments/kidney-biopsy/ (accessed 05 September 2022).

Gonzalez-Vallina, R., Alonso, E.A., Rand, E. et al. (1993). *Outpatient percutaneous liver biopsy in children*. Journal of Pediatric Gastroenterology and Nutrition 17: 370–375.

Grant, A. and Neuberger, J. (1999). *Guidelines on the use of liver biopsy in clinical practice*. International Journal of Gastroenterology and Hepatology 45 (suppl IV): IV1–IV11.

Gupta, A., Campion-Smith, J., Hayes, W. et al. (2016). *Positive trends in paediatric renal biopsy service provision in the UK: a national survey and re-audit of paediatric renal biopsy practice*. Pediatric Nephrology 31 (4): 613–621.

Hatfield, M.K., Beres, R.A., Sane, S.S., and Zaleski, G.X. (2008). *Percutaneous image-guided solid organ core needle biopsy: Coaxial versus noncoaxial method*. American Journal of Radiology 190: 413–417.

Health and Safety Executive (2002). Control of Substances Hazardous to Health (COSHH). London: HSE.

Hoffer, F.A. (2000). *Liver biopsy methods for paediatric oncology patients*. Paediatric Radiology 30 (7): 481–488.

Hussain, F., Watson, A., Hayes, J., and Evans, J. (2003). *Standards for renal biopsies. A comparison of inpatient and day care procedures*. Pediatric Nephrology 18: 53–56.

Hussain, F., Mallik, M., Marks, S.D. et al. (2010). *Renal biopsies in children: current practice and audit of outcomes*. Nephrology, Dialysis, Transplantation 25 (2): 485–489. https://doi.org/10.1093/ndt/gfp434.

King, L. (2003). *Subcutaneous insulin injection technique*. Nursing Standard 17 (34): 45–52, quiz 54–55.

Kupesic, S. (2017). Urgent procedures in medical practice. New Delhi: Jaypee Brothers medical publishers LTD.

Lachaux, A., Le Gall, C., Chambon, M. et al. (1995). *Complications of percutaneous liver biopsy in infants and children*. European Journal of Pediatrics 154: 621–623.

Langley, P. (1999). *Guided Imagery: a review of the effectiveness in the care of children*. Paediatric Nursing 11 (3): 18–21.

Lawson, R.A., Smart, N.G., Gudgeon, A.C., and Morton, N.S. (1995). *Evaluaton of an amethocaine gel preparation for percutaneous analgesia before venous cannulation in children*. British Journal of Anaesthesia 75 (3): 282–285.

Lindor, K.D., Jorgensen, R.A., Rakela, J. et al. (1996). *The role of ultrasonography and automated-needle biopsy in outpatient percutaneous liver biopsy*. Hepatology 23: 1079–1083.

Litchtman, S., Guzman, C., Moore, D. et al. (1987). *Morbidity after percutaneous liver biopsy*. Archives of Disease in Childhood 62 (9): 901–904.

Little, A.F., Ferris, J.V., Dodd, G.D., and Baron, R.L. (1996). *Image-guided percutaneous hepatic biopsy: Effect of ascites on the complication rate*. Radiology 199: 79–83.

Lungren, M.P., Lindquester, W.S., Seidel, F.G. et al. (2016). *Ultrasound-guided liver biopsy with gelatin sponge pledget tract embolization in infants weighing less than 10 kg*. Journal of Pediatric Gastroenterology and Nutrition 63 (6): e147–e151. https://journals.lww.com/jpgn/Fulltext/2016/12000/Ultrasound_Guided_Liver_Biopsy_With_Gelatin_Sponge.27.aspx (accessed 05 September 2022).

Marieb, E. (2012). Essentials of human anatomy and physiology. San Francisco: Pearson.

McGill, D.B., Rakela, J., Zinsmeister, A.R., and Ott, B.J. (1990). *A 21-year experience with major haemorrhage after percutaneous liver biopsy*. Gastroenterology 99: 1396–1400.

Munoz, A.T., Valdez-Ortiz, R., Gonzalez-Parra, C. et al. (2011). *Percutaneous renal biopsy of native kidneys: efficiency, safety and risk factors associated with major complications*. Archives of Medical Science 7 (5): 823–831. https://doi.org/10.5114/aoms.2011.25557.

Nilsson, A. and Hallqvist, C. (2013). *Active and passive distraction in children undergoing wound dressings*. Journal of Pediatric Nursing 28: 158–166.

Nischal, U., Nischal, K.C., and Khopkar, U. (2008). *Techniques of skin biopsy and practical considerations*. Journal of Cutaneous and Aesthetic Surgery 1 (2): 107–111.

Nobili, V., Comparcla, D., Sartorelli, M.R. et al. (2003). *Biopsy and ultrasound-guided percutaneous liver biopsy in children*. Pediatric Radiology 33: 772–775.

Nursing and Midwifery Council (NMC) (2015) The Code: Professional standards of practice and behaviour for nurses, midwives and nursing associates. London, NMC. https://www.nmc.org.uk/standards/code/ (accessed 05 September 2022).

Perraul, J., McGill, D.B., Ott, B.J., and Taylor, W.F. (1978). *Liver biopsy; Complications in 1,000 in-patients and outpatients*. Gastroenterology 74: 103–106.

Pickett, H. (2011). *Shave and punch biopsy for skin lesions*. American Family Physician 84 (5): 995–1002.

Pinkerton, C.R., Cushing, P., and Sepion, B. (1993). Impact of diagnosis on the family. In: Childhood Cancer Management (eds. C.R. Pinkerton, P. Cushing and B. Sepion), 2. London: Chapman and Hall.

Pratt, R.J., Pellowe, C.M., Wilson, J.A. et al. (2007). *epic2: National evidence-based guidelines for preventing healthcare-associated infections in NHS hospitals in England*. The Journal of Hospital Infection 65 (Suppl 1): S1–S64.

Price, D., Tomsett, A., and Gartland, C. (2000). *Preparation for renal biopsy: a play package*. Paediatric Nursing 12 (2): 38–39.

Rees, L., Brogan, P., Bockenhauer, D., and Webb, N. (2012). Paediatric Nephrology Second edition (Oxford Specialist Handbook in Paediatrics), 19–22. Oxford: Oxford University Press.

Rivera-Sanfeliz, G., Kinney, T.B., Rose, S.C. et al. (2005). *Single-pass percutaneous liver biopsy for diffuse liver disease using an automated device: experience in 154 procedures*. Cardiovascular and Interventional Radiology 28 (5): 584–588.

Robinson, S. and Collier, J. (1997). *Holding children still for procedures*. Paediatric Nursing 9 (4): 12–14.

Roebuck, D. (2008). *Focal liver lesion in children*. Paediatric Radiology 38 (Suppl 3): S518–S522.

Royal College of Nursing (RCN) (2019). Restrictive physical interventions and the clinical holding of children and young people: Guidance for nursing staff. https://www.rcn.org.uk/professional-development/publications/pub-007746 (accessed 05 September 2022).

Royal College of Nursing (RCN) (2020). Standards for infusion therapy. https://www.rcn.org.uk/clinical-topics/Infection-prevention-and-control/Standards-for-infusion-therapy (accessed 05 September 2022).

Schiemann, A.O., Barrios, J.M., Al-Tawil, Y.S. et al. (2000). *Percutaneous liver biopsy in children: impact of ultrasonography and spring-loaded biopsy needles*. Pediatric Gastroenterology Nutrition 31 (5): 536–539.

Sclare, I. and Waring, M. (1995). *Routine venipuncture: improving services*. Paediatric Nursing 7 (4): 23–27.

Sharma, P., McDonald, G.B., and Banaji, M.J. (1982). *The risk of bleeding after percutaneous liver biopsy: relation to platelet count*. Clinical Gastroenterology 4: 451–453.

Short, S.S., Papillon, S., Hunter, C.J. et al. (2013). *Percutaneous liver biopsy: pathologic diagnosis and complications in children*. Journal of Pediatric Gastroenterology and Nutrition 57 (5): 644–648.

Siegel, C.A., Silas, A.M., Suriawinata, A.A., and van Leeuwen, D.J. (2005). *Liver biopsy 2005: when and how?* Cleveland Clinic Journal of Medicine 72 (3): 199–224. https://www.ccjm.org/content/72/3/199.long (accessed 05 September 2022).

Smerdely, P., Boyages, S., and We, D. (1989). *Topical iodine containing antiseptics for neonatal hypothyroidism in very low birth weight babies*. Lancet 2: 661–664.

Smith, T.P., McDermott, V.G., Ayoub, D.M. et al. (1996). *Percutaneous transhepatic liver biopsy with tract embolization*. Radiology 198: 769–774.

Tayeb, B.O., Eidelman, A., Eidelman, C.L. et al. (2017). *Topical anaesthetics for pain control during repair of dermal laceration*. CDSR 2017 (2): CD005364. (also available free online).

Teare, J. (1997). *A home care team in paediatric wound care*. Journal of Wound Care 6 (6): 295–296.

Tickle, J. (2013). *Wound infection: a clinician's guide to assessment and management*. Wound Care 18 (suppl9): S16–S22.

Trott, A. (1997). Wound and Lacerations: Emergency Care and Closure, 2nde. St Louis: Mosby.

Wellesley, I. (2009). *Consent in children*. Anaesthesia and Intensive Care Medicine 10 (4): 196–199.

White, R. and Morris, C. (2009). *Mepitel: a non-adherent wound dressing with Safetac technology*. BJN 18 (1): 58–64.

Winslow, E.H., Jacobson, A., and Peragallo-Dittko, V. (1997). *Rethinking subcutaneous injection technique*. American Journal of Nursing 97 (5): 71–72.

Chapter 4

Administration of blood components and products

Kate Khair[1], Lisa Baldry[2], and Rachel Moss[3]

[1]RN (Adult), RN (Child), MSc, MCGI, PhD; Clinical Academic Careers Fellow, Centre for Outcomes Research and Experience in Children's Health Illness and Disability (ORCHID), Great Ormond Street Hospital, London, UK

[2]FIBMS; formerly Chief Biomedical Scientist, GOSH

[3]Senior Transfusion Practitioner, GOSH

Chapter contents

Introduction	62
An overview of blood transfusion	62
Administration of blood components	66
Coagulation factors	70
Conclusion	71
References	71

Procedure guidelines

4.1 Preparation – CYP and family (transfusion)	63
4.2 Preparation – prescription (transfusion)	63
4.3 Preparation – transfusion	63
4.4 Infuse component – identity check and administration	65
4.5 Infuse product – observations, recordings, and traceability	65
4.6 Reaction management (transfusion)	66
4.7 Infuse component (albumin)	67
4.8 Observations and recordings (albumin)	67
4.9 Preparation – CYP and family (immunoglobulin)	68
4.10 Preparation – prescription (immunoglobulin)	68
4.11 Preparation – equipment for intravenous or subcutaneous infusion of immunoglobulin	68
4.12 Procedure – intravenous infusion (immunoglobulin)	69
4.13 Procedure – subcutaneous infusion (immunoglobulin)	69
4.14 Reaction management (immunoglobulin)	70
4.15 Completing the infusion (immunoglobulin)	70

The Great Ormond Street Hospital Manual of Children and Young People's Nursing Practices, Second Edition. Edited by Elizabeth Anne Bruce, Janet Williss, and Faith Gibson.
© 2023 John Wiley & Sons Ltd. Published 2023 by John Wiley & Sons Ltd.

Introduction

Children and young people (CYPs) experience a wide range of chronic diseases, such as haemophilia, sickle cell disease or thalassaemia, leukaemia, or immune deficiency, as well as acute life-threatening episodes such as burns, or road traffic accidents, which require treatment with blood components. These may be red cells, platelets, plasma, or derivatives of plasma such as coagulation factors, immunoglobulin or albumin. The administration of these components is in itself simple; however, potential hazards such as human error, transfusion reaction, infection, antibody development, and anaphylaxis (see Chapter 2: Allergy and Anaphylaxis) may be severe (Serious Hazards of Transfusion 2019). For some families, the use of blood components is considered to be unacceptable, due to religious and/or cultural beliefs or concerns over transmission of infectious diseases.

Administration of any blood component should form part of a care-plan, involving a trained practitioner, the CYP and the family/carer. CYPs with inherited conditions such as haemophilia or immune deficiency may require life-long therapy, and their parents/carers may administer the required blood components to them at home, or when older, the young person may self-infuse. It is therefore imperative that they, their family/carers, and primary/community nurses are involved in the care planning process.

This chapter describes:

- An overview of the history of transfusion
- Nursing practice guidelines relating to:
  - Administration of red blood cells, platelets, plasma, and cryoprecipitate
  - Administration of albumin
  - Administration of immunoglobulin
  - Administration of coagulation factors.

An overview of blood transfusion

It is surprising that this relatively simple and yet life-saving procedure has become part of routine clinical care only within the last 100 years. While venesection (bloodletting) has been common practice since the times of Hippocrates (approx. 420 BC), evidence of blood transfusion did not appear until after the discovery of the blood circulation by William Harvey in 1628, with written evidence of transfusion in 1666 when, in Oxford, blood was transfused from one dog to another (Giangrande 2000).

Blundell, an obstetrician at Guys Hospital in London, performed the first recorded human blood transfusion in 1828. He recognised that women often died from postpartum haemorrhage and, having seen the results of transfusion of blood in animals, applied this technique to humans, but realised that only human blood should be used in humans following the death of a dog from transfused human blood (Blundell 1828).

Initially blood transfusion was carried out without knowledge of blood groups, and not surprisingly many recipients died. In the 1900s, in Vienna, Karl Landsteiner identified four distinct blood groups (now known as A, B, AB, and O). By the 1920s, blood grouping became universal practice and in 1921, Percy Oliver at King's College Hospital London, established the world's first blood donor service. Sister Linstead, a nurse at King's, gave blood for this patient and the first British Red Cross Transfusion Service was established (Giangrande 2000). In 1922 this service was used 13 times; in 2017 National Health Service Blood and Transplant (NHSBT) collected over 6,000 blood donations per month (National Health Service 2020).

Despite this vast number of collections, the demand for blood remains high. Whole blood is rarely used, as most recipients require only part of the donation. Almost all donations are separated into their components (red cells, platelets, fresh frozen plasma (FFP), cryoprecipitate (cryo), coagulation factors, immunoglobulin, and albumin). These are used singly or in combination as necessary; for example, a CYP with liver disease may receive individual coagulation factors as well as platelet and red cell transfusions.

Since the 1980s, the viruses that cause hepatitis A, B, and C, cytomegalovirus (CMV), human T-cell leukaemia viruses (HTLV) I and II, and human immunodeficiency virus (HIV) have been identified. In each case, tests have been developed to detect virally positive donors who are then excluded from donor panels. The risk of being infected with these viruses from UK donated blood components is now extremely low. However, blood components should still be considered to be potentially infectious and their administration should be avoided unless there is no other option. Viral inactivation processes, such as treatment with methylene blue, solvent detergent, and prion reduction technology are utilised for plasma components. Since the 1990s there have been concerns regarding the spread of variant Creutzfeldt-Jakob disease (vCJD) by transfusion of infected blood components. The prion protein responsible for vCJD is detectable in white cells, platelets, and plasma (Lefrère and Hewitt 2009), suggesting that transmission via transfusion is possible (Peden et al. 2004). However, although nearly two million blood components are transfused annually, only a very small number of recipients have become infected. Several steps have been introduced in the UK to minimise the risk of transmission of vCJD.

Since 1999, all NHSBT components are white cell depleted (leucodepleted). Since 2004, potential donors who have themselves been transfused are no longer able to donate and FFP for use by CYPs has been sourced from outside the UK. Non-UK cryoprecipitate has been readily available in the UK since 2009.

Since 2017 the Hepatitis B vaccination is included in the infant vaccination schedule, however children born before 2017 who are likely to require a life long transfusion support programme may be given Hepatitis B immunisation. For more information see Chapter 12: Immunisations (Public Health England 2017).

In 1996, the Serious Hazards of Transfusion (SHOT) committee was established to monitor blood transfusion safety. Since 2007 the Annual SHOT report has contained a chapter relating to paediatric cases and summarises reported incidents involving CYPs. These are most commonly incidents of incorrect blood component transfusion and are due to:

- Failure to meet special requirements such as irradiated or CMV negative products.
- Failure to use correct units or volume for transfusion.
- Failure of correct patient identification process.

The most important role that nurses have is ensuring that the correct blood component is being given to the right CYP by following hospital procedure, checking the blood component against the prescription, AND the wristband, which MUST be attached to the CYP and not to their cot or bed. The wristband is the final identifying protector of a CYP who cannot identify themselves. In the community or in exceptional cases, where CYPs are not wearing hospital identity bracelets, local policy for checking their identity must be in place. In some hospitals electronic bedside devices have been installed to perform patient identification checks between the blood component and the wristband.

Cultural and religious beliefs may affect a CYP's blood component treatment options. The most common group who fall into this category are Jehovah's Witnesses, who refuse to accept blood transfusion based on literal interpretation of a number of passages in The Bible (Genesis 9:4, Leviticus 17:14, and Acts 15:20, 15:29 and 21:25). Some may accept fractionated blood products (albumin, immunoglobulin, coagulation factors) and these with careful surgical techniques may negate the need for blood transfusion. In CYPs with life-threatening bleeding or diseases where blood or platelet transfusion is unavoidable it might be necessary to apply for a court order (see Chapter 17: Intellectual (Learning) Difficulties, 18: Mental Health, 31: Safeguarding).

All decisions to transfuse a CYP should be underpinned by the principles of Patient Blood Management (PBM), an evidence-based, multi-disciplinary approach to optimising the care of patients who need a transfusion (National Blood Authority (NBA) 2016; NHS Blood Transfusion (NHSBT) 2021). CYPs with haemophilia are now treated with genetically engineered factor VIII and IX. Recombinant technology will continue to affect 'blood' component therapy in the future.

Chapter 4 Administration of blood components and products

Procedure guideline 4.1 Preparation – CYP and family (transfusion)

Statement	Rationale
1 a) Inform the CYP and family of the following: • That a blood component transfusion is necessary • The reason for the transfusion • What it entails • The likely duration of the process • Any potential risks and complications b) Obtain and document informed consent	1 a) To inform them of risks, benefits, and alternatives and address any issues or concerns they may have. b) To obtain informed consent.
2 Ensure the CYP is wearing an identity wristband.	2 To enable positive patient identification.
3 Ensure pretransfusion vital signs are recorded (no more than 60 minutes before commencement of transfusion): • Temperature • Respiration rate • Pulse • Blood pressure	3 To establish baseline parameters; these may alter if a reaction occurs.
4 Ensure venous access has been established.	4 To enable infusion to commence.

Procedure guideline 4.2 Preparation – prescription (transfusion)

Statement	Rationale
1 Blood products must be administered only if prescribed on a dedicated blood product prescription chart. Blood components must be prescribed by an appropriately trained, competent, and locally authorised practitioner.	1 To ensure the correct treatment. To comply with the Guideline on the Administration of Blood Components (BCSH 2009, addendum 2012).
2 The prescription should include: a) Patient demographics: • First name and family name • Hospital number • Date of birth b) Date and time infusion required c) Type of blood component to be administered d) Any special requirements, e.g. gamma-irradiation, CMV-seronegative e) Volume in ml to be transfused f) A suitable infusion rate for the CYP g) An infusion time of 4 hours or less	2 To ensure the correct volume of the correct product is administered to the correct CYP. g) To reduce risk of infection.
3 Ensure there is sufficient blood component supplied to meet the prescription requirements.	3 To enable Blood Bank and the clinical area to plan adequately.
4 If administering an intravenous pre-medication of an antihistamine and steroid, do so prior to commencing transfusion.	4 To prevent reactions in CYPs who have reacted previously.
5 Ensure there are instructions for what should happen after the transfusion.	5 To ensure planning takes place.

Procedure guideline 4.3 Preparation – transfusion

Statement	Rationale
1 Arrange for the collection of the blood component from storage.	1 To ensure blood component is in optimum condition for use.
2 The person collecting the component must have documentation containing the CYP's: • First name and family name • NHS/Hospital number • Date of birth It must also contain the type of component and amount to be collected. The details on the documentation must match the details on the blood component label.	2 To ensure the correct component is collected for the correct CYP.

(continued)

Procedure guideline 4.3 Preparation – transfusion *(continued)*

Statement	Rationale
3 When a blood component is collected it must be checked out, stating date and time of removal from storage, according to local systems in use. Documentation of receipt of component on the ward should be returned to Blood Bank.	3 To enable blood component traceability and documentation of 'cold chain' in order to comply with the Blood Safety and Quality Regulations (DH 2005).
4 Check the CYP's details are the same on the blood component label, prescription and report form, i.e.: • First name and family name • NHS/Hospital number • Date of birth	4 To ensure correct component is given to the correct CYP.
5 During administration, ensure that: a) An appropriate blood component administration set, which has an integral 170–200 μm micro-aggregate filter, should be used. b) Paediatric blood administration sets, with a smaller priming volume, are used for small volume transfusions. c) Infusion pumps and syringe drivers can be used, provided they are verified as safe for this purpose. d) Blood components administered using a syringe driver require an administration system that should incorporate an integral three-way system. However, care should be taken as this system carries an inherent risk. When using an administration set of this type: e) The component bag must remain attached throughout the procedure. f) The transfer of patient and blood component details to the syringe is not advised. g) The three-way system must be checked prior to transfusion. h) A new syringe and administration set should be used when administering different components. i) Blood components from more than one donation should not be mixed in the syringe, but given sequentially using a new syringe.	5 a) To remove particulate matter, e.g. fibrin, and to prevent cell damage to blood products. b, c) To reduce wastage in the administration set. d) To ensure the component is administered from the syringe and not allowed to flow freely from the component bag. e) To identify the relevant donation in case of a reaction. f, g) To minimise documentation and administration errors. i) To identify the relevant donation in case of a reaction.

6 When preparing the transfusion:
• Check that the CYP's details are the same on the component bag and prescription:
  – First name and family name
  – NHS/Hospital number
  – Date of birth
• If a blood report form is issued with the blood it must NOT be used as part of the bedside check.
• Check the blood group on the component is compatible with that of the CYP.
• Check the expiry date of the component
• Check any special requirements are met, e.g. CMV negative, irradiated components
• Check the bag is intact.
	6 To ensure the correct component is given to the correct CYP, preventing incompatibility, administration of out-of-date components, or infection.

7 Prime the administration set using standard precautions and aseptic nontouch technique.	7 To minimise the risk of infection, prevent air embolism and ensure the set is patent.
8 If the transfusion is cancelled at this point, inform the Blood Transfusion Laboratory and return the component immediately to the Laboratory.	8 To ensure the Blood Transfusion Laboratory records are accurate and to avoid wastage if possible.

Chapter 4 Administration of blood components and products

Procedure guideline 4.4 Infuse component – identity check and administration

Statement	Rationale
1 Check the identity wristband and prescription chart match.	1 To ensure the components are being administered to the correct CYP.
2 Check the details on the component label and prescription chart match for: • First name and family name • NHS/Hospital number • Date of birth	2 To ensure the component is being administered to the correct CYP.
3 Check that the details on the component label and wristband match and perform positive patient identification by asking the CYP and parent/carer to identify him/herself and the child (take extra care for unconscious patients).	3 To ensure correct patient identification.
4 Connect the prepared blood component to the CYP according to the relevant intravenous therapy guidelines using the general principles of IV administration.	4 To reduce risk of infection.
5 Set the infusion rate according to the prescription **but** ensure the infusion is completed within four hours of removal of blood component from appropriate storage.	5 To ensure it is administered within four hours to reduce risk of infection.

Procedure guideline 4.5 Infuse product – observations, recordings and traceability

Statement	Rationale
1 Closely monitor the CYP for the first 30 minutes of transfusion. This should be negotiated with any family members in attendance. Regular visual observations should continue throughout the transfusion at least hourly.	1 This is when reactions are most likely to occur.
2 Record the date and time of starting the infusion in the CYP's medical records and sign that you are responsible for its administration.	2 To ensure accuracy of records and determine accountability for the infusion.
3 To maintain traceability for each blood component the donation number must be recorded in the CYP's transfusion record, and/or the transfusion tag returned to the transfusion laboratory.	3 To comply with current legislation.

4 Observations should be undertaken and clearly documented for every unit transfused. Minimum monitoring must include:
• Pulse rate, blood pressure, temperature and respiration rate:
  – No more than 60 minutes prior to the start of the transfusion
  – 15 minutes after the start of the transfusion
  – No more than 60 minutes after the completion of the transfusion
• If the CYP becomes unwell or shows signs or symptoms of a transfusion reaction further observations should be undertaken, recorded, and appropriate action taken.
• Routine patient observations, as defined by the clinical area, should be continued throughout the transfusion period.
	4 To monitor for any potential complications and comply with the British Committee for Standards in Haematology (BCSH) guidelines (BCSH 2017).

5 Check cannula site half-hourly for: • Redness, swelling/inflammation • Pallor • Leakage/oozing • Skin temperature change • Tenderness If **ANY** appear **STOP** the transfusion.	5 To monitor for extravasation and phlebitis.
6 Record the following hourly: • Transfusion rate • Volume infused • Total volume infused	6 To ensure the rate remains correct, prevent overtransfusion, and ensure the pump or syringe driver (if used) is working correctly.

(continued)

Procedure guideline 4.5 Infuse product – observations, recordings and traceability (continued)

Statement	Rationale
7 Observe the CYP throughout the transfusion for signs of transfusion reactions: • Sweating/fever • Rash/mottled appearance • Dizziness • Flushing • Tachycardia • Nausea • Chills/rigours • Laboured breathing/wheezing • Chest or loin pain • Loss of consciousness • Sudden collapse	7 To detect any adverse reaction to the transfusion as early as possible.

Procedure guideline 4.6 Reaction management (transfusion)

Statement	Rationale
1 If the CYP shows signs of a mild reaction: • Stop the transfusion • Maintain IV access • Inform doctor • Record vital signs • Give prescribed steroid and antihistamine • Record incident in the healthcare records • Continue transfusion when they have recovered, if appropriate • Inform Blood Transfusion Laboratory • **Remember the 4-hour rule** • Report incident according to local trust protocol.	1 To stop/reduce the reaction, maintain accurate records, and maintain patency of IV line.

2 If a moderate or severe reaction occurs:
• Stop transfusion immediately
• Maintain IV access
• Seek **urgent** medical assistance
• Give steroid and antihistamine if prescribed
• Record vital signs
• Record incident in CYP's healthcare records
• **Do not recommence transfusion**
• Inform Blood Transfusion Laboratory and:
  – Return blood component and administration set to the laboratory
  – Send a full blood count
  – Send a sample to Blood Transfusion (for transfusion reaction assessment)
  – Obtain a urine sample collected after the reaction
• Report the incident according to local trust protocol.
	2 To stop the reaction and minimise the impact, maintain accurate records, maintain patency of IV line, and assist in investigation of the incident.

Administration of blood components

The general principles for IV administration are covered in Chapter 14: Intravenous and Intra-arterial Access and Infusions and also Chapter 17: Administration of Medicines. The following additional procedures and information are related to the specifics regarding the administration of blood components and related products. Blood must only be administered in clinical areas where it has been agreed it is safe to do so with adequate staffing and the availability of resuscitation equipment.

Before any blood component is administered to a CYP, they and their parents/carers should have the opportunity to discuss the implications of treatment, the potential risks and benefits, and the practical aspects of treatment. Appropriate information leaflets should be provided and consent/assent should be obtained and recorded in the CYP's health care record.

Red cells

The term 'red cells' describes several components, which are available for transfusion and which are used in different circumstances. Red cells in additive solution (saline-adenine-glucose-mannitol [SAGM]) are used for CYPs with blood loss, anaemia, or leukaemia, where transfusion of 4 ml/kg will raise the haemoglobin by 10 g/l.

Platelets

Platelets are produced by two processes; single donor (apheresis), or pooled from four donors. Both pooled and apheresis platelets are used in CYPs, with apheresis platelets split into neonatal packs for smaller volume transfusions. Human leukocyte antigen (HLA) matched platelets are available on a named patient basis for CYPs who have either developed or are at risk of developing HLA antibodies. Platelets in PAS (platelet additive solution) are platelets where most of the plasma has been removed; these are used for CYPs who react to plasma components, e.g. for those who have allergic reactions to HLA-matched platelets or those with some immune deficiencies.

Fresh frozen plasma (FFP)

In September 2019 the UK stopped importing plasma or treating it with methylene-blue and all plasma components issued to CYPs are UK sourced (New et al. 2020). FFP is used to correct abnormal clotting, disseminated intravascular coagulation, in liver disease and cardiac surgery, or when there is a known single coagulation factor deficiency for which a coagulation factor concentrate is unavailable, e.g. factor V deficiency. Some paediatric centres use OctaplasLG® as an alternative to UK sourced FFP. This is a clinical decision made by the transfusion team; however, both components are used and transfused in the same way.

Cryoprecipitate

Cryoprecipitate is produced by freezing and thawing FFP. The precipitate contains significant quantities of factor VIII and fibrinogen, which is used to treat abnormal clotting and low fibrinogen levels.

Albumin

Albumin is available in three strengths: 4.5% or 5% is used to increase the serum albumin levels and to expand plasma; 20% is used when there are problems of fluid overload and when sodium levels are either high or low. 20% albumin is available in 50–100 ml doses, while 4.5% is available in 50–500 ml and 5% in 100–500 ml doses. Albumin is most commonly used in hypovolaemia to restore volume, in hypoproteinaemia and in hypoalbuminaemia to replace protein, and to maintain blood pressure. It is most commonly used in CYPs with renal and liver disease. Albumin is administered as an intravenous infusion (IVI).

Immunoglobulin

Immunoglobulin is a blood product prepared from pooled human plasma, which carries a degree of risk from viral transmission. To minimise the risk of transmitting infections such as hepatitis, all plasma is obtained from selected screened donors, and then undergoes validated, virus inactivation processes during the manufacturing designed to inactivate most common viruses, including HIV, hepatitis B, and hepatitis C.

Immunoglobulin is used in the treatment of CYPs with inherited primary antibody deficiency or other complex immunodeficiency disorders to prevent life-threatening infections. In addition, it can be used as supportive therapy for secondary immunodeficiencies where intensive treatments, such as chemotherapy, have caused temporary damage to the immune system, e.g. during stem cell transplantation. The aim of treatment is prevention of infection by providing passive immunity through antibody replacement from plasma; this provides some degree of protection from common infections such as measles and chickenpox and many other viral and bacterial infections. CYPs receiving immunoglobulin replacement therefore do not need the routine childhood immunisations.

Immunoglobulin therapy has also been shown to be effective in a wide range of other diseases, e.g. Kawasaki's disease and idiopathic thrombocytopenic purpura, where 'modulation' of the immune system is required, although the exact mechanism of action is not understood.

Procedure guideline 4.7 Infuse component (albumin)

Statement	Rationale
1 Set infusion rate according to prescription BUT ensure infusion is completed within **3 hours** or following the manufacturer's instructions.	1 To maintain the effectiveness of the component, to meet the manufacturer's recommendations, and to minimise the risk of infection.
2 **Remember albumin may need to be changed during the infusion if the prescribed rate means that the above recommendation will be exceeded.**	
3 The intravenous administration set should be flushed with 20 ml normal saline to ensure the total amount of albumin prescribed is infused.	3 The administration set may retain up to 20 ml of albumin.
4 Give diuretic **if** prescribed at required time, according to the local Medicine Administration Policy.	4 To prevent fluid overload, especially if fluids are being restricted.

Procedure guideline 4.8 Observations and recordings (albumin)

Statement	Rationale
1 Record date and time of starting the infusion.	1 To ensure accuracy of records.
2 Sign that you are administering the albumin.	2 To determine who is accountable for the infusion.
3 Record the batch of the albumin in the CYP's notes.	3 To assist component and CYP tracing.
4 Establish the frequency and type of observations that the CYP may require during the infusion according to their clinical condition.	
5 Do not leave the CYP unattended for the first 30 minutes of the infusion.	5 This is when reactions are most likely to occur.
6 If a reaction occurs, inform pharmacy and seek advice.	6 To assist investigation of incident.
7 If more than one bottle is required, the same administration set can be used.	
8 If large volumes of albumin are required, this should be planned with the department supplying the albumin.	8 To ensure adequate stock is available.

Procedure guideline 4.9 Preparation – CYP and family (immunoglobulin)

Statement	Rationale
1 Carry out a risk assessment to ensure the family understands the need for treatment and how it is administered: a) **Intravenous** b) **Subcutaneous** – use with caution if the CYP has low platelets.	a) To inform the family and gain consent. b) To reduce the risk of severe bruising.
3 Explain the procedure to the CYP and family and include: a) The reason for treatment b) The risks and benefits c) The options for ongoing treatment.	2 To prepare them for treatment and obtain consent. c) To plan ahead and liaise with local services.
3 Assess that they are fit for treatment and perform baseline observation of temperature, blood pressure, respiration rate, heart rate.	3 To establish the normal for the CYP, ruling out pre-existing disease processes.
4 Weigh the CYP.	4 To calculate the dose.
5 Complete pretreatment blood tests and investigations: • Immunoglobulin trough levels (IgGAM) • Serum and plasma for long-term storage (store Ig) • Liver function tests • Hepatitis C screen.	5 • To monitor treatment efficacy • To enable look-back in the event of an infectious outbreak • To monitor the effectiveness of treatment.

Procedure guideline 4.10 Preparation – prescription (immunoglobulin)

Statement	Rationale
1 Immunoglobulin is a blood product and **MUST NOT** be administered unless prescribed on the CYP's prescription chart.	1 To ensure treatment is necessary and given as prescribed.
2 Calculate the dose: a) Replacement therapy: 300–500 mg/kg/3 weeks. b) Modulation: 1–2 g/kg (single dose). c) Round the dose to the nearest whole bottle.	a) To give appropriate dose. c) To prevent wastage.
2 Prescribe the **named product** to be used. Calculate the infusion rate in ml/hr (rate is product specific and should be calculated in ml/kg/hr).	3 To avoid product switching. For intravenous infusion rates the product insert should be read.
3 Prescribe premedication if required. a) Check the product dose, batch number, and expiry date. b) Record in the CYP's medical and nursing records and blood product register. c) Ensure immunoglobulin is at room temperature. d) Check the CYP's identity band and prescription according to the local medicine administration policy before starting the infusion.	4 Pre-medication is usually only given if there has been a recent infusion reaction. a) To avoid medication errors. b) This enables accurate recording of infusion details. c) This is more comfortable and avoids chilling the CYP. d) To ensure the immunoglobulin is being administered to the correct CYP.

Procedure guideline 4.11 Preparation – equipment for intravenous or subcutaneous infusion of immunoglobulin

Statement	Rationale
1 Gather equipment for intravenous or subcutaneous infusion as appropriate (see Chapter 14: Intravenous and Intra-arterial Access and Infusions).	1 To ensure safe infusion.
2 Topical local anaesthetic creams may be used. If used before insertion of a subcutaneous cannula, apply local anaesthetic cream to sites 1–2 hours prior to infusion.	2 To minimise discomfort of procedure.
3 Ensure pumps are available and working.	3 For safe subcutaneous infusion.

Procedure guideline 4.12 Procedure – intravenous infusion (immunoglobulin)

Statement	Rationale
1 If using powder/diluent read mixing instructions carefully.	1 To reconstitute as per manufacturer's instructions.
2 Prime administration set with immunoglobulin using standard precautions and an aseptic nontouch technique.	2 To minimise the risk of infection.
3 Check the CYP's identity band and prescription according to the local medicine administration policy.	3 To ensure the immunoglobulin is being connected to the right CYP.
4 Infuse immunoglobulin at the prescribed rate, starting slowly and increasing the rate every 30–minutes until the maximum rate is reached.	4 To minimise the risk of and promptly detect adverse reactions.
5 Do not leave the CYP unattended during the infusion as there is risk of adverse reactions. Ensure that the batch number is documented when the infusion is commenced.	5 To monitor for potential adverse reactions (see adverse reactions).
6 Check peripheral infusion access site half-hourly for: • Inflammation (tenderness, swelling, redness) • Leakage	6 To detect for signs of extravasation (see additional information in IV infusion guidelines).
7 Check the site and the infusion system is intact.	7 To detect signs of extravasation and ensure that the infusion pump is working correctly.
8 Record: • Infusion rate • Pressures • Hourly volume infused • Total volume infused	8 To ensure the rate remains correct and ensure that the infusion pump is working correctly.
9 The intravenous solution administration set will need flushing with 0.9% sodium chloride if the total amount of immunoglobulin infused is less than 100 ml.	9 The administration set may retain up to 20 ml of the product.

Procedure guideline 4.13 Procedure – subcutaneous infusion (immunoglobulin)

Statement	Rationale
1 Select suitable infusion sites: abdomen, thighs, or buttocks: a) Thighs are preferred in children under 2 years. b) Abdomen is preferred in older CYPs, as the thighs become more muscular.	1 a) To minimise discomfort and swelling. b) To promote steady absorption.
2 Remove local anaesthetic cream (if used) five minutes before needles are inserted.	2 To allow the skin to dry and maximise its effect.
3 Draw up the drug for the infusion in the syringe and prime the administration line using a nontouch technique.	3 To prevent infection.
4 Lift a skin fold and insert the needle into the subcutaneous tissue. The angle of insertion will depend on the needle type, length, and the amount of subcutaneous tissue present.	4 To prevent the needle going into the muscle underneath.
5 Secure the needle with tape or occlusive dressing as appropriate.	5 To prevent the infusion being dislodged.
6 Assess the CYP's subcutaneous tissue to decide on infusion rate: • 5–10 ml can be infused in babies 1–6 months old over 1 hr. • <10 ml can be infused in 40–60 minutes in children under 7 years. • 10–25 ml can be infused in 60–90 minutes in older CYPs. • >30 ml may need to be split between two sites. NB: Initial discomfort at the site is normal.	6 To maximise comfort and mobility.
7 Set the pump at the appropriate rate for the syringe size: a) Observe the CYP. b) Record details of the infusion, site, rate. c) Check the infusion site. NB: Swelling and redness at the site is normal, but will disappear 24 hrs after the infusion.	7 To observe for leakage.
8 **Do not leave the CYP unattended during the infusion as there is risk of adverse reactions. This may be negotiated with any family members in attendance.**	8 To monitor for potential adverse reactions (see reaction management, Procedure Guideline 4.14).

Procedure guideline 4.14 Reaction management (immunoglobulin)

Statement	Rationale
1 Monitor the CYP's (temperature, blood pressure, pulse, respiratory rate) throughout the infusion and for 1 hour after the first infusion or 20 minutes after subsequent infusions.	1 To ensure prompt detection of a possible reaction to the product.
2 If the reaction is mild: • Headache • Fever, chills, sweating • Flushing • Nausea Reduce the infusion rate, administer paracetamol/ibuprofen.	2 To minimise reaction and to make the CYP comfortable.

3 If the reaction is moderate:
• Vomiting
• Severe headache, dizziness
• Urticarial rash, wheals
• Mild wheezing
• Chest pain
  a) Stop the infusion.
  b) Call medical assistance.
  c) Administer antihistamine +/- paracetamol/ibuprofen
  d) Continue the infusion at a lower rate if possible.
	3
	
	a) To stop reaction.
	b, c) To minimise the reaction and make the CYP comfortable.
	
	d) To continue treatment if/when safe to do so

4 If the reaction is severe:
• Tightness of throat or chest
• Difficulty breathing or wheezing
• Back or loin pain/darkened urine
• Loss of consciousness
• Sudden collapse
  a) **Stop the infusion** and infuse 0.9% sodium chloride.
  b) Call urgent medical assistance and administer adrenaline.
  c) Record incident in CYP's healthcare records.
  d) Complete an incident report form.
	4 To minimise impact from reaction.
	
	a, b) To make the CYP comfortable while assessing and treating them.
	
	c) To maintain accurate records.
	d) To promote accurate recording of incidents.

Procedure guideline 4.15 Completing the infusion (immunoglobulin)

Statement	Rationale
1 Dispose of equipment in a sharps bin in accordance with the Trust Waste policy.	1 To reduce risk of infection by safe disposal.
2 Document in the CYP's medical and nursing healthcare records and blood products register: • The batch of the immunoglobulin. • Date and time of starting infusion. • Sign that you are responsible for its administration.	2 To ensure accuracy of records, assist product and tracing of CYP and determine accountability for the infusion.

Immunoglobulin is usually given as an intravenous infusion (IVIG) but it can also be given by subcutaneous infusion (SCIG). With new products being licenced specifically for this purpose, SCIG is becomeing increasingly popular as a safe and effective treatment, particularly in small children where venous access is difficult. It is also easy to administer at home, with parents/carers being taught how to administer this treatment.

It is considered poor practice to change products for a CYP, once they have been established on one particular product, because the components are not identical, and CYPs who tolerate one product may not tolerate another. In addition, switching products exposes the CYP to another plasma pool and increases the risk of exposure to blood-borne viruses.

Minor adverse reactions occur relatively frequently during and after the first few infusions, while more severe reactions are uncommon when the infusions are administered appropriately. Most systemic adverse reactions are associated with administration via the intravenous route and occur when infusions are given too quickly or if there is a concurrent febrile illness.

The general principles for IV therapy are covered in Chapter 14: Intravenous and Intra-arterial Infusions and Access. The specific care required for a CYP receiving intravenous immunoglobulin or subcutaneous immunoglobulin infusions follow below.

Coagulation factors

Single, plasma-derived, or genetically engineered (recombinant), coagulation factors (factors VII, VIII, IX, X, XI, XIII, fibrinogen, von-Willebrand factor, antithrombin, and protein C concentrates) are generally available in 250, 500, and 1000 IU vials and occasionally in vials of 1500, 2000, or 3000 IU. These are mainly used by CYPs with congenital bleeding disorders such as haemophilia. They can also be used in combination for CYPs with acquired coagulation disorders, such as those with liver or cardiac disease. Genetically engineered (recombinant) factors VII, VIII, IX, and XIII are available and pose no risk of transfusion of human blood-borne viruses and are generally considered 'safe' for use in any CYP.

Many CYPs with bleeding disorders require life-long replacement therapy, administered at home by their parents/carers, themselves or their community nurses. This is undertaken in partnership between the hospital, community team and family.

With the exception of fibrinogen concentrate, all coagulation factors are administered by bolus intravenous bolus through a 23 G butterfly (unless a cannula or central venous access is in situ). The guidelines for administration of IV bolus (see Chapter 14) should be followed. Fibrinogen concentrate is given as an IVIG following the guidelines in Chapter 14. Coagulation factors **MUST NOT** be filtered, as this will lead to the coagulation factors being removed by the filters, leading to the administration of a suboptimal dose and resultant bleeding.

Several new products, which 'disrupt' the coagulation pathway and reduce bleeding, are in clinical trials or are newly licensed. These include monoclonal antibodies and proteins that enhance and/or inhibit coagulation. They are given by subcutaneous injection (see Chapter 17: Administration of Medicines) as prophylaxis as infrequently as once monthly. Always seek expert haemophilia advice when caring for CYPs receiving these products as there are contraindications to concomitant treatment with some coagulation factors.

Conclusion

Administration of blood and its components is both a life-saving and potentially life-threatening procedure. It is imperative that the administration of these components and products, in hospitals and the community, is undertaken following rigorous training and following strict procedures. For many CYPs, administration of these components and products is part of their everyday lives and parental/self-administration in the community facilitates good quality of life outcomes for them and their families (Khair 2002).

References

Blundell, J. (1828). *Observations on transfused blood by Dr Blundell with a description of his gravitor. Lancet* ii: 321–324.

British Committee for Standards in Haematology (BCSH) (2017). Administration of Blood Components. https://b-s-h.org.uk/guidelines/guidelines/administration-of-blood-components/ (accessed 06 September 2022).

Department of Health (2005). The blood safety and quality regulations. www.legislation.gov.uk/uksi/2005/50/resources (accessed 06 September 2022).

Giangrande, P. (2000). *Historical review – the history of blood transfusion. British Journal of Haematology* 110: 758–767.

Khair, K. (2002). *Pilot testing of the 'Haemo-QoL' quality of life questionnaire for haemophiliac children in six European countries. Haemophilia* 8: 47–54.

Lefrère, J.J. and Hewitt, P. (2009). *From mad cows to sensible blood transfusion: the risk of prion transmission by labile blood components in the United Kingdom and in France. Transfusion* 49 (4): 797–812.

National Blood Authority (NBA) (2016). Patient Blood Management Guidelines: Module 6 - Neonatal and Paediatrics. NBA, Canberra, Australia. https://www.blood.gov.au/pubs/pbm/module6/ (accessed 06 September 2022).

New, H.V., Stanworth, S.J., et al. on behalf of the BSH Guidelines Transfusion Task Force British Society for Haematology (2020). *British society for haematology guidelines on transfusion for fetuses, neonates and older children. Br J Haematol.* 2016 (175): 784–828.

NHS Blood Transfusion Service (NHSBT) (2021). Patient Blood Management. National Blood Transfusion Committee for NHS England. https://hospital.blood.co.uk/patient-services/patient-blood-management/ (accessed 06 September 2022).

Peden, A.H., Head, M.W. et al. (2004). *Preclinical vCJD after blood transfusion in a PRNP codon 129 heterozygous patient. Lancet* 364 (9433): 527–529.

Public Health England (2017). Immunisation against infectious disease (The Green Book). https://www.gov.uk/government/collections/immunisation-against-infectious-disease-the-green-book (accessed 06 September 2022).

Serious Hazards of Transfusion (SHOT) (2019). Annual SHOT reports 1996 – 2019. Paediatric Cases chapters 2007-2019 https://www.shotuk.org/ (accessed 06 September 2022).

Chapter 5

Bowel care

Helen Johnson[1] and June Rogers[2]

[1]BSc (Hons), RN (Adult), RN (Child), ENB 216; Formerly Clinical Nurse Specialist Stoma Care, GOSH Stoma Care
[2]RN (Adult), RN (Child), BSc (Hons), MSc; Children's Bladder and Bowel Nurse Specialist, Bladder & Bowel UK, Manchester, UK

Chapter contents

Introduction	74
Diarrhoea	74
Constipation	74
Laxatives	75
Preparation for investigations or surgery	76
Treatment of faecal soiling/incontinence	76
Products to help with the management of faecal incontinence/soiling	76
Factors to note	84
Stoma pouch selection	85
References	85

Procedure guidelines

5.1 Administering a rectal suppository	78
5.2 Administering an enema	79
5.3 Rectal washout on an infant	80
5.4 Anal irrigation	80
5.5 Antegrade colonic enema (ACE washout)	81
5.6 Stoma siting	82
5.7 Changing a pouch	83

Principles tables

5.1 Stoma pouch selection	82
5.2 Potential problems with stomas	84

The Great Ormond Street Hospital Manual of Children and Young People's Nursing Practices, Second Edition. Edited by Elizabeth Anne Bruce, Janet Williss, and Faith Gibson.
© 2023 John Wiley & Sons Ltd. Published 2023 by John Wiley & Sons Ltd.

Introduction

Elimination has been cited as one of the activities of daily living (Williams 2015). It is important for nurses to understand the elimination routines of the child or young person (CYP) in their care and cater for any variations from the norm. Although elimination is a natural body function, there are a lot of 'social taboos' surrounding the subject and discussion can cause embarrassment and discomfort. Consideration must be given to religious and cultural beliefs, particularly in relation to acceptance of an altered body image following stoma formation (Black 2009a).

When required, various methods can be used to empty or clean the bowel. Different approaches are used in different circumstances. In the majority of cases it is preferable to use laxatives. However, if the CYP has a mechanical obstruction of the bowel, laxative use may be contra-indicated. Stimulating peristalsis in an obstructed bowel will cause increased discomfort and possibly perforation. Emptying or cleansing the bowel is necessary to: treat constipation, prepare the bowel for investigation or surgery, or to control faecal incontinence.

This chapter includes guidelines on the following practices:

- Management of diarrhoea
- Management of constipation
- Administering a rectal suppository
- Administering an enema
- Rectal washout (infant)
- Rectal washout (older CYP)
- Antegrade colonic enema (ACE washout)
- Stoma care

For further information, the reader is directed to the National Institute for Health and Care Excellence (NICE) guideline on the management of constipation in CYPs (NICE 2010).

Diarrhoea

There are a number of causes of diarrhoea in childhood, including infection, food allergy, disaccharide malabsorption, general malabsorption (coeliac disease and cystic fibrosis), inflammatory bowel disease, and toddler diarrhoea, which is by far the commonest cause. A careful history with an understanding of associated symptoms will give a clue as to the underlying cause and help direct the most appropriate treatment.

Toddler diarrhoea

Toddler diarrhoea is also known as chronic nonspecific diarrhoea. Affected children develop 3–10 watery loose stools per day. The stools are often more smelly and paler than usual and parents/carers may report bits of undigested vegetable food in the stools (such as bits of carrot, sweetcorn, etc.). Mild abdominal pain sometimes occurs, but apart from the loose stools the child is usually symptom free.

A child with just toddler diarrhoea is otherwise well, grows normally, plays normally and is usually not bothered about the diarrhoea. No detailed tests are usually needed if the child is otherwise well. Symptoms usually go, with or without treatment, by the age of 5–6 years.

The cause of the diarrhoea is not clear but it is **not** due to malabsorption of food or to a serious bowel problem. It is also not due to an intolerance of a type of food.

Often, no treatment is needed, particularly if symptoms are mild. Reassurance that it will ease in time may be all that is required. However, in many cases slight changes to the child's diet may be helpful. They are the 4 Fs: fat, fluid, fruit juices, and fibre. Advice to parents/carers should include the following:

1. Increase fat in the diet.
2. Decrease fluid in the diet.
3. Avoid fructose and sorbitol – decrease fruit juices.
4. Increase dietary fibre.
5. Provide normal diet for age.
6. Offer reassurance.
7. Be aware that there is no role for medications.
8. The parents/carers should be told that there are no serious sequelae, and this is not a precursor to inflammatory bowel disease.
9. Most children are better by 4 years of age, and are better by the time they become potty trained.

Constipation

Constipation is a common childhood condition and is responsible for 90–95% of all bowel problems in CYPs. In most cases the constipation develops as a result of a number of factors, which is then often made worse by the passage of a large painful stool, which perpetuates the problem when the CYP begins to associate pain with having their bowels opened (Kocaay et al. 2011).

There have been a number of definitions of constipation, but it is now generally accepted that for a diagnosis of constipation to be made it must include two or more of the following in a CYP with a developmental age of at least 4 years with insufficient criteria for diagnosis of irritable bowel syndrome (IBS):

1. Two or fewer defecations in the toilet per week.
2. At least one episode of faecal incontinence per week.
3. History of retentive posturing or excessive volitional stool retention.
4. History of painful or hard bowel movements.
5. Presence of a large faecal mass in the rectum.
6. History of large diameter stools that may obstruct the toilet.

Criteria must be fulfilled at least once per week for at least 2 months before a diagnosis can be made.

It is expected that most CYPs will open their bowels at least three times per week; however it has been shown that the consistency of the stool is of equal importance to the frequency. The awareness of stools that are difficult or painful to pass is important, as it has been identified that a high number of CYPs develop constipation as a result of experiencing pain with defecation This is obviously an important trigger factor for the development of constipation, and questions regarding stool consistency and presence of pain or discomfort should always be included in any paediatric continence assessment.

Constipation can be divided into two types: idiopathic or functional and nonidiopathic:

Idiopathic constipation

Idiopathic or functional constipation – i.e. where there is no underlying cause – is the most common type of constipation in CYPs. Constipation is referred to as 'idiopathic' if it cannot be explained by anatomical or physiological abnormalities. The exact cause of constipation is not fully understood, but factors that may contribute include pain, fever, dehydration, dietary and fluid intake, psychological issues, toilet training, medicines such as anticholinergics, and familial history of constipation. NICE (2014) has produced a set of Quality Standards based on the original NICE guidance (2010) regarding the assessment and treatment of CYPs with idiopathic constipation.

Nonidiopathic constipation

There are a number of conditions, both congenital and acquired, that can result in constipation. These include anorectal anomalies, such as imperforate anus and Hirschsprung's disease; neurological conditions such as spina bifida, sacral agenesis, and spinal cord injuries; and endocrine conditions such as hypothyroidism (Rintala 2002).

Investigations

The first and most important investigation in constipation is a detailed history of the problem, to determine cause and treatment. Areas to be questioned include:

- What is the CYP's normal bowel habit, how has it changed, and over what period of time?
- What is their normal diet and how has it changed recently?
- What medication is the CYP receiving?
- Do they have any other medical conditions?
- Have there been any changes in the CYP's normal routines – e.g. changing schools or attending for the first time? – these can disrupt toileting habits.
- Has the CYP suffered previous bowel problems or undergone abdominal surgery?

NICE (2010) produces a number of supportive documents alongside their guidance and currently there are two history-taking questionnaires (one for children under and one for those over 1 year of age) available to download from their website (www.nice.org.uk/guidance/cg99).

It is important to recognise that CYPs may perceive rectal examinations as abuse, particularly when force or coercion is used, and therefore routine digital rectal examination (DRE) is not recommended by NICE in children over the age of 1 year. NICE (2010) also makes clear recommendations regarding other investigations that are not to be carried out routinely as part of the initial assessment. As well as DRE these include abdominal X-ray, transit studies, and ultrasound. It is important, however, particularly if the symptoms have been noted from birth and if the child's symptoms do not improve with the recommended treatment, that the perianal area is inspected and the position of the anus is noted. As many of the children who present in this group are of the younger age and still in nappies, this can be done quite easily by asking the parent/carer to change the child's nappy and the area can be inspected while their bottom is exposed.

By taking a careful detailed history the diagnosis of idiopathic constipation can be confirmed and any 'red flags' easily identified. The 'red flags' findings and clues that may indicate an underlying disorder include:

- Constipation reported from birth with delayed passage of meconium
- Abnormal appearance or position of anus
- Gross abdominal distension
- Unexplained abnormal gait
- Ribbon stools
- Previously unknown/undiagnosed leg weakness or motor delay
- Abdominal distension and vomiting

Amber flags include:

- Faltering growth
- Disclosure/evidence raising concerns over maltreatment

If any 'red flags' are identified then the CYP should be referred urgently to a healthcare worker experienced in the specific aspect of health that is causing concern. It is at this stage that a more detailed examination, including a DRE, would be carried out if necessary. If any 'amber flags, including faltering growth and possible maltreatment, are identified then the constipation should be treated, and the CYP referred on for further investigation as detailed in local guidelines and policies.

Plain abdominal X-ray, to show any faecal loading or obstruction, should not be performed purely to establish a diagnosis of constipation. NICE make the following recommendation: 'Consider using a plain abdominal radiograph only if requested by specialist services in the ongoing management of intractable idiopathic constipation' (NICE 2010).

Further investigations, when underlying conditions are present/suspected, are:

- Sigmoidoscopy – allows a detailed examination of the rectum and sigmoid colon.
- Colonoscopy – allows a detailed examination of the bowel as far as the caecum.
- Barium enema – allows a clear picture of the structure of the colon.
- Rectal biopsy, suction biopsy, or full thickness biopsy to examine the presence of ganglion nerve cells, to exclude Hirschsprung's disease.
- Colonic transit studies – the CYP will be given radio-opaque markers, made up of different shapes, to swallow at intervals. Abdominal X-rays note how long it takes for the different markers to be evacuated.
- Ano-rectal manometry – measurements are taken of the pressures within the anal canal. A small tube placed in the rectum records the pressure created by contraction and relaxation of anal muscles.

Treatment of constipation

For successful treatment of constipation there needs to be a clear understanding of the various factors involved for each individual CYP, which in some cases necessitates a multidisciplinary approach to ensure all the CYP's needs are met. The general principles in managing constipation in CYPs are to soften and clear any faecal impaction, establish a regular pain-free pattern of defaecation and prevent relapse by supportive management including demystification and education for the child and family.

Laxatives

NICE recommend laxatives as first line treatment, with macrogol being the laxative of choice.

Disimpaction

It is important to clear out the bowel first if the CYP is impacted and NICE (2010) makes the following treatment regimen recommendations for disimpaction:

- Polyethylene glycol 3350 + electrolytes, e.g. Movicol Paediatric Plain (Movicol PP™), using an escalating dose regimen as the first-line treatment from 6 months of age.
- Movicol PP™ may be mixed with any cold drink.
- Add a stimulant laxative, such as sodium picosulfate, if Movicol PP™ does not lead to disimpaction after 2 weeks.
- Substitute a stimulant laxative singly or in combination with an osmotic laxative such as lactulose™ if Movicol PP™ is not tolerated.
- Inform families that disimpaction treatment can increase symptoms of soiling and abdominal pain initially.
- It is important that CYPs undergoing disimpaction are reviewed within a week to check progress and adjust dosage regime if necessary.
- NICE also advises that rectal medications, including sodium citrate enemas, should not be used unless all oral medication has failed, and that phosphate enemas should be used only under specialist supervision in hospital due to the risk of phosphate overload (Marek et al. 2015).

Maintenance

As a rough guide the suggested starting maintenance dose of macrogol for CYPs following disimpaction is roughly half the dose required during disimpaction. However, the correct dose is whatever produces the optimum results of at least three soft, easily passed stools per week with the consistency of the stool and the ease of passage being the important factors. Clinical experience has shown that the best way to reach the optimum maintenance dose is to slowly titrate the dose of Movicol PP™ down from the disimpaction dose until the optimum dose is reached.

NICE recommend the following regimen for maintenance:

- Movicol PP™ (Polyethylene glycol 3350 + electrolyte) as the first-line treatment.
- Adjust the dose of Movicol PP™ according to symptoms and response.
- Add a stimulant laxative if Movicol PP™ does not work.
- Substitute a stimulant laxative, such as sodium picosulfate, if Movicol PP™ is not tolerated by the CYP. Add another laxative such as lactulose™ or docusate™ if stools are hard.
- Continue medication at maintenance dose for several weeks after regular bowel habit is established – this may take several months.
- Children who are toilet training should remain on laxatives until toilet training is well established.
- Do not stop medication abruptly: gradually reduce the dose over a period of months in response to stool consistency and frequency.
- Some CYPs may require laxative therapy for several years with a small minority requiring continued ongoing laxative therapy.

Diet
Encourage a well-balanced, high-fibre diet along with increased fluid intake. Excessive milk drinking in later infancy should be avoided. It is generally accepted that once a child is fully weaned, milk intake should not exceed 1 pint per day.

Toileting
CYPs should be encouraged to sit on the toilet after meals. Enough time should be allowed for the bowel to empty.

Suppositories and enemas
When oral laxatives have failed, particularly if the CYP has an underlying disorder, a suppository or enema may be prescribed. It must be remembered, however, that some CYPs may find rectal administration distressful, so it is important that these procedures are undertaken only with the CYP's full cooperation.

Follow up
CYPs should be followed up with regularly to assess progress and re-evaluate laxative use. Families should also be given the contact details of a healthcare worker they can contact for advice if problems develop between appointments.

Biofeedback
This is a treatment to retrain the nerves and muscles used in evacuation. The treatment can be lengthy and needs full commitment from the CYP and their family. The evidence base, however, for the use of biofeedback is poor and it is not currently recommended by NICE (2010) as a standard treatment intervention for idiopathic constipation.

Invasive treatments
For CYPs with intractable constipation and for those whose constipation is related to an underlying disorder, further invasive treatments may be indicated and include:

- Rectal washouts such as Peristeen® (Alenezi et al. 2014; Ausili et al. 2010).
- ACE washouts (Peeraully et al. 2014).
- Bowel resection; this would be the last resort, but subtotal colectomy with ileorectal anastomosis or ileosigmoid anastomosis may be performed.

Preparation for investigations or surgery

All centres will have protocols for preparation of the bowel for investigation or surgery. These can vary in use of certain laxatives or enemas. It is important, therefore, to identify and follow local guidelines and protocols regarding bowel preparations for specific investigations/surgical interventions. However, no CYP with inflammatory bowel disease should have rectal washouts or enemas except for foam enemas, which are used for ulcerative colitis. The rectal route for suppositories, enemas or washouts should not be used in imunosuppressed CYPs as they are susceptible to infections such as necrotising fasciitis which can be fatal (Fustes-Morales et al. 2002).

Treatment of faecal soiling/incontinence

CYPs can suffer faecal soiling/incontinence for a number of reasons including:

- Constipation with overflow
- Anorectal anomalies, spina bifida
- Resection of bowel leading to a shortened gut
- Emotional difficulties (encopresis)

Nurses need to be aware of the psychological effects faecal incontinence has on the CYP and the family and their beliefs and values. These effects can be minimised more easily the earlier the problem is addressed. Whatever the cause, faecal soiling/incontinence needs to be treated. It would be hoped that some programme of management will have started before the CYP begins school.

Overflow soiling associated with constipation should stop once the constipation has resolved. For CYPs with faecal incontinence related to an underlying condition, treatment options include:

- Timed evacuations using a combination of oral/rectal preparations and a toileting programme
- Rectal washouts
- Colonic irrigation
- ACE washouts (Peeraully et al. 2014)

Sometimes further surgery, such as repeat pull-through, colonic resection, levatorplasty, colostomy, or stimulated gracilopasty, will be performed. See Figure 5.1 for a suggested pathway for proactive management of nonidiopathic bowel problems from birth.

Products to help with the management of faecal incontinence/soiling

There are a range of containment products available, both disposable and reusable to help manage faecal incontinence. The degree of soiling will dictate the most appropriate product to be used.

Further information regarding the full range of products and resources available can be obtained via PromoCon (part of the charity Disabled Living), which provides national advice and information via its website and helpline (www.promocon.co.uk, helpline: 0161 6078219).

Suppositories
NICE does not recommend suppositories as a treatment for idiopathic constipation. Suppositories can be used as a method of evacuating faeces or to administer medication. Whatever the indication, the method of administration is the same. The route of administration is normally into the rectum, but suppositories can be inserted into a colostomy using the same principles.

Ensure the environment where the procedure is to take place is private, and has a toilet, commode, or bedpan available if the suppository being administered is to evacuate the rectum.

Explanation of the procedure to the CYP and their parents/carers will alleviate anxiety. Some families regard the rectal route for

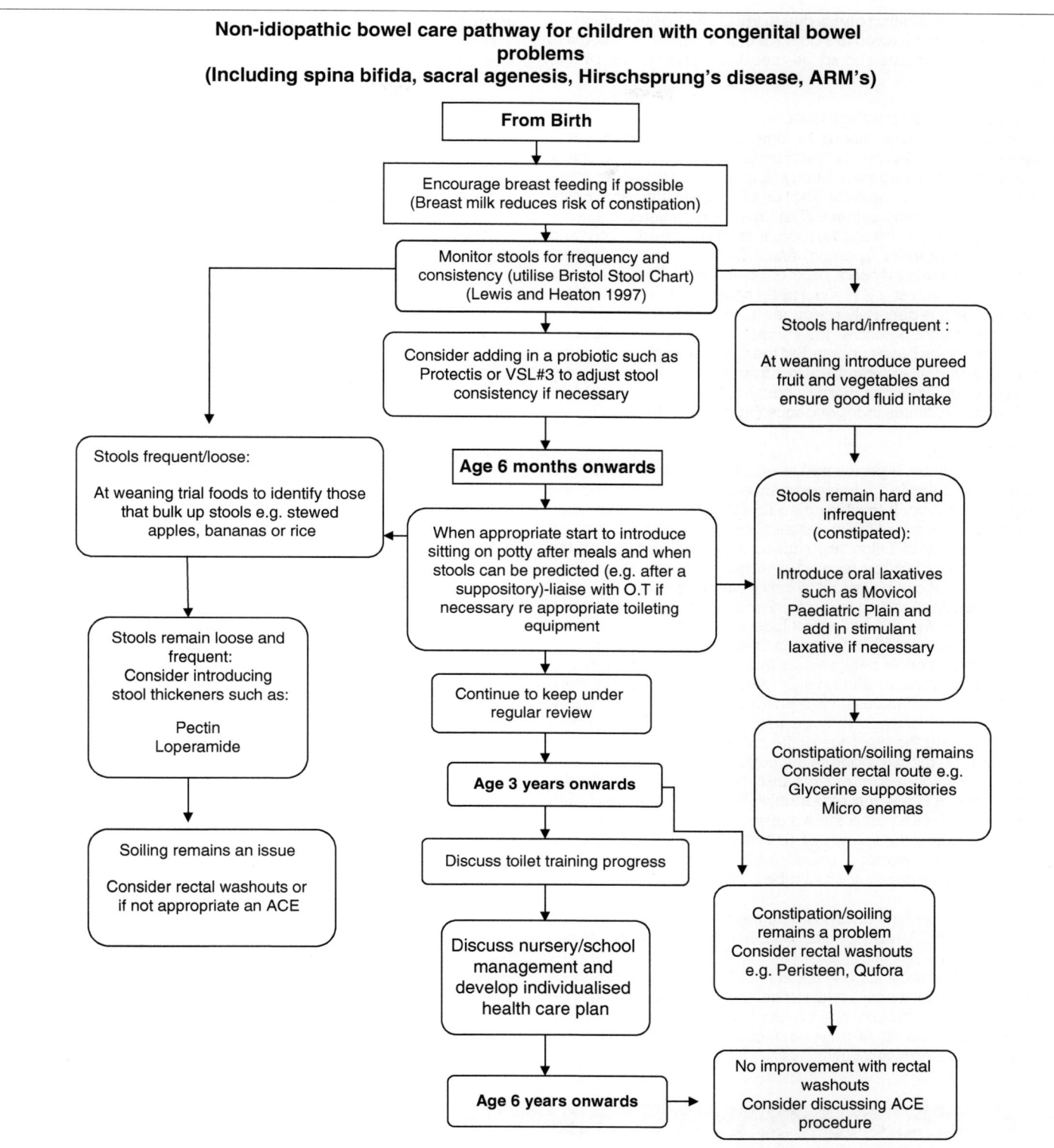

Figure 5.1 Non-idiopathic bowel care pathway for children with congenital bowel problems (including spina bifida, sacral agenesis, Hirschsprung's disease, anorectal malformations).

medication to be the least acceptable (Seth et al. 2000). Suppositories may be contraindicated in some CYPs, e.g. post rectal surgery, or those who are neutropenic.

Enemas

NICE does not recommend the administration of enemas for treatment of idiopathic constipation. This can be seen as an unpleasant and embarrassing procedure by some CYPs. Therefore, consideration must be given to certain aspects that can lessen anxiety. Ensure the environment where the procedure is to be carried out is private and has a toilet, bedpan, or commode available. CYPs who are bedbound will need to remain on the bed and will need incontinence sheets or a nappy.

Allow enough time for the procedure to be undisturbed. Generally 30–40 minutes is needed to ensure the enema and stools are evacuated. Explain the procedure to the CYP and parents/carers.

While the enema is being given, due to the CYP's position, they will not be able to see what you are doing. If only a part of the enema is prescribed, the amount should be measured prior to the procedure starting.

Transanal colonic irrigation

Colonic irrigation is a means of emptying the transverse and descending colon. This can be performed either by using a colostomy irrigation kit (a bag for holding saline with a long tube attached that has a soft plastic cone at the end) or a Peristeen trans anal washout kit, or the Shandling catheter. The Shandling catheter is a rectal catheter that has a retaining balloon; it is useful for children who have a patulous (wider opening) anus. The balloon will stop the washout from running straight back out of the anus. The catheter is rather cumbersome and CYPs will need help to perform the irrigation; as a result it is generally no longer used in practice.

New developments such as the Peristeen system and Qufora for transanal irrigation have superseded the older systems such as the Shandling catheter and can be used from the age of three years. The majority of CYPs can learn to carry out the procedure themselves, which facilitates independence (Ausili et al. 2010).

Anal irrigation

Trans anal irrigation is performed to evacuate stools from the rectum and lower colon in the management of faecal incontinence and chronic constipation. It involves introducing water into the rectum and colon via the anus. The water and contents of the rectum and descending sigmoid colon are subsequently evacuated into the toilet. Although initially performed by a parent/carer it is a procedure that the CYP can be taught to carry out independently.

This section is based on using the Peristeen anal irrigation system. The reader will need to check local policy to determine what other systems are available for use in their own area.

As this procedure is designed to take place over the toilet or commode, appropriate toileting aids (such as a seat reducer/step) should be in place if necessary to enable the CYP to sit comfortably. Distraction techniques may be useful for some CYPs to help them relax during the insertion of the rectal catheter. If the CYP is able; encourage them to operate the control unit – this will not only act as a distraction technique but also help facilitate later independence. Some CYPs may experience abdominal cramps during the procedure; try to pump the water more slowly and check the temperature. Adjust the volume of air in the balloon if there is leakage of fluid or the catheter is expelled prematurely.

The following precautions should be noted:

- The Peristeen anal irrigation is designed to be used in children over the age of 3 years; special caution must be used in children under 3 years.
- Special caution must also be taken in CYPs with recent abdominal or anal surgery, anal fissure or inflammatory bowel disease.
- Rectal irrigation should not be used when there is a known obstruction of the large bowel or acute stage of inflammatory bowel disease or diverticulitis.

Antegrade colonic enema (ACE)

The use of the antegrade colonic enema (ACE procedure) is now considered to be the follow-on option if a trial of transanal irrigation (Peristeen) is either not tolerated or not effective.

The appendix is brought out onto the abdominal wall as a small opening. This allows a catheter to be inserted directly into the caecum, through which a washout can be performed while the CYP is sitting on the toilet. The whole of the colon can be evacuated and the CYP can be clean for up to 48 hours.

If the CYP has had an appendicectomy, a caecal flap can create this channel.

Washout solutions for the ACE vary from centre to centre so it is important to always follow local policies and guidelines, but generally include an enema solution and saline. It is usual to mix equal measures of enema and saline; this is given and then followed by a saline flush.

Stoma care

The word stoma comes from the Greek meaning mouth or opening. The majority of stomas raised in childhood are formed in the neonatal period, and are usually a temporary measure in the surgical correction of congenital abnormalities. Conditions that may require stoma surgery include: imperforate anus, Hirschsprung's disease, cloacal exstrophy, bladder exstrophy, necrotising enterocolitis, ulcerative colitis, Crohn's disease, familial adenomatous polyposis, tumours, and trauma.

There are four main types of output stomas:

1. Colostomy: A portion of the colon is brought out through the abdominal wall and is normally sited in the left iliac fossa. In children the transverse, descending or sigmoid colon may be used.
2. Ileostomy: a portion of ileum is brought out through the abdominal wall and is normally sited in the right iliac fossa.
3. Jejunostomy: A portion of the jejunem is brought through the abdominal wall. This stoma has a high output and these CYPs generally require total parental nutrition.
4. Urinary diversions: These include:
   - Ileal conduit – a section of the ileum is isolated to act as a reservoir and the ureters implanted into it. This stoma can be sited in the left or right iliac fossa.
   - Ureterostomy – one or two of the ureters can be brought out onto the abdominal wall, either side by side or at either side of the abdomen.
   - Vesicostomy – the neck of the bladder is brought through the abdominal wall low down at the pelvis.

The success of any surgery is generally related to the level of understanding and the support given to the CYP and family. Families need to know what is happening, what the surgery involves, and how they will cope afterwards. It is vitally important to be honest when preparing CYPs for surgery. Meeting another family whose child has had stoma surgery can be an excellent support. They can answer questions from a personal perspective and share experiences such as what support is needed at school.

Procedure guideline 5.1 Administering a rectal suppository

Statement	Rationale
1 Gather equipment and ensure the room is warm and private: • Suppository • Lubricating jelly • Gloves and plastic apron	1 To allow the procedure to be carried out promptly without interruption.
2 Take off nappy or underwear. a) Ask the CYP to lie on left side with knees bent up to abdomen. b) Infants can lie on their back with feet and legs held up.	2 To enable access to the rectum. a) Insertion of suppository will be easier in this position. b) This position is easier to maintain in an infant.
3 Wash hands, put on nonsterile gloves and a plastic apron.	3 To minimise the risk of infection.

Procedure guideline 5.1 Administering a rectal suppository *(continued)*

Statement	Rationale
4 a) Open suppository, lubricate the end. b) Holding the suppository between index finger and thumb, locate the anus, and gently insert the suppository with the index finger. The suppository should be fully inserted into the rectum next to the rectal wall.	4 a) Lubrication will make insertion easier. b) Fully inserting the suppository against the wall of the rectum will allow it to be retained longer and therefore be more effective.
5 Ask the CYP to try and retain the suppository as long as possible.	5 The longer the suppository is retained the better the result.
6 If the suppository is used to evacuate the rectum, sit the CYP on the toilet or commode to empty the bowel.	6 Allow enough time sitting on the toilet/commode for the rectum to empty.
7 If the suppository is for medication purposes, e.g. analgesia, wipe excess lubricating jelly off perineum and replace nappy or underwear.	7 The suppository will dissolve and medication absorbed through bowel mucosa.
8 Dispose of the used or remaining equipment in accordance with local policies. Wash hands.	8 To minimise the risk of infection.
9 The suppository administration and result should be documented in the CYPs healthcare record.	9 The suppository administration and result should be documented in the CYPs healthcare record.

Procedure guideline 5.2 Administering an enema

Statement	Rationale
1 Gather equipment and ensure the room is warm and private: • Enema • Gloves and plastic apron • Lubricating jelly • Rectal catheter if needed • Incontinence sheet.	1 To allow the procedure to be carried out promptly with no interruption.
2 Take off nappy or underwear. a) Ask the CYP to lie on their left side with knees bent up to abdomen. b) Infants can lie on their back with feet and legs held up.	2 To facilitate access to rectum a) Insertion of the enema nozzle or rectal catheter is easier. b) This position is easier to maintain with an infant.
3 Wash hands, put on gloves and plastic apron.	3 To minimise the risk of infection.
4 Lubricate the end of the enema nozzle. 　If a rectal catheter is to be used, attach it to the enema nozzle and lubricate the end.	4 Lubrication ensures easier insertion. 　Using a catheter allows the enema to be instilled high up in the colon. If the rectum is loaded with faeces the tube will be able to bypass it and produce a better result.
5 Gently squeeze the enema bottle to allow the solution to prime the nozzle or rectal catheter.	5 To expel any air from the nozzle or catheter.
6 a) Identify the anus and gently insert the nozzle or catheter into anus. b) Squeeze the enema bottle until all the solution has entered the rectum. c) Continue squeezing the enema bottle as the nozzle or catheter is gently removed.	6 a) The catheter or nozzle should be inserted far enough into the rectum to stop the enema solution from running out of the anus. c) Squeezing the bottle while taking out the catheter or nozzle stops fluid from running back into the bottle.
7 Older CYPs should be asked to try and keep the enema solution in their bowel for as long as they can.	7 This allows the enema solution to be as effective as possible. If the solution is pushed out immediately it will not be as effective.
8 Sit the CYP on the toilet, commode, or bedpan, allowing time to empty the bowel.	8 Sitting on the toilet or commode offers the best position for emptying the bowel. The CYP needs to sit on the toilet/commode long enough for the bowel to empty fully.
9 Continually reassure the CYP if abdominal cramps occur.	9 The enema causes peristalsis, which can be uncomfortable. As the bowel empties the cramps lessen.
10 Dispose of the used or remaining equipment in accordance with local policies. Wash hands.	10 To minimise the risk of infection.
11 The results of the administration of the enema should be documented in the CYPs healthcare record.	11 To ensure a record of the procedure and outcome is made.

Procedure guideline 5.3 Rectal washout on an infant

Rectal washout may be requested in older CYPs prior to investigations; if so, the following guideline may be used. Larger catheters and larger volumes of saline will be needed.

Statement	Rationale

1 Gather equipment and ensure the room is warm and private.
   a) Plastic apron
   b) Disposable gloves
   c) Incontinence sheets
   d) Disposable bowls
   e) Rectal/nasogastric tube (10 or 12 Fr)
   f) Syringe (50 ml)
   g) Warm saline
   h) Lubricating jelly
	1 Having equipment ready ensures the procedure can be uninterrupted. The baby will be naked or partially naked; therefore, the room needs to be warm.
	   a–d) To adhere to universal precautions and minimise the risk of infection.

2 Explain procedure fully to parents/carers and undress infant feet to waist.	2 Can be seen as a distressing procedure; if all questions and fears are answered parents/carers will feel more relaxed.

3 a) Pour warm saline into bowl, draw up about 20 ml into syringe, and attach rectal tube.
   b) Prime the tube with saline.
	3 a) Saline is used as it will not be absorbed by the gut.
	   b) To prevent the introduction of air into the rectum, as this could cause further distension.

4 Infants are generally more content to lie on their backs during the procedure, but any position they want to assume can be accommodated. Ask parents/assistant to lift up the infant's feet and hold them still.	4 It is easier to control all equipment during the procedure if legs are supported and not kicking out. This also ensures that parents/carers are close to the infant to provide comfort.
5 Wash hands, put on disposable gloves and plastic apron. Lubricate the end of the tube. Locate the anus and gently insert the tube about 1–2 inches.	5 1–2 inches is far enough to begin with, the rectum can be emptied and the tube can then be advanced more easily if necessary.

6 a) Slowly inject the saline into the rectum.
   b) Once it has entered, gently draw back on the syringe. If any pressure is felt stop drawing back. If no saline can be drawn back, disconnect syringe from tube, gently moving the tube back and forth.
	6 a) To administer the treatment
	   b) To stimulate evacuation by gravity. Drawing back on the syringe makes the procedure quicker and will cause no problem as long as no pressure is felt. Too much suction could risk damaging or perforating the bowel wall.

7 Evacuated stool and saline should be collected in a disposable bowl. It is important to check that the amount of saline being instilled is being returned.	7 To avoid abdominal distension.
8 In infants, no more than 20 ml of saline should be instilled at one time.	8 Overfilling the rectum/sigmoid colon could cause distension and possible perforation.
9 Repeat the above steps until the abdomen is deflated (Hirschsprung's or constipation) or the saline is running clean (prior to surgery).	9 To complete treatment.
10 Medical staff may have prescribed the amount of saline to be used in total. If not, the infant's warmth dictates. When the washout has been completed gently remove the catheter, then clean and dress the infant.	10 Attempts should be made to keep the infant warm at all times. If this is unsuccessful the washout should be stopped and, if required, repeated later.
11 Dispose of the used or remaining equipment in accordance with local policies. Wash hands.	11 To minimise the risk of infection.
12 The results of the rectal washout should be documented in the CYPs healthcare record.	12 To ensure a record of the procedure and outcome is made.

Procedure guideline 5.4 Anal irrigation

Statement	Rationale

1 Gather the following equipment and ensure the room is warm and private:
   • Anal irrigation kit (Peristeen)
   • Irrigation bag and tubing
   • Control unit
   • Rectal catheter (two sizes, small/large)
   • Lukewarm (body temperature) water (approximately 20 ml per kg – but local policy/guidelines will dictate)
   • Plastic apron and gloves
	1 To ensure that the procedure can be uninterrupted.

2 Undertake a comprehensive nursing and medical assessment.	2 To identify any contraindications.
3 Performing rectal irrigation is not without risk and the decision to undertake it should be made in consultation with senior medical personnel and the CYP's GP, if the procedure is to be continued in the community.	3 To ensure the procedure is suitable and appropriate for the CYP.

Chapter 5 Bowel care

Procedure guideline 5.4 Anal irrigation (continued)

Statement	Rationale
4 Explain the procedure to the CYP.	4 To enlist the CYP's cooperation and gain consent.
5 Fill the irrigation bag with lukewarm water and run it through the system until there is sufficient water in the catheter packaging.	5 To enable the catheter to become lubricated.
6 Position the CYP as appropriate. If they are able to stand unsupported, insertion of the catheter is best carried out with the CYP standing next to the toilet. This can involve standing directly in front of the toilet facing away and leaning slightly forwards or standing to the side of the toilet depending on the space available. If the CYP is unable to stand, they should be positioned on a bed or changing mat for insertion of the catheter and inflation of the balloon. They can then be lifted onto the toilet or commode using a hoist and toileting sling if necessary.	6 To ensure the CYP is comfortable and to enable the procedure to be carried out as easily as possible.
If the CYP is confident in sitting on the toilet and has good sitting balance, then the catheter can be inserted while the CYP is sitting on the toilet. With time this is a procedure that some CYPs can be taught to do independently.	To help promote independence.
7 Wash hands, put on plastic apron and gloves.	7 To adhere to universal precautions.
8 Once the catheter has been inserted into the rectum (approx 2.5 cm past the balloon section, but this will differ depending on the size of the CYP), the catheter balloon is inflated by turning the dial to the appropriate symbol and using sufficient pumps of the balloon (usually 2–3 for the large catheter, 1–2 for the small catheter).	8 To retain the catheter and instilled fluid.
9 The dial is then turned to the water symbol and water is pumped slowly into the rectum – the exact quantity instilled will depend on the individual, but is usually 350–500 ml.	9 To commence the washout.
10 When the appropriate volume of water has been instilled the dial is turned to the air symbol and the balloon is deflated. The water and contents of the rectum and descending colon are subsequently evacuated into the toilet.	10 To allow the rectal catheter to slide out.
11 Once the evacuation is complete the CYP should be assisted to wipe their bottom if able, otherwise this should be carried out by their carer.	11 To make the CYP comfortable.
12 The rectal catheter should be disposed of as per local policy and the remaining equipment cleaned and stored away. Wash hands.	12 To minimise the risk of infection.
13 The results of the rectal irrigation should be documented in the CYP's healthcare records.	13 To ensure an accurate record of the procedure is made.

Procedure guideline 5.5 Antegrade colonic enema (ACE washout)

Statement	Rationale
1 Ensure bathroom is warm and private.	1 The CYP will be more relaxed in privacy.
2 Gather equipment: • Washout solutions • Size 10 FR catheter • Lubricating jelly • Gloves and plastic apron • 60 ml bladder syringe	2 To ensure procedure is uninterrupted.
3 Wash hands, put on gloves and plastic apron, lubricate the end of the catheter.	3 To adhere to universal precautions.
4 Gently introduce into the ACE stoma. It needs to be inserted about 3–4 inches. It is easier to insert the catheter with the CYP standing up or lying down.	4 The catheter needs to go through the appendix and into the caecum. If it is not introduced far enough, the washout solution will not enter the colon. Sitting down may make passing the catheter more difficult.
5 Draw up the half-strength enema solution into the bladder syringe. Attach the syringe into the catheter and slowly inject the solution. Continue until all the enema solution has been instilled. Keep the empty syringe attached to the catheter for a few minutes.	5 Injecting the enema solution too quickly may not produce enough stimulation for the colon to empty fully. This gives time for the enema solution to move through the colon before the saline is instilled. Otherwise it will be diluted more.
6 Bend back the catheter and remove syringe. Refill the syringe with saline and reattach to the bent catheter. Straighten the catheter and slowly inject the saline flush until all prescribed saline is given.	6 Bending back the catheter will stop the already instilled enema solution returning through the catheter. The volume of saline flush will help flush out faeces.

(continued)

The Great Ormond Street Hospital Manual of Children and Young People's Nursing Practices

Procedure guideline 5.5 Antegrade colonic enema (ACE washout) *(continued)*

Statement	Rationale
7 When all solution has been instilled, gently remove the catheter.	7 The tube needs to be removed; otherwise the fluid will run back out into the syringe.
8 The CYP needs to sit on the toilet for up to about 45 minutes or until all fluid and stool has been evacuated. They should try to push out the washout solution and stool.	8 Evacuation of the bowel can take at least 30–45 minutes. The bowel will empty more quickly if the CYP tries to evacuate their bowel.
9 Dispose the used or remaining equipment in accordance with local policies. Wash hands.	9 To minimise the risk of infection.
10 The results of the ACE washout should be documented in the CYPs healthcare record.	10 To ensure a record of the procedure and outcome is made.

Procedure guideline 5.6 Stoma siting

Statement	Rationale
1 It is generally not necessary to mark the site of the stoma in a newborn infant.	1 The stoma will usually be of a temporary nature and will be closed before the child is out of nappies. Surgery is often performed as an emergency.
2 If the CYP is older and out of nappies, or if the stoma is a more permanent treatment, the stoma should be sited prior to surgery. When marking a stoma site, the following points should be considered.	2 If the stoma is placed in the optimal position the CYP should have no problems with stoma management. This will make acceptance of the stoma a little easier.
3 The CYP should be able to see the stoma site.	3 It is important to be able to see the stoma when lying down, sitting up, and standing. Changing a pouch is extremely difficult if the stoma cannot be seen.
4 The stoma should be brought through the rectus abdominus sheath.	4 This muscle grips the bowel and will help to prevent prolapse or retraction of the stoma.
5 Any bony prominences must be avoided.	5 If the stoma is too near the hip, movement will loosen the adhesive of the pouch.
6 Any previous scars must be avoided.	6 Skin creases; folds and scars make the skin surface uneven. Loose stools will leak along these tracts.
7 The waistline of clothes should be avoided.	7 Stomas should be under the waistline both for discretion and pouch security.
8 Ensure that any prostheses or braces do not cover the site.	8 Any appliances worn can usually be adapted so as not to interfere with the pouch.
9 If the CYP uses a wheelchair, the stoma must be sited while they are in the wheelchair.	9 The stoma is usually sited higher on the abdomen, as this will make it easier to see and manage.

Principles table 5.1 Stoma pouch selection

Principle	Rationale
1 There are many different pouches produced by a number of manufacturers. However, there are basically two designs of pouch: a) A one-piece pouch, which has an adhesive flange with a pouch bonded onto it. b) A two-piece pouch, which has an adhesive flange and a separate pouch that attaches to the flange.	1 a) This pouch is designed to stay in place for 1–3 days. It also has a flat profile. b) This allows the opportunity to keep the flange on for a few days but change the pouch more frequently.
2 Both the one-piece and the two-piece pouches have either a closed end (for formed stool) or an open, drainable end (for loose stool).	2 Closed pouches need to be taken off and discarded when roughly two-thirds full. Ileostomy pouches need to be emptied roughly 3–6 times per day.
3 Urinary pouches have a tap at the end to which an overnight drainage bag can be attached. They also have a nonreturn valve in the pouch.	3 Overnight drainage bags are important to facilitate uninterrupted sleep. Nonreturn valves stop urine from tracking back up the ureters.

Principles table 5.1 Stoma pouch selection *(continued)*

Principle	Rationale
4 Older CYPs with colostomies that produce formed stools have the opportunity to use a colostomy plug. A flange is placed around the colostomy, a plug with a filter and a cap on the top is inserted into the colostomy, and then the cap snaps over the flange. The plug needs to be taken out at least every 12 hours and a pouch attached to the flange.	4 Plugs cannot be used if the stool is loose as the loose stool would probably leak out or the bowel would push out the plug. The bowel needs time to empty at least once a day.
5 The choice of pouch to be used is affected by factors such as manual dexterity, vision, and size.	5 One-piece appliances may be easier to manage for CYPs with poor vision or dexterity problems. Two piece pouches are not ideal for use with small infants, as there is often not enough room on the abdomen to attach the baseplate.
6 In the early postoperative period it is advisable to use a one-piece, clear, drainable pouch.	6 The colour of a newly formed stoma needs to be observed following surgery. A two-piece pouch will be painful to apply in the early postoperative period.

Procedure guideline 5.7 Changing a pouch

Statement	Rationale
1 Gather appropriate equipment and ensure the room is warm and private: • Receptacle to empty pouch into • Disposable gloves and plastic apron • Bowl of warm water • Gauze squares or cleansing wipes • New pouch • Bag to dispose of used pouch and cleansing materials • Scissors • Template or measuring device.	1 To be prepared to carry out the procedure without interruption.
2 Position the child/baby lying down. Older CYPs can lie down or stand up.	2 The CYP needs to be comfortable. When lying down or standing up the abdomen is smooth. When sitting upright the abdominal skin becomes wrinkled; this will compromise pouch adhesion.
3 Wash hands and put on disposable gloves and plastic apron.	3 To adhere to universal precautions.
4 If a drainable pouch is being used it needs to be emptied before removing it.	4 Unless emptied first the pouch contents will spill. Also, when parents/carers are at home they should not put full pouches in the household waste.
5 a) Remove old pouch by carefully peeling off the pouch from top to bottom with one hand, while supporting the skin with the other. b) Only silicone-based adhesive removers should be used on neonatal and infant skin.	5 a) Supporting the skin makes the procedure less uncomfortable and helps prevent the skin from tearing. b) Silicone based adhesive removers are not absorbed so do not dry out the skin, which reduces the risk of soreness.
6 The pouch can then be put into a disposable bag and discarded as per local policy for disposal of clinical waste.	6 To minimise the risk of contamination/cross-infection.
7 a) Clean the peristomal skin with warm water and gauze. b) If some residue is left on the skin from the old pouch, use a dry piece of gauze to remove it before washing. c) Do not use cotton wool. d) Ensure the skin is dried thoroughly.	7 a) Sterile water is used only in the immediate post operative period. b) The residue will spread over the skin if wet. Any residue left on the skin may interfere with the adhesion of the new pouch. c) Cotton wool will deposit strands, which may interfere with pouch adhesion.
8 Prepare the new pouch. The aperture should be cut to fit snugly around the stoma with no peristomal skin exposed.	8 It is easier to prepare the new pouch beforehand. If any skin is exposed to effluent it will become excoriated.
9 Put on the new pouch. a) If a one-piece pouch is being used, fold the adhesive backwards in half, placing the pouch on the underside of the stoma first, then flip the adhesive over the stoma and secure all around. b) If a two-piece pouch is being used. Secure the flange first and then attach the pouch. c) Pull the pouch gently. d) If a drainable pouch is being used, ensure the clip is secured correctly at the bottom of the pouch.	9 b) Two-piece pouches usually leak because the pouch has not been attached properly to the flange. c) To ensure it is attached completely. d) If the clip is not secure the pouch will fill up and subsequently leak.

(continued)

Procedure guideline 5.7 Changing a pouch (continued)

Statement	Rationale
10 Dispose the used or remaining equipment in accordance with local policies. Wash hands.	10 To minimise the risk of infection
11 The outcome of the stoma pouch change should be documented in the CYPs healthcare record.	11 To ensure a record of the procedure and outcome is made

Principles table 5.2 Potential problems with stomas

Principle	Rationale
1 A healthy stoma is red/pink in colour. It is very important, especially in the postoperative period, to check the colour of the stoma regularly. If the stoma appears darker in colour, medical advice should be sought.	1 If the blood supply is compromised the bowel will become necrosed. The stoma will become purple/black. Surgical refashioning of the stoma may be necessary.
2 In the early postoperative period all stomas will be oedematous. At 6 weeks the stoma should have shrunk to its actual size. This is important, as the parent/CYP needs to cut the pouch or flange to the exact size of the stoma. They have to be aware that the stoma will change shape and size.	2 Only one or two spare pouches should be prepared at a time. This will ensure that no abdominal skin is exposed to stoma output as the stoma shrinks. Families are advised to wait 6 weeks before arranging pre-cut pouches or having pouches/flanges cut by prescription companies.
3 Prolapse of loop stomas in infants and CYPs is common. Families need to be aware of the possibility of a prolapse, what this looks like, and when to seek medical advice. Older CYPs should be discouraged from lifting heavy weights.	3 If the prolapsed bowel remains red/pink and soft there is usually no cause for concern. If the colour changes, i.e. becomes darker, or the bowel is tense to the touch, medical advice should be sought. Some prolapses require reducing under sedation or general anaesthetic. Lifting heavy weights puts strain on the abdomen and can cause prolapse.
4 Some stomas can become retracted. This will cause more problems with an ileostomy as the output is much looser, and the stool will leak under the adhesive of the pouch. Parents/carers can seek the advice of the stoma nurse or the doctor if the stoma appears sunken.	4 Retracted stomas can be managed by using a pouch with a convex adhesive flange. This will push out the stoma. If this fails the stoma may need surgical refashioning.
5 Stenosis of the stoma can also occur. Often the narrowing of the bowel cannot be seen at the surface, but there may be a reduction in the amount of stool passed or stools may become ribbon-like.	5 Simple dilation of the stoma can solve the problem. If this does not work surgical revision of the stoma can be undertaken.
6 Over-granulation can occur if the pouch fits too tightly. Continuous rubbing on the bowel mucosa can cause a granuloma to form.	6 Granulomas can bleed easily and can be distressing. Silver nitrate can be used to treat them; if this does not work they can be surgically removed.
7 Sore peristomal skin.	7 Check correct type of pouch is fitted and the pouch has been prepared properly. Do not use any products containing alcohol on neonates or infants as the alcohol can be absorbed and skin will dry and become sore (Slater 2011).

Factors to note

Some infants who undergo surgery on the small intestine experience a temporary intolerance to lactose. Their ileostomy output will be very loose, and test positive to sugar. These babies will need special lactose-free formula milk. It is important that when these infants start weaning they are given a milk-free diet. When all corrective surgery is completed the CYP will probably be able to take a normal diet. This decision will be taken on an individual basis, with the support of a dietician.

CYPs and their parents/carers need to understand that some foodstuffs will affect stoma function. Some foods can produce more odorous stools, e.g. eggs, onions, fish, and cheese. Green vegetables, onions, beans, and fizzy drinks will increase flatus. Foods such as nuts, popcorn, or dried fruits can swell in the gastrointestinal tract and cause bowel obstructions if eaten in large amounts. However, the CYP should eat a well-balanced diet and most things can be eaten in moderation.

CYPs with urinary diversions, such as ileal conduits or mitrofanoff pouches, are encouraged to drink one to two glasses of cranberry juice daily, as this inhibits the growth of bacteria and reduces urinary infection (Goldman 2012). If they cannot drink juice it is available as a powder or pastille.

Infants and children with ileostomies are susceptible to sodium depletion. Older CYPs may complain of cramps or pins and needles in their legs, hands, or feet if sodium is low. Regular urinary sodium levels need to be taken and, if low, sodium supplements should be given. The CYP may be advised to use extra salt on their food. Foods such as marmite, cheese, or crisps are a good source of salt.

Dehydration is a potential problem for infants and children with ileostomies. Maintaining fluid balance can be difficult in small babies. Parents/carers should be aware of the usual consistency of their child's output and any increase in volume or change in consistency should be discussed with their stoma or community nurse. Advice should be given on signs of dehydration, i.e. sunken fontanel, decrease in urinary output, increase in stoma output, dark shadows under eyes, dry skin, and lethargy. Medical advice should be sought if dehydration is suspected, as infants can become very ill quickly and may need intravenous fluids.

Some older CYPs may want to try colostomy irrigation as a means of managing their colostomy. However, many of them will have tried rectal or ACE washouts in the past and want to be free of washouts. Using a colostomy plug may provide the older CYP with an alternative to wearing a pouch, especially when participating in sporting activities.

There is no doubt that surgery resulting in an altered body image is difficult to accept. For some, after many years of soiling and washouts, a stoma is a means of having control over one's bowel with less attention needed than washouts. Ongoing support is needed as the CYP goes through different stages of their life. Meeting other youngsters who have had similar surgery can be a valuable support; often CYPs feel they are the only one to have such problems. Some may need extra psychological support in coming to terms with the surgery.

Parents/carers of CYPs undergoing stoma surgery should have a discussion with the school about their child's condition. In some areas a CYP will have the support of a welfare assistant, while in other areas the parents/carers have to attend to their child's care if necessary. Older CYPs may prefer to utilise the privacy of the school nurses room to perform stoma care, as communal toilets in school are notorious for lack of privacy. Starting these discussions early will ensure as little disruption as possible to the CYP's education.

All stoma appliances are available on prescription. Prior to discharge it is usual to give the family a supply that will last until the GP prescribes more. Pharmacies may take a day or two ordering stock, therefore the family should not wait until they are using their last pouch before ordering more. Some companies offer a home delivery service but a prescription is still required from the GP. Young people who have a permanent stoma after the age of 16 will be exempt from prescription charges.

Stoma pouch selection

Many nurses ask which pouch to use. There are various factors to consider when selecting the most appropriate pouch (Black 2009b). Using an inappropriate pouch is time consuming and can cause needless discomfort and inconvenience for the CYP and their family.

Changing a pouch

When changing a pouch, especially for the first time, ensure you have enough time to perform the procedure. CYPs may be very frightened about the procedure; they will need explanations of what you are doing, and parents/carers will be trying to assimilate what they need to learn. No preparations containing alcohol should be used on premature skin, including adhesive removers and pastes. Silicone-based adhesive removers can be used. Bonding agents should not be used in preterm infants as there are limited numbers of fibrils anchoring the epidermis to the dermis in this age group. If the layer between the epidermis and dermis is weaker than the bond between the pouch adhesive and the epidermis, epidermal stripping can occur when the pouch is removed.

Potential problems with stomas

There can be problems with stoma management in paediatric patients, especially as the majority will be neonates and some will be premature and complications can be high in this age group (Patwardhan et al. 2001).

References

Alenezi, H., Alhazmi, H., Trbay, M. et al. (2014). Peristeen anal irrigation as a substitute for the MACE procedure in children who are in need of reconstructive bladder surgery. *Can Urol Assoc J.* 8 (1-2): E12–E15.

Ausili, E., Focarelli, B., Tabacco, F. et al. (2010). Transanal irrigation in myelomeningocele children: an alternative, safe and valid approach for neurogenic constipation. *Spinal Cord* 48 (7): 560–565.

Black, P. (2009a). Managing physical postoperative stoma complications. *British Journal of Nursing* 18 (7): S4–S10.

Black, P. (2009b). Choosing the correct stoma appliance. *British Journal of Nursing* 18 (4): 510, 512–514.

Fustes-Morales, A., Gutierrez-Castrellon, P., Duran-Mckinster, C. et al. (2002). Necrotizing fasciitis: report of 39 pediatric cases. *Archives of Dermatology* 138 (7): 893–899.

Goldman, R.D. (2012). Cranberry juice for urinary tract infection in children. *Canadian Family Physician* 58 (4): 398–401.

Kocaay, P., Eğrıtaş, O., Dalgıç, B. (2011). Normal defecation pattern, frequency of constipation and factors related to constipation in Turkish children 0-6 years old. *The Turkish Journal of Gastroenterology* 22(4): 369–375.

Lewis, S.J. and Heaton, K.W. (1997). Stool form scale as a useful guide to intestinal transit time. Scandinavian Journal of Gastroenterology 32 (9):920-924.

Marek, I., Benz, K., Kusnik, S. et al. (2015). Phosphate intoxication after application of enema – a life-threatening iatrogenic complication. *Klinische Pädiatrie* 227 (4): 235–238.

National Institute for Health and Care Excellence (NICE) (2010). Constipation in children and young people: diagnosis and management. www.nice.org.uk/guidance/CG99 (accessed 06 September 2022).

National Institute for Health and Care Excellence (NICE) (2014). Constipation in children and young people (QS62). Quality standard. www.nice.org.uk/guidance/qs62 (accessed 06 September 2022).

Patwardhan, N., Keily, E.M., Drake, D.P. et al. (2001). Colostomy for anorectal anomalies: high incidence of complications. *Journal of Paediatric Surgery* 36 (5): 795–798.

Peeraully, M.R., Lopes, J., Wright, A. et al. (2014). Experience of the MACE Procedure at a Regional Pediatric Surgical Unit: A 15-Year Retrospective Review. *Eur J Pediatr Surg.* 24 (1): 113–116.

Rintala, R.J. (2002). Fecal incontinence in anorectal malformations, neuropathy, and miscellaneous conditions. *Semin Pediatr Surg.* 11 (2): 75–82.

Seth, N., Llewelyn, N.E., and Howard, R.F. (2000). Parental opinions regarding the route of administration of analgesic medication in children. *Paediatric Anaesthesia* 10 (5): 537.

Slater, R. (2011). Paediatric stoma care: surgery and management. *Gastrointestinal Nursing* 9 (6): 20–26.

Williams, B.C. (2015). The Roper-Logan-Tierney model of nursing: A framework to complement the nursing process. *Nursing* 45 (3): 24–26.

Chapter 6

Burns and scalds

Brian McGowan[1] and Sally Robertson[2]

[1]RN (Child), MSc, SFHEA; Lecturer in Higher Education Practice, Ulster University, Belfast, UK
[2]MA, Pg. Cert, BA, RN Child Dip; Head of Education, Great Ormond Street Hospital, London, UK

Chapter contents

Introduction	88
Common causes of burns in CYPs	88
Overview of anatomy of the skin	88
Classification of burns	89
First aid following a burn	89
Assessment	90
Fluid resuscitation for major burns	90
Wound healing	91
Wound care	92
Choice of dressing	94
Nutrition	94
Psychological care following a burn	94
References	96

Procedure guidelines

6.1 First aid following a burn	89
6.2 Assessment of a burn	90
6.3 Dressing changes	92
6.4 Referral to the community children's nursing team	94
6.5 Ongoing care of the child	95
6.6 Health promotion and education following a burn	95

Principles table

6.1 Fluid resuscitation	91

The Great Ormond Street Hospital Manual of Children and Young People's Nursing Practices, Second Edition. Edited by Elizabeth Anne Bruce, Janet Williss, and Faith Gibson.
© 2023 John Wiley & Sons Ltd. Published 2023 by John Wiley & Sons Ltd.

Introduction

A burn[1] is a traumatic multisystem life-changing event, and the long-term care of the child or young person (CYP) who has been burned and their family can extend over several years. Effective nursing care following a burn injury is essential, as is the aftercare and ongoing treatment and prevention of scarring to promote the well-being of the child. *Note:* The terms *child* and *children*, rather than CYP(s), will be used frequently in this chapter, as burns are more common in young children. However, burns can occur at any age, including in young adults, particularly where there are physical or cognitive disabilities.)

Most burns heal without any longterm problems, but complete healing in terms of cosmetic outcome is often dependent on appropriate care, especially within the first few days after the injury. Most simple burns can be managed in primary care, but complex burns warrant a specialist and skilled multidisciplinary approach for a successful clinical outcome (Enoch et al. 2009).

It is important to remember that a burn injury can cause extreme stress for all family members. Therefore, children's nurses must ensure that the well-being of parents/carers and siblings is considered, as well as that of the child. Using a person centred model of care (Magowan and McGowan 2021) and giving consideration to the five outcomes identified within the white paper *Every Child Matters: Change for Children* (Department of Health [DH] 2004) the children's nurse should continually assess and evaluate nursing care. According to the National Burn Care Review (NBCR 2021), the goal of burn care is the restoration of form, function, and feeling and treatment should consist of seven phases (see Figure 6.1). With this in mind, this chapter will examine the process of burn management from injury through to healing and will consider the topics listed below:

- Common causes of burns
- Overview of anatomy of the skin
- Classification of burns
- First aid following a burn
- Assessment
- Fluid resuscitation for major burns
- Wound healing and wound care
- Dressing changes
- Nutrition
- Psychological care following a burn
- Referral to the Community Children's Nursing Team
- Ongoing care
- Health promotion and education following a burn

Common causes of burns in CYPs

Burns are a relatively common form of injury in childhood and can be simply defined as the death/necrosis of tissues due to exposure to or contact with a heat source. Burn injuries can usually be attributed to the following sources:

- **Scalds:** Exposure to a hot liquid or steam.
- **Fire:** Exposure to a naked flame will result in a burn.
- **Contact burns:** For example, coming into contact with an unattended iron or a radiator that is too hot.
- **Electrical burns:** These include contact with a live electrical source or lightning.
- **Radiation:** CYPs who have been inadequately protected from the sun can suffer from extensive sun burn.
- **Chemical burns:** Chemical (acid and alkali) burns differ from other kinds of burns as the damage caused may be attributed to chemical changes as opposed to heat. However, many chemicals undergo exothermic reactions on contact with the skin and this will also contribute to the severity of the burn. Knowledge of the specific chemical agent involved will direct subsequent intervention.

Scalds are the most common cause of burn injury in children, representing 43% of acute burn injuries. It is estimated that on average 110 children per day are seen in emergency departments with burn injuries, 46 as a result of a hot cup of tea or coffee spill, and the most common place of injury for children is in the home, 49% of whom are burnt in the kitchen (Children's Burns Trust 2016).

Overview of anatomy of the skin

The skin is the largest organ of the human body (Taylor 2001). Whilst acting as a cover for the body, the skin provides protection from bacteria, as well as maintaining temperature and preventing water loss. In children under 2 years of age, the skin is one-fifth thinner than adult skin (Peters 2001). It is comprised of two main layers; the epidermis and dermis. The epidermis is made up of epithelial cells, split into four layers, and acts as the outermost protective shield of the body. Below this layer lies the dermis, which makes up the bulk of the skin. The dermis has two major layers comprised of connective tissue. Connective tissue is made up of three types of fibres, the most abundant of which are collagen fibres. The connective tissue gives the skin its strength. Only the dermis is vascularised and nutrients reach the epidermis by diffusing through tissue fluid from blood vessels in the dermis. The dermis is rich in nerve fibres, blood vessels, and lymphatic vessels. Below the dermis lies the hypodermis or subcutaneous layer, which is made up of adipose and connective tissue. The subcutaneous layer thus anchors the skin to underlying organs in the body. Approximately half of the body's fat stores are located in the subcutaneous layer and it acts as an effective shock absorber, as well as an insulator to prevent heat loss (Marieb 2004).

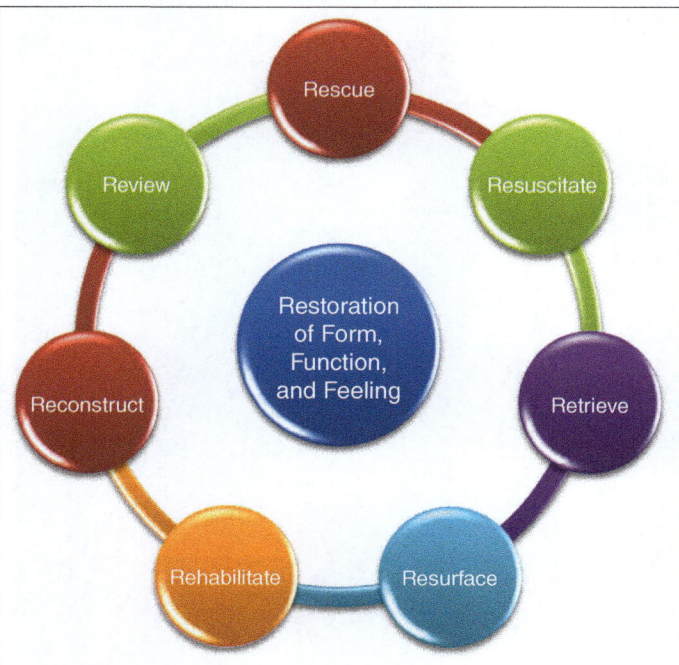

Figure 6.1 Seven phases of burn management (National Burn Care Review 2001).

---

[1] The original authors of this chapter were Lorraine Laccohee, Juanita Harrison, and Brian McGowan.

Classification of burns

Classification of a burn relies on clinical observation and this remains the 'standard for diagnosis' (Heimbach et al. 2002). The following list has been adapted from Appleby (2005).

- **Superficial burns:** Limited to the superficial epidermal layer of the skin. The appearance will be red, caused by erythema and possibly blistered. The skin will blanch on pressure and sensation will be extremely painful, as no nerve endings will have been damaged. The sun and minor scalds mainly cause superficial burns. These burns do not tend to scar.
- **Superficial partial thickness burns:** The entire epidermis will have been burnt, causing a pink surface with both open and closed blisters. The skin will blanch less quickly on pressure and will be painful for the child. Scalding to the skin mainly causes this depth of burn.
- **Deep partial thickness burns:** The epidermis and dermis will have been destroyed here, leaving some skin appendages. The burn appearance will be a cream base with blisters. The area will not blanch and will be less painful for the child as some nerve endings have been destroyed.
- **Deep or full thickness burns:** This type of burn involves the dermis and underlying fat. The appearance of the skin will be white, brown, black, leathery and waxy as a result of all layers of the skin being penetrated. These burns will not blister and are painless and numb for the child, as all nerve endings will have been destroyed.

First aid following a burn

Appropriate first aid must be used to treat any burns or scalds as soon as possible. This will limit the amount of damage to the skin (National Health Service [NHS] 2022).

The initial first aid stages for any scald/burn are:

- Stop the burning process as soon as possible. This may mean removing the person from the area, dousing flames with water, or smothering flames with a blanket. Do not put yourself at risk of getting burnt as well.
- Remove any clothing or jewellery near the burnt area of skin, including babies' nappies. However, do not try to remove anything that's stuck to the burnt skin as this could cause more damage.
- Cool the burn with cool or lukewarm running water for 20 minutes, as soon as possible after the injury. Never use ice, iced water, or any creams or greasy substances such as butter.
- Keep yourself or the person warm. Use a blanket or layers of clothing, but avoid putting them on the injured area. Keeping warm will prevent hypothermia, which is a risk when cooling a large burnt area, particularly in young children and the elderly.
- Cover the burn with cling film. Put the cling film in a layer over the burn, rather than wrapping it around a limb. A clean, clear plastic bag can be used for burns on your hand.
- Treat the pain with analgesia.
- Sit upright as much as possible if the face or eyes are burnt. Avoid lying down for as long as possible as this will help to reduce swelling (NHS 2022).

Procedure guideline 6.1 First aid following a burn

Statement	Rationale

1 Assess the child's:
  a) Airway:
    • Have they been in a house fire?
    • Are there burns around the nose, mouth, and neck?
    • Is there soot around the nose and mouth?
  b) Breathing:
    • Rate
    • Rhythm
    • Noise
    • Work.
  c) Circulation:
    • Check pulse
    • Are there any circumferential burns or full thickness burns that may restrict blood flow to periphery?
	1
	a, b) A child's airway is naturally smaller in diameter than an adult airway. A burn involving the airway may result in tracheal oedema and obstruct breathing.
	
	c) Swelling from a full thickness or circumferential burn may compromise a child's circulation. In this situation an emergency escharotomy (release of rigid burnt skin) may be performed, allowing the tissue to expand and restore blood flow to the burned area.

2 Administer first aid:
  a) Immerse affected area in or place under running cold water promptly.
    NB. Do not use ice as a cooling fluid as this will constrict capillaries.
  b) Limit application of cold water to 10 minutes or 20 minutes in the case of extensive burns or alkali burns.
  c) Elevate any limbs involved if possible and sit the child up if the burn is above the navel.
  d) Do not attempt to remove clothing unless the burn is chemical.
  e) Topical applications should be confined to wet compresses or sterile dressings while medical advice is being sought.
  f) Apply cling film as a temporary dressing or to retain a cold compress while awaiting medical intervention.
  g) Cling film should be applied in small, overlapping sections.
	2
	a) To reduce/remove heat energy from the area. Cold water rapidly cools residual heat, which will relieve pain, reduce tissue damage, and reassure the child.
	b) Excessive use of water can cause hypothermia. When the skin has been burned it is unable to prevent the loss of body fluid or keep the body at its normal temperature.
	c) Elevation of the burnt limb decreases oedema to the affected area.
	d) Removal of clothing may deroof blisters or take off skin, thus increasing distress. However, a chemical burn will continue while the material is next to the skin.
	e) A wet dressing will continue cooling and thus relieve pain. Any other substance used could hinder subsequent examination and assessment.
	f) To help relieve pain, as the burn and thus the nerve endings are not exposed to the air so readily. Applying cling film will reduce the risk of bacterial contamination in the first instance. Cling film and a compress will also prevent the child from seeing the wound, therefore helping to reduce distress.
	g) To avoid constrictions to blood flow (Fowler 1998).

Procedure guideline 6.2 Assessment of a burn

Statement	Rationale
1 a) Take a detailed chronology of how the burn occurred. b) If there is any suspicion of nonaccidental injury, then local child protection guidelines must be followed.	1 a) To ensure that treatment given is appropriate to the extent of the burn. b) To ensure consistency and identify any discrepancies that might be indicative of a nonaccidental injury.
2 a) Establish the timescale of when the burn happened and the length of time the child was in contact with the source of the burn. b) Establish what first aid measures, if any, were taken.	2 a) To aid with the classification and depth of the burn. Fluid resuscitation begins from the time of injury, NOT the time of admission to hospital. On admission, fluid resuscitation may already be in arrears. b) To enable more accurate classification of the burn and aid health education once the wound is healing.
3 Assess the depth of the burn: a) Observe and record the colour of the skin, presence of blisters, and the texture of the skin (Fowler 1998). b) Assess the skin for capillary refill by applying pressure to affected areas. c) Assess the child's level of pain. d) The percentage of burns on the child's body must also be assessed. This can be carried out using a Lund and Browder chart (1944). e) Alternatively the extent of the burn can be assessed by using the child's own palm size. The "rule of nines" may also be used (modified for use in children) to calculate the percentage body surface area burned. f) The assessment of the size of the burn should be checked by two experienced practitioners, one of whom is usually a doctor. The assessment should be documented on the body chart (Lund and Browder 1944).	3 a) To determine the severity and extent of the burn. b) Poor capillary refill indicates a deeper burn. c) A burn is intensely painful. Deeper burns will have destroyed nerve endings but a burn is usually of mixed depth. Do not assume that a full thickness burn is painless for a child. d) The Lund and Browder charts account for both age and size differences in children. For example, the head will be proportionately larger than the limbs. The child's surface area is therefore accounted for (see Figure 6.2). e) The child's own palm size represents 1% of a burn. This can be a more difficult method unless the child is co-operative and the burn is in one small area. For more information regarding using the rule of nines to calculate total body surface area see Moore et al. (2020). f) Inaccurate estimation of burn size can occur, with small burns being overestimated and large burns being underestimated (Collis et al. 1999). This has knock-on effects for the calculation of resuscitation fluid.
5 If the child has sustained injuries to the face or neck they should be encouraged to sit up. NB: Children who have received burns to these areas should be treated at a regional burns unit and may require assessment by an anaesthetist prior to transfer.	5 To reduce oedema and thus reduce the potential for respiratory distress.

Once first aid has been administered, the course of action taken following a burn injury is dependent on a number of variables, including age, percentage of body surface area affected, depth of burn and any associated injuries. In children, a burn involving more than 10% of the total body surface area requires resuscitation and once this is commenced the child should be referred to a specialist centre. However, smaller burns may also be problematic and require treatment in specialist centres to minimise the risk of complications. The following types of burns should be referred to a specialist unit (NBCR 2021):

- Burns greater than 10% in children
- In infants under 1 year of age
- Burns of special areas – face, hands feet, genitals, perineum, and over major joints
- Circumferential burns to limbs or chest
- Full thickness burns greater than 5% of total body surface area
- Electrical burns
- Chemical burns
- Burns with associated inhalation injury
- Burns indicative of nonaccidental injury

Assessment

As with all trauma, children who have been burned should be assessed according to trauma management guidelines beginning with airway (A), breathing (B), and circulation (C). Basic trauma management appropriately performed at this stage can offset the development of complications at a later stage and will have a profound effect on eventual outcomes. The child's condition should be stabilised before treatment of the burn; for resuscitation, see Chapter 30.

Fluid resuscitation for major burns

The first 24 hours following the burn is known as the shock phase. If a child's injuries cover 10% of their body surface area they will have lost a large amount of body fluid. Fluid resuscitation is required to maintain the tissue perfusion in the early phase of burn shock, in which hypovolaemia occurs due to steady fluid extravasation from the intravascular compartment (Walker et al. 2014).

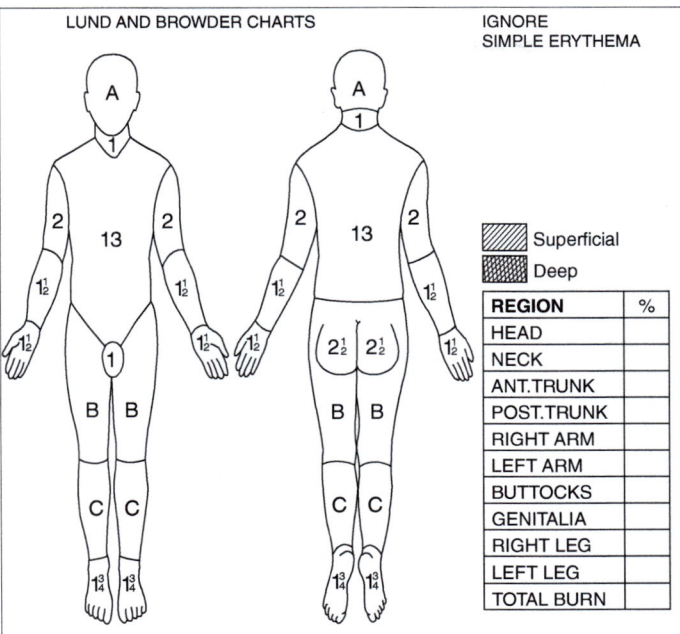

Figure 6.2 The Lund and Browder charts (Lund and Browder (1944), cited in Bosworth 1997).

Evidence suggests that timely fluid resuscitation is vital to minimise the risk of hypovolaemic shock and infection, which can significantly reduce multiorgan failure and mortality in thermally injured children (Zuo et al. 2017).

Box 6.1 Parkland Formula

> **Parkland formula for fluid replacement** (Pape et al. 2001).
> 3–4 ml Hartmann's solution × body weight (kg) × % burn
> = Total amount of resuscitation fluid to be infused in 24 hrs

Wound healing

Wound healing

As with any wound, the healing of a burn goes through several stages: the inflammatory phase, destructive phase, proliferative phase, and maturation. The healing of a burn will depend largely on the depth. The following is an approximate guideline:

Depth of Burn	Length of Healing Time
Superficial	Generally 3–7 days.
Superficial dermal burns	Up to 14 days. Skin grafting may be required if burn is over a joint.
Deep dermal burn	28 days to several months. Skin grafting is likely to be needed unless area is particularly small.
Full thickness burn	Unlikely to heal without surgical intervention. Skin grafting will be needed.

Principles table 6.1 Fluid resuscitation

Principle	Rationale
1 The majority of burns units recommend the use of crystalloids for fluid replacement (Pape et al. 2001) although colloids are also used.	1 A Cochrane review concluded that colloids are more expensive than crystalloids and have not been shown to be any more effective in fluid resuscitation (Lewis et al. 2018).
2 The Parkland formula (Pape et al. 2001) is used to replace lost fluid over 24 hours (see Box 6.1). a. Half of the calculated total is given over the first 8 hours; the second half is given over the remaining 16 hours. b. Fluid resuscitation begins from the time of the injury and NOT the time of admission.	2 To maintain blood supply to all vital organs, particularly the viscera. To prevent and treat hypovolaemic shock.
3 The child also has a metabolic water requirement. This should be given at 1.5 ml per kg per hour. Infants should receive a minimum of 30 ml per hour (Prelack et al. 2017).	
4 Regular monitoring of urea, glucose, and electrolytes; packed cell volume; and urine output during the resuscitation phase is essential.	4 To replace electrolytes lost through the burn injury. Young children may be particularly prone to hypoglycaemia.
5 Oral consumption of liquids should be encouraged if possible.	5, 6 There is a significant risk of paralytic ileus developing and early feeding offsets its development (Shields et al. 2016).
6 If the burn is >10% total body surface area (TBSA), a nasogastric tube should be passed and enteral feeding started immediately.	6 To ensure adequate hydration and nutrition, which is essential for cell growth and wound healing (Shields et al. 2016).
7 Fluid intake and output should be closely monitored. Following fluid resuscitation a child should be able to maintain an adequate urine output while fluid maintenance is decreased.	7 Urine output is the most important indicator of response to fluid resuscitation (Fowler et al. 1996). If this is not achieved, there is the potential of acute renal failure.

Wound care

Over the years there has been much debate over whether blisters from the burn should be de-roofed or remain intact before applying a dressing. Burn blisters are formed as a result of damaged capillaries leaking plasma. This leads to the heat-damaged epidermis lifting and separating from the dermis and the accumulated fluid thus causing the blister. Reseach suggests that most blisters should be debrided rather than left intact; the debridement enables better recovery for patients, involves fewer staff resources, and enables a full assessment of the wound. Any blister smaller than the patient's little fingernail can be left intact, but any larger than this should be de-roofed (Murphy and Amblum 2014).

Once a wound assessment has been made, an appropriate dressing can be chosen to enhance the healing process see Table 6.1.

Burns dressings

Burns dressings are carried out to reduce the risk of infection and to minimise pain. Cleansing of the wound should allow removal of excess exudate and previous dressing product debris. Dressings should be generous in covering the whole of the wound and should not slip. Dressing changes should be left for as long as possible, as repeated changes increase the risk of wound infection. Although the research is weak, there is some evidence to suggest that antibiotics should not be used as prophylactic treatment, as they may increase the risk of resistant bacteria developing (Barajas-Nava et al. 2013; Burch and Köpke 2016). The contact layer should be chosen to best suit the needs of the wound. A partnership approach to wound management is recommended, with the dressing of choice chosen in consultation with colleagues from the multidisciplinary team.

Burns dressings are a traumatic experience, so should be as stress free as possible. Dressing changes and wound cleansing have been identified as the most painful wound-care interventions for a child (Kammerlander and Eberlein 2002). Appropriate and sufficient pain relief is therefore essential prior to carrying out the dressing change. Following consultation with medical colleagues, appropriate prescription and administration of oral morphine should be offered 30 minutes before a dressing change is due to start. This may also be supplemented with an anxiolytic such as Midazolam (Byers et al. 2001; Hansen et al. 2001). For children who are more anxious, the use of Entonox may well be more appropriate, as it provides both analgesia and anxiolysis. Entonox can also provide distraction and requires the child to take control of their own pain relief and regulate their breathing (Bruce and Franck 2000). For more information on the use of Entonox and other pain guidelines see Chapter 24: Pain Management. The role of the family in this scenario is pivotal and their participation should be discussed in advance to ascertain what role they wish to play. Support from play staff can also be beneficial in helping to prepare the child and offer suitable distraction during the procedure (see Chapter 27: Play as a Therapeutic Tool for further information).

Table 6.1 Examples of dressing and creams

Occlusive or low adherent dressings	These are laid directly over the wound surface, allow exudate through from the wound bed, and minimise pain on removal.
Foam dressings	If blisters are present, these can be used as a secondary dressing over an occlusive or paraffin gauze dressing to soak up excess exudates and provide a comfortable cushioned layer to the wound. Foam dressings come in different depths and can be cut to shape without this affecting their function.
Soft gauze	Use over the occlusive dressing if the area is dry with no blistering and secure with a crepe bandage to provide extra cushioning protection and keep the area clean and dry.
Hydrocolloid dressings	Can be laid directly over the wound surface. These soak up exudates and form a gel that keeps the burn moist and warm. The healing wound would need to be reassessed to ensure that exudate does not leak through once its capacity has been reached.
Antimicrobial creams	May be prescribed and used with dressings. These have good hydrating properties and antimicrobial factors, thus reducing the risk of bacterial infection and promoting comfort (McKirdy 2001).

Procedure guideline 6.3 Dressing changes

For any dressing change the following equipment will be needed:

- Clean dressing trolley or suitable large clean surface.
- Sterile dressing pack and spare galley pot.
- Sterile gloves.
- Appropriate dressings to place over the wound bed – follow local guidelines.
- Gauze/foam dressings appropriate to the size that will be needed for the limb – follow local guidelines.
- Appropriate creams prescribed.
- Bandages and tape to secure dressing.
- Spatulas to decant any cream into a separate container.
- Plastic disposable apron.
- Disposable plastic bag for soiled dressings, etc.
- Wound swabs.

Statement	Rationale
1 If possible, two nurses should be available to perform the dressing change.	1 This enables one nurse to remain 'clean.'
2 The room should be warmed prior to commencing the dressing change if there is extensive skin loss.	2 Extensive skin loss can result in a rapid reduction in body heat due to convection, conduction, and radiation.

Procedure guideline 6.3 Dressing changes (continued)

Statement	Rationale
3 Explain the procedure in full to the child and the parent/carer using appropriate language that is easily understood. Give the parent/carer the option to remain in the room while the dressing change is carried out. Explanation should include how the dressing change will be done, how long it might take, and what the child might expect from the dressing change.	3 To ensure they understand the procedure fully. NB: Information and explanation should continue throughout the dressing change for the same reason.
4 If the parents/carers are staying, ensure that their role has been discussed before the procedure begins.	4 To help relieve any feelings of anxiety and promote adherance from the child by involving the parent/carer.
5 Involve the skills of a play specialist where appropriate in order to distract and occupy the child while the procedure is being carried out.	5 Distraction will capture the child's attention and imagination and help to reduce distress. Examples include the use of bubbles or water toys if in the bath (Webster 2000).
6 Assess the child's current level of pain and administer pain relief in anticipation of pain during the procedure.	6 As well as background pain a dressing change will induce significant breakthrough pain. Administration of pain relief in advance will offset the intensity and or duration of the pain and make the procedure more bearable.
7 Thoroughly wash and dry hands using soap and water (follow local handwashing policies).	7 To minimise the risk of infection.
8 Use an aseptic technique to set up the dressing trolley with the appropriate dressings, creams and bandages prior to commencing the dressing change.	8 To prevent infection. For more information on the aseptic nontouch technique (ANTT) see Chapter 14: Intravenous and Intra-arterial Access and Infusions
9 For large areas, ensure that the gauze is already rolled. The number of dressings needed must be estimated and opened before starting the dressing change.	9 To enable the burnt limb to be dressed quickly and easily, causing minimal distress to the child. Being organised and prepared will cause less anxiety for the child and parent/carer and prevent unnecessary waste.
10 If creams are being used, then use a spatula to remove cream from the pots into a separate sterile container. Ensure pots are then labelled with child's name to ensure they are not used for anyone else.	10 The use of a spatula and separate pots of cream for each individual child will avoid cross-infection.
11 For dressing changes being carried out in the bath, ensure that the bathroom is kept warm (above 27°C). Run the bath to an appropriate depth, ensuring that all limbs are covered with tepid water.	11 To minimise the risk of hyperthermia.
12 Remove old dressings from the wound. For children having a bath the majority should be removed before they enter the bath.	12 Removal of dressings allows reassessment of the burn area and any change of treatment can then be decided. Removal also allows the skin to be cleaned in order that any infection can be identified and swabbed.
13 Do not remove a dressing with force. Stubborn dressings should be soaked off in the bath or soaked off using saline or tepid water.	13 Forcing a dressing is extremely traumatic and can destroy new epithelial tissue and delay the healing process further. Children may cope better with the procedure if they are able to soak their own dressings off in the bath (Bale 1996).
14 Gently pat skin dry once the burnt area has been cleansed. Clean towels will need to be used if the child has been bathed.	14 To avoid destroying new epithelial tissue. To avoid infection of the wound area.
15 If carrying out a dressing change without bathing, use normal saline or lukewarm tap water to cleanse the area.	15 To clean the area (National Institute for Health and Care Excellence [NICE] 2020).
16 Following cleansing, apply appropriate cream or dressing to the affected area (adhere to local guidelines). The wound contact layer chosen should be determined in partnership with members of the multidisciplinary team following wound assessment.	16 All dressings act as a protective layer before application of gauze and should promote wound healing and allow skin to heal without sticking to the new dermal layer.
17 Apply generous layers of gauze or foam dressing over the initial dressing, ensuring all affected areas are covered.	17 Gauze or foam dressing will provide comfort through padding and also soaks up any exudate from blisters. This will enable the wound dressing to remain intact for some time.
18 Apply layers of crepe bandage and secure with tape, ensuring that the tape does not contract and squeeze the affected area.	18 To provide support and fix the dressing in place without affecting circulation.

Choice of dressing

The aim of a burn dressing is to keep the area clean and dry and prevent the wound from becoming infected. However, in addition to this, the dressing used will play a key role by providing the right environment to support and promote wound healing (Baranoski 2005). No one dressing is suitable for all types of wounds. Benbow (2004) identifies the following issues that will influence choice of dressing:

- The action of the dressing, i.e. what you want the dressing to do
- What the limitations of that dressing are
- How the dressing should be applied and removed.

Specifically when dressing burns, the depth, surface area and moistness need to be considered when selecting an appropriate dressing. Evidence shows that moisture plays an important part in wound healing. However, there needs to be the correct balance that will draw away excess exudate while maintaining moisture in the wound bed (Baranoski 2005). The nurse must also consider which dressings to combine together in order to promote optimum healing and be cost effective. Table 6.1 gives a few examples of how a burn wound can be dressed. However, choice of dressings will largely depend on local hospital or primary care trust guidelines for wound management and local policy should always be followed.

Nutrition

All children require a balanced diet of vitamins, minerals, and nutrients as they grow. When the skin has been damaged, nutrition plays an important role in the promotion of wound healing. Additionally, a burn injury is a major cause of catabolism and is associated with an accelerated metabolic rate and abnormalities in lipid and carbohydrate metabolism. Casey (1998) stated that children who are deficient in nutrients can be susceptible to impaired healing due to the following:

- Deficiency in vitamin C inhibits collagen synthesis and capillary development. This is due to the unique structure of this group of proteins, which require vitamin C to form stable bonds between the collagen fibres.
- Protein is also essential for wound healing. Granulation and tissue repair rely greatly on the presence of amino acids and thus a protein deficiency will inhibit these mechanisms (Wallace 1994).
- A deficiency in zinc will inhibit epithelialisation. Zinc is essential for protein synthesis and therefore will be needed wherever cell division is taking place.

In the days following a burn injury involving more than 10% of the total body surface area, the caloric need of the body is greatly increased (Wilson 2000). For this reason it is recommended that a specialist dietician should carry out an assessment of the child's nutritional state. Appropriate nutritional supplements can then be provided in order to promote wound healing. If the child is unwilling or unable to manage food orally appropriate steps will need to be taken to ensure that they are receiving adequate nutrition. In the initial stages the child might benefit from having a nasogastric tube inserted to ensure they receive the optimum nutritional intake.

Psychological care following a burn

The psychological recovery from a burn injury is a long process. The child may display signs of extreme anxiety through the initial trauma, repeated exposure to painful procedures, and possible separation from parents/carers. In addition, long-term hospitalisation can also lead to emotional problems. Parents/carers, as well, may require emotional support. Feelings of guilt over the accident or incident are common. Assessment by a psychologist may be indicated to guide care interventions. A compassionate partnership approach to psychological care is recommended from admission to discharge and requires empathy and a nonjudgemental attitude. The British Burn Association has set clear guidance within their standards, which should be adhered to when caring for the psychological needs of patients following a burn injury (National Network for Burn Care 2018).

Procedure guideline 6.4 Referral to the community children's nursing team

When preparing the child and family for discharge, the community children's nursing (CCN) team within the primary care setting may need to take over the care of the burn. Early contact with the community team is essential. Depending on the initial severity of the burn, physiotherapy and potentially occupational therapy referral may be required.

Statement	Rationale
1 Telephone the CCN team with the contact details for the family and a summary of the ongoing care requirements.	1 To ensure that the referral can be accepted by the CCN team and that they have the correct details and understand the care needs of the child
2 Complete and forward the appropriate referral form, including the child's name, date of birth, address, telephone number, name of person with parental responsibility, GP details, diagnosis, nursing care required, and any other relevant information.	2 To ensure a smooth transition from hospital to home and consistent nursing care.
5 Negotiate directly with the CCN about what dressings will be sent home with the child.	5 To ensure they are aware of the child's needs at home. It can take several days for the local team to prescribe and supply the appropriate dressings.
6 Discharge the child with appropriate analgesia for dressing changes and ensure that parents/carers know how long before the procedure to administer analgesia.	6 Parents/carers can be empowered to administer pain relief before the CCN arrives at the home.
7 Document all liaison and communication.	7 Accurate record keeping is essential (NMC 2015).

Chapter 6 Burns and scalds

Procedure guideline 6.5 Ongoing care of the child

Scar formation following a burn injury will depend on the depth of the burn. A superficial burn will usually leave minimal scarring, while deeper burns may leave more obvious scars. Redness will be evident for months following healing as the skin has formed new epithelial tissue that needs time to mature fully. At this time the new skin will be hypersensitive to both heat and cold.

Statement	Rationale
1 Educate the child and parent/carer to use total sun block on the new area of skin for at least 12 months (McKirdy 2001).	1 New skin needs time to mature and will be extremely sensitive to heat (Howell 1998).
2 Educate the family to gently massage the new area of skin using a moisturiser for sensitive skin several times every day.	2 Moisturisers help restore the skin's normal texture; minimise scar tissue; and prevent flaking and dryness that can occur in freshly healed burns (McKirdy 2001). These symptoms are due to the newly epithelialised tissue producing less skin oils.
3 Encourage the child and family to comply with programmes of occupational therapy and physiotherapy.	3 Ongoing adherence will reduce the incidence/effect of contracture formation and will help in the restoration of function. Superficial and partial thickness burns will eventually return to normal function, but full thickness burns will not recover this ability (Fowler 1998).
4 Any burn will alter the skin's makeup and has the potential to scar. Pressure garments are extremely effective in the control of scar management and should be applied immediately following wound healing (Robson et al. 1998). Silicone gels may also help in the control and management of hypertrophic scarring, reducing discomfort and irritation (Majan 2006).	4 Application of pressure to the scar area will prevent further shortening of collagen within the new skin area and help prevent excessive scarring until the scar is mature, which has been achieved when the scar is avascular, flat, and soft (Wilson 2000).
5 a) Encourage the wearing of pressure garments. The garment should be worn for 23 hours per day for 1–2 years until the scar is mature (Wilson 2000). b) Garments should be washed regularly and may need to be altered as the child grows. Children may find the garments hot and sometimes confining, so positive reinforcement of the benefits needs to be provided. However, they may also find them comforting as they cover up marking/scarring and thus draw attention away from the burn injury.	5 a) Daily adherence will ensure the best results for the child's scarring. Pressure garments work to minimise the appearance of scars but will not prevent scar formation. However, they do help to protect the newly healed skin. b) To maintain hygiene and comfort and promote concordance.

Procedure guideline 6.6 Health promotion and education following a burn

Health promotion is an essential part of the care provided to a child following a burn injury. There are two elements to consider: Firstly, the newly healed burn will be sensitive to sunlight and must be protected at all times by avoiding contact with direct sunlight and the use of high-factor or total-block sun creams. Secondly, the risk of further burns injuries can be avoided by providing education regarding the causes of burns and how these can be prevented. The following guidelines can be used as a basis for re-educating parents/carers.

Statement	Rationale
Hot water/liquids	
1 Keep hot liquid drinks out of reach of children.	1 If a hot drink is on the floor or low table, the child is more likely to knock or kick the cup over, potentially causing a burning scald. Boiling water causes superficial skin loss in just 0.1 seconds and a full thickness burn in 1 second (Clarke 1992).
2 Always check the temperature of bathwater before allowing your child to get in. Teach your children not to touch the taps. Never leave the child unsupervised in the bathtub. If possible run the cold water first and then add hot water until a suitable temperature is reached. Alternatively, thermostats can be fixed so that the water temperature does not exceed a certain limit, for example, 40 °C.	2 Scalding can occur in a matter of seconds. A fall into bath water at 42 °C results in partial thickness skin loss in just 1 second and full thickness loss within 10 seconds (Clarke 1992).
3 Turn saucepan handles toward the back of the stove when cooking. Never leave a child unsupervised in the kitchen.	3 Small children will naturally be tempted to pull a handle that is above them. This could potentially cause burns to the face and body as well as the arms and legs.

(continued)

Procedure guideline 6.6 Health promotion and education following a burn *(continued)*

Statement	Rationale
Electricity	
1 Place plastic childproof plugs into all unused electrical sockets. Always unplug equipment with a heat output when not in use (e.g. electrical heaters, hairdryers).	1 Little fingers fit very easily into plug sockets and thus potentially are at risk of an electrical burn.
2 Always keep irons out of reach even when cooling and never leave unattended.	2 Equipment like this can be easy to operate and may lead to a thermal burn if used by young children unsupervised. Irons remain hot for a period of time after switching off.
3 Keep extension cords used out of sight and to a minimum.	3 Young children may be easily able to unplug from the extension cord, which puts them at risk of an electrical burn.
Matches and candles	
1 Keep matches in a container that a child cannot open and keep them out of their reach. Remember that children can stand on chairs and climb up to shelves to obtain things.	1 To avoid accidental injury.
2 Avoid smoking in the presence of children and in particular, avoid having a child on your lap when smoking. Ensure that all cigarettes and lighters are kept out of reach.	2 To avoid accidental injury. A cigarette tip is a potential burn hazard.
3 Ensure a child is supervised near burning candles or incense. Never leave burning candles unattended.	3 A child can easily put their hand into the flame or knock the candle over, potentially causing a burn injury.
Fire safety	
1 Keep a small fire extinguisher handy in the kitchen. Ensure older children know how the extinguisher works.	1 For a small fire this might be adequate to extinguish the blaze.
2 Educate your children in how to alert the emergency services.	2 The parent or adult may not be able to access the telephone and may need to rely on someone else.
3 Educate your children to leave the house quickly and safely if there is a fire and to avoid any smoke-filled areas.	3 It may not be possible for a person to ensure everyone else is safely outside if the house is filling with smoke.

References

Appleby, T. (2005). Burns. In: *Critical Care Nursing; a Holistic Approach*, 8e (eds. P.G. Morton, D.K. Fontaine, C.M. Hudak and B.M. Gallo). Philadelphia: Lippincott Williams & Wilkins.

Bale, S. (1996). Caring for children with wounds. *Journal of Wound Care* 5 (4): 177–180.

Barajas-Nava, L.A., López-Alcalde, J., Roqué i Figuls, M. et al. (2013). Antibiotic prophylaxis for preventing burn wound infection. *Cochrane Database of Systematic Reviews* (6): CD008738. https://doi.org/10.1002/14651858.CD008738.pub2.

Baranoski, S. (2005). Wound dressings, a myriad of challenging decisions. *Home Healthcare Nurse* 23 (5): 305–315.

Benbow, M. (2004). Mixing dressings – a clinical governance issue. *Journal of Community Nursing* 18 (3): 26–32.

Bosworth, C. (1997). *Burns Trauma: Management and Nursing Care*. London: Ballière Tindall.

Bruce, E. and Franck, L. (2000). Self-administered nitrous oxide (Entonox) for the management of procedural pain. *Paediatric Nursing* 12 (7): 15–19.

Burch J. and Köpke S. (2016). Can prophylactic antibiotics prevent burn wound infection? Cochrane Clinical Answers. https://www.cochranelibrary.com/cca/doi/10.1002/cca.815/full (accessed 10 September 2022).

Byers, J.F., Bridges, S., Kijek, J., and LaBorde, P. (2001). Burn childs' pain and anxiety experiences. *Journal of Burn Care Rehabilitation* 22: 144–149.

Casey, G. (1998). The importance of nutrition in wound healing. *Nursing Standard* 13 (3): 51–54.

Children's Burns Trust (2016). www.cbtrust.org.uk (accessed 8 June 2018).

Clarke, J. (1992). *A Colour Atlas of Burn Injury*. London: Chapman and Hall.

Collis, N., Smith, G., and Fenton, O.M. (1999). Accuracy of burn size estimation and subsequent fluid resuscitation prior to arrival at the Yorkshire Regional Burns Unit. A three-year retrospective study. *Burns* 25: 345–351.

Department of Health (DH) and Department for Education and Skills (DfE) (2004). *National Service Framework for Children, Young People and Maternity Services*. London: HMSO.

Enoch, S., Roshan, A., and Shah, M. (2009). Emergency and early management of burns and scalds. *BMJ* 338: b1037. https://www.bmj.com/content/338/bmj.b1037 (accessed 10 September 2022).

Fowler, A. (1998). Nursing management of minor burn injuries. *Emergency Nurse* 6 (6): 31–37.

Fowler, A., Byers, J., and Flynn, M.B. (1996). Acute burn injury: a trauma case report. *Critical Care Nurse* 16 (4): 55–65.

Hansen, S.L., Voigt, D.W., and Paul, C.N. (2001). A retrospective study on the effectiveness of intranasal midazolam in pediatric burn child. *Journal of Burn Care Rehabilitation* 22: 6–8.

Heimbach, D., Mann, R., and Engrav, L. (2002). Evaluation of the burn wound management decisions. In: *Total Burn Care*, 2e (ed. D. Herndon), 101–108. London: Saunders.

Holt, L. (1998). Assessing and managing minor burns. *Emergency Nurse* 6 (2): 14–16.

Howell, F. (1998). Management of minor burn injuries. *Practice Nurse* 15 (4): 208–212.

Kammerlander, G. and Eberlein, T. (2002). Nurses views about pain and trauma at dressing changes: a central European perspective. *Journal of Wound Care* 11 (2): 76–79.

Lewis, S.R., Pritchard, M.W., Evans, D.J.W., Butler, A.R., Alderson, P., Smith, A.F., and Roberts, I. (2018). Colloids versus crystalloids for fluid resuscitation in critically ill patients. *Cochrane Database of Systematic Reviews* (3): https://www.cochranelibrary.com/cdsr/doi/10.1002/14651858.CD000567.pub7/full (accessed 10 September 2022).

Lund, C. and Browder, N. (1944). Estimation of areas of burns. In: *Burns Trauma: Management and Nursing Care* (ed. C. Bosworth), 1997. London: Ballière Tindall.

Magowan, R. and McGowan, B. (2021). Being person-centred in children's services. In: *Fundamentals of Person-Centred Healthcare Practice* (eds. B. McCormack, T. McCance, C.Bulley, D. Brown, A. McMillan and S. Martin) Hoboken: Wiley Blackwell.

Majan, J.I. (2006). Evaluation of a self-adherent soft silicone dressing for the treatment of hypertrophic postoperative scars. *Journal of Wound Care* 15 (5): 193–196.

Marieb, E.N. (2004). The integumentary system. In: *Human Anatomy and Physiology*, 6e (eds. E.N. Marieb, J.B. Mallatt and R.T. Hutchings). New York: Pearson/Benjamin Cummings.

McKirdy, L. (2001). Management of minor burns. *Journal of Community Nursing* 15 (10): 28–33.

Moore, R.A., Waheed, A., and Burns B. (2020). Rule of nines. StatPearls Publishing. https://www.statpearls.com/ArticleLibrary/viewarticle/28674 (accessed 10 September 2022).

Murphy, F. and Amblum, J. (2014). Treatment for burn blisters: debride or leave intact? *Emergency Nurse* 22 (2): 24–27.

National Burn Care Review (NBCR) (2021). National Burn Care Review 2021. https://www.britishburnassociation.org/national-burn-care-review/ (accessed 10 September 2022).

National Health Service (NHS) (2022). Burns and scalds. https://www.nhs.uk/conditions/burns-and-scalds/ (accessed 10 September 2022).

National Institute for Health and Care Excellence (NICE) (2020). Burns and Scalds. Clinical knowledge summaries. https://cks.nice.org.uk/burns-and-scalds#!scenario:3 (accessed 10 September 2022).

National Network for Burn Care (2018). National burn care standards. http://www.britishburnassociation.org/standards (accessed 10 September 2022).

Nursing and Midwifery Council (2015). The Code: Professional standards of practice and behaviour for nurses, midwives and nursing associates. https://www.nmc.org.uk/standards/code/ (accessed 10 September 2022).

Pape, S., Judkins, K., and Settle, J.A.D. (2001). *Burns. The First Five Days*, 2e. London: Smith & Nephew.

Peters, J. (2001). Caring for dry and damaged skin in the community. *British Journal of Nursing* 6 (12): 645–665.

Prelack, K., Yu, Y.M., Dylewski, M. et al. (2017). Measures of total energy expenditure and its components using the doubly labeled water method in rehabilitating burn children. *Journal of Parenteral and Enteral Nutrition* 41 (3): 470–480.

Robson, M.C. et al. (1998). Clinical aspects of healing in specialized tissue. In: *Wounds: Biology and Management* (eds. D.J. Leaper and K.G. Harding). Oxford: Oxford University Press.

Shields, B.A., King, B.T., and Renz, E.M. (2016). Cutting-edge forward burn nutrition: from the battlefield to the burn center. *Current Trauma Reports* 2 (2): 106–114.

Taylor, K. (2001). The management of minor burns and scalds in children. *Nursing Standard* 16 (11): 45–51.

Walker, T.L.J., Rodriguez, D.U., Coy, K. et al. (2014). Impact of reduced resuscitation fluid on outcomes of children with 10–20% body surface area scalds. *Burns* 40 (8): 1581–1586.

Wallace, E. (1994). Feeding the wound: nutrition and wound care. *British Journal of Nursing* 3 (13): 662–667.

Webster, A. (2000). The facilitating role of the play specialist. *Paediatric Nursing* 12 (7): 24–27.

Wilson, R. (2000). Massive tissue loss: Burns. In: *Acute and Chronic Wounds: Nursing Management*, 2e (ed. R. Bryant). London: Mosby.

Zuo, K.J., Medina, A., and Tredget, E.E. (2017). Important developments in burn care. *Plastic and Reconstructive* Surgery 139 (1): 120e–138e.

Chapter 7

Complementary and alternative medicine (CAM)

Jenni Hallman

RN (Adult), RN (Child), BSc (Hons) Children's Oncology Nursing; formerly Oncology Complementary Therapy Nurse Specialist; Great Ormond Street Hospital, London, UK

Chapter contents

Introduction and definitions	100	A practical example of a massage therapy service	103
A brief history of CAM and surrounding legislation	100	Case studies	109
The five most commonly used CAM	101	Conclusion	110
Disclosure of CAM to healthcare practitioners	102	References	110
Massage therapy	102		

Procedure guidelines

7.1 Massage   103

Introduction and definitions

Complementary and alternative medicine (CAM) refers to health-related therapies which are not considered to be part of conventional medicine. Although the terms 'complementary' and 'alternative' are often used as a single category, they have very distinct differences and can mean different things to different people. This chapter provides a definition and brief history of CAM and surrounding legislation, an overview of the five most commonly used CAMs in the UK, and a step-by-step guide for the use of massage, which can be incorporated into nursing care. It does not include in-depth information regarding the vast number of therapies available, which can be found elsewhere (National Centre for Complementary and Integrated Health 2015). Muscle relaxation and guided imagery are discussed in Chapter 27: Play as a Therapeutic Tool.

Complementary therapies are used alongside conventional treatments with the aim of providing some element of symptom management and psychological and emotional support.

Definitions

CAM is now increasingly defined as *holistic* and *integrated*. Holistic medicine refers to patient-centred care that encompasses the consideration of biological, psychological, spiritual, social, and environmental aspects of health. Integrated medicine is based on the relationship between patient and practitioner and promotes health for the whole person in the context of his or her family and community. Complementary therapies are nondiagnostic and are used *alongside* conventional Western medicine. These include therapies such as massage and guided imagery. Alternative therapies are used *in place of* conventional Western medicine (Kemper et al. 2011). Therapies such as osteopathy provide diagnostic information (Plant, cited in Brooker and Waugh 2007). Other alternative therapies are based on a variety of nonbiomedical beliefs and often have not been subjected to clinical research (National Center for Complementary and Integrated Health 2015).

A brief history of CAM and surrounding legislation

The history of many complementary and alternative therapies dates back thousands of years, with their origins particularly in Chinese and Indian cultures.

Interest in complementary therapies has steadily grown, and in the year 2000 the World Health Organization (WHO) defined them as:

> a broad set of health care practices that are not part of the Country's own tradition and are not integrated into the dominant health care system (WHO 2000, p. 1).

A major problem with CAM is the lack of statutory regulation. Osteopaths and chiropractors are currently the only therapists regulated by law (Tavares 2003). Acupuncturists are required to register with their local authority (DH 2003). Most complementary therapy practice is either voluntarily self-regulated or unregulated (Tavares 2003). In order to assist with understanding the regulation of CAM, they can be divided into three groups (see Box 7.1). Group 1 shows what has been commonly regarded as the 'Big 5' in CAM and are seen to have a diagnostic approach. The therapies in Group 2 are seen to complement conventional medicine without any diagnostic properties. Group 3 are those that favour a philosophical approach and are outside the realm of conventional medicine.

Use of CAM in UK

The government is committed to developing a National Health Service (NHS) that is responsive to the needs and wishes of individuals, and that enables them to play an active role in managing their health conditions. Within the hospital setting, it is becoming more and more common for patients, parents, and carers to enquire about and try to access information about complementary therapies.

The majority of CAM research has been carried out in adult settings, particularly amongst the oncology population. Complementary therapies in adult hospices and in palliative care are now commonly used (Currin and Meister 2008). The use of and the interest in these therapies is steadily growing within paediatrics (Calipel et al. 2005; Rheingans 2007).

Box 7.1 Categorisation of Complementary and Alternative Medicines

Group 1: Professionally organised alternative therapies	Group 2: Complementary therapies	Group 3: Alternative disciplines
• Acupuncture • Chiropractic • Herbal Medicine • Homoeopathy • Osteopathy	• Alexander technique • Aromatherapy • Bach remedies and other flower extracts • Body work therapies including massage • Counselling/stress therapy • Hypnotherapy • Healing • Maharishi Ayurvedic medicine • Meditation • Reflexology • Shiatsu • Nutritional medicine • Yoga	**3a. *Long established/ traditional*** • Anthroposophical medicine • Ayurvedic medicine • Chinese herbal medicine • Eastern medicine (Tibb) • Naturopathy • Traditional Chinese medicine **3b. *Other alternative disciplines*** • Crystal therapy • Dowsing • Iridology • Kinesiology • Radionics

Source: Adapted from House of Lords (2000).

Many children's hospices now offer some form of complementary therapies to children and young people (CYPs) and their families as part of their care. In an ever-changing environment, healthcare practitioners need to be able to provide the answers to any questions we may be asked.

There are a large number of complementary therapies on offer, not all of which are evidence based. Some therapies are more common than others and therefore more research and evidence is available. Lack of evidence does not necessarily mean lack of effectiveness. Across surveys of CAM in general the average one year prevalence of use is 41.1% and the average expenditures amount to £1.6 billion each year (Posadzki et al. 2013). Approximately 33% of people with complex, chronic, or life-limiting conditions such as cancer, asthma, arthritis, and cystic fibrosis are estimated to use complementary therapies (Kemper et al. 2011). For CYPs with developmental disabilities the number is 30–70% and families expressed that they wanted their clinicians to be able to offer advice and to counsel them regarding their CAM options (Kemper et al. 2011). Recent concerns regarding the inappropriate prescribing of antibiotics and treatment-resistant organisms could also be responsible for the increased interest in CAM (Bell and Boyer 2013). Families are often reluctant to disclose their use of CAM to the medical profession (McDonough et al. 2007). In fact very few referrals are made from general practitioners (GP's) and 74% of those who access CAM self-refer (Crawford et al. 2006).

The five most commonly used CAM

Acupuncture
Acupuncture has been used therapeutically in China for thousands of years and its prominence in Western medicine is growing (Jindal and Mansky 2008). Over the years, acupuncture has evolved and spread through the different regions in China and throughout the world. This has resulted in a number of different and unique types and forms of the practice being developed. Traditional Chinese acupuncture is the original form from which others have derived, although even this varies from region to region depending on the different schools of thought and approaches.

Acupuncture is based on the notion of energy or Qi (pronounced *chee*), which is distributed throughout the body via a complex network of channels known as meridians (Adams and Cheng 2011). Acupuncturists believe that ill health is caused by altered or obstructed Qi. Along each meridian there are specific acupoints which serve as target points to restore the alteration or obstruction (Vickers and Zollman 1999). These acupoints are accessed with a dry needle. Acupressure is similar to acupuncture but is performed by applying pressure to the acupoints, rather than the use of needles and is therefore less invasive and traumatic for CYPs with a fear of needles.

Various studies have shown acupuncture to be beneficial in reducing symptoms of nausea and vomiting and demonstrated a reduction in required medications (Rheingans 2007; Jindal and Mansky 2008). Acupuncture has also been shown to be beneficial in the treatment of headaches (Kemper et al. 2011) and nocturnal enuresis (Libonate et al. 2008), and has been used in Germany in the treatment of both chronic and hospital-induced constipation (Anders et al. 2012). A number of hospital-based pain management clinics now offer acupuncture alongside conventional pain medication (Lewith and Robinson 2009).

Homoeopathy
Homoeopathy is based on the principle that 'like cures like'. The practice dates back to Hippocrates, the father of modern medicine, who practiced over 2,400 years ago. Its modern-day founder was the German physician Samuel Hahneman. While working as a doctor in the late eighteenth century, Hahneman was dissatisfied with the conventional medicine of his day. After trialling various substances on himself and other healthy volunteers, he deduced that illnesses could be treated with very small amounts of a substance that in larger quantities would cause that same illness (Bell and Boyer 2013). Hence the description 'like cures like' evolved.

A study of 53 children in the UK with life-limiting conditions showed that 29% of them had accessed homoeopathic medicine at some point (Wood and Finlay 2011). As discussed previously, those with life-limiting or chronic conditions are more likely to seek CAM, but it is worth noting that homoeopathy is also commonly used for children with upper respiratory tract infections, otitis media, and other conditions relating to the ears, neck, and throat, as well as for babies who are teething (Kemper et al. 2011).

Osteopathy
Osteopathy is a way of detecting, treating, and improving health problems by moving, stretching, and massaging a person's joints and muscles. Osteopathy was established in America in the late 1800s by Dr Andrew Taylor Still, who felt that there should be a better system of healing than that which was currently available. He called his system osteopathy and believed that the human body functioned as a total biological unit and possessed self-healing and self-regulatory mechanisms. He felt that the structure and function of the body were interrelated and that abnormal pressure in one part of the body would produce abnormal pressure and strains in other parts (Findley and Shalwala 2013).

A number of studies have looked at osteopathy use in neonatal intensive care units (Cerritelli et al. 2015; Lund et al. 2011; Pizzolorusso et al. 2014). One study in which 101 pre-term infants were randomised to treatment (osteopathy) or nontreatment found that those in the treatment group had a shorter hospital stay of six days on average, compared to those in the nontreatment group (Cerritelli et al. 2013).

Dr William Garner Sutherland, a student of Dr Still, pioneered cranial osteopathy in the 1900s. After looking at bones of the skull, Sutherland concluded that good physical and mental health depended not only on the bones being in the correct position, but also on the ability of the sutures or seams between the bones to allow slight movement. Sutherland referred to the movement that could be felt throughout the body, in every tissue over which we have no control, as the 'primary respiratory system' (Haines and Sumner 2010).

Aromatherapy
Aromatherapy is defined as the therapeutic use of aromatic substances extracted from plants. The most important class of these substances is essential oils, which can often be present only in small quantities; more than a ton of rose petals would be required to make 300 g of rose oil, which is why essential oils are so expensive and sold only in small quantities of 10 or 30 ml (Lawless 2012). Many oils are diluted with alcohol or synthetic substances to make up the quantities, but essential oils are undiluted and this, aromatherapists believe, is what makes them so effective. The development of modern aromatherapy is attributed to a French chemist by the name of Rene Gattefosse. While working in a perfume laboratory, Gattefosse burnt his hand and immediately doused it in some nearby lavender oil. The burn healed quickly and without scarring, which led him to study the potential curative powers of plant oils. In 1937, he named his findings aromatherapy (Ernst et al. 2006). Essential oils have three distinct modes of action; pharmacological, physiological, and psychological (see Box 7.2). Essential oils can be used as compresses, can be inhaled, or can be massaged onto the skin. All three of these methods will result in the oils penetrating the blood stream (Price and Price 2011).

Aromatherapy is often delivered in the form of a massage. The use of an aromatherapy massage has been shown to decrease anxiety and increase relaxation of muscle due to the aroma used (Kuriyama et al. 2005). Patients receiving aromatherapy massages have described greater improvement in self-reported anxiety for up to

Box 7.2 Modes of Action of Essential Oils

Pharmacological	Chemical changes take place when an essential oil enters the bloodstream.
Physiological	Essential oils affect all the systems of the body; they can sedate or stimulate individual systems, resulting in different effects. For example, lavender promotes relaxation, while basil, peppermint, or rosemary stimulate and improve concentration.
Psychological	The effect that takes place when the essence is inhaled and the individual responds to that odour.

Source: Price and Price (2011), Lawless (2012)

two weeks after the intervention (Wilkinson et al. 2007). An observational study of 71 CYPs being treated with aromatherapy massage for burns in a hospital in South Africa found that they had a reduction in heart rate and respiratory rate and often fell asleep (O'Flaherty et al. 2012).

Herbal medicine

Herbal medicine is probably one of the oldest of health cares. The first documented evidence of it was in India over 5,000 years ago. In ancient Egypt, herbs were used for religious purposes and for cosmetics and healing. They were also used extensively in the mummification process (Pittman 1994). Ginger is one of the most frequently used herbal medicines to treat nausea and vomiting. Although the exact mechanism of action is unknown it is proven in reducing the symptoms of morning sickness and motion sickness, as well as nausea and vomiting associated with surgery (Quimby 2007). Herbal medicines are traditionally used more commonly in eastern than in western cultures, but were found to be the most popular type of CAM by one study looking at published surveys of CAM usage in the UK paediatric population (Posadzki et al. 2013). Germany also reports a high use of herbal medicine; one study found that nearly half of the herbal medicine taken by CYPs were prescribed by the medical profession, with the majority being used for the treatment of coughs and colds (Du et al. 2014). Parents often initiate herbal medicine use, with most of the information gathered from the internet, magazines or advertisements or from long standing family held beliefs and traditions. The WHO has expressed long standing concerns over herbal medicines; they argue that there is a potential for adverse effects due to a lack of regulation, quality control systems and the loose distribution channels, for example being able to order products on line (WHO 2000). Herbal therapies have the potential to interact with other treatments: St John's wort, a common over-the-counter remedy for depression, can react with a number of drugs, including theophylline, cyclosporine, warfarin, and some antibiotics and chemotherapy (Quimby 2007; Multum 2022).

Disclosure of CAM to healthcare practitioners

All of the above CAMs are available to both health practitioners and families. It is important that families feel able to communicate to healthcare practitioners (HCPs) if they are interested in or have accessed any CAM. A thorough nursing and medical history is essential. If families do want to pursue CAM, then appropriate referrals should be made to ensure specialist advice and there should then be open communication between families, health practitioners, and CAM practitioners. It is recognised that the majority of families do not inform HCPs about their use of CAM (Crawford et al. 2006; Kemper et al. 2011; McDonough et al. 2007). Direct questioning may not only provide answers as to what CAMs have been accessed, but also why they have been sought. As mentioned, some herbal medicines can interact with conventional medication. Caution should also be used with therapies such as aromatherapy, where oils such as German chamomile can affect the metabolism of codeine and may increase the risk of bleeding if used alongside anticoagulants, and it can also lower the blood pressure (http://patient.info/doctor/complementary-and-alternative-medicine).

Massage therapy

Modern massage is based on the techniques of Per Henrik Ling, a Swedish physiologist and fencing master who developed the Swedish Gymnastic Movement. In 1838, the Swedish Institute opened in London, and in 1895 a society of trained masseurs was formed to increase the standard of training. In 1899 Sir William Bennett inaugurated a massage department in St Georges Hospital London, and later, during the First World War, massage was used to treat soldiers suffering from nerve injury and shell shock (Tucker 2008). During the latter part of the twentieth century, massage went into its greatest period of decline, but now once again we are beginning to see its benefits and it is slowly being reintroduced into hospital settings.

There are a number of benefits of massage. The one most commonly supported by CYPs in hospital is that it is a distraction from their illness or pain, and also in the cases of many, from the boredom associated with being an in-patient (Bayliss et al. 2014). Many conditions can cause the skin to become dry, and using oils or creams can help prevent this. CYPs who are immobile are also at risk from pressure ulcers, and massage increases the blood flow, therefore reducing the risk of these developing. Parents have also stated that they view massage and other CAM as calming and soothing, and that this experience is often contrary to that of conventional medicine which can be perceived as rushed and enforced; this alone is seen as a benefit to both parent and CYP (Bayliss et al. 2014; Wood and Finlay 2011).

CYPs can become stressed or angry about their illness and the need for a hospital admission. Being hospitalised means conforming to being a patient, with very little choice or control over what is happening. School-age CYPs especially, are known to have concerns over hospitalisation and illness, and unfamiliar surroundings are known to increase anxiety (Coyne 2006). Massage can act as a distraction and something that they can control themselves. Simple measures, such as choosing which area of their body they want to be massaged or the cream they want to use, can all help a CYP to regain a sense of control.

Parents can also suffer from high levels of anxiety when their child is hospitalised and in some cases they can become afraid to touch their child for fear of hurting them; this is especially prevalent when they have had surgery or have external lines such as cannulas, central lines or nasogastric tubes inserted (Dunn and Board 2011). Parents of chronically ill CYPs have also expressed concerns that they feel more like nurses than parents and they describe a sense of resentment over their nursing role dominating their parenting experience (Kirk et al. 2005). Recently in America, parents of hospitalised children were taught Reiki and reported benefits of enhanced comfort and relaxation and improved pain relief for their children (Kundu et al. 2013). Parents can also be taught simple massage techniques to soothe or calm their child and help reinstate normal physical contact between parent and child. Massage is now regularly used in neonatal intensive care units to promote bonding between parent and baby (Vickers et al. 2004). It has been shown to improve weight-gain, lessen stressor behaviours and have positive effects on the neurological and neuromotor development in preterm babies, (Kulkarni et al. 2010). Massage has also proved to be beneficial in alleviating symptoms of pain, headache, attention deficit hyperactivity disorder (ADHD), asthma and colic (Synder and Brown 2012).

A practical example of a massage therapy service

Nurse-led massage was introduced on the oncology wards at Great Ormond Street Hospital (GOSH) in 2011. Following completion of an International Therapy Examination Council (ITEC) holistic body massage course, the service was gradually introduced with the support of the Nottingham Complementary Therapy Nurse Specialist. This nurse-led service provided massage, distraction and relaxation therapies to CYPs in a specially designed complementary therapy room or at the bedside. The massage used is gentle sweeping, relaxing and stroking movements, called effleurage, rather than the usual percussion or petrissage that is used for adults. Percussion involves striking the body using brisk, invigorating and stimulating strokes; petrissage means kneading or rubbing with force to manipulate tissues and muscles (Tucker 2008). Both percussion and petrissage could be potentially harmful if used on children.

For many CYPs who experience side effects of their cancer treatment, symptoms are often heightened at night when they are trying to rest or sleep. As well as providing massage, the nurse can teach simple self-help techniques, such as regulating breathing, which they can use either in hospital or at home at any time of the day or night. Nursing staff are also formally taught about the service, how it was set up and how it is benefitting CYPs, so that they are able to provide information to other families and refer them if appropriate.

The complementary therapy nurse (CTN) introduces herself to all families within a few days of their admission to the oncology wards. It is recognised that the time of admission and diagnosis is incredibly stressful and for this reason the CTN often reintroduces herself a few days later. Both the service and the CTN's nursing and oncology background are explained to the family, as they can be reassured that her oncology background provides an understanding of the diagnosis and the protocols that the CYP will be following and the potential and actual side effects of both their disease and treatment. Families also know that due to the nursing background of the CTN she will be able to answer questions and provide support. The CTN links closely with ward physiotherapists and occupational therapists and reports any changes or concerns regarding a CYP's muscle tone or condition to them, the ward nurses, and the doctors in charge of their care. Referrals are also made to psychosocial services if the CTN feels, when talking to the CYP or a parent, that additional support may be needed.

Parents and CYPs are informed that massage can help them to feel relaxed and that if they are well enough it can be provided in the complementary therapy room, thus providing a change of scenery and a safe environment within the hospital setting. Massage can be introduced and incorporated into nursing care and can be safely taught to CYPs, parents, and carers by anyone holding a holistic massage qualification.

Basic massage techniques

Basic massage techniques can be applied by one person consistently in post or incorporated into daily care. Whoever is performing the procedure, time needs to be allowed for the session to ensure that it is not rushed and that interruptions are kept to a minimum.

Procedure guideline 7.1 Massage

Statement	Rationale
1 Check blood results and any infectious precautions prior to arranging the massage.	1 To check platelet count – if less than 30×10^9/l. the CYP will require a much gentler massage to avoid any potential bruising. Usual hospital policy should be adhered to if the CYP is infectious, for example, use of aprons, gloves, and masks if required.
2 Explain to the CYP and family what you are going to do. Ask what area they would like you to massage (e.g. legs, feet, hands).	2 To ensure understanding and gain consent. To give choice and involve the CYP in the decision making.
3 Aim for a time when there will be no or very minimal interruptions.	3 To ensure privacy and maximum relaxation.
4 Make sure that: a) The CYP is comfortable. b) The room is warm enough. c) Spare blankets are available.	4 a) To ensure maximum relaxation. b) To prevent the CYP from getting cold when oils/creams are used. c) Spare blankets can be used both to cover and to place under the CYP to protect bedding.
5 Mute or switch off TV and any computer games, and dim the lights in room. Play music of the CYP's choice if they want.	5 To create a relaxing environment, give the CYP control over the session and minimise distraction.
6 Wash hands.	6 To prevent infection.
7 Distribute oil or cream into small container that will be single-patient use only.	7 To prevent cross-infection.
8 Expose only the area of body to be massaged; keep the rest of the body covered.	8 To prevent the CYP getting cold and maintain comfort and dignity.
9 Warm oil or cream by rubbing hands together before applying to the CYP's skin.	9 To bring oil/cream to room temperature.
10 Begin massage by placing hands gently on the CYP's skin or by gently holding area to be massaged.	10 To acclimatise the CYP to your touch.
11 If the CYP becomes upset or anxious, stop massage and return to gentle holding	11 To minimise anxiety.

The Great Ormond Street Hospital Manual of Children and Young People's Nursing Practices

1. To massage legs and feet:

Apply oil/cream to legs and feet:

1.1 Using one hand, gently 'pick-up' muscle at front of thigh working up from knee to top of thigh. When you reach the top of the thigh use a smooth stroking action back to the knee. (Repeat ×3)

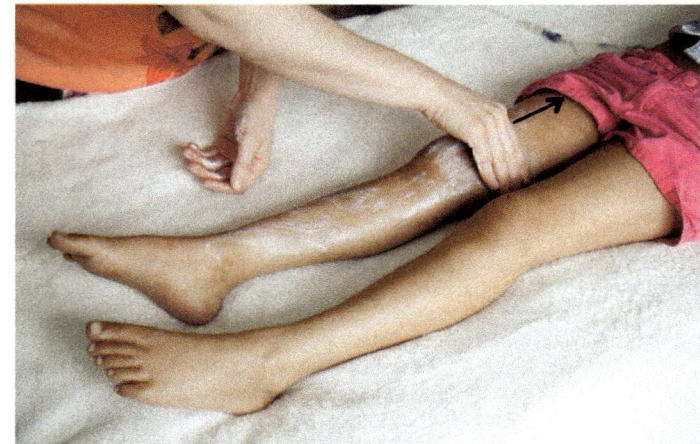

1.2. Use thumbs to gently circle around the knee. (Repeat ×3)

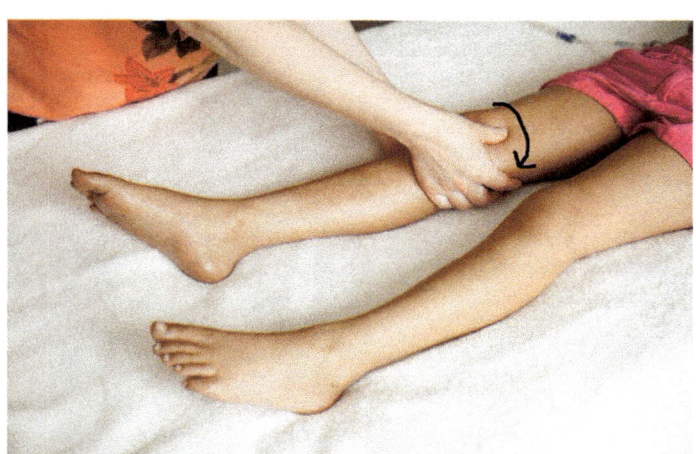

1.3. Use both hands to alternate strokes along the back of calf, keeping hand in full contact with leg at all times. (Repeat ×3)

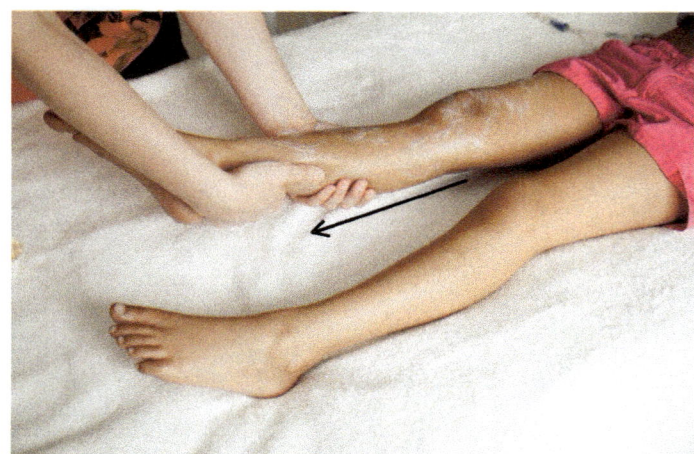

1.4. Use fingers to gently knead calf area, using circular motions. (Repeat ×3)

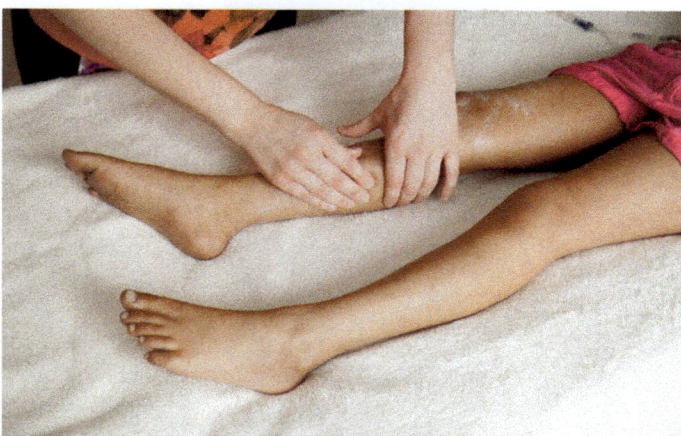

1.5. Use thumbs to gently circle sole of foot. (Repeat ×3)

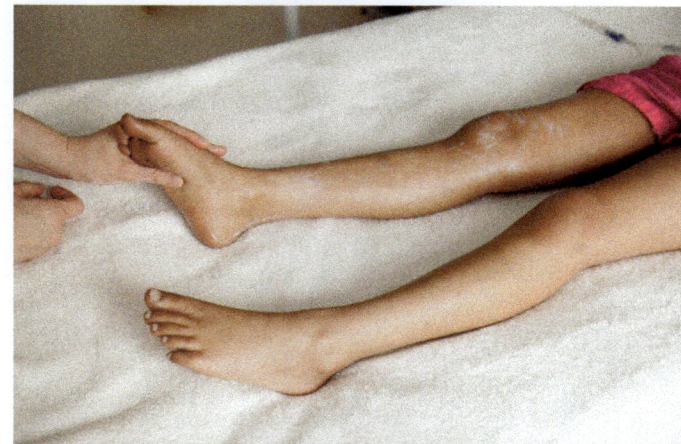

1.6. Use finger and thumb to gently circle each joint of the big toe, then stroke full length of big toe. (Repeat above move on all toes)

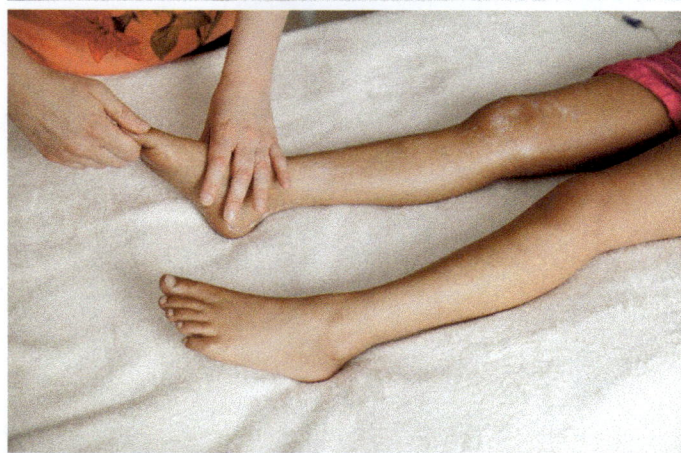

1.7. Use finger or thumb to slowly and gently squeeze between toes.

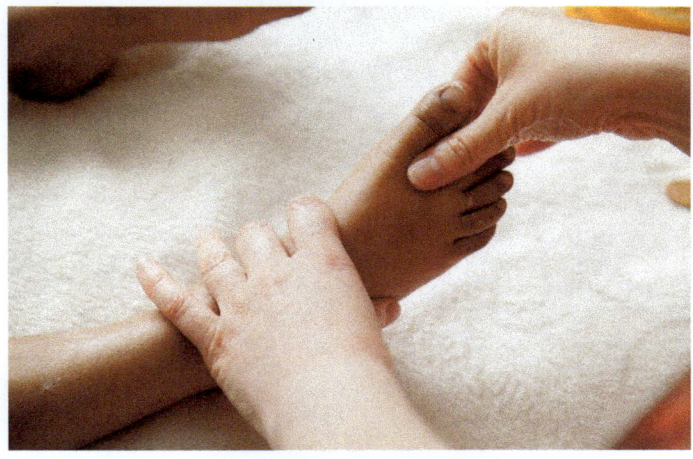

1.8. Hold foot firmly to finish and then cover leg and foot with blanket.

2. To massage hands and arms:
Apply oil/cream to hands and arms.

2.1 With one hand, gently 'pick up' muscle on upper arm and forearm, working up from wrist to shoulder. When you reach the shoulder use a smooth stroking action back to the wrist. (Repeat ×3)

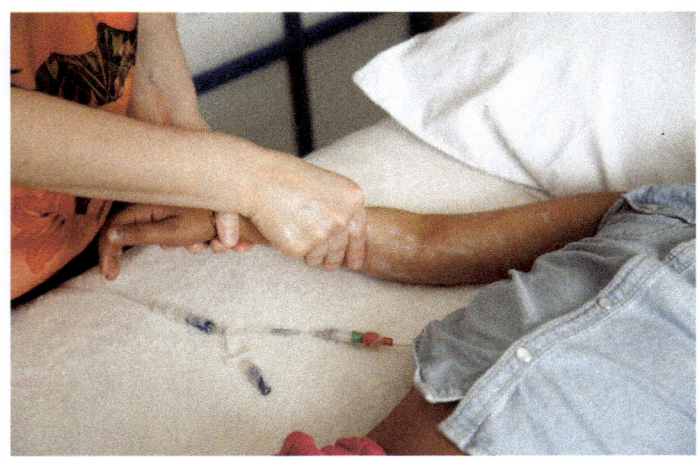

2.2 Use finger or thumb to gently circle each joint of each finger then stroke full length of each finger.

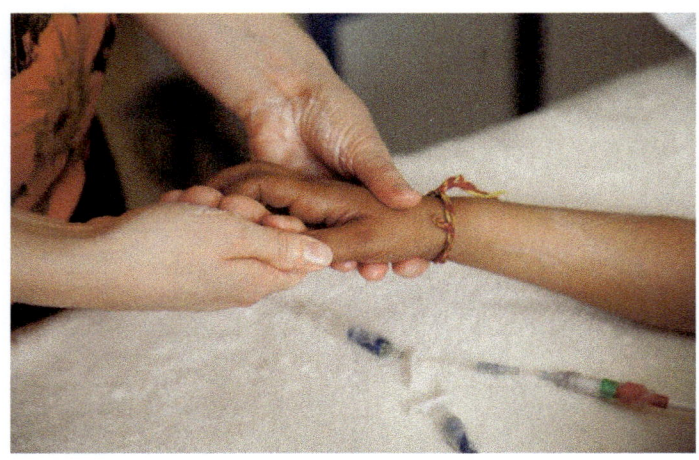

2.3 Use finger or thumb to gently squeeze pad between each finger.

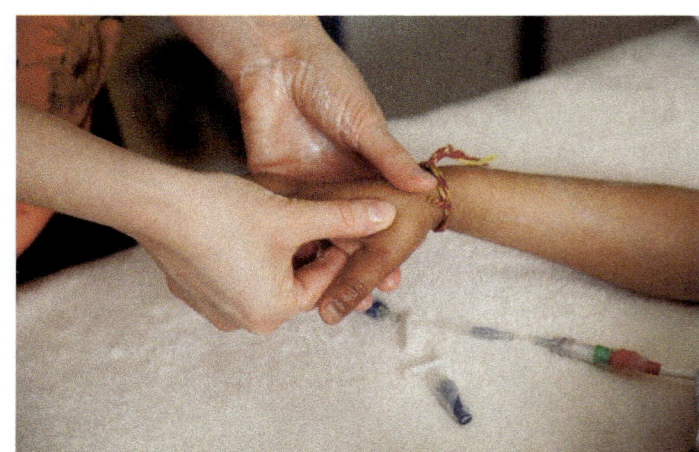

Chapter 7 Complementary and alternative medicine (CAM)

2.4 Turn hand over and support in one hand, use fingers/thumb to gently circle palm of hand. (Repeat ×3)

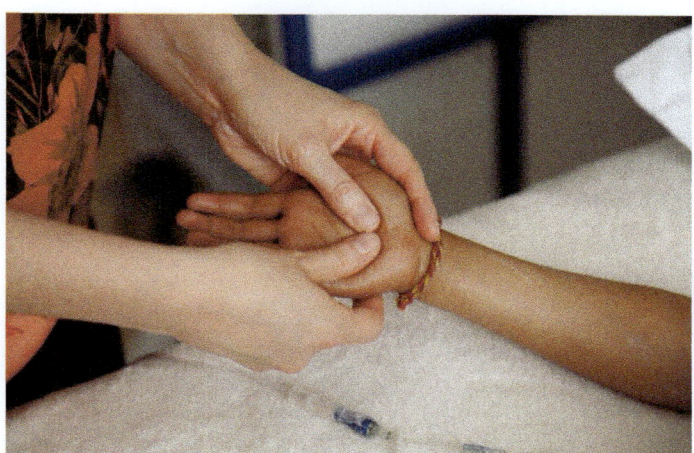

2.5 Hold hand flat between both hands to finish.

3. To massage abdomen:

Apply oil/cream to abdomen.

3.1 Place hand flat on abdomen and hold still for 30 seconds.

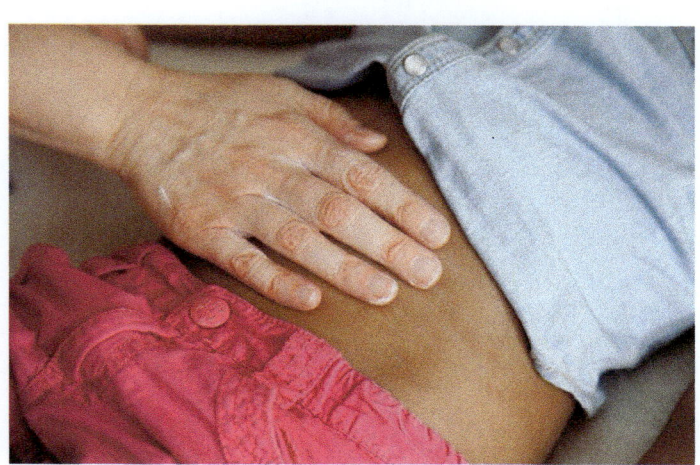

3.2 Using fingers, gently make circles in a CLOCKWISE direction, ensuring you cover the entire abdomen, making a square shape around the navel.

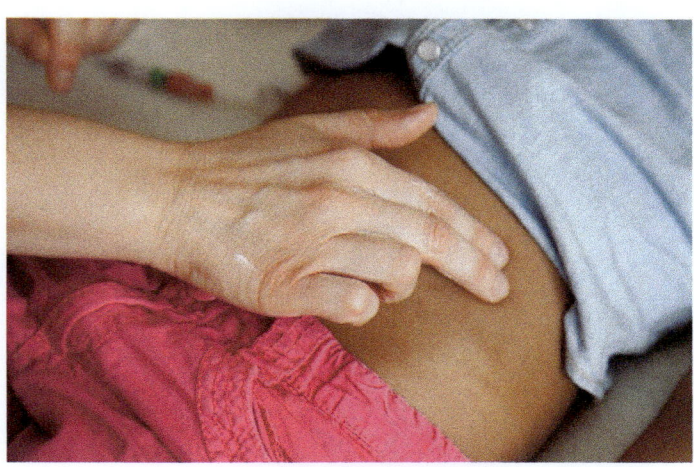

3.3 Place hand flat on the abdomen and hold for at least five seconds to finish.

4. To massage face:

If using, apply oil/cream to your fingertips (you do not have to use oil/cream for face).
Gently place hands flat at side of face.

4.1 Using thumbs, gently stroke out 'worry' lines **across** forehead, working from hairline to eyebrows. (Repeat ×3)

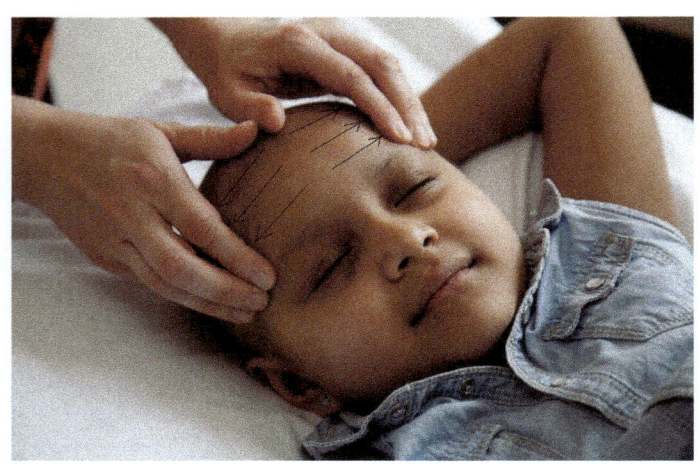

4.2 Use fingertips to press at side of nostrils then sweep under cheekbones round to the temples and up to the hairline. (Repeat ×3)

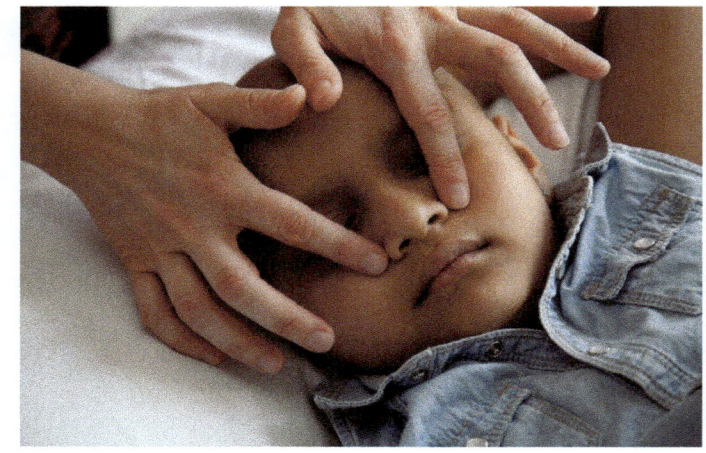

4.3 Place thumbs at hairline and hold applying light/moderate pressure.

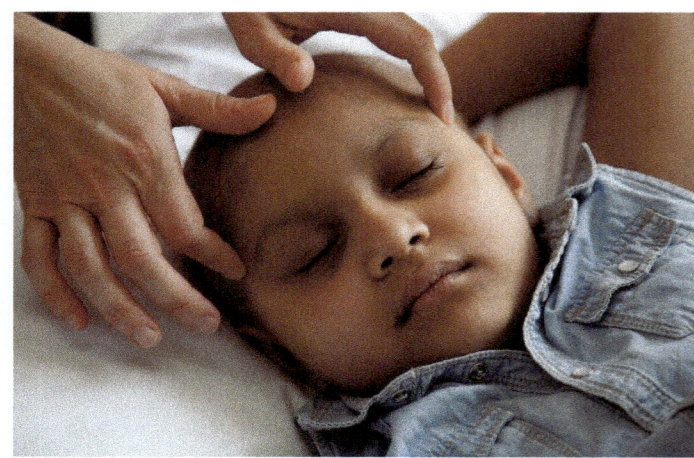

4.4 Use fingertips to circle and very gently pinch jawline from chin to ears.

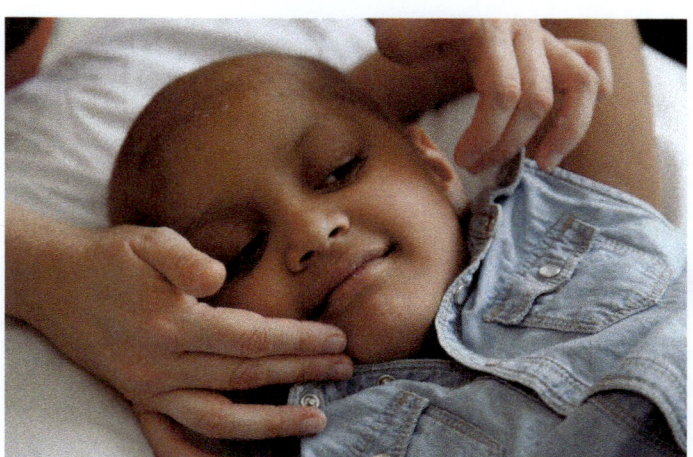

4.5 Use fingers to circle jawbone/cheek area.

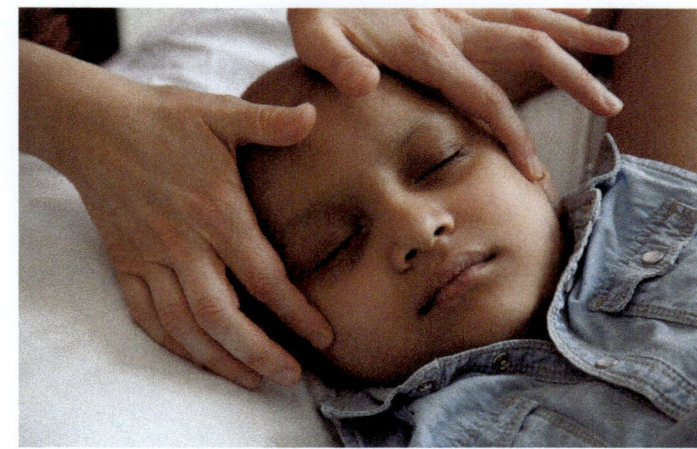

4.6 Finish by repeating stroking of worry lines, then place hands at side of face to end.

Case studies

The following case studies give examples of how massage has been used and has benefitted CYPs at GOSH. Names have been changed to ensure confidentiality. CYPs on the oncology wards can suffer from a range of symptoms depending on their disease and numerous side-effects from treatment. Case Study 1 looks at how massage helped to relax an 11-year-old boy and improve his sleep pattern.

The person providing the massage or any CAM should be a familiar, safe person that the CYP knows they can trust. For patients who are in hospital for long periods of time this allows a therapeutic relationship to develop. This extends beyond the benefits of the massage by providing a relaxed environment for ongoing, informal psychosocial support (see Case Study 2). The formation of a trusting relationship is cited as one of the main reasons why CAM are seen as beneficial; the therapist is seen as having time to care and therefore a trusting partnership is allowed to form, whereby the needs and wants of the patient are first and foremost (Smith et al. 2009).

Case study 1

Matthew was an 11-year-old boy suffering from posterior fossa syndrome post brain surgery; he was unable to mobilise or communicate. Matthew had regular massage sessions alongside intensive rehabilitation. Initially massage was used to desensitise and then to relax his muscles post physiotherapy. After spending several weeks in hospital, both in the Paediatric Intensive Care Unit (PICU) and on the wards, Matthew was finding it difficult to sleep for long periods and was requiring medication in order to sleep at night. Matthew often fell asleep during or shortly after his massages and, by providing massage treatments later in the day, his sleep pattern gradually improved. His parents, who stayed with him during the sessions, also reported that they felt a sense of calm both from the atmosphere the massages created and from seeing their son relax both physically and emotionally.

Case study 2

Hannah was a 15-year-old girl who had been unwell for most of her life; she had chronic lung disease and was receiving palliative care. Hannah had episodes of severe and debilitating pain and due to her lung disease was no longer able to walk and could speak only in short sentences. Hannah was desperately worried about her family and how they would cope when she was no longer here. Hannah would ask her mum and any other family members to leave when she had a massage and the sessions became a time for her to talk about her life and her worries and fears or to ask questions, not only about what was happening to her, but about world events and things she felt she wanted to do for herself and for others in the time she had. Hannah would often fall asleep toward the end of her massages and it was a huge privilege, as a nurse, to be able to give Hannah this time.

Studies have shown that symptoms of pain can be improved by massage (Sng et al. 2013; Ucuzal and Kanan 2014). Pain is unique to the individual experiencing it and is not easy to measure. It is affected by a number of factors, including mood and memory of painful experiences (Lindholm et al. 2009). Finding ways to manage pain is an ongoing medical dilemma, especially in paediatrics where a child's perception of and ability to communicate pain makes managing it even more challenging (Kortesluoma et al. 2008). Case Study 3 shows how the use of massage helped to both distract and to relieve pain related to peripheral nerve damage.

Studies have shown that complementary therapies help a person cope with their illness and that therapies undertaken in a hospital setting appear to have a longer lasting positive effect compared to those accessed as an outpatient (Fox et al. 2013; Landier and Tse 2010). Research carried out at GOSH showed improvement in patients' moods. The sessions gave them something to look forward to and a high percentage of those interviewed also reported how massage sessions would help them to relax or fall asleep (Bayliss et al. 2014), as Case Study 4 also demonstrates.

Case study 3

Joe was a 12-year-old boy with a metastatic rhabdomyosarcoma; he suffered severe and debilitating pain both from his disease and from the chemotherapy that was given to try to halt its progress. Joe was able to move his upper body but not his lower and due to his risk of pathological fractures he was bedbound. Although his feet hurt to touch due to peripheral neuropathy, he always wanted them to be massaged as he said 'it gave him a different feeling from the constant pain and made them feel better'. Joe was receiving large quantities of pain relief via a patient controlled analgesia (PCA) pump, which he self-administered every five minutes. During his massages he would often fall asleep and his use of his PCA while sleeping and immediately after waking would often be far less than prior to his massage. Joe's dad described his massages as the only thing he had to look forward in his day and also felt that it gave him the opportunity to talk to someone who had the time to listen.

Case study 4

Sam was an 11-year-old boy with a brain tumour; as a result he suffered from ataxia and, although determined to walk, was often frustrated by what he thought of as his clumsiness and lack of fine motor skills. Sam hated being in hospital and was often withdrawn and tearful. Initially, massage sessions for Sam allowed him to relax and to sleep, but just as importantly they gave him something to look forward to and to structure his day around. Sam said after his treatment that he 'didn't know how he would have got through it without the massages'. When he was well enough, Sam came to the therapy room, and he said the room made him think he wasn't in hospital. His father described the therapy room as 'Sam's sanctuary'. Sam said that even if he didn't fall asleep he could dream about being elsewhere and doing things he liked to do. On days when Sam struggled with his anxiety or felt tearful he said he would try to imagine how he felt when he was having a massage and that this would help him to relax.

Conclusion

CAM are increasing in popularity among the general population and as this interest gathers momentum, it is highly likely that HCPs will meet CYPs and families who are already accessing or have questions about them. Advice and guidance is vitally important for families and this can be sought from homoeopathic hospitals and hospices, where CAM are more widely used (National Association of Complementary Therapists in Hospice and Palliative Care 2020). Thorough history taking and open communication channels will help to provide a safe environment, where the needs of CYPs and their families can be met, and CAM can work safely alongside conventional medicine. As one patient stated, 'having a massage allowed me to dream': In a place of uncertainty and at a time of illness, sometimes dreams can be the most important things.

References

Adams, D. and Cheng, F. (2011). The safety of pediatric acupuncture: a systematic review. *Pediatrics* 128 (6): 1575–1587.

Anders, E.F., Findeisen, A., Nowak, A., and Rudiger, U.T.I. (2012). Acupuncture for treatment of hospital-induced constipation in children: a retrospective case series study. *Acupuncture in Medicine* 30 (4): 258–260.

Bayliss, J., Bluebond-Langner, M., Hallman, J. et al. (2014). Patient and Family Experience of Massage during Cancer Therapies: The Massage Study. Final Report submitted to Nelsons (unpublished; available from julie.bayliss@gosh.nhs.uk)

Bell, I. and Boyer, N. (2013). Homeopathic medications as clinical alternatives for symptomatic care of acute otitis media and upper respiratory infections in children. *Global Advances in Health and Medicine* 2 (1): 32–43.

Brooker, C. and Waugh, A. (2007). *Sleep, Rest, Relaxation, Complementary Therapies and Alternative 4 Therapies Foundations of Nursing Practice: Fundamentals of Holistic Care*. London, New York, Toronto, Sydney: Mosby and Elsevier.

Calipel, S., Lucus-Polomeni, M., Wodey, E., and Ecoffey, C. (2005). Is hypnosis as effective as midazolam as preoperative medication in children? *Focus on Alternative and Complementary Therapies* 10 (4): 313–314.

Cerritelli, F., Pizzolorusso, G., Ciadardelli, F. et al. (2013). Effect of osteopathic manipulative treatment on length of stay in a population of preterm infants: a randomised control trial. *BMC Pediatrics* 13: 65.

Cerritelli, F., Cicchitti, L., Martelli, M. et al. (2015). Osteopathic manipulative treatment in pre-terms: study protocol for a randomised controlled trial. *Trials* 16: 84.

Coyne, I. (2006). Children's experience of hospitalization. *Journal of Child Health Care* 10: 326–336.

Crawford, N., Cincotta, D., and Powell, C. (2006). A cross-sectional survey of complementary and alternative medicine use by children and adolescents attending the university hospital of Lim a Wales. *BMC Complementary and Alternative Medicine* 6 (16).

Currin, J. and Meister, E. (2008). A hospital-based intervention using massage to reduce distress among oncology patients. *Cancer Nursing* 31 (3): 214–221.

Department of Health (DH) (2003). *National Guidelines for the Use of Complementary Therapies in Supportive and Palliative Care*. London: Department of Health.

Du, Y.I.K., Zhuang, W., Bodemann, S. et al. (2014). Use of herbal medicine products in children and adolescents in wolf Germany BMC. *Complementary and Alternative Medicine* 14: 218.

Dunn, K. and Board, K. (2011). Parents and technology in the in-patient pediatric setting: a beginning model for study. *Pediatric Nursing* 37 (2): 75–85.

Ernst, E., Pittler, M.H., and Wider, M.A. (2006). *The Desktop Guide to Complementary and Alternative Medicine: An Evidence-Based Approach*, 2e. Philadelphia: Mosby.

Findley, T.W. and Shalwala, M. (2013). Fascia research congress: evidence from 10-year perspective of Andrew still Taylor. *Bodywork and Movement Therapies* 17 (3): 356–364.

Fox, P., Butler, M., Coughlan, B. et al. (2013). Using a mixed method research design to investigate complementary alternative medicine (CAM) use among women with breast cancer in Ireland. *European Journal of Oncology Nursing* 17: 490–497.

Haines, S. and Sumner, G. (2010). *A Practical Guide to Biodynamic Craniosacral Therapy*. London, Philadelphia: Singing Dragon.

House of Lords Select Committee on Science and Technology (2000). *Complementary and Alternative Medicine*. London: The Stationary Office.

Jindal, V. and Mansky, G.A. (2008). Safety and efficacy of acupuncture in children – a review of the evidence. *Journal of Pediatric Hematology/Oncology* 30 (6): 431–442.

Kemper, K., Vohra, S., and Walls, R. (2011). The use of complementary and alternative medicine in pediatrics. *Pediatrics* 122 (6): 1374–1386.

Kirk, S., Glendinning, C., and Callery, P. (2005). Parent or nurse? The experience of being the parent of a technology-Dependant child. *Journal of Advanced Nursing* 51 (5): 456–464.

Kortesluoma, R., Nikkonen, M., and Serlo, W. (2008). "You just have to make the pain go away" – children's experiences of pain management. *Pain Management Nursing* 9 (4): 143–149.

Kulkarni, A., Kaushik, J., Gupta, P. et al. (2010). Massage and touch therapy in neonates: the current evidence. *Indian Pediatrics* 47: 771–776.

Kundu A, Dolan-Oves R, Dimmers M, Towle C, Doorenbos A (2013) Reiki training for caregivers of hospitalized pediatric patients: a pilot program *Complementary Therapies in Clinical Practice* 19 50–54

Kuriyama, H., Watanabe, S., Nakaya, T. et al. (2005). Immunological and psychological benefits of aromatherapy massage. *Evidence-based Complementary and Alternative Medicine* 2: 179–184.

Landier, W. and Tse, A. (2010). Use of complementary and alternative medical interventions for the management of procedure-related pain, anxiety and distress in pediatric oncology: an integrative review. *Journal of Pediatric Nursing* 25 (6): 566–579.

Lawless, J. (2012). *Encyclopaedia of Essential Oils: The Complete Guide to the Use of Aromatic Oils in Aromatherapy, Herbalism, Health and Well-Being*. London: Thornsons.

Lewith, G. and Robinson, N. (2009). Complementary and alternative medicine: what the public want and how it may be delivered safely and effectively. *Journal of the Royal Society of Medicine* 102 (10): 411–414.

Libonate, J., Evans, S., and Tsao, J. (2008). Efficacy of acupuncture for health conditions in children: a review. *The Scientific World Journal* 8: 670–682.

Lindholm, T., Sjoberg, R., Pedroletti, C. et al. (2009). Infants and Toddlers' remembering and forgetting of a stressful. Medical procedure. *Journal of Pediatric Psychology* 34 (2): 205–216.

Lund, G., Edwrads, G., Medlin, B. et al. (2011). Osteopathic manipulative treatment for the treatment of hospitalised pre-term infants with nipple-feeding dysfunction. *The Journal of the American Osteopathic Association* 111 (1): 44–48.

McDonough, S., Northern Devine, P., and Baxter, D. (2007) Complementary and Alternative Medicine: Patterns of Use in Ireland. Research Update (50). www.ark.ac.uk (accessed 21 July 2020)

Multum, C. (2022). St John's wort. www.drugs.com/mtm/st-john-s-wort.html (accessed 29 September 2022).

National Association of Complementary Therapists in Hospice and Palliative Care (2020). www.nacthpc.org.uk (accessed 21 July 2020).

National Center for Complementary and Integrative Health (2015). nccih.nih.gov (accessed 2 November 2018).

O'Flaherty, L., Van Dijk, M., Albertyn, R. et al. (2012). Aromatherapy massage seems to enhanced relaxation in children with burns: an observational pilot study. *Burns* 38 (6): 840–845.

Pittman, V. (1994). *Herbal Medicine: The Use of Herbs for Health and Healing*. Massachusetts Queensland: Element Dorset.

Pizzolorusso, G., Cerritelli, F., Accorsi, A. et al. (2014). The effects of optimally timed osteopathic manipulative treatment on the length of hospital stay in moderate and late pre-term infants: results from a randomised controlled trial evidence-based complementary and alternative medicine. https://www.ncbi.nlm.nih.gov/pmc/articles/PMC4260368 (accessed 26 September 2022).

Posadzki, P., Watson, L.K., Alotaibi, A., and Ernst, E. (2013). Prevalence of the use of complementary and alternative medicine (CAM) by patients/comsumers in the UK: systemic review of surveys. *Clinical Medicine* 13 (2): 126–131.

Price, S. and Price, L. (2011). *Aromatherapy for Health Professionals*. London: Churchill Livingstone Elsevier.

Quimby, E. (2007). The use of herbal therapies in pediatric oncology patients: treating symptoms of cancer and side effects of standard therapies. *Journal of Pediatric Oncology Nursing* 24 (1): 35–40.

Rheingans, J. (2007). A systematic review of nonpharmacologic adjunctive therapies for symptom management in children with cancer. *Journal of Pediatric Oncology Nursing* 24 (2): 81–94.

Smith, J., Sullivan, S.J., and Baxter, G. (2009). The culture of massage therapy: valued elements and the role of comfort, contact, connection and caring. *Complementary Therapies in Medicine* 17 (4): 181–189.

Sng, Q.W., Taylor, B., Liam, J.L. et al. (2013). Post-operative pain management experiences among school-aged. Children: a qualitative study. *Journal of Clinical Nursing* 22: 958–968.

Synder, J. and Brown, P. (2012). Complementary and alternative medicine in children: an analysis of the recent literature. *Current Opinion in Pediatrics* 24 (4): 539–546.

Tavares, M. (2003). *National Guidelines for the Use of Complementary Therapies in Supportive and Palliative Care*. London: The Prince of Wales's Foundation for Integrated Health.

Tucker, L. (2008). *An Introductory Guide to Massage*. London: EMS Publishing.

Ucuzal, M. and Kanan, N. (2014). Foot massage: effectiveness on post-operative pain in breast surgery patients. *Pain Management Nursing* 15 (2): 458–465.

Vickers, A. and Zollman, C. (1999). ABC of complementary medicine. Acupuncture. *BMJ* 319: 973–976.

Vickers, A., Ohlsson, A., Lacy, J.B., and Horsley, A. (2004). Massage for promoting growth and development for pre-term and/or. Low birth-weight infants. *Cochrane Database of Systematic Reviews* 2000 (2): CD000390. https://doi.org/10.1002/14651858.CD000390.

Wilkinson, S.M., Love, S.B., Westcombe, S.E. et al. (2007). Effectiveness of aromatherapy massage in the management of anxiety and depression in patients with cancer: a multi-centred randomised controlled trial. *Journal of Clinical Oncology* 25 (5): 532–539.

Wood, D. and Finlay, F. (2011). Complementary and alternative medicine use in children with life-limiting conditions. *Nursing Children and Young People* 23 (4): 31–34.

World Health Organization (WHO) (2000). *General Guidelines for Methodologies on Research and Evaluation of Traditional Medicine*. Geneva: World Health Organization.

Chapter 8

Administration of systemic anti-cancer treatment (SACT)

Emily Baker[1], Nicky Farrell[2], Bhumik Patel[3], Cindy Sparkes[4], and Julie Bayliss[5]

[1]DipHE Nursing Child Branch, BSc (Hons) Children's Cancer Nursing, MA Practice Education; Senior Clinical Research Nurse Haematology/Oncology, Great Ormond Street Hospital, London, UK

[2]RN (Adult), RN (Child), BSc (Hons) Nursing, DipHE Child Health, ENB 998, ENB 240; Macmillan Clinical Nurse Specialist, Neuro-Oncology-Endocrinology, GOSH

[3]MPharm, MSc, PGCert; Senior Specialist Pharmacist in Paediatric Palliative Care, GOSH

[4]MSc, PGCE, RN (Child); Lead Educator, Haematology and Oncology, GOSH

[5]RN (Adult), RN (Child), BSc, MSc, ANP, NMP; Consultant Nurse, Paediatric Palliative Care, GOSH

Chapter contents

Introduction	114	Personal protective equipment (PPE)	115
Legislation and recommendations	114	Work practices	115
Consent	114	Safe administration of SACT	115
Safe handling	114	Routes of administration	116
Reconstitution and preparation of chemotherapeutic agents	114	References	122

Procedure guideline

8.1 Administration of SACT via the intravenous route	118	8.3 Extravasation (Adapted from EONS 2012)	121
8.2 Administration of SACT via the oral route	121		

Principles tables

8.1 Prescribing cytotoxic therapy	117

The Great Ormond Street Hospital Manual of Children and Young People's Nursing Practices, Second Edition. Edited by Elizabeth Anne Bruce, Janet Williss, and Faith Gibson.
© 2023 John Wiley & Sons Ltd. Published 2023 by John Wiley & Sons Ltd.

Introduction

This chapter provides a brief overview of safe practice in the administration of systemic anticancer treatment (SACT). It is intended to ensure that children and young people (CYPs), and staff are safeguarded by defining best practice, and should be read in conjunction with national policies and relevant local policies in each individual Trust. This chapter also has links with other chapters within this book, including Chapter 14: Intravenous and Intra-arterial Access and Infusions and Chapter 17: Administration of Medicines. National policy is intended to safeguard patients and staff by defining best practice for all disciplines involved in the delivery of SACT. The term *SACT* covers any therapy used in the treatment of a malignancy, which includes targeted therapies (e.g. Imatinib), as well as conventional cytotoxic chemotherapy. The term *cytotoxic* generally refers to any agent that may be genotoxic, oncogenic, mutagenic, or teratogenic. *Cytotoxic drug* is a term used to refer to all drugs with direct or indirect antitumour activity including anticancer drugs, monoclonal antibodies, partially targeted treatments, and immunosuppressive drugs. The health risk from cytotoxic drugs comes from the inherent toxicity of the drug and the extent to which the healthcare worker (HCW), CYP or carer is exposed.

Legislation and recommendations

The principle legislation and best practice guidelines relating to the administration of SACT that HCWs involved should be aware of are:

1. London Cancer Alliance (2015), *Integrated Care Systems (ICSs): Guidelines for safe prescribing, handling, and administration of systemic anticancer therapy.*
2. National Cancer Peer Review National Cancer Action Team (NCAT) (2013a), *The Manual for Cancer Services*: Supports quality assurance of cancer services and enables quality improvement. This strategy incorporates a national programme of peer review for cancer services, assessing all aspects of cancer services, and aiming to improve care for people with cancer and their families.
3. National Confidential Enquiry into Patient Outcome and Death (NCEPOD) (2018), *On the Right Course?*: Reviewed the care of CYPs who died within 30 days of receiving SACT, highlighting concerns regarding the quality and safety of SACT.
4. Department of Health (DH) (2011), *Improving Outcomes: A Strategy for Cancer*.
5. National Chemotherapy Advisory Group (2009), *Chemotherapy Services in England: Ensuring Quality and Safety*: Report ensuring the quality and safety of chemotherapy services in England. Issued a number of key recommendations aimed not only at reducing the risk of administration errors occurring, but also ensuring that each service has robust policies and procedures in place in relation to the safety and quality of chemotherapy administration.
6. Medicines and Healthcare products Regulatory Authority (MHRA) (2019).
7. EU Directives (2019), *Legal Framework Governing Medicinal Products for Human Use in the EU*.
8. Health and Safety Executive (2019), *Safe Handling of Cytotoxic Drugs in the Workplace*.
9. COSHH (2013), *Control of Substances Hazardous to Health Regulations 2002. Approved Code of Practice and Guidance*.
10. British Oncology Pharmacy Association (BOPA) (2015), *Standards for Reducing Risks Associated with E-prescribing Systems for Chemotherapy*.

Awareness of these legislations and regulatory standards ensures best quality care and practices are adhered to and maintained.

Consent

In accordance with the Department of Health (DH) guidance on informed consent (DH 2001), written consent must be obtained from a person with parental responsibility prior to commencing SACT or participating in any clinical trial. For SACT administered outside clinical trials the standard NHS consent form dictates the amount of information necessary in order to obtain a valid consent. For CYPs participating in clinical trials a trial-specific consent form must be completed as mandated by the European Medicines Agency (2018) and UK and European legislation Medicines for Human Use (Clinical Trials) Regulations (2004); European Parliament 2001).

Any individual with decision making responsibility for CYPs receiving SACT should be fully informed of the treatment and must have given full written consent. Practice may vary in individual Trusts regarding who ensures the consent is documented, but this should be defined by local policy. It is good practice to give families a copy of their consent form.

In order to demonstrate adherence with the Children's Cancer Measures (National Cancer Action Team [NCAT] 2013b), any consent form that CYPs or carers sign prior to starting SACT should enable them to confirm that they have received generic written information covering the action they should take if they experience any problems, who they should contact for advice, and the symptoms that should prompt this.

Safe handling

Safety of the CYP, staff and environment should be paramount when using SACT to minimise the risks of contamination. Direct exposure to cytotoxic and/or cytostatic drugs can occur during transport, preparation, administration, or disposal, and can be a result of inadvertent inhalation, ingestion, or absorption through the skin and/or mucous membranes, or via accidental self-administration, e.g. needle stick injury. Contamination may occur under differing circumstances, such as during drug preparation and administration, or when dealing with contaminated waste. Employers and practitioners working in areas where cytotoxic drugs are prepared, administered, handled, transported, and disposed of must ensure they are aware of and comply with all relevant legislation relating to safe handling of these substances. Employers must ensure standard operating procedures are in place for all activities involving cytotoxic drugs and that these describe safe systems of work that meet all current applicable legislative requirements, including:

- Health and Safety Executive (HSE) (2019), safe handling of cytotoxic drugs in the workplace.
- Control of Substances Hazardous to Health Regulations (COSHH 2013).
- Reporting of Injuries, Diseases and Dangerous Occurrences Regulations (RIDDOR 2013).
- HSE (2013) – Personal Protective Equipment at Work.

Employees have a responsibility to carry out any potentially hazardous activity only when suitably trained and when they are confident and competent to do so; hence all staff involved in the delivery of services to CYPs with cancer must be aware of all health and safety procedures. Staff who are pregnant or planning to conceive must seek advice before handling any of these drugs.

Reconstitution and preparation of chemotherapeutic agents

Knowledge of safety precautions and risks associated with administering chemotherapy begins at the point of reconstitution. Guidelines recommend that preparation of cytotoxic medicines should be centralised in the pharmacy or in a pharmacy-controlled facility in a clinical area. Preparation is most appropriately undertaken by trained pharmacy staff using an isolator in a controlled environment (London Cancer Alliance 2015).

Personal protective equipment (PPE)

It is important to ensure that personal protective equipment (PPE) offers adequate protection and is specifically designed to handle SACT. An important aspect of safety when administering chemotherapy is the use of PPE for all staff. The employer should provide PPE to all staff involved in administering cytotoxic drugs (HSE 2013). A risk assessment should be carried out for each handling activity that might result in exposure. The correct use of PPE can shield staff from exposure to SACT and minimise the health risks, but only if the following criteria are met: The PPE must be suitable for the tasks, suited to the wearer and the environment, compatible with other PPE in use, in good condition, and worn correctly (London Cancer Alliance 2015).

Pharmacy staff preparing cytotoxic drugs within pharmacy preparation units should wear personal protection as defined by local standard operating procedure. The following recommendations are considered to be the absolute minimum regarding the protective clothing/equipment that should be worn in clinical areas for defined tasks. Local policy or specific and individual staff needs may dictate the use of further protection.

PPE worn during administration and disposal of cytotoxic medication and when dealing with SACT spillage should include:

- Hand protection (gloves). No one type of glove has been found to give unlimited protection against cytotoxic contamination; there is now some evidence to suggest that nitrile gloves offer good operator protection (Capron et al. 2012).
- Disposable gowns or aprons are preferable PPE when handling cytotoxic drugs and should be made of low permeability fabric and have:
  - Closed front
  - Long sleeves
  - Elastic or knit cuffs (London Cancer Alliance 2015)
- Eye protection should be worn during disposal of waste, when dealing with a cytotoxic spillage and during administration if there is a risk of spraying, splashing or aerosols (London Cancer Alliance 2015).
- Eye protection should fully enclose the eyes, meet British Standard (2002) BS EN 166 and, where possible, should be disposable or capable of undergoing decontamination cleaning.
- Respiratory protection FFP2 or FFP3 masks should be worn during administration and when managing a spillage if there is a risk of spraying, splashing, or aerosol spray.

Disposable PPE must be disposed of in a designated cytotoxic waste bag. Visors and glasses are reusable and must be rinsed with warm soapy water, dried, and then stored safely in the chemotherapy preparation room.

Work practices

Disposal of waste

All areas providing SACT (inpatient and outpatient) should have a policy detailing the disposal of cytotoxic waste products in accordance with the guidelines for safe prescribing, handling, and administration of SACT drugs. Cytotoxic waste includes:

- All equipment and materials used for cytotoxic spillage.
- 'Frank' chemotherapy such as a syringe, infusion set, and/or bags of cytotoxic chemotherapy not administered.
- All equipment and materials used to prepare chemotherapy.
- Empty syringes.
- Disposable PPE.
- Infusion sets; once a noncytotoxic flush has been administered the entire set must be disposed of in a designated cytotoxic waste bag/bin.
- Nappies.
- Any used ampoules, vials, or needles used in the preparation of 'frank' chemotherapy; these should be disposed of in a designated cytotoxic sharps bin.

In the hospital setting, staff dealing with excreta (urine, vomit, faeces) should always wear gloves and aprons and dispose of these and any nappies in a designated cytotoxic waste bin or bags. Cytotoxic waste may contain high concentrations of cytotoxic drugs or metabolites (active or inactive but toxic) both during administration and up to seven days after treatment has ceased. Families/caregivers should be advised to wear gloves when handling their child's excreta for the same period of time.

Any doses prepared by pharmacy cytotoxic/aseptic units which are not required or have expired must be returned to the unit for disposal in the designated delivery container or as per local policy. Any expired doses must be returned before a replacement supply is provided.

Spillage and contamination

Cytotoxic spillage kits must be available, and all staff working in areas where SACT medications are administered must know where a cytotoxic spillage kit is located. In order to ensure the safety of all staff working in clinical areas where cytotoxic medication is administered and to comply with relevant health and safety legislation, standard operating procedures detailing the appropriate actions staff should take in the event of a cytotoxic spillage. All staff should be familiar with local standard operating procedures and be regularly trained to deal with cytotoxic spillages. Cytotoxic spill kits should include:

- Absorbent granules/pads/sheets/paper towels
- Two pairs of powder-free gloves (gloves containing powder may enhance absorption of cytotoxic materials)
- Protective gown
- Disposable shoe coverings
- FFP2 or FFP3 filtered face piece respirator (not surgical mask)
- Safety glasses BS EN 166
- Clinical hazardous waste bag
- Cytotoxic waste disposal bag
- 1 large sharps bin with purple lid
- Plastic tweezers (to pick up any sharp materials or broken glass)
- Sign to identify the spill
- Atomizer
- Water for injection

The spillage kit should also contain detailed instructions for dealing with both large and small spillages. The spillage should be recorded on an accident/incident reporting form as soon after the event as is practicable and the occupational health team informed of the names of the staff involved. New or expectant mothers should never be involved in the management of a cytotoxic spillage. If chemotherapy spills onto clothes, the individual should be advised to remove their clothes and thoroughly wash the affected area with soap and water. The contaminated clothing should then be washed at a high temperature and ideally should be washed separately from other noncontaminated clothes. Parents/carers who administer home chemotherapy for their child should be provided with this information (written/verbal).

Safe administration of SACT

SACT administration should be provided by a multidisciplinary team of doctors, nurses, and pharmacists working to approved protocols or treatment pathways. All staff involved in the administration of

SACT to CYPs must have undergone appropriate training and be listed on a local register of staff assessed as competent in administration of SACT. Training should be updated annually. The administration of cytotoxic drugs must be in accordance with the local trust medicine administration policy and the cytotoxic medicines policy and guidance, i.e. the policy for the safe handling of hazardous medicines and guidelines for the safe prescribing, handling, and administration of cytotoxic drugs.

Following training and successful assessment of competence, nursing staff may administer SACT via all routes other than via the intrathecal or intrareservoir routes. HCWs administering SACT drugs are required to be competent in intravenous drugs administration before they can begin training in administration of SACT medication.

Training

The *Manual for Cancer Services* indicates that a nurse training programme in oncology skills and chemotherapy administration should be agreed by the Children's Cancer Network (CCN) Chemotherapy Group (NCAT 2013a, b). Training requirements for nurses working in different settings (e.g. primary treatment centres, paediatric oncology shared care units, community) vary but should, as a minimum, meet the following requirements. Further detailed information on the competencies that should be included within each 'type' of training, along with specifications detailing minimum requirements for the types of training and numbers of trained nurses by location and setting are available within the manual (NCAT 2013a, b).

The Royal College of Nursing (RCN) states that the nurse managing chemotherapy should have knowledge of and technical expertise in both administration and specific interventions associated with chemotherapy agents and should have received education and training (RCN 2016).

Assessment

Prior to administering SACT, a thorough nursing assessment must be undertaken and should consider:

- The CYP's diagnosis and disease presentation.
- Pre-existing conditions.
- Existing SACT-induced toxicity.
- The CYP's past experience with the prescribed drugs.
- Anticipation of side effects; probability, timing, prevention strategies, previous successes, failures, and assessment methods.
- Preparation of the CYP and family.
- Identifying the family's desired level of involvement in care.
- Record preassessment and level of family involvement.

Preparation

Treatment protocols specify investigations and tests that should be carried out before the administration of specific drugs to establish a results baseline. Treatment records should be maintained for each CYP, detailing any investigations necessary prior to starting chemotherapy, and investigations that should be performed serially during the course (to detect/monitor any toxicity and response), and their intended frequency should be verified and recorded. Any short-term side effects as a result of the drug can be monitored and if necessary, modifications to the drug dosage or even the drugs being given can be made before the next block of treatment. Failure to verify that the results of recent tests are satisfactory prior to the commencement of further chemotherapy can lead to increased toxicity, which may, in some instances, result in permanent disability or even death. Nausea and vomiting, one of the most common side effects of chemotherapy, is potentially avoidable. It is therefore imperative to give appropriate antiemetics before chemotherapy and to plan patient care accordingly. Follow local and national antiemetic guidelines for chemotherapy-induced nausea and vomiting (Children's Cancer and Leukaemia Group [CCLG] 2019). Written guidelines/protocols should be agreed by the head of the chemotherapy service for the treatment and/or prevention of regimen-specific complications, such as the use of mesna with ifosfamide, or cyclophosphamide and sodium bicarbonate and folinic acid rescue with high-dose methotrexate (NCAT 2013a, b). Accurate recording and monitoring of fluid balance is vital in order to prevent and/or detect toxic complications of chemotherapy treatment.

Routes of administration

The oral route

Some SACT used in the treatment of children's cancers may be given via the oral route. Oral administration is generally economical, convenient, and less invasive than other routes. However, it may also be unreliable and impractical in CYPs for whom swallowing tablets is difficult and/or adherence or compliance may be an issue. In these cases alternate preparations should be discussed with the pharmacy. Staff handling oral cytotoxic agents should ensure adequate safety precautions are taken. Appropriate gloves should always be worn when administering oral chemotherapy. Crushing or cutting of oral chemotherapy should be avoided if at all possible. Staff administering oral cytotoxic medicine should be assessed as competent to administer cytotoxic medication. Appropriate PPE should be worn, such as plastic aprons, nonsterile gloves, visors/goggles and chemical repellent armlets. All cytotoxic medicine checks require two registered practitioners to undertake a high-risk check in accordance with local medicine administration policies. For more information see Chapter 17: Administration of Medicines.

The intravenous route

It is generally accepted that CYPs who are to receive long-term cytotoxic treatment should have a central venous access device (CVAD) inserted to facilitate treatment (RCN 2016). Hickman™ and Broviac™ catheters are commonly used in CYPs, along with implantable ports and peripherally inserted central catheters (PICCs) (Cowley 2004; Abedin and Kapoor 2008). Peripheral cannulae are used very rarely in children receiving SACT and extreme care must be taken when administering any chemotherapy via this route (London Cancer Alliances 2015).

Extravasation

Extravasation is defined as the accidental leakage of medication from its intended compartment (the vein) into the surrounding tissue (European Oncology Nursing Society [EONS] 2012). Depending on the substance that extravasates into the tissues and its physicochemical nature (vesicant, exfoliant, irritant) the degree of injury can range from a very mild skin reaction to severe necrosis (EONS 2012). Extravasation injuries are well documented within the field of haematology/oncology as many of the cytotoxic drugs used are classified as vesicants (Schulmeister 2011). Vesicants are drugs that have the potential to cause blistering and ulceration, which when left untreated can lead to more serious side effects of extravasation, including tissue destruction and necrosis (Ener et al. 2004). Additional precautions should be taken when administering vesicant chemotherapy to ensure the procedure is completed safely. Trusts should have policies and guidelines in place for staff as to the best practice when administering vesicant chemotherapy, and these should be reviewed and updated regularly. The policies/guidelines should detail the procedure to follow should an extravasation injury occur, and a policy for the treatment of extravasation injuries should also be available. Vesicant drugs can cause serious damage if inadvertently administered into the subcutaneous tissue, and for this reason are not usually administered by nurses via the peripheral route (National Institute for Occupational Safety and Health (NIOSH) 2016). Nursing staff who administer cytotoxic vesicant drugs peripherally should have received additional training and be competent to do so. They should also gain consent of the medical and management teams to undertake these extended practices to ensure they are adequately covered by local Trust policies.

Extravasation can be difficult to determine in some instances, as signs and symptoms can be similar to phlebitis and/or infection. CYPs may not always experience pain or discomfort if vesicant cytotoxic drugs extravasate (EONS 2012). Consequently, all HCWs involved in the administration of vesicant drugs should possess skills to assess possible incidents. While there is some controversy regarding the specific treatment of extravasation of some vesicants, extravasation guidelines published by EONS (2012) recommend the same initial treatment regardless of the nature of the drug.

Intrathecal route

A number of chemotherapy protocols used in the treatment of childhood leukaemia, lymphoma, and brain tumours involve the use of cytotoxic drugs injected intrathecally (see Chapter 17: Administration of Medicines). Only a small number of cytotoxic drugs can be safely administered into the intrathecal space. At least 55 incidents are known to have occurred around the world (a number in England) where the intravenous vinca alkaloid drug vincristine has been injected intrathecally during chemotherapy treatment (DH 2008). These incidents have resulted in the paralysis or death of the patients involved. The UK Government agreed on a target to reduce the number of patients dying or being paralysed by intrathecal injections of vinca alkaloids to zero by the end of 2001 (DH 2008). Updated national guidance on the safe administration of intrathecal chemotherapy, issued in 2008, built on that issued in 2001 (DH 2001, 2008). The key requirements are as follows:

- A written local policy covering all aspects of the national guidance.
- A register of all trained and competent staff.
- An annual review of competence.
- A designated area for the administration of intrathecal injections.
- Under normal circumstances intrathecal chemotherapy should be administered only within normal working hours.
- Intrathecal chemotherapy must be administered separately from any intravenous chemotherapy. Where chemotherapy protocols state that intravenous chemotherapy is due on the same day as intrathecal chemotherapy:
  - Intrathecal chemotherapy will be retained in pharmacy until confirmation of administration of intravenous chemotherapy, through written or electronic verification of prescription charts, following which the intrathecal may be released from pharmacy for administration to a designated area or person(s).
  - Intravenous chemotherapy will be retained in pharmacy until confirmation of administration of intrathecal chemotherapy through written or electronic verification of prescription charts, after which intravenous chemotherapy will be released.
- Where intravenous chemotherapy has been commenced prior to intrathecal chemotherapy being due, confirmation of administration must be seen and any remaining chemotherapy returned to pharmacy for storage prior to release of intrathecal chemotherapy. Intravenous chemotherapy will then be released only following confirmation of administration of intrathecal chemotherapy.
- If a regimen involves intrathecal chemotherapy combined with continuous intravenous chemotherapy, it is only acceptable to issue intrathecal chemotherapy once there is evidence that the infusional intravenous chemotherapy has started.
- Vinca alkaloids must NOT be given on the same day as intrathecal chemotherapy except in the case of a life-threatening clinical emergency, following a proper formal risk assessment.

Any nurse involved in checking intrathecal chemotherapy prior to administration must have undergone a designated training programme and appear on a local register of staff designated as competent to check intrathecal chemotherapy.

Principles table 8.1 Prescribing cytotoxic therapy

Principle	Rationale
1a) Prescribers must have received appropriate in-house education and training in order to be able to prescribe cytotoxic therapy.	1a) To ensure those prescribing have appropriate knowledge of the use of cytotoxic therapy, including side effects and supportive care.
b) The decision to initiate the first course of cytotoxic therapy for a malignant disease must be made by a consultant. The prescription can then be written by either a consultant or a specialist registrar.	b) To ensure the decision to treat is co-ordinated by a senior clinician alongside the multidisciplinary team.
c) Subsequent cycles of cytotoxic therapy can be prescribed by those with appropriate training.	
d) As a result of a number of adverse incidents involving the maladministration of cytotoxic therapy via the intrathecal route, the Department of Health declared that junior and trainee doctors must play no part in the prescribing of intrathecal cytotoxic therapy (DH 2008).	d) To minimise the risk of a prescription error.
2a) Cytotoxic therapy for CYPs is usually calculated using body surface area. This is can be calculated by a nomogram, which requires height and weight measurements. However, most centres in the United Kingdom use the chart provided by the Children's Cancer and Leukaemia Group (CCLG) for estimation of body surface area in infants and children (CCLG 2008).	2a)–c) To ensure accurate dosing for CYPs and minimise the risk of cytotoxic drug toxicity.
b) Care must be taken with CYPs who are overweight or underweight, taking into consideration the possible need for a calculation of ideal body weight. Individual protocol guidelines should always be followed. Where CYPs are noted to have a BMI that falls beyond the 98th centile or below the 2nd centile, the need to use either the ideal body weight or the calculation of dosing weight should be discussed and agreed.	

(continued)

Principles table 8.1 Prescribing cytotoxic therapy *(continued)*

Principle	Rationale
c) Some protocols may require doses to be prescribed in mg/kg or may require a dose amendment according to age or bodyweight. Again, individual protocol guidelines should always be followed.	
3a) Cytotoxic therapy for malignant diseases in CYPs should be prescribed according to a recognised (CCLG) protocol. Each Principal Treatment Centre is responsible for keeping a list of approved regimes.	3a) To ensure the most appropriate and consistent treatment is given.
b) If a CYP requires a treatment not on the approved regime list, the consultant must provide an 'off protocol' form, using dedicated paperwork and documented clearly in their health record. The information provided should include: • The reason for off-protocol prescribing. • The SACT drugs required and detail of how they are to be administered. • Criteria for toxicity evaluation, both at baseline and prior to each subsequent cycle. • Number of intended cycles and time to re-evaluation. • Supportive care requirements and appropriate supporting references.	b) To ensure there is an audit trail of treatment and communication is clear for all involved.
4a) Cytotoxic prescriptions should be produced using a recognised electronic prescribing system where possible.	4a) To minimise the risk of errors (National Institute for Health and Care Excellence (NICE) (2014).
b) Intrathecal SACT medication must always be prescribed on a designated intrathecal chemotherapy prescription chart. This may not be electronic.	b) To comply with the DH guidance (2008) and minimise the risk of an error.
5a) The usual demographic details required for prescriptions include: full name, date of birth, hospital number and/or NHS number, weight, height (if appropriate), body surface area, allergy status, ward/clinic, consultant's name.	5a) To minimise the risk of any errors and follow the legal requirements for prescription writing.
b) Prescriptions for cytotoxic therapy for malignant disease must also include: • Name of the drug • Dosage • Frequency, including the number of days of treatment • Route of administration • Treatment regime/protocol • Cycle and/or course number as appropriate For infusions: • Details of the diluent/solution and volume. • Duration of infusion and any other administration instructions. • Any additives to the fluids must be clearly indicated.	b) To minimise the risk of errors.
c) Supportive therapies for the particular chemotherapy cycle must be prescribed at the same time on the relevant system, i.e.: • Mesna bolus • Folinic acid rescue • Antiemetic therapy, following national/local policy in regards to the emetic potential of the regime/drugs	c) To minimise the risk of errors, such as supportive therapy being missed, and to aim for good control of nausea and vomiting.

Procedure guideline 8.1 Administration of SACT via the intravenous route

Statement	Rationale
1 Staff must receive education and training in the administration of SACT, and therefore only those who have been assessed as competent can administer SACT unsupervised. In order to be able to administer SACT intravenously they must also be deemed competent in intravenous therapy.	1 To ensure staff have adequate knowledge about the drugs being given, their side effects, and any supportive care required. This includes the management of infiltration and extravasation.

Administration: Prior to bedside

2 Inform the CYP and family/carer that you are about to prepare their medication for administration.	2 To prevent any delays in administration, and allow them time to prepare.

Chapter 8 Administration of systemic anti-cancer treatment (SACT)

Procedure guideline 8.1 Administration of SACT via the intravenous route *(continued)*

Statement	Rationale
3 When preparing to administer intravenous SACT the professional doing so must ensure they have the following to hand: • CYP's medical notes • Consent form for treatment • A recent weight • Access to the CCLG body surface area chart (if being used) • Results of any recent tests/investigations • Prescription (ideally on an electronic system) • Access to the CYP's treatment protocol • The cytotoxic drugs • Any supportive therapies being given at the same time (i.e. fluids, bolus meds, anti-emetics) • All equipment required for administration • Volumetric pump/syringe driver • Appropriate PPE	3 To ensure all relevant information for checking and all the necessary equipment is to hand to minimise delays.
4 The checking of cytotoxic therapy can be seen as high risk, so requires a check by two registered nurses (or one registered nurse and a competent medical staff member).	4 To minimise the risk of errors.
5 The nurse/person administering the medication is responsible for checking the 6Rs: 1 Right drug 2 Right patient 3 Right route 4 Right time 5 Right dose 6 Right documentation. In addition to this they are responsible for checking that: • The CYP is not allergic to the drug. • There has been the appropriate interval between treatment days/cycles. • Safety checks according to the protocol have been completed (i.e. full blood count, GFR). • The CYP has been examined and has been deemed fit to receive this cycle of cytotoxic therapy.	5 To minimise the risk of error.
6 a) Intravenous cytotoxic medications should be prepared following an aseptic nontouch technique (ANTT). b) PPE required: • Gloves • Disposable apron/gown • Chemical repellent armlets • Visor/goggles • Respiratory protection, if required	6 a) To minimise the risk of infection to the CYP and to follow national guidance. b) To minimise the risk of exposure of the administrator to the cytotoxic medication being prepared.
7 a) For infusional SACT a volumetric infusion pump should be used. b) A 'closed system' IV infusion set should be used and primed with a compatible solution prior to attaching the cytotoxic medication. The priming volume should be the volume for the appropriate particular set being used. c) Where the volume to be administered is less than 50 ml a syringe driver may be used, particularly if the rate of infusion is very slow and the length of infusion is long (i.e. <5 ml/hr over 48 hours). However, this should be discussed with the pharmacist/chemotherapy lead nurse. d) The giving set for the syringe driver should also be primed with a compatible noncytotoxic solution following the priming volume for that particular set.	7 a) In order to ensure the medication is given over the correct time. b) To minimise the risk of any spillage and therefore exposure to cytotoxic medication spilling/splashing from the end of the infusion set, and to allow early identification of potential problems with the set. A 'closed system' infusion set also allows the medication to be flushed through without removing the completed bag of cytotoxic medicine from the top of the set, therefore minimising the risk of exposure. c) To prevent over-running of the medication, allowing for changing of the syringe at 24 hours in line with the ANTT guidelines. d) To minimise the risk of any spillage and risk of exposure to cytotoxic medication spilling/splashing from the end of the set.

(continued)

Procedure guideline 8.1 Administration of sact via the intravenous route *(continued)*

Statement	Rationale
7 e) When attaching the cytotoxic bag to the giving set this should be done at waist height, over the prepared plastic tray.	7 e) To minimise the risk of splashing or spillage if the bag splits, or if there are any issues during attachment.

Administration: At the bedside

Statement	Rationale
8 Once at the bedside: a) Check the CYP's identity against their identity bracelet b) This should be done by the same two people who checked the medication.	8 To comply with the 6Rs and prevent any errors.
9 Prior to administering intravenous cytotoxics, the patency of the intravenous access device in use must be established by checking for blood return, and flushing the device with an appropriate solution (i.e. 0.9% sodium chloride/glucose 5%).	9 Ensuring patency by checking for blood return greatly reduces the risk of infiltration or extravasation.

Bolus administration

Statement	Rationale
10 When administering a bolus SACT it is advisable to: a) Administer vesicants first (after any required premedication). b) If being given peripherally, vesicants should be given via a newly inserted cannula. The cannula site should be placed to avoid joints, and the antecubital fossa). c) In the child population vesicant boluses may be given via syringe, but in the adolescent population vesicant boluses may be given in the same way as in the adult setting, via a fast-drip. d) Vinca alkaloids in the adolescent setting may be given using a 50ml minibag (as in the adult setting). In the child population vinca alkaloids may be given in a minimum of 10ml, via a syringe. Vinca alkaloids given in volumes of less than 10ml must be subject to diligent risk assessment as determined by pharmacy/lead chemotherapy nurse and consultant. e) When administering vesicant medications via bolus, whether via the peripheral or central route, blood flow from the device should be checked after every 2–5ml during the administration.	10 a), b) To ensure the integrity of the vein/device is at its greatest to minimise the risk of an extravasation. c) As children tend to have smaller veins and may require closer fluid monitoring administering via a fast-running drip can minimise irritation caused by the drug. d) To minimise the risk of maladministration of cytotoxic therapy via the intrathecal route and comply with the DH guidelines (2008). e) To allow early identification of, and minimise the risk of extravasation.
11 Once the medication has been administered, flush the device with a compatible solution and dispose of all waste as per local policy for cytotoxic waste.	11 To ensure there is no drug left in the device and that all waste is disposed of safely.

Infusion administration

Statement	Rationale
12 a) When administering an infusional SACT medication, attach the set using ANTT following appropriate checks of device patency. b) Once attached, initially set the volume to be infused limit to the priming volume of the set and set a flow rate faster than the infusion rate (e.g. 100–200 ml/hr). c) Set the pump pressures to 50mmHg (or 25mmHg if a vesicant medication). d) Run the infusion until the volume to be infused alarms, then set the pump at the prescribed rate for the infusion and set the volume to be infused for the whole prescribed volume of medication indicated. e) When the infusion is complete, flush the line with a compatible solution using the volume of the line again, as per priming.	12 a) To minimise the risk of infection. b) To prevent any over-running of the medication due to the primed giving set c) To allow early identification of any problems with the device and minimise the risk of infiltration or extravasation. d) To allow the solution in the primed line to fast-run to the CYP, bringing the cytotoxic medication to the end of the giving set, allowing for more accurate timing of administration. e) To ensure all the medication is given to the CYP and none remains in the giving set.
13 a) If adminstering an infusional vesicant via a peripheral cannula the above steps should be followed but extra care should be taken to prevent extravasation. b) The CYP's peripheral cannula should be left without a bandage throughout the infusion, to allow the site to be monitored easily. c) Visual checks of the site should take place every 10–15 minutes and be documented.	13 To allow early identification of any signs of extravasation.

Chapter 8 Administration of systemic anti-cancer treatment (SACT)

Procedure guideline 8.1 Administration of SACT via the intravenous route *(continued)*

Statement	Rationale
14 When the infusion is complete, flush the line with a compatible solution, using the volume of the line again as per priming.	14 To ensure all the medication is given to the CYP and none remains in the giving set.
15 Dispose of the giving set and other waste following local guidelines for disposal of cytotoxic waste.	15 To ensure waste is disposed of safely.
16 The plastic tray and reusable PPE should be washed with soap and water and dried before storing away.	16 To reduce the risk of contamination / infection and follow ANTT guidelines.

Procedure guideline 8.2 Administration of SACT via the oral route

Statement	Rationale
1 Appropriate PPE should be worn: • Plastic apron • Nonsterile gloves • Chemical repellent armlets • Visor/goggles.	1 To minimise the risk of exposure to the cytotoxic medication.
2 a) Oral suspensions/liquids should be drawn up into an oral syringe over a plastic tray. b) A cap should then be placed on the end of the syringe.	2 a) To contain any spillage that may occur when drawing up the medication and therefore minimise the risk of exposure. b) To prevent any spillage of the medication and minimise the risk of exposure.
3 a) Tablets should not be crushed or split wherever possible and should be either given whole or dissolved. b) Capsules should not be opened.	3 a), b) To prevent the risk of inhalation of cytotoxic medication and the risk of misdistribution of the drug once crushed/split/opened.
4 a) Once the drug has been administered, dispose of waste as per local policy on cytotoxic waste. b) The plastic tray should be washed with soap and water and dried before storing away.	4 a) To ensure waste is disposed of safely. b) To follow ANTT guidelines and minimise the risk of contamination.

Procedure guideline 8.3 Extravasation (Adapted from EONS 2012)

Statement	Rationale
1 If extravasation is suspected, stop the infusion or bolus injection immediately. DO NOT remove the cannula at this point.	1 To allow the cannula to be used to withdraw the vesicant medication.
2 Disconnect the infusion or syringe (not the cannula/needle).	
3 Leave the cannula/needle in place and try to aspirate as much of the drug as possible with a 10 ml syringe. Avoid applying direct manual pressure to the suspected extravasation site.	3 To prevent any further extravasation of the vesicant. By withdrawing as much of the vesicant from the site as possible the extent of the extravasation injury may be minimised. Avoiding direct manual pressure may also minimise injury by preventing spread of the vesicant within the tissues.
4 Mark the affected area and take digital images of the site.	4 To enable ongoing assessment of the injury.
5 Do not remove the cannula/needle until after medical review.	5 To ensure local access remains; it may be necessary to use an antidote or irrigate the extravasation site with fluid.
6 Collect the extravasation kit, notify the medical team, and seek advice from local experts.	6 Expert advice is essential when treating extravasation injuries in order to prevent further damage to the site. Every clinical area should hold a local policy regarding the recognition and treatment of extravasation (NCAT 2013a, b).
7 Complete an incident report form as per local policy and document in the healthcare record.	7 To ensure an accurate record is provided.
8 a) Administer pain relief if required. b) Complete required documentation.	8 a) To manage localised pain. b) CYP may require follow up care.

References

Abedin, S. and Kapoor, G. (2008). Peripherally inserted central venous catheters are a good option for prolonged venous access in children with cancer. *Pediatric Blood & Cancer* 51 (2): 251–255.

British Oncology Pharmacy Association (BOPA) (2015). Standards for reducing risks associated with e-prescribing systems for chemotherapy. Version 1.0. http://www.bopawebsite.org (members-only section) (accessed April 2019).

British Standards (2002). Personal eye protection. Specifications. BS EN 166:2002. ISBN 0 580 38916 2

Capron, A., Destree, J., Jacobs, P., and Wallemacq, P. (2012). Permeability of gloves to selected chemotherapeutic agents after treatment with alcohol or isopropyl alcohol. *American Journal of Health-System Pharmacy* 69: 1665–1670.

Children's Cancer and Leukaemia Group (CCLG) (2008). Estimation of body-surface area in infants and children. Chemotherapy Standardisation Group. https://www.ouh.nhs.uk/oxparc/professionals/documents/Body-surfaceareaCCLGChart1.pdf (accessed May 2019).

Children's Cancer and Leukaemia Group (CCLG) (2019). National framework guideline for the prevention and management of chemotherapy induced nausea and vomiting. www.cclg.org.uk/News/a-national-framework-guideline-for-the-prevention-and-management-of-chemotherapy-induced-nausea-and-vomiting-/197715 (accessed May 2019).

Control of Substances Hazardous to Health (COSHH) (2013). The Control of Substances Hazardous to Health Regulations 2002. Approved Code of Practice and Guidance, 6th edition. www.hse.gov.uk/pubns/books/l5.htm (accessed April 2019).

Cowley, K. (2004). Make the right choice of vascular access device. *Professional Nurse* 19 (10): 43–46.

Department of Health (DH) (2001). HSC/2001/023 Good practice in consent: achieving the NHS Plan Commitment to Patient-centred Consent Practice. London, DH. https://webarchive.nationalarchives.gov.uk/20121105174045/www.dh.gov.uk/en/PublicationsAndStatistics/LettersAndCirculars/HealthServiceCirculars/DH_4003736 (accessed May 2019).

Department of Health (DH) (2008). HSC 2008/001 Updated National Guidance on the Safe Administration of Intrathecal Chemotherapy. London, DH.

Department of Health (DH) (2011). Improving Outcomes: A Strategy for Cancer, London, DH. https://assets.publishing.service.gov.uk/government/uploads/system/uploads/attachment_data/file/213785/dh_123394.pdf (accessed April 2019).

Ener, R.A., Meglathery, S.B., and Styler, M. (2004). Extravasation of systemic hemato-oncological therapy. *Annals of Oncology* 15: 858–862.

EU Directives (2019). Legal framework governing medicinal products for human use in the EU. https://ec.europa.eu/health/human-use/legal-framework_en (accessed June 2019).

European Medicines Agency (2018). Guideline for good clinical practice E6(R2) EMA/CHMP/ICH/135/1995. http://academy.gmp-compliance.org/guidemgr/files/WC500002874.PDF (accessed May 2019).

European Oncology Nursing Society (EONS) (2012). Extravasation guidelines. http://www.cancernurse.eu/education/guidelines-recommendations.html (accessed February 2019).

European Parliament (2001). Clinical Trials Directive (EC2001/20). https://ec.europa.eu/health/human-use/clinical-trials/directive_en (accessed May 2019).

Health and Safety Executive (HSE) (2013). Personal protective equipment (PPE) at work: a brief guide. www.hse.gov.uk/pubns/indg174.pdf (accessed April 2019).

Health and Safety Executive (HSE) (2019). Safe Handling of Cytotoxic Drugs. London, DH www.hse.gov.uk/healthservices/safe-use-cytotoxic-drugs.htm (accessed April 2019).

London Cancer Alliance (2015). Integrated care systems (ICSs): guidelines for safe prescribing, handling and administration of systemic anticancer therapy, version 2.0. http://www.londoncancer.org/media/144228/Appendix20D_Pan-london-cytotoxic-handbook-july-2015.pdf (accessed April 2019).

Medicines and Healthcare Products Regulatory Authority (MHRA) (2019). http://www.gov.uk/government/organisations/medicines-and-healthcare-products-regulatory-agency (accessed March 2019).

Medicines for Human Use (Clinical Trials) Regulations (2004). No. 1031. www.legislation.gov.uk/uksi/2004/1031/contents/made (accessed May 2019).

National Cancer Action Team (NCAT) (2013a). National Cancer Peer Review Programme Manual for Cancer Services: Children's Cancer Measures v3. London, DH. http://www.londoncancer.org/media/58824/ccncg_measures-april2013.pdf) (accessed April 2019).

National Cancer Action Team (NCAT) (2013b). National Cancer Peer Review Programme Manual for Cancer Services: Chemotherapy Measures v2. London, DH.

National Chemotherapy Advisory Group (2009). Chemotherapy services in England: ensuring quality and safety. London, DH. www.theacp.org.uk/news/22-aug-2009-ncag-report-published.asp (accessed April 2019).

National Confidential Enquiry into Patient Outcome and Death (NCEPOD) (2018). On the right course? www.ncepod.org.uk/2018cictya.html (accessed April 2019).

National Institute for Health and Care Excellence (NICE) (2014). Cancer services for children and young people. Quality standard [QS55]. https://www.nice.org.uk/guidance/qs55 (accessed 10 April 2021).

National Institute for Occupational Safety and Health (NIOSH) (2016). Llist of antineoplastic and other hazardous drugs in healthcare settings, 2016. https://www.cdc.gov/niosh/docs/2016-161/default.html (accessed May 2019).

Reporting of Injuries, Diseases and Dangerous Occurrences Regulations (RIDDOR) (2013). www.hse.gov.uk/healthservices/safe-use-cytotoxic-drugs.htm (accessed March 2019).

Royal College of Nursing IV Therapy Forum (2016). *Standards for Infusion Therapy*, 4e. London: RCN.

Schulmeister, L. (2011). Vesicant chemotherapy extravasation management. *British Journal of Nursing (Intravenous Supplement)* 20 (19): S6–S12. United Kingdom Oncology Nursing Society.

Chapter 9

Early recognition and management of the seriously ill child

Denise Welsby[1] and Liesje Andre[2]

[1] RN (Adult); EPALs Subcommittee faculty member, instructor and course director, Resuscitation Council UK; Head of Resuscitation Services, Great Ormond Street Hospital, London, UK

[2] RN (Adult), RN (Child), PGCME; formerly Lead Nurse, Resuscitation, GOSH

Chapter contents

Introduction	124	'Just in case'/'just in time' training and situational awareness	127
Prevention: The 'chain of prevention'	124	AVPU (neurological observations)	127
Early recognition of the seriously ill child	124	Supporting the CYP using the structured A-E assessment tool	127
Rapid assessment using the A-E assessment tool	125	References	130

The Great Ormond Street Hospital Manual of Children and Young People's Nursing Practices, Second Edition. Edited by Elizabeth Anne Bruce, Janet Williss, and Faith Gibson.
© 2023 John Wiley & Sons Ltd. Published 2023 by John Wiley & Sons Ltd.

For the purposes of this chapter, the term 'child' refers to anyone under 12 years of age and "young person" refers to 12-17 year olds. For any patient aged 18 years or over, see Resuscitation Council (UK) guidance for the management of the deteriorating adult.

Introduction

In the UK on average, 5300 children and young people (CYPs) between the ages of 0 and 19 years die each year. Around three in five of these deaths occur in infancy and one in five occurs between the ages of 15 and 19 years (Wolfe et al. 2014). Many of these deaths are in the community and are often preventable. Greater attention is needed to address public health issues of poverty, inequality, and mental health for CYPs. While the child mortality rate has declined in recent years, statistics continue to highlight the UK as having one of the worst rates of death among children in Europe (Maconochie and Bingham 2014).

This chapter focuses on the *rapid assessment* of the CYP whose condition is deteriorating when time is of the essence. It has links with several other chapters in this book: For history taking, observations, and a thorough admission assessment see Chapter 1: Assessment. For resuscitation practices, see Chapter 30: Resuscitation.

Prevention: The 'chain of prevention'

While many childhood deaths occur in the community, CYPs also die in acute care settings. Some of these deaths may be preventable with effective early identification and response to the early warning signs of deterioration (Bottiger and Van Aken 2015).

The chain of prevention (Figure 9.1) was devised and reviewed by the European Resuscitation Council and the Resuscitation Council UK and helps structure the processes required to detect and prevent deterioration and cardiorespiratory arrest. The principles included in the chain are education, monitoring, recognition, calling for help, and response (Pitcher et al. 2015; Smith 2010).

Education
The teaching of 'early warning signs' to help staff recognise the deteriorating CYP, alongside the teaching of resuscitation skills, is now mandatory education for health care professionals in NHS Trusts (NHS Health Education England (2021). In the past, hospital staff were taught only resuscitation skills and their application during a cardiac arrest. Now, resuscitation training includes this important first step towards the recognition of the acutely ill CYP through interpretation of observed early warning signs, which are charted against nationally approved physiological parameters. The recognition of these signs in the ill CYP, in conjunction with a systematic approach, parental information, and gut feeling helps to alert staff to potential deterioration (Morrison and Berg 2016; Thim et al. 2010).

Figure 9.1 Chain of prevention. *Source:* Courtesy of the Resuscitation Council UK (RC UK).

Education includes:

- Use of a structured 'Airway, Breathing, Circulation, Disability, and Exposure' (ABCDE). approach (Figure 9.2) to recognise potentially life-threatening problems and manage these in order of priority.
- Simulation training to identify any theory practice gaps (O'Leary et al. 2016).
- Application of Resuscitation Council approved treatment algorithms (Greif et al. 2015; Skellet et al. 2021a).

Monitoring
For observations, see Chapter 1: Assessment. ECG monitoring is covered in Chapter 15: Investigations. Neurological observations are covered in Chapter 21: Neurological Care.

Recognition
The ultimate goal of early recognition is to quickly identify those CYPs at risk of deteriorating, whether it is as a result of their presenting condition, a new problem, or a complication of the healthcare provided, so that interventions and management strategies can be established early to reduce the risk of morbidity and or mortality (Austen et al. 2012). Early detection safeguards the CYP by providing appropriate clinical intervention in the most appropriate clinical environment (Armstrong et al. 2017).

Healthcare settings where 'early warning scoring systems' (EWS) have been introduced have made a significant impact in identifying the unwell CYP and preventing deterioration (Alam et al. 2014). When used in conjunction with an ABCDE (A-E) approach (Figure 9.2), an EWS helps to avert further deterioration and initiates prompt management of the deteriorating CYP (Bannister et al. 2016). It may be necessary to consider transferring the CYP to a high-dependency unit (HDU), where they can be more closely observed, to ensure effective treatment and management during this phase of their illness.

Early recognition of the seriously ill child

Children have a tremendous ability for physiological compensation when acutely unwell and it is important to remember that some of the early signs of deterioration may not be obvious (Churpek et al. 2016).

The rapid assessment of the seriously ill CYP should follow a structured format to identify those elements that would cause the greatest risk of cardiopulmonary arrest. This structured approach follows a simple aide-mémoire called the A-E assessment tool (Figure 9.2). All healthcare professionals should follow this structured approach in order to systematically assess and manage the elements of deterioration that are considered life threatening. In children, cardiorespiratory arrest is usually secondary to profound hypoxia, reflecting the end of the body's ability to compensate for the effects of the underlying illness or injury. The initial problem may originate from the airway, breathing, or circulation. It should be noted however, that irrespective of the primary underlying aetiology, cardiorespiratory arrest in children is rarely a sudden event. It represents a progressive deterioration, as the respiratory system and/or circulatory systems fail as the body loses its ability to compensate for the underlying illness or disease process (Skellet et al. 2021b).

Early recognition and effective management of both respiratory and/or circulatory failure will prevent the majority of paediatric cardiorespiratory arrests and thus reduce both morbidity and mortality (Bannard-Smith et al. 2016). A deteriorating child pathway (Figure 9.3) has been developed at GOSH, which includes the use of the communication tool SBARD – **S**ituation, **B**ackground, **A**ssessment, **R**ecommendation, **D**ecision – to facilitate prompt and appropriate communication (Thomas et al. 2009). Other tools include RSVP (Reason, Story, Vital signs, and Plan) (Featherstone et al. 2008).

> **PRIMARY SURVEY AND RESUSCITATION**
> Quickly Assess the Patients A.V.P.U
> **Alert, Verbal, Pain, Unresponsive**
>
> **A AIRWAY:**
>   Assessment
>   - Ascertain Patency
>   - Is the airway at risk?
>   - Rapidly assess for airway obstruction
>   - Management
>   - Establish a patient airway AVPU= P or U (8 or less on GCS
>   - Perform chin lift or jaw trust manoeuvres if required
>   - Insert an oropharyngeal airway
>   - Consider definitive airway: oraltracheal or nasotracheal intubation
>
> **B BREATHING VENTILATION AND OXYGENATION:**
>   Assessment
>   - Expose the neck and chest
>   - Determine the rate and depth of respirations
>   - Inspect the chest for unilateral and bilateral chest movement, use of accessory muscles and signs of injury
>   - Auscultate and percuss the chest bilaterally
>   Management
>   - Administer high flow oxygen
>   - Ventilate with BVM if AVPU P or U (8 or less on the GCS)
>   - Attach CO_2 monitoring device to endotracheal tube if tube in situ
>   - Attach patient to pulse oxmieter.
>
> **C CIRCULATION:**
>   Assessment
>   - Skin colour
>   - Capillary refill, peripheral and central
>   - Peripheral and central pulses; rate, rhythm, regularity and volume
>   - BP
>   Management
>   - Attach 3 lead ECG monitor
>   - IV/IO access obtained, check FBC, U&E, and Glucose
>   - Consider fluids 0.9% Nacl
>   - Prevent hypothermia
>
> **D DISABILITY:**
>   - Determine AVPU score and reassess frequently
>   - Pupils; size, equality, and reaction
>   - Past medical history, meds, allergies, last ate or drank
>
> **E EXPOSURE:**
>   - Expose but prevent hypothermia

Figure 9.2 Example of the A-E assessment tool.

Rapid assessment using the A-E assessment tool

Early recognition and effective initial treatment prevents deterioration and buys time for a definitive diagnosis to be made. Focused treatments can then be instituted while using the 'A-E' assessment tool (see Figure 9.2).

In summary the A-E tool aims to provide life-saving treatment:

- To break down complex clinical situations into more manageable parts.
- To serve as an assessment and treatment algorithm.
- To establish common situational awareness among all treatment providers.
- To buy time to establish a final diagnosis and treatment.

(Jones et al. 2013)

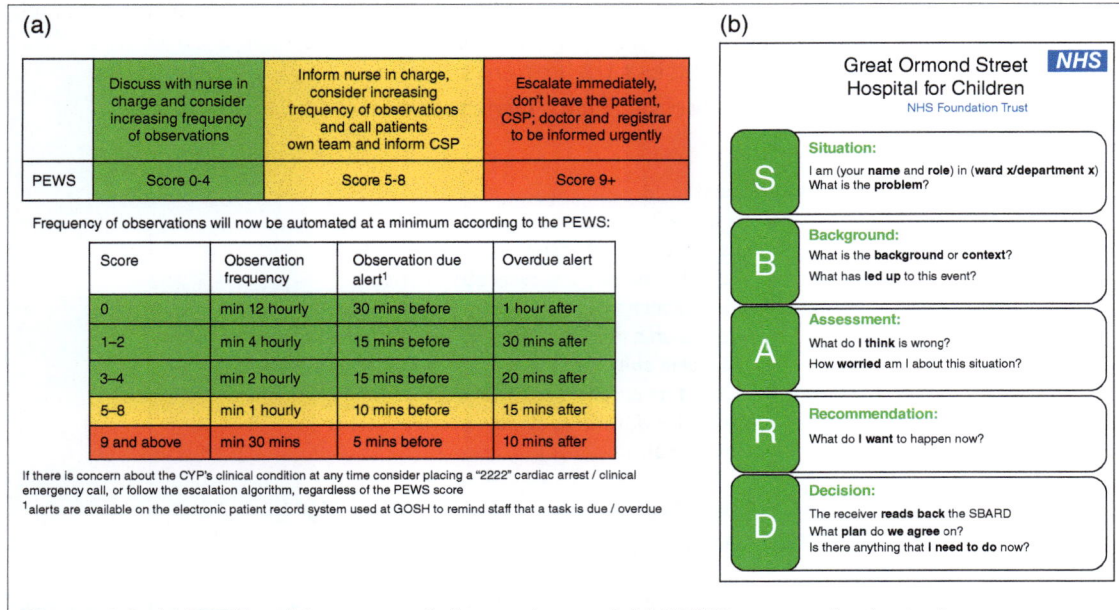

Figure 9.3 (a) PEWS and frequency of observations and (b) SBARD communication tool.

In all circumstances, life-threatening airway problems are assessed and treated first; second, life-threatening breathing problems are identified and treated; and so on through-out the A-E assessment.

Using this structured approach will ensure that vital interventions and treatments are commenced promptly and safely. With practice and confidence, this rapid assessment can be completed within one to two minutes (Jafarpour et al. 2014). Assistance and support may be required from a clinical expert, a specialist, or an outreach team within the hospital, (e.g. medical emergency team), so it is vital that staff are aware of whom to contact in the clinical setting they are working in. To improve awareness of deteriorating CYPs, many hospitals have introduced 'safety huddles'; a communication strategy utilised by ward-based clinical staff and medical emergency teams (Brady and Goldenhar 2014). Most importantly, if in doubt, ask for help as soon as possible (Figure 9.4). Clinical experts can offer clear guidance to clarify any concerns regarding the CYPs illness and current presentation. Improved outcome is most often based on a team effort (Nolan et al. 2016).

On completion of the initial A-E assessment and the delivery of interventions to reverse the signs of deterioration, further reassessments should be carried out until the CYP is stable, as it may take a few minutes for the effects of an intervention to become evident (Jarvis et al. 2015a).

When to perform an A-E assessment

The A-E assessment tool is used for both CYPs and adults. The clinical signs of critical illness are similar, regardless of the underlying cause. This makes exact knowledge of the underlying cause or specialist disease process unnecessary when performing the initial assessment and treatment.

Remember: Treat first which kills first; **A**irway, **B**reathing, **C**irculation, etc.

The A-E approach should be used for all CYP assessments and whenever critical illness is suspected. Cardiac arrest is often preceded by adverse clinical signs and these can be recognised and treated with the A-E approach to potentially prevent cardiac arrest (Smith 2010) and is recommended as the first step in managing the post resuscitation child upon the return of spontaneous circulation (ROSC) (Mandell et al. 2015).

When followed, the A-E assessment along with clinical observations, clinical history, physical examination and the collation of information from an early warning system can assist in the detection

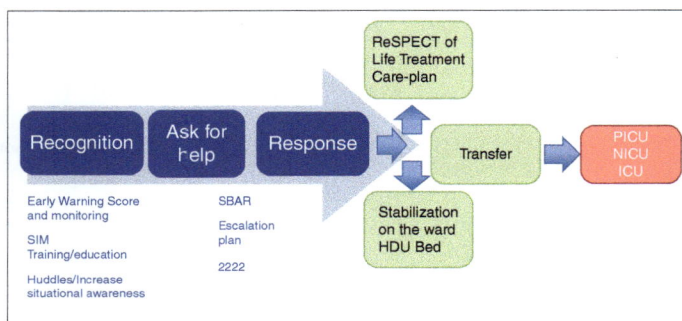

Figure 9.4 Deteriorating child pathway. *Source:* Courtesy of Liesje Andre, former Lead nurse in Resuscitation at GOSH. [1]SIM: Simulation Training. [2]SBARD: mnemonic used to communicate important facts about a child. [3]ReSPECT: Recommendation on Emergency Summary Plan and End of Life care and Treatment.

of serious illness and ensure a robust escalation strategy with approximately 90% sensitivity (Jarvis et al. 2015b). Each component of the evaluation is effective in identifying serious illness and reflects changes in a CYP's physical and emotional condition.

It is important to note that the A-E approach focuses on the general deterioration of a CYP who is still displaying signs of life, and does not include specific clinical management for the acutely injured CYP, e.g. trauma management. It can *only* be used for a CYP who is still displaying signs of life and should not be used if cardiopulmonary arrest is suspected. In the arrest situation, the paediatric advanced resuscitation algorithm should be followed (see Chapter 30: Resuscitation).

Advanced life support algorithms are available online at www.resus.org.uk.

Combining the A-E assessment with an early warning score (EWS)

On admission to any hospital setting the CYP's clinical vital signs are observed and documented as a base line while carrying out a systemic assessment using A-E (Olgers et al. 2017; Sefton et al. 2017). These physiological readings are concurrently applied to an early warning scoring system such as the national Paediatric Early

Table 9.1 Observations to be completed for Paediatric Early Warning Score (PEWS) documentation.

- AVPU (Alert, Verbal, Pain, Unresponsive)/conscious level
- Respirations
- Heart rate
- Capillary refill time
- Work of breathing
- Blood pressure
- Saturations
- Supplemental oxygen

Warning Score (PEWS), children's early warning system (CEWS), or medical emergency team criteria (MET), which are set physiological criteria based on acceptable values for the child's age (Table 9.1). In combination with the child's neurological status, the total Early Warning Score (EWS) highlights to the clinical team the level of intervention required, and whether an immediate call for help should be activated to prevent further deterioration or cardiopulmonary arrest (McLellan et al. 2017).

Given that children have a natural ability to compensate for being unwell, it is important to note that the EWS alone must never be the only trigger to call for support. Trends of physiological readings are more important than isolated readings. In addition, it must be noted that for some children, an abnormal EWS may be normal for them. Should this be the case, clear rational of the abnormality should be documented in the medical notes and communicated to all care providers. Extra caution should prevail when managing these children, as recognition of deterioration can be more challenging. In this situation, parental concern, or the healthcare worker's gut feelings are extremely beneficial to identify that something is not quite right. In all cases, if there is a belief that the child is deteriorating and/or their conscious level is dropping, it is important to call for help and support early, rather than waiting for the observations to trigger a specific early warning score (Akre et al. 2010).

'Just in case'/'just in time' training and situational awareness

For all CYPs, planning ahead for any potential deterioration will enable swift, prompt management of any airway, breathing, circulatory or neurological compromise. Putting in place simple, yet strategic planning for the worst-case scenario ahead of time heightens awareness of those CYPs who may be at risk and require watching. It mentally prepares staff to identify equipment and their ability to use it safely, the underpinning specific skills and knowledge to assist in managing an emergency event, and to check the environment for any hazards around the bed space which could cause injury to the CYP or rescuer.

Some hospitals have already introduced a system called 'Just-in-case', 'Just in time'; training that encourages all staff to do just that by:

- Placing a BMV apparatus in the room and having a refresher on how to use it.
- Removing all unnecessary clutter and informing parents/carers to do the same.
- Checking oxygen ports are functional.
- Ensuring suction is set up and ready for use.
- Refreshing their knowledge of the advanced life support algorithm (child specific).

- Ensuring that relevant clinical staff, such as the Outreach and Resuscitation teams, are aware of potential chance of child deterioration (Schuller et al. 2015).

AVPU (neurological observations)

The CYP's conscious level can be quickly assessed by using the AVPU scale which uses four simple categories; **A**lert; **V**erbal response; responds to **P**ain; **U**nresponsive (Figure 9.5). It can be assessed by simply speaking to the CYP and looking for appropriate normal reactions for their age, or if necessary, by applying a small painful stimulus to determine the response. One recommendation of how to assess for a response is to try and wake the CYP up. For example, in small babies, tapping the soles of the feet or calling their name loudly, or for older children, gentle tactile stimulation and calling their name may be enough to elicit a response. If there is a decreased level of consciousness, or the CYP does not appear to be breathing normally, airway compromise must be considered and supportive measures taken, such as airway and ventilatory support (Hoffmann et al. 2016).

As a modified version of the Glasgow Coma Scale, the AVPU (Figure 9.5) helps to assess and interpret the level of consciousness. This can be achieved within a few moments of meeting the child and supported by questioning the parents or named nurse as to what is normal behaviour for them. It is good practice to review the AVPU level repeatedly during the assessment to determine if this had improved or become more compromised since the initial assessment was made. It is considered formally in the A-E assessment under D for neurological disability ABC**D**E.

If the neurological level has worsened, help should be called for (if not already summoned) without delay, as advanced airway management and the clinical emergency team may be required. For more information regarding neurological assessment, AVPU, and the Glasgow Coma Scale see Chapter 21: Neurological Care.

Supporting the CYP using the structured A-E assessment tool

'Airway, Breathing, Circulation, Disability, and Exposure'

A: Airway

Airway obstruction can be partial or complete. Partial airway obstruction can lead to respiratory failure, exhaustion, cyanosis, apnoea, and eventually hypoxic brain injury. If left untreated, partial obstruction can become complete and the CYP will deteriorate into respiratory failure, then cardiopulmonary arrest. Airway compromise should be considered in CYPs with congenital abnormalities such as Pierre Robin syndrome, and those with central nervous system depression, e.g. head trauma, metabolic disorders.

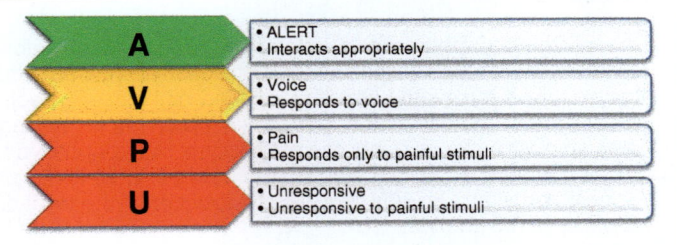

Figure 9.5 AVPU level. A = 15, V = 12, P = 8, U = 3. (*Source:* devised from the Resuscitation Council [UK] 2016).

> **Causes of airway obstruction**
> - Congenital abnormalities, e.g. choanal atresia, Pierre Robin syndrome
> - Secretions, vomit, blood, foreign body
> - Nasal tubes (feeding and naso-pharyngeal airway tubes)
> - Oxygen via nasal cannula
> - Central nervous system depression
> - Epiglottitis
> - Croup
> - Facial/head/throat trauma

If the CYP is verbally responsive, e.g. talking or crying, this indicates that the airway is currently patent and they can breathe on their own. This should be continuously re-assessed. Oxygen saturation levels (SPo2) should be recorded with the view to commencing the CYP on supplemental oxygen to maintain blood oxygenation saturations between 94–98% (Van de Voorde et al. 2021). Oxygen saturations should not be interpreted alone, as some CYPs with underlying cardiovascular disease may have a normally low saturation reading, which is considered acceptable given their underlying condition. It is always recommended to use additional observations such as, distal perfusion, extremity temperature and blood gas analysis to support the use of oxygen.

B: Breathing

The most noticeable sign that the CYP is struggling to compensate for their underlying disease process is their work of breathing. A simple approach involves using the 'look, listen, and feel' approach.

Look

Viewing the CYP initially from the bottom of the bed will give an overview of bilateral chest expansion and accessory muscle involvement such as the use of the abdomen, neck, and intercostal muscles.

Signs of increasing respiratory effort in respiratory distressed CYPs include:

- Increased use of intercostal muscles
- Increased use of subcostal muscles
- Increased use of sternocleidomastoid muscles
- Sternal recession
- Nasal flaring
- Head bobbing.

Listen

Auditory clues of inadequate breathing/ventilation include the following sounds:

- Muffled or hoarse speech
- Snoring
- Stridor
- Grunting
- Wheezing.

These sounds are audible without a stethoscope and provide information about the location of any airway obstruction and the amount of effort required to breathe. Snoring, muffled or hoarse speech, and stridor are all indicative of upper airway obstruction. Snoring suggests an obstruction in either the oropharynx or hypopharynx. Muffled or hoarse speech indicates obstruction at or near the level of the vocal cords, and stridor suggests obstruction at the level of the larynx or in the trachea.

Auscultating the chest during a period of deterioration does not require a lengthy a process. In this situation, listening to the chest is simply to confirm the degree of normal air entry to both lung fields. A more definitive assessment of both lungs can be completed later by the clinician once the CYP is stabilised. Beware of the silent chest; this indicates that very little air is going in and out, and that emergency airway support is needed (McLellan et al. 2014).

Feel

After observing for effort of breathing and bilateral chest expansion, confirmation of lung movement can be made by placing both hands on the chest, with thumbs together over the sternum and the hands around the circumference of the chest wall, to feel for chest wall expansion and/or recession. Intercostal recession, sub-sternal recession, and sub-costal recession will all indicate a child who is working hard to maintain adequate oxygen saturations for end organ perfusion. Only when the respiratory muscles begin to tire, or the airway becomes obstructed, does the child engage their abdominal muscles to further support respiratory drive and oxygenation. This is an ominous sign and should be managed promptly with anaesthetic support.

Once completed, the above findings, together with the airway assessment, will determine if additional treatments are necessary to support better oxygenation. Treatments such as suction, humidified oxygen, saline nebulization, and bronchodilators, should be considered at this time.

> **NOTE:** Irrespective of the degree of airway and breathing difficulty, it is good practice to plan for the worst-case scenario, "Just in Case" there is further deterioration, as discussed earlier. Ensure a bag mask valve device (BMV) with supplemental oxygen (see *Chapter 30: Resuscitation*) is in close proximity to the CYP and that suction is available, set up, and ready for use.

Ongoing respiratory compromise will rapidly affect other vital organs/systems. The hypoxic state causes a cardiac response, where the heart rate increases to assist the body to drive more circulating volume, to support respiratory muscle wall function, and to maintain breathing. Lack of perfusion to the extremities occurs as the skin's circulating blood flow is shifted back to the central core to support vital organ perfusion. The skin may become ashen and mottled before central cyanosis (blue lips) is apparent.

As circulating blood oxygen decreases, the hypoxic or hypercapnic state may lead to agitation or drowsiness and alterations in level of consciousness (AVPU, see Figure 9.5). If interventions are not carried out promptly to reverse the hypoxic state, loss of consciousness will follow. High-flow oxygen should be administered using a non-rebreathing face mask if breathing is inadequate. Supplemental oxygen delivery is guided by the CYP's clinical state, age, saturations, and neurological level (see Figure 9.5). Ultimately, when the CYP is exhausted and requiring ongoing respiratory support, anaesthetic support is essential. This should be sought early, as the potential for an endotracheal tube intubation is heightened. In the event of cardiopulmonary resuscitation, always use 100% oxygen to maximise oxygen delivery to the tissues. For more information see Chapter 30: Resuscitation.

C: Circulation

Once the airway and breathing have been assessed and appropriate management introduced the process moves on to circulation. Knowing how the CYP's cardiovascular system is responding haemodynamically to the underlying illness will indicate whether they are able to 'compensate' during this acute phase of their illness, or if they are in a 'decompensated state' or shock, and at risk of cardiopulmonary arrest due to circulatory failure.

> Shock is defined as a condition which occurs when the circulatory system is unable to provide sufficient blood carrying oxygen and nutrients to meet the metabolic demand of vital organs.
>
> In the seriously ill child, it is important to identify if they are in a compensated or decompensated shocked state, as this will guide immediate treatment. (Skellet et al. 2021b).

Compensated shocked state

In a compensated state, the CYP is still conscious and able to increase their cardiac output to meet the demand of vital organ perfusion and function. In children this is most likely seen when both the respiratory rate and heart rate increase in response to oxygen demand for perfusion of vital organs.

Signs of compensation
- Mild to moderate irritability
- Mild to moderate tachypnea
- Decreased urine output
- Delayed capillary refill
- Decreased skin turgor
- Normal blood pressure (within normal parameters for age)

The lowest systolic and diastolic perfusion pressure required to maintain a compensated state can be measured by using a formula calculated using the child's age (Figure 9.6).

Decompensated shocked state

This state develops as the blood pressure begins to drop and vital organ perfusion becomes profoundly compromised. Clinical signs of inadequate organ perfusion become more apparent.

Signs of decompensation
- Neurological level drops as brain perfusion is compromised (AVPU [P-U])
- Respiratory exhaustion
- Bradycardia
- Hypotension
- Unconsciousness.

Completing a structured A-E assessment and noting all clinical signs and symptoms in relation to the CYP's haemodynamic state is invaluable for determining whether they are in a compensated or decompensated state (Jones et al. 2013). Frequency of haemodynamic monitoring should be increased if the CYP triggers an early warning score of 5 or above, or if there is an element of 'gut feeling', or suspicion which has not yet been identified by the EWS (McLellan et al. 2017). **Stay vigilant**.

Determining the colour and temperature of the skin, in particular the hands and feet, will identify any poor circulation or tissue perfusion. Identify any cyanosis, mottling, or coldness and perform a capillary refill check on the foot, back of the hand, and in the centre of the chest in babies.

Normal capillary refill time should be less than two seconds; anything longer indicates poor perfusion. If not already in situ, obtain prompt venous access (IV), or request support to obtain intraosseous access (IO) so that supportive intravenous fluids can be delivered (Rosenberg and Cheung 2013). For insertion and use of an intraosseous cannula see Chapter 30: Resuscitation.

In general, the rule of thumb when choosing fluids in the management of a seriously ill CYP is to replace like for like; i.e. blood products for severe blood loss, plasmalyte and/or normal saline for dehydration, and dextrose for hypoglycemia (Van de Voorde et al. 2021).

Confirm both radial and central pulses based on the CYP's age to determine the rate, rhythm, regularity and the strength of the beat. This is also called stroke volume (Latham et al. 2017). In the ill CYP, a palpable pulse felt in the peripheral circulation indicates that they are currently able to compensate for the underlying illness and maintain an adequate systolic blood pressure to maintain end organ perfusion. The integrity of the pulse pressure should be appreciated: Barely palpable pulses suggest poor cardiac output or loss of stroke volume and circulating volume. A bounding pulse would suggest a condition such as sepsis. In all instances additional advice should be sought immediately.

Stroke volume
- The amount of volume ejected from the left ventricle with each heartbeat.
- This is dependent on heart rate, myocardial contractility, and circulating blood volume.

Vascular (IV) access

Intravenous access should be considered early in all CYPs showing signs of deterioration, as fluids are usually required to support them in maintaining circulating volume and perfusion. In addition, achieving access in the cold shocked CYP is extremely difficult due to peripheral circulation shutdown. The common sites for achieving IV access are the dorsum of the hand or antecubital fossa of the elbow. Whichever site is chosen, success will be determined by the ability to palpate a suitable vein given the clinical state of the CYP. If a peripheral vein is not evident, or if three attempts to achieve IV access have failed (over 60 seconds), time should not be lost to further attempts (Rosenberg and Cheung 2013). Clear indication that the CYP is cold and peripherally shut down should result in rapid intraosseous needle (IO) insertion, even in the CYP who is still conscious (see Chapter 30: Resuscitation).

Once IV/IO access is obtained, routine bloods should be taken for baseline biochemistry (urea and electrolytes), haematology (full blood count), and blood glucose before any fluids are infused. Additional blood tests, such as coagulation screen, microbiological screen, group, save, and cross match, can be requested based on the presentation. Fluid resuscitation volumes are based on body weight, at 10mls/kg. If the child's exact body weight is unknown, approved formulas can be used to guide fluid volumes.

This should be administered as a bolus via the IV/IO route. However, where it is suspected that large volumes may result in pulmonary oedema (heart failure) or cerebral oedema (diabetic ketoacidosis) fluids should be adjusted to 5–10ml/kg (Urbano et al. 2012) and the CYP reassessed frequently and after every intervention.

Some signs of fluid overload
- Dyspnoea
- Increased heart rate (age adjusted)
- Raised jugular venous pressure
- Pulmonary crackles on auscultation.

Age in years x 2 + 70 = lowest systolic BP acceptable to maintain organ perfusion
Age in years x 1.5 + 40 = lowest mean diastolic BP to maintain myocardial oxygenation.

Figure 9.6 Lowest acceptable systolic and diastolic blood pressure (BP).
Source: European Resuscitation Council and RC UK, p. 4.

If in doubt, seek expert advice (e.g. anaesthetist/intensivist) to identify alternative means of improving tissue perfusion, as inotropes or vasopressors may be necessary (Garcia-Canales et al. 2017).

Cardiac monitoring

Three-lead electrocardiographic monitoring (ECG) should be established in order to appreciate if the CYP's heart is beating adequately to support their underlying illness or disease. Monitoring by this simple approach will display three fundamental elements of the ECG – rate, rhythm, and regularity – with the additional benefit of appreciating the morphology (i.e. size, shape, and width of PQRST complexes and the ECG rhythm pattern) of the cardiac presentation. This information can be helpful in the diagnosis of any metabolic, hypoxic, or systemic abnormalities as a causative factor of the deterioration. If left untreated, these abnormalities are life threatening and therefore must be treated promptly. For more information on performing an ECG see Chapter 15: Investigations.

Some ECG abnormalities

Ventricular ectopic = Hypokalemia
Bradycardia = Hypoxic state
Tachycardia = Pain, anxiety, sepsis, structural heart damage

D: Disability

This element of the assessment relates to the CYP's neurological status and overall level of consciousness and takes into consideration the following information:

- AVPU
- Pupils
- Posturing or limb movement
- Past medical history
- Current medications
- Allergies
- Last intake
- Last urine output
- When bowels last opened
- Any parental concerns.

Urine output

Look for other signs of reduced cardiac output such as oliguria or reduced urinary output, as the kidneys are reliant on an adequate blood pressure to function normally. A urine output of less than 1 ml/kg/hr in children and less than 2 ml/kg/h in infants indicates inadequate renal perfusion during a shocked state. Asking questions of parents such as 'When did your baby last have a wet nappy?' are helpful in appreciating how unwell the child potentially is.

AVPU (neurological disability)

Formal assessments of all elements of the CYP's neurological state are made. Having initially appreciated the level of consciousness on first examination, the neurological level of the CYP should be reassessed more formally to identify if the level of consciousness may have worsened. If there is any indication that the CYP is becoming less responsive, help (if not already summoned) should be called for without delay, as advanced airway management may be required. For further information on neurological assessment see Chapter 1: Assessment and Chapter 21: Neurological Care. Disability assessment should include pupil size and reaction time (whether sluggish, brisk, or nonreactive), as this may highlight whether a neurological event has caused the deterioration. It is important to enquire whether the CYP is displaying any abnormal limb tone or movements. Any abnormalities should be recorded and reported to the on-call doctors (Waterhouse 2017).

Past medical history

Knowing the past medical history and which medications the CYP is receiving will also help to manage the situation. It is important to identify if the deterioration was as a result of the underlying disease process and could therefore be predicted and prevented in future, or was due to the introduction of specific medicines that caused sensitivity and an adverse reaction needing re-evaluation, adjustment, or stopping.

Glucose

An estimation of the CYP's glucose levels can be obtained at the bedside and requested when blood sampling is taken once an IV/IO cannula is inserted. In the ill child an increase in the body's metabolism demand results in an increase demand for glucose. Children do not have large reserves of glycogen in the liver to break down to meet this demand, so when ill they can become hypoglycemic very quickly. This is normally between 4 and 7 mmols.

E: Exposure

It is important to fully expose the CYP when completing a clinical examination, to appreciate any signs of limb discoloration, bruising/rash, cyanosis, loss of body fluids, or blood from orifices, wounds, or drains. These can indicate other concerns such as dehydration, trauma, internal bleeding, and sepsis. Be wary however, that children may become hypothermic due to exposure and interventions. Dignity and comfort must always be maintained, irrespective of age (Thim et al. 2012).

Check a formal core temperature to identify any indication of hot sepsis, although in some septic children a pyrexia may not be evident, yet they may still be septic (Freitag et al. 2016).

The A-E assessment in the ill CYP is a rapid assessment and it is important to remember that continuous reassessment is necessary to identify any significant change, be it positive or negative.

References

Akre, M., Finkelstein, M., Erickson, M. et al. (2010). Sensitivity of the pediatric early warning score to identify patient deterioration. *Pediatrics* 125: e763–e769.

Alam, N., Hobbelink, E.L., Van Tienhoven, A.J. et al. (2014). The impact of the use of the early warning score (EWS) on patient outcomes: a systematic review. *Resuscitation* 85 (5): 587–594.

Armstrong, L., Shepherd, A., and Harris, F. (2017). An evaluation of approaches used to teach quality improvement to pre-registration healthcare professionals: an integrative review. *Int. J. Nurs. Stud.* 73: 70–84.

Austen, C., Patterson, C., Poots, A. et al. (2012). Using a local early warning scoring system as a model for the introduction of a national system. *Acute Med* 11: 66–73.

Bannard-Smith, J., Lighthall, G.K., Subbe, C.P. et al. (2016). Clinical outcomes of patients seen by rapid response teams: a template for benchmarking international teams. *Resuscitation* 107: 7–12.

Bannister, M., Trotter, P., Jawad, A., and Veitch, D.Y. (2016). Airway and head and neck high dependency unit: a single-centre experience. *J. Laryngol. Otol.* 130: 777–730.

Bottiger, B.W. and Van Aken, H. (2015). Kids save lives – training school children in cardiopulmonary resuscitation worldwide is now endorsed by the World Health Organization (WHO). *Resuscitation* 94: A5–A7.

Brady, P.W. and Goldenhar, L.M. (2014). A qualitative study examining the influences on situation awareness and the identification, mitigation and escalation of recognised patient risk. *BMJ Qual. Saf.* 23: 153–161.

Churpek, M.M., Adhikari, R., and Edelson, D.P. (2016). The value of vital sign trends for detecting clinical deterioration on the wards. *Resuscitation* 102: 1–5.

European Resuscitation Council and the Resuscitation Council (UK) (2016). European Paediatric Advanced Life Support, 4e. Resuscitation Council UK.

Featherstone, P., Chalmers, T., and Smith, G.B. (2008). RSVP: a system for communication of deterioration in hospital patients. *Br J Nurs* 17 (13): 860–864.

Freitag, A., Constanti, M., O'Flynn, N. et al. (2016). Suspected sepsis: summary of NICE guidance. *BMJ* 354: i4030.

Garcia-Canales, A., Pena-Juarez, R.A., and Sandoval-Franco, L.M. (2017). Vasopressors and inotropes: use in pediatrics. *Arch. Cardiol. Mex.* 88 (1): 39–50.

Greif, R., Lockey, A.S., Conaghan, P. et al. (2015). European Resuscitation Council guidelines for resuscitation 2015: Section 10. Education and implementation of resuscitation. *Resuscitation* 95: 288–301.

Hoffmann, F., Schmalhofer, M., Lehner, M. et al. (2016). Comparison of the AVPU Scale and the Pediatric GCS in prehospital setting. *Prehosp. Emerg. Care* 20: 493–498.

Jafarpour, S., Nassiri, S.J., Bidari, A. et al. (2014). Principles of primary survey and resuscitation in cases of pediatric trauma. *Acta Med. Iran* 52: 943–946.

Jarvis, S., Kovacs, C., Briggs, J. et al. (2015a). Aggregate National Early Warning Score (NEWS) values are more important than high scores for a single vital signs parameter for discriminating the risk of adverse outcomes. *Resuscitation* 87: 75–80.

Jarvis, S., Kovacs, C., Briggs, J. et al. (2015b). Are observation selection methods important when comparing early warning score performance? *Resuscitation* 90: 1–6.

Jones, D., Mitchell, I., Hillman, K., and Story, D. (2013). Defining clinical deterioration. *Resuscitation* 84: 1029–1034.

Latham, H.E., Bengtson, C.D., Satterwhite, L. et al. (2017). Stroke volume guided resuscitation in severe sepsis and septic shock improves outcomes. *J. Crit. Care* 42: 42–46.

Maconochie, I.K. and Bingham, R. (2014). Paediatric resuscitation. *BMJ* 348: g1732.

Mandell, I.M., Bynum, F., Marshall, L. et al. (2015). Pediatric early warning score and unplanned readmission to the pediatric intensive care unit. *J. Crit. Care* 30: 1090–1095.

McLellan, K.E., Schwarze, J., and Beattie, T. (2014). Chest auscultatory signs in infants presenting to A&E with bronchiolitis. *Eur. J. Emerg. Med.* 21: 436–441.

McLellan, M.C., Gauvreau, K., and Connor, J.A. (2017). Validation of the Children's Hospital Early Warning System for critical deterioration recognition. *J. Pediatr. Nurs.* 32: 52–58.

Morrison, W.E. and Berg, R.A. (2016). Caring for the team is caring for the patient (and the future). *Pediatr. Crit. Care Med.* 17: 703–704.

Nolan, J.P., Ornato, J.P., Parr, M.J. et al. (2016). Resuscitation highlights in 2015. *Resuscitation* 100: A1–A8.

NHS Health Education England (2021). Core Skills Training Framework (CSTF) and Enabling Staff Movement in NHS Trusts in England. https://skillsforhealth.org.uk/info-hub/core-skills-training-framework-cstf-and-enabling-staff-movement-in-nhs-trusts-in-england/ (accessed 11 March 2021).

O'Leary, J., Nash, R., and Lewis, P. (2016). Standard instruction versus simulation: educating registered nurses in the early recognition of patient deterioration in paediatric critical care. *Nurse Educ. Today* 36: 287–292.

Olgers, T.J., Dijkstra, R.S., Drost-De Klerck, A.M., and Ter Maaten, J.C. (2017). The ABCDE primary assessment in the emergency department in medically ill patients: an observational pilot study. *Neth J Med* 75: 106–111.

Pitcher, D., Gwinnutt, C., and Lockey, A. (2015). Education for cardiac arrest – prevention and treatment. *Resuscitation* 96: e7.

Rosenberg, H. and Cheung, W.J. (2013). Intraosseous access. *CMAJ* 185: E238.

Schuller, M.C., Darosa, D.A., and Crandall, M.L. (2015). Using just-in-time teaching and peer instruction in a residency program's core curriculum: enhancing satisfaction, engagement, and retention. *Acad. Med.* 90: 384–391.

Sefton, G., Lane, S., Killen, R. et al. (2017). Accuracy and efficiency of recording Pediatric early warning scores using an electronic physiological surveillance system compared with traditional paper-based documentation. *Comput. Inform. Nurs.* 35: 228–236.

Skellett, S., Maconochie, I., Bingham, B et al. (2021a). Paediatric basic life support guidelines. Resuscitation Council (RC) UK. https://www.resus.org.uk/library/2021-resuscitation-guidelines/paediatric-basic-life-support-guidelines (accessed 31 May 2022).

Skellett, S., Maconochie, I., Bingham, B et al. (2021b). Paediatric advanced life support guidelines. Resuscitation Council (RC) UK. https://www.resus.org.uk/library/2021-resuscitation-guidelines/paediatric-advanced-life-support-guidelines (accessed 31 May 2022).

Smith, G.B. (2010). In-hospital cardiac arrest: is it time for an in-hospital 'chain of prevention'? *Resuscitation* 81: 1209–1211.

Thim, T., Krarup, N.H., Grove, E.L., and Lofgren, B. (2010). ABCDE – a systematic approach to critically ill patients. *Ugeskr. Laeger* 172: 3264–3266.

Thim, T., Krarup, N.H., Grove, E.L. et al. (2012). Initial assessment and treatment with the airway, breathing, circulation, disability, exposure (ABCDE) approach. *Int. J. Gen. Med.* 5: 117–121.

Thomas, C.M., Bertram, E., and Johnson, D. (2009). The SBAR communication technique: teaching nursing students professional communication skills. *Nurse Educ.* 34: 176–180.

Urbano, J., Lopez-Herce, J., Solana, M.J. et al. (2012). Comparison of normal saline, hypertonic saline and hypertonic saline colloid resuscitation fluids in an infant animal model of hypovolemic shock. *Resuscitation* 83: 1159–1165.

Van de Voorde, P., Turner, N.M., Djakow, J. et al. (2021). European Resuscitation Council Guidelines 2021: Paediatric Life Support. *Resuscitation* 161: 327–387. https://cprguidelines.eu/ (accessed 31 May 2022).

Waterhouse, C. (2017). Practical aspects of performing Glasgow coma scale observations. *Nurs. Stand.* 31: 40–46.

Chapter 10

Fluid balance

Eileen Brennan[1], John Courtney[2], and Josephine Jim[3]

[1] RN (Child), RN (Adult), ENB 147, MSc; Formerly Nurse Consultant in Paediatric Nephrology, Great Ormond Street Hospital, London, UK
[2] Formerly Assistant Chief Nurse, Great Ormond Street Hospital for Children NHS, Foundation Trust, London, UK
[3] RN (Child), BSc (hons), ENB 415; Paediatric intensive care Sister & CRRT/ Renal lead nurse PICU, GOSH

Chapter contents

Introduction	134
Maintenance of fluid requirements	134
Fluid balance in the ill CYP	134
Renal replacement therapy (RRT)	134
Vascular access	136
Haemofiltration (HF)	136
Haemodialysis (HD)	136
Dialysis fluid for HD	137
Haemofiltration	139
Peritoneal dialysis (PD)	139
Types of PD	139
Preparing the CYP for dialysis access	141
References	154
Further reading	155

Procedure guidelines

10.1 Fluid input/output	141
10.2 Preparation of the CYP and family for HD/HF	142
10.3 Inserting a catheter (HD/HF)	142
10.4 Preparing the equipment (HF)	143
10.5 Preparation for HF	144
10.6 Starting CRRT	144
10.7 Monitoring and maintaining CRRT	146
10.8 Discontinuing CRRT	147
10.9 Commencing HD	149
10.10 Discontinuing HD	150
10.11 Preparation (PD)	150
10.12 Preparation for surgery (PD)	151
10.13 Starting PD for AKI	151
10.14 Care of the CYP on PD	153
10.15 Special considerations (PD)	153
10.16 Discontinuing PD	154

Principles table

10.1 Assessing fluid balance in the ill child	140

The Great Ormond Street Hospital Manual of Children and Young People's Nursing Practices, Second Edition. Edited by Elizabeth Anne Bruce, Janet Williss, and Faith Gibson.
© 2023 John Wiley & Sons Ltd. Published 2023 by John Wiley & Sons Ltd.

Introduction

Fluid and electrolyte homeostasis is an essential requirement for optimal cellular and organ function. The kidneys play an essential role in maintaining this balance; in health they regulate the volume and composition of body fluids by actively absorbing and excreting fluids, electrolytes, and the unwanted end-products of metabolism. Correction and maintenance of fluids and electrolytes in children and young people (CYPs) presents unique challenges. The content and distribution of total body water changes with age (Willock and Jewkes 2000). To assess these changes, it is important to note that body fluids are split into two main compartments; intracellular and extracellular fluid. Extracellular fluid is further divided into intravascular (plasma), interstitial (fluid surrounding tissues), and transcellular (cerebrospinal fluid, sinovial, pleural, peritoneal). It is important to remember that age-related changes affect both body water content and distribution (Table 10.1). Three-quarters of water distribution of extracellular fluid is located in the interstitial space and one-quarter in the plasma (Willock and Jewkes 2000).

This chapter deals primarily with the treatment of advanced stages of renal impairment and disease and covers renal replacement therapy. For more detailed information regarding the general principles for managing IV fluids in CYPs see National Institute of Health and Care Excellence (NICE 2015) guidelines.

Maintenance of fluid requirements

Fluid loss consists mainly of urine, insensible losses (skin and respiratory tract), sweat, vomit, and stool. Fluid balance is normally achieved in infants by maintaining adequate fluids, nutrition, and warmth. The mechanisms to maintain homeostasis are highly sophisticated and finely balanced by many complex systems of movement of fluids and electrolytes between the vascular space and the body tissues. This involves osmosis and diffusion, with a complex process of oncotic and hydrostatic forces moving fluid around the body compartments.

Infants and preterm babies are particularly vulnerable to any imbalance of fluids and electrolytes; this is partly due to their large percentage of extracellular fluid, immature compensatory mechanisms, and high metabolic rate during the first few months of life. Any small insult during this time can upset this fine balance, resulting in impaired renal function. Fluid and electrolyte maintenance or replacement will depend on the type and amount of fluid being lost. This must be calculated on an individual basis according to the CYP's fluid status and electrolytes. Different laboratories often have different reference ranges for blood levels due to different methods of testing specimens. For this reason it is important to use local hospital or laboratory guidelines when checking reference ranges (Phadke et al. 2014). Fluid requirements to maintain health are listed in Table 10.2.

A fluid imbalance can lead to or indicate mild, moderate, or severe renal failure, requiring some form of intervention. The most common causes of paediatric acute kidney injury (AKI) are trauma, sepsis, haemolytic uremic syndrome (HUS), glomerular diseases such as glomerulonephritis, obstructive uropathy within

Table 10.1 Approximate total body water (% of body weight)

Approximate total body water (% of body wt)	Pre-term	Term	1–2 years	Adult male
Water content	90%	70–80%	64%	60%
ICF	48%	48%	34%	40%
ECF	27%	27%	30%	20%

Source: Modified from Metheny and Snively (1983).

Table 10.2 Daily total water intake, including water contained in food. (These recommendations are for adequate intakes and should not be interpreted as a specific requirement)

Age (years)	Total daily intake (ml)
Infants 0–6 months	700 ml (assumed to be from milk)
7–12 months	800 ml (from milk and complementary foods and beverages)
1–3 years	1300 ml
4–8	1000–1400
9–13	1200–2100 girls
	1400–2300 boys
14–18	1400–2500 girls
	2100–3200 boys

Source: Gordon et al. (2010) and Rees et al. (2012).

the urinary tract, major surgery, and side effects of medicines such as chemotherapy and antibiotics (Table 10.7). The treatment of AKI may include renal replacement therapy in the form of peritoneal dialysis (PD), continuous renal replacement therapy (CRRT), haemodialysis (HD), or haemodiafiltration (HDF). The focus of this chapter will be fluid balance and the treatment of AKI.

Fluid balance in the ill CYP

Fluid balance (fluid input/output) must be measured and calculated according to clinical condition. Weight and height measurements are required to calculate fluid requirements by surface area (400 ml/m^2/day or 30 ml/kg/day) (Rees et al. 2012). This may need to be estimated if a CYP is critically ill. Fluid status and baseline observations should be assessed. Table 10.2 indicates the recommended daily fluid intake for a healthy CYP and Table 10.3 is a reference table (modified from the advance life support group) to assess the level of hydration in CYPs. Samples for blood and urine electrolytes may be required if severe dehydration or bloody diarrhoea is present. The severity of dehydration in relation to weight loss is shown in Table 10.5.

Renal replacement therapy (RRT)

Monitoring fluid balance in ill CYPs is a basic requirement, as they are often at high risk of developing a fluid imbalance secondary to their illness or treatment intervention. Early recognition and replacement of fluids during this time can reduce the risk of AKI and the need for renal replacement therapy (RRT). RRT may be a transient or a permanent requirement depending on the severity or cause of kidney failure; recovery of renal function after a period of therapy is never guaranteed. The choice of renal replacement therapy will depend on the expertise and resources available in the area and may be intermittent or continuous. Dialysis is used as a supportive therapy until kidney function recovers; however, in end-stage renal failure (ESRF) the loss of renal function is irreversible and dialysis replaces renal function. Dialysis is a 'term used to describe the removal of solutes and water from the blood across a semipermeable membrane' (Challinor 2014, p. 165). To clear waste products from the blood, all renal replacement modalities use diffusion across a semipermeable membrane, either the peritoneal membrane or haemodialyser/haemofilter membrane, plus ultrafiltration to remove excess fluid from the body. CYPs requiring dialysis are

Table 10.3 Assessing hydration (modified from Advanced Life Support Group (2012) and Davenport (1996)

Assessment	Normal hydration	Mild dehydration <5%	Moderate dehydration 5–10%	Severe dehydration >10%	Hypervolaemia
General appearance	Alert, good muscle tone	Alert, good muscle tone. May be thirsty	May be irritable or lethargic, sunken eyes, sunken anterior fontanelle	Confused, floppy, sunken eyes, reduced eyeball turgor, sunken anterior fontanelle	Lethargic, puffy
Colour	Consistent, pink lips, palms of hands, nail beds	Pink lips, palms of hands	Pale	Mottled/pale/grey	Normal
Temperature of extremities (in warm environment)	Warm	Normal or cool	Cool	Cold	Cool or warm depending on degree of overload
Peripheral pulses	Strong	Strong	May be weak	Weak	May be strong
Mucous membranes	Pink, moist	May be dry	Dry	Pale, dry	Pink, moist
Capillary refill time (in warm environment)	1–2 seconds	1–2 seconds	May be > 2 seconds	>2 seconds	1–2 seconds
Respiration	Normal for age	Normal for age	Normal or elevated	Elevated	May be elevated
Skin turgor/observable oedema	Pinched skin immediately falls back to normal	Pinched skin immediately falls back to normal	Pinched skin slowly falls back to normal	Pinched skin remains tented	May have peri-orbital/abdominal/leg oedema
Heart rate	Normal for age	Normal for age	May be raised	Marked tachycardia	May be normal or tachycardia
Urine output	Infant 2 ml/kg/hr; Child 1 ml/kg/hr; Adolescent 0.5 ml/kg/hr	Reduced	Reduced	Reduced or anuric	Reduced or anuric
Urine S.G	1.005–1.020	May be >1.020	>1.020	>1.020	<1.005 before treatment of diuretics
Blood pressure	Normal for age	Normal	Normal	May be normal or low	Usually raised
Temperature gap	<2°C in warm environment	<2°C	May be wide	Wide	Usually >2
SPO_2	97–100%	97–100%	97–100% if recordable	May not be recordable	May be low
Chest X-ray	Clear	Clear	Clear	Clear	May show pulmonary oedema/enlarged heart
Abdominal X-ray	Normal	Normal	Normal	Normal	May show ascites/hepatomegaly
CVP (Rt. Atrium)	0–5 mmHg	Normal	Normal	Normal or low	>5 mmHg
Body weight	Fairly stable (<1% body weight gain or loss per day)	Weight loss <50 g/kg	Weight loss 50–100 g/kg	Weight loss >100 g/kg	Weight gain >1%

usually transferred to specialised renal units or to a paediatric intensive care unit. All forms of replacement therapy require a high level of clinical expertise and are not available in all paediatric units. PD is performed via a catheter inserted into the peritoneum; HD or haemofiltration (HF) requires vascular access.

Vascular access

Central venous catheters can be single or dual lumen and should be of sufficient diameter size to allow for high blood flows. However, use of a single lumen catheter requires a larger blood circuit, which may be less optimal for young children. An uncuffed central venous catheter can be sited if treatment will be short term; otherwise a cuffed catheter is placed.

An arterio-venous (AV) fistula is a permanent form of access used in CYPs receiving long-term HD. This is created by the surgical anastomosis of an artery and a vein in the arm, most commonly the radial artery and cephalic vein. An AV fistula can be used for acute dialysis. Most fistulas are formed for long-term treatment.

Haemofiltration (HF)

HF is an extracorporeal blood purification therapy that mimics work done by the kidneys, paralleling what occurs in the human glomerulus, in order to improve the chances of renal recovery usually for CYPs with acute kidney insufficiency (AKI) (Hanson and Moist 2003; D'Intini et al. 2004; Drummond and Bellamy 2010; Ronco et al. 2015). It is used predominantly in paediatric intensive care units (PICU) as one of the continuous modalities of renal replacement therapy referred to as CRRT, (Shaheen et al. 2009). It has become the front line therapy and treatment of choice in many PICU's because the consensus is that CRRT offers optimal treatment for haemodynamically unstable CYPs when compared to standard intermittent HD, (Brophy 2008; Lyndon et al. 2012; Prowle and Bellomo 2010; Rewa et al. 2015). The modalities within CRRT are preferred because they are generally less aggressive than HD as they allow for slow, isotonic fluid removal, which results in better haemodynamic tolerance, avoiding rapid electrolytes and fluid shifts in critically ill CYPs with shock and severe fluid overload (Askenazi et al. 2013; John and Eckardt 2007; Sefton et al. 2001; Symons et al. 2003). The multiple CRRT modalities include continuous veno-venous haemofiltration (CVVH), continuous veno-venous haemodialysis (CVVHD), continous veno-venous haemodiafiltration (CVVHDF), and slow continuous ultra-filtration (SCUF). The solute clearing mechanisms have determined the nomenclature of these modalities (MacLaren and Butt 2009).

Haemodialysis (HD)

HD is a procedure in which blood is pumped out of the body, from a specially created vascular access, and around an extracorporeal circuit, where it passes through the haemodialyser before it is returned to the CYP. The haemodialyser consists of a semipermeable membrane across which bloods flows on one side and dialysis fluid on the other. The process of diffusion allows excess solutes to be removed from the blood; excess water is removed by the process of ultrafiltration. HD is a very effective method of renal replacement therapy for both acute and ESRF in CYPs.

Commencing extracorporeal treatments HD/HF
Calculation of extracorporeal volume (ECV)

The nurse must first estimate the CYP's total blood volume (Table 10.8), before the extracorporeal volume (ECV) can be calculated. The ECV is estimated as being 8–10% of the total blood volume (Mactier et al. 2009). Once the ECV has been calculated, suitably sized dialysis lines and HD/HF can be selected to ensure this volume is not exceeded. If the CYP is grossly oedematous, allowances should be made to their weight to avoid over estimation of the ECV, which could result in a larger than required circuit being selected. A range of circuit sizes (neonatal, paediatric and adult) are available (Rees et al. 2012). In cases when the smallest circuit available is near to or greater than the CYP's ECV it is necessary to prime the circuit with bank blood. As a rule, children and infants less than 10 kg will receive a blood prime. This minimises any potential adverse cardiovascular effects and allows for safe dialysis. Usually the blood is not returned at the end of the session as it is extra to their circulating volume. For example, a child of 10 kg will have a TBV of 800 ml (wt × 80) and an ECV of 64–80 ml (8–10% of TBV). Therefore, the volume of blood in the dialyser and circuit must not exceed 80 ml (Table 10.8).

The haemodialyser

The haemodialyser/filter is composed of a modified cellulose membrane or synthetic material. Variations in dialyser membrane design, size and thickness result in different solute and fluid clearances. The haemodialyser/filter is selected according to the CYP's body surface area, which is calculated using a standard nomogram (see Figure 10.1). The surface area of the membrane in the dialyser should not exceed that of the CYP (Mactier et al. 2009) and varying sized dialysers, ranging from $0.2\,m^2$ to $1.7\,m^2$ and greater are available. The ECV also indicates the blood pump speed for the dialysis session. Thus, the 10-kg child will have a maximum blood pump speed of 80 ml/min (Rees et al. 2012).

Anticoagulation of the circuit

To prevent clotting in the dialyser membrane or the circuit itself the dialysis circuit is routinely anticoagulated with unfractionated heparin (Mactier et al. 2009). The dose of heparin is titrated to the CYP's weight and their individual requirements. Doses range from 0 to 25 units/kg/hr (Rees et al. 2012). It is given continuously during dialysis and a bolus dose may also be given at the start of the session. Heparin-free dialysis is possible for those CYPs who have just had or who are about to have surgery. The circuit is flushed with saline regularly to help keep the fibres clear (Mactier et al. 2009). Alternatively, low molecular weight heparin, such as dalteparin, can be given as a single bolus at the start of dialysis.

Table 10.4 Fluid replacement choice for hypovolaemia

Fluid choice	
Isotonic crystalloid fluid	Colloid fluids
0.9% sodium chloride	4.5% albumin
Plasma-Lyte	Gelofusine
Hartmann's solution	Haemaccel

Plasma-Lyte is isotonic to plasma and has less chloride than other solutions, so causes less hyperchloraemic acidosis. It is a more balance solution than Hartmann's (Weinberg et al. 2016).

Table 10.5 Degree of dehydration

Degree of dehydration	Estimated loss of body weight in a child/infant	Approximate loss of body weight (ml/kg) in infant	Estimated loss of body weight in older children and adolescents	Approximate loss of body weight (ml/kg) older children and adolescents
Mild	<5%	50 ml/kg	3%	30 ml/kg
Moderate	5–10%	100 ml/kg	6%	60 ml/kg
Severe	10–15%	150 ml/kg	9%	90 ml/kg

Source: Willock and Jewkes (2000).

Table 10.6 IV fluid and electrolytes requirements in AKI

	Initial management for rehydration in AKI		
Dehydrated	0.9% sodium chloride	**Fluid resuscitation** 10–20 ml/kg over 30 minutes, assess urine output and repeat as necessary	
Hypovolaemia	Hartmann's (APLS guidelines) or 4.5% albumin	10–20 ml/kg isotonic solution	
Fluid overload AKI	Frusemide 2–4 mg/kg IV	Dialysis if no response	
Sodium, potassium, and chloride requirements			
Weight:	**<10 kg**	**11–30 kg**	**>30 kg**
Sodium, potassium, and chloride daily requirement	2.5 mmols/kg	2 mmols/kg	1.5 mmols/kg

Source: Rees et al. (2012).

Table 10.7 Causes of AKI

Pre-renal	Renal	Post renal
Diarrhoea and vomiting	Bloody diarrhoea (HUS)	Urethral obstruction, e.g. PRV
Cardiac impairment	Hypovolaemia	Polydipsia and polyuria
Birth asphyxia	Hypovolaemia	Poor urinary output
Umbilical catheters	Infection	Poor urinary output
Bilateral renal arterial or venous thrombosis	Poor blood supply	Poor urinary output
Drugs	Drugs	

Source: Rees et al. (2012).

Table 10.8 Estimated blood volumes

	Estimated blood volumes			
Age	Neonates	Infant	Child	Adult
Blood ml/kg	90	80	70	65

Source: Davenport (1996).

Dialysis fluid for HD

Water is required to dilute the dialysis fluid and must meet national standards for microbiological and chemical purity (Rees et al. 2012). Water is softened and filtered and passed through a reverse osmosis membrane before it is used. The dialysis fluid, or dialysate, enables diffusion to take place across the dialyser. The HD machine dilutes concentrated bicarbonate and acidic component with the purified water and ensures the correct concentration is produced. It warms it to 37°C and pumps it around the dialyser allowing diffusion to occur. Sodium, bicarbonate, potassium, glucose, and calcium levels can be adjusted to ensure an appropriate concentration and optimal mix for the CYP. The selection of dialysate values should be made in conjunction with the biochemical results. For example, a CYP with a serum potassium level of 3.0 mmol/l would lose more potassium through diffusion if the standard solution of 2 mmol/l was used, but this can be prevented or reversed if a higher potassium containing solution is selected.

Dialysis treatment sessions

CYPs with AKI may require daily dialysis to cope with fluid gains and provide adequate solute clearance (Table 10.9). Sessions vary in length, for example, in CYPs with a serum urea >40 umol/l it is necessary to limit dialysis length to less than two hours to avoid the risk of solute disequilibrium (Rees et al. 2012). Disequilibrium occurs if there is a discrepancy between the serum urea and the urea level in the brain, which can occur if the serum urea is reduced too quickly. To compensate, water moves across the blood–brain barrier to lower the brain urea, causing swelling with potentially catastrophic neurological effects. Conversely, a CYP needing to be dialysed for the hyperkalaemia and hyperphosphataemia resulting from tumour lysis will be dialysed until the rate of lysing falls and their own renal function can cope.

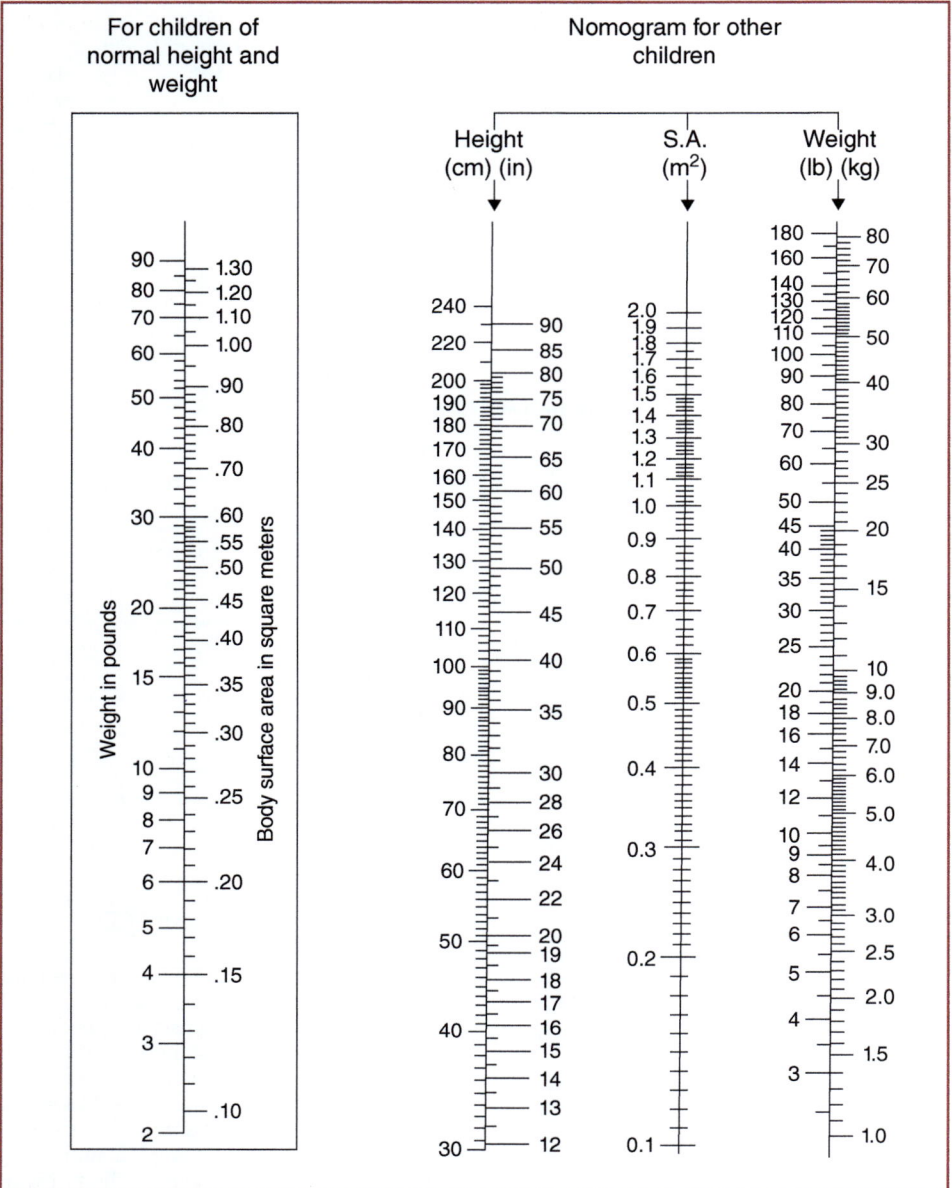

Figure 10.1 Body surface area in children. For children of average size, you can estimate body surface area (BSA) by using the nomogram on the left. Simply find the child's weight in pounds and then read across to the corresponding BSA on the right. For other children, use the nomogram on the right. With a straight edge, connect the patient's weight in the right column with height in the left column; the point of intersection in the middle column is the BSA. Modified from https://www.uncp.edu/sites/default/files/2017-11/Nomogram.pdf.

Table 10.9 Indications for dialysis

Indications for dialysis	
Hyperkalaemia	K > 6.5 mmol/l
Severe fluid overload	Not responding to furosemide
Urea	Ur > 40 mmol/l
Severe hyper/hyponatraemia	>150 < 118 mmol/l or
Acidosis	$HCO_3 < 16$ mmol/l
Multisystem failure	
Prolonged oliguria	<1 ml/kg/hr

Source: Rees et al. (2012).

Fluid loss

The amount of fluid to be removed during the dialysis session is calculated every session. The saline used to prime the lines at the start and at the end of the session is known as the wash-back. This should be added to total fluid removal as its volume can be as much as 400 ml.

Fluid input, output and balance of the previous day in addition to the previous day's weight and current blood pressure will help in the calculation of the amount of fluid that needs to be removed. The maximum amount of fluid removed should not exceed 5% of body weight (Rees et al. 2012).

Complications associated with haemodialysis

The commonest complication associated with HD is hypotension (20–30%), followed by cramps, nausea, and vomiting and headaches (Sherman et al. 2007). This occurs if too much fluid (ultrafiltrate) is removed during the HD session or it is removed too rapidly. For the fluid to be removed, it must be within the vascular space if the rate of fluid removal is greater than the rate of vascular refill then hypotension results.

The ideal weight is called the 'dry' or 'target' weight. At this weight the blood pressure should be within normal limits for age and the fluid balance deemed isovolaemic (Rees et al. 2012). Clinical features of dehydration include hypotension, yawning, light-headedness, tachycardia, pallor, nausea and vomiting, cramp, and cold and clammy peripheries. If left untreated the CYP can destabilise. A bolus infusion of 0.9% sodium chloride will instantly increase the circulating volume and correct the signs and symptoms. If a CYP is severely affected and collapses, administration of saline is the first priority.

Haemofiltration

The fundamental principle behind CRRT is continuous removal of water and unwanted solutes through a semipermeable membrane or filter, (Deepa and Muralidhar 2012; Shaheen et al. 2009). Blood is drained from a large calibre double lumen central catheter, propelled through the circuit, which contains a hollow filter where some fluid and small to medium-sized solutes – such as urea, creatinine, potassium, sodium, ionised calcium, phosphate, glucose, and drugs not bound to proteins – will pass through the membrane, but not large molecule substances such as blood cells and plasma proteins (Baldwin and Fealy 2009; Goldstein, 2011a,b; MacLaren and Butt 2009; Ricci et al. 2006). The three main depurative mechanisms, such as diffusion, convection, and ultrafiltration, occur before the blood is returned to the venous circulation (Cerdá and Ronco 2009; MacLaren and Butt 2009). During CVVH, fluids move across the semipermeable membrane down a hydrostatic pressure gradient, dragging dissolved solutes with them (solvent drag) (D'Intini et al. 2004; MacLaren and Butt 2009). Solute clearance is determined by particle size, where small and medium molecules are sieved out across a pressure gradient. Solute clearance is also determined by percentage of blood flowing through the extracorporeal circuit, hydrostatic pressure across the semipermeable membrane, and the ratio of ultrafiltrate production to filter blood flow, which is referred to as filtration fraction (FF) (MacLaren and Butt 2009). FF is also impacted on by haematocrit and plasma oncotic pressure and, on the effluent side of the membrane, ultrafiltration forms as water is driven across a membrane by a pressure gradient (Murray and Hall 2000; Ronco et al. 2015). Furthermore, in CVVH replacement fluids are infused into the extracoporeal circuit either before (predilution) or after (postdilution) the filter. It is thought that predilution provides the added advantage of prolonging filter life by diluting the blood haematocrit (Dirkes 2000; Faber and Klein 2009; Foot and Fraser 2005; Prowle and Bellomo 2010). Replacement solutions must have near physiological levels of electrolytes and buffer to prevent electrolyte imbalance and iatrogenic acidosis (Brophy 2008; D'Intini et al. 2004; Faber and Klein 2009; Murray and Hall 2000). Replacement fluids administered postdilution result in an increased haemo-concentration, which can cause early filter blockage (Faber and Klein 2009; Ronco et al. 2015).

The depurative process of diffusion occurs in modalities such as CVVHD, where solutes move across a semipermeable membrane down a concentration gradient (Brophy 2008; MacLaren and Butt 2009). In this mode a dialysate solution is administered counter current to the blood flow, which will increase the movement of toxic waste and small molecules such as urea across the membrane through the process of diffusion with no substitution fluid (Baldwin and Fealy 2009; Faber and Klein 2009). The dialysate fluid does not mix with the blood in this mode. Both convective and diffusive mechanisms can be combined in CVVHDF to remove toxins via convection and diffusion, using both dialysate and replacement fluid (MacLaren and Butt 2009). CVVHDF may be more suitable for the highly catabolic CYP and has also become popular because it has the advantage of excellent solute clearance as well as a gently hemodynamic profile (Drummond and Bellamy, 2010; Goldstein 2011a,b; Prowle and Bellomo 2010; Saudan et al. 2006). CVVHDF has the benefits of incorporating both diffusive and convective principles to remove both small and medium-sized molecules of waste products, utilising both dialysate and substitution solution.

Ultrafiltration and adsorption occurs in all therapies (D'Intini et al. 2004). During ultrafiltration there is movement of fluid through a semipermeable membrane along a pressure gradient where positive pressure is generated on the blood side of the membrane, while negative pressure is generated on the fluid side. It is this gradient that drives the fluid from the blood side into the fluid side, which results in net removal of fluids from the CYP (Dirkes and Hodge 2007). The net removal of fluid is dependent on the pressure applied to the filter inside and outside the fibres. In this mode there is minimal solute clearance through convection (Nikkiso Europe GmbH 2012). This is the main mechanism of SCUF and can be used to manage fluid overload in cases such as congestive cardiac failure.

Challenges and complications associated with CRRT in CYP

CRRT predisposes the CYP to some major complications such as haemodynamic instability, haemorrhage, hypothermia, electrolyte and acid base imbalance, infection, and inappropriate drug dosage (Dirkes and Hodge 2007), and impaired vascular access drainage and thrombosis (Goldstein 2011a,b; MacLaren and Butt 2009). One of the challenges of introducing CRRT, particularly in children, is the difficulty of venous catheterization with large-calibre catheters required for small vessels (Santiago et al. 2009). Functional vascular access is a prerequisite to achieve the blood flow needed to obtain solute clearance (Goldstein 2011a,b; MacLaren and Butt 2009). It is the vital determinant of successful and effective RRT (Ronco et al. 2015). Poor patency affects treatment as it is not delivered continuously without interruptions. Some of the complications arise from the fact that 10–15% of total blood volume is pumped through the extracorporeal circuit, which predisposes the child to hypotension, especially at the time of connection (Goldstein 2009; Santiago et al. 2009; Shaheen et al. 2009). The large extracorporeal circuit can also lead to thermodynamic instability (Basu et al. 2011; Goldstein 2011a,b), which is particularly pertinent in small infants and neonates who have limited thermoregulatory capacity, which predisposes them to hypothermia (MacLaren and Butt 2009).

Peritoneal dialysis (PD)

PD requires the insertion of a dialysis catheter into the peritoneum. This is then used to flush dialysate solution into and out of the peritoneum. The peritoneum is used as an autogenic semipermeable membrane, filtering waste products and electrolytes from the blood via diffusion. As the dialysate used is glucose-based, it also allows fluid to be drawn from the blood into dialysate via osmosis and waste products, electrolytes, and excess fluid are then removed via the catheter.

PD is the preferred treatment for CYPs, primarily because of the difficulties accessing and maintaining vascular access for HD and HF, especially in small children (Rees et al. 2012). There are instances where PD may not be viable and HD or HF may be required; for example, following extensive abdominal surgery, adhesions, peritonitis, or significant gut involvement in haemolytic ureamic syndrome, pancreatitis, and ascites.

Types of PD

PD may be used in the management of both acute and chronic renal failure within the hospital or home environment. PD can be further divided into different modalities such as automated peritoneal dialysis (APD) used for overnight dialysis; continuous cycling PD (CCPD) used for AKI or chronic overload; tidal dialysis, which is cycling overnight with a constant volume of fluid left in the peritoneum; optichoice, which is APD with an additional exchange during the day for CYPs who require additional dialysis; and continuous ambulatory peritoneal dialysis (CAPD), which is a manual method of dialysis for ESRF.

Manual PD is often used in CYPs with AKI in nondialysis units and in the neonatal period as initial fill volumes are too small for the automated machines. It is an extremely time-consuming treatment and has the potential for high infection rates because of the type of connections within the circuit. When PD machines are available the infant can be switched from manual to automated dialysis when they can tolerate fill volumes of 60 ml per cycle.

CAPD is a system that is not dependent on a machine; requires minimal equipment; and is a very simple procedure to learn. The CYP usually requires four manual exchanges during the day. This type of dialysis is usually only suitable for adolescents who still have reasonable urine output. It can be used in the management of ESRF at home.

Assessment of a CYP requiring PD

There are many factors that are taken into consideration when assessing the requirement for dialysis. Blood values (specifically creatinine, potassium, sodium and urea), weight, fluid status, blood pressure, and urine output are the main areas for consideration. Once all other medication interventions have failed to resolve the anuric phase, dialysis of some form will be indicated. The type of dialysis suitable will be dependent on the CYP's vital signs and the availability of PD. A full physical assessment and accurate history is essential at this stage.

PD prescription

Collation of blood pressure, respiratory rate, and pulse, U&Es, weight, and clinical assessment dictates the dialysis regimen and concentration and the type of fluids required. The dialysis fill volume in AKI starts at 10 ml/kg and can be increased up to 30–50 ml/kg over the next 48 hours if the catheter does not leak. The dwell time starts at 30 minutes for manual dialysis and is then changed according to the CYP's individual clinical needs. Ultrafiltration in small babies is normally more rapid than in older CYPs. This is due to the large surface area of the peritoneum; for this reason they require a shorter dwell time to ultrafiltrate effectively. Ultrafiltration (UF) in PD is the process whereby fluid (mostly water and electrolytes) moves across the peritoneal membrane as a result of a pressure gradient. The glucose concentrations come in 1.36, 2.27, and 3.86% (Table 10.10). In general, high glucose concentration removes greater amounts of fluids (Rees et al. 2012).

Table 10.10 Choice of PD fluids available

Type of dialysis fluid	Glucose dianeal	Bicarbonate/lactate physioneal	Starch derived glucose polymer icodextrin 7.5%	Amino acid neutrineal
	PD4-Ca 1.25 mmol/l	Physioneal 40 Ca-1.25 mmol/l		
	PD1-Ca 1.75 mmol/l	Physioneal 35 Ca-1.7 5 mmol/l	Extraneal Ca-1.75	
Concentration	1.36% 2.27% 3.86%	1.36% 2.27%	One concentration used only for last bag fill or long dwell periods	1.36% only
Bag size	0.25–5 l bags	2.5 l only		2 L only

Principles table 10.1 Assessing fluid balance in the ill child

Statement	Rationale
1 General observations (Table 10.3): a) Assessment of general well-being. b) Dry mouth and skin. c) Sunken eyes and fontanelle, skin colour that appears mottled	1 a) Unusual but often subtle behaviours, e.g. very still, slightly confused, hallucinations. b) Dry mucous membranes and skin are signs of dehydration. c) Indicate a moderate to severe level of dehydration (Table 10.3).
2 Vital signs: the frequency of measurement will be dependent on clinical condition: a) Capillary refill b) Respiratory rate c) Heart rate d) Blood pressure e) Peripheral and core temperature gap f) Pulse oximetry g) Central venous pressure (CVP) h) Observe the child for oedema. This is often seen around the eyes, ankles, abdomen and scrotal area.	2 Measurement and interpretation of vital signs are tools to help assess fluid status. a) 1–2 seconds would indicate that hydration status may be normal; >2 seconds may indicate a level of dehydration. b) Can be elevated with dehydration. c) Often elevated during dehydration as peripheral blood supply is reduced to maintain blood supply to the vital organs. d) May be low in dehydration. As the condition deteriorates, a slight elevation may be seen as the body tries to compensate for the fluid loss (flight or fight response). Severe hypertension with a low urine output and warm peripheries are signs of fluid overload and AKI (Rees et al. 2012). e) If this is >2 °C in a child who has been well wrapped in a blanket, this may indicate dehydration (vasoconstriction). f) A low oxygen saturation may indicate dehydration, fluid overload, and pulmonary oedema g) CVP is generally low in dehydration and high in fluid overload. h) In odema, fluid is leaking from the tissues. A low serum albumin indicates intravascular depletion. Care should be taken to distinguish the difference between the two (Table 10.3).

Principles table 10.1 Assessing fluid balance in the ill child *(continued)*

Statement	Rationale
3 Once the fluid status has been ascertained, a careful plan of fluid replacement may be calculated; the choice of solution replacing the salt and water is critical in dehydrated CYPs (Tables 10.4 and 10.6).	3 To adequately hydrate the CYP.
4 Weight should be recorded daily during the acute stage. Bed scales can be useful if the child is unstable. If the child is in renal failure, a weight should be taken before and after any renal replacement intervention.	4 Weight gain/loss is age and condition dependent and is an important requirement for assessing fluid balance.
5 An early morning urine should be sent for urinary electrolytes, protein, specific gravity, and osmolarity.	5 To assist in the assessment of fluid requirements. The body attempts to reabsorb fluids by retaining sodium. This results in reduced sodium in the urine and can be a sign of dehydration. Measuring the specific gravity and osmolarity can assist in the assessment of fluid requirements, and protein in the urine may indicate a more serious renal disease, such as congenital nephrotic syndrome.
6 Perform blood test (urea and electrolytes [U&Es]/FBC/blood glucose/blood gases as required). Haematocrit, serum osmolarity, and plasma sodium and potassium are particularly useful when assessing levels of fluid and electrolyte imbalance.	6 To help guide the experienced clinician to prescribe the appropriate fluid and electrolyte requirement.

Procedure guideline 10.1 Fluid input/output

Statement	Rationale
1 Record an accurate fluid balance.	1 To assess fluid status, and enable an early detection of positive or negative balance.
2 There are a number of ways to calculate fluid requirements: a) Insensible losses (400 ml/m²/24 hr) plus previous day's urine output. b) A basic calculation of ml/kg (Table 10.2): Babies prescribed phototherapy or overhead heating will require additional fluids. Ensure monitoring of weight (daily) and weigh nappies.	2 To enable good renal perfusion and a well-hydrated child. a) This calculation is required if a child is on renal replacement therapy as they often do not have a urine output. b) To maintain homeostasis as babies receiving phototherapy have increased insensible losses.
3 Assess fluid status hourly during the acute stage.	3 Early recognition of oliguria/anuria indicates fluid depletion or acute kidney injury <1 ml/kg.
4 Administer IV fluids and assess type of fluid and volume requirements before administration (Table 10.4).	4 To rehydrate and expand the intravascular space and prevent potential fluid overload.
5 All fluid loss should be recorded as total output including vomit/nasogastric aspirate and stool/colostomy fluid and urine.	5 >1 ml/kg/hr. of urine output should be expected if the child is adequately hydrated. A reduction of urine output could indicate dehydration or AKI.
6 Urine output may be accurately measured by: Weighing nappies (wet weight minus dry weight) Monitoring output from a urinary catheter Collecting and measuring contents of urinary bottles and bedpans.	6 Accurate fluid output is essential during the acute phase of illness to monitor fluid status. A urinary catheter can be considered to be a high-risk infection risk in CYPs who are oliguric or anuric.
7 Calculate hourly urine output as ml/kg/hr. based on a child's normal weight.	7 A urinary output of >2 ml/kg/hr. in infants and 1 ml/kg/hr. in CYPs is within normal limits (Glasper et al. 2016).

Preparing the CYP for dialysis access

All forms of dialysis need venous access, which is usually inserted under anaesthetic. The CYP needing dialysis will have deranged electrolytes (hyperkalaemia and acidosis) stabilised prior to theatre. This is essential for the safety of the child. The first-line treatments for hyperkalaemia and acidosis are:

- Calcium resonium (oral/rectal)
- Nebulized ventolin; repeat as required
- Intravenous sodium bicarbonate
- Insulin
- Calcium gluconate

These are effective methods of reducing the serum potassium and/or forcing extracellular potassium into the cells, thereby lowering the serum potassium temporally to enable the child to undergo line insertion. Administering IV sodium bicarbonate can lower calcium levels, which affect muscle contraction, cardiac function and blood clotting. Before correcting acidosis the ionised calcium levels must be measured and corrected.

Care must be taken when giving calcium. Ideally this should be given as an infusion over 30 minutes by a central line. if the CYP has only peripheral access the calcium needs to be diluted to 20 mg in 1 ml to avoid extravasation, as calcium salts can cause serious tissue necrosis.

Procedure guideline 10.2 Preparation of the CYP and family for HD/HF

Statement	Rationale
1 HD and HF must be performed only by staff who are: • Confident in caring for the acutely ill CYP. • Able to develop expertise in HF and or HD and maintain competence. • Familiar with the equipment • Able to manage the side-effects of HF/HD. (Clevenger 1998; and Sefton et al. 2001.	1 To ensure that the treatment is performed safely and effectively, and to reduce the likelihood of side effects and complications.
2 Ensure the CYP and family are prepared for the procedure using • written information, • verbal explanation, and • visual demonstration of the procedure where possible.	2 To minimise anxiety and to clarify their understanding of the procedure. To ensure effective communication between staff and parents/carers. To ensure participation and family-centred care (Kuo et al. 2012).
3 Introduce play and appropriate literature. If the CYP is well enough, encourage play and distraction. If appropriate, young adults can access the information leaflets found on the GOSH web.	3 To provide information that will prepare the CYP, minimise anxiety, and increase concordance (www.gosh.nhs.uk/medical-information-0/procedures-and-treatments/peritoneal-dialysis).
4 The CYP should be assessed and the therapy planned around their individual needs, taking into account underlying illness, severity of illness, and the advantages and disadvantages of the therapies that are available (Schetz 2001; Flynn 2002). This should be clearly documented.	4 To ensure that the treatment prescribed is appropriate for the CYP's needs and in the best interest of the child and family (Bunchman 2002; Flynn 2002; Kuo et al. 2012).
5 Ensure that the child and family understand the need for the choice of treatment and are aware of the risks and benefits of the procedure.	5 To minimise anxiety and facilitate informed consent to treatment.

Procedure guideline 10.3 Inserting a catheter (HD/HF)

Statement	Rationale
1 Appropriate vascular access should be inserted following local guidelines. The type of catheter should be designed for this purpose to achieve good blood flows, i.e. not PICC or Hickman lines. Acceptable lines include: a) Cuffed central venous catheter (CVC). OR b) Uncuffed CVC, which is held in place by sutures.	1 Good vascular access is essential for all extracorporeal treatments and is one of the most important determinants in ensuring effective treatment (Headrick 1998; Bunchman 2002; MacLaren and Butt 2009; Goldstein 2011a,b; Ronco et al. 2015). Inadequate blood flow will result in suboptimal dialysis. a) Cuffed lines last longer and the risk of displacement is reduced. However, they will need a GA to be removed once dialysis is no longer required. b) Uncuffed central venous catheters are for short-term use of two weeks or less. The risk of infection is high and displacement is higher; however, they do not require a general anaesthetic to be removed.
2 Cuffed CVC should be used if HF or HD treatment required for long periods, i.e. for more than 10 days.	2 Risk of displacement or accidental removal is reduced in cuffed catheters.
3 The catheter should be placed into the jugular vein with the tip sited in the right atrium. Femoral veins are also accessed for haemofiltration. The site and position of the catheter should be noted.	3 Optimal placement is essential for achieving adequate dialysis.
4 The catheter is tunnelled percutaneously under the skin.	4 The cuff acts as a physical barrier to external microbial entry and anchors the catheter in place.
5 Care should be taken when placing catheters in CYPs who may require long-term dialysis.	5 The subclavian vein should never be used for catheter placement in ESRF, as this causes a high incidence of vessel stenosis as well as compromising the formation and use of a fistula in that side (Mactier et al. 2009).
6 Careful handling of the line is required. An aseptic nontouch technique should be used every time the line is accessed and usage should be confined to dialysis only.	6 To minimise the risk of infection (Goldstein et al. 1997; Sharma et al. 1999; de Jonge et al. 2005).
7 The catheter usage should be restricted to dialysis only if possible.	7 To reduce the risk of line infection.

Chapter 10 Fluid balance

Procedure guideline 10.3 Inserting a catheter (HD/HF) *(continued)*

Statement	Rationale
8 If the child suffers a persistent pyrexia, the catheter may need to be removed, with replacement into a new access site. Follow local policy for culture of line and prescribing of antibiotic therapy.	8 If a central venous catheter becomes infected, the bacteria can form a film around the plastic, which is impossible to eradicate.
9 It should be possible to withdraw blood freely out of either catheter lumen and reinfuse it back with minimal resistance.	9 A blockage can be due to thrombosis stenosis.
10 If a catheter has poor flow or has a high resistance to re-infusion, instillation of tissue plasminogen activator (TPA) or urokinase can be used. Follow local procedure.	10 This helps to dissolve thrombus.
11 The CYP's pretreatment status should be assessed and documented. This includes: • Vital sign recording, accurate blood pressure, and core and peripheral temperature • Fluid balance • Weight • Biochemical, haematological, and blood gas results • General overall condition.	11 To assess if they are well enough for the procedure and provide a baseline for future monitoring. In the acute, possibly life-threatening situation it may be necessary to assess the risks of treatment v nontreatment and make an informed decision on the information.

Procedure guideline 10.4 Preparing the equipment (HF)

Statement	Rationale
1 An appropriate haemofiltration machine should be selected and checked according to local policy and manufacturers' recommendations. It should be cleaned and decontaminated between patients.	1 To ensure effective treatment and prevent equipment malfunction and complications.
2 a) Suitable haemofiltration equipment should be selected based on the child's weight and clinical condition. b) The haemofiltration circuit should be assembled according to the manufacturer's recommendations and local policy and machine self-tests performed.	2 a) To minimise complications and ensure that the technique is delivered safely. b) With some machines this allows for recalibration, reducing error alarms.
3 The circuit should be primed according to the manufacturer's recommendations and local policy. Priming fluid should be based on clinical need and documented.	3 To detect circuit leaks or malfunctions. To remove air and traces of sterilising agents, reducing the risk of air emboli and anaphylaxis.
4 The amount and type of anticoagulant should be assessed, prescribed and prepared for use, taking into consideration any underlying contraindications in the CYP's condition.	4 To reduce the risk of circuit clotting and anticoagulation of the CYP.
5 The type of haemofiltration fluid should be assessed and prepared for use. The type may be changed during the procedure. Factors to take into account include the CYP's blood chemistry, age, diagnosis, metabolic status, and liver function.	5 Incorrect choice of haemofiltration fluid can lead to ineffective treatment and deterioration of the CYP. Complications include metabolic, electrolyte, and acid–base imbalances (Ellis et al. 1997; Soysal et al. 2007). CYPs with liver dysfunction cannot metabolise the lactate present in most replacement fluids and a bicarbonate base solution should be selected (Naka and Bellomo 2004). This should also be considered in severe metabolic derangement (particularly acidosis).
6 The need for further electrolyte supplements (such as potassium or phosphate) should be assessed and administered as per prescription.	6 To reduce complications and potential electrolyte imbalance as a result of haemofiltration.
7 Therapy goals should be agreed, taking into consideration the rate of fluid exchange and the amount of fluid loss per hour.	7 To calculate the settings needed after treatment has commenced.
8 a) If the circuit volume exceeds more than 10% of the total circulating blood volume, the circuit should be primed with whole blood just before the start of treatment (Headrick 1998; Dirkes and Hodge 2007). b) The blood should be as 'fresh' as possible. Local policy for administration of blood products must be followed (Parshuram and Cox 2002).	8 a) To prevent haemodilution and cardiovascular instability. b) Blood that has been stored for longer periods may have elevated potassium levels, especially if irradiated and the rapid administration of large volumes, which is required in haemofiltration, may cause hyperkalaemia. Hypocalcaemia may also be a complication due to the use of citrate in blood bank storage (Parshuram and Cox 2002).

Procedure guideline 10.5 Preparation for HF

Statement	Rationale
1 Ensure that all equipment is prepared and assembled for use and the haemofiltration machine is primed and ready in recirculation mode.	1 To ensure the procedure goes smoothly and to minimise complications.
2 Using aseptic nontouch technique, clean the catheter in accordance with local policy.	2 To minimise the risk of infection.
3 Attach a 10ml syringe to each lumen, remove the heparin and a small amount of waste from each lumen, and discard.	3 To prevent heparin being administered and to check for clots in the CVC.
4 Attach another 10ml syringe, release the CVC clamps and check each lumen for patency by withdrawing blood. Switching lumens is not advisable as this will increase recirculation of blood and reduce the effectiveness of treatment by up to 30%. Discuss repositioning of device if it is considered close to the vessel wall.	4 To establish that the CVC is patent. Adequate fluid removal and dialysis are dependent on adequate flow rates.
5 Attach a three-way tap (primed with saline) to each lumen and flush with 0.9% sodium chloride solution.	5 To establish if both lumens are patent and allow each lumen to be clamped independently.
6 If either lumen is blocked, follow local guidelines for checking and re-establishing patency (as above for HD).	6 Two patent IV access ports are required to perform haemofiltration.
7 Using the three-way taps and lumen clamps, ensure both lumens are securely clamped.	7 To prevent blood loss from the CVC and prepare to start haemofiltration.

Procedure guideline 10.6 Starting CRRT

Statement	Rationale
1 Commencing haemofiltration is a two-person procedure. At least one member should be a competent haemofiltration practitioner. Staff should closely monitor the access, the machine, and the CYP for any respiratory and/or cardiovascular changes and take appropriate action.	1 To maintain patient safety.
2 Resuscitation equipment and appropriate intravenous fluid and a unit of blood should be available regardless of whether a blood prime is needed. The nurse should ensure this is ordered and available.	2 Commencing haemofiltration can cause clinical instability, which requires prompt intervention and resuscitation (Dirkes 2000; Dirkes and Hodge 2007; Uchino et al. 2007; Santiago et al. 2009). An allergic reaction to the membrane of the haemofilter can cause severe hypotension (Flynn 2002).
3 Administer oxygen for two minutes prior to starting haemofiltration. If the CYP is receiving artificial ventilation, increase the oxygen level as agreed with the medical team.	3 To prevent hypoxia, a known complication when starting haemofiltration, especially in younger children.
4 a) If the CYP is receiving vasoactive or inotropic drugs, discuss with the medical team and CRRT primary user in order to titrate drugs to minimise complications. b) Children weighing less than 10kg have blood volumes of approx. 80ml/kg. If the patient's circuit volume is in excess of 10% of the patient's total blood volume, blood priming is necessary. Children under 10kg are at a higher risk because the large extracorporeal volume predisposes them to complications such as hypotension, hypothermia, which are more common in this group (Santiago et al. 2009).	4 a) Due to the presence of the extracorporeal circuit and large fluid/blood shifts, haemofiltration can lead to reduced plasma levels of drugs, which may need to be increased to maintain stability (Uchino et al. 2007). b) The extra-corporeal circuit holds a significant level of the patient's blood which will need to be replaced to prevent hypotension and anaemia (Goldstein 2009). The circuit holds about 100ml of blood and a neonate's circulating volume is 80ml/kg. The estimated blood volume of a neonate weighing 3kg is 240ml; 100ml is 41% of the CYP's circulating volume.
5 Prime the circuit with 1 litre of sodium chloride mixed with 5000 units of heparin sodium followed by 500 ml of plain 0.9% sodium chloride to remove the heparin. Recirculate for 5–10 minutes, and when ready to commence treatment, blood prime if necessary.	5 Priming the circuit helps to eliminate any air within the circuit to prevent air embolism and the initial heparinisation of the circuit helps to reduce blood clotting. Recirculation helps prolong filter life since filter fibres are hydrophilic and will be saturated and able to clear more solutes (Nikkiso Europe GmbH 2012).

Procedure guideline 10.6 Starting CRRT *(continued)*

Statement	Rationale

6 Check the CYP for any signs of clinical instability before proceeding. Vital signs should be observed throughout the 'start-up' process (Uchino et al. 2007).
  a) Check blood gas and blood results especially U&Es, FBC for haemaglobin levels, and ammonia or other toxin levels before commencing.
  b) Utilise a pressure transducer and X-ray to confirm position of the catheter especially if it's in the subclavian veins.
	6 To minimise complications as haemofiltration can exacerbate instability.
	  a) To maintain a baseline to work from and be able to monitor effectiveness of therapy especially in clearing toxins, such as ammonia, urea, and creatinine levels.
	  b) For detection of incorrect position of the catheter and to prevent complications such as pneumothorax (Santiago et al. 2009).

7
  a) After recirculation choose single or double connection option to connect the patient onto the machine. Two CRRT competent nurses are required to connect and commence CRRT.
  b) Using an aseptic nontouch technique, aspirate and discard heparin from the lines.
  c) Flush both lumens using a luer lock syringe, accessing for patency. Stop the haemofiltration pump and clamp both the arterial and venous lines close to the tip and attach the circuit to catheter lumens.
	7
	  a) At least two nurses are required so that one nurse can focus on the machine and the other nurses can focus on the access and the patient.
	  b) To reduce/prevent infection and aspirate and discard blood in order to prevent administering a bolus of heparin to the patient.
	  c) Use luer lock syringe to prevent infection and air emboli.

8 Release the clamps from both lumens. Turn the 3-way tap so that the access line is open to the circuit and the return line empties into a 20 ml syringe.	8 To allow blood to flow in/out of the catheter and prevent any air entering the machine or patient.
9 Start the blood pump using the minimum rate for the weight and if tolerated build up to recommended optimum speed following CRRT hospital guidelines. Observe the return lumen closely for air and be prepared to clamp the lumen to prevent it entering the patient. Open the three-way tap to the machine once a few milliliters have collected into the syringe and there is no possibility of air in the circuit.	9 To detect air and minimise complications. Any air in the circuit will enter via the venous lumen.
10 If prescribed, administer a bolus of heparin into the haemofiltration circuit just after the blood pump is started as per local policy.	10 To maintain/promote the integrity of the circuit and prevent clotting (Schetz 2001; Bouman et al. 2006; Dirkes and Hodge 2007).
11 Reassess and monitor vital signs and, if stable, increase the pump speed to the appropriate level for the CYP's weight.	11 To minimise any respiratory or cardiovascular complications.
12 Commence the anticoagulant infusion if prescribed.	12 Anticoagulate the extra-corporeal circuit to maximise CRRT circuit life and prevent premature filter clotting. (Bouman et al. 2006; Ricci et al. 2006; Uchino et al. 2007).
13 Set the fluid exchange rate termed predilution/turnover, according to the calculated values based on the pump speed and filtration fraction, the CYP's clinical condition, local policy, and multidisciplinary team guidance.	13 This determines the level of the treatment the patient receives. The calculation will enable the machine to determine the rate of convection required to remove solutes.
14 Set the amount of fluid loss to be achieved during the haemofiltration session.	14 To commence the therapy and reduce fluid overload.
15 Set alarm parameters/limits in accordance with manufacturer's instructions.	15 To alert staff to problems and minimise complications.

Procedure guideline 10.7 Monitoring and maintaining CRRT

Statement	Rationale
1 A competent haemofiltration nurse should be present at the bedside at all times.	1 The CYP is at risk of significant blood loss/air emboli if the circuit becomes accidentally disconnected or ruptures. The machine may alarm and require troubleshooting or the CYP may become unstable.
2 The CYP should be fully monitored before, during and after CRRT. a) Cardiovascular assessment: continuous ECG, invasive blood pressure every hour. b) Respiratory assessment: Oxygen saturations, capnography, ventilator settings, respiratory rate and effort, and blood gases every hour. c) Gastrointestinal assessment: function and nutritional status. d) Renal/fluid volume assessment. Assess for oedema, fluid losses, blood glucose, and CRRT fluid balance. e) Neurological assessment: pain score, GCS, and medication effects, especially the effects of sedatives, paralysing agents, and toxins every hour. f) Monitor body temperature for hyperthermia/hypothermia. Children under 10 kg on CRRT are prone to hypothermia due to their immature body temperature control (Askenazi et al. 2013). Core temperature monitoring is mandatory for all children under 10 kg on CRRT (Dirkes and Hodge 2007). g) Monitor biochemical values, and other levels as required e.g. ammonia, as well as FBC and clotting. 1 hour after haemofiltration has commenced and 4–6 hourly thereafter.	2 To ensure early detection of complications and side effects and maintain safety (Dirkes and Hodge 2007). a) Cardiac status highlights effects of fluid removal and tolerance to therapy; excessive fluid removal can result in hypotension. b) Respiratory status can highlight positive or negative effects of CRRT. For example overhydration can increase pulmonary pressures. c) Optimum nutrition is an essential component for healthy growth and development. d) Assessment determines tolerance to and effectiveness of therapy. e) High toxin levels can cause altered level of consciousness, confusion, and dizziness due to hyperammonia or high or low serum urea, nitrogen levels. f) Hypothermia is a common complication of CRRT, especially in children under 10 kg, and can result in arrhythmias (Santiago et al. 2009). g) Monitoring levels can detect abnormalities and ensure prompt intervention (Dirkes and Hodge 2007). Hypophosphataemia frequently occurs during CRRT, as small molecules pass through filter, so monitoring and administration of replacement is vital (Bellomo and Ronco, 2000).
5 Monitor the vascath insertion site at least hourly and document.	5 To detect catheter dislodgment earlier and avoid exsanguinations and early signs of circuit clotting (Ejaz et al. 2007). For early detection of complications such as haematoma, altered venous drainage at lower limbs, and catheter-related infections (Santiago et al. 2009; Basu et al. 2011).
6 Monitor circuit: observe and document hourly: • Blood pump speed • Arterial pressures • Return pressures • Pressure drop • Turnover/pre-dilution • Substitution • Dialysate if on CVVHDF mode • Transmembrane pressure (TMP) • Fluid type • Hourly fluid loss and fluid loss after each four-hourly cycle • Colour of ultrafiltrate	6 Hourly documentation provides a trend that may identify early signs of circuit clotting, rupture of the filter and alert nurses of catheter dysfunction/disconnection/haemorrhage thus maintain patient safety (Dirkes and Hodge 2007; Ejaz et al. 2007).
7 If heparin is being used, the circuit activated clotting time (ACT) should be assessed one hour after starting haemofiltration and four hourly thereafter, as well as adverse effects of anticoagulation such as hematomas, thrombocytopenia, and allergic reaction (Dirkes and Hodge, 2007).	7 To monitor anticoagulation of the circuit and ensure patient safety.
8 If the ACT is below the recommended level (generally 140–160 if clotting is deranged or 160–180 if clotting is normal) the dose of heparin should be increased in line with local guidelines (Bunchman 2002).	8 A low ACT indicates that the circuit is at risk of clotting.
9 If the ACT is above the recommended level, the dose of heparin should be decreased in line with local guidelines.	9 A high ACT indicates that the circuit is over-anti-coagulated, which increases the risk of complications, such as bleeding (Bouman et al. 2006; Monchi et al. 2004; Schetz 2001).

Procedure guideline 10.8 Discontinuing CRRT

Statement	Rationale
1 Once the treatment goal has been achieved, or if the circuit becomes clotted, haemofiltration can be discontinued.	1 To complete or restart treatment.
2 Assess whether the CYP can be disconnected from the circuit immediately or needs to have the extracorporeal blood 'washed back.' Influencing factors include weight, current haemoglobin level, overall clinical condition, current fluid balance, and state of the circuit, e.g. if the circuit has been in use for a long time and has visible clots.	2 'Washing back' the extracorporeal blood may be beneficial in increasing the haemoglobin level without the need for another blood transfusion. This needs to be balanced against the additional fluid volume administered as a result. It may be beneficial for a smaller CYP, as the volume of blood in the circuit can account for a significant amount of the overall circulating volume.
3 Discontinue haemofiltration following specific step-by-step guidelines highlighted in the CRRT hospital guidelines (Nikkiso Europe GmbH 2012). a) Ensure that the person removing the circuit and others nearby are wearing personal protective equipment (PPE), including goggles. b) Discontinue haemofiltration, stop the blood pump and clamp the arterial and venous lines and the catheter lumens.	3 To maintain safety of the CYP (see Figure 10.2). a) To prevent contamination and protect the HCW. The circuit is at risk of rupturing if it is removed under high pressure. b) To ensure no bleeding occurs.
4 If the circuit blood is to be washed back, disconnect the arterial end from the catheter and attach a bag of 0.9% sodium chloride. Follow instructions on the machine for blood wash back. Release all clamps and start the blood pump slowly.	4 To draw 0.9% sodium chloride solution into the circuit to flush out the blood and return to the CYP. Follow instructions on the machine, which calculates volume of blood washed back to the CYP.
5 Continue the blood pump until the circuit is coloured 'salmon pink.'	5 This indicates that most of the red blood cells have been returned to the CYP.
6 Once the wash back is complete, remove the circuit from the machine following specific step-by-step CRRT hospital guidelines, then switch off the machine.	6 To prevent infection and blood leakage.
7 a) Using an aseptic technique, remove the three-way taps and flush both access and return lines of the catheter with 0.9% saline, then inject 1000 units heparin to fill the exact volume of each lumen and reclamp. Close off each lumen with an IV device cap and label the lines to show heparin is in situ. b) For both wash-back and discontinuation techniques, disconnect the lines from the catheter using aseptic nontouch technique. Attach a 10ml syringe with 0.9% sodium chloride to each lumen.	7 a) To maintain catheter patency for future use and warn staff of the presence of heparin in the line. b) To disconnect the extracorporeal circuit and maintain catheter patency.

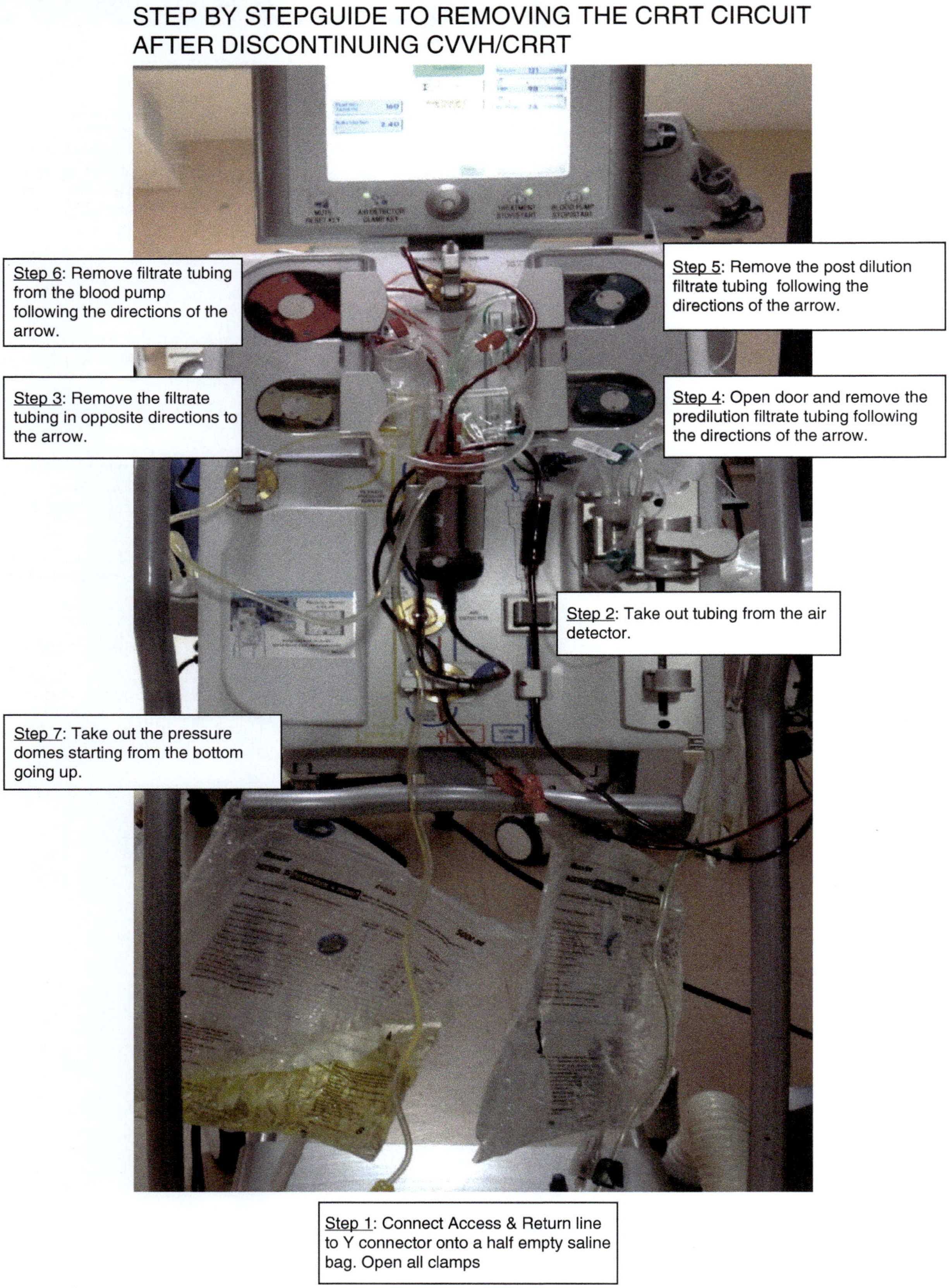

Figure 10.2 Step-by-step guide to removing the CRRT circuit after discontinuing CVVH/CRRT.

Procedure guideline 10.9 Commencing HD

Statement	Rationale
1 Wash hands.	1 Following local hand hygiene policy.
2 Start the cleaning cycle of the HD machine.	2 To ensure the machine is disinfected prior to use in accordance with manufacturer's instructions. This cycle can take 40 minutes.
3 Gather equipment together.	3 To be efficient undertaking the procedure.
4 When the cleaning cycle is completed, select the dialysis mode and connect the bicarbonate and acidic dialysis concentrates once the initial safety function check has been carried out.	4 To confirm the finish of the clean cycle and to signify the intention to start a new HD cycle. The machine performs safety checks and begins to prepare the dialysis concentrate for delivery.
5 To assemble the circuit and dialyser: a) Place the dialyser in the holder. b) Connect the arterial line to the arterial (red) end of the dialyser. c) Clamp the patient end of the line and spike an IV bag of 0.9% sodium chloride. d) Connect the venous line to the venous (blue) end of the dialyser and hang the waste bag on the IV pole. e) Feed the pump segment into the pump; ensure the luer lock connections on the dialyser and the pressure transducers are securely attached.	5 To assemble the circuit and dialyser and place correctly on the machine. Always refer to manufacturer's instructions for further guidance. c) The saline will prime from the IV bag, through the arterial line, through the dialyser, into the venous line, and collect in the waste bag. d) During priming the blue end is uppermost to facilitate air removal.
6 Unclamp the arterial line and start the blood pump to commence priming the air from the circuit. Raise the level of saline in the venous drip chamber to three-quarter full and activate the air detector.	6 To expel air from the circuit and ready the fibres in the dialyser for blood.
7 Attach 500 ml bag of sodium chloride 0.9% to infusion giving set. Prime the infusion line and then attach to the arterial infusion port.	7 This is used to allow infusion of saline to the circuit during recirculation and later enable the return of blood to the CYP.
8 Gently clamp the venous line to expel air bubbles.	8 To de-aerate the dialyser to enhance diffusional area.
9 Attach the dialysate ports to the dialyser when the function checks are complete and the dialysis fluid is ready.	9 To allow dialysis fluid to come into contact with the dialyser. This can only be done once the function checks are complete.
10 Prepare the heparin/saline solution. The heparin is drawn up according to individual requirements, dose approximately 10–25 units/kg/ml. Label and attach the syringe to the arterial circuit and place in the syringe driver.	10 To facilitate heparin delivery during the procedure to prevent clotting of the circuit.
11 Using an aseptic nontouch technique, connect the vascular access to arterial and venous lines of the circuit.	11 To minimise the risk of infection.
12 Set the session length, required fluid loss, and heparin rate and infusion stop time (if required). Start HD.	12 Once these are entered, the machine is ready to start dialysis.
13 The following should be documented hourly: • Blood pump speed • Arterial pressure • Venous pressure • Transmembrane pressure (TMP) • Fluid type.	13 To maintain patient safety and to detect trends that may identify the early signs of circuit clotting (Ejaz et al. 2007).
14 Also record: • Temperature • Pulse rate • Respiratory rate • Blood pressure • Pre- and postdialysis and hourly blood pressure and heart rate measurement during the dialysis session • Paediatric Early Warning Score (PEWS) should be performed/scored with each set of observations and scoring grid followed. Respond and escalate PEWS according to local policy.	14 To detect if an alteration in their current care or treatment regime is required. To detect dehydration, fluid overload, or infection. To ensure changes in condition are appropriately escalated.
15 If the CYP has a fistula do not record their blood pressure on the same limb. If the CYP is experiencing dizziness, nausea, or cramps, he or she may need to lie down and may need a drink. b) If the symptoms persist, consider giving them an extra drink (outside of their fluid restriction) c) The length of time that a CYP is on HD is dependent on their overall clinical condition. Usually two-to-four hour sessions are sufficient for safe HD.	15 To avoid damaging the fistula. Haemodialysis causes fluid shifts and rapid fluid removal can result in transient hypovolaemia. b) Persistence of the problem may indicate clinical dehydration c) At the end of HD the nurse needs to decide if the CYP requires extra dialysis. This is based on factors that include weight, blood pressure, haemoglobin level, condition, and fluid balance.

Procedure guideline 10.10 Discontinuing HD

Statement	Rationale
1 When the dialysis session has been completed the blood pump is stopped and the circuit clamped.	1 In preparation for the blood in the circuit to be returned to the CYP.
2 Using 0.9% sodium chloride, 'wash-back' or return the blood in the circuit, then stop the pump and clamp the access and circuit tubing.	2 This ensures all the blood is returned to the CYP to prevent anaemia.
3 Disconnect the circuit from the vascular access using aseptic non-touch technique.	3 To minimise the risk of infection.
4 Instil appropriate anticoagulant agent, e.g. heparin into vascular access, then cap off.	4 To maintain patency of the access between sessions.
5 Dispose of circuit and equipment in accordance with local and national guidelines.	5 To reduce the risk of cross-infection.
6 Evaluate the procedure and record the information in the CYP's healthcare records.	6 To aid communication and ensure continuity of care.
7 Where possible weigh the CYP and complete the record of the dialysis session.	7 The post-HD weight is part of the information that will help the team assess the effectiveness of the HD session.
8 Remove the lines and empty the dialyser from the machine according to manufacturer's instructions before commencing the cleaning programme.	8 The machine should be disinfected between CYP to minimise risks of cross-infection.
9 Discard equipment appropriately.	9 To observe local and national policies on correct disposal of clinical waste.

Procedure guideline 10.11 Preparation (PD)

Statement	Rationale
1 Assess the need for dialysis (Table 10.9).	1 To ensure that the infant/CYP is suitable for PD and that all other medical treatments for anuria/oliguria have been explored prior to insertion of the PD catheter.
2 Prepare the CYP and family for the procedure: using verbal, visual, and written information, dolls and toys if appropriate, offering time for questions and discussion.	2 To minimise anxiety and to clarify their understanding of and consent to the procedure.
3 Choose an appropriate-sized Tenckhoff catheter (three sizes available suitable for infants of 1 kg and above).	3 PD is dependent on a functioning Tenckhoff catheter.
4 If the CYP is constipated they should be given laxatives before going for surgery.	4 To minimise complications of catheter displacement and mechanical problems with the catheter drainage.
5 Dietary assessment made and a nasogastric tube inserted at the same time as the Tenckhoff catheter if necessary.	5 Adequate nutrition and good albumen levels are vital to the efficiency of fluid removal on PD. Adequate nutrition will help reduce the urea level and lead to a faster recovery.
6 Monitor vital signs as often as condition requires. If vital signs or blood levels are outside the normal range they must be continually monitored.	6 Abnormal vital signs usually require the team to change the dialysis prescription.
7 Interpretation of vital signs preperitoneal dialysis: a) An increasing peripheral/core temperature gap. b) An increasing pulse rate and respiratory rate. c) Hypertension. d) Weight gain/loss.	7 a) Temperature gap should be less than 2°C when the infant is adequately wrapped up; more than 2°C may be a sign of peripheral shutdown due to hypovolaemia or sepsis. b) Potential sepsis, pain or pulmonary oedema, anaemia. c) Fluid overload. d) Weight loss usually indicates good ultrafiltration/improved urine output, weight gain can indicate inadequate dialysis.

Chapter 10 Fluid balance

Procedure guideline 10.12 Preparation for surgery (PD)

Statement	Rationale
1 As for other forms of dialysis, psychological preparation and support is extremely important in the early stages of the process. Provide written and verbal information as appropriate and liaise with a play specialist.	1 To provide information, minimise anxiety and ensure informed consent and concordance. For more information, see Procedure Guideline 10.2
2 Preinsertion of PD catheter: a) Ensure that the CYP is safely prepared and transferred to theatre following local policies and protocols. b) Ensure antibiotic cover is prescribed. c) Supply theatres with necessary equipment needed for insertion of catheter and dressing of the new catheter.	2 To ensure that care is standardised and meets the CYP's needs. b) To reduce the risk of infection. c) To ensure the correct catheter is inserted and that the site is dressed appropriately to ensure that PD can be performed effectively and reduce the risk of infection at the exit site.

Procedure guideline 10.13 Starting PD for AKI

Statement	Rationale
Manual	
1 Setting up manual PD, collect the following equipment: • Dialysis prescription and record chart • Drip stand • Heater for PD fluid • Manual PD giving set neonatal/paediatric • Dialysis fluid (Table 10.10) • Povidone–iodine or alternative disinfectant • Antimicrobial handwash • Dressing pack • Sterile gloves • Trolley • Alcohol wipes • Apron	1 To ensure the procedure goes smoothly and to minimise complications.
2 Explain the procedure to CYP and family.	2 To minimise anxiety and to clarify their understanding of and consent to the procedure.
3 Wash hands for one minute.	3 To reduce the risk of infection.
4 Collect equipment.	4 To ensure the procedure goes smoothly and minimise complications.
5 Clean trolley with hard surface wipes, wash hands for one minute.	5 To reduce the risk of infection.
6 Open PD giving set, dressing pack, onto a sterile field and open the PD fluid bag into a sterile field.	6 Maintaining a sterile field can reduce the risk of cross-contamination.
7 Open sterile gloves onto cleaned work surface.	7 Reduce the risk of contaminating the sterile field with your hands.
8 Wash hands for 1 minute and put on sterile gloves.	8 To reduce the risk of infection.
9 Clamp clamps of giving set, spike fluid bag with end of giving set and hang the bags of fluid onto stand.	9 If the fluid runs through the giving set before it is hanging on a stand the filters may become wet and this will affect the efficiency of the dialysis.
10 Prime set with dialysis fluid, keep the burette upright when full. Care must be taken not to wet the air filters of the burette as this will cause problems when filling and draining the burettes.	10 If the filter becomes wet, a vacuum is produced inside the burette and it will be impossible to fill or drain the burette. In this situation the PD giving set may need to be changed. An air inlet placed into the filter may be helpful in this situation.
11 The tubing containing fluid is normally warmed by the fluid bag being placed on a warmer	11 For comfort and to prevent a drop in the CYP's core temperature.
12 Place sterile field under catheter, place cleaning fluid solution into the pot, submerge catheter for three minutes.	12 Cleaning fluid used as per hospital policy is used to disinfectant the catheter and prevent infections by pathogens.
13 Connect set to PD catheter.	13 To start dialysis.

(continued)

Procedure guideline 10.13 Starting PD for AKI (continued)

Statement	Rationale
14 Hang drain bag below the level of the CYP.	14 Drainage from the peritoneum is dependent on gravitational force.
15 Take and record BP.	15 It is important to have a base line BP before starting dialysis, as blood pressure is one of the most important observations to accurately assess fluid balance.
16 Open drain clamp and allow any fluid in situ to drain for 10 minutes and then clamp.	16 To ensure the peritoneum is empty.
17 Fill chamber with the prescribed amount of fluid required by the CYP.	17 The fluid prescription should start at 10 ml/kg and be increased as tolerated.
18 If the drainage is blood stained the catheters should be flushed continuously, with 10 ml/kg of 1.36% dialysis fluid (with 200 units/l heparin added), until the dialysate clears becomes clear, cycling can then begin.	18 Placing of a PD catheter can cause a small amount of trauma to the tissues and bleeding occurs. Flushing will prevent the formation of a clot in the catheter.
19 Open clamp to allow the fluid to fill over approximately 10 minutes and reclamp. When starting PD it is important to administer fluid slowly.	19 To reduce discomfort and minimise the risk of leakage. The dialysis settings are adjusted according to age, condition, biochemistry, and vital signs. Young children are usually high transporters, so fluid and electrolytes move across the peritoneum faster and their cycles are shorter. If a CYP presents with a very high urea, slow dialysis is recommended as reducing the urea too quickly can cause disequilibrium (Rees et al. 2012).
20 Leave fill in situ for prescribed length of time starting with dwells of 30 minutes. Care should be taken at this time to observe for leaking around the catheter; if this occurs, the fill volume may need to be reduced.	20 A dwell time of 30 minutes is usually sufficient for good clearance of electrolytes and fluid removal. However, a fill of 30–50 ml/kg is usually required for adequate acute dialysis; the rate at which the fill can increase is dependent on the success of the catheter. If the catheter leaks, the risk of infection increases and therefore the fill volume should be increased with caution.
21 Open drain clamp and allow to drain for 10 minutes; fluid from the peritoneum should drain by gravity.	21 Fluid should drain freely from the CYP when the clamps are open.
22 Start to record the dialysis in, out and UF. UF is the fluid removed by dialysis. The amount of fluid removed will be dependent of the CYP's fluid balance.	22 Accurate recording of dialysis fluid in and out is essential to determine fluid balance.

Automated machine (home choice)

1 Standard prescription: fill volumes for a newly inserted PD catheter should start on 10 ml per kg of 1.36% dialysis fluid, increasing to 40–50 ml/kg or 800 ml/m² in children less than two years and 1.1–1.4 l/m² from over two years of age. The fluid volume is increased as tolerated over a 48-hour period in AKI.	1 Increasing the fill time gradually reduces the risk of complications of pain on filling and potential leakage.
2 **Starting automated dialysis:** Programme: Total volume of fluid: 800 ml–1.4 l/m² Start with continuous cycles Length of cycles.	2 The dialysis programme is adjusted according to age, condition, biochemistry, and vital signs. As a rule young children are high transporters, so fluid and electrolytes move across the peritoneum faster and their cycles are shorter. If a CYP presents with a very high urea, slow dialysis is recommended, as reducing the urea too quickly can cause disequilibrium (Rees et al. 2012).
3 Dwell time of 30–40 minutes for babies. 50–80 minutes depending on clinical condition.	3 The dwell time influences the process of osmosis and diffusion. This needs to be titrated according to the CYP's blood results and vital signs.
4 Set up machines for peritoneal dialysis according to manufacturers' instructions and hospital policy for aseptic nontouch technique. Prime circuit with dialysis fluid according to manufacturers' instructions.	4 All equipment used in the delivery of therapies should comply with standards for medical equipment and hospital policy if good practice is to be maintained.
5 Connect PD: Using an aseptic nontouch technique, access PD catheter and connect circuit. Open all clamps and initiate dialysis; always flushing postdrain prior to filling.	5 The aseptic nontouch technique reduces the risk of infection.
6 Ensure that the CYP is comfortable.	6 To minimise distress and ensure the dialysis is running effectively before leaving the bedside.

Procedure guideline 10.14 Care of the CYP on PD

Statement	Rationale
1 Accurate fluid balance is essential. Record the ultrafiltration (UF), fluid input/output hourly during the acute phase.	1 UF is the fluid removed by dialysis. The amount of fluid removed will be dependent of the CYP's fluid balance.
2 Calculate the fluid restriction daily based on the urine output + UF + insensible loss of the previous day.	2 Fluid restrictions are essential to prevent the CYP becoming fluid-overloaded (Rees et al. 2012).
3 The following observations are preformed four hourly on stable CYPs and hourly if unstable: • Core and peripheral temperature • CVP is sometimes required in ITU • Blood pressure • Neurological observations for Haemolytic Uraemic Syndrome • Pulse • Respiratory rate • ECG monitoring • Bloods for U&E and FBC daily once stable • Blood sugars	3 To help assess fluid balance. Hyperglycaemia can develop due to the high concentration of glucose in the dialysis fluid or as a secondary complication to HUS.
4 Provide adequate nutrition by TPN or nasogastric tube feeding.	4 To lower the urea and speed up recovery (Rees et al. 2012).
5 Monitor the weight twice daily.	5 To assess the effectiveness of the dialysis prescription.

Procedure guideline 10.15 Special considerations (PD)

Statement	Rationale
1 Signs and symptoms of infection are: • Cloudy PD effluent • Abdominal pain • Pyrexia • Vomiting • Hypotension	1 Early detection of peritonitis. If the only symptom is cloudy fluid, the sample should be sent to haematology for analysis as cloudy fluid can result from an allergic response post insertion of the catheter or in response to the PD fluid. In this situation a raised esoinophil count is usually detected in the PD specimen and full blood count.
2 Observe the exit site regularly for signs of inflamed or exudate, swabs should be taken if necessary. Should a tunnel infection be suspected, this should be confirmed on ultrasound scan and treated with appropriate antibiotic treatment.	2 To enable prompt treatment of exit site infections and prevent tunnel infection and peritonitis.
3 Signs and symptoms of disequilibrium are observed: confusion, convulsion, drowsy.	3 A rapid fall in the urea level can result in cerebral oedema due to failure to equalise the blood brain barrier. The dialysis should be reduced at this point by significantly increasing the dwell time (Rees et al. 2008).
4 Constipation should be avoided and laxatives prescribed if necessary.	4 This causes problems with drainage, reducing efficiency of dialysis and leading to overload. Constipation also leads to discomfort and pain on dialysis.
5 If the waste fluid contains long white fibres (fibrin), monitor closely and treat with heparin if the quantity increases.	5 To prevent catheters becoming blocked, thus reducing efficiency of dialysis and leading to overload.
6 **Alarms:** Low UF can be caused by a number of factors: • Kinked lines • Failing peritoneum • Hypotension • Leakage • Need for a more concentrated dialysis • Fluid retention • Constipation • Low albumin	6 It is necessary to identify the reason for a failing dialysis session and resolve the problem to prevent a life-threatening situation (Rees et al. 2012).

Procedure guideline 10.16 Discontinuing PD

Statement	Rationale
1 Follow the procedure below: Wash hands for one minute.	1 Reduce the risk of infection.
2 Collect equipment • Clean trolley with hard surface wipes. • Wash hands for 1 minute. • Open PD cap. • Open sterile gloves onto cleaned work surface. • Wash hands for one minute and put on sterile gloves. • Close clamps of PD catheter and set. • Place connection into povidone–iodine solution. • Disconnect. • Replace cap onto catheter. • Disconnect set and dispose of used dialysis set. • Record in health care record.	2 On completion of dialysis equipment should be available close to the dialysis machine to ensure the CYP is disconnected from the dialysis machine safely and prevent the risk of infections. Disposable equipment should be disposed of according to your hospital policy.
3 Disconnection of all PD lines should be done with great care according to hospital policy. Aseptic nontouch technique should be used every time the line is accessed.	3 To minimise the risk of infection.
4 PD specimens should be taken if the CYP becomes pyrexial or if the fluid in the drainage bag appears cloudy.	4 To avoid high risk of infection. If white cell count is $>100 \times 10^6/l$ indicates a possible peritonitis.
5 The wound dressings for acute sites should be kept clean and dry, only change if exudate is observed.	5 Exit site infections can lead to infections and peritonitis.

References

Advanced Life Support Group (2012). *Advanced Paediatric Life Support: The Practical Approach*, 5e London: BMJ Publishing Group.

Askenazi, D.J., Goldstein, S.L., Koralkar, R. et al. (2013). Continuous renal replacement therapy < 10kg: a report from the prospective pediatric continuous renal replacement therapy registry. *The Journal of Pediatrics* 162 (3): 587–592.

Baldwin, I. and Fealy, N. (2009). Nursing for renal replacement therapies in the intensive care unit: historical, educational, and protocol review. *Blood Purification* 27: 174–181.

Basu, R.J., Wheeler, D.S., Goldstein, S., and Doughty, L. (2011). Acute renal replacement therapy in pediatrics. *International Journal of Nephrology* 2011: 785392. https://doi.org/10.4061/2011/785392.

Bellomo, R. and Ronco, C. (2000). Continuous haemofiltration in the intensive care unit. *Critical Care* 4 (6): 339–345.

Bouman, C.S., De Pont, A.C.J., Meijers, J.C. et al. (2006). The effects of continuous venovenous hemofiltration on coagulation activation. *Critical Care* 10 (5): 1.

Brophy, P.D. (2008). Renal supportive therapy for pediatric acute kidney injury in the setting of multiorgan dysfunction syndrome/sepsis. *Seminars in Nephrology* 28 (5): 457–469. WB Saunders.

Bunchman, T.E. (2002). Plasmapheresis and renal replacement therapy in children. *Current Opinion in Pediatrics* 14 (3): 310–314.

Cerdá, J. and Ronco, C. (2009). The clinical application of CRRT – current status: modalities of continuous renal replacement therapy: technical and clinical considerations. *Seminars in Dialysis* 22 (2): 114–122. Blackwell Publishing Ltd.

Challinor, P. (2014). Chapter 8: Haemodialysis. In: *Renal Nursing*, 4e (ed. N. Thomas), 165. Chichester: Wiley.

Clevenger, K. (1998). Setting up a continuous venovenous hemofiltration educational program. A case study in program development. *Critical Care Nursing Clinics of North America* 10 (2): 235–244.

Davenport, M. (1996). Paediatric fluid balance. *Care of the Critically Ill* 12 (1): 26–31.

Deepa, C. and Muralidhar, K. (2012). Renal replacement therapy in the ICU. *Journal of Anaesthesiology Clinical Pharmacology* 28 (3): 386–396.

D'Intini, V., Ronco, C., Bonello, M., and Bonello, R. (2004). Renal replacement therapy in acute renal failure. *Best Practice & Research. Clinical Anaesthesiology* 18 (1): 145–157.

Dirkes, S.M. (2000). Continuous renal replacement therapy: dialytic therapy for acute renal failure in intensive care. *Nephrology Nursing Journal* 27 (6): 581.

Dirkes, S. and Hodge, K. (2007). Continuous renal replacement therapy in the adult intensive care unit: history and current trends. *Critical Care Nurse* 27 (2): 61–80.

Drummond, A.D. and Bellamy, M.C. (2010). Renal replacement therapy in the intensive care unit. *Current Anaesthesia and Critical Care* 21 (2): 69–74.

Ejaz, A.A., Komorski, R.M., Ellis, G.H., and Munjal, S. (2007). Extracorporeal circuit pressure profiles during continuous venovenous haemofiltration. *Nursing in Critical Care* 12 (2): 81–85.

Ellis, E.N., Pearson, D., Belsha, C.W., and Berry, P.L. (1997). Use of pump-assisted hemofiltration in children with acute renal failure. *Pediatric Nephrology* 11 (2): 196–200.

Faber, P. and Klein, A. (2009). Acute kidney injury and renal replacement therapy in intensive care unit. *Nursing in Critical Care* 14 (4): 207–212.

Flynn, J.T. (2002). Choice of dialysis modality for management of pediatric acute renal failure. *Pediatric Nephrology* 17 (1): 61–69.

Foot, C.L. and Fraser, J.F. (2005). So you need to start renal replacement therapy on your ICU patient? *Current Anaesthesia and Critical Care* 16 (6): 321–329.

Glasper, E.A., McEwing, G., and Richardson, J. (2016). *The Oxford Handbook of Children's and Young People's Nursing*, 2e. Oxford: Oxford University Press.

Goldstein, S.L. (2009). The clinical application of CRRT – current status: overview of pediatric renal replacement therapy in acute kidney injury. *Seminars in Dialysis* 22 (2): 180–184. Blackwell Publishing Ltd.

Goldstein, S.L. (2011a). Continuous renal replacement therapy: mechanism of clearance, fluid removal, indications and outcomes. *Current Opinion in Pediatrics* 23 (2): 181–185.

Goldstein, S.L. (2011b). Advances in pediatric renal replacement therapy for acute kidney injury. *Seminars in Dialysis* 24 (2): 187–191. Blackwell Publishing Ltd.

Goldstein, S.L., Macierowski, C.T., and Jabs, K. (1997). Hemodialysis catheter survival and complications in children and adolescents. *Pediatric Nephrology* 11 (1): 74–77.

Gordon, J., Blakeley, K., Blannin, J. et al. (2010). Constipation in children and young people: diagnosis and management. NICE clinical guideline 99.

NICE Publications, London, UK. www.nice.org.uk/guidance/cg99/evidence (accessed 2 June 2022).

Hanson, G. and Moist, L. (2003). Acute renal failure in the ICU: assessing the utility of continuous renal replacement. *Journal of Critical Care* 18 (1): 48–51.

Headrick, C.L. (1998). Adult/pediatric CVVH. The pump, the patient, the circuit. *Critical Care Nursing Clinics of North America* 10 (2): 197.

John, S. and Eckardt, K.U. (2007). Renal replacement strategies in the ICU. *Chest Journal* 132 (4): 1379–1388.

de Jonge, R.C.J., Polderman, K.H., and Gemke, R.J.B.J. (2005). Review article. Central venous catheter use in the pediatric patient: mechanical and infectious complications. *Pediatric Critical Care Medicine* 6 (3): 329–339.

Kuo, D.Z., Houtrow, A.J., Arango, P. et al. (2012). Family-centered care: current applications and future directions in pediatric health care. *Maternal and Child Health Journal* 16 (2): 297–305.

Lyndon, W.D., Wille, K.M., and Tolwani, A.J. (2012). Solute clearance in CRRT: prescribed dose versus actual delivered dose. *Nephrology, Dialysis, Transplantation* 27 (3): 952–956.

MacLaren, G. and Butt, W. (2009). Controversies in paediatric continuous renal replacement therapy. *Intensive Care Medicine* 35 (4): 596–602.

Mactier, R., Hoenich, N., and Breen, C. (2009). *Clinical Practice Guidelines for Haemodialysis*, 5e. Petersfield, UK: Renal Association.

Metheny, N.M. and Snively, W.D. (1983). *Nurses Handbook of Fluid Balance*, 4e. London: J. B. Lippincott.

Monchi, M., Berghmans, D., Ledoux, D. et al. (2004). Citrate vs. heparin for anticoagulation in continuous venovenous hemofiltration: a prospective randomized study. *Intensive Care Medicine* 30 (2): 260–265.

Murray, P. and Hall, J. (2000). Renal replacement therapy for acute renal failure. *American Journal of Respiratory and Critical Care Medicine* 162: 777–781.

Naka, T. and Bellomo, R. (2004). Bench-to-bedside review: treating acid–base abnormalities in the intensive care unit-the role of renal replacement therapy. *Critical Care* 8 (2): 108.

National Institute of Health and Care Excellence (NICE 2015) Intravenous fluid therapy in children and young people in hospital. NICE guideline [NG29]. https://www.nice.org.uk/guidance/ng29 (accessed 11 February 2022).

Nikkiso Europe GmbH (2012). Advance Module 2 Aquarius System Training. Instructions For Use – Aquarius System Platinum Software Version 6.02, Rev. 4.0 (09/2012) Nikkiso Europe GmbH, Desbrocksriede 1, 30855. Langenhagen, Germany.

Parshuram, C.S. and Cox, P.N. (2002). Neonatal hyperkalemic-hypocalcemic cardiac arrest associated with initiation of blood-primed continuous venovenous hemofiltration. *Pediatric Critical Care Medicine* 3 (1): 67–69.

Phadke, K.D., Goodyer, P., and Bitzan, M. (eds.) (2014). *Manual of Paediatric Nephrology*. Heidelberg and New York: Springer.

Prowle, J.R. and Bellomo, R. (2010). Continuous renal replacement therapy: recent advances and future research. *Nature Reviews Nephrology* 6 (9): 521–529.

Rees, L., Feather, S., Shroff, R. (2008). Haemodialysis Clinical Practice Guidelines for Children and Adolescents. British Association for Paediatric Nephrology. https://www.erknet.org/fileadmin/files/user_upload/British_Association_for_Paediatric_Nephrology._Haemodialysis_clinical_practice_guidelines_for_children_and_adolescents.pdf (accessed 30 June 2022).

Rees, L., Brogan, P.A., Bockenhauer, D., and Webb, N.J. (2012). *Paediatric Nephrology*. Oxford University Press.

Rewa, O., Villeneuve, P.M., Eurich, D.T. et al. (2015). Quality indicators in continuous renal replacement therapy (CRRT) care in critically ill patients: protocol for a systematic review. *Systematic Reviews* 4 (1): 1.

Ricci, Z., Ronco, C., Bachetoni, A. et al. (2006). Solute removal during continuous renal replacement therapy in critically ill patients: convection versus diffusion. *Critical Care* 10: R67.

Ronco, C., Ricci, Z., De Backer, D. et al. (2015). Renal replacement therapy in acute kidney injury: controversy and consensus. *Critical Care* 19 (1): 1.

Santiago, M.J., López-Herce, J., Urbano, J. et al. (2009). Complications of continuous renal replacement therapy in critically ill children: a prospective observational evaluation study. *Critical Care* 13 (6): R184.

Saudan, P., Niederberger, M., De Seigneux, S. et al. (2006). Adding a dialysis dose to continuous hemofiltration increases survival in patients with acute renal failure. *Kidney International* 70 (7): 1312–1317.

Schetz, M. (2001). Anticoagulation for continuous renal replacement therapy. *Current Opinion in Anaesthesiology* 14 (2): 143–149.

Sefton, G., Farrell, M., and Noyes, J. (2001). The perceived learning needs of paediatric intensive care nurses caring for children requiring haemofiltration. *Intensive & Critical Care Nursing* 17 (1): 40–50.

Shaheen, I., Harvey, B., and Watson, A.R. (2009). Haemofiltration therapy. *Paediatrics and Child Health* 19 (3): 121–126.

Sharma, A., Zilleruelo, G., Abitbol, C. et al. (1999). Survival and complications of cuffed catheters in children on chronic hemodialysis. *Pediatric Nephrology* 13 (3): 245–248.

Sherman, R., Daugirdas, J., and Ing, T. (2007). Complications during hemodialysis. In: *Handbook of Dialysis*, 4e (eds. J.T. Daugirdas, P.G. Blake and T.S. Ing), 170–191. Philadelphia: Lippincott Williams and Wilkins.

Soysal, D.D., Karaböcüoğlu, M., Çıtak, A. et al. (2007). Metabolic disturbances following the use of inadequate solutions for hemofiltration in acute renal failure. *Pediatric Nephrology* 22 (5): 715–719.

Symons, J.M., Brophy, P.D., Gregory, M.J. et al. (2003). Continuous renal replacement therapy in children up to 10 kg. *American Journal of Kidney Diseases* 41 (5): 984–989.

Uchino, S., Bellomo, R., Morimatsu, H. et al. (2007). Continuous renal replacement therapy: a worldwide practice survey. *Intensive Care Medicine* 33 (9): 1563–1570.

Willock, J. and Jewkes, F. (2000). Making sense of fluid balance in children. *Paediatric Nursing* 12 (7): 37–42.

Further reading

National Collaborating Centre for Women's and Children's Health (2009) Diarrhoea and vomiting caused by gastroenteritis; diagnosis, assessment and management in children younger than 5 years. Royal College of Obstetricians and Gynaecologists. London. www.nice.org.uk/guidance/cg84/evidence/full-guideline-243546877 (accessed 2 June 2022).

Quinlan, C., Cantwell, M., and Rees, L. (2010). Eosinophilic peritonitis in children on chronic peritoneal dialysis. *Pediatric Nephrology* 25 (3): 517–522.

Ring, P.A. and Camille, C.J. (2018). Chapter 25. The Child with Renal Dysfunction. In: *Wong's Nursing Care of Infants and Children*, 11e (eds. M.J. Hockenberry and D. Wilson), 996–1050. Elsevier.

Walters, S., Porter, C., and Brophy, P.D. (2009). Dialysis and pediatric acute kidney injury (AKI): choice of renal support modality. *Pediatric Nephrology* 24 (1): 37–48.

Weinberg, L., Collins, N., Van Mourik, K., and Bellomo, R. (2016). Plasma-Lyte 148: a clinical review. *World Journal of Critical Care Medicine* 5 (4): 235–250.

Chapter 11

Personal hygiene and pressure ulcer prevention

Sarah Kipps[1], Rachel Allaway[2], and Sarah Carmichael[2]

[1]Formerly Practice Educator, Nursing Quality
[2]BSc (Hons), Children's Nursing; Clinical Nurse Specialist, Tissue Viability, Great Ormond Street Hospital, London, UK

Chapter contents

Introduction	158
Bathing	158
Toileting	159
Nappy and incontinence pad care	161
Nail care	165
Oral hygiene	165
Oral assessment	166
Eye care	169
Ear care	170
Pressure ulcer prevention and management	171
Management of pressure ulcers	176
Conclusion	177
References	197

Procedure guidelines

11.1	Assessment for bathing	178
11.2	Baby bathing	178
11.3	Topping and tailing	180
11.4	Washing and bathing the CYP	180
11.5	Bed bathing	181
11.6	Bathing the CYP with special needs	182
11.7	Assessment of toileting needs	182
11.8	Toileting the CYP	183
11.9	Assessing nappy rashes	185
11.10	Routine nappy care	185
11.11	Nail assessment	187
11.12	Nail care	187
11.13	Oral assessment	188
11.14	Oral hygiene tools	189
11.15	Performing oral care	191
11.16	Oral health promotion	192
11.17	Oral care during compromised health	192
11.18	Eye Care	194
11.19	Administration of eye drops	195
11.20	Insertion of contact lenses	196
11.21	Removal of soft contact lenses	196
11.22	Removal of gas permeable contact lenses and all contact lenses	196
11.23	Care of contact lenses	196
11.24	Administration of ear drops	197

The Great Ormond Street Hospital Manual of Children and Young People's Nursing Practices, Second Edition. Edited by Elizabeth Anne Bruce, Janet Williss, and Faith Gibson.
© 2023 John Wiley & Sons Ltd. Published 2023 by John Wiley & Sons Ltd.

Introduction

Personal hygiene is an important consideration in the holistic care of both healthy children and young people (CYPs) and in those with specific needs and/or compromised due to illness, surgery, and hospitalisation. A good standard of hygiene is an integral component of daily life and/or is necessary to maintain dignity and self-esteem, as well as to prevent infection. It is essential that maintaining such a standard continues during a CYP's time in hospital. Maintaining hygiene can also assist to promote normality in the sick CYP, enhance comfort, and aid psychological well-being.

For any admission to hospital, the importance of involving the family is paramount in relation to all areas of care (Hockenberry and Wilson 2010; Turnbull and Petty 2013), including the personal and hygiene needs of the CYP. Parents/carers should be encouraged to participate in the general care of their child as much as their condition allows. The CYP's usual routine should be discussed on admission and continued as much as possible to facilitate family interaction and participation (Davis et al. 2003; Peate and Whiting 2006; POPPY Parents of Premature Babies Project 2009; Tran et al. 2009) in line with a 'partnership' approach. The nurse has a role in facilitating the involvement of the CYP and family in undertaking as much care as they are able, or indeed, wish to do. This role also extends to support through teaching and advising on matters such as hygiene. Moreover, the nurse should teach and guide support workers and students both by example in delivering best practice and by providing theory to support practice. Integral to this is the need to ensure that practice remains evidence based, even for fundamental aspects of care such as personal hygiene.

There are many factors that influence how often care-giving practices are carried out, including individual preference, normal routine, age, culture, and, most importantly in the sick CYP, the physiological state relating to illness. Healthy CYPs will continue their normal routine as much as possible in hospital. However, in those with an acute illness in high-dependency, intensive care or following surgery, reducing any further physiological stress or unnecessary handling should take precedence and personal hygiene often occurs less frequently than normal. The sick CYP should be assessed for their ability to cope with care procedures on a regular basis and if they are not able to tolerate these, they should be kept to an absolute minimum or left until later.

Due to their size and/or gestation, low-birth-weight or premature babies are less able to tolerate prolonged and frequent episodes of handling, as this can cause temperature instability and stress (Cleveland 2008; Ellis 2005; Knobel and Holditch-Davis 2007; Sherman et al. 2006; Thomas 2003a; Waldron and MacKinnon 2007), hence the concept of 'minimal handling'; i.e. long periods of rest with minimal stimulation (Bauer 2005; Khurana et al. 2005) is commonplace. For more information see Chapter 20: Neonatal Care. The same principle can apply to any CYP who is acutely unwell. For these reasons, there are no firm guidelines on how often caregiving is performed as this should be individualised and based on on-going assessment and evaluation.

Cultural considerations, including norms and variations, also need attention and are incorporated into both the assessment process and individual care regimes. Girls who are Muslim for example, may wish to request assistance from female carers only and it may not be appropriate to perform bathing and other routines on particular religious days such as the Sabbath within the Jewish population.

Attending to hygiene needs should be made as fun and enjoyable as possible with the use of appropriate toys. In the older CYP, independence should be encouraged, particularly in adolescence, when self-consciousness and body image issues are more common. Maintaining privacy and dignity is paramount for the CYP at any age, particularly with regard to personal matters. An example is illustrated in relation to elimination, where lack of privacy can lead to embarrassment, which could result in retention of faeces and constipation.

Overall, it is imperative that individual, family, cultural and societal needs are considered and acknowledged for all the previously mentioned areas of personal hygiene (Hewitt 2000) as well as both physical and emotional needs.

Standard precautions should be applied whenever the carer comes into contact with body fluids to minimise cross-infection (Lawson 2001); for example, the use of gloves and aprons during nappy care, correct disposal of body fluids and hand washing, or the use of alcohol hand-rub between patients (Moralejo and Jull 2003). For more information see Chapter 13: Infection Prevention and Control.

Bathing

Bathing and/or washing are essential elements of personal hygiene (Trigg and Mohammed 2006), which both promote a CYP's comfort and well-being and minimise infection via the skin.

The skin forms a structural boundary and interface for any organism (Visscher et al. 2002). It consists of three layers – epidermis, dermis, and subcutaneous tissue (Tortora and Derrikson 2013). The subcutaneous layer is comprised of fatty tissue for insulation and serves as fuel for heat production. The middle layer – dermis – is composed of elastin fibres, collagen, and fibrous protein. The top layer, the epidermis, is the most important for infection control, as this is the protective layer with

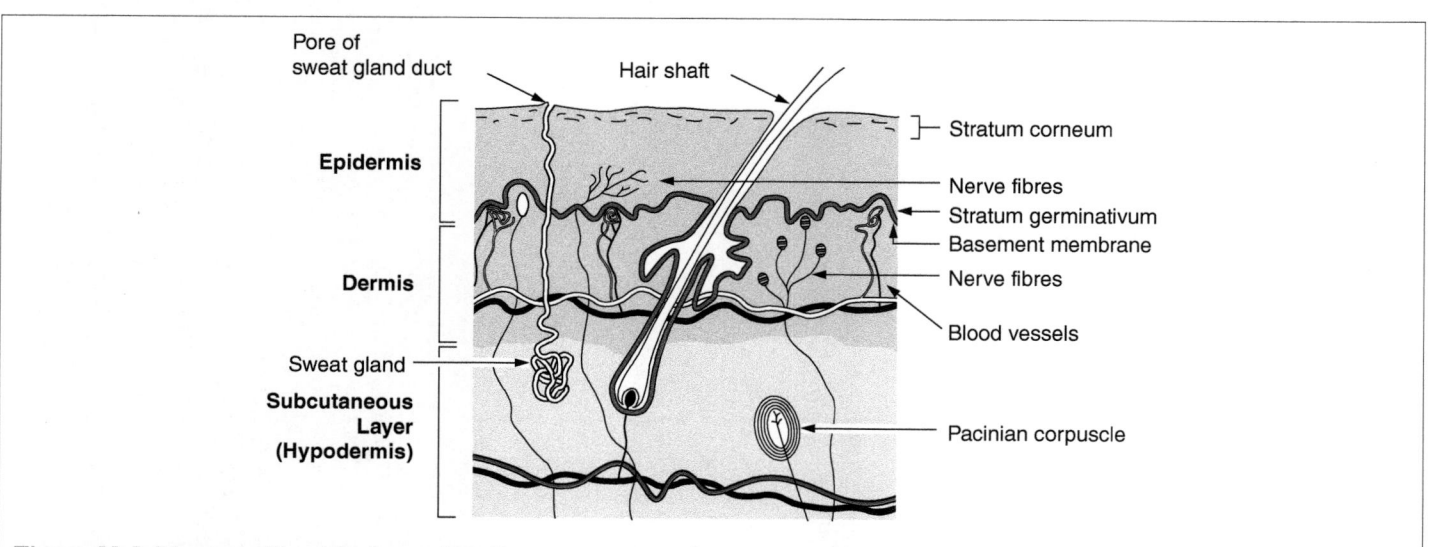

Figure 11.1 Diagram of the skin. *Source:* http://www.nurse-prescriber.co.uk/visual_library.htm © 2005 Cambridge University Press, UK.

impermeability to both water and bacteria, the stratum corneum (Jackson 2008; Tortora and Derrikson 2013) (Figure 11.1).

Resistance to substances and bacteria relies on the skin being both intact and sufficiently developed. From birth, the skin of a term neonate has a well-developed stratum corneum complete with keratin formation. At birth, the full-term neonate has a skin pH of 6.4, which falls to 4.9 (adult value) in the first four days (Irving 2001). This acidity creates an 'acid mantle' providing natural protection against infection (Blincoe 2006a, 2006b; Hale 2007). Bathing within the first 24 hours of life and daily bathing thereafter up to 10–14 days old can mean this process is delayed and can slow the separation of the umbilical cord due to the delay of normal skin flora colonisation (Franck et al. 2000; Hopkins 2004; Mainstone 2005). In addition, it is widely recognised that the newborn baby can lose body heat rapidly in the first days of life and exposure for bathing can potentially cause the body temperature to drop (Bergstrom et al. 2005; Medves and O'Brien 2004). 'Topping and tailing' (in other words, washing the face, body, and nappy area separately) can be carried out on days when bathing is not performed. In addition, the preterm neonate has physiological differences in their skin compared with the full term infant (Walker et al. 2005a, b). The neonate born at less than 34 weeks gestation lacks sufficient keratin and so the barrier function is limited in the first 10–14 days after birth (Irving et al. 2006; Jackson 2008; Walker et al. 2005a). Moreover, skin acidity takes significantly longer to fall, often taking weeks rather than days, and delaying the acid mantle formation (Blincoe 2006a, b; Mancini 2004; Quinn et al. 2005). Skin frailty and susceptibility to damage and infection, along with greater physiological and temperature instability means that bathing is not appropriate until weight and condition allow and the neonate can maintain their body temperature sufficiently outside an incubator (Mainstone 2005; Hale 2007). Bathing is also not recommended in healthy, very low-birth-weight babies (<1.5 kg) for at least seven days after birth (Behring et al. 2003; Medves and O'Brien 2004; Quinn et al. 2005) for the same reasons. Again, 'topping and tailing' is recommended until condition, weight and temperature stability allow. In the older CYP, systemic illness and immobility may prevent bathing due to safety issues involved in transferring the CYP and excessive handling during illness. Bed bathing or washing the skin gently is recommended in line with physiological stability. In addition, showering can be a suitable or preferred alternative for the older CYP.

Whatever method of cleansing is appropriate, it is important to assess the skin's integrity and cleanliness (McGurk et al. 2004). Close observation of the skin is paramount, particularly in the sick CYP, as skin breakdown can occur due to a variety of factors including oedema, pressure, friction, immobility, malnutrition and obesity. Washing or bathing a CYP provides a good opportunity to observe the skin and attend to other aspects such as response to stimulation, movements, pressure areas, and elimination function.

Washing and bathing are often appropriate times to communicate with a CYP of any age. Baby bathing, for example, is a time for promoting parent–baby interaction by tactile communication and can be a positive experience for both. The baby's behaviour and the bath experience are used to engage parents/carers with their neonate (Hockenberry and Wilson 2010). In the toddler or pre-school child, the nurse and/or family can use this time to teach hygiene practices, reinforcing behaviours such as cleaning, hair washing, drying, and dressing. In the older CYP, assistance with washing or bathing is a chance to give advice and teach health promotion in relation to hygiene; for example, appropriate frequency and use of products like deodorant and shampoo. It is important to remember that there may be individual cultural norms to address with respect to frequency, which should assist with hygiene and the issue of privacy.

For a child of any age, bathing is an ideal opportunity to involve parents/carers in caregiving and to facilitate parent–child interaction. For many children, normal bathing routines at home include elements of play, learning, and close physical contact with their parents and carers.

N.B. All CYPs having procedures or undergoing surgery should have a bath or shower using soap within the preceding 24 hours, to reduce the risk of surgical site infections (National Institute for Health and Care Excellence [NICE] 2019, Department of Health (DH) 2011).

Washing and bathing the child or young person

Assessment and preparation are an important part of bathing. Assessment applies to readiness of the CYP for bathing as well as assessing the environment and safety aspects. The toddler or preschool child may only require a bath every two to three days. The older CYP may require a daily bath or shower and hair wash and should be encouraged to maintain their own independence where possible. Teeth and nail care are also pertinent areas of hygiene, as is hair washing. The latter gives an opportunity to inspect the condition of the head and check for head lice. As the child gets older, the potential for self-consciousness and embarrassment may arise and this should be minimised by ensuring privacy and dignity is maintained at all times, taking cultural factors into account.

CYPs are developing independence and need to be taught care procedures appropriate to their age and development. Parents/carers have a central role to play in a ward environment, where busy schedules and time constraints may make encouraging independence difficult. This is an ideal chance to reinforce partnership and negotiation. Unless there are good clinical reasons for changes to the CYP's normal daily routine, every effort should be made to keep practices as normal as possible while in hospital. Full independence with self-care develops over time in most CYPs, providing they are able-bodied and well. Individuality in development also needs to be recognised in relation to growing independence with bathing or dressing ability. Choice should also be allowed, for example the older child or adolescent may prefer showering or washing to bathing. Bath time is usually a time of fun and an opportunity to play. This should not be any different for a sick, immobile or disabled CYP although the physiological condition of the CYP will influence when and how this is carried out.

Some CYPs may require additional help with bathing. If the CYP is not fully able-bodied or sick, then a bed bath may be necessary. Parents/carers can be taught this procedure. For the CYP with special needs, personal cleaning and bathing should continue as close to their normal routine as possible. Equipment or adaptations, such as bath lifts, hoists or supports may be necessary for those who are difficult to mobilise. For more information see Chapter 19: Moving and Handling.

Toileting

Attaining continence is a developmental milestone, which generally takes place over the first few years of life. For some, reaching this milestone comes later than expected; for others, continence may never be achieved for a specific reason, such as cognitive impairment, severe learning difficulties, neurogenic bladder, trauma, congenital malformation, or surgical intervention. There may also be a loss of continence at some later point in development, be it transient or permanent (Sanders 2002). In order to attain continence, children must learn to attend to their own elimination needs. This ability develops over time as independence and cognitive maturity increases (Schum et al. 2002). Continence, both urinary and bowel, is learnt and develops over time as a complex sequence of events. Generally, achievement of 'normal' milestones for complete toilet training occurs from 18 months up to 3–4 years but it must be emphasised that significant variations exist between individual children. It is more important to observe for stages rather than ages. However, the following serves as a guide.

In infancy, the bladder is controlled by a spinal reflex arc as part of the autonomic nervous system. As the bladder fills, the

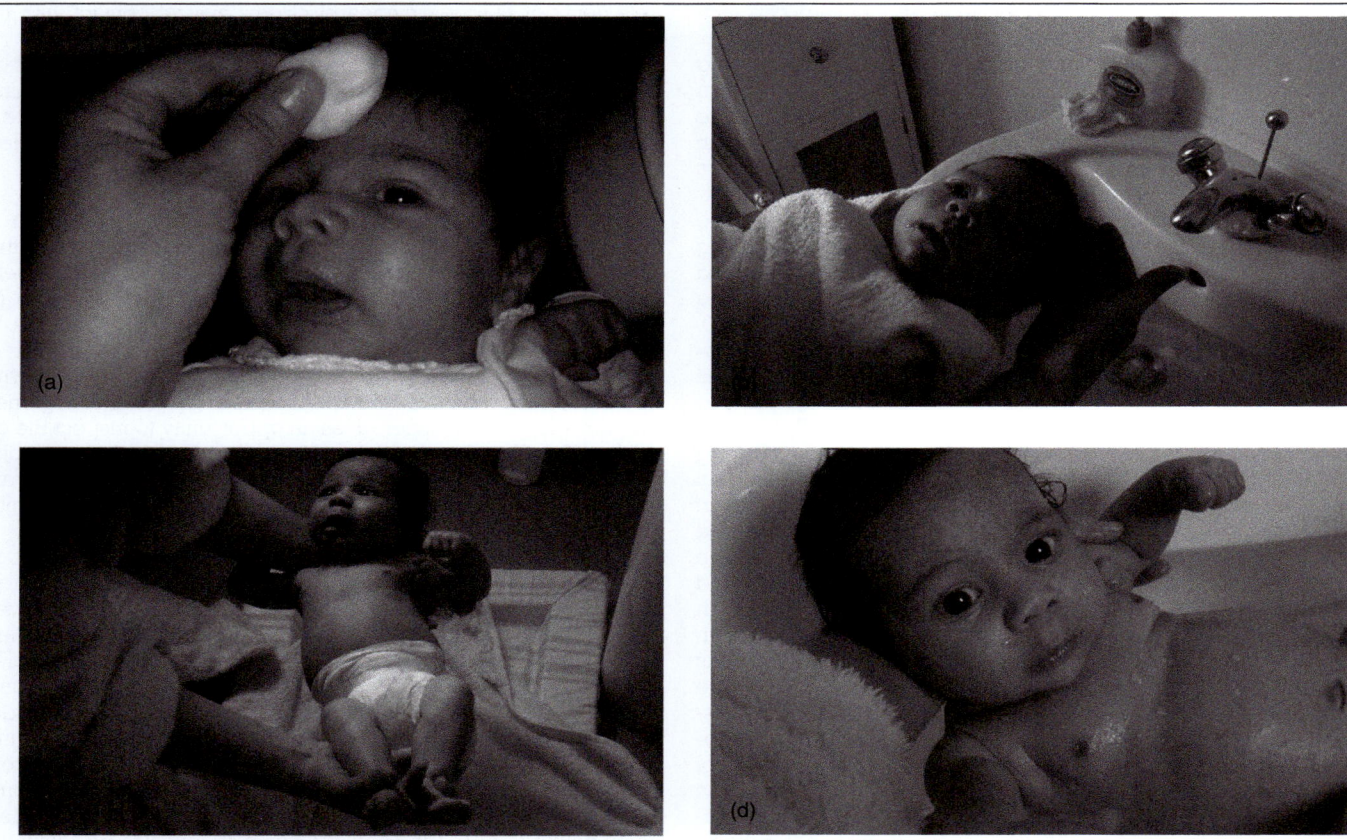

Figure 11.2 (a–d) Baby bathing. *Source:* Photograph courtesy of Julie Petty.

detrusor muscle sends sensory messages to the sacral bladder zone within the spinal cord. When the bladder is empty, impulses return to the muscle of the bladder to cause relaxation while the sphincter is closed. When the bladder is full, motor impulses cause the detrusor muscle to contract, the sphincter relaxes and urine can be passed (Dewar 2010; Mota and Barros 2008; Tennant 2010; Wu 2010). Over time, a child comes to learn to interpret the feelings of having a full bladder and inhibit urination until an appropriate time (Rogers 2000). Development of this pathway occurs over the first 18–20 months of life. From two years of age, a child's cognitive maturity develops, so that the interpretation of signals and the self-control of voiding are linked together and co-ordinated. From two years, a child should have commenced co-operation in toilet training and by three years should have daytime bladder control. Night bladder control should also start to mature from three years of age.

Bowel control is based on relaxation of the internal anal sphincter and simultaneous increased activity of the external sphincter in response to faeces within the rectum, again under reflexive control. During toilet training, the child will come to voluntarily contract the external sphincter until an appropriate time for elimination.

In the healthy child, the aim is to achieve self-toileting at an expected stage of development in line with the physical development of urinary and bowel function. The child is then deemed 'toilet trained' (Rogers 2002). Even a child who is not continent for physical reasons can still be taught to be independent, e.g. to attend to a stoma or intermittent catheterisation. Most children, even those with learning difficulties can, with patience, be toilet trained (Rogers 2002). The concept of early and thorough child and family education is of utmost importance here (Boucke 2003).

When a CYP is unable to attend to their own toileting needs the nurse must assist with toileting in the appropriate way, maintaining privacy and dignity at all times and with consideration of cultural and societal norms to provide individualised care for the CYP.

Assessment of toileting needs

Assessment of toileting needs should be carried out in children of all ages to identify CYPs' bladder and bowel function. This assessment will help identify any potential problems. It is important that appropriate care can be given according to normal routine and stage of development. In order to assess the normal toileting pattern of a child, it is important to understand how continence and toilet training develops as described previously. Privacy and dignity should be maintained at all times, particularly, for example, for adolescent girls during menstruation.

It should be remembered that the complex pattern of continence does not always occur as expected. Certain situations may alter normal elimination; for example, illness, infection, medication, immobility, fear and anxiety, lack of privacy, and loss of consciousness. If continence problems are not managed and become chronic, they may result in referral, treatment and/or surgery in secondary care (NICE 2010a, b).

CYPs with special needs or disabilities may differ widely in terms of their developmental level. Assessment of toileting patterns unique to their specific needs is the key to deciding what management strategy to implement for these CYPs (Barone et al. 2009; Dewar 2010; Horn et al. 2006; Rogers 2002; Schmidt 2004).

Bedwetting and constipation are two common childhood continence difficulties. NICE guidelines have been published with details of assessment, treatment, and information for support for CYPs and families (NICE 2010a, b). The overall aim is to help the CYP to achieve complete continence, or to manage the condition discreetly and effectively. If full control is not clinically possible the service should respond effectively to the child's physical, psychological and social needs (The Paediatric Continence Forum 2014).

Bedwetting is a widespread and distressing condition that can have a deep impact on a CYP's behaviour, emotional well-being and social life. It is also very stressful for the parents or carers. The prevalence of bedwetting decreases with age. Bedwetting that occurs fewer than two nights a week has a prevalence of 21% at about four and a half years and 8% at nine and a half years. More frequent bedwetting is less common and has a prevalence of 8% at four and a half years and 1.5% at nine and a half years (Butler and Heron 2008).

The causes of bedwetting are not fully understood. Bedwetting can be considered to be a symptom that may result from a combination of different predisposing factors. There are a number of different disturbances of physiology that may be associated with bedwetting. These include sleep arousal difficulties, polyuria, and bladder dysfunction. Bedwetting also often runs in families.

Constipation is common in childhood (see Chapter 5: Bowel Care). It is prevalent in around 5–30% of the child population, depending on the criteria used for diagnosis. Symptoms become chronic in more than one third of patients and constipation is a common reason for referral to secondary care. Morbidity may be under-reported because people may not seek advice because they are embarrassed (NICE 2010a). The exact cause of constipation is not fully understood but factors that may contribute include pain, fever, dehydration, dietary and fluid intake, psychological issues, toilet training, medicines, and familial history of constipation. Constipation is referred to as 'idiopathic' if it cannot be explained by anatomical or physiological abnormalities (NICE 2010a).

Toileting the child or young person

For the continent CYP, individual toileting routine should be maintained as much as possible during hospital stay. For those with special needs, incontinence may be an issue and this should be dealt with sensitively and within a multidisciplinary framework. Incontinence results from many different 'special needs' and may relate to a physical problem such as neuropathic bladder or congenital malformation, or to a learning difficulty, leading to developmental delay. In addition to assessment of toileting needs it is worth noting that children who are anxious or fearful may regress and day and/or night wetting may occur. Nurses and the family must be aware of these changes and act accordingly. Other issues that may affect toileting include constipation, diarrhoea, the presence of a stoma, and enuresis (Rhodes 2000). For more information see Chapter 5: Bowel Care.

Nappy and incontinence pad care

Nappy and incontinence pad care (excluding incontinence sheets) applies to the neonate, infant and toddler up to the point of completed toilet training. The principles also apply to the use of incontinence pads in the older CYP. In addition, some children who have developmental delay and have not yet reached this stage, or those with incontinence during the day and/or at night may require nappies. The principles described in this section will cover both nappy and pad care but for ease will refer to nappy care throughout.

A newborn baby will pass urine between 5 and 20 times a day and can have a bowel movement following each feed. During illness and in certain medical and surgical conditions CYPs may experience increased frequency of micturition (Philipp et al. 1997; Price 2000; Turner 2000). Skin integrity in the neonate and young infant may make them physically more susceptible to skin irritation, breakdown, and attack from infective agents (Adam 2008; Adam et al. 2009; Borkowski 2004; Prasad et al. 2003; Scheinfeld 2005) particularly when they are unwell. Any infant, CYP who is incontinent and requiring the use of nappies, is at risk of developing nappy rash (Atherton 2004, 2005; Atherton and Mill 2004). When skin is exposed to urine and faeces for prolonged periods an excess of moisture builds up and skin becomes waterlogged. This then becomes soft and fragile with an increased friction coefficient, making it vulnerable to frictional damage (Irving et al. 2006). In addition, the combination of ammonia in urine, and bacteria in faeces creates a chemical cocktail that increases skin pH and releases proteolytic enzymes, causing irritation. This results in the painful redness and rawness (inflammation) known as nappy rash (Coughlin et al. 2014; Merrill 2015; NICE 2020). Skin damage and increased skin pH affect the body's natural defence mechanisms against harmful micro-organisms. In extreme cases, a secondary infection can occur, complicating the condition and its treatment and resulting in further skin breakdown. In the hospital environment any skin breakdown increases the risk of hospital acquired infection.

In general the incidence of nappy rash relates to the length of time skin is in contact with dampness, urine, and faeces, and the susceptibility of an individual's skin to these factors (Allison 2000). When dealing with a complex system such as the skin, which is affected by both internal and external stressors as well as emotional and systemic factors, identification of cause can sometimes be extremely difficult. There will always be situations where a causative agent cannot be found, and despite the best care, nappy rash may still occur. The aim of nursing care is to prevent nappy rash through regular and thorough cleaning, drying, and airing and, should the condition arise, the application of protective, medicated, or soothing creams (Blincoe 2005, 2006a, b; Camm 2006; Jackson 2008; Trotter 2006).

Choice of nappies/pads

The choice of nappy system, whether disposable or reusable, makes little difference to the incidence of nappy rash if used correctly. Individual limitations should be considered when planning frequency of nappy changes and assessing the causes of nappy rash (Blincoe 2005, 2006a, b). It is important when making a choice that the correct size of nappy is selected for comfort, avoidance of spillage (too large), and avoidance of possible pressure injury (too small). Correct sizing will help avoid the overuse of unnecessary incontinence sheets. The overuse of incontinence sheets places the CYP's skin at risk of moisture-associated skin damage due to moisture trapping between the incontinence sheet and the patient's skin, which in turn causes excess moisture layers between the mattress and the sheet.

Modern disposable nappies use gel technology to effectively draw fluid away from the skin and can be changed less frequently in the absence of stools, making regular application of barrier creams unnecessary in most children. A Cochrane review found that there was not enough evidence from good-quality randomised controlled trials to support or refute the use and type of disposable nappies for the prevention of nappy dermatitis in infants (Baer et al. 2006). If used, creams should be applied sparingly in a thin invisible layer with the skin remaining visible through the cream. This will reduce the risk of skin/nappy transfer, which can block the nappy lining and compromise absorbency and function (Price 2000).

Cloth nappies are less efficient at keeping moisture away from skin and therefore may require more frequent changing and the regular use of a barrier cream. Careful laundering is required to kill bacteria and ensure removal of possible irritant washing agents. Fabric conditioner should not be used, as this will reduce nappy absorbency, as well as being a potential irritant to infant skin (Allison 2000). Modern re-useable nappies are popular but are not recommended for use in hospital (Oakley and Gomez 2017). Parents who do use these may need initial guidance when switching to the use of disposable nappies.

All nappies can be preweighed to enable monitoring of urine or fluid output using the conversion of 1 g weight = 1 ml urine/stool output (Gardner et al. 2010).

Skin cleansers

For normal unbroken skin, water alone (avoiding the use of soap) applied with cotton wool or a soft cloth, is adequate for cleaning the skin of the nappy area (Trotter 2008), as it is least likely to cause irritation, sensitivity, or disrupt the pH of the skin. If alternatives to water for cleansing are sought, the use of emollient cream, liquid paraffin, or oil (e.g. olive oil) as cleaning agents are less abrasive than soap, will not affect skin pH, and are recommended for children with nappy rash. However, nurses should be aware that they may affect the adherence of certain barrier creams. Use of nut-based oils (e.g. arachis or peanut oil) is not generally recommended, as its use has been shown to be a possible causative factor in the development of peanut allergy (Lack et al. 2003). Gentle cleansing technique reducing friction is of upmost importance for children with nappy rash.

Some brands of baby wipes have been shown to cleanse as gently as water and may contain additives that may help to maintain the barrier properties of the skin (Atherton 2009; Jones 2000; Turner 2000). Alcohol-based wipes should be avoided as they will cause obvious distress if used on broken or irritated skin. It is not recommended to use baby wipes on inflamed or broken skin.

Assessment for nappy rash

The cornerstone of successful treatment of any episode of nappy rash is the accurate assessment of various possible etiological factors and the treatment of precipitating or perpetuating causes (Atherton 2004, 2005; Atherton and Mill 2004). The nurse should be aware of predisposing factors (Box 11.1). During the initial nursing history assessment, potential 'at risk' CYPs can be identified before rashes occur and appropriate preventative measures can be implemented (Adam 2008; Adam et al. 2009).

Episodes can vary considerably between individuals (Allison 2000) so careful assessment, evaluation, and recording of any rash and subsequent treatment are vital.

As well as assessing rash severity and response to treatment the nurse should be able to distinguish between nappy rash and other common skin conditions (Adam 2008; Atherton 2004; Cooper 2000; Jordan et al. 1986) (Table 11.1). The use of a nappy rash- and incontinence-associated dermatitis grading scale is useful and allows the multi-disciplinary team and parents to assess and implement an appropriate treatment strategy and identify any improvement or deterioration of an existing rash (Figure 11.4).

Clinicians must know how to prevent nappy rash and how to best manage this if the skin breaks down, depending on the severity of the damage. A severity rating scale and clear guideline for the prevention and care of nappy rash and incontinence associated dermatitis is useful in practice to support assessment, clinical management, and onwards referral to inpatient Tissue Viability Clinical Nurse Specialists for CYPs while in hospital.

Table 11.1 Types of nappy rash, their aetiology, and appearance

Type of nappy rash	Aetiology	Appearance
Contact (irritant) early stage	Moisture, friction, prolonged contact with urine and stool.	Generalised superficial red rash (erythematous), commonly sparing skin folds.
Jaques napkin rash/eruption	Acidic urine or stool output, chronic diarrhoea, or urinary dribbling with associated genitourinary abnormality or malformation (Allison 2000). Sometimes complicated with secondary infection.	Acute irritant nappy rash with open raw sore areas, punctuate sores, eruption or rashes.
Bacterial	*Staphylococcus, Streptococcus*	Warm, broken, scratched skin, weeping shallow ulcers with collaret of scale with oedema/swelling. Other symptoms include pyrexia and irritability (Allison 2000, Zsolway et al. 2002).
Intertrigo	Moisture trapped in skin folds. Commonly seen in children with watery/loose diarrhoea or inadequate cleaning/drying (Allison 2000).	Redness, soreness, or rash limited to areas where two surfaces of the skin are in close contact, e.g. inner walls of buttocks, near the anus.
Fungal	*Candida albicans*	Bright/beefy red/angry looking, sometimes scaly and sharply demarcated rash; satellite lesions spreading into skin creases or beyond the margins of the nappy area. Can also present as contact irritant rash, which is unresponsive to treatment or becomes suddenly worse. Classical white patches surrounded by red skin are less common but possible.
Refractory nappy rash	Nutritional deficiencies of essential fatty acids, biotin, riboflavin, pyridoxine, copper or zinc (possibly presenting with a low alkaline phosphatase, which is a zinc dependant enzyme) (Zsolway et al. 2002).	Unresolving nappy rash, unresponsive to antifungal treatments, in hospitalised or generally unwell patient (Zsolway et al. 2002).
Atopic dermatitis	Unknown aetiology (Zsolway et al. 2002).	Scaly rash, which may also appear on other areas of body including face and flexures of arms and legs with evidence of rubbing or scratching in older infants (Zsolway et al. 2002).
Allergic dermatitis	Babies' skins can develop a sensitivity reaction to any products used for nappy care.	Starts with a red area, which can become raised and itchy (can be confused with eczema). Long-term eruptions have whitened central areas surrounded by reddened skin.
Seborrhoea eczema	Inflammatory condition, unknown aetiology.	Erythematous, greasy, salmon-coloured, well-demarcated, scaly plaques.
Psoriasis		Rarely affecting children under four years. Irritant rash, salmon-pink lesions with clearly defined edges and covered in silvery scale, possibly with symptoms of psoriasis on other skin areas.

Chapter 11 Personal hygiene and pressure ulcer prevention

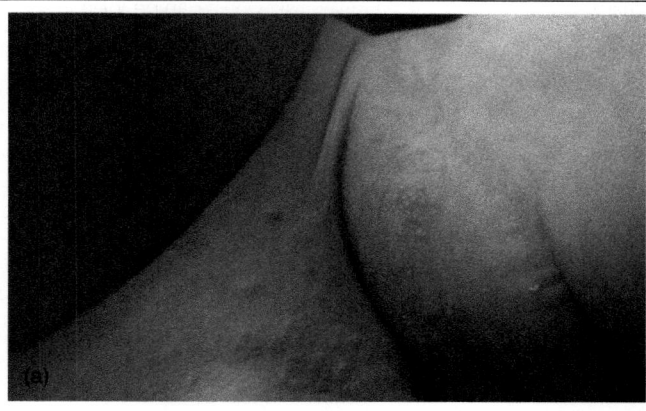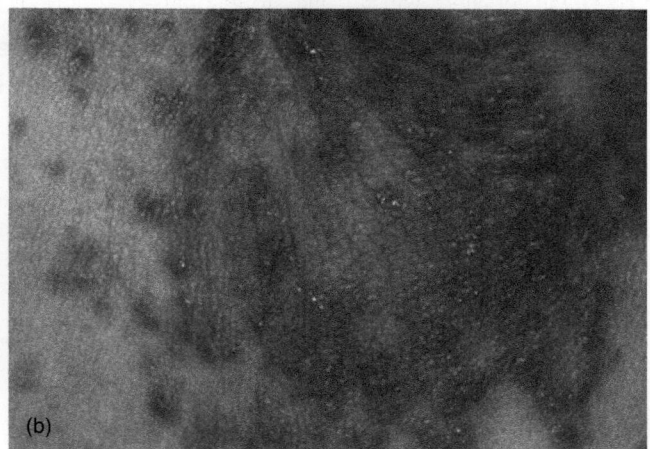

Figure 11.3 (a, b) Typical nappy rash. *Source:* Photograph courtesy of Julie Petty.

Treating nappy rash

Nappies cause the skin to become fragile by increasing its hydration and pH. Prolonged contact with urine and faeces/faecal enzymes damages the delicate skin, resulting in contact dermatitis. A gentle dabbing motion should be used to clean and dry the skin to prevent frictional damage caused by overzealous scrubbing and wiping

Periods of skin airing should be introduced during nappy changes and for more prolonged periods in severe cases, as this promotes dryness and allows skin repair to occur. While infants or children are asleep you are able to lay them on an open nappy to allow for sufficient air to circulate with minimal mess but allowing for protection. During the day the infant can be placed without a nappy in a towel/protective lined bath or play pen for periods of directly supervised play. The careful selection and application of barrier creams may be beneficial when nappy rash is present (Walker et al. 2005a, b). Encouraging a good nutritional intake will provide essential vitamins to aid cell repair.

In all cases of nappy rash an appropriate pain assessment should be carried out and adequate analgesia prescribed and administered.

Creams, lotions, topical medications/applications

There is agreement in the literature that water alone is sufficient for skin cleansing and products are generally avoided (Johnson and Taylor 2010; Stokowski 2006; Trotter 2004, 2006, 2007a, b, 2008; Trigg and Mohammed 2006). However, there are some conditions that require topical application, either as a treatment or to provide a skin barrier, to prevent further excoriation. The majority of barrier creams contain either water repellent silicones such as dimethicone, or waterproof ingredients such as petroleum, which creates a protective layer between skin and nappy contents. Barrier creams are less effective when applied to broken skin and should be ideally used as a preventative measure (Atherton and Mill 2004) or in the early stages of irritation. They require frequent application to be effective, some adhering more effectively than others and trials to find one that suits the needs of an individual CYP may be required (Maxwell and Sinclair 2012). Creams may also include ingredients with known soothing, antiseptic, or astringent properties (Allison 2000; Price 2000; Williams 2001). It is important to follow manufacturer's instructions.

CYPs with bowel disruptions related to medical treatment, or who are undergoing surgery resulting in a period of altered bowel activity, may benefit from a regimen of preventative application of barrier products and periods of airing as a routine precaution to prevent outbreaks.

Creams and sprays designed to protect skin against watery irritant stoma output may be beneficial for use in CYPs whose causative irritant is watery diarrhoea, or for use in those who require minimal handling or are too unwell to tolerate repeated frequent changes. These preparations are designed to adhere to the skin for long periods to enable the fixture of stoma bags. They are nongreasy and less likely to rub off the skin during nappy changes or cause nappy lining blockage. They have the advantage of creating a tough barrier requiring less frequent application. These are indicated for moderate to severe nappy rash and incontinence associated dermatitis (see Figure 11.3).

Hydrocolloid pastes and treatment pastes, e.g. Ilex Paste which, due to their impermeable nature, facilitate rehydration and promote granulation, form an occlusive or complete seal over sore skin and repel harmful fluids and bacteria. If skilfully applied can be used to protect raw areas of skin from irritant output (Ilex Health 2013; Scardillo and Aronovitch 1999). Corticosteroids are powerful anti-inflammatory agents, which can accelerate healing and consequently may be of benefit for treating severe nappy rash (Borkowski 2004).

Topical hydrocortisone is widely recommended by experts to settle inflammation causing discomfort (Joint Formulary Committee 2020; Paige et al. 2010; Ravanfar et al. 2012). On this basis, NICE (2020) recommends the short-term use of topical hydrocortisone for nappy rash unresponsive to simple measures, once-daily application for no more than a week.

Infants and children are more susceptible than adults to the adverse effects of corticosteroids (localised effects include skin atrophy; systemic effects include growth retardation). The manufacturers of hydrocortisone cream 1% state that 'extreme caution is required in dermatoses of infancy especially napkin eruption where the napkin can act as an occlusive dressing and increase absorption. In infants and children, courses of treatment should therefore not normally exceed 7 days' (Association of the British Pharmaceutical Industry (ABPI) Medicines Compendium 2013).

The recommendation to prescribe topical hydrocortisone preparations only for children one month of age or older is based on information in the British National Formulary which states that, for nappy rash, a mild topical corticosteroid can be used, but should be avoided in neonates (Joint Formulary Committee 2020). They are more readily absorbed in infants, especially when applied in the occluded environment of the nappy, and therefore a low potency formula should be applied very sparingly. Professionals remain divided on their use because of their associated immunosuppressive properties, which decrease the skin's ability to fight infection and increase the risk of developing *Candida dermatitis*. The use of corticosteroid creams for this purpose should always be under the

Prevention and Care of Nappy Rash and Incontinence Associated dermatitis (IAD)

Great Ormond Street Hospital for Children — NHS Foundation Trust

Cleanse for Nappy Rash and IAD with both emollient (Aquamax or other equivalent) mixed in water

- Use gauze squares to gently cleanse sore nappy/ pad areas
- To dry skin pat gently with dry gauze or leave to air dry
- Use a pat and roll technique to reduce friction
- Demonstrate the technique to parents and carers

Severity	Description	Cleanse	Barrier
Normal	Intact skin with no erythema	Water or own baby wipes	Parent or carer's cream of choice or small sachet of hospital cream until own cream is available.
Mild & At Risk	Erythema of the skin with no broken areas & intact skin at risk of breakdown. Including therapy that might alter bowel habit or pH of urine, children prone to IAD i.e. chemotherapy, reversal of stoma.	Water & gauze	LBF Barrier Cream (apply a thin invisible layer). If no improvement after 48 hours change to LBF Sterile barrier film sticks/spray.
Moderate	Erythema of skin with small broken areas	Water & gauze	LBF Sterile barrier film sticks/spray. Apply spray daily, increase frequency of spray application as necessary.
Severe	Erythema with large areas of broken skin extending to dermis classified as moisture lesion.	(Emollin if in pain)	LBF Barrier film sticks/spray to moisture lesions. For deep lesions **ILEX paste** to be prescribed and used as per instruction leaflet. **If no improvement after 48 hours make TVN referral**
Candida	Bright red rash with satellite lesions/pustules at margins that may extend into groins and skin folds. Other presentations to consider include cellulitis.	(Emollin if in pain)	Send skin swab for MC&S. Apply anti-fungal cream as per prescribing guidelines. Then use once absorbed use **Medihoney Barrier cream**.

Choice of Creams- The first line product recommended by the Tissue Viability Team for the prevention of Nappy Rash/IAD is LBF barrier cream. The second line product is Medihoney barrier cream.

Other barrier creams i.e. Metanium, Proshield will still be available within the Trust to order for specific patient groups. i.e. patients with EB or patients whom LBF is not working well and this decision will be made on an individual recommendation.

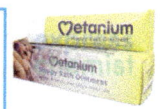
Available from pharmacy

For Tissue Viability Referrals please call extension 5524 or bleep 2234

Pictures used with permission of Wounds UK

Figure 11.4 Guidelines for the prevention and care of nappy rash and incontinence associated dermatitis.

supervision of the treating medical team or specialist review and be prescribed on the patient's medicine prescription chart.

Antifungal creams, used most commonly for *Candida* rashes (thrush), should be considered in cases that are not responsive to standard nappy rash treatment (Borkowski 2004). Care must be taken not to use creams or sprays that create a barrier to absorption of the antifungal cream.

During bouts of nappy rash there is a disruption of the normal skin barrier and irritant or allergic contact dermatitis may occur more readily. It is important to remember that any topical application contains preservatives and ingredients that may be potential sensitizers and in turn can result in skin irritation (Allison 2000; Scardillo and Aronovitch 1999). The possibility of peanut oil allergy arises again, as some common topical nappy creams may contain as much as 30% arachis oil as a base (Lack et al. 2003). Parents/carers should be aware of these issues and check ingredients in a pharmaceutical formulary and in 'product supplied' information when selecting a cream for patient use. Evaluation of any products used is essential and should be carried out following three to four days of continuous use, unless obvious reaction or deterioration occurs beforehand.

Nail care

The nails are horny plates of modified epithelium that serve to protect the tips of the fingers and toes (Watson 2005). The nail apparatus is composed of several parts including the nail matrix, the plate or the actual nail itself, and the surrounding proximal and lateral nail folds. The areas underneath the nail comprise the nail bed, the hyponychium, where the nail plate separates from the nail matrix and the subungual space underneath the whole nail (Figure 11.5).

Finger and toenails can be a potential source of infection and personal hygiene principles must apply to these areas in the CYP who is either healthy or sick. Transient flora is acquired from the environment, which is carried on the hands, feet and nails and then transferred to other parts of the body by cross transmission (Lawson 2001). The subungual space under the nail is particularly prone to harbouring micro-organisms and there may be a higher concentration at this site than elsewhere. It is therefore important to consider nail care when attending to the holistic personal hygiene needs of any CYP. In addition, there are specific times when nail cleanliness is paramount, for example when attending to other procedures such as wound care, during mealtimes, after outside play in mud or sand, and as part of preoperative preparation, when infection risk must be minimised as much as possible.

Although the main focus here is on the CYP, nail cleanliness in relation to the hands is also an essential component of general hygiene for staff (Arrowsmith and Taylor 2014; World Health Organisation [WHO] 2009); for more information see Chapter 13: Infection Prevention and Control. Micro-organisms carried on hands and nails can be transferred between patients by cross-transmission if adequate handwashing policies are not adhered to (Lawson 2001). Normal handwashing, the aim of which is to remove dirt, organic debris, and microorganisms as quickly as possible (Boyd 2003), may be ineffective to remove the pathogens from nails and subungual space.

Nail assessment

As part of the general assessment of hygiene status of a CYP, the nails should be observed carefully so that appropriate care can be given. Nail assessment needs to include the changing presentation of finger and toenails as a child grows. Baby nails are much softer and thinner and grow from a more fragile nail bed. This needs to be taken into account when caring for the delicate nails of the newborn and infant. In the older CYP, nails are thicker and more robust, and there may be cultural and age specific decorations such as varnish, false nails, and jewellery. Note that all nail varnish and decorations from fingers and toes, must be removed preoperatively.

Prevention of nail problems is based on thorough assessment and good nail hygiene. Both the finger and toenails must be included in the assessment.

Nail hygiene
Nail hygiene is an important hygiene consideration for CYPs of all ages and is best carried out during bathing or wash time.

Oral hygiene

The mouth is important for eating, drinking, speech, communication, taste, breathing, and defence against infection. Oral hygiene is an integral part of total care in which nurses play a pivotal role (Gibson and Nelson 2000). Systematic assessment forms the basis of all care undertaken and is essential to ensure any changes are monitored and appropriate treatment implemented. Planned interventions help to minimise or reverse changes in the oral cavity. The frequency of oral care and the 'tools' used to perform safe and effective care, are often debated in the literature. Nonetheless there is evidence that states that oral care and dental hygiene should begin as the primary teeth erupt. National guidelines verify the importance of good oral hygiene from as early an age as possible (DH/ British Association for the Study of Community Dentistry 2014; Devalia et al 2019), which is further supported by emerging guidance and advice through online resources such as NHS (2013). Babies with no teeth require consideration, as erupting primary teeth can decay like permanent teeth if not looked after properly.

The principle objective of oral hygiene is to maintain the mouth in a good condition (Gibson and Nelson 2000). It specifically aims to:

- Achieve and maintain a clean, healthy oral cavity
- Prevent the buildup of plaque on oral surfaces, thus helping prevent dental caries
- Keep oral mucosa moist
- Maintain mucosal integrity and promote healing
- Prevent infection
- Prevent broken or chapped lips
- Promote patient comfort and well-being
- Maintain normal oral function

For the nurse to provide a good standard of oral hygiene, knowledge and understanding of the normal anatomy and physiology of the mouth, teeth, gums, tongue, and lips is required (Figure 11.6).

The anatomy and physiology of the mouth is complex. There are two major functions of the mouth; digestion and defence. The oral cavity is the first part of the gastrointestinal tract. The structures visible on examination are the mucosal lining, the lips, the tongue, and the teeth.

The **mucosal lining** is continuous with the gastrointestinal tract and protects the underlying tissues. The mucous membranes, via the salivary glands, secrete mucus and saliva. Saliva is formed mainly of water (99% of total) and normally has a pH of 6.8–7.0. It does, however, become more alkaline as the secretory rate increases during chewing. Saliva contains lysozyme, which has an antiseptic action; immunoglobulin (IgA), which has a defensive function; and salivary amylase, which is a digestive enzyme. These properties result in keeping the oral mucosa moist, smooth, clean, and shiny, with the buffering capacity to minimise change in overall Ph, maintaining the balance of the microbial flora.

The **lips** form a muscular entrance to the mouth; they are covered by squamous, keratinized epithelial tissue, which is vascular and very sensitive. They are necessary for ingestion of food,

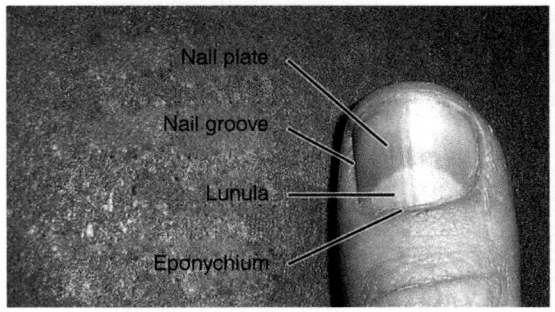

Figure 11.5 A sagittal view of the nail demonstrating the structure of the nail unit and the underlying tissues and bone.

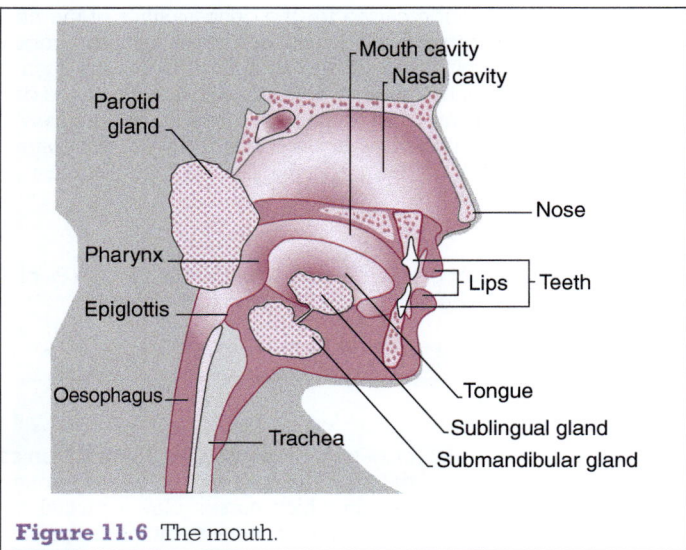

Figure 11.6 The mouth.

enunciation of words, and to convey the mood of a person, e.g. smiling and grimacing.

The **tongue** is covered with mucous membrane from which project numerous papillae and taste buds on the upper surface. The tongue plays an important part in mastication (chewing), deglutition (swallowing), speech, and taste (Waugh and Grant 2001). The muscles of the tongue afford it great mobility, which is essential for speech and swallowing; its other main function is interpreting taste sensations.

The **teeth** consist of enamel, dentine, cementum, and pulp. The first tooth normally erupts around six months of age with the full complement of 20 deciduous primary teeth being acquired by the age of two and a half years.

Permanent dentition begins between five and six years and the full number of 28 teeth have normally appeared by 13–15 years. The four wisdom teeth erupt later, usually by the age of 25, making the full complement of 32 teeth (Waugh and Grant 2001).

In addition to this knowledge, nurses must also understand the importance of adequate hydration and nutrition, microbiology, and oral infections and the effects of various drugs treatments and diseases on the oral mucosa (Thurgood 1994). For example, antibiotics alter the flora in the mouth and increase the risk of opportunistic infections, antihistamines reduce salivary production, a fever may result in halitosis, and thumb-sucking may alter the position of the teeth.

CYPs with a number of conditions may have compromised oral well-being, for example, those with cerebral palsy or other disability and those with epidermolysis bullosa. Special consideration is required to identify the optimum method for oral hygiene (DH 2007) (see later section on compromised oral health).

The CYP with an immunodeficiency may experience persistent Candida infections and is at increased risk of bacteraemia/septicaemia. They may also have reduced production of protective immunoglobulins in their saliva, which increases the risk of infection.

Assessing and identifying the 'usual' oral care is crucial in CYPs with special needs or other long-term conditions that may compromise oral health to determine the assistance they might require to maintain normal oral hygiene, which must be made explicit in a plan of care. As far as possible, the CYP should be assisted to maintain their normal pattern of care. Consideration will need to be given to identify the optimum method for oral hygiene to be performed.

Oral assessment

Oral assessment is considered to be central to planning effective care and begins with a history of previous dental care. This includes recording the CYP's usual brushing and cleaning regimen, as well as any previous oral problems. A thorough oral assessment is required to enable appropriate mouth care to be planned and implemented. The oral assessment represents the vital first step in planning effective oral care (Gibson et al. 2006) and should be explained to the CYP and their family, including why the assessment is necessary and what it entails. Based on this assessment, an individualised care plan can be developed that identifies either prophylactic or treatment specific measures. The use of an oral assessment tool can facilitate the development of a care plan. Assessment has the potential to provide baseline data, predict, prevent or minimise oral complications, and evaluate nursing interventions (Coyne et al. 2010; Hockenberry and Wilson 2010).

Oral hygiene 'tools' for children and young people with primary/secondary teeth

A regular teeth-cleaning regime is essential for good dental health (NHS 2013). The overall aim is to prevent tooth decay, which is preventable when there is good oral hygiene with fluoride toothpaste, a reduced sugar intake and regular dental checkups (Great Ormond Street Hospital (GOSH) 2017, Public Health England 2017). Regular brushing is imperative in plaque removal. There is general agreement that a small-headed, soft toothbrush, with nylon bristles and round-ended filaments, should be used to brush or clean teeth and massage the gingiva (British Dental Health Foundation (BDHF) 2014; DH 2014). Teeth should be cleaned effectively twice a day, as soon as possible after a meal if eating, and before bedtime, with a soft toothbrush and toothpaste. The more frequently and the longer teeth are cleaned the greater the probability of effective plaque removal. Even when the CYP is not eating, regular and thorough mouth care is vital. However, as the bristles are hard, they are not advisable for those with a fragile mucosa. Foam sponges are useful as a temporary measure, especially when the gingiva is bleeding and swollen, but must be used with care, following advice released by the Medicines and Healthcare Regulatory Agency (MHRA 2012). However, there may be times when an optimal oral hygiene regimen is sacrificed for patient comfort.

Rinsing the oral cavity after brushing is also important. This activity removes loose debris and further irrigates the tissues (Madeya 1996). It also reduces the likelihood of ingestion of toothpaste, which can lead to fluorosis. Tap water, or for some, sterile water, is the most common mouth rinse. Chlorhexidine is not recommended for the prevention or treatment of radiotherapy- or chemotherapy-induced mucositis, or the prevention of candidiasis in CYPs with cancer unless they are unable to brush their teeth, when foam sponges moistened with water or diluted chlorhexidine may be used (UKCCSG-PONF Mouth Care Group 2006). The mouth should be rinsed with the mouthwash, which should remain in contact with the mucosal membrane for at least 30–90 seconds to be effective (British Medical Association (BMA)/Royal Pharmaceutical Society of Great Britain (RPSGB) 2010). The mouth should not be rinsed with water after using mouthwash. The rationale for using an antibacterial mouth rinse in this small group of CYPs is that many of the micro-organisms responsible for causing systemic infections can be isolated from the oral cavity. In addition to toothbrushing and rinsing with water/chlorhexidine, CYPs who are profoundly neutropenic and at risk of developing fungal infections should use a prophylactic antifungal agent.

The general guidelines of oral hygiene outlined in this section and throughout this chapter are examples of best practice that should be taught to all CYPs and their families. Underpinning this practice is the need to explore and document the CYP's 'usual' oral hygiene routine (DH 2014).

Preparation and performing oral care

One of the most effective means of preventing dental caries is a regimen of proper oral health tailored to the individual CYP by the dentist (Hockenberry and Wilson 2010). CYPs should be taught to carry out their own oral care under the supervision and guidance of parents/carers. In some situations, parents/carers may need to be taught proper brushing techniques along with their children. Young children will need to have their teeth brushed for them up to an age when the parent or carer feels they have the dexterity to do it properly for themselves. The easiest and most effective way is for the adult to sit down and have the child stand in front with the child's head against the adult's chest and brush the teeth (Lloyd 1994). Neonates and very young children may lie in the adult's lap. In the case of an ill CYP who is confined to their bed or sofa, it is more appropriate to find a position that is most comfortable for them.

In the very young child, in CYPs who have not been used to regular dental care, and in CYPs with learning disabilities, play therapy can be a useful medium through which to introduce a regular regimen. Allowing the child to handle the mouth-care products in a nonthreatening environment that includes performing mouth care on a favourite toy, their parent/carer or a nurse, are useful techniques to reduce anxiety. Play specialists can help provide a supportive role in this aspect of care. Aids such as specially designed brushes or electric toothbrushes may be required in order for the CYP with special needs to be enabled to undertake effective cleaning of their teeth. For more information see Chapter 27: Play as a Therapeutic Tool.

Older CYPs may need to be reminded that mouth care should remain part of their daily hygiene routine. This group have increased concern regarding body image and sexuality and may be anxious or embarrassed by changes in their oral cavity such as: gingival enlargement; increased salivation; inability to swallow or speak effectively; halitosis. They may be angry about these changes and direct their anger toward staff or even reject treatment measures. The following good practices should always be considered for this group:

- Where possible allow them control; for example, let them choose the timing of mouth care.
- Respect their need for privacy when undertaking any aspect of oral care.
- Involve them in planning their oral care so that they will understand its importance and thus be more receptive to health teaching; ideally, they should be accepted as a vital member of the healthcare team.

Ensure explanations are age appropriate and reinforced with written information.

Health promotion and oral care

Healthcare workers have an important role in informing, advising, helping with the acquisition of skills, assisting with the process of clarifying beliefs, enabling the adaptation of lifestyle, and promoting change in the structures and organisations that influence health status (Coutts and Hardy 1995). Dental decay is one of the most common childhood diseases. From newborn, to toddler, to the young and older child, every childcare health professional has an important role in encouraging and shaping good oral healthcare practices (Daly et al. 2002; DH 2004a, b; NICE 2004), by keeping up to date with all the latest guidance (Cochrane Oral Health Group 2022). The main cause of dental decay is sugar in the diet. While any simple sugars, in theory, can be metabolised by plaque bacteria to generate acid, those most implicated are the nonmilk extrinsic sugars, such as those added during processing or preparation, or prior to consumption of food and beverages. Honey is also in this category. Nonmilk extrinsic sugars do not include lactose in milk, dairy products or fructose found naturally within fruit and vegetables (intrinsic sugars). Starch products such as bread are only slowly degraded in the mouth to sugars, and together with fruit, vegetables and dairy products are not strongly linked to caries (Scottish Dental Clinical Effectiveness Programme (SDCEP) 2018). It is both the presence of nonextrinsic sugars in the diet and the frequency of their consumption that are the basic cause of dental caries (Moynihan 2002; Watt and McGlone 2003). The factors associated with caries incidence include:

- Amount of fermentable carbohydrate consumed
- Sugar concentration of food
- Physical form of carbohydrate
- Length of time teeth are exposed to decreased plaque pH
- Frequency of eating meals and snacks
- Length of interval between eating
- Sequence of food consumption

(SIGN 2014; Levine and Stillman-Lowe 2009)

To produce tooth decay three factors are required; a susceptible tooth, bacteria and sugar. Establishing good oral care and dental practices early in life encourages children to believe in the importance of healthy teeth. Healthcare workers and schoolteachers have an important role to play in the ongoing education of children and the whole family (see http://www.teethtlc.co.uk/).

Compromised health and oral care

CYPs with an underlying condition or illness may be more susceptible to poor oral health and subsequent caries development (see Table 11.3, taken from Gibson and Nelson 2000).

For these patients, assessment of the mouth using a recognised tool, e.g. the Oral Assessment Guide (Table 11.2) is important. The focus of an individualised mouth care regimen will be minimising

Table 11.2 Oral assessment guide for children

Category	Method of assessment	1	2	3
Swallow	Ask the child to swallow or observe the swallowing process. Ask the parent/carer if there are any notable changes.	Normal Without difficulty	Difficulty in swallowing	Unable to swallow at all. Pooling, dribbling of secretions.
Lips and corner of mouth	Observe appearance of tissue.	Normal Smooth, pink, and moist	Dry, cracked, or swollen	Ulcerated or bleeding
Tongue	Observe the appearance of the tongue using a pen-torch to illuminate the oral cavity.	Normal Firm without fissures (cracking or splitting) or prominent papilla Pink and moist	Coated or loss of papillae with a shiny appearance with or without redness and/or oral *Candida*	Ulcerated, sloughing, or cracked
Saliva	Observe consistency and quality of saliva.	Normal Thin and watery	Excess amount of saliva, drooling	Thick, ropy, or absent

(continued)

Table 11.2 Oral assessment guide for children *(continued)*

Category	Method of assessment	1	2	3
Mucous membrane	Observe the appearance of tissue using a pen-torch to illuminate the oral cavity.	Normal Pink and moist	Reddened or coated without ulceration and/or oral *Candida*	Ulceration and sloughing, with or without bleeding
Gingivae	Observe the appearance of tissue using a pen-torch to illuminate the oral cavity.	Normal Pink or coral with a stippled (dotted) surface. Gum margins tight and well defined, no swelling.	Oedematous with or without redness, smooth	Spontaneous bleeding
Teeth (If no teeth score 1)	Observe the appearance of teeth using a pen-torch to illuminate the oral cavity.	Normal Clean and no debris	Plaque or debris in localised areas	Plaque or debris generalised along gum line
Voice	Talk and listen to the child. Ask the parent/carer if there are any notable changes.	Normal tone and quality when talking or crying	Deeper or raspy	Difficult to talk, cry, or not talking at all

Source: Adapted from Eilers et al. (1988). © Great Ormond Street Hospital. NB: If score > 8, introduce pain assessment instrument.

Table 11.3 General conditions that may compromise oral well-being

General conditions that may compromise oral well-being	Specific examples	Oral complications that may be experienced
Impaired/altered physical dexterity	Cerebral palsy Accidents or other illness causing: • Neurological damage • Unconsciousness • Loss of limb maxillofacial injury	Difficulty or inability to perform oral hygiene resulting in: • Build-up of plaque • Dental caries • Halitosis Ataxia or spasticity may increase risk of damage to mucosa and soft tissue structures
Physical complications	Restricted oral access due to: • Orthodontic or maxillofacial surgery • Enlarged, protruding tongue • Respiratory problems • Epidermolysis bullosa • Restricted movement of tongue due to surgery or pain • Chronic constipation • Cleft palate (may have prosthesis) Intubated and nursed in the intensive care environment particularly for neonates or infants that are orally intubated	May cause difficulty in performing oral hygiene (as above) Mouth breathing, causing dry mucosa Increased risk of mucosal deterioration Ineffective removal of debris Foul mouth and odour Lips, gums, palate prone to pressure sores; retention of food debris under prosthesis
Fragile mucosa	Effects of chemo/radiotherapy Epidermolysis bullosa Preterm neonate	Mucositis, ulceration, causing: • Pain • Infection • Bleeding
Children and young people with special needs	Down syndrome and other disabling conditions	Tendency towards thick, ropy, sticky saliva which adheres to the surface of teeth and forms plaque Deformed teeth may retain plaque
	Habitual licking or biting of lips	Dry, cracked, or inflamed lips Discomfort
	Teeth alignment abnormalities	Require effective cleaning to avoid build-up of debris
Children and young people with reduced level of consciousness	Child or young person who is dying Following epileptic seizure Head injury Post-surgical procedure Physical injury Infection Toxic injury Sedation during intensive care and intubation for mechanical ventilation	Oral care should be performed twice daily by healthcare worker/parent/carer, since the mouth can become dry or coated with mucus

Table 11.3 General conditions that may compromise oral well-being (continued)

General conditions that may compromise oral well-being	Specific examples	Oral complications that may be experienced
Immunodeficiencies	HIV Postcytotoxic therapy	Reduced production of protective immunoglobulins in saliva resulting in increased risk of infection
	Combined immune deficiency	Persistent *Candida* infections
Common childhood illnesses and dental habits	Measles Fever Grinding of teeth Thumb-sucking	Koplik, white spots Dryness, coated tongue, halitosis Mild/severe loss of tooth surface Alteration to position of teeth (upper, anterior)
Poor nutritional intake	Anorexia Dehydration Chronic disorders requiring high intake of refined oral carbohydrates, e.g. glycogen storage disease	Vitamin deficiency, tissue vulnerability Dryness, halitosis Increase in dental caries Oral ulceration
Foreign body in nose	Commonly inserted are peas, peanuts, and small toys	Sudden foul odour in the mouth
Drugs	Antibiotics	Altered oral flora, increased risk of opportunistic infections
	Antihistamine Atropine Chlorhexidine-based mouthwash	Reduced salivary production Reduced salivary production Temporary brown staining of teeth Stinging/burning sensation Bitter taste, altered after taste
	Corticosteroids Cyclosporine Cytotoxic agents Diuretics Insulin Iron supplements Long-term, high sugar content medication, e.g. Lactulose Morphine Nifedipine Oxygen therapy Phenytoin	Delayed healing of tissue Gum hyperplasia Altered taste perception (often metallic) Saliva absent or ropy Altered salivary function Altered salivary function Temporary green/black staining of teeth Increased incidence of dental caries Dry mucosa Gingival enlargement Dry mucosa Gingival hypertrophy

Source: From Gibson and Nelson (2000).

trauma, reducing risk of infection, ensuring oral comfort and maximising oral health. This includes those with:

- Cardiac disease
- Immunosuppression, as a result of cancer therapies and HIV
- Haemophilia and other bleeding disorders
- Reduced level of consciousness
- Developmental delay/learning disability
- Impaired dexterity
- Health disorders requiring medium to long-term use of medication
- Conditions necessitating intensive care/artificial ventilation by oral intubation

Eye care

The eyes should generally be clean and free of any discharge or debris. Cleaning of the eyes should not be routine, but restricted to certain conditions such as suspected or actual infection, encrustation, excessive stickiness, or any other known specific disease. In addition, eye care may be necessary to prevent dryness and damage when the CYP is unable to naturally lubricate the eyes themselves, such as following surgery or when receiving muscle relaxants. However, it must be acknowledged that parents/carers may incorporate eye care into their hygiene routine at home. If appropriate, gentle cleansing can be performed unless there is any reason for the eyes not to be touched, such as existing damage or avoidance of unnecessary handling in an unstable patient. This should be discussed with the parents/carers and reasons explained. If eye care is performed, a clean technique should always be adhered to, with appropriate hand washing and the use of clean products. In healthy and older CYP, where cleaning the eyes is part of the overall washing routine, this should be continued and the use of tap water suffices.

Administration of eye drops

Topical drug delivery for the treatment of eye disease remains the preferred route, as many regions of the eye are relatively inaccessible to systemically administered drugs. Drugs are delivered to treat infections, to provide intraocular treatment for diseases such as glaucoma, and pre- and postsurgical procedures (see Chapter 17: Administration of Medicines).

Topical drug delivery is itself complicated by effective removal mechanisms that include the blinking reflex, tear turnover, and low corneal permeability. Further complications include patient anxiety and the difficulty found in administering them.

Drugs administered as eye drops penetrate directly into the cornea. The cornea is considered to be the main pathway for the permeation of drugs into the eye. It is an optically transparent tissue that conveys images to the back of the eye and covers about one-sixth of the total surface area of the eyeball (Agarwal et al. 2002; Bartlett and Jaanes 2008; Wilson et al. 2005). The concentration of drug in the precorneal area provides the driving force for its transport across the cornea via passive diffusion. Thus, efficient ocular drug absorption requires good corneal penetration as well as prolonged contact with the corneal tissue.

As previously mentioned, eye drops are used to treat conditions such as glaucoma and conjunctivitis, and are used pre and post-surgical procedures for conditions such as cataracts, glaucoma and squints.

Glaucoma refers to increased pressure on the inside of the eyeball. The increased pressure is usually caused by an obstruction to or the absence of the aqueous drainage system. Conservative treatment usually consists of anti-inflammatory eye drops such as Betoptic, which works by decreasing the production of aqueous humour. Surgical management aims to create a drainage system through performing a goniotomy or a trabeculectomy, following which steroid and antibiotic eye drops would be administered (Agarwal et al. 2002; Bartlett and Jaanes 2008; Wilson et al. 2005).

Squint repair involves surgery that moves the muscles back to their correct alignment through resecting the muscles of the eyeball. Maxitrol drops are given post operatively to reduce the swelling and assist prevention of infection in the newly repaired squint.

Types of drops used for eye treatment include:

- Mydriatic-cycloplegic
- Coricosteroids
- Antibiotics

A mydriatic drug dilates the pupil and is used for pre surgical procedures that require visualisation of structures behind the iris such as cataract extraction and vitrectomy. Drugs used include atropine or cyclopentolate.

Combinations of corticosteroids and antibiotics are used to suppress inflammation following ophthalmic surgery. Examples include betamethasone (Betnesol) and dexamethasone (Maxitrol) (Agarwal et al. 2002; Bartlett and Jaanes 2008; BMA/RPSGB 2010; Wilson et al. 2005).

Contact lenses

Contact lenses are small, thin optical lenses worn on the front surface of the eye to correct refractive eye problems, such as myopia, hyperopia, and astigmatism. There are two types of contact lenses; soft lenses and rigid gas permeable (RGP) lenses. Soft lenses are larger than the diameter of the cornea, whereas RGPs have a diameter smaller than that of the cornea. Contact lenses must not be worn while asleep, as this can cause irreversible changes to the cornea.

CYPs may have to wear contact lenses as a consequence of surgical removal of congenital cataracts, high refractive error, or congenital anterior segment abnormalities. They may have very high prescription soft lenses or they may have a cosmetic lens with a painted iris to camouflage an abnormal iris. As well as fitting lenses to help improve the eyesight, contact lenses are occasionally used to act as a bandage on the eye for example after surgery or injury. These lenses may be thinner and larger than standard contact lenses. They are inserted and removed in the same way as other soft lenses but this may be more difficult as the eye can be particularly uncomfortable.

Inserting and removing the lenses is usually undertaken by the patient or parent/carer, but at times the lens may need to be dealt with by the nursing staff; for example, if a CYP is going to theatre. In a young child who is upset by the procedure, it is easier to insert and remove the lenses when they are asleep.

Some CYPs may wear daily disposable lenses that are discarded after every use and require no solutions, just instructions to always wash the hands before touching either the eyes or the lenses and never to reuse the lens on a second day. If the lenses are not daily disposable, there are likely to be between one and three special solutions that are used to clean and disinfect contact lenses. Tap water should never be used on the lenses as it may contain organisms that can cause eye infections.

Maintaining contact lens hygiene is paramount. Any questions about wearing contact lenses should be posed to the eye care specialist. The parents/carers and CYP should have been made aware of the importance of keeping the contact lenses clean, since eye infections associated with contact lenses can result in the vision being affected, and in rare instances, can lead to blindness (College of Optometrists 2014).

In an emergency, soft lenses can be removed using a pair of round-ended forceps and rigid lenses can be removed using a rubber sucker (if available). This should be performed by a skilled practitioner.

CYPs of all ages may wear contact lenses instead of spectacles although children less than eight years old are likely to have had their lenses fitted in a hospital eye department. Interest in contact lenses starts at an early age and their use is widely suited to all age groups. The average age at which children are first fitted with contact lenses is currently 13 years although studies have shown that even young children can be very successful in wearing, handling and looking after contact lenses Contact lenses also have a very high satisfaction rate among young wearers, rated as high as 97% among eight to 12-year-olds and 99% among 13–17 year olds. Both groups benefit from significant improvements in their quality of life (College of Optometrists 2014).

Ear care

Eardrops may need to be administered to a CYP with an obstruction in the ear such as wax or dried blood (postsurgery), or to treat an infection. The drops may be simple softening drops or may contain antibiotics, with or without anti-inflammatory properties. Foreign objects, such as cotton buds, should never be put into the ear.

Eardrops can be used if there is an infection of the outer ear canal (otitis externa) or the middle ear (otitis media) if the eardrum is perforated.

Otitis externa

This is an inflammation of the ear canal between the eardrum and the outside of the ear. Because of its warm dark environment, the ear canal is a perfect medium for bacteria and fungus to grow. CYPs with otitis externa will complain of an 'itchy ear,' which feels full or plugged up. Following this the ear will become red, swollen, and extremely painful. This can be treated by cleaning out the ear and administering eardrops.

Otitis media

Normally the middle ear is filled with air and relies on three tiny bones to transmit sound signals to the inner ear. In the case of infection, pus, fluid, and inflammation are produced in the middle ear, the area behind the eardrum. With otitis media, older CYPs will complain of ear pain, ear fullness, dizziness, or hearing loss. Younger children may demonstrate irritability, fussiness, tugging of the ear, or have difficulty in sleeping, feeding, or hearing. CYPs of any age may have a high temperature.

Antibiotics are an effective treatment for otitis media if it is caused by bacterial infection and Augmentin would be the drug of choice. In association with these oral medications, eardrops can be employed after medical assessment. If there is a perforation of the eardrum, Ciprofloxacin hydrochloride is used, primarily because of its anti-inflammatory properties. If the eardrum is unperforated, Sofradex can be useful. In situations where the otitis media is not caused by a bacterial infection, symptomatic treatment is undertaken, namely analgesia and eardrops.

Pressure ulcer prevention and management

Pressure ulcers are areas of localised damage to the skin, which can extend to underlying structures such as muscle and bone (Allman 1997; Allman et al. 1995). Damage is believed to be caused by a combination of factors including pressure, shear, friction, and moisture (Allman et al. 1995). Pressure ulcers are not commonly associated with very young babies and children. However, they do occur within paediatric practice. CYPs continue to be vulnerable to this type of skin injury and the resultant pain and discomfort (Kipps and Maxwell 2013; Wounds 2013). Pressure ulcers are, in most cases, avoidable, provided adequate early assessment takes place and preventative measures are implemented. The factors associated with increased risk of pressure injury are illustrated in Figure 11.7.

It is extremely important to work with parents, carers and CYPs using a family-centred care approach to help reduce anxiety and involve them in repositioning and reporting skin care issues where possible. An age-appropriate approach to care is also essential; for example, encouraging young people to self-report skin integrity and discussion about early mobilisation and the implications of staying in bed.

Groeneveld et al. (2004) cite the most common sites for pressure ulcer development in CYPs as the occiput, sacrum, buttocks, heels, ears, malleolus and lumbar spine. This is supported by Butler (2006). However in children younger than 36 months, the occipital region is at greatest risk of pressure damage as the head carries a larger proportion of the total body weight and surface area (Butler 2006; Parnham 2012).

SSKIN care bundle approach

One approach that has been used successfully for pressure ulcer prevention is the SSKIN care bundle, which includes five essential elements and highlights the importance of monitoring patients for signs of skin damage and using suitable equipment to prevent pressure ulcers (Gibbons et al. 2006; Wounds 2013) (see Figure 11.8).

The five elements of the SSKIN Bundle are:

- **Skin inspection**: Performing regular assessment of the entire skin of the CYP, with emphasis over bony prominences to identify fragile or vulnerable skin or patient's at-risk status.
- **Support surface**: Ensuring appropriate pressure relieving/ redistribution equipment or devices are selected. For example, this may include the use of a high specification support surface and/or dermal pads.
- **Keep moving:** Implementing a repositioning schedule that optimises independent movement.
- **Incontinence and moisture:** Ensuring appropriate management of incontinence, perspiration or exudates in conjunction with a skin care routine to keep the skin clean and dry.
- **Nutrition and hydration:** Encouraging individuals to eat and drink regularly and assisting patients when necessary to maintain good nutritional status.

Risk assessment

Regularly assessing risk is part of the process of supporting CYPs and maintaining safety in the hospital setting. The risk assessment process acts as an aid and an adjunct to clinical care, but does not replace clinical judgment and should not be used in isolation of other clinical features. NICE (2014, 2015) recommend carrying out and documenting an assessment within six hours of admission of pressure ulcer risk for neonates, infants, and CYPs:-

- Being admitted to secondary care or tertiary care, or
- Receiving NHS care in other settings (such as primary and community care and emergency departments) if they have a risk factor, for example:
    - Significantly limited mobility (for example, people with a spinal cord injury)
    - Significant loss of sensation
    - A previous or current pressure ulcer
    - Nutritional deficiency
    - The inability to reposition themselves
    - Significant cognitive impairment

Extrinsic Risk Factors
- Pressure e.g. lying in bed
- Medical device related pressure injury, e.g. splints, endotracheal tubes, chest braces, probes, or catheters
- Shear
- Friction
- Reduced or restricted mobility and activity, e.g. children and young people undergoing surgery or in critical care
- Tolerance of the skin
- Moisture e.g. oedema, sweat, wound exudates
- Incontinence, urinary or faecal (inappropriate to age and/or developmental stage) and other sources of moisture
- Changes in environment, carer, or equipment

Intrinsic Risk Factors
- Nutrition, e.g. malnutrition and dehydration
- Tissue perfusion and oxygenation
- Sensory impairment, cognition, and psychosocial status
- Reduced level of consciousness
- Reduced skin/tissue perfusion secondary to disease process or medication, e.g. inotropes
- Previous history of pressure ulceration
- Comorbidity, e.g. systemic signs of infection, blood supply, pain, medication
- Disease processes, i.e. depression and mental illness
- Infection
- Emotional disturbance affecting motivation and the ability to self-care (NICE, 2014)

Figure 11.7 Intrinsic and extrinsic pressure ulcer risk factors.

Glamorgan Paediatric Pressure Ulcer Risk Assessment

Risk Factor (If data such as serum albumin or haemoglobin is not available, write NK – not known and score 0)	Score	Instructions
MOBILITY Child cannot be moved without great difficulty or deterioration in condition / under general anaesthetic >2	20	Assign one score for the patients mobility (the other 3 will be scored 0).
Unable to change his/her position without assistance / cannot control body movement	15	
Some mobility, but reduced for age	10	
Normal mobility for age	0	
OTHER Significant anaemia (Hb <9g/dl)	1	Assign one score for the patients with each risk factor.
Persistent pyrexia (temperature > 38.0°C for more than 4 hours)	1	
Poor peripheral perfusion (cold extremities/ capillary refill > 2 seconds / cool mottled skin)	1	
Inadequate nutrition/ identified at risk of malnutrition	2	
Low serum albumin (< 35 g/l)t	1	
Incontinence (inappropriate for age)	1	
Equipment /objects/hard surface pressing or rubbing on skin (enough to cause pressure damage e.g NG tube secured without duoderm, close fitting devices (BIPAP masks, neck collars) or TED stockings	15	Ensure all equipment is checked regularly to prevent pressure ulcers

Paediatric Pressure Ulcer Prevention Strategies

Risk of developing pressure ulcers	Prevention Strategies (if concerned please call tissue viability team for support)
0 Low Risk	■ Daily risk assessment score ■ Daily Skin inspection either by nurse, report from parent or discussion with young person ■ Foam mattress (unless indicated otherwise) ■ Encourage child to move or carer to reposition regularly ■ Assess risk of malnutrition weekly
10+ At Risk	■ Daily risk assessment score ■ Twice daily skin inspection ■ Foam mattress (unless indicated otherwise) ■ Encourage child to move or carer to reposition regularly ■ Regular repositioning if unable to move independently ■ Assess risk of malnutrition weekly
15+ High Risk	■ Daily risk assessment score ■ Two hourly skin inspection ■ Repose mattress or Alternating air mattress should be used if patients skin is marking or has erythema despite regular repositioning (unless indicated otherwise) ■ Encourage child to move or carer to reposition regularly ■ Regular 2 hourly repositioning if unable to move independently ■ If unable to reposition highlight to nurse in charge and refer to TVN if necessary ■ Assess risk of malnutrition weekly
20+ Very High Risk	■ Daily risk assessment score ■ Hourly skin inspection if possible (document if unable to move or check skin integrity) ■ Alternating air mattress (unless unsafe to do so based on local guidelines or clinical condition) Use ADERMA dermal pads to reduce pressure (not on open wounds/broken skin) ■ Minimum 2 hourly repositioning ensure all pressure areas are protected ■ Assess risk of malnutrition weekly ■ If unable to reposition highlight to nurse in charge and refer to TVN if necessary
15+ Equipment Related	**Equipment related pressure damage** Equipment which might cause pressure injury or secured in a way which might cause excessive pressure, shear or friction must be moved frequently if safe to do so. Protective dressings should be used if indicated. If it can not be moved please document.

Pressure Ulcer Record (indicate on body map)

Ulcer number	Date Ulcer first Observed	Grade, Location and details of ulcers (use notes page on reverse to document further if required)	Referral to Tissue Viability Team	Incident form	Prevention plan reviewed and changed if necessary	Sign, print and date

Pressure Ulcer Prevention, Repositioning, and Nutrition Screening Documentation Record

Date	Before Admission	Day of Admission					KEY
Time							
Glamorgan Score (Reassess Daily)							**Y**=Yes **N**=No
Glamorgan Equipment Risk level							

Admission
- Any pre existing pressure ulcers?
- Do they require referral to TVN?
- Parent/patient given information

Overall skin integrity on admission (description):-

Skin Inspection: Head, Ears, Shoulders/elbows, Hips, Sacrum, Buttock, Heels, Nose, Other (Specify), Pressure areas above all checked & intact?, Referral to TVN indicated and complete?

Key:
- ✓ = skin intact
- **A** = patient/carer reports skin intact
- **B** = Redness/skin marking
- **C** = covered by dressing/cast
- **U** = unable to visualize (document reasons)
- **PU** = Pressure Ulcer (1–4) & Documented on the Pressure Ulcer record

Surface: Foam, Repose or Alternating Air Mattress; Use of barrier dressing i.e. ADERMA; Slide sheets to prevent friction

- **F** = Foam (purple memaflex)
- **R** = Repose
- **Air** = Alternating Air

Keep Moving: Frequency of Repositioning 1hrly 2hrly 3hrly 4hrly; Body Position; Head repositioned; Child not lying on tubing & catheters; Facemask and cannula checked for skin Integrity; Probes repositioned

- **P** = Prone
- **L** = Left
- **S** = Supine
- **R** = Right
- **Sit** = Sitting in bed/chair
- **U** = unable to move due to patients physiological deterioration
- **Ref** = patient refused
- **I** = Patient moving independently

Incontinence: Barrier cream applied; Nappy/ Pad change

- **N/A** = not applicable

Nutrition: See Nutrition Screening Flowchart Algorithm for children under and over 1 year. Is patient at risk of malnutrition?; Referral to dietitian; Fluid/Food Chart Commenced and Updated

- **O** = (other variation please specify in comments section)

Staff Member's initials

Figure 11.8 International NPUAP/EPUAP pressure ulcer classification system. *Source:* National Pressure Ulcer Advisory Panel, European Pressure Ulcer Advisory Panel, and Pan Pacific Pressure Injury Alliance (NPUAP/EPUAP/PPPUIA) (2014), pp. 12–13.

Daily documentation of risk assessments ensures communication within the multidisciplinary team, provides evidence that care planning is appropriate, and serves as a benchmark for monitoring progress (National Pressure Ulcer Advisory Panel, European Pressure Ulcer Advisory Panel and Pan Pacific Pressure Injury Alliance (NPUAP/ EPUAP/ PPPUIA) 2014).

There are different risk assessment tools available for use in the paediatric population, for example, Braden Q, Garvin and Glamorgan (Noonan et al. 2011; Willock et al. 2009). However, the NICE guideline development group (NICE 2015) agreed that it was not possible to recommend a pressure ulcer risk assessment tool and that further risk assessment tools in this population may be available in the future. Pressure ulcer risk assessment is an essential component of the admission procedure, not only to identify risk, but also to ensure that effective preventive strategies can be implemented. Early recognition of risk factors is the precursor to planning preventive care (Parnham 2012). While the development of reliable and valid assessment tools based on evidence is ongoing, hospitals should choose risk assessment tools based on validity and reliability demonstrated by existing evidence. The Glamorgan Risk assessment tool is used at GOSH, due to the reliability and interrater reliability demonstrated in preliminary data, the ease of use and the inclusion of a medical equipment risk section.

While the preliminary data indicates that the risk assessment scale is reliable, more research on the reliability and validity of this tool with specific paediatric patient groups is required, ideally comparing the performance of this tool with other published paediatric pressure ulcer risk assessment tools.

The GOSH Adapted Glamorgan Pressure Ulcer Risk Assessment tool is documented in the Combined Mandatory Risk Assessment on the SSKIN Care Record (see Figure 11.8). All risk assessments must be documented, signed, and dated by the assessor, stored with the nursing documentation, and kept at the bedside at all times.

The Glamorgan Risk Assessment Score must be completed and documented in the medical notes for all CYPs, including those attending daycare, at the following time points:

- On admission within six hours
- Daily reassessment for all CYPs
- When a CYP's condition, care, treatment, or situation changes, for example, on return from surgery
- Daycare stays of more than two hours
- When the CYP is transferred from one ward or department to another, for example, return from intensive care
- Prior to discharge

Skin assessment

Skin status is the most significant early indicator of the skin's response to pressure exposure and the on-going risk of pressure injury. A thorough systematic approach to skin assessment is essential. Particular attention should be paid to bony prominences, for example heels, elbows, hips, and shoulder blades, which are areas at increased risk of pressure injury due to pressure, friction, and shearing forces. Particular attention should be given to the head, including temporal region of the skull and the back of head, especially in infants less than 36 months of age. Any areas of skin in contact with any equipment or devices must be checked and devices re-sited regularly.

Identifying the early signs of pressure ulcer formation allows healthcare workers to intervene quickly, preventing significant loss of tissue and associated complications. Early signs of tissue damage include:

- Persistent erythema (redness of the skin)
- Nonblanching erythema (red skin that does not go white and return to red following the application of light finger pressure)
- Blisters
- Discolouration
- Localised heat, oedema or induration (hardness of skin)

Very careful assessment is required for CYPs with darkly pigmented skin. The following signs may indicate pressure damage in darkly pigmented skin:

- **Early stages:**
  - Purplish or bluish localised areas of skin localised heat
- **More advanced:**
  - Localised coolness
  - Localised oedema and induration

Pressure Ulcers in CYPs are graded using the International Pressure Ulcer Grading Classification System (National Pressure Ulcer Advisory Panel, European Pressure Ulcer Advisory Panel, and Pan Pacific Pressure Injury Alliance 2014) and are categorised one to four (Figure 11.9), although some hospitals use the additional categories of deep tissue injury and unstageable pressure ulcers.

On admission to hospital, including Accident and Emergency departments, the CYP's general skin condition, integrity, and any pre-existing damage should be assessed at the earliest possible opportunity (e.g. dryness, cracking, erythema, maceration, excoriation, fragility, temperature) and the findings should be documented in the medical notes. It is important to obtain a baseline skin assessment when a CYP arrives in a clinical area so that any skin damage present can be identified and treated promptly (Royal College of Nursing [RCN] 2005).

Early skin assessment will also avoid confusion regarding when and how the damage occurred if it is later the subject of a complaint or clinical incident. In certain instances this may not be possible due to the nature of the presenting illness, objection of CYP/carer, religious/cultural reasons, and issues related to the maintenance of privacy and dignity. If the skin is not assessed the reason for this must be documented in the CYP's notes. If appropriate a member of staff, ideally of the same gender, may assess the CYP's skin integrity. If the CYP is unstable upon arrival to the hospital a full skin assessment must be documented at the safest and earliest opportunity when they have been stabilised.

Parent and carer education

The parent/carer will often be the first to notice any skin changes given their level of interaction with the CYP and their familiarity with the skin through dressing, changing nappies, bathing, etc. Education regarding the early signs of pressure damage will assist the parent/carer in protecting their child long term from such complications. Families and carers need to be aware of the hospitals commitment to reducing the occurrence of pressure ulcers and the severity of those that do occur. All parents/carers should have ready access to information about pressure damage prevention such as, e.g. the GOSH information leaflet 'Looking after Your Child's Skin during Your Hospital Stay' (GOSH 2016).

Care planning

A score of 15 or above on the Glamorgan assessment tool constitutes a CYP being at high risk.

Care for a CYP scoring 15 or above, must include:

- Daily inspection of skin and bony prominences.
- The prophylactic use of a barrier film for those in nappies or pads. Barrier films protect the skin from moisture, shear, and friction, which can contribute to pressure ulcer development.
- A plan for repositioning at least every two hours, except when the CYP cannot physiologically tolerate position changes (NICE 2014). If the CYP cannot be turned, an appropriately trained healthcare worker should explain the reason for this to the family and document this in the CYP's medical record.
- Use of a repositioning record chart. Early assessment should identify the potential exposure to these forces and allow for intervention before damage occurs in vulnerable CYPs (Quigley and Curley 1996).
- Use of specialist mattresses, e.g. Repose® mattress: Pressure-reducing base mattresses have been demonstrated to significantly reduce the incidence of pressure ulceration (McInnes et al. 2015). The mattress should be impervious to body fluids, cleaned regularly, and checked annually for cover damage in order to avoid cross-contamination between patients (Cullum et al. 2000). The mattress should not impact on any CYP's ability to rest or sleep.
- Completed moving and handling assessment to reduce friction and shear.

Category/Stage I: Nonblanchable Erythema

Intact skin with non-blanchable redness of a localized area usually over a bony prominence. Darkly pigmented skin may not have visible blanching; its color may differ from the surrounding area.

The area may be painful, firm, soft, warmer or cooler as compared to adjacent tissue. Category/Stage I may be difficult to detect in individuals with dark skin tones. May indicate "at risk" individuals (a heralding sign of risk).

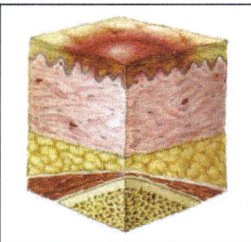 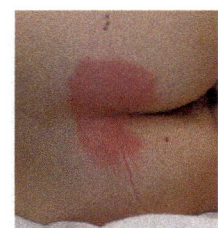

Category/Stage II: Partial Thickness Skin Loss

Partial thickness loss of dermis presenting as a shallow open ulcer with a red pink wound bed, without slough. May also present as an intact or open/ruptured serum-filled blister.

Presents as a shiny or dry shallow ulcer without slough or bruising. * This Category/Stage should not be used to describe skin tears, tape burns, perineal dermatitis, maceration or excoriation.

*Bruising indicates suspected deep tissue injury.

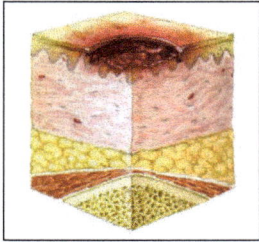 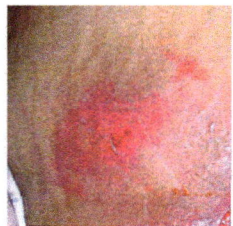

Category/Stage III: Full Thickness Skin Loss

Full thickness tissue loss. Subcutaneous fat may be visible but bone, tendon or muscle are not exposed. Slough may be present but does not obscure the depth of tissue loss. May include undermining and tunneling.

The depth of a Category/Stage III pressure ulcer varies by anatomical location. The bridge of the nose, ear, occiput and malleolus do not have subcutaneous tissue and Category/Stage III ulcers can be shallow. In contrast, areas of significant adiposity can develop extremely deep Category/Stage III pressure ulcers. Bone/tendon is not visible or directly palpable.

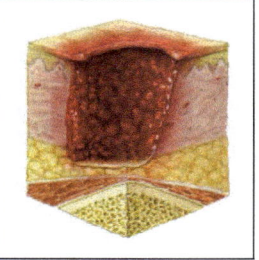 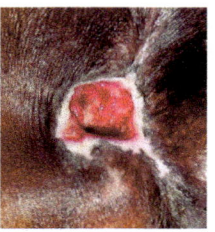

Category/Stage IV: Full Thickness Tissue Loss

Full thickness tissue loss with exposed bone, tendon or muscle. Slough or eschar may be present on some parts of the wound bed. Often include undermining and tunneling.

The depth of a Category/Stage IV pressure ulcer varies by anatomical location. The bridge of the nose, ear, occiput and malleolus do not have subcutaneous tissue and these ulcers can be shallow. Category/Stage IV ulcers can extend into muscle and/or supporting structures (e.g., fascia, tendon or joint capsule) making osteomyelitis possible. Exposed bone/tendon is visible or directly palpable.

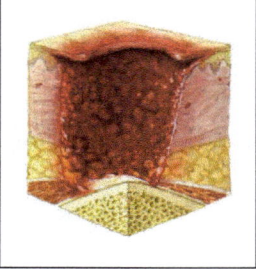 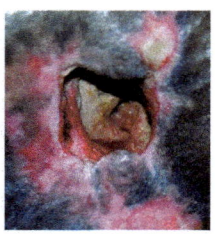

Unstageable: Depth Unknown

Full thickness tissue loss in which the base of the ulcer is covered by slough (yellow, tan, gray, green or brown) and/or eschar (tan, brown or black) in the wound bed.

Until enough slough and/or eschar is removed to expose the base of the wound, the true depth, and therefore Category/Stage, cannot be determined. Stable (dry, adherent, intact without erythema or fluctuance) eschar on the heels serves as 'the body's natural (biological) cover' and should not be removed.

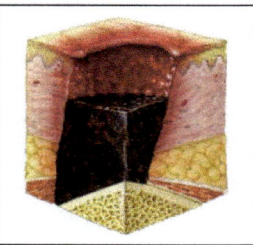 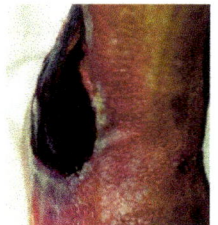

Suspected Deep Tissue Injury: Depth Unknown

Purple or maroon localized area of discolored intact skin or blood-filled blister due to damage of underlying soft tissue from pressure and/or shear. The area may be preceded by tissue that is painful, firm, mushy, boggy, warmer or cooler as compared to adjacent tissue.

Deep tissue injury may be difficult to detect in individuals with dark skin tones. Evolution may include a thin blister over a dark wound bed. The wound may further evolve and become covered by thin eschar. Evolution may be rapid exposing additional layers of tissue even with optimal treatment.

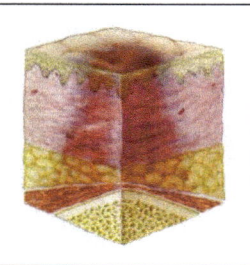 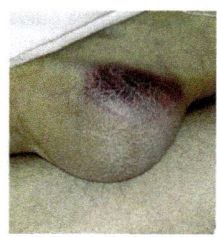

Figure 11.9 Risk assessment document: adapted glamorgan paediatric risk assessment, paediatric pressure ulcer risk assessment strategies, and pressure ulcer risk assessment and paediatric SKIN care bundle.

Chapter 11 Personal hygiene and pressure ulcer prevention

- Completed nutritional assessment to identify adequate dietary intake.
- Give family/carer a copy of the local information leaflet, e.g. Looking after your child's skin advice leaflet (GOSH 2016).
- CYPs at significant risk of pressure ulcer development should be identified at shift changes and when transferred to another ward area, unit or healthcare provider. This ensures prevention strategies are maintained.

Repositioning to prevent pressure ulcers

Keeping all CYPs moving regularly and safely, whether in bed or a chair, is the key to pressure ulcer prevention. Careful consideration should be paid to safe mobilisation and repositioning for all CYPs in order to minimise pressure on bony prominences and avoid positioning on any existing pressure ulcer (NICE 2014). For more information see *Chapter 19: Moving and Handling*. CYPs who are unable to be turned frequently are more susceptible to pressure ulcers. While care that is acceptable to the CYP, and the needs of the parent/carer must be considered (NICE 2014), nurses have a duty of care to prevent harm. Some will find repositioning painful or difficult and will need support and encouragement. It is important to find out the reasons why a CYP is reluctant to be moved in order to give the support needed, e.g. through engagement of play specialists and providing adequate analgesia (NICE 2014).

Any CYP who is assessed to be at risk of developing pressure ulcers should be repositioned if it is medically safe to do so (NPUAP/EPUAP/PPPUIA 2014). Frequency of repositioning may be restricted by medical condition, level of comfort and attached medical devices, e.g. IV cannulae and external fixators. In cases where CYPs cannot be adequately repositioned a suitable support surface should be used.

The suggested time interval between repositioning in many cases is two hours. However, this should be adjusted according to the response of the CYP's skin to pressure, i.e. if the skin reddens after two hours reduce the time interval and reassess (NPUAP/EPUAP/PPPUIA 2014). Capillary pressure varies between individuals (NICE 2014). Dermal capillary pressure may be compromised by impaired cardiac function, peripheral shutdown, ambient temperature and drug therapies, etc. An ill CYP may have significantly reduced dermal capillary pressure when compared to a healthy CYP. If there is no evidence of erythema then turning may not be necessary, but a CYP must be assessed every two hours. If it is medically unsafe to move a CYP as frequently as indicated by the risk assessment this must be documented and regularly reassessed and they must be mobilised at the safest and earliest opportunity.

Three of the possible positions and tilts used are shown in Figure 11.10a–c. The term '30° tilt' describes the use of pillows to position a patient off their bony prominences (hips and sacrum) so that weight is redistributed over the larger surface area of the buttocks. The tilt positions should not be used exclusively but to offer alternative positions to the traditional side-to-side turns. By having five alternative positions, the time period any part of the body is exposed to pressure is reduced (Figure 11.10d–e). It may be

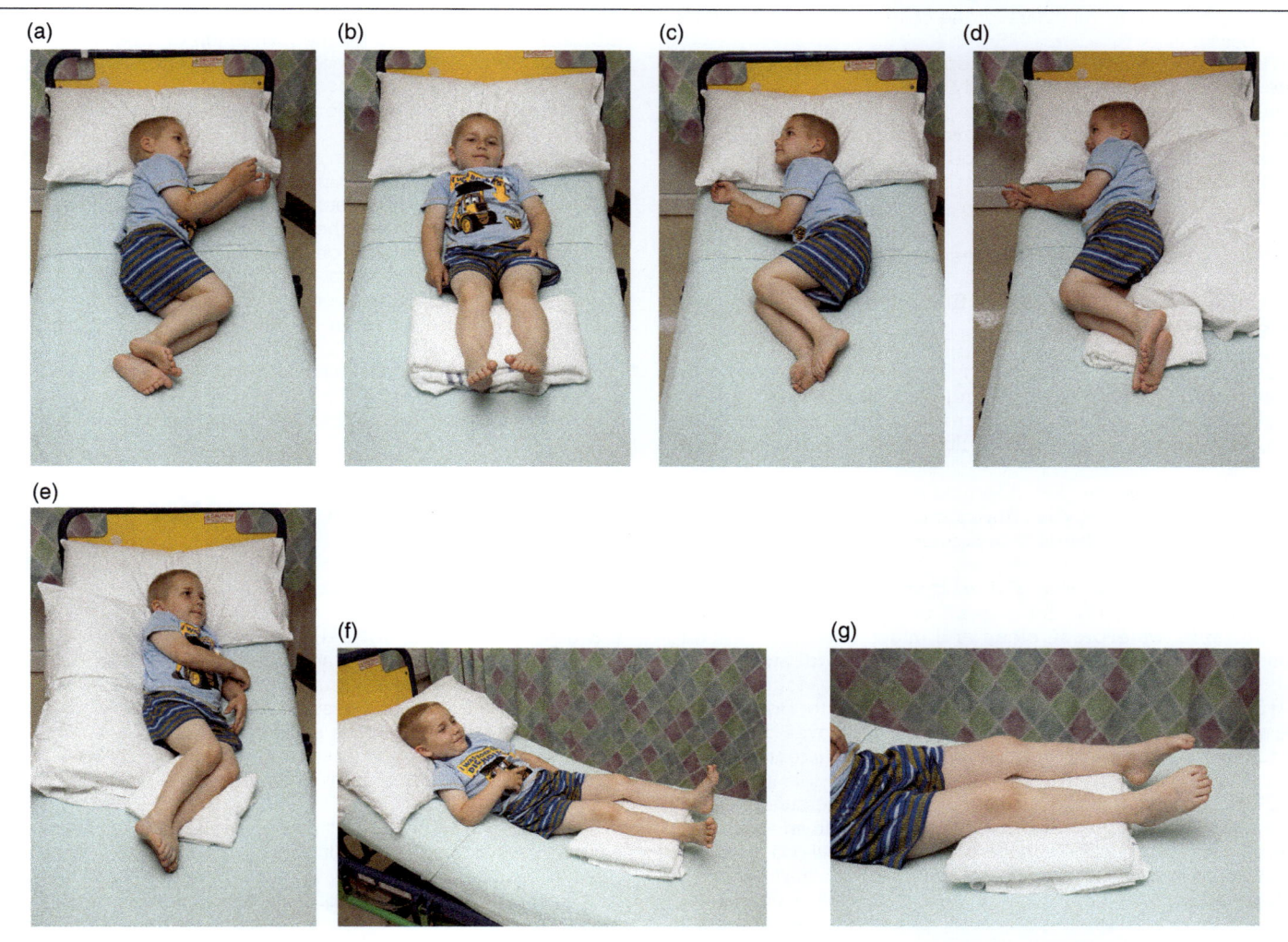

Figure 11.10 (a–g) Various positions and tilts.

possible to extend the time period between 30° tilt positions as the pressure is spread over a greater surface area. Also because the CYP does not need to be physically rolled it is often possible to reposition them without assistance. It can be useful to put towels or pillow in between knees to aid positioning and comfort.

Having placed the CYP in the 30° tilt position it should be possible to place a hand beneath them and touch the sacrum to ensure that it is free of pressure (Figure 11.10d–e). Limb elevation is integral to 30° tilt. One or two pillows or alternatively towels should be used (depending on limb size) to elevate the lower limbs, leaving the heels extended over the end completely free of pressure (Figure 11.10f–g). This position should be adopted routinely for all at risk patients, even if they are on a pressure-relieving mattress, as most of these provide inadequate pressure relief at the heel.

Tilting the foot end of the bed up by 10–15° will prevent the CYP slipping down the bed. This has the dual effect of reducing exposure of the skin to shear and friction, thereby limiting the need for moving and handling by nursing staff. Nursing staff should be aware that this may increase pressure over the sacrum/buttocks, which may require more frequent observation.

It is important to recognise the effects of manual handling on the skin and to minimise friction and shear by limiting the potential for rubbing or dragging the CYP's skin during repositioning. Devices to assist manual handling, e.g. sliding sheets, hoists, should be used where possible to reduce the potential of skin damage to the CYP and injury to parents, carers and staff.

Young children are encouraged to sit out of bed on their parent/carer's laps. This should not be discouraged in those at risk of pressure damage. Sitting out on the parent/carer's lap provides a positional change and is important for the child as it provides comfort and reassurance.

The sitting position places susceptible CYPs at particular risk due to the concentration of body weight upon the relatively small surface area of the buttocks. Older CYPs at risk of pressure ulcer development should avoid sitting in chairs for prolonged periods. The agreed period of time should be recorded in the care plan and will generally be no longer than two hours (NICE 2014).

Support surfaces, mattresses, and cushions

Pressure relieving mattresses fit into two main categories:

1 Continuous low pressure (CLP): The surface contours to the shape of the user thus spreading pressure over a larger surface area and reducing pressure at bony prominences. The surface may be air, gel, foam or fluid filled (or a combination of these).
2 Alternating pressure (AP): Alternate air cells inflate and deflate over a 7–10 minute cycle. The inflated cells support the user's weight while the deflated cells provide pressure relief.

All CYPs, irrespective of risk or medical status, are entitled to a base mattress (for cot or bed) that is pressure reducing, comfortable, waterproof, clean and intact. Pressure-reducing base mattresses have been demonstrated to significantly reduce the incidence of pressure ulceration (McInnes et al. 2015). The mattress should be impervious to body fluids, cleaned regularly and checked annually for cover damage in order to avoid cross-contamination between patients (Cullum et al. 2000).

CYPs identified as being at risk of developing pressure ulcers but who cannot be repositioned should be supplied with an appropriate pressure relieving support surface. Consult your local policy for alternative mattresses and for the rental of specialist beds/mattresses.

Comfort and the promotion of rest is a primary objective in respect to most disease processes; provision of equipment to support this goal is therefore justified. Pillows, foam wedges, gamgee, etc. can be used to help maintain position, but care should be taken that these do not interfere with the action of any other support surface in use. Many CYPs by virtue of their disease process or developmental stage may have difficulty maintaining position (Ndawula and Brown 1990).

Pressure relieving mattresses should be covered by no more than a single, unfolded sheet, which is not tucked in, in order to ensure effectiveness. Layers of bed linen between the CYP and a CLP support surface will prevent the surface contouring to their body shape, which creates increased interface pressures. In the case of AP, excess bed linen can fill the space vacated by the deflated cells, limiting the delivery of pressure relief. Tucking sheets in can, in both cases, cause problems. The taut bed sheet either limits contouring (CLP) or forms a bridge between inflated cells limiting the pressure relief provided by the deflated cells (AP).

There is no evidence that any of the following items listed are able to relieve pressure effectively and they may in some circumstances increase interface pressures (EPUAP 2019):

- Synthetic/genuine sheepskins
- Water filled gloves
- Doughnut-type devices
- Fibre-filled overlay mattresses, e.g. 'Spenco'

In rare circumstances it is acceptable to use genuine/synthetic sheepskin or fibre-filled overlays, but only to promote comfort, not as, or in place of a pressure-relieving device (EPUAP 2019)

Staff education

Educational programmes for the prevention of pressure damage should be structured, organised, and comprehensive, and made available to all levels of healthcare providers.

The educational programme should include information on:

- Skin; the largest organ in the body (including differences between premature babies, neonates and older children).
- Pathophysiology and risk factors for pressure damage.
- Risk assessment tools and their application.
- Principles of positioning to decrease risk of pressure damage.
- Documentation of assessment (the CYP, risk status and condition of skin), planning, implementation and evaluation of subsequent care.
- Selection and instruction in the use of pressure relieving and other devices.
- Clarification of responsibilities for all concerned with this problem.
- Development and implementation of guidelines.

Management of pressure ulcers

In the event that a pressure ulcer is identified by hospital staff the following actions should be taken.

Catagory 1–4 pressure ulcer

- Record in the nursing notes and inform nurse in charge.
- Review pressure risk assessment and SSKIN care bundle.
- Referral to the specialist tissue viability nurse for wound management advice or plastics surgery team for all categories of pressure ulcer where necessary.
- Full skin assessment of bony prominences to check for further skin injury.
- Ensure CYP is on the correct pressure relieving mattress.
- Review positioning and turning frequency. Increase frequency of repositioning.
- Offload pressure from area of pressure damage.
- Involve parents/carers in care if possible, ensuring that they have the local information leaflet.

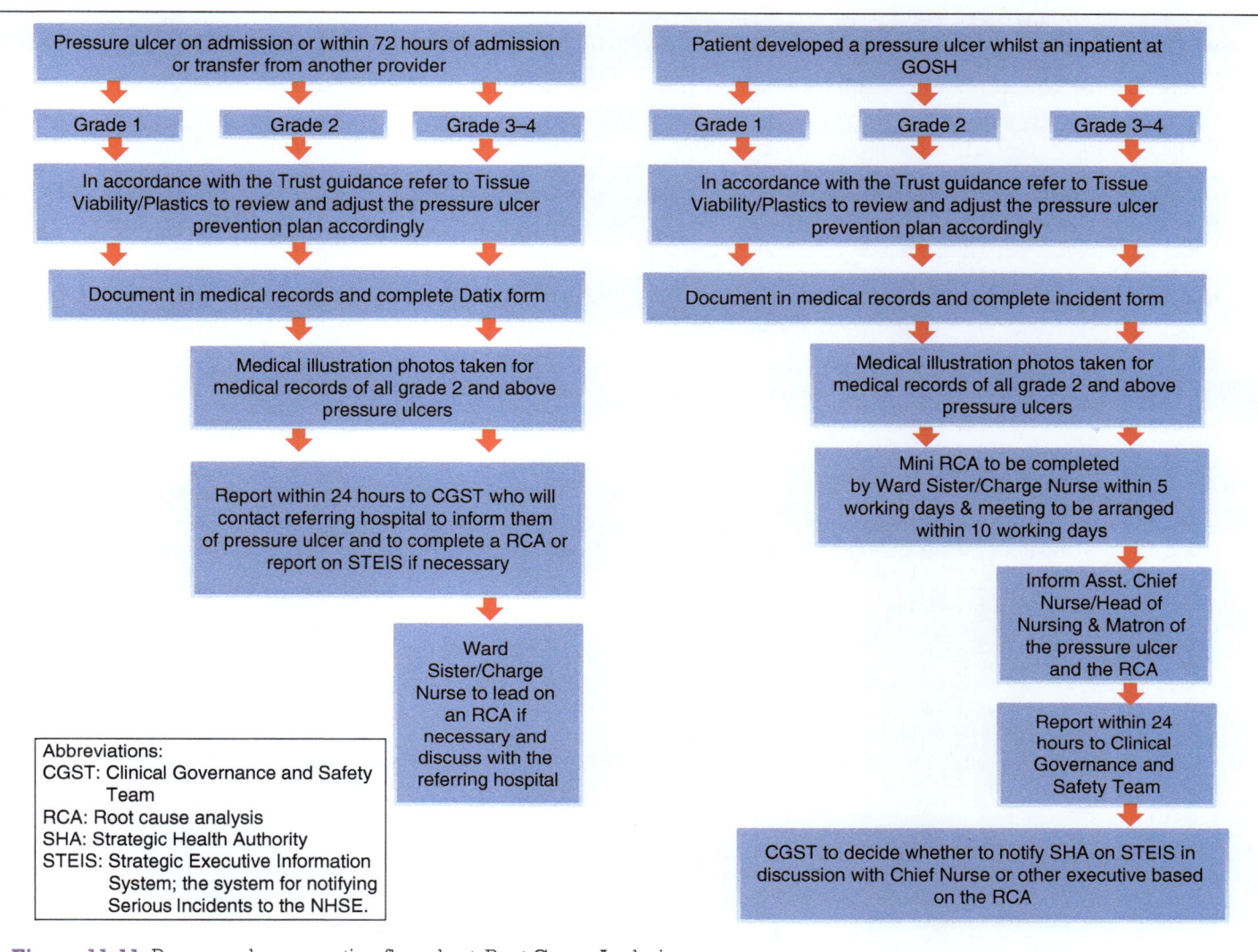

Figure 11.11 Pressure ulcer reporting flow chart. Root Cause Analysis

- Continue to observe, being aware that the extent of the pressure damage may not be clear for up to 72 hours.
- Complete clinical incident form; include category, site of injury, specialty, and all requested information.

Category 2–4 pressure ulcer, in addition to the above

- Request medical illustration to provide photographic evidence of current condition of pressure ulcer.
- Follow the local guidance for reporting for Grade 3 and 4 pressure ulcers.
- Refer to Plastic Surgery team if necessary.
- Pressure ulcers must be reported as Clinical Incidents and a root cause analysis undertaken (see Figure 11.11).

Pressure ulcer identified on admission to hospital

In the event that a category 1–4 pressure ulcer is identified by hospital staff on admission, follow the steps listed above. Careful liaison with the hospital risk teams must be taken with reporting and recording of pressure ulcer incidents in line with local policies.

Management after discharge

If a CYP is ready for discharge from hospital and a pressure ulcer has not completely healed, a referral to the GP or community team should be made, giving background and details of care required.

Conclusion

This chapter has provided general information and guidance on a range of personal hygiene issues and pressure ulcer prevention to ensure the care of both the well and the sick CYP in hospital. Health professionals and parents/carers alike must strive to give the best possible care in these basic but essential areas, recognising the individuality of each CYP in relation to the sex, age, culture, religion, and clinical condition. Care planning should be adjusted accordingly to such specific needs with parents/carers being mindful of privacy and dignity at all times. Finally, child care professionals and parents/carers should work together to facilitate best practice in these fundamental aspects of nursing care.

The Great Ormond Street Hospital Manual of Children and Young People's Nursing Practices

Procedure guideline 11.1 Assessment for bathing

Statement	Rationale
General	
1 For all ages, assess the CYP and family's normal routine in order to incorporate this into care as much as is appropriate within the hospital setting. Discuss washing/bathing and caregiving routines with the CYP and family and any specific requirements that are needed.	1 To continue hygiene routine as normal for the family. However, some practices are not appropriate in the hospital environment, e.g. some parents bathe with their children at home.
2 Document the CYP's normal routine and specific needs in the nursing notes.	2 To encourage a partnership approach to care between nurse and family. For all carers to be aware of the CYP's needs.
3 Assess and observe for any culture-specific variations in practices.	3 It is imperative that cultural and societal norms are incorporated into care regimes within the hospital setting.
The neonate and infant (up to age 1 year)	
1 In the term neonate less than 24 hours old, bathing is not absolutely necessary unless the baby is covered in thick meconium or blood (Trigg and Mohammed 2006).	1 To minimise the potential for temperature instability and avoid the disruption of normal skin mantle/acidity (Johnson and Taylor 2010). This acidity along with vernix (Hale 2007, Hoath 1997, Tollin et al. 2005) allows protection from pathogens.
2 If a newborn is bathed in the first 24 hours (e.g. if meconium/blood covered) the body temperature must be greater than 36.5°C, once stabilised after 2–4 hours of life.	2 To minimise the risk of hypothermia. A central (axilla) temperature of > 36.5°C is safe (Odio et al. 2001).
3 In the neonate greater than 24 hours old, body temperature must be stable at the normal range of 36.6–37.2°C (Fellows 2010).	3 To avoid thermal instability from exposure and excess heat loss.
4 Assess the baby's readiness for a bath (physiological state and temperature stability) and consider environmental factors such as safety and room temperature (see below).	4 For maintenance of safety and to minimise risk (Behring et al. 2003; Jackson 2008).
5 Room temperature must be at 20–25°C with no draughts (Odio et al. 2001).	5 Allows a thermal balance to be achieved with minimal energy spent on heat production (Gardner et al. 2010).
6 Note weight of the baby. If less than 1250–1500 g, bathing should not be done for the first week of life.	6 To avoid thermal instability.
7 Assess the behavioural state of the baby. He / she should be awake, alert and calm. Bathing should take place before feeding (Trigg and Mohammed 2006).	7 For the baby to be safe and to facilitate appropriate stimulation and interaction.
CYPs	
1 Assess the CYP and their family's ability for self-care with consideration of age, illness, and mobility.	1 To promote self-care and independence as appropriate for age and stage of development.
2 Assess ease of movement and mobility.	2 CYPs unable to move easily get cold very quickly when undressed due to skin exposure and immobility.
3 Assess and ensure normal body temperature of 36.6–37.2°C in a room temperature of at least 20°C.	3 To avoid thermal instability (Gardner et al. 2010; Hockenberry and Wilson 2010).
4 In cold rooms, apply additional safe heating.	4 For room temperature to be adequate as stated above.
5 Assess the need for support aids.	5 CYPs who require support to sit will require aids.
6 Assess the bath height and the weight of the CYP and adjust as necessary.	6 To ascertain whether aids are required for lifting and to avoid back injuries.

Procedure guideline 11.2 Baby bathing

Statement	Rationale
1 Assemble equipment required, depending on the age and needs of the CYP. This may include: • Baby bath • Soft cloth • Towel(s) • Nappy • Soap • Shampoo • Creams • Baby wipes • Clean clothes	1 For adequate preparation, readiness and ease of procedure.

Procedure guideline 11.2 Baby bathing *(continued)*

Statement	Rationale
2 Use water to clean the skin. Soap, shampoo, or baby bath is not necessary in the first one to two months unless parents/carers specifically request.	2 Although there are some differing opinions in the literature as to whether products or water alone should be used (Blincoe 2005, 2006a, 2006b; Walker et al. 2005b), it is generally accepted that cleaning skin with water is as effective as other skin cleansing solutions in neonates (Johnson and Taylor 2010; Stokowski 2006; Trigg and Mohammed 2006; Trotter 2004, 2006, 2007a, 2007b, 2008).
3 If parents/carers choose to use one of the wide variety of skin care products available, this should be discussed with the relevant health professional. The latter should check that all products are suitable for use in neonates.	3 Parents/carers may have preferences for the use of specific preparations, which should be recommended for use in the neonate (Walker et al. 2005b).
4 If soap or emollients are used, they should have a neutral pH and only be used two to three times/week (Camm 2006, Hale 2007, Mainstone 2005, Walker et al. 2005a, b).	4 To prevent the loss of acid mantle of the skin and minimise infection (Hale 2007).
5 Avoid the use of talcum powder unless medically indicated. Advise parents/carers, that adequate drying is enough to keep a baby's skin dry.	5 Talcum powder can be an infection risk and so parents/carers should be advised of this.
6 Place bath at a comfortable height on a safe, secure stand or place on the floor.	6 To avoid back injury and strain and to avoid the bath becoming unstable or falling.
7 Fill baby bath one-quarter to one-half full with water that feels comfortably warm (29–32°C) to the skin, using the elbow to test the temperature. Fill with cold water first, and then apply hot water.	7 To avoid extremes of temperature that could harm the baby.
8 Undress the baby to the nappy and wrap in a towel.	8 To keep the baby warm.
9 Firstly, clean the face, starting with the area around the eyes with clean or sterile water and dry (Figure 11.2a).	9 As stated above, water is an effective cleaning agent and soap is not recommended for the delicate skin of the face (Johnson and Taylor 2010).
10 Only perform eye care if there is discharge. This need not be done routinely (see guidelines on Eye Care). However, if there is encrustation, discharge, or a known eye problem, perform eye care at this stage.	10 Routine eye care can be traumatic and is unnecessary unless there is evidence of a known condition that requires attention. However, parents/carers may choose to incorporate eye care into the normal hygiene routine.
11 Do not use cotton wool for the face.	11 Cotton wool may leave strands on the face and eyes.
12 Clean the face including the nose, the skin creases around the neck, and under the chin, and the contours of the ears. In neonates, there is no need to attempt to clean inside the ear canal. Remove ear wax only once it is easily accessible.	12 Debris such as milk and saliva can collect in certain areas such as skin creases and may cause soreness or harbour infection if not cleaned away. The ear will naturally rid itself of any wax over time.
13 Wash hair if necessary, holding baby over the bath, and use corner of towel to dry (Figure 11.2b).	
14 Unwrap the towel, remove nappy and, holding securely, place baby gently into the bath. This is done by using one of your arms to place underneath to support the baby's neck/shoulders and by holding the upper arm of the baby on opposite side. Your other arm should grasp the baby's feet or placed underneath the buttocks (Figure 11.2c). This hand becomes free when the baby is in the bath (Figure 11.2d).	14 For adequate support for the baby's head and neck and for maintenance of safety.
15 Do not leave the baby unsupported until they are able to sit without support. Never leave an infant or young child unsupervised in a bath. They must be observed at all times. The use of nonslip mats is recommended.	15 To maintain the safety and well-being of the infant or child at all times.
16 Use a soft cloth or wash wipe to wash the baby with free hand, attending to skin creases.	16 Skin creases are more likely to harbour micro-organisms.
17 Watch for signs of stress in the baby such as increased agitation, colour changes, muscle tone changes, increased respiratory rate, excessive crying, and jitteriness (Boxwell 2010; Gardner et al. 2010; Thomas 2003a). Also watch for heat loss by observing colour and temperature of the skin (Thomas 2003b). Stop the bath if signs of stress or cooling are evident.	17 To maintain safety for the baby.
18 Wrap the baby in a towel and dry body thoroughly.	18 To maintain temperature, comfort, and skin integrity.

(continued)

The Great Ormond Street Hospital Manual of Children and Young People's Nursing Practices

Procedure guideline 11.2 Baby bathing *(continued)*

Statement	Rationale
19 a) During the whole procedure, observe for rashes, marks or other abnormalities. b) If dry skin and/or a 'cradle cap' are observed, apply baby oil or olive oil gently to affected parts.	19 a) To identify any skin condition that may require attention. b) Baby oil or olive oil can help maintain soft, moist skin and prevent flakiness and excessive dryness (Trotter 2004).
20 Apply a clean nappy, fastening this underneath the umbilical cord if this is still attached.	20 To facilitate drying of the cord (see section on nappy care and Chapter 20: Neonatal Care).

Procedure guideline 11.3 Topping and tailing

Statement	Rationale
1 Assemble equipment: • bowl of warm water, • soft flannel or cloth, • towel • clean nappy • nappy creams and other products if used (see Statements 2–5 in Procedure Guideline 11.10 Nappy care) and if necessary clean clothes.	1 For adequate preparation.
2 Fill bowl with water at 29–32°C (baby bathing guidelines).	2 For safe temperature and to avoid thermal stress.
3 Place baby on towel and keep wrapped or keep the baby dressed.	3 To maintain body temperature.
4 Repeat statements 9–13 in baby bathing section for washing the face, neck, eyes and ears using warm water. Dry face.	4 As for baby bathing.
5 Clean hands and nails, under arms and around the umbilical cord stump, again using water only.	5 For care of umbilical cord care, see Chapter 20: Neonatal Care. Water alone is recommended for cleaning the cord stump (Dunn 2009; Trotter 2008; Zupan et al. 2004).
6 Unwrap or undress the baby and remove nappy.	6 To prevent heat loss from exposing the body for too long.
7 Clean baby's body with warm water and a soft cloth observing for rashes, marks, etc. (for use of soap and shampoo, see baby bathing guidelines).	7 To ensure that the skin in clean and intact. Warm water is sufficient to clean the skin.
8 Clean nappy area last, cleaning from the front to the back in females (away from the genitalia toward the anus); see section on nappy care for greater detail.	8 To prevent cross-infection from stool or bowel bacteria to the urinary tract.
9 Dry the body thoroughly.	
10 Place clean nappy on, securing under the umbilical cord stump and dress the baby.	10 See nappy care section for more detail.

Procedure guideline 11.4 Washing and bathing the CYP

Statement	Rationale
Toddler and preschool child	
1 Accompany the child at all times during bathing.	1 To ensure safety of the child at all times.
2 The face and body can be cleaned with gentle soap and flannels/cloths and a shampoo recommended for use in children for the hair.	2 Milder products that are recommended for use in children are less likely to cause skin reactions.
3 Ears should be gently cleaned when necessary using a soft cotton bud to gently remove any earwax that is accessible outside the ear canal. Never insert a cotton bud into the ear canal.	3 To clean away visible earwax. To prevent damage or pushing ear wax further into the canal and causing blockage and loss of hearing.
4 Nails should also be cleaned (see section on nail care).	4 Nails are a particular source of colonisation for bacteria.
5 Clean teeth twice a day – morning and evening with recommended child's soft toothbrush.	5 See guidelines on Oral Hygiene Tools.
6 Use play, toys, and involve siblings as appropriate.	6 To make bath time an enjoyable experience.
7 Use nonslip mats in the bath.	7 To ensure safety of the child at all times.

Chapter 11 Personal hygiene and pressure ulcer prevention

Procedure guideline 11.4 Washing and bathing the CYP *(continued)*

Statement	Rationale
School age	
1 Older children (generally over the age of seven years but variations do exist) will be taught and will become able, in time, to perform their own personal hygiene. This should include such activities as cleaning teeth, drying and dressing independently with supervision (Hockenberry and Wilson 2010).	1 To encourage good hygiene practices and independence.
The older child/adolescent	
1 The older CYP may be self-caring, if fully mobile and well, for all aspects of hygiene. This may include independent showering and hair washing practices.	1 To encourage good hygiene practices and independence.
2 Maintain privacy at all times and continue individual hygiene routines as well as cultural considerations.	2 To respect the CYP's dignity and avoid embarrassment.

Procedure guideline 11.5 Bed bathing

Statement	Rationale
1 Discuss the bed bath with the CYP.	1 To facilitate consent, understanding, and cooperation.
2 Provide a warm, private environment for the procedure and ensure that the bed is a comfortable height.	2 To ensure the environment is conducive to protecting privacy, dignity, and safety considerations.
3 Ensure a surface is cleared for equipment.	3 For good preparation, safety, and ease.
4 Assist the CYP to undress and cover with towels.	4 To ensure privacy and dignity and prevention of exposure before necessary.
5 Clean eyes (see guidelines on Eye Care), face, and teeth.	
6 Expose and wash/dry upper body while legs and feet are covered.	6 As above.
7 Then vice versa: cover upper body and clean and dry legs and feet.	7 As above.
8 Observe particular parts of the body that may warrant greater attention such as ears, axilla, groin, skin creases, and genitalia (see below).	8 Certain body areas harbour more dirt, debris, and pathogens.
9 Check the pressure areas and general skin condition.	9 To ensure early detection of any bruised or broken skin. This is an easy and appropriate time to check.
10 Change washcloth and water if it is very dirty. Then clean genitalia prior to the anal area.	10 To prevent cross-infection from stool and bowel bacteria.
11 For boys aged one year and over, ensure the foreskin is clean and retract very gently if necessary to clean.	11 Care must be taken with retracting the foreskin during infancy but this can be done in the older boy to ensure cleanliness in this area.
12 For girls, wipe the genitalia from front to back followed by anal area.	12 To prevent cross-infection from stool and bowel bacteria to the genitalia.
13 Assistance may be needed to roll the large / heavy CYP safely to gain access to the back of the body.	13 To prevent injury to the CYP and care giver, by the use of correct patient handling techniques. For more information see Chapter 19: Moving and Handling.
14 Dry thoroughly and cover.	14 To maintain dignity at all times
15 Assist to dress as necessary.	
16 Change the sheet, with assistance if necessary, to roll CYP from side to side.	16 As above, to prevent injury to oneself and the CYP.
17 Hair can be washed over the end of the bed as needed.	
18 Perform passive limb exercises if appropriate or recommended according to guidelines.	18 In the immobile CYP, this may be an ideal time to perform such manoeuvres in order to exercise the limbs, encourage circulation, and prevent complications associated with immobility.
19 Talk/interact and/or play with the CYP as appropriate.	19 To put them at ease and encourage interaction.
20 Throughout the procedure, observe the CYP's vital signs.	20 To ensure they have not been compromised physiologically by the procedure.

Procedure guideline 11.6 Bathing the CYP with special needs

Statement	Rationale
1 Assess the need for equipment in CYP with special needs (see guidelines on Assessment for Bathing) and check the bath is the correct size to take any supportive bathing equipment required.	1 To ensure readiness and ensure safety.
2 If the CYP is not able to mobilise, it may be preferable to bath/wash as quickly as possible and play after the bath.	2 To avoid delays and the potential for heat loss that this may cause.
3 Consider safety for CYPs with poor head control or epilepsy.	3 To maintain patient safety.
4 Consider equipment to lift the CYP in and out of the bath, e.g. bath stands, bath overlays, bath lifts and hoists, adjustable height baths, bath boards, and seats.	4 To minimise risk and injury to CYP and parent/carer. See Chapter 19: Moving and Handling.
5 Use appropriate bathing equipment for the CYP who needs support in a semi-reclined or sitting position, e.g. foam supports, hammock supports, bath cushions and inserts, mouldable supports, and grab bars	5 As above.
6 Liaise and gain advice from other members of the multidisciplinary team, e.g. occupational therapists, physiotherapists, play specialists if needed. Parents/carers can also advise on the effective bathing methods used at home.	6 To ensure the correct equipment, mobilising and distraction techniques are employed during the procedure
7 Bed bathing is a safe alternative for immobile, heavier CYPs (see previous section) or a shower may be easier.	7 To maintain safety by selecting an appropriate method of bathing.
8 Ensure manual handling techniques are maintained.	8 To minimise risk and injury.

Procedure guideline 11.7 Assessment of toileting needs

Statement	Rationale
1 Ascertain the CYP's developmental level in relation to toileting ability and the stage of toilet training attained.	1 To facilitate and continue the normal pattern as much as possible.
2 Assessment should be thorough and systematic and should include the following: • Medical history of elimination problems (e.g. urinary tract infections, constipation, presence of pre-existing stomas, catheters) • Factors that alter normal elimination (illness and hospitalisation, infection, medication, immobility, fear and anxiety, lack of privacy, and loss of consciousness) • Details of age-appropriate milestones • Language development and delay • Mobility level • Presence of any existing problems such as bedwetting; daytime enuresis (Rogers 2000)	2 For complete and holistic care of the CYP.
3 It may be valuable to assess level of continence using a specific tool/checklist if necessary, such as that proposed by Rogers (2002). Consider: **a) Motor development** • Nonmobile child: can they sit with or without support? • Mobile child: does the child attempt to squat without losing balance? Is independent walking developing? **b) Cognitive development** • Does the child search actively and appropriately for toys by means such as eye? Do they initiate an action? • Do they engage in make-believe play, e.g. sitting a doll on a potty. **c) Language development** • Does the child understand a simple request such as 'Where's Mummy/Daddy?' • Are they able to communicate needs with words, signs, and/or gestures **d) Toileting ability** • Does the child stay dry for at least an hour? • Is he/she aware of what a potty or toilet is for? • Does he/she show awareness of when they are wet or soiled?	3 To account for the many factors that may influence toileting ability while the CYP is hospitalised. In addition, a tool/checklist may assist the nurse to assess level of continence more thoroughly and ensure that no important elements are forgotten. a–c) It is vital that toileting procedures and expectations on behaviour are applicable to the current level of development in relation to motor, cognitive, and language domains. d) If toilet training has commenced at home, it is important to continue as much as possible. Assistance with toileting can then be tailored to the individual child and their developmental level.

Procedure guideline 11.7 Assessment of toileting needs *(continued)*

Statement	Rationale
4 If the CYP is known to be incontinent or has a specific toileting problem, the nurse needs to find out as much as possible about the condition as part of the assessment process. Again, a tool or checklist can be used for this considering, for example: • Onset of incontinence. • Frequency of micturition and opening bowels, fluid intake, and necessity for particular medication, e.g. laxatives for constipation. • Symptoms such as urgency, nocturia, poor urinary stream, pain, warning of the need to void. • Method of continence management, e.g. frequent toileting, use of pads, urine collection devices. • Environmental factors; for example, accessibility of toilet and availability of assistance. • Impact on the individual and family including effect on mood, self-esteem, social activity. • Identification of conditions that might exacerbate incontinence.	4 Again, as above, a tool/checklist may assist the nurse to assess the level of incontinence and what the specific problems are (Rigby 2001).
5 Assess the CYP's ability for self-care as well as the ability to verbalise the need for voiding.	5 To determine the level of dependency on parents/carers.
6 Assess their need for privacy in line with specific cultural and societal requirements.	6 To minimise embarrassment and loss of dignity/self-consciousness.
7 Following initial assessment of needs, regular and ongoing assessment is required particularly if the CYP is dependent on parents/carers, nonverbal or immobilised.	7 The more dependent and vulnerable CYP will require parents/carers to assess when to assist with toileting.
8 During assisting with toileting, the urine and stool can be observed for normality and any potential problems. Specimens can be taken as required during toileting sessions (see Chapter 15: Investigations).	8 To assess for normality along with any potential problems related to alteration to normal elimination as brought about by illness, hospitalisation, medication, and infection to give some examples.
9 At any age, assess the normal routine and incorporate this as much as is appropriate within the hospital setting. Discuss toileting routine with the CYP and their family and any specific requirements that are needed.	9 To continue hygiene routine as normal for the family.
10 Document the CYP's normal routine and specific needs in the nursing notes.	10 To encourage a partnership approach to care between nurse and family and ensure that parents/carers are aware of their child's needs.
11 Assess and observe for any culture-specific requirements or variations in practices.	11 It is imperative that cultural and societal norms are incorporated into care regimes within the hospital setting.

Procedure guideline 11.8 Toileting the CYP

Statement	Rationale
Toileting the continent CYP	
1 Assess the CYP's age and developmental level in relation to toilet training – see section on assessment of toileting needs.	1 To ensure that toilet training and normality is continued as much as possible within the hospital setting.
2 Acknowledge the possibility of developmental regression in CYP who are hospitalised, e.g. temporary loss of continence, particularly in children with recently acquired skills in this area.	2 To ensure the effects of hospitalisation are recognised and minimised.
3 Continue with toilet training programme as much as possible within the constraints of hospital routine and current treatment, e.g. sitting on potty as certain times, use of a reward system when a potty is used successfully (Bakker et al. 2002; Barone et al. 2009; Dewar 2010; Horn et al. 2006; Schmidt 2004).	3 As for rationale 1 above.
4 If the CYP is continent but immobile, support the parents/carers to assist with the use of a bedpan, helping the CYP to roll onto the bedpan or to sit up onto it.	4 To facilitate toileting while the CYP is to unwell or immobile to self-care.

(continued)

Procedure guideline 11.8 Toileting the CYP (continued)

Statement	Rationale
5 Follow manual handling guidelines at all times (e.g. do not bend over or stretch beyond normal capability, ensure the bed is the correct height). See Chapter 19: Moving and Handling.	5 To prevent injury to staff.
6 Ensure a private environment by the use of curtains or screens if the CYP is not in a cubicle.	6 To maintain privacy and dignity.
7 Encourage the CYP and/or family to verbalise the need for assistance if appropriate.	7 To ensure that assistance is provided swiftly when required.
8 Wear nonsterile gloves and aprons when handling and disposing of body fluids.	8 To minimise the risk of infection. See Chapter 13: Infection Prevention and Control.

Toileting the CYP with a disability or specific need

Statement	Rationale
1 Following assessment, ascertain any individual toileting problems and formulate a plan in discussion with parents/carers.	1 To continue the CYP's normal routine, in line with a partnership approach.
2 Follow local or national guidelines, if applicable, for the management of specific problems, e.g. catheter care (Simpson 2001), constipation (NICE 2010a) and stoma care.	2 For safe, evidence based practice. See Chapter 33: Urinary Catheter Care and Chapter 5: Bowel Care).
3 Liaise with the multidisciplinary team, e.g. occupational therapist, physiotherapist, stoma nurse, and incontinence advisor, in relation to the management of specific problems.	3 For holistic and thorough assessment of the CYP's special needs and to utilise expert assistance for best practice.
4 Administer relevant prescribed medication as necessary, e.g. laxatives, antibiotics, drugs to increase motility.	4 Certain drugs may be part of the CYP's care and may also have side effects that may affect toileting, e.g. loose stools.
5 Gain advice on products and special equipment from the multidisciplinary team, e.g. occupational therapist, social services, or community teams.	5 To facilitate best practice.

Box 11.1 Predisposing Factors to Development of Nappy Rash

Contact with ammonia in urine or bacteria in faeces
Abrasion (chafing on clothes or nappy)
Infrequent nappy changes
Fungal infections (e.g. thrush or *Candida*)
Plastic pants
Sensitivity to:

- Household chemicals, e.g. fabric conditioner/washing powders
- Creams, lotions, and bath additives
- Materials (e.g. elastic/latex)
- New foods/dietary changes (e.g. when weaning)
- Prescribed medication

Immunisation
Teething
Cold or infection
Incorrectly washed reusable nappies
Over application of creams blocking pores in nappy linings
High body temperature increasing humidity in wet nappy
Riboflavin deficiency (causing scrotal or vulval dermatitis, inflammation in genital region)
Watery stool (Zsolway et al. 2002).
Zinc deficiency (Zsolway et al. 2002)
Immunological deficiency conditions and immune suppressed patients

Procedure guideline 11.9 Assessing nappy rashes

Statement	Rationale
1 Establish how long the patient has been suffering with nappy rash.	1 To identify acute nature and severity of rash, and possible presence of secondary bacterial and fungal infections.
2 Does the baby look generally well? For what condition/treatment is the CYP in hospital?	2 Nappy rash, which fails to respond to conventional treatment in the presence of other conditions, may have a more complex diagnosis attributable to gut function, or nutritional deficiencies.
3 Check for links with any predisposing factors (see Box 11.1).	3 Identification of predisposing factors can aid treatment and be used to prevent further outbreaks.
4 Obtain history of pre-existing skin conditions. Examine other skin areas for rashes including trunk, head, knee, elbow, and neck crevices.	4 To identify general skin condition such as eczema or psoriasis as opposed to nappy rash and determine treatment regime/need for medical input.
5 Establish frequency of nappy changes	5 To assess skin sensitivity to rash outbreaks and to determine frequency of nappy changes during treatment.
6 Ascertain if discomfort is limited to nappy changes.	6 To differentiate between infected and irritant nappy rash and systemic infection. To enable assessment of type and regularity of pain relief required.
7 What does the rash look like? Is the skin intact?	7 To enable identification and differentiation of nappy rash from other skin conditions / skin infections.
8 Note any spots; size and colour, whether they are raised or flat, have a head, are weeping or crusting (Figure 11.3).	8 To determine treatment / need for medical input.
9 Choose appropriate cream, emollient or gel.	9 To aid skin repair and recovery.
10 Where treatment is already implemented, assess for improvement or deterioration.	10 To evaluate treatment success or identify need to change product or call for specialist advice.
11 Document severity and extent of rash using an appropriate tool if available.	11 To enable assessment and evaluation of subsequent care/treatment.
12 To hand over current assessment of nappy rash to nursing team and patients named nurse.	12 To provide continuity of care.
13 Swab unresolving/severe rashes for bacterial and fungal organisms.	13 To aid diagnosis.

Procedure guideline 11.10 Routine nappy care

Statement	Rationale
1 Nappy care should be carried out as soon as possible after soiling: • After feeds • Before long periods of sleep • In the hospital setting check nappy area three to four hourly unless otherwise indicated • Six to eight hourly in the case of premature infants At first sign of nappy rash increase frequency of changing	1 To prevent prolonged periods of skin contact with irritants known to cause nappy rash. To ensure nappy area is checked regularly in the absence of family carer. Sick, premature neonates require minimal handling. To combat further skin damage. Increased frequency of nappy changes has been shown to decrease outbreaks and speed up recovery and resolution of condition.
2 Ensure you have everything ready before starting: • Nappy • Gloves, apron • A toy/mobile • A warm, dry and clean environment • A changing mat, or towel to lay the baby on • Any creams that you wish to use • Bag/bin for disposal of the old nappy • Wash and dry your hands	2 To prevent having to leave baby unattended during procedure, minimise the risk of contamination and to distract the baby.
3 Lay the baby on a towel or changing mat. Undo the bottom half of the baby's clothes and lift them out of the way.	3 To prevent soiling.
4 Unfasten nappy tabs and fasten them back onto the nappy, fold nappy over and underneath bottom.	4 To prevent tabs sticking to the baby's skin.

(continued)

Procedure guideline 11.10 Routine nappy care *(continued)*

Statement	Rationale
5 As for bathing guidelines, using water and gauze, clean the front of the nappy area first (the genital area before the anal area).	5 To reduce the possibility of bacteria from the bowel/anal area being transferred to the urethra, which could cause a urinary tract infection.
6 For girls, always wipe from front to back, away from the vagina toward the perineal area and anus. For boys, clean the penis. Do not retract the foreskin in infants in the first year. From age 1 year upwards, gentle retraction can be done to check for cleanliness.	6 As above.
7 Clean between the folds of the groin and thighs thoroughly.	7 These are common areas where nappy rash occurs.
8 Lift both legs by the ankles and clean the bottom.	
9 Dry the bottom thoroughly from front to back.	
10 Apply a clean nappy.	
11 As stated in the guidelines on Bathing, water alone can be used to clean the nappy area without the necessity for skin products. This also applies to the routine use of barrier creams on the skin. The skin can be left without a barrier cream unless parents/carers request a particular product, which should be checked for suitability in neonates (Walker et al. 2005a, b). In the case of a rash developing however, it may be necessary to use a specific product.	11 Water alone has been shown to be sufficient for cleansing the skin in the first 1–2 months and the benefits of routine barrier creams have not been agreed on.
12 If applying creams in the case of nappy rash or other skin conditions requiring topical treatment, loosely tape up the nappy and wash your hands before applying; alternatively measure out cream prior to nappy change.	12 To prevent introduction of micro-organisms into cream pot/tube.
13 Carefully apply cream, taking special care around the vagina and any creases, applying from front to back.	13 To prevent transfer of bowel bacteria to urethra.
14 In newborns, the umbilical cord stump should be observed at each nappy change and cleaned if necessary with water.	14 Water has been shown to be effective for cleaning the cord stump (Zupan et al. 2004).
15 As stated in the Bathing section, avoid covering the umbilical cord with the nappy until the stump has separated and has been removed. A notch can be cut at the front top edge of the nappy if necessary or the nappy can be folded at the top).	15 To prevent the cord becoming moist, aiding drying of the stump and reducing risk of infection (Dunn 2009). See Chapter 13; Infection Prevention and Control.
16 In boys tuck the penis facing downwards.	16 To prevent upward leaks.
17 Fasten the nappy at both sides with the tapes, making sure it is snug, but not so tight that it pinches the skin.	17 A nappy that is too tight can cause chaffing, abrasive friction, and discomfort.
18 a) Retape the soiled nappy around the contents and put in plastic bag or bin. b) Remove faecal matter from reusable nappies and place in sanitising bin. c) Wash hands thoroughly.	18 To prevent contamination.
19 a) Re-dress baby. b) In all cases of nappy rash ensure appropriate pain relief is prescribed and given.	19 To ensure that the baby is comfortable.

Procedure guideline 11.11 Nail assessment

Statement	Rationale
1 Assess nails as part of the CYP's overall hygiene routine alongside the parents/carers if present.	1 To incorporate nail care into daily routine of the CYP and family.
2 Observe all aspects of the nails and nail bed, including the subungual area of both fingers and toes.	2 For holistic and thorough assessment of hygiene status of the nails.
3 Observe for dirt and debris on and under the nail.	3 Presence of dirt serves as an infection source.
4 Observe nail for length and for the presence of jagged or broken edges.	4 Long, jagged/broken nails can further increase infection risk and cause trauma (Boyd 2003).
5 Observe and note the presence of nail varnish, false nails, and jewellery.	5 Nail decorations increase the risk of infection (Boyd 2003).
6 Observe whether there is any evidence of nail-biting or damage to the skin around the nail area.	6 Loss of continuity between skin and nail can harbour micro-organisms (Watson 2000).
7 Observe the colour of the subungual area, checking that it is pink, with adequate capillary refill without presence of cyanosis.	7 Colour of the nail beds provides useful information on oxygenation and perfusion.
8 Assessment must be carried out preoperatively.	8 To minimise the risk of infection intraoperatively.
9 Assess for presence of disease such as fungal infection, redness, swelling, abnormal growth, trauma, hardened nails that may indicate skin conditions as well as any gross abnormalities that may affect appearance and growth of the nails.	9 To facilitate swift detection and treatment of any potential problems. Nail problems can stem from many sources on fingers and/or toes.
10 For all ages, assess the CYP and family's normal routine. Incorporate this into care as much as is appropriate within the hospital setting. Discuss and document care-giving routine in relation to nail care with the CYP and family and any specific requirements that are needed.	10 To continue hygiene routine as normal for the family. However, some practices may not be appropriate in the hospital environment; for example, some parents/carers bite their infants/child's nails to shorten them at home. Therefore alternative advice should be offered. To encourage a partnership approach to care between nurse and family. To ensure all parents/carers are aware of the child's needs.
11 Assess and observe for any culture-specific variations in practices; for example, the colour of the subungual and surrounding area, presence of rings.	11 In some cultures, discolouration may be due to different foodstuffs or substances, e.g. henna. It is imperative that cultural and societal norms are incorporated into care regimes within the hospital setting wherever possible.

Procedure guideline 11.12 Nail care

Statement	Rationale
1 For all ages, assess nails at bath or hand wash times according to assessment criteria in the previous section.	1 Assessment is the first stage in order to plan subsequent care.
2 It may be necessary to teach the parents/carers nail care by performing the practice then supervising them.	2 Some parents/carers (for example, those with a first baby) may be unsure and require teaching and support for even the most basic of care tasks.
3 For all CYPs, if nails require cutting, discuss with the parents/carers and gain consent or support them to carry out the procedure.	3 This aids the negotiation of care in the context of a partnership between nurse and family.
4 In the neonate/baby, check and clean nails during bathing or topping and tailing using water and a soft flannel/cloth.	4 For the integration of care practices.
5 Check the neonate's fingernails and cut to the level of the top of the finger using small baby nail scissors or clippers. Alternatively, nails can be gently filed using a soft, small emery board.	5 Cutting too close to the skin may cause trauma and damage to the nail bed. Equipment specially designed for babies should be used to minimise such damage.
6 For the preschool child, wash the child's hands and nails or assist them to do so, during hand washing and/or bathing, using a soft brush if necessary.	6 As above, for the integration of care practices.

(continued)

Procedure guideline 11.12 Nail care (continued)

Statement	Rationale
7 a) In CYPs of any age, cut nails using nail scissors, paying particular attention to jagged edges. b) Cut/trim or file nails straight across. c) Provide reassurance at all times.	7 a), b) To minimise the risk of damage to the nail. c) The CYP may be fearful of the procedure and so continual reassurance may be required)
8 Teach the CYP hand and nail care during the procedure if appropriate.	8 To encourage independence and health promotion.
9 For the older CYP, observe hand and nail washing technique, teaching and giving guidance as necessary.	9 Generally speaking, children over the age of five will be able to perform their own hygiene if able and healthy.
10 If the older child is unable to perform nail care due to special needs, illness, immobility, lack of dexterity, perform the procedure during bed bathing/washing.	
11 Prior to surgery, remove any nail varnish with recommended solution, any jewellery and false nail and cut the nails as stated before.	11 To minimise infection intraoperatively and to be able to observe the perfusion of the fingertips.
12 Emphasise the importance of cleaning under the nail with the use of a brush.	12 The area underneath the nail is a potential source for pathogens to harbour.
13 Attend to, and clean, both fingernails and toenails.	13 Toenails in particular are a potential source of infection in certain conditions and so should not be missed.

Procedure guideline 11.13 Oral assessment

Statement	Rationale
1 Use an oral assessment tool such as the Oral Assessment Guide (OAG) (Table 11.2), to record the status of the oral cavity (Gibson et al. 2010). An effective oral assessment should involve the examination of the eight aspects of the mouth.	1 To identify specific problems. To enable appropriate advice to be given. To facilitate effective management. To promote oral health.
2 The eight subscale scores are added together to obtain an overall assessment score (minimum 8, maximum 24) (Gibson et al. 2006, 2010). 1 = normal, 2 = mild alterations without severe compromise of either epithelial integrity or systemic functioning 3 = definite compromise.	2 A risk assessment score allows for a consistent approach to care to be applied by all healthcare workers. A plan of care is then instituted as a result of the score obtained.
3 Assessment of the oral cavity must be performed thoroughly, regularly, and systematically.	3 To monitor changes and prescribe appropriate interventions.
4 The assessment procedure should be explained to the CYP and family, including why the assessment is necessary and what it entails.	4 To obtain informed consent. Communication helps to ensure success.
5 Whenever possible the CYP should be involved in the assessment. When assessing the mouth of a young child it is advisable to have a second adult present to support the child's head.	5 To help ensure success. To teach good mouth care. For comfort and reassurance.
6 A good source of light is required to examine the oral cavity, e.g. pen torch.	6 To enable good visualisation of the mouth.
7 Standard precautions should be adopted and nonsterile gloves worn.	7 To minimise the risk of cross-infection.
8 The teeth should, if possible, be cleaned prior to examining the oral cavity.	8 To remove plaque and debris. To aid observation and assessment.
9 It is important to accurately record the assessment in the CYP's healthcare record and on the oral assessment score sheet.	9 To monitor any changes. To implement appropriate treatment. To ensure continuity. To evaluate care.
10 Special skills of observing 'in an instant' maybe required when undertaking oral assessment in CYPs with special needs.	10 To undertake assessment quickly To explain and gain collaboration to undertake the assessment.

Procedure guideline 11.14 Oral hygiene tools

Principle	Rationale
Toothbrushes	
1 A small-headed, soft, nylon-bristled toothbrush, with round-ended filaments should be used to brush/clean teeth (BDHF 2014; DH 2014).	1 These provide the most effective method for removing plaque.
2 CYPs at risk of low platelet count should use a soft toothbrush.	2 To minimise the risk of damage to the mucosa.
3 Toothbrushes are for single patient use and should be kept clean. They should therefore be rinsed and stored once dry and be changed: • Daily while undergoing bone marrow transplantation • Every 2–3 months or sooner if the bristles become splayed (BDHF 2014; UKCCSG-PONF Mouth Care Group 2006).	3 To minimise the risk of infection.
Powered toothbrushes	
1 These have a rotating, oscillating, and vibratory action.	1 Brushes that work with a rotation oscillation action remove more plaque and reduce gingivitis more effectively than a manual tooth brush (Robinson et al. 2005).
2 The bristles of the powered toothbrush are hard and are not advisable for CYPs with a fragile mucosa.	2 Their efficacy is not yet proven in cancer care.
3 Powered toothbrushes are useful for physically impaired CYPs, e.g. in conditions that cause upper limb disability such as juvenile idiopathic arthritis (Foster and Fitzgerald 2005) or those who find it difficult to use a manual toothbrush (DH 2014).	3 To facilitate effective brushing.
Fluoride toothpaste	
1 Fluoride toothpaste strengthens tooth enamel and decreases risk of dental caries.	1 Clear evidence exists that fluoride toothpaste is efficacious in preventing caries (Walsh et al. 2019; BDHF 2014).
2 For children up to the age of three you should use a smear of toothpaste containing no less than 1000 ppm fluoride; for three to six year olds a pea-sized blob of 1350–1500 ppm fluoride toothpaste and for the 7 years and over, 1350 ppm fluoride toothpaste or above (BDHF 2014).	2 Using the correct amount of fluoride toothpaste is important. It can have a drying effect if left in contact with oral mucosa and excessive fluoride may result in very tough teeth and produce unsightly spotting, i.e. fluorosis.
Foam cleaning sponges	
1 When a child has no teeth, – moisten sponges with water (UKCCSG-PONF Mouth Care Group 2006). These may be used as a temporary measure, or combined with a toothbrush to remove debris and cleanse the mouth when the CYP: • Has no teeth or is unable to lubricate their own mouth • Has a reduced level of consciousness • Has severe mucositis that prevents them from brushing their teeth. Foam sponges can be moistened with water or diluted Chlorhexidine (UKCCSG-PONF Mouth Care Group 2006). They can also be used in the terminal stages of illness when comfort is the only intended outcome.	1 Sponges are: • Ineffective at removing plaque (Pearson and Hutton 2002) • Soft, unthreatening and easy to use • Able to be squeezed into difficult places • Able to deliver fluids to specific places
2 In the neonate/infant prior to appearance of teeth, foam sponges soaked in clean water (use sterile water in the neonate) can be used to clean and moisten the lips, tongue, and inside the mouth. For the very small neonate, cotton wool buds can provide an alternative. Liquid paraffin or Vaseline can also be applied in this way.	2 To moisten dry lips when the neonate/infant is unable to lubricate their own lips; e.g. when intubated or sedated in intensive care.
3 Mouth care packs should be disposed of once opened.	3 To avoid the risk of infection, discard oral swabs after use (MHRA 2012).
4 Take care at all times when using foam sponges and follow the manufacturer's instructions for use. Check that the foam head is firmly attached to the stick before use.	4 Foam heads of oral swabs may detach from the stick and present a choking hazards.

(continued)

Procedure guideline 11.14 Oral hygiene tools *(continued)*

Principle	Rationale
5 Do not leave the swabs soaking in liquid prior to use. If necessary moisten the swab immediately before use.	5 Soaking the swabs can affect the strength of the foam head attachment, causing it to detach.
6 If the patient is likely to bite down on the swab, consider using an alternative, e.g. a small-headed toothbrush with soft bristles.	
7 Ensure that all CYPs and carers are aware of this advice and the manufacturer's instructions for use.	6 To ensure that foam sponges are used safely (MHRA 2012).

Dental floss

1 Combined with a toothbrush, dental floss is the most effective method of removing plaque. It reaches parts that toothbrush bristles are unable to reach.	1 Dexterity is needed to manipulate floss. It is difficult to floss someone else's teeth.
2 It must be used with care and is not advised in children younger than 10 years old (Lloyd 1992).	2 Some conditions may cause bleeding and increase the risk of infection.
3 For CYPs with reduced immunity, flossing should only be used following a risk assessment by a dental practitioner (UKCCSG-PONF Mouth Care Group 2006).	3 Some conditions may cause bleeding and increase the risk of infection.

Vaseline

1 Vaseline can be applied to the lips to soothe dryness.	1 It is the most acceptable method to prevent dry, cracked lips (Campbell et al. 1995). It provides an occlusive barrier, which retains moisture, is easy to apply, and will remain in place for many hours if not licked off!
2 It should not be used in the following circumstances: • Oxygen therapy • Near a naked flame/cigarettes • Babies under phototherapy	2 It is highly flammable and traps bacteria (National Pharmacy Association 2020).

Chlorhexidine based mouthwash (0.2% solution)

1 Chlorhexidine can be used as an adjunct to other oral hygiene measures for secondary infection in mucosal ulceration and for control of gingivitis,. It can be used prophylactically and therapeutically for high-risk patients and is available as a mouthwash, spray, or gel.	1 These preparations may be used in place of toothbrushing for painful periodontal conditions, e.g. primary herpetic stomatitis, if the CYP has a haemorrhagic disorder, or is disabled (Paediatric Formulary Committee 2022).
2 Rinse the mouth thoroughly with water between using toothpaste and Chlorhexidine containing products (Paediatric Formulary Committee 2022).	2 Prolonged use of Chlorhexidine causes reversible brown staining of the teeth and tongue. It can be incompatible with some ingredients in toothpaste.
3 Chlorhexidine should remain in contact with the mucous membranes for 30–90 seconds and then be spat out.	3 This allows it to be absorbed into the cell wall of micro-organisms. It is active against yeast, fungi, and gram-negative and gram-positive organisms.
4 Unless the CYP is unable to brush their teeth, Chlorhexidine is not recommended for the prevention or treatment of radiotherapy/chemotherapy-induced mucositis, nor the prevention of candidiasis in CYPs with cancer.	4 Foam sponges moistened with water or diluted Chlorhexidine may be used (UKCCSG-PONF Mouth Care Group 2006) if the CYP is unable to brush their teeth.

Anti-fungal agents and the treatment of oral candidiasis

1 Administer antifungals as prescribed and in accordance with local and/or national protocols and guidelines.	1 The antifungal treatment comes into contact with the oral mucosa, hence directly treating oropharyngeal candidiasis for a CYP with a normal immune system. Drug doses for antifungal agents should be prescribed according to the current version of the Paediatric Formulary Committee (2022).
2 It should be given an hour after the use of Chlorhexidine or other medicated mouthwash and 20–30 minutes after eating and drinking. (Gibson and Nelson 2000).	2 To allow for effective absorption of the antifungal treatment.
3 Following the administration of any antifungal agent reassess the mouth using the OAG assessment tool (Table 11.2). If the oral mucosa is deteriorating seek medical attention.	3 To monitor response to treatment. Specialist advice should be sought if the CYP has extensive or severe candidiasis (NICE 2022)

Chapter 11 Personal hygiene and pressure ulcer prevention

Procedure guideline 11.15 Performing oral care

Statement	Rationale
1 Whenever possible oral care should be performed by the CYP and/or family member/carer.	1 To reduce anxiety. To allow time for questions.
2 Whenever possible encourage the child/young person to take control of their mouth care, e.g. choosing the time to do it.	2 To increase adherence and support self-management of oral care.
3 In the case of a well neonate, oral care will simply involve observation of the mouth, tongue and lips. If clean and moist, no further intervention is required. As stated earlier, liquid paraffin or Vaseline can be applied to the neonate's dry lips if necessary. If the neonate is unwell, it may be necessary to perform more regular mouth care to lubricate the mouth and lips (see guidelines on Oral Care during Compromised Health).	3 A neonate prior to the appearance of teeth does not need routine mouth care unless there is an indication to do so (e.g. dryness or presence of any Candida or other conditions). A well neonate will be able to lubricate their own mouth and lips.
4 Once teeth start to appear within the first year, gentle cleaning with a soft toothbrush and low-fluoride toothpaste, both suitable for use in babies, should be carried out on a daily basis.	4 To prevent any potential for tooth decay at the earliest possible age. Good teeth-cleaning habits benefit the CYP for life (Lloyd 1994).
5 The child should be encouraged to handle the mouth care products in a nonthreatening environment and perform mouth care on a favourite toy, parent/carer, or nurse. Play specialists can help prepare older children for mouth care procedures.	5 To ensure age appropriate preparation. To reduce anxiety.
6 Ensure explanations are age appropriate and reinforced with written information.	6 To ensure that the child understands why mouth care is important.
7 The need for privacy must be respected when undertaking any aspect of oral care.	7 To decrease anxiety or embarrassment from changes in their oral cavity, e.g. gingival enlargement, increased salivation, inability to swallow or speak effectively, or halitosis.
8 Normal practice from home may be continued if appropriate. Teeth should be cleaned effectively twice a day.	8 Bedtime brushing is especially important, as there is more time for interaction between oral bacteria and unremoved substrate on the tooth substance.
9 The CYP's mouth should be assessed daily using an oral assessment guide and appropriate mouth care given.	9 An oral assessment guide will allow for the consistent assessment of improvement or deterioration and allow for the implementation of management strategies.
10 Prior to performing oral hygiene the nurse should: a) Put on an apron b) Perform a clinical handwash. c) Put on a pair of nonsterile gloves. d) Gloves should be powder and latex free.	a–c) To minimise the risk of cross-infection. Oral fungal infections are often asymptomatic. *Candida albicans* can be transmitted between patients on the hands of staff. d) To prevent an allergic reaction.
11 Children under 7 years should position their heads so that parents/carers can access their mouth while stabilising their head. This is achieved by the child having their back to the adult, while the adult cups their chin with one hand and brushes the child's teeth with the other. This is known as the 'Starkey' position.	11 The teeth of children under 7 years are most effectively cleaned if it is done by their parents/carers (Lloyd 1994). To facilitate access, ensuring effectiveness of cleaning.
12 Fluoride toothpaste should be used as follows: • Use a small pea-sized amount on a toothbrush. • Supervise use of toothpaste to prevent swallowing of excessive amounts. • It should be spat out and rinsed thoroughly with water.	12 Fluoride can build into the enamel to increase resistance to decay.
13 The toothbrush should be used by: • Placing the tips of bristles at 45° against teeth and gums. • Moving the brush backwards and forwards in a gentle but vibratory motion. • To clean the inner (lingual) surfaces place toothbrush vertical to teeth and move up and down against the gums. • Always start and finish in the same spot. • It is important that the gums as well as the teeth are cleaned. • Teeth should be cleaned for 2–3 minutes.	13 To ensure adequate cleaning action. To ensure a thorough and complete cleaning.

(continued)

Procedure guideline 11.15 Performing oral care *(continued)*

Statement	Rationale
14 Using an electric toothbrush requires less dexterity.	14 The bristles do the action and therefore the brush needs to be moved around all areas of the mouth.
15 Using a toothbrush with timer is more effective.	15 Ensures teeth are cleaned for a recommended effective period.
16 Dental floss is used by pulling gently downwards and upwards against each tooth to clean both above and below the gum.	16 Flossing removes bacteria that escape normal toothbrushing. Daily use recommended.
17 If the CYP has been assessed as having dry, cracked, or ulcerated lips apply Vaseline. Vaseline if required should be used sparingly and applied with a gloved finger.	17 To maintain integrity and comfort.
18 Each container of Vaseline is for single patient use.	18 To prevent cross-contamination.
19 All used equipment should be cleaned, disinfected, and stored safely.	19 As above.

Procedure guideline 11.16 Oral health promotion

Principle	Rationale
1 For snacks between meals encourage non-sugary foods, e.g. cheese, fresh vegetables, or water.	1 Sugar promotes dental caries. Frequent exposure to sugar increases the incidence of caries.
2 If sugary foods are consumed, ensure they are part of main meals and completed before teeth are brushed.	2 Sugar can contribute to dental caries, especially when given at night. Saliva flow is greatly reduced at night so the sugar remains in contact with the teeth for longer periods.
3 Involve the dietician in the CYP's care. Many CYPs with chronic illness require a diet high in refined carbohydrates to ensure adequate energy intake. Liaise with the dietician before advising any reduction in sugar content.	3 To ensure that the CYP is receiving an adequate energy intake.
4 Avoid sugary medicines.	4 Most commonly used paediatric medicines and are available sugar free.
5 Encourage regular dental checkups; at least annually. This should begin around 1 year of age. CYPs at increased risk of oral problems should have checkups more frequently.	5 Should begin around 1 year of age. Dentists can assess manipulative skills and special needs of children to prescribe the best brushing technique and regimen. Good dental habits are important to family health.
6 Do not leave a child unattended while brushing their teeth.	6 To prevent injury as an inpatient. Trauma to the teeth is not uncommon in childhood.

Procedure guideline 11.17 Oral care during compromised health

Principle	Rationale
1 If the CYP has been assessed as having swallowing difficulties: a) Commence a fluid balance chart. b) Consider monitoring their weight. c) Contact the dietician. d) Use a local anaesthetic spray if prescribed. e) Discuss pain management with appropriate personnel.	1 a–c) To maintain adequate hydration. To ensure nutritional adequacy. d–e) To minimise pain.
2. If the CYP has been assessed as having plaque or debris on their teeth: a) Consider referral to the dentist. b) Consider a dietary referral. c) Commence health education as and when appropriate.	2 Risk factors are available against which to assess CYPs (SIGN 2014).

Procedure guideline 11.17 Oral care during compromised health *(continued)*

Principle	Rationale
Immuno-compromised CYPs	
1 All CYPs undergoing chemotherapy, regardless of diagnosis, should use a soft toothbrush and toothpaste twice a day.	1 To ensure that they receive appropriate mouth care.
2 An oral care protocol should be in place.	2 Ensures standardised and appropriate care is given (Gibson et al. 1997; Nelson et al. 2001).
3 When the oral cavity lies within the treatment field, radiotherapy will exert a direct effect, decreasing cell renewal with the resulting complications.	3 Decreased cell renewal results in: • Epithelial thinning • Inflammation • Ulceration • An increased risk of secondary infection
4 A number of the chemotherapy agents used are known to cause oral stomatitis.	4 Reduced bone-marrow activity results in an increased risk of: • Bleeding due to thrombocytopenia • Infection due to neutropenia
Oral phobia	
1 Children who have been, or who are intubated can experience problems having oral hygiene performed, leading to oral phobia	
2 Oral care should be assessed on an individual basis, but intubated CYPs should: • Have their teeth cleaned as normal. • Have Vaseline applied to their lips.	2 To increase comfort and reduce the risk of oral infection and cracked lips.
3 The endotracheal tube will need to be repositioned to the opposite side of their mouth if they are intubated orally, and it is safe to do so. Liaise with appropriate nurse specialist.	3 To reduce the risk of pressure ulcers of the mouth.
CYPs with epidermolysis bullosa	
1 Only the use of a mouthwash, rather than toothbrush or mouth care foam, may be possible.	1 To ensure the mucosal integrity is maintained where the mucosa is very fragile and easily damaged.
2 If possible a small toothbrush or foam cleaning sponges may be used.	2 To prevent infection.
3 An electric toothbrush (small, round oscillating head) may be used for front teeth and wherever access permits.	3 To maintain comfort and dignity of the patient.
Stomatitis due to *Candida albicans*	
1 This is quite common in childhood and is treated with oral nystatin. *Candida albicans* appears as slightly raised white patches, generally starting on the tongue, spreading to the mucous membranes of the gums, cheeks, and palate.	1 It may be associated with: • Gastrointestinal disturbances when children are cutting teeth • Antibiotic therapy • Immunosuppression • A lack of cleanliness
The neonate/infant in high dependency or intensive care	
1 Neonates and infants within the intensive care environment may be intubated orally or may be receiving oxygen therapy. Regular cleaning and moistening of the lips and all parts of the mouth should be done using foam sponges or cotton wool buds soaked in sterile water followed by liquid paraffin (see guidelines on Performing Oral Care).	1 Oral intubation and the presence of an artificial tube renders lubrication of the mouth and lips difficult and debris may build up. Oxygen is also likely to cause further dryness of the lips, tongue, and mucous membranes.
2 This should be done at regular intervals depending on age and gestation and how the sick neonate tolerates interventions; ideally four to six hourly if condition allows. This will be less frequent in the preterm/low-birth-weight neonate (eight hourly).	2 The sick preterm neonate is more prone to physiological stress during interventions and the concept of 'minimal handling' should be considered (Bauer 2005 Khurana et al. 2005).
3 The neonate/infant who is compromised in this way should have close observation of their lips and mouth for excoriation from the presence of tubes as well as for the presence of *Candida* inside the mouth.	3 Artificial tubes (endotracheal or feeding) can cause friction, particularly during movement or if they are in place for significant time periods. In addition, any such tube in place is a potential infection risk.

Procedure guideline 11.18 Eye care

Statement	Rationale
General eye cleansing (aseptic)	
1 Prepare all equipment: • Sterile or boiled, cool tap water • Sterile gauze swabs, and galipot, or • An eye care pack • Gloves	1 For adequate preparation.
2 a) Reassure and explain the procedure to the parents/carers and the CYP if they are able to understand. b) Ensure the baby/ CYP is in an appropriate position and is stable enough to undergo the procedure – e.g. is not stressed from too much handling and is exhibiting vital signs within normal limits.	2 a) The child/parent may be fearful of the procedure so reassurance is essential to minimise anxiety. b) For ease of procedure and accessibility. To prevent causing any undue or further stress.
3 Pour sterile water or cooled, boiled water into a sterile galipot.	3 To prevent infection from bacteria present in nonsterile water.
4 Wet sterile gauze swabs, one by one, and gently wipe across bottom lid of eye from inner to outer corner. Use one swab for each swipe and discard. Clean until discharge has been removed.	4 To avoid cross-infection between each eye.
5 Clean both eyes in this way, ensuring that separate swabs are used for each eye.	5 As above.
6 Repeat as necessary. Eye cleansing is usually carried out during hygiene/care sessions (Johnson and Taylor 2010). This will be determined by the condition of the eyes and the baby/CYP's normal routine as discussed.	6 Frequency should be individualised to each baby/CYP.
7 During eye care, assess and observe eyes for stickiness, discharge, encrustation, dryness, trauma, and redness.	7 To identify potential infection, damage, or other condition that warrants specific eye care/treatment.
Specific eye care	
1 If the above occurs, specific eye treatment is necessary. Firstly, if there is discharge or excess stickiness present, take a swab for culture and sensitivity and send to the microbiology laboratory. Consider if it may be a viral infection and take appropriate sample (see Chapter 15: Investigations).	1 For appropriate antibiotics to be commenced following culture.
2 In the presence of infection or other known disease, apply prescribed eye cream to the bottom of each eyelid, using a separate pack for each eye. Similarly, eye drops may be prescribed – one vial for each eye. Apply by gently retracting the upper and lower eyelid and dropping one drop to each eye. For more information on the administration of eye drops see Chapter 17: Administration of Medicines.	2 Eye creams may have antibiotic properties and should form part of the total eye care regimen. Having separate vials/packs avoids cross-infection between each eye. Gentle application is necessary to avoid damage to the delicate area around the eyes.
3 Eye ointment or drops should be applied in the same way to the baby / CYP who is receiving muscle relaxants or requires care for excessive dryness. In a baby/CYP who is totally immobilised, moist, lubricating gel pads can be used and replaced regularly according to recommended guidelines for use.	3 Some eye preparations are designed for lubrication of the eye to prevent dryness and corneal damage.
4 If there is discharge with persistent tearing but no infection is diagnosed, there may be a blocked tear duct (dacryostenosis). Discharge should be wiped away (as above for general cleansing) when this builds up, and the side of the nose can be gently massaged.	4 This condition is common in newborns and infants and should diminish within the first year of life.
5 If cleaning is required more than four to six times a day, antibiotics may be required.	5 Infection may be a secondary occurrence.
6 In any CYP, specific eye diseases will warrant individual care regimes as prescribed (see Box 11.2).	6 To ensure that the correct treatment is provided for the condition.

Procedure guideline 11.18 Eye care *(continued)*

Statement	Rationale
7 For eye care in relation to any of the conditions mentioned above, repeat as necessary with subsequent care sessions (Johnson and Taylor 2010) or as conditions warrants. If prescribed drops or ointments are administered, continue according to pharmacists' recommendations.	
8 When no further discharge, infection, or immobility is present, review and assess the eyes for continuing problems, discontinuing treatment on consultation with the medical team.	

Box 11.2 Eye diseases and their treatments

Eye condition	Treatment
Contagious conjunctivitis (bacterial or viral)	Antibiotics/antiviral agents will be required.
Allergic reaction resulting in redness, swelling, itching and tearing	Antihistamines or drops will be required and possibly steroids.
Stye (infection at the base of the eyelash)	Treat with warm compress and antibiotics.
Corneal abrasions	These will require lubricating and antibiotic ointment.
Trauma, chemical burns, lacerations, and cuts	These will require immediate medical attention.

Procedure guideline 11.19 Administration of eye drops

Statement	Rationale
1 Ensure that the drops have been prescribed correctly on the CYP's prescription chart.	1 To adhere to hospital drug policy.
2 Prepare the CYP and family by explaining the procedure, including information about the drops.	2 To relieve anxiety and determine the level of cooperation.
3 Liaise with the family as to how the CYP will be positioned, i.e. whether someone is needed to help hold the CYP in a safe position or if a younger child needs to be wrapped in a blanket.	3 To ensure the safety of the child and accurate instillation.
4 Ensure a separate bottle of drops is available for each eye if both eyes require treatment.	4 To prevent cross-infection.
5 Ensure the drops used are for the named CYP only and have not been used for other patients.	5 To prevent cross-infection.
6 Advise parents/carers of the importance of correct instillation.	6 To enhance their understanding of effective technique.
7 Wash your hands thoroughly.	7 To adhere to hospital infection control policy and to prevent infection.
8 Tilt the CYP's head back or lie them flat.	8 To ensure accurate instillation.
9 With your forefinger, gently pull down the lower eyelid to form a pocket.	9 To ensure accurate instillation.
10 Place the dropper close to the CYP's eye (avoid touching the eye, eye lashes, or any other surface) and administer the correct amount of drops into the lower eyelid.	10 To ensure accurate instillation.
11 Release the lower eyelid and allow the CYP to blink.	11 To ensure the whole eye is covered by the drug.
12 Wipe away any excess fluid.	12 To prevent irritation to the surrounding area.
13 If another drop or another type of drug is required repeat the same process, waiting for a few minutes before proceeding.	13 The fornix can only accommodate one drop. Extra will overspill, possibly leading to systemic absorption.
14 If an ointment is required, prepare the CYP as above and apply by squeezing a thin line of the ointment, starting at the inside corner of the eye and allow them to blink.	14 To ensure accurate administration.
15 If using drops and ointments, use the drop first then wait five minutes before applying the ointment.	15 To prevent overspill and ensure accurate administration.

Procedure guideline 11.20 Insertion of contact lenses

Statement	Rationale
1 Wash hands thoroughly.	1 To reduce risk of lens contamination.
2 Remove the lens from the case and make sure it is clean.	
3 Position the lens on the tip of the index finger of your right hand (left hand if left-handed). Make sure the lens is right side out.	3 To ensure accurate insertion.
4 Hold upper eyelid with your left hand. Pull lower lid downward with the middle finger of right hand.	4 To ensure accurate insertion.
5 Place the lens gently on the eye. If inserting a lens in a CYP's eye, you may need to push the lens under the upper lid first. The lens will naturally centre on the eye once the lids are closed.	5 To ensure accurate insertion.
6 Release lower eyelid first and then gradually release the upper eyelid.	6 To ensure lens is not blinked out.

Procedure guideline 11.21 Removal of soft contact lenses

Statement	Rationale
1 Wash your hands thoroughly.	1 To reduce risk of lens contamination.
2 Hold the upper eyelid with your left hand. Pull the lower lid downward with the middle finger of your right hand.	2 To ensure accurate removal.
3 Use the index finger and thumb of your right hand to pinch the lens gently out of the eye. To remove soft contact lenses from a young child, see directions in next section.	3 To ensure accurate removal.

Procedure guideline 11.22 Removal of gas permeable contact lenses and all contact lenses

Statement	Rationale
1 Wash your hands thoroughly.	1 To reduce risk of lens contamination.
2 Hold upper eyelid with your left hand. Pull lower lid downward with a finger or thumb of your right hand.	2 To ensure accurate removal.
3 Push both lids against globe and toward each other. The lens will be pushed out by the pressure from the lids.	3 To ensure accurate removal.

Procedure guideline 11.23 Care of contact lenses

Statement	Rationale
1 Cleaning: immediately after removing the lens from the eye, rub in the palm of the hand with cleaning solution.	1 To remove buildup of daily debris.
2 Rinsing: after cleaning the lens, rinse the lens with saline.	2 To ensure cleaning solution has been removed.
3 Disinfecting: place the clean lens in a clean lens container filled with fresh disinfecting solution to store the lens.	3 To prevent infection. The case should be cleaned, rinsed, and air-dried before new disinfecting solution is used. Contact lens cases are a common source of infection and need to be cleaned inside and out after each use.
4 Ensure that the right and left contact lenses are placed in appropriate sections of case.	4 To ensure correct lens is used.

Procedure guideline 11.24 Administration of ear drops

Statement	Rationale
1 Inform the parent/carer and CYP if they are able to understand, that you are going to administer the eardrops.	1 To obtain verbal consent for the procedure. To obtain their cooperation if they are old enough.
2 Answer any questions they may have about their eardrops.	2 To allay any worries that they may have. To address their information needs.
3 Check that the eardrops are prescribed according to local policy.	3 To minimise risk of drug error.
4 Ensure that: • The correct eardrops are prescribed. • The correct route and instructions, i.e. one or both ears are prescribed. • The correct strength is stated. • The number of drops is stated. • The frequency is stated.	4 To minimise risk of drug error.
5 Prepare the drug.	
6 Prepare the equipment to administer the drops: • Eardrops • Cotton wool or gauze swabs • A tray	
7 Prior to the procedure, wash your hands.	7 To minimise the risk of cross-infection.
8 The procedure: • Check that the name and hospital number on the CYP's identity bracelet matches that on the prescription chart and that their name is also on the bottles of drops. • Tilt the head to one side making sure the CYP is comfortable, ensuring their head is supported. • Gently pull the ear lobe out and upwards to straighten the ear canal. • Place the eardrops in the ear canal. If necessary, squeeze the bottle gently to allow the drops to fall. • Keep the head tilted for at least two minutes to allow the drops to reach the area required. • If required, repeat for the other ear. • If there is any oozing from the ear, dab it dry with the cotton wool or gauze. • Rewash hands after the eardrops have been administered.	8 To ensure the drops are given to the correct patient. Single-patient use bottles must be used to prevent cross-contamination.
9 Sign the CYP's drug prescription chart.	9 To determine responsibility for administration.
10 Record the administration of the drug in the CYP's healthcare records.	10 To maintain an accurate record.

References

Adam, R. (2008). Skin care of the nappy area. Pediatric Dermatology 25 (4): 427–433.

Adam, R., Schnetz, B., Mathey, P. et al. (2009). Clinical demonstration of skin mildness and suitability for sensitive infant skin of a new baby wipe. Pediatric Dermatology 26 (5): 506–513.

Agarwal, S., Agarwal, A., Apple, D.J., and Buratto, L. (2002). Textbook of Ophthalmology, vol. 1. Philadelphia: Lippincott Williams and Wilkins.

Allman, R.M. (1997). Pressure ulcer prevalence, incidence, risk factors and impact. Clinical Geriatric Medicine 13 (3): 421–436.

Allison, F. (2000) Nappy rash: an overview. Practice Nursing 11(17): 17-19.

Allman, R.M., Goode, P.S., Patrick, M.M. et al. (1995). Pressure ulcer risk factors among hospitalized patients with activity limitation. Journal of the American Medical Association 273 (11): 865–870.

Arrowsmith, V.A., Taylor, R. (2014). Removal of nail polish and finger rings to prevent surgical infection (Review). Cochrane Database Syst Rev. 2014 Aug 4; 2014(8):CD003325 https://pubmed.ncbi.nlm.nih.gov/25089848 (accessed 28 June 2022).

Association of the British Pharmaceutical Industry (ABPI) Medicines Compendium (2013). Summary of product characteristics for hydrocortisone cream 1%. Electronic Medicines Compendium Datapharm Communications Ltd. www.medicines.org.uk/emc/medicine/24557 (accessed 28 June 2022).

Atherton, D.J. (2004). A review of the pathophysiology, prevention and treatment of irritant nappy dermatitis. Current Medical Research and Opinion 20 (5): 645–649.

Atherton, D. (2005). Maintaining healthy skin in infancy using prevention of irritant napkin dermatitis as a model. Community Practitioner 78 (7): 255–257.

Atherton, D.J. (2009). Managing healthy skin for babies. Infant 5 (4): 130–132.

Atherton, D. and Mill, K. (2004). What can be done to keep babies' skin healthy? RCM Midwives 7 (7): 288–290.

Baer, E.L., Davies, M., Easterbrook, K. (2006). Disposable nappies for preventing nappy rash in babies and infants. http://www.cochrane.org/CD004262/SKIN_diposable-nappies-for-preventing-nappy-rash-in-babies-and-infants (accessed 28 June 2022).

Bakker, E., van Gool, J.D., van Sprundel, M. et al. (2002). Results of a questionnaire evaluating the effects of different methods of toilet training on achieving bladder control. British Journal of Urology 90: 456–461.

Barone, J.G., Jasutkar, N., and Schneider, D. (2009). Later toilet training is associated with urge incontinence in children. Journal of Pediatric Urology 5 (6): 458–461.

Bartlett, J.D. and Jaanes, S.D. (2008). Clinical Ocular Pharmacology, 5e. Oxford: Butterworth Heineman.

Bauer, K. (2005). Effects of positioning and handling on preterm infants in the neonatal intensive care unit. In: Research on Early Developmental Care for Preterm Neonates (eds. J. Sizun and J.V. Browne). Paris: John Libbey Eurotext.

Behring, A., Vezeau, T.M., and Fink, R. (2003). Timing of the newborn first bath: a replication. Neonatal network. The Journal of Neonatal Nursing 22 (1): 39–46.

Bergstrom, A., Byaruhanga, R., and Okong, P. (2005). The impact of newborn bathing on the prevalence of neonatal hypothermia in Uganda: a randomized, controlled trial. Acta Paediatrica 94 (10): 1462–1467.

Blincoe, A.J. (2005). Cleansing and caring for the skin of neonates. British Journal of Midwifery 13 (4): 244–247.

Blincoe, A.J. (2006a). Protecting neonatal skin: cream or water. British Journal of Midwifery 14 (12): 731–732, 734.

Blincoe, A.J. (2006b). Caring for neonatal skin and common infant skin problems. British Journal of Midwifery 14 (4): 213–216.

Borkowski, S. (2004). Nappy rash care and management. Pediatric Nursing 30 (6): 467–470.

Boucke, L. (2003). Infant Potty Basics. Lafayette, CO: White-Boucke Publishing.

Boxwell, G. (2010). Neonatal Intensive Care Nursing, 2e. London: Routledge.

Boyd, S. (2003). Hands that rock the cradle: nail hygiene in the NICU. Journal of Neonatal Nursing 9 (2): 41–44.

British Dental Health Foundation (2022). http://www.dentalhealth.org (accessed 4 July 2022).

British Medical Association (BMA)/Royal Pharmaceutical Society of Great Britain (RPSGB) (2010) Pharmaceutical Press; 59th revised edition.Butler, C.T. (2006). Pediatric skin care: guidelines for assessment, prevention and treatment. Pediatric Nursing 32 (5): 443–450.

Butler, R.J. and Heron, J. (2008). The prevalence of infrequent bedwetting and nocturnal enuresis in childhood: a large British cohort. Scandinavian Journal of Urology and Nephrology 42: 257–264.

Camm, J. (2006). Skincare for newborns: guidelines and advice. RCM Midwives 9: 126.

Campbell, S.T., Evans, M.A., and Mactavish, F. (1995). Paediatric Oncology Nursing Forum Guidelines for Mouth Care. London: Royal College of Nursing.

Cleveland, J. (2008). Parenting in the neonatal intensive care unit. Journal of Obstetric, Gynecologic, and Neonatal Nursing 37 (6): 666–691.

Cochrane Oral Health Group (2022). International oral healthcare guideline repository. https://oralhealth.cochrane.org/international-oral-health-guideline-repository (accessed 28 June 2022).

College of Optometrists (2014). A survey of UK contact lens practice for children and young people. Optometry in Practice 15(3).

Cooper, P. (2000). The use of Clinisan in the skin care of the incontinent patient. British Journal of Nursing 9 (7): 445–448.

Coughlin, C., Eichenfield, L.F., and Frieden, I. (2014). Diaper dermatitis: clinical characteristics and differential diagnosis, Pediatric Dermatology 31 (S1): 19–24.

Coutts, L. and Hardy, L. (1995). Teaching for Health, 2e. Edinburgh: Churchill Livingstone.

Coyne, I., Neill, F., and Timmins, F. (2010). Clinical Skills in Childrens Nursing. Oxford: OUP.

Cullum N. Deeks J. Sheldon TA. Song F. Fletcher AW. (2000). Beds, mattresses and cushions for preventing and treating pressure sores (Cochrane Review (2):CD001735.). Oxford, Cochrane Library Issue 1. http://www.ncbi.nlm.nih.gov/pubmed/10796662 (accessed 28 June 2022).

Daly, B., Watt, R., Batchelor, P., and Treasure, E. (2002). Essential Dental Public Health. Oxford: Oxford University Press.

Davis, L., Mohay, H., and Edwards, H. (2003). Mothers involvement in caring for their premature infants: an historical overview. Journal of Advanced Nursing 42 (6): 578–586.

Department of Health (DH) (2004a). Choosing Health: Making Healthy Choices Easier – Executive Summary. London: Department of Health.

Department of Health (DH) (2004b). NHS Dentistry: Delivering Change –Report by the Chief Dental Officer (England) July. London: Department of Health.

Department of Health (DH) (2007). Valuing people's Oral Health: A Good Practice Guidance for Improving the Oral Health of Disabled Children and Adults. London: Department of Health.

Department of Health(DH)/British Association for the Study of Community Dentisty, 2 (2014, April). Delivering better oral health. from An evidence based toolkit for prevention, https://www.gov.uk/government/publications/delivering-better-oral-health-an-evidence-based-toolkit-for-prevention (accessed 28 June 2022).

Department of Health (DH) (2011). High impact intervention Care bundle to prevent surgical site infection. www.cmccn.nhs.uk/files/7614/1381/8478/high-impact-intervention-no4.pdf (accessed 4 July 2022).

Devalia, U., Tomlinson, S., Lau, K., Bolooki, H., Johnson King, O., Liu, C. (2019). Mini mouthcare matters. A guide for hospital healthcare professionals. NHS Health Education England. http://mouthcarematters.hee.nhs.uk/wp-content/uploads/sites/6/2020/01/MINI-MCM-GUIDE-2019-final.pdf (accessed 28 June 2022).

Dewar, G. (2010). The right potty training age; what's best for your child. http://parentingscience.com/potty-training-age.html (17 September 2018).

Dunn, P.M. (2009). Managing the umbilical cord at birth. Infant 5 (3): 73.

Eilers, J., Berger, A.M., and Petersen, M.C. (1988). Development, testing, and application of the oral assessment guide. Oncology Nursing Forum 15 (3): 325–330.

Ellis, J. (2005). Neonatal hypothermia. Journal of Neonatal Nursing 11: 76–82.

European Pressure Ulcer Advisory Panel (EPUAP) (2019). Pressure Ulcer Prevention Guidelines, 3e. Oxford: EPUAP. www.epuap.org (accessed 4 July 2022).

Fellows, P. (2010). Management of thermal stability. In: Neonatal Intensive Care Nursing, 2e (ed. G. Boxwell), 86–112. London: Routledge.

Foster, H. and Fitzgerald, J. (2005). Dental disease in children with chronic illness. Archives of Disease in Childhood 90 (7): 703–708.

Franck, L., Quinn, D., and Zahr, L. (2000). Effect of less frequent bathing of preterm infants on skin flora and pathogen colorization. Journal of Obstetric, Gynecologic, and Neonatal Nursing 29 (6): 584–589.

Gardner, S.L., Carter, B.S., Enzman-Hines, M.I., and Hernandez, J.A. (2010). Merenstein and Gardners Handbook of Neonatal Intensive Care, 7e. St Louis: Mosby.

Gibbons, W., Shanks, H.T., Kleinhelter, P., and Jones, P. (2006). Eliminating facility-acquired pressure ulcers at Ascension health. Joint Commission Journal on Quality and Patient Safety 32 (9): 488–496.

Gibson, F. and Nelson, W. (2000). Mouth care for children with cancer. Paediatric Nurse 12 (1): 18–22.

Gibson, F., Horsford, J., and Nelson, W. (1997). Oral care: practice reconsidered within a framework of action research. Journal of Cancer Nursing 1 (4): 183–190.

Gibson, F., Cargill, J., Allison, J. et al. (2006). Establishing content validity of the oral assessment guide in children and young people. European Journal of Cancer 42 (12): 1817–1825.

Gibson, F., Auld, E.M., Bryan, G. et al. (2010). A systematic review of oral assessment instruments. Cancer Nursing 33 (4): E1–E19.

Great Ormond Street Hospital for Children (GOSH) (2016). Looking after your child's skin during a hospital stay. http://www.gosh.nhs.uk/medical-information/procedures-and-treatments/looking-after-your-childs-skin-during-a-hospital-stay (accessed 21 February 2022).

Great Ormond Street Hospital for Children (GOSH) (2017) Tooth Decay Information. http://www.gosh.nhs.uk/medical-information/search-medical-conditions/tooth-decay (accessed 21 February 2022).

Groeneveld, A., Anderson, M., Allen, S. et al. (2004). The prevalence of pressure ulcers in a tertiary care pediatric and adult hospital. Journal of Wound, Ostomy, and Continence Nursing 31 (3): 108–120.

Hale, R. (2007). Protecting neonates' delicate skin. British Journal of Midwifery 15 (4): 231–232, 234–235.

Hewitt, D. (2000). Child-centred care; ethno friendly or ethnocentric? Paediatric Nursing 12 (6): 6–8.

Hoath, S.B. (1997). The stickiness of newborn skin: bioadhesion and the epidermal barrier. Journal of Pediatrics 131: 338–346.

Hockenberry, M.J. and Wilson, D. (2010). Wong's Nursing Care of Infants and Children, 9e. St Louis: Mosby.

Hopkins, J. (2004). Essentials of newborn skin care. British Journal of Midwifery 12 (5): 314–317.

Horn, I.B., Brenner, R., Rao, M., and Cheng, T.L. (2006). Beliefs about the appropriate age for initiating toilet training: are their racial and socioeconomic differences? Journal of Pediatrics 149: 165–168.

Ilex Health (2013). Ilex Skin Protectant. https://ilexhealthproducts.com/collections/ilex-skin-protection (accessed 28 June 2022).

Irving, V. (2001). Caring for and protecting the skin of preterm neonates. Journal of Wound Care 10: 253–256.

Irving, V., Bethell, E., and Burton, F. (2006). Neonatal wound care – Minimising trauma and pain. Journal of Wound Care 2 (1): 33–41.

Jackson, A. (2008). Time to review neonatal skin care. Infant 4 (5): 166–168.

Johnson, R. and Taylor, W. (2010). Skills in Midwifery Practice, 3e. Edinburgh: Churchill Livingstone.

Joint Formulary Committee (2020). BNF 79 (British National Formulary). March–September. London: Pharmaceutical Press.

Jones, K. (2000). Baby skincare wipes pass no more tears mildness test. British Journal of Midwifery 8 (9): 577–580.

Jordan, W.E., Lawson, K.D., Berg, R.W. et al. (1986). Nappy dermatitis: frequency and severity among a general infant population. Pediatric Dermatology 3 (3): 198–207.

Khurana, S., Whit Hall, R., and Anand, K.J.S. (2005). Treatment of pain and stress in the neonate. NeoReviews 6 (2): e76.

Kipps, S., Maxwell, J. (2013). Head, shoulders and heels. A multimodal approach to the reduction of pressure ulcers in infants, children and young people. Poster presentation, European Pressure Ulcer Advisory Panel conference, Vienna.

Knobel, R. and Holditch-Davis, D. (2007). Thermoregulation and heat loss prevention after birth and during neonatal intensive-care unit stabilization of extremely low-birthweight infants. Journal of Obstetric, Gynecologic, and Neonatal Nursing 36: 280–287.

Lack, G., Fox, D., Northstone, K., and Golding, J. (2003). Factors associated with the development of peanut allergy in childhood. New England Journal of Medicine 348 (11): 977–985.

Lawson, L.G. (2001). Handwashing: a neonatal perspective. Journal of Neonatal Nursing 7 (2): 42–46.

Levine, R. and Stillman-Lowe, C. (2009). The Scientific Basis of Oral Health Education, 6e. London: British Dental Journal/British Dental Association.

Lloyd, S. (1992). Brushing up on children's mouth care. Professional Care of Mother and Child 2 (1): 16–17.

Lloyd, S. (1994). Teaching parents to look after children's teeth. Professional Care of Mother and Child 4 (2): 34–36.

Madeya, M.L. (1996). Oral complications from cancer therapy: part 2-nursing implications for assessment and treatment. Oncology Nurses Forum 23 (5): 808–820.

Mainstone, A. (2005). Maintaining infant skin health and hygiene. British Journal of Midwifery 13 (1): 44–47.

Mancini, A.J. (2004). Skin. Pediatrics 113 (4): 1114–1119.

Maxwell, J., Sinclair, D. (2012). Treatment of moisture related lesions in children. hr.247printhub.com/downloads/proshield/hrprc006.pdf (accessed 28 June 2022).

McGurk, V., Holloway, B., and Crutchley, A. (2004). Skin integrity assessment in neonates and children. Paediatric Nursing 16 (3): 15–18.

McInnes E., Jammali-Blasi, A., Bell-Syer, S.E.M., Dumville, J.C., Middleton, V., Cullum, N. (2015). Support surfaces for pressure ulcer prevention. Cochrane Database of Systematic Reviews. https://www.cochranelibrary.com/cdsr/doi/10.1002/14651858.CD001735.pub5/full (accessed 28 June 2022).

Medves, J.M. and O'Brien, B. (2004). The effect of bather and location of first bath on maintaining thermal stability in newborns. Journal of Obstetric, Gynecologic, and Neonatal Nursing 33 (2): 175–182.

Medicines and Healthcare Regulatory Agency (MHRA) (2012). Oral swabs with a foam head – heads may detach during use MDA/2012/020. MHRA: London. https://www.gov.uk/drug-device-alerts/medical-device-alert-oral-swabs-with-a-foam-head-heads-may-detach-during-use (accessed 28 June 2022).

Merrill, L. (2015). Prevention, treatment and parent education for diaper dermatitis. Nursing for Women's Health 19 (4): 324–336.

Moralejo, D. and Jull, A. (2003). Hand rubbing with an alcohol based solution reduced healthcare workers' hand contamination more than hand washing with antiseptic soap. Evidence-Based Nursing 6 (2): 54.

Mota, D.M. and Barros, A.J. (2008). Toilet training; methods, parental expectations and associated dysfunctions. Journal of Pediatrics 64 (1): 9–17.

Moynihan, P.J. (2002). Dietary advice in dental practice. British Dental Journal 193: 563–568.

NHS (2013). Healthy body; children's teeth. https://www.nhs.uk/live-well/healthy-teeth-and-gums/taking-care-of-childrens-teeth/ (accessed 28 June 2022).

National Institute for Health and Care Excellence (NICE) (2004). Dental Recall: Recall Interval between Routine Dental Examinations, Clinical Guideline 19. London: National Institute of Clinical Excellence.

National Institute for Health and Care Excellence (NICE) (2010a). Constipation in children and young people: diagnosis and management. Clinical guideline 99. London NICE. (updated 2017). www.nice.org.uk/guidance/CG99 (accessed 28 June 2022).

National Institute for Health and Care Excellence (NICE) (2010b). Bedwetting in under 19s. Clinical guideline [CG111]. www.nice.org.uk/guidance/cg111 (accessed 28 June 2022).

National Institute for Health and Care Excellence (NICE) (2014). Pressure ulcers: prevention and management. Clinical guideline [CG179]. www.nice.org.uk/guidance/cg179 (accessed 28 June 2022).

National Institute for Health and Care Excellence (NICE) (2015). Pressure ulcers. NICE quality standard [QS89]. www.nice.org.uk/guidance/qs89 (accessed 28 June 2022).

National Institute for Health and Care Excellence (NICE) (2020). Clinical knowledge summaries; Nappy rash http://cks.nice.org.uk/nappy-rash/ (accessed 28 June 2022).

National Institute for Health and Care Excellence (NICE) (2019). Surgical site infections: Prevention and treatment. NICE Clinical Guideline 125. NICE. London www.nice.org.uk/guidance/ng125 (accessed 4 July 2022).

National Institute for Health and Care Excellence (NICE) (2022). Scenario: Adults and young people (not immunocompromised). London, National Institute of Health and Care Excellence. https://cks.nice.org.uk/topics/candida-oral/managment/adults-young-people-not-immunocompromised/ (accessed 4 July 2022)

National Pharmacy Association. (2020). SOP: Supplying Paraffin-Based and Paraffin-Free Products. https://www.npa.co.uk/information-and-guidance/supplying-paraffin-based-skin-products/(accessed 28 June 2022).

National Pressure Ulcer Advisory Panel, European Pressure Ulcer Advisory Panel and Pan Pacific Pressure Injury Alliance (NPUAP/EPUAP/PPPUIA) (2014). Prevention and Treatment of Pressure Ulcers: Quick Reference Guide (ed. E. Haesler). Osborne Park, Australia: Cambridge Media http://www.epuap.org/wp-content/uploads/2016/10/quick-reference-guide-digital-npuap-epuap-pppia-jan2016.pdf (accessed 5 July 2022).

Ndawula, E. and Brown, L. (1990). Matresses as reservoirs of epidemic methicillin-resistant staphylococcus aureus. Lancet 337: 448.

Nelson, W., Gibson, F., Hayden, S., and Morgan, N. (2001). Using action research in paediatric oncology to develop an oral care algorithm. European Journal of Oncology Nursing 5 (3): 180–189.

Noonan, C., Quigley, S., and Curley, M.A. (2011). Using the Braden Q scale to predict pressure ulcer risk in paediatric patients. Journal of Pediatric Nursing 26 (6): 566–575. https://doi.org/10.1016/j.pedn.2010.07.006.

Oakley, A., and Gomez, J. (2017). Napkin dermatitis. DermNet NZ. httsp://dermnetnz.org/topics/napkin-dermatitis (accessed 4 July 2022).

Odio, M., Streicher-Scott, J., and Hansen, R.C. (2001). The interactive newborn bath: using infant neurobehaviour to correct parents and newborns. The American Journal of Maternal and Child Nursing 24 (6): 280–286.

Paediatric Formulary Committee (2022). British National Formulary for children. https://bnfc.nice.org.uk/about/paediatric-formulary-committee/ (accessed 2022).

Paige, D.G., Gennery, A.R., and Cant, A.J. (2010). The neonate. In: Rook's Textbook of Dermatology, 8e (eds. T. Burns, S. Breathnach, N. Cox and C. Griffiths), 17.1–17.85. Chichester: Wiley-Blackwell.

Paediatric Continence Forum (2014). Paediatric continence commissioning guide – A handbook for the commissioning and running of paediatric continence services. http://www.paediatriccontinenceforum.org/wp-content/uploads/2013/09/PCF-Commissioning-Guidance-for-NICE-11-August-2014-Final.pdf (accessed 4 July 2022).

Parnham, A. (2012). Pressure ulcer risk assessment and prevention in children. Nursing Children and Young People 24 (2): 24–29.

Pearson, L.S. and Hutton, J.L. (2002). A controlled trial to compare the ability of foam swabs and toothbrushes to remove dental plaque. Journal of Advanced Nursing 39 (5): 480–489.

Peate, F. and Whiting, P. (2006). Caring for Children and Families. Chichester: Wiley.

Philipp, R., Hughs, P., and Golding, J. (1997). Getting to the bottom of nappy rash. British Journal of General Practice 47 (421): 493–497.

POPPY Parents of Premature babies Project (2009). We Were there… Parents' Experiences of Having a Premature Baby. London: NCT.

Prasad, H.R., Srivastava, P., and Verma, K.K. (2003). Nappy dermatitis – an overview. Indian Journal of Pediatrics 70 (8): 635–637.

Price, S. (2000). A practical guide to preventing and treating nappy rash. British Journal of Midwifery 8 (11): 702–704.

Public Health England (2017). Delivering better oral health: an evidence-based toolkit for prevention. https://www.gov.uk/government/publications/delivering-better-oral-health-an-evidence-based-toolkit-for-prevention (accessed 4 July 2022).

Quinn, D., Newton, N., and Piecuch, R. (2005). Effect of less frequent bathing on premature infant skin. Journal of Obstetric, Gynecologic, and Neonatal Nursing 34 (6): 741–746.

Quigley, S.M. and Curley, M.A. (1996). Skin integrity in the pediatric population: preventing and managing pressure ulcers. Journal of Society Pediatric Nursing 1 (1): 7–18.

Ravanfar, P., Wallace, J.S., and Pace, N.C. (2012). Nappy dermatitis: a review and update. Current Opinion in Pediatrics 24 (4): 472–479.

Rhodes, C. (2000). Effective management of daytime wetting. Paediatric Nursing 12 (2): 14–17.

Rigby, D. (2001). Integrated continence services. Nursing Standard 16 (8): 46–55.

Robinson, P.G., Deacon, S.A., Deery, C. et al. (2005). Manual versus powered toothbrushing for oral health. Cochrane Database of Systematic Reviews 2 (CD002281): 1–68.

Rogers, J.M. (2000). Promoting continence; the child with special needs. Paediatric Nursing 12 (4): 37–42.

Rogers, J.M. (2002). Learning disability nursing; continence care award; solving the enigma: toilet training children with learning disabilities. British Journal of Nursing 11 (14): 958–962.

Royal College of Nursing (2005) Pressure ulcer risk assessment and prevention: clinical practice guidelines.

Sanders, C. (2002). Choosing continence products for children. Nursing Standard 16 (32): 39–43.

Scardillo, J. and Aronovitch, S.A. (1999). Successfully managing incontinence-related irritant dermatitis across the lifespan. Ostomy/Wound Management 45 (4): 36–44.

Scheinfeld, N. (2005). Nappy dermatitis; a review and brief survey of eruptions of the nappy area. American Journal of Dermatology 6 (5): 273–281.

Schmidt, B.A. (2004). Toilet training: getting it right the first time. Contemporary Pediatrics 21: 105–119.

Scottish Intercollegiate Guidelines Network (SIGN) (2014) Dental interventions to prevent caries in children. A national clinical guideline. http://www.scottishdental.org/wp-content/uploads/2014/04/SIGN138.pdf (accessed 4 July 2022).

Scottish Dental Clinical Effectiveness Programme (SDCEP) (2018). Prevention and Management of Dental Caries in Children, 2nd Edition. Edinburgh: https://www.sdcep.org.uk/published-guidance/caries-in-children/ (accessed 4 July 2022).

Schum, T.R., Kolb, T.M., McAuliffe, T.L. et al. (2002). Sequential acquisition of toilet-training skills: a descriptive study of gender and age differences in normal children. Pediatrics 109 (3): 48–54.

Sherman, T.I., Greenspan, J.S., St Clair, N. et al. (2006). Optimising the neonatal thermal environment. Neonatal Network 25 (4): 251–260.

Simpson, L. (2001). Indwelling urethral catheters. Nursing Standard 15 (46): 47–54.

Stokowski, L.A. (2006). Neonatal skin: back to nature? Midwifery Today 78: 34–35.

Tennant S. (2010) Toilet training more beneficial when started early. Urology Times, April, 22–25.

Thomas, K.A. (2003a). Preterm infant thermal responses to care giving differ by incubator control mode. Journal of Perinatology 23 (8): 640–645.

Thomas, K.A. (2003b). Infant weight and gestational age effects on thermoneutrality in the home environment. Journal of Obstetric, Gynecologic, and Neonatal Nursing 32 (6): 745–752.

Thurgood, G. (1994). Nurse maintenance of oral hygiene. British Journal of Nursing 3 (7): 332–353.

Tollin, M., Bergsson, G., Kai-Larsen, Y. et al. (2005). Vernix caseosa as a multicomponent defence system based on polypeptides, lipids and their interactions. Cellular and Molecular Life Sciences 62 (19–20): 2390–2399.

Tortora, G.J. and Derrikson, B.H. (2013). Principles of Anatomy and Physiology, 14e. Chichester: Wiley.

Tran, C., Medhurst, A., and OConnell, B. (2009). Support needs of parents of sick and/or preterm infants admitted to a neonatal unit. Neonatal, Paediatric and Child Health Nursing 12 (2): 12–17.

Trigg, E. and Mohammed, T.A. (2006). Practices in children's Nursing – Guidelines for Hospital and Community, 2e. Edinburgh: Churchill Livingstone.

Trotter, S. (2004). Care of the newborn: proposed new guidelines. British Journal of Midwifery 12 (3): 152–157.

Trotter, S. (2006). Neonatal skincare: why change is vital. RCM Midwives Journal 9 (4): 134–138.

Trotter, S. (2007a). Baby products – it's all in the labelling. MIDIRS Midwifery Digest 17 (2): 263–266.

Trotter, S. (2007b). Baby Care – Back to Basics & Trade. TIPS Limited Scotland.

Trotter, S. (2008). Neonatal skin and cord care – the way forward. Nursing Practice 40: 40–45.

Turnbull and Petty (2013). Evidence-based thermal care of low birthweight neonates. Part two: family-centred care principles. Nursing Children and Young People, 25 (3): 26–29.

Turner, A. (2000). Healthy infant skin: focus on nappy rash and sensitive skin. British Journal of Midwifery 8 (5): 306–310.

UKCCSG-PONF Mouth Care Group (2006). Mouth care for children and young people with cancer: evidence-based guidelines. https://www.cclg.org.uk/write/MediaUploads/Members%20area/Treatment%20guidelines/Mouth-Care-at-a-Glance.pdf (accessed 4 July 2022).

Visscher, M.O., Chatterjee, R., Ebel, J.P. et al. (2002). Biomedical assessment and instrumental evaluation of healthy infant skin. Pediatric Dermatology 19 (6): 473–481.

Waldron, S. and MacKinnon, R. (2007). Neonatal thermoregulation. Infant 3 (3): 101–104.

Walker, L., Downe, S., and Gomez, L. (2005a). Skin care in the well-term newborn: two systematic reviews. Birth 32 (3): 224–228.

Walker, L., Downe, S., and Gomez, L. (2005b). A survey of soap and skin care product provision for well term neonates. British Journal of Midwifery 13 (12): 768–772.

Walsh, T., Worthington, H.V., Glenny, A. et al. (2019). Fluoride toothpastes of different concentrations for preventing dental caries. Cochrane Systematic Review. https://doi.org/10.1002/14651858.CD007868.pub3.

Watson, R. (2000). Anatomy and Physiology for Nurses, 11e. London: Baillière Tindall.

Watson, R. (2005). Anatomy and Physiology for Nurses, 12e. London: Baillière Tindall.

Watt, R.G. and McGlone, P. (2003). Prevention. Part 2. Dietary advice in the dental surgery. British Dental Journal 195: 27–31.

Waugh, A. and Grant, A. (2001). The Digestive System Waugh a Grant a in: Anatomy and Physiology in Health and Illness. Edinburgh: Churchill Livingstone.

World Health Organisation (2009). WHO Guidelines on Hand Hygiene in Health Care. https://www.org.int/publications/i/item/9789241597906 (accessed 4 July 2022).

Wounds UK (2013). Pressure ulcer prevention in the acute setting: using AdermaTM in practice. Wounds UK, 2013; https://www.smith-nephew.com/global/assets/pdf/products/wound/approved%20aderma%20in%20practice%20wounds%20uk%20nov%202012%20final.pdf (accessed 4 July 2022).

Williams, C. (2001). 3M Cavilon durable barrier cream in skin problem management. British Journal of Nursing 10 (7): 469–472.

Willock, J., Baharestani, M.M., and Anthony, D. (2009). The development of the Glamorgan paediatric pressure ulcer risk assessment scale. Journal of Wound Care 18 (1): 17–21.

Wilson, E., Trivedi, R., and Pandey, S.K. (2005). Pediatric Cataract Surgery; Techniques, Complications and Management. Philadelphia: Lippincott Williams and Wilkins.

Wu, H.Y. (2010). Achieving urinary continence in children. Nature Reviews Urology 7 (7): 371–377.

Zsolway, K., Harrison, A., and Honig, P. (2002). Nappy rash in a young infant. Pediatric Case Reviews 2 (4): 220–225.

Zupan J, Gardner P, Omari AA. (2004). Topical umbilical cord care at birth. Cochrane Review, Issue 3, Oxford, update software.

Chapter 12

Immunisation

Helen Bedford

RN (Adult), RHV, PhD, MSc (Nursing Studies), BSc Nursing (Hons), FFPH, FRCPCH, Professor of Children's Health, UCL Great Ormond Street Institute of Child Health, London, UK

Chapter contents

Introduction	202
Routine immunisation schedule for CYPs in the UK	202
Special risk groups	203
Immunity	203
Types of vaccine	204
General considerations	204
Specific diseases and the vaccines	206
Vaccines not in general use in UK	213
Storage and administration of vaccines	213
Ensuring good uptake	213
Vaccine safety scares	214
Immunisation of healthcare workers	214
Conclusion	215
References	215
Further reading	216

Procedure guideline

12.1 Administration of vaccines — 205

Introduction

This chapter focuses on vaccines included in the UK childhood routine vaccination schedule. COVID-19 vaccines for children and young people are not covered due to the rapidly changing nature of recommendations for vaccination against SARS-CoV-2. For guidance see https://www.gov.uk/government/publications/covid-19-the-green-book-chapter-14a. Immunisation has proved to be one of the most successful public health interventions. In countries with effective immunisation programmes there has been a significant decline in the incidence of vaccine-preventable infectious diseases. Globally, smallpox was declared eradicated in 1979. Huge progress has been made toward achieving the goal of worldwide eradication of poliomyelitis, with the disease remaining endemic in only two countries: Afghanistan and Pakistan (The Global Polio Eradication Initiative 2020). Unfortunately, further progress is currently being hampered by conflict in these and other previously polio-free countries. In Finland, where a two-dose policy of measles, mumps, and rubella (MMR) vaccine has been in place since 1982, indigenous measles was eliminated in 1996 and mumps and rubella in 1997 (Peltola et al. 2008). In the UK, high uptake of childhood vaccines has resulted in an all-time low incidence of most vaccine-preventable diseases with some remarkable achievements. Within a few years of introducing the new conjugate vaccines, Haemophilus influenzae type b (Hib) in 1991 and meningococcal C (MenC) in 1999, there was a dramatic decline in invasive disease caused by these organisms (Campbell et al. 2009; Collins et al. 2013). Based on an analysis of notifiable diseases in US cities and states from 1888 to 2011 it was reported that since vaccines were introduced, about 35 million cases of measles and 103 million cases of diphtheria, tetanus, and pertussis combined have been prevented in the United States (Van Panhuis et al. 2013). This confirms the significance of immunisation as the most effective and cost-effective public health intervention after the provision of clean water.

Perhaps ironically, this reduction in childhood infectious disease has created new challenges and has led some parents/carers and professionals, who no longer have routine experience of the diseases, to question the value of immunisation and focus more on the risks attached to vaccines rather than on the complications of disease. This has resulted in some parents/carers rejecting specific vaccines (Campbell et al. 2017) or being hesitant about the vaccination decision (Larson et al. 2014). This is a cause for concern and vaccine safety scares in the past such as the debacle over the safety of MMR vaccine triggered by a now-discredited study which was widely interpreted as showing a link between MMR vaccine and development of autism and bowel disease, provide a sharp reminder of how a dent in the confidence of vaccines can result in a rapid decline in vaccine uptake, followed by a resurgence of disease. All professionals involved in giving immunisations should be fully informed of the benefits and, where they exist, the side effects of vaccines, so that they can advise parents/carers appropriately. The actual administration of the vaccine is only a minor part of the process. The overwhelming majority of vaccines in the UK are given in the community setting, primarily by practice nurses, school nurses, immunisation teams, and some health visitors. However, hospital staff must be familiar with the routine schedule, indications, contraindications, and current issues, as they will often be asked for advice by parents/carers. It should also be standard practice for staff to review the immunisation status of children and young people (CYPs) seen in Accident and Emergency and outpatients' departments, as well as those admitted. For some children, often the most vulnerable, this will provide an important opportunity to catch up on incomplete immunisations or remind parents/carers that further immunisations are due and to advise primary care accordingly (Walton et al. 2007; Gandhi et al. 2011). The UK has a highly organised and successful vaccination programme for CYPs, but frequent developments can make it challenging to keep up to date. Promoting immunisation should be a core component for all those involved in the provision of children's healthcare.

Routine immunisation schedule for CYPs in the UK

The routine schedule in the UK is based on advice from the Joint Committee on Vaccination and Immunisation (JCVI) and published in the online publication 'Immunisation Against Infectious Diseases' (*The Green Book*) by the UK Health Security Agency (2020a), previously Public Health England, and letters from the Chief Medical Officer (CMO) and Chief Nursing Officer (CNO), see Table 12.1. There have been significant changes to the routine schedule in the past decade. These include the introduction of new vaccine programmes: rotavirus vaccine (2013), routine influenza vaccine (2014), meningococcal B vaccine (2015), hepatitis B (2017), and HPV for boys (2019) and also, changes to the number and timing of doses of some vaccines. As changes to the schedule are made regularly it is important to always check the latest guidance on the UK Health Security Agency immunisation website (https://www.gov.uk/government/collections/immunisation).

Table 12.1 Routine immunisation schedule for CYPs in the UK (UK Health Security Agency 2022a).

Age due	Vaccines offered	How given
8 weeks	Diphtheria, tetanus, pertussis, polio, Haemophilus influenzae type b, hepatitis B (DTaP/IPV/Hib/HepB)	One injection
	Meningococcal B	One injection
	Rotavirus vaccine	By mouth
12 weeks	DTaP/IPV/Hib/HepB	One injection
	Pneumococcal vaccine (PCV)	One injection
	Rotavirus	By mouth
16 weeks	DTaP/IPV/Hib/HepB	One injection
	Meningococcal B	One injection
12–13 months	Hib/MenC	One injection
	Meningococcal B	One injection
	PCV	One injection
	Measles, mumps, and rubella (MMR)	One injection
Annually from 2 years	Influenza	Nasal spray
Three years four months or soon after	DTaP/IPV	One injection
	MMR	One injection
12–13 years (girls and boys)	Human papillomavirus vaccine (HPV)	One injection (two doses at least six months apart)
Around 14 years	dT/IPV	One injection
	MenACWY	One injection

Special risk groups

Some CYPs with chronic disorders are at increased risk of complications from infectious diseases. Not only is it important that they receive the 'routine' vaccines, but they may also require extra doses of these, as well as vaccines not given universally. Table 12.2 indicates the conditions where this applies. For more details see Chapter 7 of the *Green Book* (UK Health Security Agency 2020).

In addition, bacillus Calmette-Guerin (BCG) is indicated for:

- All infants born in areas where the incidence of TB is 40 per 100 000 or greater.
- Children whose parents/carers or grandparents were born in a country with a high incidence of TB.
- Previously unvaccinated new immigrants from a high prevalence country.

Extra doses of hepatitis B vaccine are indicated for:

- Children born to women who are carriers of hepatitis B virus or who had acute hepatitis B infection during pregnancy require additional doses of hepatitis B vaccine.

Some occupational groups and some people with particular lifestyles may also need extra vaccines. In particular, healthcare workers (HCWs) should have influenza and hepatitis B vaccines, and chickenpox vaccine, if not already immune. Pertussis vaccine is also indicated in some groups of HCWs (UK Health Security Agency 2019). More details regarding all indications are available in the online *Green Book* (UK Health Security Agency 2020).

Immunity

For almost as long as diseases have been studied, it has been noted that there are some diseases that very rarely recur in the same person. After the first attack, the body seems to become immune. This is due to the presence of primed memory cells that are able to respond rapidly to a second attack so that the causative organism cannot multiply and produce the disease. Immunity from infection can be induced by either active or passive means.

Passive immunity

Passive immunity follows when an injection of preformed antibodies is administered or a baby acquires antibodies transplacentally. Injected antibodies are usually in the form of an immunoglobulin preparation derived from the plasma of individuals who have either encountered a particular infection or who have been vaccinated. The immunity acquired is immediate but short lasting, usually three to six months. A number of forms of immunoglobulin are available:

- Human normal immunoglobulin – given to immunosuppressed individuals in contact with measles
- Specific immunoglobulins against:
  - Herpes zoster; given to pregnant women, some neonates and immunosuppressed individuals after exposure to chicken pox
  - Hepatitis B, rabies, and tetanus; given to normal individuals after exposure to these infections.
  - RSV monoclonal antibodies; given to infants at risk of severe complications of bronchiolitis. This is produced using recombinant DNA techniques.

Further details can be obtained from UK Health Security Agency (UK Health Security Agency 2022b).

Active immunity

Active immunity results when the body is stimulated by an antigen to produce antibodies and/or memory cells specific to a particular infection. This may be achieved either by natural infection or by immunisation. Although the protection against future disease acquired from natural infection may in a few cases be greater than that from a vaccine, the disadvantage is that it puts an individual at risk from the complications of disease and may even result in death. When a vaccine is administered it stimulates the production of memory cells and usually antibodies. If the organism is encountered, immunological memory enables the body to produce antibodies or

Table 12.2 Additional vaccines recommended for individuals with chronic conditions.

Condition	Haemophilus influenzae type b	Hepatitis A	Hepatitis B	Influenza	Meningococcal	Pneumococcal
Asplenia or dysfunction of the spleen (including sickle cell and coeliac disease)	+			+	+	+
Cerebrospinal fluid leaks						+
Chronic heart disease				+		+
Chronic kidney disease (including haemodialysis patients)			+	+		+
Chronic liver disease		+	+	+		+
Chronic neurological disease				+		+
Chronic respiratory disease				+		+
Cochlear implants						+
Complement disorders (including those receiving complement inhibitor therapy)	+				+	+
Diabetes				+		+
Haemophilia		+	+			
Immunosuppression				+		+
Morbid obesity				+		

cells specific to that infection, which then neutralise the infecting organisms or their toxin. Active immunity is usually long lasting, although a booster may be required at intervals following some killed vaccines such as diphtheria, tetanus, and polio.

Types of vaccine

Vaccines can be categorised as to whether they are viral or bacterial, live or 'killed'; killed whole organism, toxoids, or components (Table 12.3). On the basis of knowing the type of vaccine, one can predict both the likely contraindications and adverse effects.

Live vaccines

These contain live but attenuated (weakened) organisms. To produce an immune response, the organism replicates over a period of a few days or weeks after being administered. Although live attenuated virus vaccines such as polio and rotavirus vaccine have the potential for transmission of the vaccine-derived virus to others the risk is low. Live polio vaccine is now rarely used outside resource-poor countries. Despite concerns about the potential for the transmission of vaccine viruses to vulnerable infants, it is recommended that rotavirus vaccine is administered to infants in neonatal intensive care unit settings (Ladhani and Ramsay 2014). LAIV should not be given to children or adolescents who are clinically severely immunocompromised due to conditions or immunosuppressive therapy. Immunity from live vaccines is usually long lasting, possibly even for life, and a mild form of the disease can occur as a result of vaccination. For example, fever, rash, and loss of appetite have been reported in about 5% of recipients of MMR 7–10 days after its administration, with about 1% having parotitis 21 days following the vaccine. After BCG, a live bacterial vaccine, disseminated BCG may occur in immunosuppressed individuals with serious disorders such as Severe Combined Immunodeficiency Syndrome (SCIDS).

Toxoids

These are vaccines prepared from the toxin produced by the organism. It has been chemically and heat inactivated, so that although it still produces an immune response it is not capable of causing disease.

Whole cell vaccines

These vaccines are prepared from the complete organism, which has been killed and rendered nonpathogenic. They are not commonly used now. An example is the previously used whole-cell pertussis vaccine.

Conjugate vaccines

These are prepared by taking the polysaccharide (sugar) capsule of the organism and attaching a protein. The polysaccharide by itself is poorly immunogenic in young children, but the addition of the protein renders it highly immunogenic. Examples of conjugate vaccines in routine use are Hib, meningococcal ACWY vaccines, and the pneumococcal vaccines given to young children. The meningococcal B vaccine is not a conjugate vaccine.

Component vaccines

These are prepared from components of the organisms. Examples are acellular pertussis and some influenza vaccines.

Genetically engineered vaccines

Hepatitis B, HPV, and rotavirus vaccines are manufactured using recombinant technology. A strain of yeast or similar organism is used to produce the antigen. It is likely that in the future more vaccines will be produced in this way.

General considerations

Contraindications to childhood immunisation

Contraindications to all vaccines are detailed in the guidance produced by the Department of Health (UK Health Security Agency 2020a). There are very few genuine contraindications to vaccines and most CYPs who have permanent contraindications will be under the care of a paediatrician. There are general contraindications that apply to all vaccines and those that apply only to specific vaccines or to CYPs with specific conditions:

1 Immunisation should not be carried out in anyone with a history of an anaphylactic reaction to a preceding dose of the same vaccine or its contents.
2 Immunisation should be postponed in anyone suffering from a significant acute illness. This does not include minor illnesses, such as coughs and colds without fever or systemic upset, which are not sufficient reasons to postpone immunisation.
3 Most vaccines should be postponed in the presence of an evolving neurological disorder.

The latter two are to avoid wrongly attributing the progression of the disorder to the vaccine. Arrangements should be put in place to ensure immunisation takes place once the CYP has recovered, or the disorder has stabilised.

In addition to these general contraindications, some live vaccines may pose a risk to individuals with altered immunity. A best

Table 12.3 Types of vaccines.

	Live (Attenuated)	**Inactivated or component**	**Toxoid**
Viral	Influenza Measles/mumps/rubella (MMR) Polio (oral – OPV) Rotavirus Varicella Yellow fever	Hepatitis A and B Human papillomavirus vaccine (HPV) Influenza Japanese encephalitis Polio (inactivated – IPV) Tick-borne encephalitis	
Bacterial	BCG Typhoid (oral)	Anthrax *Haemophilus influenzae* type b (Hib) Meningococcal B Meningococcal C (conjugate) Meningococcal ACWY (conjugate) Pertussis (acellular) Plague Pneumococcal (plain and conjugate) Typhoid (inactivated)	Diphtheria Tetanus

Procedure guideline 12.1 Administration of vaccines

Statement	Rationale
1 Before embarking on the vaccination process, informed consent should be sought from someone with parental responsibility, or from the young person, if 'Fraser/Gillick' competent. Whether or not the latter applies, the procedure should be explained in an age-appropriate manner. Written consent is not required, but it must be fully informed.	1 Consent should be obtained for any treatment including vaccination. Full details may be obtained from "Consent: Immunisation Against Infectious Diseases" (UK Health Security Agency 2021, 2013b, ch. 2).
2 a) After consent has been obtained, the presence of any contraindications should be excluded and then the vaccine prepared. b) The individual vaccine container and where appropriate, diluent should be checked to ensure it is the right vaccine, of the right strength, and that it is within its expiry date.	2 a) To ensure that the CYP has no valid contraindications. b) To protect the CYP and to ensure the vaccine is potent.
3 a) It is not necessary or practical to attempt to sterilise the skin, however, it should be visibly clean – using soap and water only. b) If alcohol is used to clean the skin, it should be allowed to dry before the injection is given. c) With the exception of BCG vaccine, injections should normally be given by deep subcutaneous or intramuscular (IM) injection, using a 23G needle, 25mm in length. A 16mm long needle should be reserved for premature or very small babies only.	3 a) To minimise the risk of infection. There is evidence that disinfecting makes no difference to the incidence of bacterial complications of injections. b) Cleaning the skin with alcohol that is not allowed to dry may make the injection more painful and could inactivate a live vaccine. c) To ensure the vaccine gives the best immunity with the least local reaction.
4 a) CYPs with bleeding disorders should not be given IM injections. b) Intramuscular and subcutaneous injections should be given in the deltoid or anterolateral thigh. Vaccines should not be given in the buttock, unless a large volume injection of immunoglobulin is needed, in which case the buttock may be used. c) BCG vaccine is given intradermally at the insertion of the left deltoid, using a 26G needle 10mm long	4 a) IM injections may increase the risk of bleeding in this group. b) For infants the anterolateral aspect of the thigh is preferred as it provides a large muscle mass. Immunisations should not be given into the buttock, due to the risk of sciatic nerve damage and the possibility of injecting the vaccine into fat rather than muscle. c) Intradermal administration ensures the best possible protection with the least possible local reactions.
5 Once the vaccine has been given, the name of the vaccine, its batch number, the dose, and the site of immunisation should all be recorded. This information should be given to the parent/carer in the child's personal child health record or other immunisation record, the GP, and whatever local agency is responsible for providing immunisation statistics.	5 To ensure that: • The individual child receives the correct number of all the necessary immunisations, in a timely fashion. • Any local reaction after one of two injections can be attributed to the correct vaccine. • If there is a problem with one or more batches of vaccine, the recipients can be traced. • Parents/carers and GPs should have an accurate record of the CYP's immunisation status. • Coverage of vaccination can be monitored and appropriate action taken if it is inadequate. This is an important component of monitoring vaccinations programmes.

practice statement on immunisation of the immunocompromised CYP has been developed by the Royal College of Paediatrics and Child Health (RCPCH 2002). This provides detailed guidance on children with primary immunodeficiency, those being treated with standard and intensive chemotherapy, solid organ recipients, children being treated with immunosuppressive drugs for inflammatory disease and children with HIV infection. This document is currently being updated; go to https://stateofchildhealth.rcpch.ac.uk/evidence/prevention-of-ill-health/immunisations/ to ensure you have the most recent version. Guidance is also available online from UK Health Security Agency (2020). It is often appropriate to consult the CYP's consultant.

The guidance on the recommended intervals between administration of live vaccines has been reviewed and most can be administered at any interval before or after each other. However, current recommendations should be consulted (UK Health Security Agency 2022a). Immunoglobulin may reduce the response to a live vaccine. As a generalisation, if a live vaccine is given before immunoglobulin, an interval of four weeks should be left; if immunoglobulin precedes a live vaccine, an interval of three months should be allowed.

Adverse reactions and safety of vaccines

All vaccines can give rise to side effects. These are usually mild and self-limiting. For example, swelling and redness at the injection site are common. By remembering whether a vaccine is live or 'dead,' it is possible to predict, in general terms, the likely adverse effects and contraindications. In addition to mild local reactions, most vaccines can cause systemic upset of varying degrees. Live vaccines may also produce the disease, but almost always in a mild form.

It may be difficult to distinguish a coincidental illness from an adverse reaction and often the tendency is to assume the latter. Following the first dose of MMR vaccine a proportion of children develop mild measles, mumps, or rubella. In a study involving 581 pairs of twins, one twin received MMR vaccine and the other a placebo. Three weeks later the roles were reversed. Low rates of systemic effects thought due to the vaccine were reported. Fever greater than 38.5°C occurred at a maximum rate 9–10 days after the vaccine among 4.9% of vaccinees compared with 1.0% after placebo. After the same interval, 4.3% of vaccinees developed a rash, compared with 3.0% given placebo. Children who received the vaccine were more likely to be irritable and drowsy, although cough and/or cold were more common following the placebo (Peltola and Heinonen 1986).

Other studies have confirmed these findings. For MMR and most other combined vaccines there is evidence that there is little, if any increase in the rate of reactions in comparison with giving the antigens separately. A notable exception is MMRV (measles, mumps, rubella, varicella combined vaccine), which is associated with an increased risk of convulsions after the first dose given at 12–23 months, compared with MMR and V given on the same day. Combining some antigens may change the immune response for better or worse, depending on the combination.

Serious adverse reactions following vaccination are rare. Studies involving large numbers of CYPs are necessary to determine the frequency of such reactions. These are usually performed after the vaccine has been in use for some time and are part of postmarketing surveillance. Studies linking hospital records with immunisation records have reported that 1 in 3000 children have a febrile convulsion due to the MMR vaccine (Farrington et al. 1995) and 1 in 32000 developed idiopathic thrombocytopenic purpura due to it (Miller et al. 2001). These are roughly a tenth of the rates after the diseases. Before the introduction of rotavirus vaccine to the routine immunisation schedule for children in the UK large studies were conducted among more than 63000 infants to determine its safety and efficacy (Ruiz-Palacios et al. 2006). Following the introduction of rotavirus vaccine it has been shown that intussusception occurs at a rate of about 1 or 2 for every 100000 first doses of rotavirus vaccine given.

All significant adverse events following immunisation (AEFIs) should be reported to the local immunisation lead and to the Medicines and Healthcare products Regulatory Agency (MHRA) using the 'Yellow Card' system (MHRA 2020).

Efficacy of vaccines

No vaccine is 100% effective; however, disease developing in immunised children is usually milder than that without immunisation. Before any vaccine is introduced, trials are conducted to ensure it is of high efficacy. After a first injection of combined MMR vaccine about 5–10% of children are not protected against measles (Uzicanin and Zimmerman 2011). A higher proportion, perhaps as high as 30%, are not protected against mumps (Demicheli et al. 2012) and a smaller proportion, 1–2%, are not protected against rubella. This means that there will always be some cases of disease if only one dose is given. It is important to remember that not all preparations of a vaccine are the same. Although there is little variation in the measles vaccines used in the developed world, the efficacy of different pertussis vaccines varies enormously. Trials in the 1990s showed that one variety of whole cell pertussis vaccine had an efficacy of 35–40%, whereas the whole cell vaccine that was used in the UK had an efficacy of 90% (Miller 1999). The Jeryl Lynn mumps vaccine used in the UK has an efficacy of 70–90%, whereas studies have shown that the Rubini strain offers no protection (Elliman et al. 2009). The efficacy of the BCG vaccine has also been found to vary widely (Mangtani et al. 2014). To monitor the effectiveness of vaccines, all cases of most routine vaccine-preventable diseases should be notified to the local authority or local Health Protection Team. Some, such as tuberculosis, Hib, pneumococcal, and meningococcal infections, are also the subject of enhanced surveillance schemes. These are more accurate and allow detailed study of the characteristics of cases of the diseases.

Herd immunity

If a high enough rate of protection can be achieved by high vaccine uptake with an effective vaccine a disease becomes so uncommon that even those still susceptible are at little risk. This is known as 'herd immunity' or 'community immunity' and provides protection not only to immunised individuals, but also to those who have not been immunised. This is an important way of protecting CYPs who cannot be immunised because they are either too young, have a contraindication, or have been immunised but still remain unprotected due to 'vaccine failure'. The uptake needed to attain herd immunity will depend on the disease, the vaccine and the population. The more infectious the disease and the more mixing within the population, the greater the level of immunisation that will be required to achieve herd immunity. The exception to this is tetanus, as the disease is not transmitted from person to person, so individuals need their own immunity to be protected and there is no herd immunity.

The aim of any vaccination programme is to reduce the incidence of disease. However, characteristics of the disease, the population and the vaccine will determine to what extent this is possible and how it might be achieved. The options for vaccination programmes are:

- **Eradication**: Where the disease and its causal agent are completely and permanently removed worldwide. The only example of a human disease that has been eradicated is naturally occurring smallpox.
- **Elimination**: Reduction to zero (or a very low defined target rate) of new cases in a defined geographical area. Elimination requires continued measures to prevent re-establishment of disease transmission.
- **Containment**: Reduction of morbidity and mortality to levels that are no longer considered to be a public health problem.

The aim of the MMR vaccination programme is to eliminate these infections. To achieve this, very high levels of immunity are needed. For example, in the case of measles, which is highly infectious, 95% of the population needs to be immune to prevent circulation of the disease. Since the vaccine is about 90% effective against measles, if 88% of children are given MMR vaccine, only 79% of each birth cohort would be protected against measles. It is therefore recommended that children receive two doses of MMR vaccine. The second dose is needed to protect those who did not respond to the first dose. High rates of protection against measles (99%) are achieved with a two-dose schedule (Uzicanin and Zimmerman 2011).

Specific diseases and the vaccines

Diphtheria

Organism:	*Corynebacterium diphtheriae* and *Corynebacterium ulcerans*. Most isolates do not produce toxin, i.e. are nontoxigenic.
Disease:	Significant disease only results from infection with a strain producing the toxin, i.e. a 'toxigenic' strain. After an incubation period of two to four days, one of three clinical pictures may occur – nasal, tonsillar, or laryngeal. In each case an exudate appears at the relevant site. There may or may not be constitutional upset. As the name suggests, *Corynebacterium ulcerans* presents with a skin ulcer. The main complications of infection with either organism are respiratory obstruction, myocarditis and muscle paralysis. Treatment is with antitoxin, antibiotics, and supportive therapy.

Morbidity:	Between 2012 and 2021 there were 50 isolations of toxigenic organisms.
Mortality:	Approximately 5% – the last death in the UK in childhood was in 2008 in an unimmunised school aged child (Wagner et al. 2010). Between 2012 and 2021, there were three adult deaths. All were due to *Corynebacterium ulcerans*.
Vaccination:	The toxin is chemically and heat treated to produce a toxoid. When used as a vaccine it prevents the complications of the disease, but does not prevent infection. The vaccine is not available separately.
Efficacy:	87–96%.
Contraindications:	As for any killed vaccine.
Adverse effects:	Local reactions and mild systemic upset are fairly common. More severe effects are rare. The low-dose vaccine denoted by a lowercase 'd' must be used in individuals who are 10 years of age or older.

Haemophilus influenzae type b (Hib)

Organism:	*Haemophilus influenzae* type b (Hib). Other serotypes rarely cause invasive disease.
Disease:	Following a short incubation period, meningitis, epiglottitis, septic arthritis, pneumonia, pericarditis, bacteraemia, or cellulitis may occur. The disease is less common after the fourth birthday but still sufficiently common for the vaccine to be recommended for all children up to their 10th birthday. Treatment with antibiotics and supportive therapy is usually effective. Between 10 and 30% of children with meningitis are left with a significant neurological or auditory disability.
Morbidity:	Prior to the introduction of immunisation, there was a 1 in 600 chance of contracting the disease before the age of 5. The disease is now rare and between 2012 and 2018 the annual Hib incidence was less than 1 per million population with only two cases of Hib meningitis. A cohort of children under 4 years were offered a booster dose of vaccine in 2003 and since 2006, all children are offered a booster dose at 12 months of age.
Mortality:	Approximately 5% for meningitis and higher for epiglottitis. There used to be 65 deaths per year. The last death in a child was in 2011 and in an adult in 2015.
Vaccination:	Nature of vaccine: the polysaccharide (sugar) capsule is attached ('conjugated') to a protein (tetanus toxoid or diphtheria toxoid derivative). The vaccine is not available separately.
Efficacy:	Over 95% – in areas where it is part of the universal immunisation programme, disease is very uncommon.
Contraindications:	As for any killed vaccine.
Adverse effects:	Other than mild local reactions, these are very uncommon.

Hepatitis B

Organism:	A virus of the genus *Hepadnavirus*
Disease:	Acute infection may be symptomatic with evidence of varying degrees of liver dysfunction or entirely asymptomatic. Some infections are cleared, while in other cases it persists and patients are known as 'carriers'. The carrier state is commoner the younger a person is when they are infected. Carriers are at high risk of developing potentially fatal liver disease – cancer and cirrhosis. The infection may be passed from mother to infant around the time of delivery (vertical spread), or by blood products or from person to person during sexual intercourse (horizontal spread). There is also some spread within families, the mode of transmission not always being clear. When acquired vertically the infant is usually asymptomatic but about 90% become a carrier and have a 25% risk of developing liver disease later in life.
Morbidity:	Depends on the population. The carrier state is noted in 1 in 1500 blood donors in the UK, but in 1 in 100 mothers in some inner city areas. There were 292 reports of acute Hepatitis B in England in 2018.
Mortality:	Accurate figures are not available.
Vaccination:	Nature of vaccine: Recombinant DNA product prepared from yeast.
Efficacy:	Depends on the age and general health of the recipient. It is very effective in infants, but less so in adults or those with chronic illnesses, such as renal failure. It is available as a separate vaccine.
Contraindications:	As for any killed vaccine.
Adverse effects:	Uncommon.

Human papillomavirus

Organism:	A double-stranded DNA virus with over 200 strains. HPV viruses are classified as either 'high-risk' or 'low-risk' depending on whether or not they are oncogenic (cancer-causing) strains.
Disease:	HPV is extremely prevalent and most people are infected in their life-time. The virus infects squamous epithelia, including the skin and mucosae of the upper respiratory and anogenital tracts. Most infections are self-limiting and asymptomatic. Persistent genital infection with a high-risk strain can result in cancer of the cervix. About 40 strains infect the genital tract, with 70% of cervical cancers being caused by two strains: HPV16 and HPV18. Of genital warts over 90% are caused by two types, HPV6 and HPV11. The viruses that cause problems in the genital area are usually spread by sexual intercourse. HPV is the precipitant of a proportion of a number of other cancers including those of the anus, vulva, penis, vagina and head and neck. HPV can also cause laryngeal papillomatosis (polyps in the voice box), but this is rare.

Mortality:	Each year, in spite of the screening programme, there are about 850 deaths due to cervical cancer (680 in 2019). In 2009, there were over 91 000 new cases of genital warts. But this has fallen to just over 24,000 in 2019.
Vaccination:	Two vaccines have been used in the UK: Cervarix®, with two strains of the virus (16 and 18), which was used routinely in the UK from 2008 to 2012, and Gardasil®, with four strains of the virus (6, 11,16, and 18), which has been in use since 2012. Both are produced using recombinant technology. It was recommended that from September 2014, two doses of the vaccine should be offered to 12- to –13-year-old girls instead of the previous three doses. From 2019, the vaccine has also been offered to 12- to 13-year-old boys. For maximum benefit, the vaccine needs to be given before infection has occurred, i.e. before sexual debut. A vaccine against nine strains of HPV has been licensed and is being introduced to UK in 2022, but at the time of writing, is not part of the national programme.
Efficacy:	The vaccine is highly effective (over 99%) at preventing infection with the included strains and has been shown to reduce the risk of cervical cancer and anogenital warts. Current studies suggest protection is maintained for at least 10 years.
Adverse effects:	Most common side effects are pain and swelling at the injection site.

Influenza

Organism:	There are three types of influenza virus that infect humans: A, B, and C. Influenza A and influenza B are responsible for most clinical illness. Changes in the principal surface antigens of influenza A make these viruses antigenically labile. Minor changes (antigenic drift) occur progressively from season to season. Major changes (antigenic shift) occur periodically, resulting in the emergence of a new subtype. In 2009, a new influenza virus H1N1 was detected. This was referred to as 'swine flu', as the virus showed some similarities to the virus that infects pigs. This virus spread quickly from person to person worldwide and H1N1 vaccines were developed rapidly. There were estimated to be 280,000 deaths worldwide but fortunately the disease was mild in most people.
Disease:	The organism is highly infectious and transmitted by aerosol, droplets, or direct contact with respiratory secretions of someone with the infection. The incubation period is one to three days. The infection spreads rapidly, especially in closed communities. Most cases in the UK tend to occur during a six- to eight-week period during the winter. The timing, extent, and severity of this 'seasonal' influenza can all vary. Symptoms include sudden onset of fever, chills, headache, myalgia, and extreme fatigue. Other common symptoms include a dry cough, sore throat, and stuffy nose.
Mortality:	In healthy individuals, influenza is an unpleasant but usually self-limiting disease with recovery in two to seven days. Serious illness and mortality from influenza are highest among neonates, older people, and those with underlying disease, particularly chronic respiratory and cardiac disease, or those who are immunosuppressed.
Morbidity:	Even in a low incidence year, 3000–4000 deaths have been attributed to influenza. On average about 50 deaths a year are in children.
Vaccination:	The World Health Organization (WHO) monitors influenza viruses throughout the world. Each year WHO makes recommendations about the strains to be included in seasonal flu vaccines for the forthcoming winter. To provide continuing protection, annual immunisation with vaccine against the currently prevalent strains is necessary. Influenza vaccines are prepared using virus strains in line with the WHO recommendations. Current vaccines are trivalent or quadrivalent, i.e. contain two subtypes of influenza A and one or two types of B viruses. Two types of influenza vaccine are available: inactivated influenza vaccines and live attenuated influenza vaccine (LAIV). Most of the vaccines are grown in embryonated hens' eggs. Viruses in inactivated vaccines are chemically inactivated and then further treated and purified, while the live viruses are cold treated so that although they can replicate in the nasal passages and produce antibodies, they are unable to do so in the warmer lower respiratory tissues. The antibodies are present in the lining of the airways. Eligible children aged six months up to two years should be offered an inactivated quadrivalent vaccine; for those 2 years to 17 years inclusive, in whom a vaccine is indicated, the first choice is the live attenuated quadrivalent vaccine. Eligible adults under 65 should be offered inactivated quadrivalent vaccine. Recently a trivalent vaccine containing an aluminium adjuvant has been introduced for those 65 and over. It is important to check with current guidance as to which individuals are eligible for vaccine and which vaccine is indicated. The advice is updated annually.
Efficacy:	This varies year on year. In 2019/20, 40–60% protection for inactivated influenza vaccine and about 50% for LAIV. The unadjuvenated trivalent vaccine has little beneficial effect in those aged 65 or more.
Contraindications:	Inactivated influenza vaccine: As for any killed vaccine. LAIV – as for any live vaccine and in addition should not be given to children with active wheezing at the time of vaccination or with a history of severe asthma. If this is not available, expert advice should be sought. It should not be given to someone taking salicylates. A risk assessment should be made before giving the vaccine to children who have had anaphylactic reaction to eggs.
Adverse effects:	Inactivated influenza vaccine: pain, swelling or redness at the injection site, low grade fever, malaise, shivering, fatigue, headache, myalgia, and arthralgia are among the commonly reported symptoms of vaccination. These symptoms are also similar to those of influenza infection and some individuals claim that the vaccine has given them 'flu' but as the vaccine is killed this is not plausible. LAIV: nasal congestion, decreased appetite, headache and malaise.

Measles

Organism:	A virus of genus *Morbillivirus* of the Paramyxoviridae family
Disease:	After an incubation period of about a week, sore eyes, a dry cough, and rash develop. Complications occur in 1 in 15 cases, with convulsions in 1% and encephalitis in 1 in 1000. A fatal progressive neurological disorder, subacute sclerosing panencephalitis (SSPE), may develop many years later. Prior to the introduction of immunisation measles, epidemics occurred every two years.
Morbidity:	There were almost 80 000 notified cases a year in the 1980s. Since many cases of notified measles are not later confirmed to be the disease, oral fluid testing on all notified cases of measles, mumps, and rubella has been in place since 1995. This allows laboratory confirmation of the initial clinical diagnosis. In 2005 there were 2114 notified cases of measles but fewer than 5% were confirmed. As a result of a decline in uptake of MMR vaccine, confirmed cases of measles increased from 56 in 1998 to a peak of 2030 in 2012. In 2019 there were 797 confirmed cases in the UK. However, in recent years, there have been global increases in measles cases due to gaps in immunity, with 83 540 cases and 74 deaths in Europe in 2018.
Mortality:	120 people died from measles in the 1980s, but only 18 in 1990–1999, and most of these were due to the late effects. Until 2006 the last confirmed deaths due to acute measles was in 1992. However, a child with an underlying immunological problem died acutely from measles in 2006. Subsequently, up to 2020, there have been 18 deaths from measles, of which five were acute deaths, three were due to SSPE (two children) and the rest were due to other late effects in adults.
Vaccination:	Live attenuated vaccine given as MMR.
Efficacy:	90–95% for the measles component. For this reason, and because measles is highly infectious, from October 1996 the standard immunisation schedule has included two doses of MMR. The second dose is usually given at three years four months but can be given routinely as young as 18 months. For mumps, the efficacy is usually quoted as 85–90%. However, it may be as low as 64%. The immunity from mumps vaccine wanes over time. In contrast, the efficacy of the rubella component is greater than 95%.
Contraindications:	As for any live vaccine. It can be given to anyone who has well-controlled HIV infection, but advice should be sought from their specialist team. MMR vaccines in use in most countries may contain trace quantities of egg protein, and so there has been concern about giving the vaccine to children who are allergic to egg for fear that they might have a serious reaction to it. However, there is a lot of experience of using the vaccine in such children without any untoward effects. Therefore, the UK Health Security Agency advises that all children with egg allergy (even anaphylaxis) should receive MMR vaccine as a routine in primary care. There is no good evidence that skin testing helps in the management of these children. Children who have had a documented anaphylactic reaction to a previous dose of the vaccine should be assessed by an allergist.
Adverse effects:	Mild measles occurs in about 5%, at 5–11 days after immunisation. Mild mumps or rubella occurs somewhat later. None is infectious. Vaccination is complicated by convulsions after 1 in every 3000 doses and idiopathic thrombocytopenic purpura (ITP) after 1 in every 32 000. Adverse reactions are much less frequent after revaccination than after the first dose (Virtanen et al. 2000). Two brands of vaccine were withdrawn in 1992 because the mumps strain used ('Urabe') gave rise to a mild meningoencephalitis, but with no long-term sequelae. The strains of mumps vaccine virus now used in UK do not give rise to this complication.

Meningococcal B

Organism	*Neisseria meningitides* serogroup B
Disease	Meningitis and/or septicaemia are the most serious manifestations of the infection. Multiorgan failure with gangrene of extremities, which may require amputation, can occur. Treatment is with antibiotics and general organ support.
Morbidity	In England in 2014–2015, before the vaccine was introduced, there were 418 cases of invasive MenB disease and 15 deaths In England. 25% of these cases were in infants (< one-year-olds) and 25% in toddlers (one- to four-year-olds).
Mortality	High mortality
Vaccination	The vaccine used in the UK is made from four proteins from group B *Neisseria meningitides* bacteria.
Efficacy	After two doses of vaccine there is 53% protection against all strains of Meningococcal B disease and 64% against vaccine strains. After three doses of vaccine, the corresponding figures were 59% and 71%
Contraindications	As for any killed vaccine.
Adverse effects	When given concomitantly with other routine vaccines, MenB vaccine gives rise to high rates of fever with about 51–61% infants experiencing a fever > 38 °C after vaccination. In view of this it is recommended that infants are given prophylactic paracetamol around the time of vaccination with two further doses at four- to eight-hour intervals (UK Health Security Agency 2022a). Pain and swelling at the injection site, irritability, diarrhoea and vomiting, and development of a rash are also common. Following MenB vaccination some children are seen in A&E and admitted to hospital for investigation as it may be difficult to distinguish the adverse effects of the vaccine from more serious conditions.

Meningococcal C

Organism:	*Neisseria meningitidis* serogroup C
Disease:	Meningitis and/or septicaemia are the most serious manifestations of the infection. Multiorgan failure with gangrene of extremities, which may require amputation, can occur. Treatment is with antibiotics and general organ support.
Morbidity:	Amputations of digits or limbs, epilepsy, brain damage, and deafness.
Mortality:	Even with intensive treatment there is a high mortality. When the vaccine was introduced in 1999 there were 578 cases in under-19-year-olds, in England and Wales about 10% of whom died. Since 1999 there has been a 99% decrease in the number of laboratory-confirmed cases in people under 20 and also a fall in the case fatality rate. In 2018/19, in England there were only 43 confirmed cases, of whom only 12 were in CYPs.
Vaccination:	Polysaccharide conjugate vaccine, along the same lines as Hib. The UK was the first country to introduce the conjugate vaccine in November 1999.
Efficacy:	95%+ in the first year of life, but wanes rapidly. Since 2016, MenC vaccine has not been given to infants under a year as disease had become so uncommon they were protected by herd (community) immunity. One dose is given at 12 months (Hib/MenC) and again at about 14 years (MenACWY). Available as MenC, Hib/MenC, and Men ACWY vaccines.
Contraindications:	As for any killed vaccine.
Adverse effects:	Local, fever general malaise, etc. Significant adverse effects are rare.

Meningococcal ACWY

Organism:	*Neisseria meningitidis* serogroups A, C, W and Y
Disease:	Meningitis and/or septicaemia are the most serious manifestations of the infection. Multiorgan failure with gangrene of extremities, which may require amputation, can occur. Treatment is with antibiotics and general organ support. Meningococcal W infection may present as a gastrointestinal infection.
Morbidity:	Amputations of digits or limbs, epilepsy, brain damage, and deafness. It may present as a gastrointestinal infection.
Mortality:	Even with intensive treatment there is a high mortality of approximately 12%. The incidence of Meningococcal W disease increased from 18 cases in England in 2008/2009 to 189 cases in 2014/2015 and reached a peak of 225 in 2016/2017. There were 83 cases in 2019/2020.
Vaccination:	Polysaccharide conjugate vaccine, along the same lines as Hib. The vaccine was introduced for CYPs at 13–14 years old in August 2015.
Efficacy:	95%+
Contraindications:	As for any killed vaccine.
Adverse effects:	Local, fever general malaise, etc. Significant adverse effects are rare.

Mumps

Organism:	A virus of the paramyxovirus group
Disease:	The most common presentations are parotitis and pancreatitis. It used to be the commonest form of viral meningoencephalitis in CYPs and was a significant cause of sensorineural deafness.
Morbidity:	Mumps only became officially notifiable with the introduction of the MMR vaccine in 1988. There were 20 713 cases notified in 1989. Since 1996, confirmation of cases has been sought using salivary antibodies. There were only 500 confirmed cases in 2002 in England and Wales. Cases started to increase in 2004, and peaked in 2005 when there were 43 378 confirmed cases. These occurred mainly among older adolescents and young adults who had either never received MMR vaccine or received only one dose. The epidemic highlighted the need for two doses of MMR vaccine. There were 5558 cases confirmed in 2019.
Mortality:	Before the vaccine came into use there were two to five deaths each year.
Vaccination:	See measles.

Pertussis

Organism:	*Bordetella pertussis*
Disease:	Varies from a cold to frequent bouts of coughing terminated by vomiting and the characteristic whoop. Convulsions and permanent neurological sequelae occur. It may be an unrecognised cause of cot death as young babies often do not whoop. It is underdiagnosed in adults.

Morbidity:	A total of 3510 confirmed notifications between 2000 and 2008, although probably under notified. In 2012 there were 9367 confirmed notifications, representing an increase of cases in all groups, but particularly in infants less than three months of age. The increase in pertussis cases in 2012 resulted in the introduction of what was initially a temporary pertussis vaccine programme for pregnant women. The aim is to prevent severe infection in young infants. Boosting the pregnant woman's antibodies protects her from catching whooping cough and the high level of antibodies are transferred transplacentally to her baby, providing protection until the child's own vaccination schedule begins at eight weeks. Pertussis vaccine in pregnancy has been shown to be safe and highly effective in protecting infants from the infection (Amirthalingam et al. 2014; Gkentzi et al. 2017).
Mortality:	There were 34 official notifications of deaths between 2000 and 2008, but there is reason to think that this was an underestimate and that about nine children a year died from pertussis. Most deaths from pertussis are in babies under the age of six months. In 2012, 14 babies died from pertussis. Since the vaccination programme started, there have been 20 deaths in babies with confirmed pertussis, including one death reported in 2019; 18 of the mothers had not been immunised and for the two mothers who had been immunised, it was too late in pregnancy for the baby to receive passive immunity.
Vaccination:	The main vaccine used in infants in the UK was changed in 2004 from a killed whole bacterial preparation ('whole cell' vaccine) to an acellular vaccine. The acellular vaccines contain a limited number of components as opposed to the whole cell vaccines which, as the name suggests, contain the whole but inactivated bacterium, with approximately 3000 components. Acellular or 'component' vaccines have been shown to have a reduction in the incidence of side effects compared with the used whole cell vaccine when given at two, three, and four months. In older children these vaccines have even fewer side effects than the conventional vaccine.
Efficacy:	Over 90% for the traditional whole cell vaccines used in UK and the five-component acellular vaccine. However, there is evidence of waning of immunity after both disease and vaccination, particularly the acellular, hence the need for one or more boosters in childhood.
Contraindications:	As for any inactivated vaccine. If prone to convulsions, special care should be taken to advise about the management of pyrexia and convulsions. The vaccine, as with other childhood vaccines, should be withheld in those children with an evolving neurological disorder.
Adverse effects:	Local reactions and pyrexia are common within 48 hours after vaccination. Convulsions occur in approximately 1 in every 60 000 doses after whole cell vaccine, when given at 8, 12, and 16 weeks. These are far less common after acellular vaccine (Le Saux et al. 2003). Long-term damage occurs rarely if ever.

Pneumococcal disease

Organism:	*Streptococcus pneumoniae* has over 90 serotypes. About 20–30 account for the majority of disease. Prior to the introduction of a vaccine, seven serotypes were responsible for 82% of invasive disease in UK children under four years old.
Disease:	Pneumonia, bacteraemia, and meningitis are the most life-threatening forms of invasive disease. A significant number of cases of acute otitis media are also caused by pneumococcal infection.
Morbidity:	In 2004/5, there were 252 cases of meninigitis, of which 104 were in children less than five years old; 6287 cases of bacteraemia of which 731 were in children under five years old; and about 70–80 000 cases of pneumonia. Approximately one in three infants has otitis media each year, 25–30% of which are due to the pneumococcus. Approximately 25% of those who survive meningitis have a significant disability.
Mortality:	15–20% for those with meningitis and about 7% for those with other invasive disease.
Vaccination:	A plain polysaccharide vaccine is prepared from 23 serotypes and a conjugate vaccine (PCV) from 13 serotypes (when PCV was introduced in 2006, it was a 7-serotype vaccine). These are available only as separate vaccines. Invasive pneumococcal disease (IPD) caused by the serotypes in the 7-serotype vaccine had decreased by 90% in 2009–10. Following a rise in nonvaccine serotypes, it was replaced by a 13-valent vaccine in 2010. This was highly effective against the vaccine strains and overall there has been a reduction in IPD of about 40% in all age groups, though this rose to 70% in under-twos.
Efficacy:	The plain polysaccharide vaccine, as with any such vaccine, is ineffective in young children, whereas the conjugate vaccine is highly effective, but, if given to infants, needs a booster to maintain immunity.
Contraindications:	As for any killed vaccine.
Adverse effects:	As for any killed vaccine.

Poliomyelitis

Organism:	An enterovirus with three antigenically distinct types.
Disease:	Most polio infections are asymptomatic, but it may cause meningitis or paralysis.
Morbidity:	The last case of wild polio acquired in UK was in 1984. 10 cases, 1994–2003, were all vaccine-associated. The disease has nearly been eradicated worldwide. In 2020 it was announced that polio had been eliminated from Africa; cases are now confined to Pakistan and Afghanistan. From an all-time low of 22 cases in 2017, there were 143 in 2019, 117 of which were in Pakistan.
Mortality:	Rare in the UK.

Vaccination:	Injected killed (IPV) replaced oral live attenuated (OPV) vaccine in the UK in 2004.
Efficacy:	Very high.
Contraindications:	As for any killed vaccine.
Adverse effects:	Killed vaccine – local reactions and fever occasionally. Oral vaccine – paralytic polio in one in two to three million recipients or unimmunised contacts.

Rotavirus

Organism:	Ribonucleic acid (RNA) viruses of which there are a number of strains.
Disease:	Causes gastroenteritis, characterised by mild fever with severe diarrhoea, vomiting, stomach cramps, and can lead to dehydration.
Morbidity:	Ubiquitous; by the age of five years most children will have encountered one or more strains of it.
Mortality:	Rare in the UK.
Vaccination:	A live attenuated human strain virus vaccine. Administered by mouth. Rotavirus vaccine was introduced into the United States in 2006 and in other countries including Canada and Australia. A previous vaccine had been withdrawn after being found to be associated with an increased incidence of intussusception. Trials on the current vaccine did not show this. However, from the post-marketing surveillance, there is evidence that the Rotarix® vaccine may be associated with a very small increased risk of intussusception, of the order of 2 per 100 000 first doses given. Despite the small increased risk, the benefits of the vaccine outweigh the risks. As the vaccine may hasten the onset of intussusception, it is important that the first dose is given no later than 15 weeks of age and the vaccine not given at all once the child is 24 weeks of age to avoid temporal association between the vaccine and intussusception which peaks at this age.
Efficacy:	Rotarix used in the UK is over 85% effective at protecting against severe rotavirus gastroenteritis infection in the first two years of life. In England in 2013–2014 it is estimated that 87 376 healthcare visits for acute gastroenteritis in young children were prevented as a result of vaccination.
Contraindications:	As with any vaccine, it should not be given to infants with a confirmed anaphylactic reaction to a previous dose of the vaccine or to any components of the vaccines. It is also contraindicated in infants with a previous history of intussusception or with malformations of the gastrointestinal tract that could predispose them to intussusception. It should not be given to infants aged 24 weeks or older. Although live vaccines are generally contraindicated in individuals with immunosuppression, with the exception of severe combined immunodeficiency (SCID) disorder, the benefits of the vaccine may outweigh the risk in infants with other forms of immunosuppression. Rare contraindications include infants with hereditary problems of fructose intolerance, glucose-galactose malabsorption or sucrase-isomaltase insufficiency.
Adverse effects:	The most common adverse effects are diarrhoea and irritability. Intussusception has been reported to occur once or twice after every 100 000 doses.

Rubella

Organism:	The rubivirus is a togavirus of the Togaviridae family.
Disease:	In most people, the illness is mild, although idiopathic thrombocytopenic purpura and encephalitis may occur. However, if acquired in the first trimester of pregnancy, it gives rise to numerous malformations in the majority of foetuses.
Morbidity:	Only became notifiable with the introduction of the MMR vaccine. There were 104 confirmed cases in the five-year period 2009–2013. Between 2016 and 2019 there was a total of 11 confirmed cases of rubella per year in England and cases of congenital rubella syndrome are very uncommon.
Mortality:	Uncommon.
Vaccination:	See measles.

Tetanus

Organism:	*Clostridium tetani*
Disease:	Also known as 'lockjaw', the disease is usually acquired from dirt contaminated with animal faeces, in a skin wound. It is not spread from person to person and so herd immunity is not possible. It causes painful spasms, which may affect the respiratory muscles.
Morbidity:	Between 2000 and 2019, there were 129 cases and 12 deaths in England and Wales from tetanus, mainly affecting unimmunised older adults. During 2003–2004 a cluster of 25 tetanus cases occurred in young injecting drug users. Two of these patients died.
Mortality:	In England in 2019, there were two reported cases of tetanus and no deaths.
Vaccination:	A purified toxoid prepared using the same principles as diphtheria toxoid. Not available separately.

Efficacy:	Highly effective.
Adverse effects:	Local reactions, fever, and general malaise occur in a small proportion of recipients. Significant adverse effects are rare.

Tuberculosis (TB)

Organism:	*Mycobacterium tuberculosis*, a slow growing bacterium.
Disease:	Spread is from person to person and can affect almost any organ in the body. The prevalence of disease is higher in association with HIV infection and deprivation. Treatment is with antitubercular drugs.
Morbidity:	Between 1991 and 2000 there were 53 236 cases notified in England and Wales – an average of 5323 per year. There was a steady increase to 8280 cases in 2011, but more recently there has been a steady decline to 4805 cases in 2018, the lowest ever recorded.
Mortality:	4080 deaths between 1991 and 2000. The number of deaths due to TB fell to less than 120 in 2018.
Vaccination:	The vaccine is not prepared from the TB organism (*Mycobacterium tuberculosis*), but from a related bovine organism (*Mycobacterium bovis*). Bacillus Calmette-Guérin (BCG) is a live attenuated vaccine.
Efficacy:	Studies have had very variable outcomes, but in UK schoolchildren it was about 80%. The dominant effect is to prevent dissemination of the disease and severe forms of disease such as meningitis, rather than infection per se.
Contraindications:	As for any live vaccine. In addition, it should not be given to anyone with a positive tuberculin test, a history of previous BCG and a scar, or a history of TB, itself. In the absence of other contraindications, a Mantoux test should be performed before offering BCG to anyone aged six years or older.
Adverse effects:	An ulcer occurs frequently at the site of immunisation and occasionally the organism may become disseminated, especially in the immunosuppressed.

Vaccines not in general use in UK

- Varicella zoster virus (VZV): A live attenuated vaccine against chickenpox is in use in the United States and a number of other countries. Although it is licenced in the UK, it is not in routine use and remains under consideration. It should be given to susceptible household contacts of immunosuppressed patients.
- Respiratory syncytial virus (RSV): Passive immunisation (monoclonal antibodies) is available and used in high-risk infants, although there is still controversy as to its value.

Storage and administration of vaccines

Storage

All vaccines are temperature and light sensitive to varying degrees. If stored outside the optimum temperature range, usually 2–8°C, the efficacy of the vaccine may decline and less commonly, may give rise to more adverse reactions. If a glass vial of vaccine is frozen it may develop hairline cracks, allowing pathogens to enter, which can cause injection site infections. All vaccines must be kept in special refrigerators where temperature is recorded at least once and ideally twice each day. This should be done with a maximum and minimum thermometer so that extremes of temperature can be noted. From the time a vaccine leaves the manufacturer to the time it enters the patient – the 'cold chain' – the temperature at which it is stored should be checked and recorded at least once every working day. Vaccines should spend the least possible time out of the refrigerator.

Ensuring good uptake

As discussed earlier in the chapter, it is important that high uptake of vaccines is achieved and maintained to ensure the protection of individual children, as well as to achieve herd immunity. In the UK over 90% of one-year-old children have received the full primary course of vaccines. However, there is a considerable range in uptake between areas, and even in high uptake areas there may be pockets of lower coverage. Children who are less likely to be fully immunised include low birthweight children, those born prematurely (Jessop et al. 2010), those with disabilities or chronic conditions, hospitalised children (Samad et al. 2006) and children in the care of the local authority (looked after children) (Walton and Bedford 2017). These are also the groups of children who are more likely to be seriously affected by an infectious disease. Poor immunisation uptake among these children is likely to be due to a combination of frequent hospitalisations, which can lead to routine care being overlooked, or the belief held by health professionals or parents/carers that vaccines are contraindicated because of the condition. This is rarely the case.

One of the most important factors affecting uptake is parental attitudes and beliefs about vaccine safety and efficacy and the seriousness of diseases (Peckham et al. 1989). These are shaped by a range of influences including previous experience, the advice of family and friends, general attitudes to health, the media and health professionals, who are consistently reported to be the most important source of advice (Stefanoff et al. 2010). A more recent additional influence is social media. Its particular potency is the speed at which messages, both positive and negative, about vaccines can spread worldwide. The sheer quantity of information readily available has increased exponentially. However, this information includes not only high-quality evidence-based material, but poorer quality, anecdotal evidence and pseudoscience. Although not of equal validity, this may not be apparent to parents seeking information (Larson et al. 2011). This makes advice from health professionals even more important.

The first part of the immunisation discussion with a vaccine-hesitant or resistant parent consists of exploring with them the nature of their concerns and the source of their information. Only in this way is it possible to ensure that the information provided meets their specific needs (Leask et al. 2012; Bedford and Elliman 2020). Some have reported that lack of information is not the major factor among parents who decide not to immunise their child; rather, it is mistrust of the information or of the professionals providing it (Yaqub et al. 2014). Clearly, trusting the source of advice is vital and has been reported to be a key component in interacting effectively with parents; this in turn can be a pivotal factor in acceptance of previously declined or delayed vaccines (Gust et al. 2008). HCWs need to be well informed to respond appropriately and accurately to parents' questions. Resources that can support HCWs in their discussions as well as being useful for parents/carers include the UK Health Security Agency Immunisation website (UK Health Security Agency 2022), the Vaccine Knowledge Project (http://www.ovg.ox.ac.uk/vaccine-knowledge-home), and NHS.uk (https://www.nhs.uk/conditions/vaccinations/?tabname=all-about-vaccinations).

One important strategy for ensuring that CYPs are protected is to check immunisation status whenever they have contact with HCWs for other reasons, whether attending accident and emergency departments, outpatients' departments, or on admission to hospital. Although it may not always be feasible or acceptable to parents to offer opportunistic immunisation, it is good practice to remind them and to follow this up with a letter to the GP and/or health visitor. CYPs with complex health needs often have their immunisation status overlooked and nurses have a particularly important role in ensuring that this group and all CYPs have the opportunity to be fully immunised (Walton et al. 2007; RCPCH 2020).

The Personal Child Health Record (PCHR), which is issued to parents/carers for all children at or soon after birth, should contain a record of all immunisations that the child has received and all serious conditions from which the child suffers. This is a valuable tool for parents/carers as well as for health professionals reviewing a CYP's immunisation status.

In September 2009, the National Institute for Health and Care Excellence (NICE) issued guidance on improving the uptake of vaccines. The guidance focused on increasing immunisation uptake among CYPs aged under 19 years in groups and settings where immunisation coverage is low and on improving uptake of the hepatitis B vaccination programme for babies born to mothers infected with hepatitis B.

The guidance emphasised the importance of the following areas:

- Good immunisation programmes (provision, access, and support)
- Accurate information systems
- Training for professionals
- The contribution of nurseries, schools, colleges of further education
- Targeting groups at risk of not being fully immunised
- The organisation of programmes for hepatitis B immunisation of high-risk infants.

The importance of opportunistic immunisation in hospital settings was also endorsed in these guidelines (NICE 2009). New guidance is expected in 2022.

Vaccine safety scares

It is often difficult to distinguish a coincidental event *following* a vaccine from an adverse reaction *due* to a vaccine (temporal vs. causal connection), which has led to major scares in relation to pertussis and MMR vaccines. A paper published in 1974 suggested that in some children, brain damage could result from the administration of whole-cell pertussis vaccine (Kulenkampff et al. 1974). Following adverse media coverage, the uptake of the vaccine plummeted to 30% and lower in some areas. As a result, there was a resurgence of whooping cough, with thousands of extra cases and many tragically avoidable deaths (Baker 2003). It took at least 15 years and millions of pounds spent on research which disproved the link for uptake rates to return to their previous level. More recently, a paper linking autism and bowel problems was widely interpreted as suggesting a possible link with MMR. However the authors were very clear in stating: 'We did not prove an association between MMR vaccine and the syndrome described' (Wakefield et al. 1998 [retracted]). The issue attracted media attention, which at times was intense. Not surprisingly, some parents and carers rejected the vaccine. The research that triggered these concerns was subsequently discredited, and a significant body of more recent research shows no evidence for such a link (Taylor et al. 2014; Hviid et al., 2019), but the fall in vaccine uptake rates left its legacy and resulted in dramatic increases in numbers of cases of measles, with two deaths being reported toward the end of the first decade of the 2000s (Ramsay 2013). Uptake rates of MMR vaccine in young children have now recovered and are even higher than before the vaccine controversy.

These examples show how easy it is, on the basis of poor research and media attention, to destroy confidence in the vaccine programme. It is therefore essential that health professionals are properly informed before advising parents/carers. Once the seeds of doubt have been sown, it is very difficult to reverse the effects.

Immunisation of healthcare workers

Healthcare workers (HCWs), by the nature of their jobs, are exposed to many infections, but they may also act as a source of infection for colleagues, parents and carers, patients, and well CYPs. It is important that all possible measures are taken to prevent infection. Immunisation plays an important part in this – see Chapter 12 of the *Green Book* (Public Health England 2013a). All healthcare workers should have up to date knowledge of the routine immunisations and also be aware of their own immunisation status. This includes tetanus, diphtheria, polio and MMR. The MMR vaccine is of particular importance as staff may transmit measles or rubella infections to vulnerable groups; it is also important for their own protection. A doctor working on an oncology unit in 2008 was confirmed as having measles (Health Protection Agency 2008). Satisfactory evidence of protection would include documentation of having received two doses of MMR or having had positive antibody tests for measles and rubella. However, the protection from the mumps component is not long lasting. Following suspected mumps cases in an acute hospital setting, investigations showed that only 7% of 42 healthcare worker contacts had a documented history of two doses of MMR vaccine (Williams et al. 2010).

BCG, if not previously given, is indicated for tuberculin negative healthcare workers who have close contact with infectious patients. This is particularly important for staff working in maternity and paediatric departments and departments in which the children are likely to be immunocompromised. In the absence of a BCG scar and a history of receiving the vaccine, the HCW or student should have a tuberculin skin test and if negative (and there is no reason to assume impaired immunity), they should be given BCG.

All HCWs and students who are likely to be exposed to blood, blood-stained body fluids, or patients' body tissues should be offered hepatitis B vaccine if not already immune. Boosters are not necessary for HCWs after a successful primary course as judged by a good antibody response.

Chickenpox is more serious in adults and immunosuppressed individuals than in children. All HCWs without a clinical history of chickenpox or herpes zoster should have serology performed. If not immune, and in the absence of contraindications, they should receive a course of the vaccine (two doses as opposed to the one required for children).

Annual influenza vaccination is recommended for HCWs directly involved in patient care as it not only helps to prevent influenza among staff, but may also reduce transmission of the infection to vulnerable patients. Uptake of the vaccine among frontline health and social care workers was 74.3% in 2019–2020, representing an increase in recent years, but there is still room for further improvement.

A programme of offering pertussis vaccine to HCWs who have regular contact with pregnant women and/or infants under three months old is being rolled out. Currently the vaccine is offered to "clinical staff working with women in the last month of pregnancy (e.g. in midwifery, obstetrics and maternity settings) and neonatal and paediatric intensive care staff who are likely to have close and/or prolonged clinical contact with severely ill young infants" (Public Health England 2019).

Conclusion

Immunisation is a highly effective intervention, which has protected millions of CYPs worldwide from disability and death. Although it is largely carried out in the community, hospital staff also have an important role to play in ensuring that CYPs are fully protected. This may involve offering vaccines in a hospital setting, or reminding parents/carers of the importance of vaccines. In the case of CYPs with complex conditions, primary care staff may value advice on the CYP's suitability for immunisation. In an era when vaccine preventable diseases are uncommon, and the public has forgotten how serious they can be, hospital staff may be the only group with experience of the diseases. This can be a valuable asset in discussing the importance of immunisation. It is also imperative that healthcare workers ensure that they too are fully immunised for their own protection, and for the protection of the CYPs, families, and staff whom they work with.

References

Amirthalingam, G., Andrews, N., Campbell, H. et al. (2014). Effectiveness of maternal pertussis vaccination in England: an observational study. *The Lancet* 384: 521–1528.

Baker, J.P. (2003). The pertussis vaccine controversy in Great Britain, 1974–1986. *Vaccine* 21: 4003–4010.

Bedford, H.E. and Elliman, D.A. (2020). Fifteen-minute consultation: Vaccine-hesitant parents. *Archives of Disease in Childhood – Education and Practice* 105 (4): 194–199.

Campbell, H., Borrow, R., Salisbury, D., and Miller, E. (2009). Meningococcal C conjugate vaccine: the experience in England and Wales. *Vaccine* 27: B20–B29.

Campbell, H., Edwards, A., Letley, L. et al. (2017). Changing attitudes to childhood immunisation in English parents. *Vaccine* 35 (22): 2979–2985.

Collins, S., Ramsay, M., Campbell, H. et al. (2013). Invasive Haemophilus influenzae type b (Hib) disease in England and Wales: who is at risk after two decades of routine childhood vaccination? *Clinical Infectious Diseases* 57 (12): 1715–1721.

Demicheli, V., Rivetti, A., Debalini, M.G., and Di Pietrantonj, C. (2012). Vaccines for measles, mumps and rubella in children. *Cochrane Database of Systematic Reviews* 2012 (2): CD004407. https://doi.org/10.1002/14651858.CD004407.pub3.

Elliman, D., Sengupta, N., El Bashir, H., and Bedford, H. (2009). Measles, mumps, and rubella: prevention. *Clinical Evidence* 12: 316.

Farrington, P., Pugh, S., Colville, A. et al. (1995). A new method for active surveillance of adverse events from diphtheria/tetanus/pertussis and measles/mumps/rubella vaccines. *Lancet* 345: 567–569.

Gandhi, M., McKenna, S., Geraets, A. et al. (2011). Establishing an opportunistic catch up immunisation service for children attending an acute trust in London. *Archives of Disease in Childhood* 96 (8): 780–781.

Gkentzi, D., Katsakiori, P., Marangos, M. et al. (2017). Maternal vaccination against pertussis: a systematic review of the recent literature. *Archives of Disease in Childhood. Fetal and Neonatal Edition* 102 (5): F456–F463.

Global Polio Eradication Initiative (2020). http://polioeradication.org/polio-today/polio-now (accessed 20 July 2022).

Gust, D.A., Darling, N., Kennedy, A., and Schwartz, B. (2008). Parents with doubts about vaccines: which vaccines and reasons why. *Pediatrics* 122 (4): 718–725.

Health Protection Agency (2008). Confirmed measles cases in England and Wales – an update to end may – 2008. *Health Protection Report* 2 (25): 20.

Hviid, A., Hansen, J.V., Frisch, M., and Melbye, M. (2019). Measles, mumps, rubella vaccination and autism: a nationwide cohort study. *Annals of Internal Medicine* 170 (8): 513–520.

Jessop, L.J., Kelleher, C.C., Murrin, C. et al. (2010). Determinants of partial or no primary immunisations. *Archives of Diseases of Childhood* 95 (8): 603–605.

Kulenkampff, M.M., Schwartzman, J.S., and Wilson, J. (1974). Neurological complications of pertussis inoculation. *Archives of Diseases of Childhood* 49: 46–49.

Ladhani, S.N. and Ramsay, M.E. (2014). Timely immunisation of premature infants against rotavirus in the neonatal intensive care unit. *Archives of Disease in Childhood. Fetal and Neonatal Edition* 99 (6): F445–F447.

Larson, H.J., Cooper, L.Z., Eskola, J. et al. (2011). Addressing the vaccine confidence gap. *The Lancet* 378 (9790): 526–535.

Larson, H.J., Jarrett, C., Eckersberger, E. et al. (2014). Understanding vaccine hesitancy around vaccines and vaccination from a global perspective: a systematic review of published literature, 2007–2012. *Vaccine* 32 (19): 2150–2159.

Le Saux, N., Barrowman, N.J., Moore, D.L. et al. (2003). Canadian Paediatric society/ Health Canada immunization monitoring program-active (IMPACT). Decrease in hospital admissions for febrile seizures and reports of hypotonic-hyporesponsive episodes presenting to hospital emergency departments since switching to acellular pertussis vaccine in Canada: a report from IMPACT. *Pediatrics* 112 (5): e348.

Leask, J., Kinnersley, P., Jackson, C. et al. (2012). Communicating with parents about vaccination: a framework for health professionals. *BMC Pediatrics* 12 (1): 154.

Mangtani, P., Abubakar, I., Ariti, C. et al. (2014). Protection by BCG vaccine against tuberculosis: a systematic review of randomized controlled trials. *Clinical Infectious Diseases* 58 (4): 470–480.

Medicines and Healthcare products Regulatory Agency (MHRA) (2020). Yellow card. https://yellowcard.mhra.gov.uk (accessed 20 July 2022).

Miller, E. (1999). Overview of recent clinical trials of acellular pertussis vaccines. *Biologicals* 27: 79–86.

Miller, E., Waight, P., Farrington, C.P. et al. (2001). Idiopathic thrombocytopenic purpura and MMR vaccine. *Archives of Diseases of Childhood* 84: 227–229.

National Institute for Health and Clinical Excellence (NICE) (2009) PH 21 Reducing the differences in the uptake of immunisations. https://www.nice.org.uk/guidance/PH21 (accessed 20 July 2022).

Peckham, C., Bedford, H., Senturia, Y., Ades, A. (1989). The Peckham Report. National Immunisation Study: Factors affecting immunisation in childhood. Horsham, Action Research.

Peltola, H. and Heinonen, O.P. (1986). Frequency of true adverse reactions to measles-mumps-rubella vaccine. A double-blind placebo-controlled trial in twins. *Lancet* 1: 939–942.

Peltola, H., Jokinen, S., Paunio, M. et al. (2008). Measles, mumps, and rubella in Finland: 25 years of a nationwide elimination programme. *The Lancet Infectious Diseases* 8 (12): 796–803.

Public Health England (2013a). Immunisation against Infectious Diseases: Chapter 12. Immunisation of healthcare and laboratory staff. https://www.gov.uk/government/publications/immunisation-of-healthcare-and-laboratory-staff-the-green-book-chapter-12 (accessed 20 July 2022).

Public Health England (2013b). Immunisation against Infectious Diseases: Chapter 2. Consent. https://www.gov.uk/government/publications/consent-the-green-book-chapter-2 (accessed 18 July 2022).

Public Health England (2017c). Immunisation against Infectious Diseases: Chapter 6. Contraindications and special considerations. https://www.gov.uk/government/uploads/system/uploads/attachment_data/file/655225/Greenbook_chapter_6.pdf (accessed 20 July 2022).

Public Health England (2019). Occupational pertussis vaccination of healthcare workers. https://www.gov.uk/government/publications/pertussis-occupational-vaccination-of-healthcare-workers/pertussis-occupational-vaccination-of-healthcare-workers (accessed 18 July 2022).

Ramsay, M. E. (2013). Measles: the legacy of low vaccine coverage. Archives of Disease in Childhood 98(10):752–754. https://adc.bmj.com/content/archdischild/98/10/752.full.pdf (accessed 10 September 2020).

Royal College of Paediatrics and Child Health (RCPCH) (2002). Immunisation of the immunocompromised Child: Best Practice Statement. London, RCPCH.

RCPCH (2020) Vaccination in the UK - position statement. https://www.rcpch.ac.uk/resources/vaccination-uk-position-statement (accessed 18 July 2022).

Ruiz-Palacios, G.M., Pérez-Schael, I., Velázquez, F.R. et al. (2006). Safety and efficacy of an attenuated vaccine against severe rotavirus gastroenteritis. *The New England Journal of Medicine* 354: 11–22.

Samad, L., Tate, A.R., Dezateux, C. et al. (2006). Differences in risk factors for partial and no immunisation in the first year of life: prospective cohort study. *British Medical Journal* 332: 1312–1313.

Stefanoff, P., Mamelund, S.E., Robinson, M. et al. (2010). Tracking parental attitudes on vaccination across countries: the vaccine safety, attitudes, training and communication project (VACSATC). *Vaccine* 28 (35): 5731–5737.

Taylor, L.E., Swerdfeger, A.L., and Eslick, G.D. (2014). Vaccines are not associated with autism: an evidence-based meta-analysis of case-control and cohort studies. *Vaccine* 32 (29): 3623–3629.

UK Health Security Agency (2020). Immunisation against Infectious Diseases: Chapter 7. Immunisation of individuals with underlying medical conditions. https://www.gov.uk/government/publications/immunisation-of-individuals-with-underlying-medical-conditions-the-green-book-chapter-7 (accessed 4 July 2022).

UK Health Security Agency (2020). Immunisation of individuals with underlying medical conditions: the green book, chapter 7. https://www.gov.uk/government/publications/immunisation-of-individuals-with-underlying-medical-conditions-the-green-book-chapter-7 (accessed 18 July 2022).

UK Health Security Agency (2022). Information for immunisation practitioners and other health professionals. https://www.gov.uk/government/collections/immunisation. (accessed 4 July 2022). *Contains information on all the vaccines, the Green Book (Immunisation Against Infectious Diseases), Vaccine Update, the newsletter for immunisation professionals, links to leaflets for parents, factsheets, and training slide sets.*

UK Health Security Agency (2022). Vaccination of individuals with uncertain or incomplete immunisation status https://www.gov.uk/government/publications/vaccination-of-individuals-with-uncertain-or-incomplete-immunisation-status (accessed 4 July 2022).

UK Health Security Agency (2022a). Immunisation against Infectious Diseases: Chapter 11. The UK Immunisation Schedule. https://www.gov.uk/government/publications/immunisation-schedule-the-green-bookchapter-11 (accessed 4 July 2022).

UK Health Security Agency (2022b). Immunoglobulin: when to use. https://www.gov.uk/government/publications/immunoglobulin-when-to-use (accessed 4 July 2022).

Uzicanin, A. and Zimmerman, L. (2011). Field effectiveness of live attenuated measles-containing vaccines: a review of published literature. *Journal of Infectious Diseases* 204 (suppl 1): S133–S149.

Van Panhuis, W.G., Grefenstette, J., Jung, S.Y. et al. (2013). Contagious diseases in the United States from 1888 to the present. *The New England Journal of Medicine* 369 (22): 2152–2158.

Virtanen, M., Peltola, H., Paunio, M., and Heinonen, O.P. (2000). Day-to-day reactogenicity and the healthy vaccine effect of measles-mumps-rubella vaccination. *Pediatrics* 106 (5): E62.

Wagner, K.S., White, J.M., Crowcroft, N.S. et al. (2010). Diphtheria in the United Kingdom, 1986–2008: the increasing role of Corynebacterium ulcerans. *Epidemiology and Infection* 138 (11): 1519–1530.

Wakefield, A.J., Murch, S.H., Anthony, A. et al. (1998). Ileal-lymphoid-nodular hyperplasia, non-specific colitis, and pervasive developmental disorder in children. *Lancet* 351 (9103): 637–641. (RETRACTED).

Walton, S., Elliman, D., and Bedford, H. (2007). Missed opportunities to vaccinate children admitted to a paediatric tertiary hospital. *Archives of Diseases of Childhood* 92 (7): 620–622.

Walton, S. and Bedford, H. (2017). Immunization of looked-after children and young people: a review of the literature. *Child: Care, Health and Development* 43 (4): 463–480.

Williams, C.J., Liebowitz, L.D., Levene, J., and Nair, P. (2010). Low measles, mumps and rubella (MMR) vaccine uptake in hospital healthcare worker contacts following suspected mumps infection. *Journal of Hospital Infection* 76 (1): 91–92.

Yaqub, O., Castle-Clarke, S., Sevdalis, N., and Chataway, J. (2014). Attitudes to vaccination: a critical review. *Social Science & Medicine* 112: 1–11.

Further reading

Centers for Disease Control. http://www.cdc.gov/vaccines/default.htm (accessed 22 March 2018). *This is a very good US website.*

Health Protection Scotland. Immunisation and vaccine preventable diseases. http://www.hps.scot.nhs.uk/immvax/index.aspx (accessed 22 March 2018).

Health Protection Wales. Immunisation and vaccine preventable diseases. http://www.wales.nhs.uk/sites3/page.cfm?orgid=457&pid=25355 (accessed 22 March 2018).

Miller, E., Andrews, N., Waight, P., and Taylor, B. (2003). Bacterial infections, immune overload, and MMR vaccine. Measles, mumps, and rubella. *Archives of Diseases of Childhood* 88 (3): 222–223. *This research study looked to see if children were more likely to get serious infections after having MMR vaccination.*

National Travel Health Network and Centre (NaTHNaC). Health Information for Overseas Travel. https://nathnac.net (accessed 22 March 2018). *The National Travel Health Network and Centre (NaTHNaC) promotes standards in travel medicine, providing travel health information for health professionals and the public*

NHS Choices. Vaccinations. https://www.nhs.uk/conditions/vaccinations (accessed 22 March 2018. *The main source of information for parents provided by the NHS.*

Northern Ireland, Public Health Agency. http://www.publichealth.hscni.net/directorate-public-health/health-protection/immunisationvaccine-preventable-diseases ().

Offit, P.A., Quarles, J., Gerber, M.A. et al. (2002). Addressing parents' concerns: do multiple vaccines overwhelm or weaken the infant's immune system? *Pediatrics* 109: 124–129. http://pediatrics.aappublications.org/cgi/reprint/109/1/124 *A review.*

Offit, P.A. and Hackett, C.J. (2003). Addressing parents' concerns: do vaccines cause allergic or autoimmune diseases? *Pediatrics* 111 (3): 653–659. http://pediatrics.aappublications.org/cgi/reprint/111/3/653. *A review.*

Offit, P.A. and Jew, R.K. (2003). Addressing parents' concerns: do vaccines contain harmful preservatives, adjuvants, additives, or residuals? *Pediatrics* 112 (6 Pt 1): 1394–1397. http://pediatrics.aappublications.org/cgi/reprint/112/6/1394 (accessed 16 April 2018). *A review.*

Offit, P.A. and Coffin, S.E. (2003). Communicating science to the public: MMR vaccine and autism. *Vaccine* 22 (1): 1–6. *A review.*

Oxford Vaccine Group. Vaccine Knowledge Project. http://www.ovg.ox.ac.uk/vaccine-knowledge-home (accessed 5 July 2022). *Provides information about vaccine preventable diseases, films about immunization decision making and FAQs.*

Royal College of Nursing. Public health – topics: immunisation. www.rcn.org.uk/development/practice/public_health/topics/immunisation (accessed 4 July 2022).

UK Health Security Agency (2020). Immunisation of individuals with underlying medical conditions: the green book, chapter 7. https://www.gov.uk/government/publications/immunisation-of-individuals-with-underlying-medical-conditions-the-green-book-chapter-7 (accessed 18 July 2022).

UK Health Security Agency (2022). Information for immunisation practitioners and other health professionals. https://www.gov.uk/government/collections/immunisation (accessed 4 July 2022). *Contains information on all the vaccines, the Green Book (Immunisation Against Infectious Diseases), Vaccine Update, the newsletter for immunisation professionals, links to leaflets for parents, factsheets, and training slide sets.*

UK Health Security Agency (2022a). Immunisation against Infectious Diseases: Chapter 11. The UK Immunisation Schedule. https://www.gov.uk/government/publications/immunisation-schedule-the-green-bookchapter-11 (accessed 4 July 2022).

UK Health Security Agency (2022b). Immunoglobulin: when to use. https://www.gov.uk/government/publications/immunoglobulin-when-to-use (accessed 4 July 2022).

World Health Organization. Immunization. https://www.who.int/health-topics/vaccines-and-immunization#tab=tab_1 (accessed 4 July 2022).

Chapter 13

Infection prevention and control

Barbara Brekle

RN (Child), BSc (Hons); Deputy Lead Nurse – Infection Prevention and Control, Great Ormond Street Hospital, London, UK

Chapter contents

Introduction	218
Financial burden of healthcare associated infections	218
The health and social care act 2008: Code of practice on the prevention and control of infections and related guidance	218
Antibiotic resistance and antimicrobial stewardship	219
The chain of infection	219
Standard precautions	221

Isolation nursing	239
Management of exposure to blood and body fluids	240
Reporting of injuries, diseases and occurrences regulations	242
Decontamination of equipment and the environment	243
References	245
Further reading	247

Procedure guidelines

13.1 Hand decontamination techniques	233	
13.2 Hand drying techniques	234	

13.3 Inoculation with blood or body fluids	242	
13.4 Dealing with spillage of blood or other body fluids	243	

Principles tables

13.1 Equipment required for handwashing	231
13.2 General hand care	231
13.3 When to perform hand hygiene	232
13.4 Choice of cleansing agent	232
13.5 Disposable gloves	236

13.6 Disposable aprons and gowns	237
13.7 Choice of facial protection	238
13.8 Principles of safe handling of laundry	244
13.9 Principles of waste disposal	245

The Great Ormond Street Hospital Manual of Children and Young People's Nursing Practices, Second Edition. Edited by Elizabeth Anne Bruce, Janet Williss, and Faith Gibson.
© 2023 John Wiley & Sons Ltd. Published 2023 by John Wiley & Sons Ltd.

Introduction

Healthcare associated infections (HCAIs), also referred to as 'nosocomial' or 'hospital' infections, are infections occurring during or after exposure to healthcare and often, but not always, as a consequence of this exposure (European Centre for Disease Prevention and Control (ECDC) are the most frequent adverse events during care delivery and are a global problem for patient safety. HCAIs can result in prolonged hospital stay, long-term disability, increased resistance of micro-organisms to antimicrobial agents, significant additional financial burden for the healthcare system, high costs for the patients and their families, and avoidable deaths.

The risk of acquiring a HCAI is universal and affects every healthcare facility and healthcare system worldwide (World Health Organization [WHO] 2011a). The assessment, prevention, and management of the risk of HCAIs is an essential part of maintaining patient safety and fundamental in any healthcare setting. Effective prevention and control of infection must be part of everyday practice and be applied consistently by everyone. Good management and organisational processes are crucial to make sure that high standards of infection prevention and control are set up and maintained (Department of Health [DH] 2015).

Financial burden of healthcare associated infections

It is estimated that 300000 patients a year in England acquire a healthcare-associated infection as a result of care within the National Health Service (NHS). In 2007, Meticillin-resistant *Staphylococcus aureus* (MRSA), bloodstream infections, and *Clostridium difficile* infections were recorded as the underlying cause of, or as a contributory factor in, approximately 9000 deaths in hospital and primary care in England. Healthcare-associated infections are estimated to cost the NHS approximately £1 billion a year, and in addition to increased costs, each one of these infections means additional use of NHS resources, greater patient discomfort, and a decrease in patient safety (National Audit Office 2009).

The health and social care act 2008: Code of practice on the prevention and control of infections and related guidance

The Health and Social Care Act 2008 (DH 2015) came into force in April 2009 and was updated in 2011. It outlines regulations for health care, social care, and mental health, helping to ensure better outcomes for the people who use these services. Initially only for hospitals and care homes, registration under the Health and Social Care Act was extended in 2008 to include all provider healthcare services, such as prison healthcare services, NHS Blood Transfusion and Transplant, independent healthcare, adult social care providers, primary dental care, private ambulance providers, and primary medical care providers (Weston 2013).

The Care Quality Commission (CQC) (see www.cqc.org.uk) is responsible for the regulation of three previous bodies (the Commission for Health Care, Audit and Inspection – known as the Healthcare Commission; The Commission for Social Care Inspection; and The Mental Health Act Commission) to ensure safety, quality and performance assessment of commissioners and providers. They ensure that regulation and inspection activity across health and social care and mental health is co-ordinated and managed under a single, integrated regulator. The regulatory system details the requirements that must be met in order to provide services (see Box 13.1). The risk-based approach means that regulation activity is targeted where action is required. If providers do not comply with the standards required, such as cleanliness and infection prevention and control, the CQC can impose specific conditions responding to these risks. This may include issuing a warning notice, or imposing conditions on registration, which range from closing a ward or service until safety requirements are met to total suspension of services where absolutely necessary. This could lead to prosecution, with heavy financial penalties for the healthcare provider.

Box 13.1 Ten criteria against which the CQC judge cleanliness and infection control requirements

1. Have systems in place to manage and monitor the prevention and control of infections.
2. Provide and maintain a clean and appropriate environment in managed premises that facilitates the prevention and control of infections.
3. Provide suitable and accurate information on infections to patients, families, and visitors.
4. Provide suitable accurate information on infections to any person concerned with providing further support or nursing/medical care in a timely fashion.
5. Ensure that people who have or develop an infection are identified promptly and receive the appropriate treatment and care to reduce the risk of passing on the infection to other people.
6. Ensure that all staff and those employed to provide care in all settings are fully involved in the process of preventing and controlling infection.
7. Provide or secure adequate isolation facilities.
8. Secure adequate access to laboratory support as appropriate.
9. Have and adhere to policies, designed for the individual's care and provider organisations, which will help to prevent and control infections.
10. Ensure, so far as is reasonably practicable, that healthcare workers (HCWs) are free of and are protected from exposure to infections that can be caught at work and that all staff are suitably educated in the prevention and control of infection associated with the provision of health and social care. For each criterion further subcriteria are included that list examples of evidence of compliance, such as policies relating to infection prevention and control, audit requirements, staff training requirements, and surveillance of HCAIs.

Antibiotic resistance and antimicrobial stewardship

Antibiotics are substances used to treat infections caused by bacteria. They can be either *bacteriostatic*, in that they do not kill bacteria but prevent them from reproducing and allow the host's defences to kill the micro-organism (e.g. tetracycline); or *bactericidal*, in that they destroy the bacteria (e.g. aminoglycosides) (Spencer 2007). Since 1950 a wide range of antibiotics have been developed and widely used in hospitals and community settings. Regarded as safe, effective, and relatively inexpensive, antibiotics had a significant role in reducing morbidity and mortality from diseases that were once widespread and untreatable. However, the effectiveness of antibiotics has become increasingly limited due to the development of resistance mechanisms that have spread in several clinically important species of bacteria (Campbell 2007).

Antimicrobial resistance has been defined as the 'resistance of a micro-organism to an antimicrobial medicine to which it was originally sensitive' (World Health Organization (WHO) 2021). Bacteria have the ability to adapt and develop resistance to antibiotics. Some strains are inherently resistant, while others may develop resistance through mutation or receipt of resistance-encoding genetic material from different strains (Acar et al. 2009). Bacteria that have the ability to resist the action of certain antibiotics have an increased chance of survival compared with bacteria that are susceptible to these drugs. Susceptible bacteria are killed or inhibited by the antibiotic, resulting in selective pressure for the survival of resistant strains of bacteria (Cohen 1992). Overuse and misuse of antibiotics have been identified as the main factors in the increase of antimicrobial resistance and some experts are concerned that due to the lack of new antibiotics in the development pipeline we may soon 'run out' of antibiotics and that classical infections will regain their status as major causes of mortality (e.g. multidrug resistant *Mycobacterium tuberculosis*) (WHO 2011b). In 2011 the Advisory Committee on Antimicrobial Resistance and HCAI (DH 2015) issued guidance on antimicrobial stewardship to help reduce inappropriate prescribing, optimise antibiotic use, and reduce the incidence of antimicrobial resistance. Nurses play a vital role in the implementation of this strategy by promoting the judicious use of antimicrobials (Ladenheim et al. 2013).

Over the last few years the development and spread of multidrug resistance, in which bacteria are resistant to several different classes of antibiotic agents, has become a particular concern and has been identified by the World Health Organization as a global threat (WHO 2011b). Gram-negative bacteria, capable of producing enzymes that destroy last-generation antibiotics, have increased in prevalence in Europe. Extended spectrum beta-lactamase (ESBL) producing *Enterobacteriaceae* or carbapenemase producing *Enterobacteriaceae* (CPE) are two examples. Infections with these organisms leave patients with few or no antimicrobial options (Huttner et al. 2013). In 2013 Public Health England (PHE 2020) published the 'Acute trust toolkit for the early detection, management, and control of carbapenemase-producing *Enterobacteriaceae*,' which highlights the importance of infection prevention and control measures, such as admission screening and isolation of colonised or infected patients to reduce the further spread of these organisms.

The chain of infection

The term 'chain of infection' is used to describe the process of the spread of infection from one individual to another. It is a circle of six links, each representing a component in the cycle. Each of the links must be present and in sequential order for infection to occur. It is important to understand each link and how the links connect to cause infection, to be able to understand how the 'chain of infection' can be 'broken' and the transmission of infections prevented (Weston 2013) (see Box 13.2).

Box 13.2 The 'Chain of Infection'

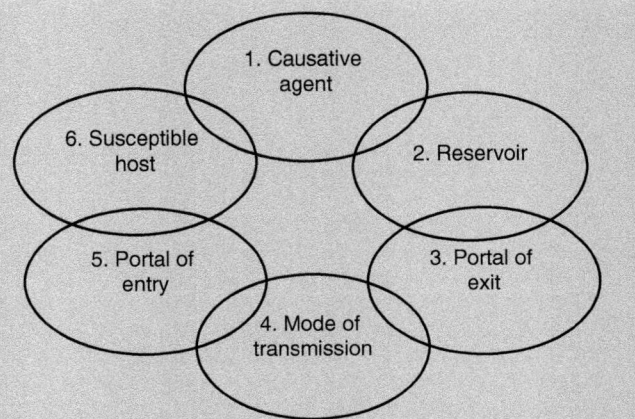

1. **Causative agent**
   Micro-organisms are mainly divided into bacteria, viruses, fungi, and parasites. To be able to produce disease, a micro-organism needs to demonstrate pathogenicity (the ability to cause disease) and virulence (the potential to cause severe disease).

2. **Reservoir**
   This is the site where a micro-organism lives. Reservoirs can be humans, animals, insects, the environment, food, or water. A human reservoir may be either an infected case or a carrier. In the healthcare setting, humans (patients, visitors, and staff) and the environment (equipment, furniture) are the most significant reservoirs.

3. **Portal of exit**
   The portal of exit is the way by which a micro-organism leaves its reservoir. In human reservoirs this is commonly the respiratory tract, the gastrointestinal tract, the genitourinary tract, the skin, and/or the mucous membranes.

4. **Mode of transmission**
   This is the route how a micro-organism spreads from one person or place to another. Some micro-organisms use more than one mode of transmission to get from their reservoir to the susceptible host.
   a) *Contact*
      This can be through either direct or indirect contact.
      Direct contact transmission occurs from body surface to another person's body surface. This may happen when lifting a child or young person (CYP) or when two CYPs play together.
      Indirect contact transmission occurs, if a healthcare worker handles one patient and fails to perform hand hygiene before handling the next patient, thus potentially transmitting micro-organisms on their hands, or through a contaminated article such as a dirty instrument or equipment (e.g. blood pressure cuff).
      This is the most common method by which micro-organisms are transmitted in a hospital environment. Examples of micro-organisms that are transmitted by this route are antibiotic-resistant bacteria (e.g. Meticillin-resistant *S. aureus* (MRSA)) or *Norovirus*.
   b) *Droplet*
      Droplets are generated through sneezing, coughing, or talking, or through procedures which generate aerosols,

(continued)

Box 13.2 The 'Chain of Infection' *(continued)*

such as suction or bronchoscopy. Transmission occurs when micro-organisms from an infected person are propelled a short distance through the air (between 1 and 2 m) onto the mucosal surfaces (conjunctiva, nasal surface, or mouth) of the new host. The droplets do not remain suspended in the air, they settle on surfaces and therefore also cause significant contamination of the environment. Most respiratory viruses (e.g. the influenza virus or respiratory syncytial virus [RSV]) remain viable on surfaces for several hours.

c) *Airborne*
Transmission occurs by dissemination of either airborne droplet nuclei (<5 μm) or dust particles that contain micro-organisms from an infected person, which are then inhaled by a susceptible host. These may remain suspended in the air and transmitted over longer distances by air currents or through air-handling units. *M. tuberculosis* or the *Varicella zoster virus* can be transmitted by this route.

d) *Faecal-oral*
Faecal-oral transmission occurs when pathogens from the gut of an infected person are ingested by a susceptible host. This can happen when drinking water has come into contact with faeces (e.g. sewage) or food has been contaminated with faecal matter (e.g. through inadequate hand and food hygiene). For example, cholera and typhoid fever can be transmitted via the faecal–oral route.

e) *Percutaneous*
Transmission occurs through the inoculation of infected blood or body fluid into the tissue of a susceptible person. Examples include infections with bloodborne viruses (e.g. human immunodeficiency virus [HIV] or Hepatitis B or C) that can be transmitted through contaminated blood products or contaminated instruments (e.g. inoculation injury).

f) *Vectorborne*
Transmission occurs through blood-sucking arthropods, either insects (e.g. mosquitoes or fleas) or arachnids (e.g. ticks). The vector transmits the micro-organisms through feeding activity to the susceptible host. Examples of infections transmitted through this mode include malaria and Lyme disease.

g) *Congenital*
This mode is also called vertical transmission. It occurs directly from the mother to the foetus or baby during pregnancy or childbirth. Examples of viruses that can be transmitted via this route are the rubella virus or cytomegalovirus.

h) *Exogenous and endogenous transmission*
All of the above described modes of transmissions are exogenous, which means that infection occurs because of the transfer of micro-organisms from one person (or creature) to another. However, some infections may also spread endogenously. This means that the infection causing micro-organisms originate from the same individual and are transferred from one body site to another, e.g. pneumonia resulting from aspiration of oral secretions in a sedated CYP.

5 Portal of entry
This is the path by which an infectious agent invades a susceptible host. It can be the same as the portal of exit through the respiratory tract, the gastrointestinal tract, the genitourinary tract, the skin and/or the mucous membranes. It can also be through indwelling devices (e.g. central venous catheters or urinary catheters) or damaged skin (e.g. trauma or surgical wounds).

6 Susceptible host
This is the individual who is at risk of becoming infected and the final link in the chain of infection. The human body has several defence mechanisms for resisting the entry and multiplication of pathogenic micro-organisms. When all these defence mechanisms function normally, infection is unlikely to occur. However, there are several factors that contribute to a compromised or deficient immune system:

a) *Gestational age*
Premature babies are particularly susceptible to infection, as they have no immunological memory and a reduced ability to develop specific antibodies against micro-organisms that they are exposed to. Their protection against infections is mostly dependent upon innate immune defences. However, due to their prematurity, natural barriers such as the mucosa and skin are weakened. Premature babies have an immature and underdeveloped population of T-lymphocytes and decreased neutrophil efficiency. Even though the neutrophil count rises abruptly within the first 24 hours after birth and stabilises within 72 hours, the neutrophil production in response to an infection is still underwhelming (Petrova and Mehta 2007) and they are deficient in some components of the complement cascade.

b) *Low birth weight*
The risk of infection is significantly increased in neonates weighing less than 1000 g.

c) *Method of nutrition*
Infection occurs less frequently in breast-fed babies because of protection from maternal antibody transference. Infection occurs more frequently in bottle-fed babies because they do not benefit from the transference of maternal antibodies and because of the risks associated with any lack of hygiene in equipment, preparation, and storage of feeds.

d) *Umbilical stump*
The risk of infection is increased by delay in cord separation, inadequate sterilised equipment used for cutting and clamping the cord, or the placement of umbilical catheters.

e) *Congenital abnormalities and congenital infections*
The risk of infection increases with cardiac and renal abnormalities, congenital infections such as rubella, cytomegalovirus (CMV), hepatitis or HIV, and in syndromes associated with abnormal immune function, such as Di-George syndrome, Down syndrome, and severe combined immune deficiency (SCID).

f) *Drug therapy*
CYPs undergoing chemotherapy and/or radiotherapy are immunocompromised as a result of their treatment. Due to the suppression of the bone marrow, neutrophils can become severely depleted. This leaves the CYP at severe risk of a potentially life-threating neutropenic sepsis, as neutrophils serve as a primary defence of the body by destroying bacteria in the blood. Other side effects of cytotoxic treatment include damage to the mucosal barriers in the mouth and the gastrointestinal tract, which can lead to inflammation, infection, ulceration, and diarrhoea.

g) *Indwelling/implanted devices*
Invasive indwelling or implanted devices are associated with a definite risk of bacterial and fungal infections and contribute significantly to the problem of HCAIs. All of these devices either breach the skin (e.g. central venous catheter) or a sterile organ (e.g. ventriculoperitoneal shunt). *Staphylococci* account for the majority of infections associated with these devices. While a variety of micro-organisms may be involved as pathogens, *Staphylococci* have the ability to adhere to materials and to promote the formation of biofilms, which is the most important feature of their pathogenicity.

Colonisation and infection

When an individual is exposed to a micro-organism such as MRSA, they can become colonised. This means that the micro-organism establishes itself (e.g. in the nose or on the skin) without invading the individual's tissue and causing damage. The length of time in which someone remains colonised is variable and may continue harmlessly indefinitely, clear spontaneously, or develop into an infection. Infection occurs when pathogens invade, live, and multiply in or on the host's bodily tissue and so cause tissue damage. Infection manifests itself both physically and physiologically and the symptoms that appear after an incubation period may either be localised (e.g. redness or pus) or systemic (e.g. fever). It is possible for individuals to become carriers, which means that without manifesting colonisation or infection they can harbour micro-organisms and may serve as a reservoir of transmission. Carriage can be transient, intermittent, or persistent.

Standard precautions

In the mid-1980s 'universal precautions' were introduced by the Centers for Disease Control (CDC 1987) in response to the HIV/AIDS epidemic with the aim to protect healthcare workers from exposure to blood and body fluids. Initially the focus was on the protection from bloodborne viruses, but the CDC later revised the recommendations to include all pathogens. The term 'universal precautions' has now been replaced by 'standard precautions', as the precautions should be part of the routine care for all patients at all times, regardless of suspected or confirmed infection status, and in any setting in which healthcare is delivered (including outpatient and community settings).

Standard precautions include:

- Hand hygiene
- The use of personal protective equipment (PPE)
- The safe handling and disposal of sharps (including the management of sharps injuries)
- Cleaning and decontamination of equipment and the environment
- The management of blood and body fluid spillages
- The handling and disposal of waste
- The handling and disposal of linen and laundry
- Pest control

In addition to standard precautions, isolation (or transmission-based) precautions are applied for patients suspected or known to be colonised or infected with a pathogen (see Table 13.1).

Hand hygiene

HCAIs can spread from patient to patient through the contamination of the hands of healthcare workers by pathogens. Contamination occurs through direct contact with patients or contaminated surfaces. Hand hygiene is considered to be the primary measure proven to be effective in the prevention of disease transmission and by cleaning hands at the right times and in the right way, most HCAIs can be prevented.

Despite comprehensive evidence of the efficacy of hand hygiene (WHO 2009), studies have repeatedly shown poor compliance with hand hygiene by healthcare workers (Pittet 2001).

In 2009 the WHO (2009) published new evidence-based guidelines, which recommend the following to improve compliance:

- The provision of alcohol gel dispensers at the point of care.
- The provision of sufficient and conveniently located handwashing sinks in clinical areas.
- Encourage patients to challenge noncompliant staff.
- Staff to challenge noncompliant colleagues.
- Role models in good hand hygiene amongst all disciplines of healthcare workers.
- Monitoring and feedback of hand hygiene compliance.
- Clear and easily accessible hand hygiene policies and procedures.
- Posters educating and reminding staff of the importance of hand hygiene and the correct techniques.

Well-defined hand hygiene programmes have demonstrated a change in behaviour and sustained adherence to long-term follow up (Boyce and Pittet 2002).

Table 13.1 Isolation precautions required for specific infections or clinical conditions (Siegel et al. 2007; Török et al. 2009; American Academy of Pediatrics 2015; PHE 2015)

Infection/condition	Isolation precautions	Incubation and duration	Infective material	Comments
Adenovirus				
Gastroenteritis	Contact	Incubation: 3–10 days. Contagious: duration of virus shedding.	Faeces	
Keratoconjunctivitis	Contact	Incubation: 4–24 days. Contagious: duration of symptoms.	Eye secretions	Can be transmitted through contaminated towels and ophthalmic solutions.
Respiratory tract disease	Contact; droplet	Incubation: 4–5 days. Contagious: duration of virus shedding.	Respiratory secretions Wear mask/respirator when in close contact with the patient (<2 m).	
Aspergillosis	Standard	Incubation: unknown.		**Contact** precautions and **airborne** precautions if massive soft tissue infection with copious drainage and repeated irrigations required. Prevention of aspergillosis in immunocompromised patients is paramount.
Bronchiolitis				(See specific viral agents)
Brucellosis	Standard; contact precautions for patients with draining wounds.	Varies from less than one week to several months. Most patients become ill within three to four weeks of exposure.	Infected animals; unpasteurised milk or milk products from infected animals.	UK statutory notifiable disease. Not transmitted from person to person except rarely via banked spermatozoa and sexual contact. Provision antimicrobial prophylaxis following laboratory exposure recommended.
Campylobacter	Contact	Incubation: 1–11 days. Contagious: Infective organisms may be excreted in the stool for up to three weeks after resolution of diarrhoea.	Infected domestic animals. Unpasteurised milk. Raw or undercooked meat.	UK statutory notifiable disease.
Chickenpox (varicella)	(See varicella)			
Clostridium difficile	Contact	Incubation: unknown. Contagious: duration of symptoms.	Faeces	Soap and water must be used to decontaminate hands, as alcohol hand gel is ineffective for removing *Clostridium difficile* spores.
Covid-19 (Coronavirus disease 2019)	Contact; Droplet	Incubation: 2–14 days (average of six days) Contagious: up to 48 hours before onset of symptoms until up to ten days after onset of symptoms	Respiratory secretions; Faeces	FFP2 or FFP3 respirators to be worn; plus visors when performing aerosol generating procedures. SARS-CoV2 is a novel pandemic virus. For current advice and guidance see https://www.gov.uk/government/organisations/uk-health-security-agency UK Health Security Agency - GOV.UK (www.gov.uk)
Creutzfeldt-Jakob disease	Standard	1.5 years to more than 30 years.	Brain, cerebro-spinal fluid, eyes, spinal cord, tonsils	No person-to-person transmission reported. Use disposable instruments for contact with tissues associated with high levels of infectivity. For current information, see: https://www.gov.uk/government/collections/creutzfeldt-jakob-disease-cjd-guidance-data-and-analysis.
Croup (acute laryngotracheobronchitis)				(See specific viral agents)
Cryptosporidium	Contact	Incubation: 2–14 days. Contagious: until 7 days after	Faeces; Faeces of infected	Oocysts resist standard chlorination. People with a diagnosis of cryptosporidiosis should not use swimming

Cytomegalovirus (CMV) Infection	Standard		Blood, breast milk, cervical secretions, saliva, semen, tears, urine	No additional precautions for pregnant healthcare workers (HCWs) required.
Epstein–Barr virus infection	Standard	Incubation: 3–12 weeks. Contagious: the virus can be shed for months to years following infection or reactivation of infection.	Saliva, blood, respiratory secretions	
E. coli (enterovirulent, including E. coli O157 (including haemolytic uraemic syndrome)	Contact	Incubation: 30–50 days. Contagious: Intermittent excretion is lifelong.	Faeces, contaminated food	UK statutory notifiable disease for haemolytic uraemic syndrome (HUS).
Giardia lamblia	Contact	Incubation: 10 hours to six days. Contagious: duration of symptoms.	Faeces	
German measles	(See Rubella)	Incubation: 5–25 days. Contagious: duration of symptoms.		
Haemophilus influenza	(See Meningitis; Pneumonia)			
Hand, foot, and mouth disease	Contact; droplet	Incubation: three to six days. Contagious: duration of symptoms.	Nasopharyngeal secretions, faeces	
Head lice	(See Pediculosis)			
Hepatitis:				
Type A	Contact	Incubation: 15–50 days.	Blood, faeces	
Type B	Standard	Incubation: 45–160 days.	Blood, body fluids	
Type C	Standard	Incubation: two weeks to six months.	Blood, body fluids contaminated with blood	
Type D	Standard	Incubation: two to eight weeks.	Blood	Requires co-infection with Hepatitis B virus
Type E	Contact	Incubation: unknown.	Faeces	
Type G	Standard	Incubation: unknown.	Blood	
Herpes simplex:				
Mucocutaneous, disseminated or primary, severe	Contact	Contagious: until lesions dry and crusted.	Skin lesions	
Neonatal	Contact	Contagious: until lesions dry and crusted – see comments.	Skin lesions	Contact precautions also required for asymptomatic, exposed infants delivered vaginally or by C-section and if mother has active infection and membranes have been ruptured for more than four to six hours until infant surface cultures obtained at 24–36 hours of age after 48 hours incubation.

(continued)

Table 13.1 Isolation precautions required for specific infections or clinical conditions (continued)

Infection/condition	Isolation precautions	Incubation and duration	Infective material	Comments
Human metapneumovirus (hMPV)	Droplet contact	Incubation: three to five days. Contagious: duration of symptoms; prolonged shedding possible in immunosuppressed patients	Respiratory secretions	Wear mask/respirator when in close contact with the patient (< 2m).
Impetigo	Contact	Incubation: Streptococcal: one to three days. Staphylococcal: 4–10 days. Contagious: until 24 hours after initiation of effective therapy.	Skin lesions	Infection is usually caused by *Staphylococcus* or *Streptococcus* bacteria. Avoid communal use of towels, flannels, bed linen, or clothes, as highly infectious.
Infectious mononucleosis (glandular fever)	Contact	Incubation: four to six weeks. Contagious: for six weeks following infection, possibly longer.	Saliva, blood	80–90% of cases are due to Epstein–Barr virus, most of the remainder are caused by Cytomegalovirus.
Influenza:				
Human (seasonal influenza, including H1N1 strain)	Droplet; contact	Incubation: one to three days. Contagious: duration of symptoms.	Nasopharyngeal secretions	FFP2 or FFP3 respirators to be worn; plus visors when performing aerosol-generating procedures.
Avian (e.g. H5N1 strain)	Droplet, contact	Incubation: three to seven days.	Faeces and secretions of infected birds	Limited evidence that suggests person-to-person transmission; See https://www.gov.uk/government/collections/avian-influenza-guidance-data-and-analysis for current avian influenza guidance.
Pandemic influenza	Droplet; contact	Incubation: one to three days. Contagious: duration of symptoms.	Nasopharyngeal secretions	FFP3 respirators, visors, gowns and gloves to be worn; See https://www.gov.uk/pandemic-flu for current pandemic influenza guidance.
Lice	(See Pediculosis)			
Malaria	Standard	Incubation: *Plasmodium falciparum*: 7–14 days. *Plasmodium vivax*: 8–14 days. *Plasmodium ovale*: 8–14 days. *Plasmodium malariae*: 7–30 days.	Mosquito bite, blood transfusion (rare)	Not transmitted from person-to-person.
Measles (rubeola)	Airborne	Incubation: 8–12 days. Contagious: 4 days before until 4 days after onset of rash; duration of symptoms in immunocompromised patients.	Respiratory droplets	Nonimmune HCWs should not enter the room.
Meningitis:				
Bacterial	Droplet	(see specific bacterial agents)		

Fungal	Standard			Not transmitted person-to-person; usually the result of spread of a fungus through blood to the spinal cord.
Haemophilus influenzae type B	Droplet	Incubation: unknown. Contagious: until 24 hours after initiation of effective treatment.	Respiratory droplets	See https://www.gov.uk/government/collections/haemophilus-influenzae-guidance-data-and-analysis for recommendations for prevention of secondary cases of *Haemophilus influenzae* (Hib) disease.
Neisseria meningitidis	Droplet	Incubation: average four days, but can range between 2 and 10 days. Contagious: until 24 hours after initiation of effective treatment.	Respiratory droplets	See https://www.gov.uk/government/collections/meningococcal-disease-guidance-data-and-analysis for current guidance on postexposure prophylaxis for contacts.
Meningitis tuberculosis	Standard; airborne (see comment)			UK statutory notifiable disease. Airborne precautions if concurrent active pulmonary disease and until active tuberculosis ruled out in family members. See https://www.gov.uk/government/collections/tuberculosis-and-other-mycobacterial-diseases-diagnosis-screening-management-and-data for current information and follow-up of contacts.
Viral	Contact; droplet (depending on viral agent)	Incubation: variable. Contagious: variable. (depending on viral agent)		Coxsackie or Echovirus groups of enteroviruses are the most common cause. Other viruses that can cause meningitis are herpes viruses, mumps virus, measles virus, and arboviruses.
Meningococcal disease (sepsis, pneumonia, meningitis)	Droplet	Incubation: 1–10 days Contagious: until 24 hours after initiation of effective treatment	Respiratory secretions	UK statutory notifiable disease for meningococcal septicaemia. See https://www.gov.uk/government/collections/meningococcal-disease-guidance-data-and-analysis for current guidance on post-exposure prophylaxis for contacts.
MERS (Middle East Respiratory Syndrome)	Airborne; droplet; contact	Incubation: 2–14 days. Contagious: duration of symptoms	Respiratory secretions	UK statutory notifiable disease. FFP3 respirators, visors, gowns and gloves to be worn in suspected and confirmed cases. See https://www.gov.uk/government/collections/middle-east-respiratory-syndrome-coronavirus-mers-cov-clinical-management-and-guidance for current MERS guidance.
Molluscum contagiosum	Contact	Incubation: two weeks to six months. Contagious: duration of symptoms.	Skin lesions	

(continued)

Table 13.1 Isolation precautions required for specific infections or clinical conditions (continued)

Infection/condition	Isolation precautions	Incubation and duration	Infective material	Comments
MRSA (Meticillin-resistant *Staphylococcus aureus*)	Contact		From people who are infected or carriers or contaminated environment	See https://www.gov.uk/government/collections/staphylococcus-aureus-guidance-data-and-analysis for guidance on MRSA screening of patients. All CYPs coming into a hospital should be screened for MRSA on admission.
Multi-drug-resistant organisms (e.g. Carbapenemase producers, extended spectrum beta lactamases (ESBL) producers, Vancomycin-resistant enterococci (VRE)	Contact		From people who are carriers or contaminated environment	See https://www.gov.uk/government/collections/antimicrobial-resistance-amr-information-and-resources for current guidance on admission screening and isolation precautions.
Mumps (infectious parotitis)	Droplet	Incubation: usually 16 to 18 days; cases may occur from 12 to 25 days. Contagious: from two days before until nine days after onset of parotid swelling.	Respiratory secretions	UK statutory notifiable disease. Nonimmune HCWs should not enter the room.
Mycobacteria, nontuberculosis	Standard	Incubation: variable.	Soil, food, water, animals	Can cause a variety of diseases (pulmonary, skin, soft tissues, joint infections) particularly in immunodeficient patients.
Necrotising enterocolitis	Standard		Faeces	
Norovirus	Contact; droplet (if projectile vomiting)	Incubation: 12–72 hours.	Faeces, vomit	Also known as 'winter vomiting disease'. Highly infectious with person-to-person transmission or through contaminated environment. Hands must be decontaminated with soap and water as alcohol gel is ineffective against norovirus.
Parainfluenza virus	Contact; droplet	Incubation: two to six days. Contagious: duration of illness.	Respiratory droplets	Wear mask/respirator when in close contact with the patient (< 2m).
Parvovirus B 19 (Erythema infectiosum)	Contact; droplet	Incubation: 4–21 days. Contagious: duration of illness.	Respiratory droplets	Pregnant HCWs should not provide care.
Pediculosis (head lice)	Contact	Incubation: 6 to 10 days. Contagious: until treated effectively.	Hair	See https://www.gov.uk/head-lice-pediculosis for current information.
Pertussis (whooping cough)	Droplet	Incubation: 6–21 days, usually 7–10 days. Contagious: five days after initiation of effective treatment.	Respiratory droplets	UK statutory notifiable disease. Wear FFP2 or FFP3 respirators. See https://www.gov.uk/government/collections/pertussis-guidance-data-and-analysis for current guidance on postexposure prophylaxis for contacts.
Pinworm infection (enterobiasis)	Contact	Incubation: one to two months. Contagious: duration of illness.		High reinfection rate. Good hand hygiene is most effective method of prevention.

Pneumonia:

Adenovirus	Contact; droplet	Contagious: duration of virus shedding.	
Bacterial (not listed elsewhere)	Standard		
Burkholderia cepacia (in patients with cystic fibrosis, including respiratory tract colonisation)	Standard		Avoid exposure to other patients with cystic fibrosis.
Fungal	Standard		
Haemophilus influenzae Type B	Droplet	Incubation: unknown. Contagious: 24 hours after initiation of effective treatment.	Respiratory droplets	See https://www.gov.uk/government/collections/haemophilus-influenzae-guidance-data-and-analysis for recommendations for prevention of secondary cases of *Haemophilus influenzae* (Hib) disease.
Meningococcal			(See Meningococcal disease)
Mycoplasma (primary atypical pneumonia)	Droplet	Incubation: two to three weeks. Contagious: duration of illness.	Respiratory droplets	
Pneumococcal pneumonia	Contact			Use droplet precautions if evidence of transmission within patient care facility.
Pneumocystis jiroveci (prev. *Pneumocystis carinii*)	Standard			Avoid placement in same room with immunocompromised patients.
Staphylococcus aureus	Droplet	Contagious: until 24 hours after initiation of effective treatment	Respiratory droplets	
Streptococcus Group A	Droplet	Contagious: until 24 hours after initiation of effective treatment.	Respiratory droplets	Contact precautions also recommended if skin lesions present.
Viral				(see specific viral agent)
Poliomyelitis	Contact	Incubation: 7–21 days. Contagious: duration of illness.	Faeces	UK statutory notifiable disease for acute polio.
Prion disease				(see Creutzfeld-Jakob disease)
Respiratory Syncytial Virus (RSV)	Contact, Droplet	Incubation: two to eight days Contagious: duration of illness.	Respiratory secretions.	Wear respiratory protection when in close contact with the patient (< 2m).
Rhinovirus	Contact; Droplet	Incubation: two to three days, occasionally up to 7 days Contagious: duration of illness	Respiratory secretions	Transmission occurs predominantly by person-to-person contact with self-inoculation through contaminated secretions on hands. Wear mask/respirator when in close contact with patient (< 2m).
Ringworm	(See Tinea)			
Rotavirus	Contact	Incubation: two to four days Contagious: duration of illness	Faeces	
Rubella (German measles)	Droplet	Incubation: 14 to 23 days. Contagious: seven days before until seven days after the onset of the rash.	Nasopharyngeal secretions	UK statutory notifiable disease. Nonimmune HCWs should not enter the room. Nonimmune pregnant women should not enter the room. Administer vaccine within three days of exposure to nonpregnant susceptible individuals.

(continued)

Table 13.1 Isolation precautions required for specific infections or clinical conditions (continued)

Infection/condition	Isolation precautions	Incubation and duration	Infective material	Comments
Salmonella	Contact	Incubation: for gastroenteritis: 6–48 hours; for enteric fever: 3–60 days (usually 7–14 days). Contagious: duration of illness.	Faeces, infected animals, contaminated food	UK statutory notifiable disease if associated with food poisoning. Children with typhoid fever: contact precautions should be continued until three negative stool cultures were obtained at least 48 hours after cessation of antimicrobial therapy.
SARS-CoV2	(see COVID-19 disease)			
Scabies	Contact	Incubation: four to six weeks. Contagious: until 24 hours after initiation of effective treatment.	Skin	Rash may persist for several weeks after treatment.
Scarlet fever	(See Streptococcal disease)			
Severe acute respiratory syndrome (SARS)	Airborne; Droplet; contact	Incubation: 2–10 days. Contagious: duration of illness.	Respiratory secretions	UK statutory notifiable disease. FFP3 respirators, visors, gowns, and gloves to be worn in suspected and confirmed cases. See https://www.gov.uk/topic/health-protection/infectious-diseases for current SARS guidance.
Shigella	Contact	Incubation: one to seven days Contagious: duration of illness	Faeces	UK statutory notifiable disease if associated with food poisoning.
Shingles	(see Varicella zsoster)			
Staphylococcal disease:				
Food poisoning	Contact	Incubation: 30 min–8 hours. Contagious: duration of illness	Contaminated food	UK statutory notifiable disease.
Pneumonia	Droplet	Contagious: until 24 hours after initiation of effective treatment.	Respiratory secretions	
Scalded skin syndrome	Contact	Contagious: duration of illness.	Wound secretions	
Skin, wound, burn	Contact	Contagious: duration of illness.	Wound secretions	
Streptococcal disease (group A):				
Skin, wound or burn	Contact	Contagious: until 24 hours after initiation of effective treatment.		
Pharyngitis	Droplet	Contagious: until 24 hours after initiation of effective treatment.	Respiratory secretions	
Pneumonia	Droplet	Contagious: until 24 hours after initiation of effective treatment.	Respiratory secretions	
Scarlet fever	Droplet	Incubation: one to seven days Contagious: until 24 hours after initiation of effective treatment.	Respiratory secretions	UK statutory notifiable disease.
Streptococcal disease (group B):				
Neonatal	Standard			All pregnant women should be screened for vaginal/rectal colonisation. Intrapartum chemophrophylaxis as indicated.

Tapeworm disease	Contact	Contagious: duration of illness.	Faeces, infected meat	
Tetanus	Standard	Incubation: two days to months, most cases within 14 days.		UK statutory notifiable disease. Not transmitted from person-to-person.
Tinea (Ringworm)	Contact	Incubation: unknown. Contagious: duration of illness.		
Toxoplasmosis	Standard	Incubation: 4 to 21 days.		Transmission from person-to-person is rare.
Toxic Shock Syndrome *Streptococcus pyogenes* mediated:	Contact; droplet	Contagious: until 24 hours after initiation of effective treatment.		
Staphylococcus aureus mediated:	Contact			
Tuberculosis:				UK statutory notifiable disease
Extrapulmonary, draining lesion	Airborne; contact	Incubation: from infection to a positive tuberculin skin test (TST) result: 2 to 12 weeks. Risk of developing tuberculosis highest during six months after infection and remains high for two years. Contagious: until three sputum smears for AAFB negative.	Lesion	Isolate patient in negative pressure room; wear FFP3 respirators.
Cavitary pulmonary, laryngeal disease; positive sputum alcohol and acid-fast bacilli (AAFB) smears	Airborne		Sputum, respiratory secretions	Isolate patient in negative pressure room and wear FFP3 respirators. See https://www.gov.uk/government/collections/tuberculosis-and-other-mycobacterial-diseases-diagnosis-screening-management-and-data for current guidance.
Extrapulmonary, no draining lesion	Standard			
Skin-test positive with no evidence of current active disease	Standard			
Typhoid fever	Contact			UK statutory notifiable disease (see *Salmonella*).
Varicella (Chickenpox)	Airborne; Contact	Incubation: 8–21 days (after use of after use of Aciclovir prophylaxis or varicella zoster immunoglobulin [VZIg] extend up to 28 days. Contagious: 24 hours before appearance of the first lesions until lesions are crusted.	Skin lesions, respiratory secretions	Nonimmune HCWs should not enter the room. Consider Aciclovir prophylaxis or VZIg for exposed immunocompromised persons for exposed immunocompromised persons. https://www.gov.uk/government/publications/post-exposure-prophylaxis-for-chickenpox-and-shingles guidance.
Varicella zoster (Shingles)				
Disseminated disease in any patient Localised disease in immunocompromised patient until disseminated infection ruled out	Airborne; contact	Contagious: when lesions appear until crusted over.	Skin lesions; respiratory	Nonimmune HCWs should not enter the room.
Localised in patient with intact immune system with lesions that can be contained/covered	Contact	Contagious: when lesions appear until crusted over.	Skin lesions	Nonimmune HCWs should not enter the room.

(continued)

Table 13.1 Isolation precautions required for specific infections or clinical conditions (continued)

Infection/condition	Isolation precautions	Incubation and duration	Infective material	Comments
Viral haemorrhagic fevers (due to Ebola virus, Lassa virus, or Marburg virus)	Contact; Droplet	Incubation: Ebola: 2–21 days; Lassa: 6–21 days; Marburg: 3–9 days. Contagious: duration of illness; largest viral load in final stages of illness when haemorrhage may occur.	Blood and other body fluids are highly infectious	UK statutory notifiable disease. Isolate confirmed cases in high secure infectious disease unit (HSIDU). For suspected cases use FFP3 respirators, visor, impermeable gown and double gloves; appropriate laboratory specimen and waste handling. See https://www.gov.uk/government/collections/ebola-virus-disease-clinical-management-and-guidance for current guidance.
Whooping cough (Pertussis)				(See Pertussis)

Chapter 13 Infection prevention and control

Principles table 13.1 Equipment required for handwashing

Principle	Rationale
1 It is essential that hand hygiene facilities are easily available in all patient areas, treatment rooms, sluices, and kitchens.	1 To encourage personnel to wash their hands.
2 a) Basins should have elbow-operated or foot-operated mixer taps. b) The use of sensor-operated mixer taps is discouraged.	2 a) This minimises recontamination of hands when turning off the tap. b) Sensor-operated mixer taps are associated with higher levels of *Pseudomonas aeruginosa* and *Legionella spp.* in the water (Halabi et al. 2001; Walker et al. 2014).
3 Liquid soap or antiseptic soap dispensers should hold disposable cartridges to avoid being 'topped up' and should be elbow, foot, or electronically operated.	3 Dispensers have been associated with contamination of contents and containers causing cross infection (Archibald et al. 1997).
4 In the clinical setting disposable paper towels should be used.	4 Cloth hand towels and air dryers are a source of contamination (Huang et al. 2012). Disposable paper towels are quicker and less noisy than hot-air hand dryers (Redway et al. 1994). Soft paper towels are preferred by nurses (Gould 1995).
5 Waste bins should have a foot-operated lid.	5 To avoid recontamination of the hands when lifting the lid.

Principles table 13.2 General hand care

Some detergents may cause dermatitis (Health and Safety Executive [HSC] 2007). Any forms of contact dermatitis should be reported to the Occupational Health Department in order to provide the individual with alternative agents and to monitor possible side effects of hospital antiseptics/detergents.

Principle	Rationale
1 Healthcare workers are prone to sore hands due to the number of times they are required to wash their hands. Adherence to good hand care reduces this risk.	1 Bacterial counts increase when the skin is damaged.
2 Always wet hands before applying soap and rinse and dry well.	2 This minimises the risk of contact dermatitis or allergic reaction occurring.
3 a) Hand creams should be used before breaks and at the end of the shift. b) It is preferable to use hand cream dispensers.	3 a) Hand creams containing an emollient are useful for maintaining skin integrity and hydration (Pratt et al. 2007). b) Communal jars or tubes may become contaminated with micro-organisms (Gould 1995).
4 Open cuts or abrasions should be covered with a waterproof plaster.	4 To prevent micro-organisms from entering or leaving the wound.
5 Soap and alcohol hand gel should not be used concomitantly on a routine basis (Kampf and Loeffler 2003).	5 Using both soap and alcohol gel routinely is unnecessary and may lead to dermatitis.
6 Allow hands to dry completely from soap and water or alcohol hand gel before donning gloves.	6 Donning gloves while hands are still wet increases the risk of skin irritation (WHO 2009).
7 Healthcare workers who suffer from chronic skin diseases, such as eczema, should consult with Occupational Health for advice when working in the clinical situation. Healthcare workers with chronic skin disease should avoid those invasive procedures that involve sharp instruments or needles when their skin lesions are active, or if there are extensive breaks in the skin surface.	7 A nonintact skin surface provides a potential route for bloodborne virus transmission, and blood–skin contact is common through glove puncture that may go unnoticed (United Kingdom Health Security Agency (UK HSA) 2021).
8. **Other points to consider:** a) Nails should be kept short and clean. If nails can be seen above the fingertips when looking at the palm of the hand then they are too long. b) Healthcare workers who have direct patient contact should not wear nail polish or artificial nails. c) The wearing of rings, watches, bracelets, and fit-tracker bracelets is discouraged. d) Healthcare workers that have direct patient contact should be 'Bare below the elbows' (DH 2020).	a) To avoid scratching the CYP. Microbes found beneath the fingernails have caused cross infection (Jeanes and Green 2001). b) Long or sharp fingernails can puncture gloves. c) Several studies have shown that skin underneath rings is more heavily colonised than comparable areas of skin on fingers (Hoffman et al. 1985; Jacobson et al. 1985 with stones can damage gloves. Bracelets and watches impede compliance with full hand hygiene. d) Cuffs of long-sleeved garments may become contaminated during patient care and prevent effective hand hygiene, which can lead to recontamination (WHO 2009).

Principles table 13.3 When to perform hand hygiene

The times at which hand hygiene should be performed have been summarised into the '5 Moments for Hand Hygiene': These are considered the most fundamental points during care delivery and daily routines when hand hygiene should be undertaken (National Patient Safety Agency [NPSA] 2004; Sax et al. 2007; WHO 2009) (see Figure 13.1). Alcohol hand gel is the preferred means for routine hand hygiene. The exceptions when hands should be washed with soap and water instead of using alcohol hand gel are listed below (see item 2: Wash hands with soap and water).

Principle	Rationale
1 **Decontaminate hands with alcohol hand gel** (WHO 2009) • Before and after touching the patient. • Before handling an invasive device for patient care, regardless of whether or not gloves are used. • If moving from a contaminated body site to another body site during the care of the same patient. • After contact with equipment in the vicinity of the patient. • After contact with the patient's surroundings. • Before handling medication. • Before preparing food. • After handling contaminated laundry or waste. • After the removal of gloves.	1 To prevent transient micro-organisms, which are likely to contaminate hands, from touching the CYP or the environment in which they are nursed. Transient micro-organisms are located under the surface of the skin and beneath the superficial cells of the stratum corneum. They are termed 'transient' because direct contact with other people, equipment, or body sites all result in the transfer of micro-organisms to and from the hands (Mackintosh and Hoffman 1984). To avoid contaminating clean areas such as the sites of indwelling devices, surgical wounds, equipment, or the environment.
2 **Wash hands with soap and water** (WHO 2009) • When visibly soiled. • After contact with blood, body fluids, mucous membranes, nonintact skin, and wound dressings. • After using the toilet. • After exposure to spore-forming pathogens (e.g. *Clostridium difficile*) or nonenveloped viruses (e.g. *Norovirus*).	2 • Alcohol hand gel should be used only on visibly clean hands. • It is less effective against spore-forming pathogens (e.g. *Clostridium difficile*) and nonenveloped viruses (e.g. *Norovirus*).

Principles table 13.4 Choice of cleansing agent

Principle	Rationale
1 Liquid soap containing an emollient and water should be available in all clinical and nonclinical areas for routine handwashing.	1 Staff are more likely to wash their hands with a product that does less harm to the skin. Liquid soap removes most transient micro-organisms (Chadwick et al. 2000, Health Protection Agency [HPA], 2007).
2 Bar soap should not be used in clinical areas.	2 Bar soap stored in wet areas contains more micro-organisms than liquid soap (Kabara and Brady 1984).
3 Alcohol hand gel should be used only on visibly clean hands.	3 It is easily available at the point of care and is the preferred means for routine hand antisepsis (WHO 2009). *NB:* Alcohol gel is less effective against spore-forming pathogens (e.g. *Clostridium difficile*) and nonenveloped viruses (e.g. norovirus). After exposure to these pathogens, hands should always be washed with soap and water.
4 Antiseptic detergents must be used for surgical hand preparation (see Box 13.3):	4 These will further reduce bacterial counts on the skin and destroy transient micro-organisms. They can be used when a higher level of disinfection is required, such as in surgery.

Box 13.3 Types of antiseptic detergents and their uses

Solution	Advantages and disadvantages
a) Chlorhexidine gluconate (most commonly used)	• Intermediate range of activity • Initially slow-acting • Has prolonged chemical activity (up to six hours) • Minimally affected by organic matter • Less irritating than povidone iodine
b) Povidone iodine	• Wide range of microbial activity • Persistent chemical activity • Neutralised in the presence of organic material (e.g. blood) • Can cause skin irritation • Frequently used for surgical scrubbing

Procedure guideline 13.1 Hand decontamination techniques

Statement	Rationale
1 All healthcare workers must be 'bare below the elbows' before washing their hands.	
2 Washing hands with soap and water: a) Wet hands under warm running water. b) Dispense one dose of soap in a cupped hand and apply, covering all surfaces. Vigorously rub all surfaces of lathered hands (see Figure 13.2): • Rub hands palm to palm. • Rub back of each hand with the palm of the other hand with fingers interlaced. • Rub palm to palm with fingers interlaced. • Rub with backs of fingers to opposing palms with fingers interlaced. • Rub each thumb clasped in opposite hand using rotational movement. • Rub tips of fingers in opposite palm in a circular motion. • Rub each wrist with opposite hand. c) Rinse hands under running water to remove residual soap. d) Dry hands thoroughly with a paper towel. e) The duration of the entire procedure should take 40–60 seconds.	a) Avoid using hot water as this may increase the risk of dermatitis (Berardesca et al. 1995). b) To ensure that all surfaces of the hands are washed. c) This helps prevent dermatitis or allergic reactions.
3 Decontaminating hands with alcohol hand gel: a) Dispense one dose of alcohol hand gel in a cupped hand and apply, covering all surfaces (see Figure 13.3): • Rub hands palm to palm. • Rub back of each hand with the palm of the other hand with fingers interlaced. • Rub palm to palm with fingers interlaced. • Rub with backs of fingers to opposing palms with fingers interlaced. • Rub each thumb clasped in opposite hand using rotational movement. • Rub tips of fingers in opposite palm in a circular motion. • Rub each wrist with opposite hand. b) Rub until hands are dry. c) The duration of the entire procedure should take 20–30 seconds.	a) Follow manufacturer's instructions.

4 Surgical hand preparation.
This is essential before all surgical and invasive procedures.
a) Use elbow or foot operated taps.
b) Rinse with water, apply antiseptic detergent to the hands and wrists, and wash for at least one minute up to the elbow. The level of your hands should always remain above your elbow when performing a surgical scrub.
c) A sterile brush may be used for the first application of the day but continual use is inadvisable. Using a prepacked sterile brush, clean under the nails (only) of both hands and discard.
d) Rinse thoroughly.
e) Apply a second application of antiseptic detergent and wash hands and two-thirds of the forearms with either:
  i) Chlorhexidine gluconate for at least two minutes.
  ii) Povidone iodine for at least one minute.
f) Rinse thoroughly.
g) One sterile towel should be used to blot dry your first hand and arm and another sterile towel for the second hand and arm.
h) After the initial surgical scrub, an alternative method is the application of an alcoholic solution, with or without an antiseptic solution. The solution is applied to the hands and wrists using standardised technique and rubbed completely dry (National Association of Theatre Nurses 2004).
	4 To remove or destroy transient micro-organisms and substantially reduce detachable resident micro-organisms. To reduce the risk of wound infections should surgical gloves become damaged.
	a) To avoid recontaminating hands after washing. The use of sensor-operated mixer taps is discouraged as it may lead to higher levels of *Pseudomonas aeruginosa* and *Legionella spp.* in the water (Halabi et al. 2001; Walker et al. 2014).
	b) To prevent contaminated water from the arms running onto the hands (National Association of Theatre Nurses 2004).
	c) Damage to the skin may occur if scrubbing too often, thus increasing the microbial colonisation of the skin.
	d) Follow manufacturer's guidelines.
	e) Skin scales could be disturbed if a rubbing action is used (National Association of Theatre Nurses 2004).
	f) Follow manufacturer's guidelines.

The Great Ormond Street Hospital Manual of Children and Young People's Nursing Practices

Procedure guideline 13.2 Hand drying techniques

Statement	Rationale
1 Always dry hands thoroughly using disposable paper towels.	1 Wet hands transfer micro-organisms more effectively than dry ones. Paper towels rub away transient micro-organisms and old, dead skin cells loosely attached to the surface of the hands.
2 Used paper towels should be disposed in pedal bins with foot-operated lids.	2 To prevent re-contamination of hands by touching the lid of the bin.

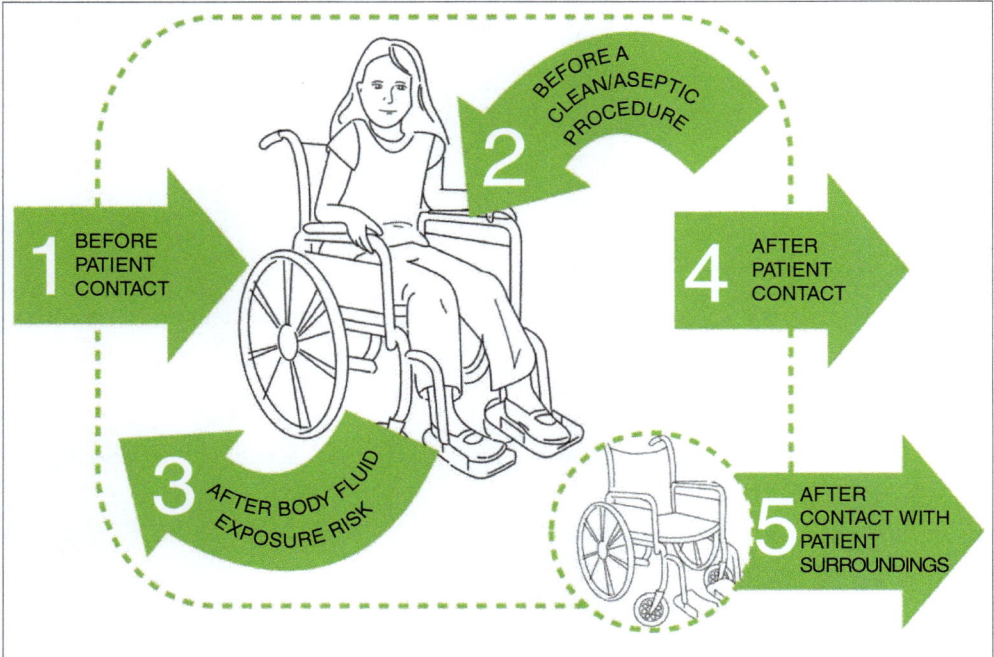

Figure 13.1 '5 Moments for Hand Hygiene' (*Source*: ©NHS England – reproduction with kind permission).

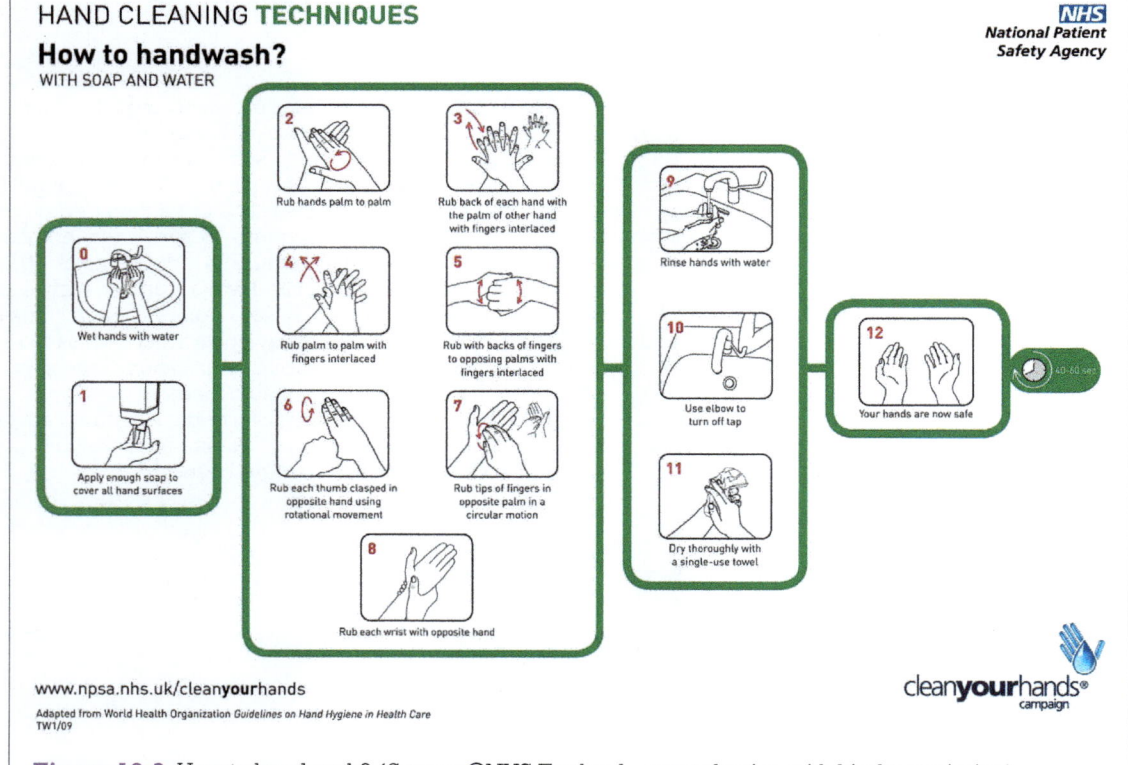

Figure 13.2 How to handwash? (*Source*: ©NHS England – reproduction with kind permission).

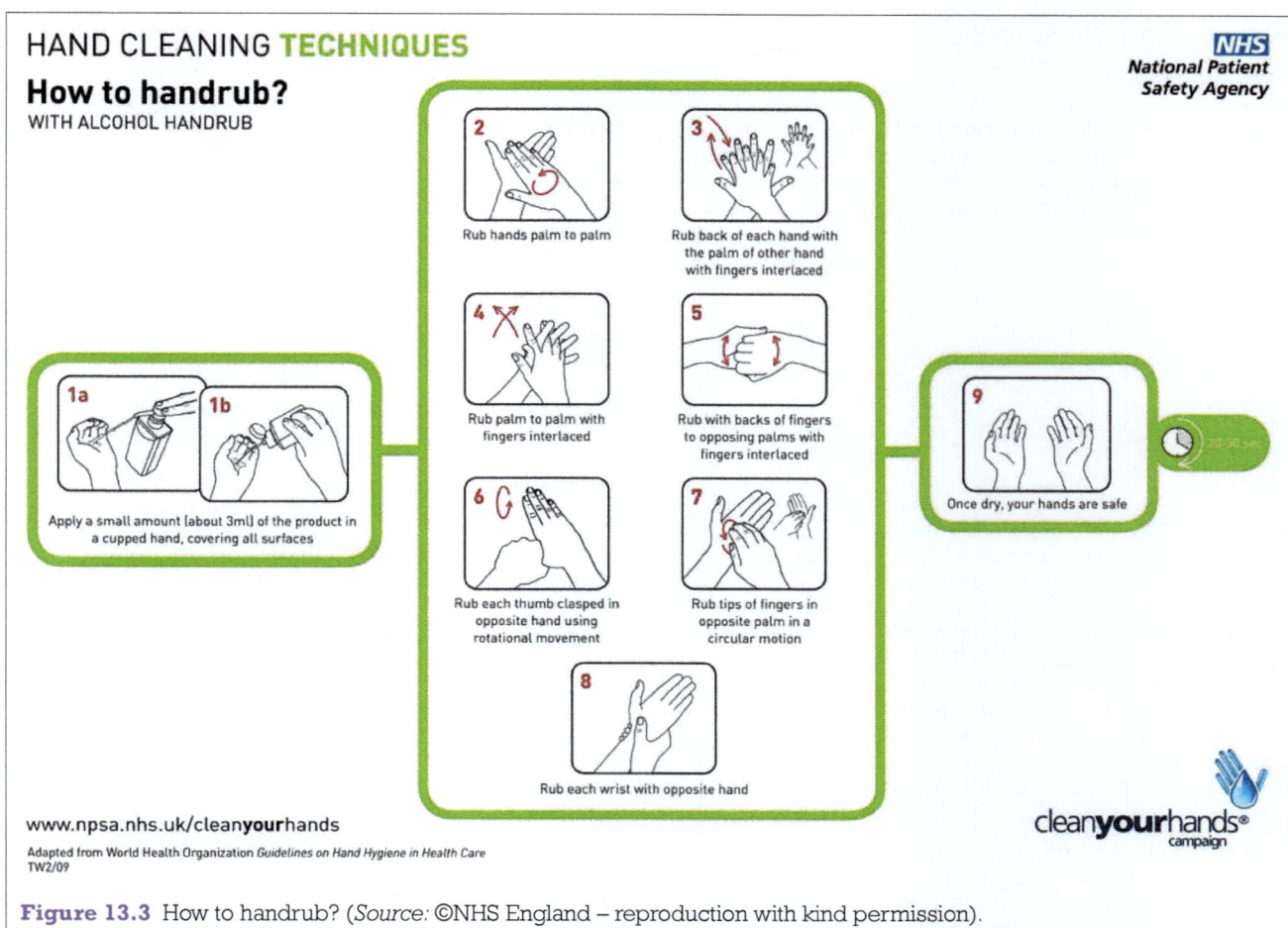

Figure 13.3 How to handrub? (*Source:* ©NHS England – reproduction with kind permission).

Personal protective equipment

PPE is defined as equipment that will protect the user against health or safety risks at work (HSE 2020). Employers are required to provide PPE free of charge where there are risks to health and safety that cannot be adequately controlled by other means.

In healthcare settings, the primary purpose of using PPE is to protect the skin and mucous membranes of healthcare workers from exposure to blood and/or body fluids. PPE also prevents clothing from contamination and therefore reduces the risk of cross-transmission. PPE includes items such as gloves, aprons, uniforms, masks/respirators, goggles, and visors.

The decision regarding the appropriate PPE to wear should be based on the assessment of the likelihood of contamination with blood and/or body fluids carried out prior to patient contact or a procedure. The assessment should be based on:

- The healthcare worker's knowledge or experience of the situation or procedure.
- The CYP's ability to cooperate throughout the procedure; e.g. wriggling during venepuncture may increase the risk of the healthcare worker becoming exposed to blood.

PPE – Good practice points

- PPE should be appropriate, fit for purpose, and suitable for the person using/wearing it.
- All staff required to wear PPE should be given training (theoretical and practical) on when and how to use PPE safely and correctly.
- PPE should not be a source of further contamination, e.g. by being removed or disposed of inappropriately by the wearer and as such contaminating the hands, the uniform worn underneath, or the environment.
- The integrity of the PPE must not be compromised during procedures, as this could potentially lead to exposure to blood and/or body fluids.
- Stocks of PPE must be in date and should be stored in appropriate areas, e.g. on shelves and off the floor to avoid contamination prior to use.
- Single-use items should not be reused and manufacturers' instructions should be followed.
- All PPE must conform to European Union (EU) standards to ensure it is of acceptable standard and safety quality.

Disposable gloves

In healthcare there are two main reasons for the wearing of disposable gloves; to protect patients and to protect healthcare workers (Dunn et al, 2019). Healthcare workers primarily wear disposable gloves as part of standard and isolation precautions to protect themselves from exposure to blood, body fluids, and mucous membranes. Other indications not related to infection prevention are the wearing of gloves to prevent exposure to medications (e.g. cytotoxic drugs) or chemicals (e.g. cleaning products). As a general rule, gloves that are worn to protect patients (e.g. during surgical procedures) must be sterile, and gloves that are required to protect healthcare workers should be non-sterile (Royal College of Nursing (RCN), 2022).

To prevent gloves being worn unnecessarily, it is important that healthcare workers are able to differentiate between specific clinical situations when gloves should be worn (e.g. when there is a risk of exposure to blood or body fluids) and those when their use is not required (e.g. when taking a blood pressure). The use of gloves in situations when their use is not recommended represents a waste of resources without necessarily leading to a reduction of cross-transmission and may also result in missed opportunities for hand hygiene (WHO, 2009).

Principles table 13.5 Disposable gloves

Principle	Rationale
1 Disposable gloves for clinical use are available in latex and synthetic materials (vinyl, nitrile, neoprene, polythene), in sterile and nonsterile form, and with or without powder. It is important that the most appropriate material for the purpose should be selected (Damani 2012).	1 **Latex:** Strong and a good fit, but carries risk of sensitisation due to latex. **Vinyl:** Fit is not as good as latex, but less risk of sensitisation. While there is little difference in the barrier properties of unused intact gloves, studies have shown repeatedly that vinyl gloves have higher failure rates than latex or nitrile gloves when tested under simulated and actual clinical conditions (Siegel et al. 2007). **Nitrile:** More expensive than latex, but carries less risk of sensitisation. The material molecular structure is very similar to that of latex. **Neoprene:** More expensive than latex. Is available as surgical gloves and can be worn by individuals who are sensitive to latex. **Polythene:** Not suitable for clinical use due to the permeability and tendency to damage easily (Damani 2012).
2 Latex is classed as a hazardous substance. Under the Control of Substances Hazardous to Health (COSHH) regulations (HSE 2009) organisations have a duty to eliminate, substitute, and limit and control exposure to latex, unless there is a need to use it (NPSA 2005). Latex gloves should have low levels of extractable proteins and residual accelerators. Evidence indicates that glove powder aerosolises latex proteins, causing the allergens to be inhaled by both the glove wearer and others in the immediate environment (Damani 2012).	2 To minimise the risk of latex allergy in healthcare workers and patients. This is becoming increasingly common.
3 Healthcare workers (up to 17%) or patients (up to 65% in CYPs with spina bifida) exposed to latex or other synthetic materials found in gloves may display signs of skin rashes, hives, flushing, itching, nasal, eye or sinus symptoms, asthma, and, rarely, anaphylactic shock (Royal College of Physicians (RCP) 2008).	3 Some CYPs are more likely to become latex sensitive such as those who have frequent exposure to latex from medical/surgical procedures. These include CYPs born with spina bifida, anomalies of the urinary tract and those who have multiple surgery. CYPs with certain food allergies may be prone to latex allergy (RCP 2008).
4 Alternatives to natural rubber latex (NRL) gloves must be available for use by healthcare workers and patients with NRL sensitivity.	4 To avoid sensitisation and allergic reactions.
5 **Sterile gloves** must be worn for all surgical and aseptic procedures, e.g.: • All surgical procedures. • Insertion of indwelling devices (e.g. chest drains, central venous catheters, urinary catheters). • Lumbar punctures and intrathecal drug administration. • Invasive diagnostic procedures.	5 • To prevent transfer of micro-organisms from healthcare workers to patients. • To protect the healthcare worker from exposure to blood and/or body fluids during surgical and invasive procedures.
6 **Nonsterile gloves** should be worn whenever there is a potential for coming in to contact with blood and/or body fluids, secretions, excretions, or contact with infectious micro-organisms both from direct and indirect contact with patients, items, instruments, equipment or the environment (Damani 2012).	6 To protect healthcare workers from acquiring micro-organisms from patients or contaminated equipment/environment.
7 Gloves should be worn as single-use items. Gloves must not be washed for subsequent reuse, nor should alcohol hand gel be used on the gloves.	7 Micro-organisms cannot be removed reliably from glove surfaces and continued glove integrity cannot be ensured (Doebbeling et al. 1988).
8 Jewellery (e.g. rings) should not be worn under gloves (WHO 2009).	8 The gloves may become damaged.
9 When gloves are worn in combination with other PPE, such as a gown, they are put on last.	9 Gloves that fit snugly around the wrist are preferred for use with a gown because they will cover the gown cuff and provide a more reliable continuous barrier for the arms, wrists, and hands.

Principles table 13.5 Disposable gloves (*continued*)

Principle	Rationale
10 It may be necessary to change gloves between tasks on the same patient.	10 To prevent cross-contamination, e.g. after suctioning a patient and before doing a dressing. Work with the principle of 'clean' to 'dirty'. Failure to change gloves between patients is an infection control hazard.
11 Gloves that have become torn, punctured, or otherwise damaged should be removed and replaced immediately (safety permitting) if this occurs during a procedure.	11 To maintain standard precautions.
12 Gloves must be removed promptly after use and before touching clean surfaces, oneself, and other persons. Gloves that have been worn for a procedure should not be worn to handle or write charts. Immediately after the removal of gloves, hands should be washed or alcohol gel applied.	12 To prevent cross-contamination.
13 Care should be taken when removing used gloves. The wrist end of the glove should be handled and the glove should be pulled down gently over the hand, turning the outer contaminated surface inward while doing so, i.e. the gloves are then disposed of inside out, preferably with the second glove also pulled over the first while removing it so that they are wrapped together.	13 To avoid contamination.
14 Gloves must be disposed of as clinical waste in the hospital setting. Follow the local waste policy.	14 To minimise the risk of contamination
15 Hands must be decontaminated after removing gloves.	15 Wearing gloves does not replace the need for hand hygiene. Gloves may have small unapparent defects or become torn during use and hands can become contaminated during the removal of gloves.

Disposable aprons and gowns

Disposable aprons or gowns are worn to prevent contamination of clothing and to protect the skin of healthcare workers from exposure to blood and body fluids. They are also worn by healthcare workers during the care of patients infected with epidemiologically important micro-organisms to reduce the opportunity for transmission of pathogens from patients or items in their environment to other patients or environments.

CDC guidelines advocate the use of gowns (Siegel et al. 2007). However, there is not sufficient evidence to support the total use of gowns instead of aprons (Health Protection Scotland 2008). The use of gowns versus aprons is dependent on the nature of the situation and therefore good practice, including a risk assessment of the situation, should dictate whether exposure to a high degree of environmental and surface contamination is expected. If gross contamination is likely, then waterproof gowns or those with waterproof panels should be worn.

Principles table 13.6 Disposable aprons and gowns

Principle	Rationale
1 It is good practice to wear disposable aprons, both in the hospital and community setting, for all care episodes where the risk of contamination exists.	1 To prevent contamination of the healthcare workers' clothing with blood and body fluids, skin scales, colonisation with antibiotic resistant micro-organisms or other infectious agents.
2 Nonpermeable long-sleeved gowns should be worn whenever there is a risk of splashing with blood and/or body fluids. In addition the use of a nonpermeable long-sleeved gown should be considered where the risk of transmission of micro-organisms is increased, such as in desquamating skin diseases in patients colonised with MRSA.	2 To prevent contamination of the healthcare workers' clothing with blood and body fluids, skin scales, or colonisation with antibiotic resistant micro-organisms or other infectious agents.
3. The routine donning of aprons or gowns on entry into an intensive care unit or other high-risk area is not necessary.	3 Evidence suggests this does not prevent or influence potential colonisation or infection of patients in these areas (Siegel et al. 2007).
4 Apron or gowns should be single use and be removed before leaving the patient's environment.	4 To prevent cross-contamination.
5 The gown should be peeled away from neck and shoulder, the contaminated outside turned toward the inside, and then rolled into a bundle before being discarded appropriately. The same principle is used for removal of plastic aprons.	5 To prevent contamination of the healthcare worker or the environment.
6 Aprons or gowns must be disposed of as clinical waste as per local waste management policy.	6 To minimise the risk of contamination.
7 Wash hands after disposal of the apron/gown.	7 To prevent cross-contamination.

Facial protection – masks, respirators, goggles, and visors

A mask/respirator, eye protection, or face shield should be worn to protect mucous membranes of the mouth, eyes, and nose of the healthcare worker if there is a risk of aerosols, sprays, splashes of blood, other body fluid, or respiratory secretions.

Full facial protection should be worn:

- When there is a risk of splashing/ spraying of blood or body fluids into mucosal surfaces (nose, mouth, eyes) or broken skin areas on the face. This poses a risk of infectious agents, including bloodborne viruses, being absorbed through mucosal surfaces and broken skin. Accidents with splashing/spraying may occur when attending to CYPs involved in trauma, those receiving dialysis (highest risk is when putting them on and when taking off the machine), during intensive care, if bleeding occurs, or when taking a blood sample.
- If a CYP has a respiratory infection and aerosolised procedures are being performed. Procedures that stimulate coughing and promote the generation of aerosols include aerosolised or nebulised medication administration, diagnostic sputum induction, bronchoscopy, airway suctioning, endotracheal intubation, positive pressure ventilation via a face mask (e.g. Continuous Positive Airway Pressure ([CPAP], Bi-level Positive Airway Pressure [BiPAP] or Variable Positive Airway Pressure [VPAP]), and high-frequency oscillatory ventilation. Droplet nuclei may land on mucosal surfaces of the healthcare worker, increasing the risk of infection.
- During surgery when drilling bone or using diathermy. Surgical smoke is produced by thermal destruction of tissue. The smoke produced has been shown to be mutagenic and can contain bacteria and viruses (papilloma virus, hepatitis, and HIV). These particles are small enough to penetrate deep within the respiratory tract (Spearman et al. 2007).

The choice of facial protection depends on the risk factors. Healthcare workers must be aware of the risks of infection to themselves as well as, if infected, the risk to others, including patients. Personal eyeglasses and contact lenses are not considered adequate eye protection. Eyeglasses do not shield the eye completely and contact lenses do not cover the entire mucosal surface.

Principles table 13.7 Choice of facial protection

Principle	Rationale
1 Eye protection, such as goggles, should be available. These should be appropriately fitted, indirectly vented with antifog coating, and should provide good peripheral vision.	1 Goggles should be available in different sizes to aid a snug fit for all shapes/sizes of face for best protection. These provide the most reliable practical protection from splashes, sprays, and respiratory droplets. Some goggles fit over prescription glasses with minimal gaps. Goggles do not protect other mucosal surfaces of the face.
2 Visors are commonly used as an infection control alternative to goggles and protect the eyes, nose, and mouth.	2 To provide better face and eye protection from splashes and sprays, a visor should have crown and chin protection and wrap around the face to the point of the ear, which reduces the likelihood that a splash could go around the edge of the visor and reach the eyes. Disposable visors made of lightweight films attached to a surgical mask or fit loosely around the face should not be relied on as optimal protection.
3 Safety glasses provide impact protection but do not provide the same level of splash or droplet protection as goggles and generally should not be used for infection control purposes.	
4 Surgical masks are plain masks that cover the nose and mouth and are held in place by straps around the head. In healthcare settings, they are normally worn during medical procedures to protect not only the CYP but also the healthcare worker from the transfer of micro-organisms, body fluids, and particulate matter generated from any splash and splatter. While they will provide a physical barrier to large projected droplets, they do not provide full respiratory protection against smaller suspended droplets and aerosols.	4 These are not regarded as personal protective equipment under the European Directive (2002).
5 The European Standard EN149:2001 (HSE 2013a) defines the following classes of filtering face pieces (FFP), that is respirators that are entirely or substantially constructed of filtering material: • FFP1 filters at least 80% of airborne particles with < 22% inward leakage • FFP2 filters at least 94% of airborne particles with < 8% inward leakage • FFP3 filters a least 99.95% of airborne particles with < 2% inward leakage. Most respirators remain efficient for up to eight hours and are single use only (check manufacturer's recommendations).	5 Generally, FFP2 respirators should be worn when attending a CYP with an airborne or droplet infection. FFP3 respirators should be worn if performing aerosol-generating procedures in this group of patients. Healthcare workers who wear an FFP3 respirator must undergo fit testing prior to use (HSE 2019). Refer to Table 13.1 to select the appropriate respirator.
6 Full-face-piece elastomeric respirators and powered air-purifying respirators (some with high-efficiency particulate air (HEPA) filters are designed and used for respiratory protection, but because of their design incidentally provide highly effective eye protection as well.	6 Selection of this type of PPE should be based on an assessment of the respiratory hazard in an infection control situation, but will also provide, as an additional benefit, optimal eye protection. They may be used when performing aerosolised procedures for CYP with, e.g. influenza.

Principles table 13.7 Choice of facial protection (*continued*)

Principle	Rationale
7 How to put on a respirator: • Select the appropriate respirator. • Respirators should be put on before entering the room or bed space of the patient. • Place respirator over nose, mouth, and chin. • Fit flexible nose piece over nose bridge. • Secure on head with elastic. • Adjust to fit. • Perform a fit-check: inhale and the respirator should collapse - exhale and check for leakage around face.	7 A good fit of the respirator is essential to provide adequate protection of the healthcare worker. If patients are cohorted in a common area or in several rooms on a nursing unit, such as in RSV or pandemic influenza cases, and multiple patients must be visited over a short time, it may be practical to wear one respirator for the duration of the activity; however, other PPE (e.g. gloves, gown, aprons) must be removed between patients, and hand hygiene must be performed between each patient episode of care.
8 How to remove a respirator: • Respirators must be removed after leaving the room or bed space. • Grasp the lower elastic of the respirator at the bottom of your head, pull it up an over and release. • Then hold the upper elastic with both hands, pull away from head and, keeping tension of the elastic, gently remove the mask forward away from your face. • Remove from face without touching the outside of the respirator. • Discard the respirator in a clinical waste bin. • Perform hand hygiene.	8 To prevent contamination of the healthcare worker or the environment.
9 Points to remember: • Masks/respirators should be changed when they become moist. • Masks/respirators should not be hung around the neck or kept in the pocket. • The outside of a worn mask/respirator is contaminated and should not be touched. • Masks/respirators are single use only and should not be reused. • Most FFP2/FFP3 respirators can be worn for eight hours continuously (check manufacturer's recommendations).	9 To prevent contamination of the healthcare worker or the environment.

Foot protection

Plastic disposable shoe covers are not recommended. Where there is a need for foot protection then individual clogs or boots should be used. These must be antistatic and slip resistant, and a procedure for regular cleaning/decontamination must be in place.

Isolation nursing

The CDC cites numerous studies of the epidemiology of HCAIs in CYPs and has identified unique infection control issues in this population (Siegel et al. 2007). Additionally, there is a high prevalence of community-acquired infections among hospitalised infants and young children who have not yet become immune, either by vaccination or by natural infection. The result is more patients and their sibling visitors with transmissible infections present in paediatric healthcare settings. Seasonal infections, such as RSV, influenza, varicella (chickenpox) and viral gastroenteritis such as *Norovirus*, cause regular outbreaks.

Close physical contact between healthcare personnel and infants and young children (e.g. cuddling, feeding, playing, changing soiled nappies, and cleaning copious amounts of uncontrolled respiratory secretions) provides abundant opportunities for transmission of infectious material. Practices and behaviours, such as congregation of CYPs in play areas where toys and bodily secretions are easily shared and family members living-in with infants and young children, can further increase the risk of transmission. CYPs in chronic care settings or in nurseries may have increased rates of colonisation with resistant micro-organisms and may be sources of introduction of resistant organisms to acute care settings.

Infection prevention and control management and the need for isolation is dependent on local decisions, which are informed by the risk to the population at the time, data regarding institutional experience/epidemiology, trends in community and institutional HCAIs, local, regional, and national epidemiology, and emerging infectious disease threats (see Table 12.1).

For CYPs with suspected or confirmed infections there are three types of isolation precautions:

1 **Contact isolation precautions:** For patients known or suspected to be infected or colonised with epidemiologically important micro-organisms that can be transmitted by direct contact with the patient or indirect contact with contaminated surfaces or equipment in the patient's environment. This isolation category requires the use of gloves and plastic apron or gown to enter the room regardless of patient contact. Nursing the CYP in a single room is preferred.

2 **Droplet isolation precautions:** For a CYP known or suspected to be infected with micro-organisms transmitted by droplets (large-particle droplets larger than 5 μm in size) that can be generated by the CYP during coughing, sneezing, talking, or during intubation and aerosol-generating procedures. Micro-organisms can be acquired by direct contact, by contact with droplets over distances of 1–2 m, and by contact with the environment, objects, or clothes recently contaminated with respiratory secretions. This isolation category requires a plastic apron or gown, FFP2 or FFP3 respirator, and gloves to enter the room. The CYP should be nursed in a single room with the door

closed. If this is not possible, spatial separation of at least 2 m between the infected patient and other patients must be maintained. This must be individually risk-assessed if respiratory oscillators are used.

3 **Airborne isolation precautions:** For patients known or suspected to be infected with micro-organisms transmitted by airborne droplet nuclei (small-particle residue – 5 μm or smaller in size – of evaporated droplets containing micro-organisms that remain suspended in the air and that can be dispersed widely by air currents within a room or over a long distance). This isolation category requires a plastic apron or gown, FFP2 or FFP3 respirator, and gloves to enter the room. The CYP should preferably be nursed in a single room that has monitored air pressure in relation to the surrounding area, a minimum of 6–12 air changes per hour and appropriate discharge of air outdoors or monitored high-efficiency filtration of room air before the air is circulated to other areas in the hospital.

Hospitals need to have a bed management system that not only helps to find the most appropriate bed for a CYP but also helps to prevent cross-infection by tracking the use of single rooms for potentially infected CYPs. Insufficient single rooms will lead to CYPs with infections being 'housed' in open ward areas. If insufficient single rooms are available, cohort nursing, i.e. placing CYPs with the same infection but no other infection, in a discrete clinical area where they are cared for by staff who are restricted to those CYPs, helps to prevent the spread of infection to other clinical areas. This is more easily achieved where wards are divided into small bays of two to four beds that can be isolated further by the closure of doors at the entrance/exit and which have en-suite sanitary facilities. Areas must be kept uncluttered, free from unnecessary equipment and have a high standard of cleanliness maintained.

Health Building Note (HBN) 04–01: (HBN 2013) outlines requirements for isolation facilities with separate air management systems, an ante-room, and en-suite facilities.

The main reasons for isolation rooms are:

- **Source isolation** (contact, droplet or airborne precautions – see above) to separate an infected CYP from other CYPs and visitors in a single room to help prevent the spread of infection.
- **Protective isolation** to separate an immunosuppressed CYP to minimise the acquisition of an exogenous infection.
- **Cohort source isolation** to segregate a number of CYPs with the same infection together in one area or ward when there are inadequate numbers of single rooms, to help prevent the spread of infection.

Single rooms are often used as an alternative for isolating CYPs with an infection depending on the risk assessment. The air flow should be neutral or slightly negative to the corridor to minimise cross-transmission.

If en-suite facilities are not available then, where necessary, a designated toilet facility should be made accessible. This will depend on the type of infection and mode of spread. The use of electric fans should be carefully reviewed as this may increase the risk of cross-transmission with micro-organisms such as varicella, MRSA or *M. tuberculosis*.

The Communicable Disease Centre sets out guidelines for Environmental Infection Control in Healthcare Facilities (Morbidity and Mortality Weekly Report [MMWR] 2003). For severely immunosuppressed CYPs, such as those undergoing bone marrow transplant, the risk of environmental micro-organisms, such as *Aspergillus spp.* must be considered. These CYPs must be nursed in mechanically ventilated single rooms or areas with a HEPA filter. This is an air filter that removes > 99.97% of particles > 0.3 μm (the most penetrating particle size) at a specified flow rate of air. HEPA filters may be integrated into the central air handling systems, installed at the point of use above the ceiling of a room, or used as portable units (MMWR 2003).

The following points should be considered when isolating CYPs in hospital:

- Does the CYP and parent/carer know why they are being isolated and have they been given the opportunity to ask questions?
- Do all staff understand about the infection and the mode of transmission?
- Do all staff know what PPE to wear, when to wear it, how to wear it, and how to dispose of it safely?
- Do visitors have to wear aprons and gloves or any other PPE?
- Does the isolation room door need to be closed all the time or can it be left open (e.g. when the CYP has an infection that is not transmitted through droplets or airborne?
- Can all staff explain the need for isolation clearly and consistently so confusing messages are not given?
- Does the CYP have their own examination equipment, weighing scales, and any other relevant equipment and, if not, do the staff know how to decontaminate the equipment?
- Do staff know to keep charts, notes, and tablet computers outside the cubicle?
- Can the CYP leave their room for short walks?
- Is access for nonessential staff restricted?
- Are the family and the CYP if appropriate, asked each day how they feel?
- Is the care plan up to date and relevant play therapy or school work built into the day plan?
- Is the need for isolation being reviewed on a daily basis?

Management of exposure to blood and body fluids

This section deals with the management of exposure to blood and body fluid spillages, including inoculation injuries. Injuries due to needles and other sharps have been associated with transmission of hepatitis B virus (HBV), hepatitis C virus (HCV), and human immune deficiency virus (HIV) to healthcare personnel (UK Health Departments 1998). The prevention of sharps injuries has always been an essential element of standard precautions. These include measures to handle needles and other sharp devices in a manner that will prevent injury to the user and to others who may encounter the device during or after a procedure. Sharps injuries occur when a needle or other sharp instrument accidentally penetrates the skin. This can happen during or after use, during or after disposal, or while resheathing or recapping a needle (HPA 2012).

In May 2010 the EU Council adopted a new EU directive, which stipulates the use of needles and intravenous cannulae with 'safety-engineered protection mechanisms' to reduce the risk of inoculation injuries to healthcare workers. This directive was transposed into UK Regulations in May 2013 (HSE 2013a). The regulations apply to all healthcare employers and compliance is mandatory.

The main requirements of these regulations are that unnecessary use of sharps must be avoided and, where it is not reasonably practical to avoid their use, sharps safety-engineered devices should be used, where reasonably practicable to do so. The regulation also stipulates that control measures should be taken to prevent the re-capping of needles, as well as placing secure containers and instructions for safe disposal of medical sharps close to work areas.

The following principles for the safe handling and disposal of sharps and the prevention of sharps injuries should be applied:

- All clinical staff must receive training in regards to the safe handling and disposal of sharps, as well as the risk, management, and reporting of sharps injuries.
- Never bend, break, or resheath a used needle or cannula.
- Sharps must never be passed by hand.
- Used needles and syringes must not be disassembled.
- The person using the sharp is responsible for its safe disposal.
- Ensure that sharps containers comply with British Standards Institute (BSI) specifications (BSI 2019).
- Sharps bins should be assembled safely according to manufacturer's instructions, to prevent spillage if the sharps bin accidentally dismantles. The appropriate written information should be completed on the bin label to ensure a record of the audit trail.
- Sharps bins must never be filled above the 'full line' on the bin. Users are responsible for locking the bin when full and for ensuring the correct identification of the source area is on the bin (ward/unit area, hospital/source building, date of disposal and the signature of the person disposing the bin).
- Staff must not push down sharps in the bin or attempt to retrieve an article from the bin as this increases the risk of injury. The temporary closure of the bin after each use should prevent accidental access.
- Sharps bins should be located at an appropriate height, never on the floor or above shoulder height. Brackets can be used, as appropriate, to secure sharps bins. They should be out of access to the general public and kept in a safe place out of reach when in use.
- Filled and sealed sharps bins waiting for disposal should be kept in a locked and safe place.
- Staff transporting filled sharps bins must wear suitable protective clothing, carry the container by the handle, and avoid carrying the bin close to their body.

'The Eye of the Needle' (HPA 2012), a report on surveillance of significant occupational exposure to bloodborne viruses in healthcare workers, indicated percutaneous injury was the most commonly reported type of exposure (67% of injuries) and that between 2002 and 2011 most occupational exposures involved members of the nursing professions. Injuries occurring after a procedure and during disposal of equipment were predominately related to failure to comply with procedures for the safe handling and disposal of sharps and clinical waste and were mostly preventable.

Ongoing surveillance of inoculation injuries in healthcare workers and the risk of bloodborne virus transmission can be obtained from the Public Health England (PHE) website (http://www.gov.uk/government/organisations/public-health-england).

Approximate transmission rates are as follows:

1 For HBV, approximately 300 per 1000 (30%) after percutaneous exposure from a donor who is HBeAg positive, for nonimmune healthcare workers.
2 For HCV, approximately 30 per 1000 (3%) after percutaneous exposure from a HCV positive donor.
3 For HIV, approximately 3 per 1000 (0.32%) after percutaneous exposure and less than 1 per 1000 (0.1%) after mucocutaneous exposure result in transmission from an HIV positive donor. The last case of an HIV sero-conversion in an occupationally exposed healthcare worker was reported in 1999 (HPA 2012).

See Box 13.4 for list of body fluids that pose a risk for HIV transmission.

Box 13.4 Body fluids that pose a risk for HIV transmission

Below is a list of body fluids and materials that may pose a risk of HIV transmission if significant occupational exposure occurs (Guidance from the UK Chief Medical Officers' Expert Advisory Group on AIDS [DH 2008] HIV Post-Exposure Prophylaxis).

Amniotic fluid
Blood
Cerebrospinal fluid
Exudative or other tissue fluid from burns or skin lesions
Human breast milk
Pericardial fluid
Peritoneal fluid
Pleural fluid
Saliva in association with dentistry (likely to be contaminated with blood, even when not obviously so)
Semen
Synovial fluid
Unfixed human tissues and organs
Vaginal secretions
Any other body fluid if visibly blood-stained

It has been considered that there is no risk of HIV transmission where intact skin is exposed to HIV-infected blood (DH 2008). Testing and follow-up for other infections (hepatitis B and C) as appropriate should be undertaken, and the need for postexposure prophylaxis for hepatitis B should be considered.

In the event of nonblood contamination through medications, information can be obtained by accessing the toxicology database of the National Poisons Information Service (www.toxbase.org).

If a CYP has been exposed, specialist advice from a paediatrician experienced in the field of HIV should be sought. Postexposure prophylaxis guidelines for CYPs exposed to bloodborne viruses can be found on the website of the Children's HIV Association of UK and Ireland (www.chiva.org.uk/protocols/pep.htlm).

Decisions about testing the infection status of CYPs or incapacitated patients after a needle-stick or other injury to a healthcare worker must take account of the current legal framework governing capacity issues and the use of human tissue. In England, Wales, and Northern Ireland this is covered by the Human Tissue Act (UK Government 2004) and the Mental Capacity (England and Wales) Act (UK Government 2005). In Scotland, this area is covered by the Adults with Incapacity (Scotland) Act (UK Government 2000) and the Human Tissue (Scotland) Act (UK Government 2006). Updated advice should be followed according to guidance from the UK Chief Medical Officers' Expert Advisory Group on AIDS (DH 2008). No blood from a CYP should be tested for bloodborne viruses without consent when investigating an inoculation injury.

Procedure guideline 13.3 Inoculation with blood or body fluids

Statement	Rationale
1 In case of any incident involving inoculation with blood or body fluids, splashes to broken skin, eyes, mouth, or nose, or a bite, perform first aid immediately: • Encourage free bleeding of any wound but DO NOT suck the wound. • Wash skin wounds with soap and copious running water. DO NOT scrub. • Flush mucosal contamination such as eyes, nose, and mouth with copious amounts of running water. If contact lenses are used, flush before and after removal.	1 This reduces the risk of infection to the recipient.
2 The line manager of the injured healthcare worker should ensure that a risk assessment occurs immediately and follow local policy, which may include: a) Sending staff to Occupational Health Department (OHD) during normal hours or b) Discussion with on-call Microbiologist/Infectious Disease Doctor (outside of OHD hours) or c) Sending staff to their local A&E department d) Completing an incident form and the Reporting of Injuries, Diseases and Dangerous Occurrences Regulations (RIDDOR) form (form F2508).	2 All healthcare workers should have immediate 24-hour access to advice on postexposure prophylaxis (PEP) and to appropriate drugs and support. d) The RIDDOR reporting is a legal requirement to monitor accidents at work.
3 Healthcare workers must not attempt to do a risk assessment on themselves or obtain consent for testing blood samples.	3 They may not have up-to-date knowledge of current advice and obtaining consent could be seen as coercion.
4 If the source patient is known, they or their parents/carers will be counselled and if in agreement their blood will be tested for hepatitis B, hepatitis C, and HIV.	4 To ascertain their infectivity status and to plan the treatment, if necessary, for the injured healthcare worker.
5 The injured healthcare worker's blood will be taken and stored.	5 This provides a baseline for future testing if any related illness occurs in the future.
6 If postexposure prophylaxis for HIV is required, this must be started as soon as possible (preferably within one hour of the injury) but can be given up to 72 hours after the exposure (DH 2008).	6 This is the optimal time to prevent sero-conversion.
7 If the healthcare worker is not immune to hepatitis B, passive immunity in the form of specific immunoglobulin or active immunity in the form of an accelerated course of hepatitis B vaccination can be considered. Healthcare workers previously vaccinated but at risk from hepatitis B following an inoculation accident may require a booster dose of hepatitis B vaccine. They should report to the occupational health department.	7 Although all healthcare workers should be vaccinated against hepatitis B there is a small failure rate. The risk of transmission to an unvaccinated individual from a hepatitis B antigen positive source is 1:3. Healthcare workers must be aware of their immunity status.
8 Hepatitis C remains the most commonly transmitted virus through inoculation injury as there is no vaccination.	8 Follow-up of healthcare workers may be needed when the donor's results are known.
9 Occupational Health Departments should counsel the healthcare worker in terms of work activities, safe sex and blood donations during the follow-up period.	9 During the incubation period of any likely disease the healthcare worker may be infectious but asymptomatic, and may inadvertently pass the infection to others.
10 All managers must ensure their staff are aware of local policies and comply with the advice.	10 Various legislation indicates managers must ensure that all staff are aware of health and safety regulations.

Reporting of injuries, diseases and dangerous occurrences regulations

The Reporting of Injuries, Diseases, and Dangerous Occurrences Regulations (RIDDOR) (HSE 2013c) places a legal duty on an employer, self-employed people, and people in control of premises, to report certain work-related injuries, such as acute illness requiring medical treatment, where there is reason to believe that this resulted from exposure to a biological agent or its toxins or infected material. This can include inoculation injury. The information enables the Health and Safety Executive (HSE) and local authorities to identify where and how risks rise and to investigate ways to reduce injury and ill health acquired at work. The reporting system is online (see www.hse.gov.uk/riddor) and requires certain information to be reported on F2508 – Report of an Injury and on F2508A – Report of a Case of Disease. Staff must follow their local policy as the necessary information must be collated. Failure to protect staff from work-related injury can result in a financial penalty or prosecution (HSE 2013c).

Blood or body fluid spillage

Blood spillage and spillage of other body fluids should be cleared up promptly and the area decontaminated and cleaned with disinfectant and detergent. Healthcare facilities should have written protocols in place for dealing with such incidents.

Procedure guideline 13.4 Dealing with spillage of blood or other body fluids

Statement	Rationale
1 Secure the area while getting the appropriate kit to clear the spillage. Use a 'wet floor' sign until the area is safe.	1 To protect other staff and/or patients from accidentally entering the area.
2 Ensure the area is well-ventilated when using a disinfectant.	2 To prevent the inhalation of potentially harmful fumes.
3 Always wear appropriate PPE; gloves and disposable apron as a minimum. Facial protection (masks and goggles) should be worn if there is any risk of splashing.	3 To prevent contamination with blood/body fluids and/or exposure to chemicals.
4 **For small spillages:** • Cover the spillage with disposable paper towels. • Once contained, the spill and the disposable paper towels should be carefully placed into a clinical waste bag. • Disinfect the area by wiping the surface with fresh hypochlorite (1000ppm) solution and leave to dry.	4 To soak up and contain the spillage and to disinfect the contaminated surface.
5 If the spillage contains glass or other sharp objects, these should be collected using a (disposable) scoop and disposed of into a sharps bin.	5 To avoid handling the contaminated glass or sharp objects.
6 **For larger spills:** • Sprinkle the spill with hypochlorite granules until all fluid is absorbed. Leave the spill for a contact period of five minutes to allow for disinfection. • A risk assessment and Control of Substance Hazardous to Health (COSHH) assessment must be carried out if using these chemicals. • Scoop up the absorbed granules with a (disposable) scoop and discard as clinical waste according to local policy. • Clean the area with a detergent afterwards and leave to dry.	6 To clean and disinfect the area.
7 Do not use chlorine-releasing agents on urine spillages.	7 This may release toxic fumes.
8 Alternatively, 'spill wipes' or 'spill kits' specifically designed for the purpose of the cleaning and disinfection of blood and body fluid spills can be used according to the manufacturer's instructions.	8 To safely clean and disinfect blood and/or body fluid spills.
9 Remove PPE, discard as clinical waste according to local policy, and wash hands with soap and water.	9 To prevent contamination of the healthcare worker or the environment.

Decontamination of equipment and the environment

The Code of Practice for the Prevention and Control of Infections and Related Guidance (DH 2015) makes the following statements in regards to cleanliness within the healthcare environment:

- Registered providers must provide and maintain a clean and appropriate environment in managed premises to facilitate the prevention and control of infections.
- Matrons or persons of a similar standing have personal responsibility and accountability for delivering a safe and clean care environment.
- The nurse or other person in charge of any patient has direct responsibility for ensuring that cleanliness standards are maintained throughout that shift.
- All parts of the premises must be suitable for the purpose, kept clean, and maintained in good physical repair and condition.
- The cleaning arrangements detail the standards of cleanliness required in each part of its premises; a schedule of cleaning frequency should be available on request.
- There must be effective arrangements for the appropriate cleaning of equipment that is used at the point of care, e.g. hoists, beds, and commodes – these should be incorporated within appropriate cleaning, disinfection, and decontamination policies.

All institutions providing healthcare must give assurance that all decontamination of reusable devices in those institutions is carried out to an acceptable standard. There must be a designated lead for cleaning and decontamination who involves directors of nursing, matrons, and the Infection Prevention and Control Team in all aspects of cleaning services, from contract negotiation and service planning to delivery at ward and clinical level. All areas should have a service level agreement (SLA) in place.

The remit of decontamination includes:

- The environment, including cleaning and disinfection of fabric, fixtures, and fittings of a building, walls, floors, ceiling, and bathroom facilities.
- Equipment, including cleaning and disinfection of items that come into contact with the CYP or service user but are not invasive devices, e.g. beds, mattresses, incubators, commodes, hoists, and slings.
- Reusable medical devices, including cleaning, disinfection, and sterilisation of invasive medical devices, such as surgical instruments and endoscopy equipment.

There are three levels of decontamination:

1 **Cleaning:** The process that physically removes visible contamination with blood, body fluids, dust, and dirt. It is essential that instruments and equipment are cleaned *prior* to disinfection or

sterilisation, as disinfectants can be inactivated by organic matter.
2. **Disinfection:** Can occur through either heat or chemicals and will not necessarily kill all micro-organisms, but will reduce them to a level that is not harmful to health. When using disinfectant chemicals, it is important to ensure that the concentration and contact time recommended by the manufacturer is used to ensure the effectiveness of the disinfection process.
3. **Sterilisation:** Can occur through either heat or chemicals and is the process in which all micro-organisms including bacterial spores are destroyed and removed. Sterile goods should always be checked prior to use to ensure they are in date and the wrapping is intact.

If equipment is decontaminated at ward or unit level there must be a documented audit trail of the process. Outbreaks of infection have cited equipment being involved in transmission (Coovadia et al. 1992), such as bassinettes, thermometers, suction apparatus, specimen form box, sinks, and pedal bins. Other commonly used equipment, such as blood pressure cuffs, have been associated with outbreaks of *Clostridium difficile* (Manian et al. 1996). Equipment which was not fit for purpose, such as wooden tongue depressors used as IV splints in young babies, have caused serious fungal infection (Holzel et al. 1998). The environment within the incubators was moist and warm, enhancing the growth of environmental fungal spores on the wood of the tongue depressor, which had been harvested in untreated forests (normally the wood used is heated in kilns prior to use in factories).

Toys and games can easily become contaminated and can be a source of cross-infection (McKay and Gillespie 2000), so those that are to be shared in the healthcare setting should be cleanable (hard surfaces rather than fabric or fluffy toys). Cleaning of toys should be performed after a known case of infection and also on a regular basis. Any broken or difficult-to-clean toys should not be used. Computer games should have a keyboard and mouse that can be easily cleaned.

Although the environment has been cited in incidents of cross-infection, the proof that it is a direct cause is limited. However, it is important to note that hands can be contaminated by the environment and act as a vehicle for micro-organisms to the CYP. The hospital environment is different from the home and the literature indicates that a clean environment is a safer environment (Dancer 1999).

Laundry management

All healthcare providers must ensure that there is adequate segregation, transportation, decontamination, and delivery of clean laundry and linen (DH 2021). Clean and dirty linen must be stored and transported separately. Follow local hospital policies for the management of laundry arrangements.

Linen should be segregated into the following categories:

1. **Used linen:** All linen that has been used, including linen that has been contaminated with blood or body fluids from patients that are not considered to have an infection.
2. **Infectious linen:** All linen from patients with a suspected or confirmed infection. Infectious linen should be segregated at the point of generation and is usually put in water-soluble bags before being placed in dirty linen skips.
3. **Heat-labile:** Items of clothing or fabrics that may become damaged by the normal heat disinfection process (e.g. baby clothes). A separate SLA for the cleaning of these items needs to be arranged with the laundry service.

Principles table 13.8 Principles of safe handling of laundry

Principle	Rationale
1 Clean linen must be stored in a clean, dry area and protected from dust. It should not be stored in the dirty utility room.	1 Baby clothes and nappies are often stored in these areas and there is a risk of contamination.
2 Clean linen should not be dropped on the floor or be placed on waste bins or linen carts.	2 Linen can become contaminated by the high microbiological load in these areas.
3 Never shake linen when making beds.	3 This action disperses skin scales and micro-organisms into the air, which will contaminate surfaces or CYPs at risk.
4 Always put dirty laundry directly in the linen carts. Infectious linen should be segregated at the point of generation and is usually put in water-soluble bags before being placed in dirty linen carts. Never hug dirty linen to the body when carrying it as this will contaminate uniforms/clothing.	4 To minimise the risk of contamination.
5 Protective clothing such as aprons and gloves should be used when handling used or contaminated laundry.	5 This helps prevent contamination of uniforms/clothing and hands.
6 Always wash hands after handling used or contaminated laundry.	6 Hands may become heavily contaminated from soiled linen.

Uniforms

Although there is no conclusive evidence that uniforms act as vector for transmission of infections (Wilson et al. 2007), some studies show that uniforms worn by staff in clinical areas may become contaminated with pathogens and therefore potentially pose a risk of cross-contamination (Callaghan 1998, Perry et al. 2001, Wright et al. 2012). Uniforms worn by HCWs are not considered to be protective clothing and appropriate PPE should be worn to reduce contamination of the uniform during the shift (Candlin and Stark 2005). The majority of PPE is single use and disposed as clinical waste after use, whereas uniforms are laundered and reused. Therefore the correct laundering of uniforms is an important aspect of infection prevention and control. It is common for staff to launder their uniforms at home as it reduces NHS costs and is more convenient. There is little effective difference between domestic and commercial laundering in terms of removing micro-organisms from uniforms and work wear (Wilson et al. 2007). If commercial laundering facilities are not available on site, an organisation must advise staff what it considers to be appropriate in these circumstances as stipulated in local policy (RCN 2020). The following conditions for laundering uniforms at home are recommended to minimise the risk of cross-contamination (International Scientific Forum on Home Hygiene 2013, Riley et al. 2015):

- Uniforms should be kept and washed separately from other personal clothing.
- Uniforms should be machine laundered with laundry detergent at a minimum temperature of 60°C.
- Tumble-dry at 40°C or more for a minimum of 20 minutes.

Patients and the wider public expect a uniform to be clean and professional in appearance. Uniforms should be changed daily. Public attitudes to wearing uniform outside the workplace indicate that it is good practice for healthcare workers to either change at work or to cover their uniform as they travel to and from work (DH 2020).

Waste disposal

The health technical memorandum 07–01 'Management and disposal of healthcare waste' (DH 2013) outlines the definitions and management of healthcare waste. It also provides advice on waste segregation (including colour-coding) and minimisation of waste. All healthcare facilities must have clearly defined policies in place to ensure safe identification, handling and disposal of waste.

There are two main categories of healthcare waste:

Hazardous waste: Includes clinical, infectious, and anatomical waste, as well as waste contaminated with medicines, including cytotoxic or cytostatic medicines. Also included are sharps contaminated with blood, body fluid, or medicines.

Nonhazardous waste – includes noninfectious, offensive, and hygiene waste, as well as waste suitable for recycling.

It is essential that all staff are familiar with local policy and receive training in waste segregation and safe disposal of healthcare waste.

Principles table 13.9 Principles of waste disposal

Principle	Rationale
1 Waste must be disposed of immediately into the correct receptacle. This includes tissues that have been used for nasal discharge and may contain infectious agents.	1 The environment will become contaminated if waste is left lying around on surfaces or the floor.
2 Clinical waste must be segregated from other waste at point of source and at all stages of the waste disposal process.	2 To reduce accidental incidents of waste being disposed of inappropriately.
3 Healthcare workers and others handling waste must wear protective clothing according to a local risk assessment of likely contamination on the type of waste handled, e.g. clinical waste, sharps bins.	3 To avoid contamination or injury.
4 Clinical waste bins should have foot-operated or electronically operated lids. These bins must be decontaminated on a regular basis.	4 To reduce the risk of contamination of hands when disposing of paper hand towels after washing.
5 Waste bags must not be overfull and must be secured adequately to avoid spillage.	5 Overfilling increases the risk of contamination of the outside of the bag.
6 Clinical waste bags and sharps bins must be labelled and tagged.	6 To ensure an adequate audit trail in the event of an incident.
7 Receptacles containing liquid clinical waste, such as disposable chest drains, should be disposed of in rigid, leakproof clinical waste bins.	7 To avoid spillage.
8 Clinical waste awaiting collection must be stored securely away from members of the public.	8 To avoid inadvertent contamination/injury or the public searching for needles/syringes/drugs.

Pest control

Pests such as flies, cockroaches, rats, and mice can carry a wide variety of pathogenic micro-organisms and therefore pose an infection control risk. Healthcare providers are responsible for ensuring that premises are free from pests. Hospitals should have a pest control programme in place, which includes regular monitoring and treating of pests. Staff should ensure that food sources for pests are eliminated and that any sightings of pests are reported to the pest control officer in accordance with their local policy.

Pests such as cockroaches and flies are known to inhabit dirty areas and therefore may become contaminated with organisms commonly found in faeces or rotting material. Flies are known to carry organisms such as *Salmonella* and *Shigella* species (Ugbogu et al. 2006) and cause concern in places such as food premises. Cockroaches have been cited in the possible transmission of multiple antibiotic resistant micro-organisms in a neonatal unit (Cotton et al. 2000).

References

Acar J, Davies J, Buckley M. (2009). *Antibiotic resistance: an ecological perspective on an old problem*. American Academy of Microbiology. https://www.ncbi.nlm.nih.gov/books/NBK559361/ (accessed 27 June 2022).

American Academy of Pediatrics (2015). *Isolation Precautions, Red Book*. In: 30e (eds. D.W. Kimberlin, M.T. Brady, M.A. Jackson and S.S. Long), 148–157. Elk Grove Village, IL: American Academy of Pediatrics.

Archibald, L.K., Corl, A., Shah, B. et al. (1997). *Serratia marcescens outbreak associated with extrinsic contamination of 1% chlorxylenol soap*. Infection Control and Hospital Epidemiology 18 (10): 704–709.

Berardesca, E., Vignoli, G.P., Distante, F. et al. (1995). *Effects of water temperature on surfactant-induced skin irritation*. Contact Dermatitis 32: 83–87.

Boyce, J.M. and Pittet, D. (2002). *Recommendations of the healthcare infection control practice advisory committee and the HICPAC/SHEA/APIC/IDSA hand hygiene task force: guidelines for hand hygiene in health-care settings*. Infection Control and Hospital Epidemiology 23 (12): S3–S40.

British Standards Institute (BSI) (2019). *BS ISO 23907-2:2019 Sharps injury protection. Requirements and test methods. Reusable sharps containers*. https://www.iso.org/standard/72503.html (accessed 27 July 2022).

Callaghan, I. (1998). *Bacterial contamination of nurses' uniforms: a study*. Nursing Standard 13 (1): 37–42.

Campbell, S. (2007). *The need for a global response to antimicrobial resistance*. Nursing Standard 21 (44): 35–40.

Candlin, J. and Stark, S. (2005). *Plastic apron wear during direct patient care*. Nursing Standard 20 (2): 41–46.

Centers for Disease Control (CDC) (1987, 1987). *Recommendations for prevention of HIV transmission in health-care settings*. MMWR 36 (suppl no. 2S): 3S–18S.

Chadwick, P.R., Beards, G., Brown, D. et al. (2000). *Report of the public health laboratory service viral gastro-enteritis working party. Management of hospital outbreaks gastro-enteritis due to small round structured viruses*. Journal of Hospital Infection 45: 1–10.

Cohen, M.L. (1992). *Epidemiology of drug resistance: implications for a post-antimicrobial era*. Science 257 (5073): 1050–1055.

Coovadia, Y.M., Johnson, A.P., Bhana, R.H. et al. (1992). *Multiresistant Klebsiella pneumonia in a neonatal nursery: the importance of maintenance of infection control policies and procedures in the prevention of outbreaks.* Journal of Hospital Infection 22: 197–205.

Cotton, M.F., Wasserman, E., Pieper, C.H. et al. (2000). *Invasive disease due to extended spectrum beta-lactamase-producing Klebsiella pneumoniae in a neonatal unit: the possible role of cockroaches.* Journal of Hospital Infection 44: 13–17.

Damani, N. (2012). Manual of Infection Prevention and Control, 3e. Oxford: University Press.

Dancer, S.J. (1999). *Mopping up hospital infection.* Journal of Hospital Infection 43: 85–100.

Department of Health (DH) (2008). *HIV post-exposure prophylaxis guidance from the UK Chief Medical Officer's Expert Advisory Group on AIDS*: https://www.gov.uk/government/publications/eaga-guidance-on-hiv-post-exposure-prophylaxis (accessed 27 June 2022).

Department of Health (DH) (2020). *Uniforms and workwear: Guidance on uniform and workwear policies for NHS employers.* : https://www.england.nhs.uk/publication/uniforms-and-workwear-guidance-for-nhs-employers/ (accessed 27 July 2022).

Department of Health (DH) (2015). *The Health and Social Care Act 2008: The Code of Practice for the Prevention and Control of Infections and Related Guidance.* https://assets.publishing.service.gov.uk/government/uploads/system/uploads/attachment_data/file/449049/Code_of_practice_280715_acc.pdf (accessed 27 July 2022).

Department of Health (DH) (2013). *Health Technical Memorandum 07–01. Management and disposal of healthcare waste.* https://www.england.nhs.uk/publication/management-and-disposal-of-healthcare-waste-htm-07-01/ (accessed 27 June 2022).

Department of Health (DH) (2015). *Start smart – then focus. Antimicrobial stewardship toolkit for English hospitals.* https://www.gov.uk/government/publications/antimicrobial-stewardship-start-smart-then-focus (accessed 27 June 2022).

Department of Health (DH) (2021). *Decontamination of linen for health and social care.* https://www.england.nhs.uk/publication/decontamination-of-linen-for-health-and-social-care-htm-01-04/ (accessed 27 June 2022).

Doebbeling, B.N., Pfaller, M.A., Houston, A.K., and Wenzel, R.P. (1988). *Removal of nosocomial pathogens from the contaminated glove. Implications for glove reuse and handwashing.* Annals of Internal Medicine 109 (5): 394398.

Dunn, H., Wilson, N., and Leonard, A. (2019) *A programme to cut inappropriate use of non-sterile medical gloves.* Nursing Times 115: 18–20. https://www.nursingtimes.net/clinical-archive/infection-control/programme-cut-inappropriate-use-non-sterile-medical-gloves-20-08-2019/ (accessed 26 July 2022).

European Centre for Disease Prevention and Control (ECDC) (2012). Surveillance of healthcare-associated infections in Europe, 2007. https://www.ecdc.europa.eu/en/publications-data/surveillance-healthcare-associated-infections-europe-2007 (accessed 27 June 2022).

European Directive (2002). *89/686/EEC. PPE Regulations 2002 SI2002 No. 1144.* https://www.legislation.gov.uk/uksi/2002/1144/made/data.pdf (accessed 27 June 2022).

Gould, D. (1995). *Hand decontamination nurses' opinions and practices.* Nursing Times 91 (17): 42–45.

Halabi, M., Wiesholzer-Pittl, M., Schoeberl, J., and Mittermayer, H. (2001). *Non-touch fittings in hospitals: a possible source of Pseudomonas aeruginosa and Legionella spp.* Journal of Hospital Infection 49: 117–121.

Health and Safety Executive (HSE) (2007). *Preventing contact dermatitis at work.* www.hse.gov.uk/pubns/indg233.pdf (accessed 28 July 2022).

Health and Safety Executive (HSE) (2009). *Control of Substances Hazardous to Health Regulations 2002: What you need to know about COSHH.* www.hse.gov.uk/coshh (accessed 28 July 2022).

Health and Safety Executive (HSE) (2019). *Guidance on respiratory protective equipment (RPE) fit testing.* https://www.hse.gov.uk/pubns/indg479.htm (accessed 11 August 2022).

Health and Safety Executive (HSE) (2022). *Personal protective equipment (PPE) at work.* https://www.hse.gov.uk/pubns/books/l25.htm (accessed 27 July 2022).

Health and Safety Executive (HSE) (2013a). *European standards and markings for respiratory protection.* https://www.rapidwelding.com/files/EuropeanStandardsAndMarkingsForRespiratoryProtection.pdf (accessed 27 June 2022).

Health and Safety Executive (HSE) (2013b). *Health and Safety (Sharp Instruments in Healthcare Regulations 2013.* www.hse.gov.uk/pubns/hsis7.htm (accessed 27 July 2022).

Health and Safety Executive (HSE) (2013c). *RIDDOR - Reporting of Injuries, Diseases and Dangerous Occurrences Regulations.* www.hse.gov.uk/riddor - (accessed 27 June 2022).

Health Building Note (HBN) (2013). *04–01 Supplement 1 Isolation facilities for infectious patients in acute settings.* https://www.england.nhs.uk/wp-content/uploads/2021/05/HBN_04-01_Supp_1_Final.pdf (accessed 27 June 2022).

Health Protection Agency (2012). *The eye of the needle: surveillance of significant occupational exposure to bloodborne viruses in healthcare workers.* https://www.gov.uk/government/publications/bloodborne-viruses-eye-of-the-needle (accessed 27 June 2022).

Health Protection Agency (HPA) (2007). *Regional microbiology network: A good practice guide to control Clostridium difficile.* https://assets.publishing.service.gov.uk/government/uploads/system/uploads/attachment_data/file/342689/rmn_GoodPractice.pdf (accessed 27 June 2022).

Hoffman, P.N., Cooke, E.M., McCarville, M.R., and Emmerson, A.M. (1985). *Micro-organisms isolated from skin under wedding rings worn by hospital staff.* British Medical Journal (Clinical Research Ed.) 290: 206–207.

Holzel, H., Macqueen, S., MacDonald, A. et al. (1998). *Rhizopus microspores in wooden tongue depressors: a major threat or minor inconvenience?* Journal of Hospital Infection 38: 113–118.

Huang C, Ma W, Stack S. (2012). *The hygienic efficacy of different hand-drying methods: a review of the evidence.* Mayo Clinic Proceedings 87(8): 791–798. https://www.ncbi.nlm.nih.gov/pmc/articles/PMC3538484/ (accessed 27 June 2022).

Huttner, A., Harbarth, S., Carlet, J. et al. (2013). *Antimicrobial resistance: a global view from the 2013 world healthcare-associated infections forum.* Antimicrobial Resistance and Infection Control 2: 31.

International Scientific Forum on Home Hygiene (2013). *Advice sheet: clothing, household linens, laundry and home hygiene.* https://www.ifh-homehygiene.org/factsheet/clothing-household-linens-laundry-home-hygiene (accessed 27 June 2022).

Jacobson, G., Thiele, J., McCune, J., and Farrell, L. (1985). *Handwashing: ring-wearing and number of microorganisms.* Nursing Research 1985, 34: 186–188.

Jeanes, A. and Green, J. (2001). *Nail art: a review of current infection control issues.* Journal of Hospital Infection 49: 139–142.

Kabara, J.J. and Brady, M.B. (1984). *Contamination of bar soaps under 'n use' conditions.* Journal of Environmental Pathology, Toxicology and Oncology 5 (4–5): 1–14.

Kampf, G. and Loeffler, H. (2003). *Dermatological aspects of a successful introduction and continuation of alcohol-based hand rubs for hygienic hand disinfection.* Journal of Hospital Infection 55: 1–7.

Ladenheim, D., Rosembert, D., Hallam, C., and Micallef, C. (2013). *Antimicrobial stewardship: the role of the nurse.* Nursing Standard 28 (6): 46–49.

Mackintosh, C.A. and Hoffman, P.N. (1984). *An extended model for the transfer of micro-organisms and the effect of alcohol disinfection.* Journal of Hygiene 92: 345–355.

Manian, F.A., Meyer, L., and Jenne, J. (1996). *Clostridium difficile contamination of blood pressure cuffs: a call for a closer look at gloving practices in the era of universal precautions.* Infection Control and Hospital Epidemiology 17: 180–182.

McKay, J. and Gillespie, L.A. (2000). *Bacterial contamination of children's toys used in a general practitioner's surgery.* Scottish Medical Journal 45: 012–013.

Morbidity and Mortality Weekly Report (MMWR) (2003). *Guidelines for environmental infection control in healthcare facilities.* http://www.cdc.gov/mmwr/preview/mmwrhtml/rr5210a1.htm (accessed 27 June 2022).

National Association of Theatre Nurses (2004). Standards and Recommendations for Safe Peri-Operative Practice. Harrogate: National Association of Theatre Nurses.

National Audit Office (2009) Reducing Healthcare Associated Infections in Hospitals in England. London: The Stationary Office.

National Patient Safety Agency (NPSA) (2004). *Clean your hands campaign*. https://tss.org.uk/covid-19/Handwashing_techniques.pdf (accessed 27 June 2022).

National Patient Safety Agency (NPSA) (2005). *Protecting people with allergy associated* with latex. National Patient Safety Agency Information, reference NPSA/2005/8. London, NPSA.

NHS Scotland (2012). *National Infection Prevention and Control Manual*. https://www.nipcm.scot.nhs.uk/ (accessed 27 July 2022).

Perry, C., Marshall, R., and Jones, E. (2001). *Bacterial contamination of uniforms*. The Journal of Hospital Infection 48 (3): 238–241.

Petrova, A. and Mehta, R. (2007). *Dysfunction of innate immunity and associated pathology in neonates*. Indian Journal of Paediatrics 74: 185–191.

Pittet, D. (2001). *Improving adherence to hand hygiene practice: a multi-disciplinary approach*. Emerging Infectious Diseases 7 (2): 234–240.

Pratt, R.J., Pellowe, C.M., Wilson, J.A. et al. (2007). *The epic2 project: national evidence-based guidelines for preventing healthcare associated infections in NHS hospitals in England*. Journal of Hospital Infection 65 (suppl. 1 Feb): S1–S64.

Public Health England (PHE) (2020). *Framework of actions to contain carbapenemase-producing Enterobacterales*. https://assets.publishing.service.gov.uk/government/uploads/system/uploads/attachment_data/file/923385/Framework_of_actions_to_contain_CPE.pdf (accessed 27 July 2022).

Public Health England (PHE) (2015). *Infectious diseases*. https://www.gov.uk/topic/health-protection/infectious-diseases (accessed 11 August 2022).

Redway, K., Knights, B., and Bozoky, Z. (1994). Hand Drying: A Study of Bacterial Types Associated with Different Hand Drying Methods and with Hot-Air Hand Dryers. London: University of Westminster.

Riley, K., Laird, K., and Williams, J. (2015). *Washing uniforms at home: adherence to hospital policy*. Nursing Standard 29 (25): 37–43.

Royal College of Nursing (RCN) (2020). *Uniforms and work wear: Guidance for NHS employers*. https://www.england.nhs.uk/publication/uniforms-and-workwear-guidance-for-nhs-employers/ (accessed 28 July 2022).

Royal College of Nursing (RCN) (2022). *Guidance for health care staff on glove use and the prevention of work-related dermatitis*. https://www.rcn.org.uk/Professional-Development/publications/tools-of-the-trade-uk-pub-010-218 (accessed 28 July 2022).

Royal College of Physicians (RCP), NHS Plus, Faculty of Occupational Medicine (2008). *Latex allergy: occupational aspects of management*. A national guideline. www.rcplondon.ac.uk/guidelines-policy/latex-allergy-occupational-aspects-management-2008 (accessed 27 June 2022).

Sax, H., Allegranzi, B., Uckay, I. et al. (2007). *'My five moments for hand hygiene': a user-centred design approach to understand, train, monitor and report hand hygiene*. Journal of Hospital Infection 67: 9–21.

Siegel JD, Rhinehart E, Jackson M, Chiarello L, and the Healthcare Infection Control Practices Advisory Committee (2007). *Guideline for isolation precautions: preventing transmission of infectious agents in healthcare settings*. http://www.cdc.gov/hicpac/pdf/isolation/Isolation2007.pdf (accessed 27 June 2022).

Spearman, J., Tsavellas, G., and Nichols, P. (2007). *Current attitudes and practices towards diathermy smoke*. Annals of the Royal College of Surgeons of England 89: 162–165.

Spencer, R.C. (2007). Microbes, infection and immunity. In: Infection Prevention and Control (ed. C. Perry), 13–37. Oxford: Blackwell.

Török, E. et al. (2009). Oxford Handbook of Infectious Diseases and Microbiology. Oxford: University Press.

Ugbogu, O.C., Nwachukwu, N.C., and Ogbuagu, U.N. (2006). *Isolation of Salmonella and Shigella species from house flies (Musca domestica l.) in Uturu*. Nigeria. African Journal of Biotechnology 5 (11): 1090–1091.

UK Government (2000). *Adults with Incapacity Act (Scotland)*. www.legislation.gov.uk/asp/2000/4/contents (accessed 27 June 2022).

UK Government (2004). Human Tissue Act. www.legislation.gov.uk/ukpga/2004/30/contents (accessed 27 June 2022).

UK Government (2005). *Mental Capacity Act*. www.legislation.gov.uk/ukpga/2005/9/contents (accessed 27 June 2022).

UK Government (2006). *Human Tissue Act (Scotland)*. www.legislation.gov.uk/asp/2006/4/contents (accessed 27 June 2022).

UK Health Departments (1998). Guidance for Clinical Healthcare Workers: Protection against Infection with Blood Borne Viruses. London: Her Majesty's Stationary Office.

UK Health Security Agency (UKHSA) (2021). Integrated guidance on health clearance of healthcare workers and the management of healthcare workers living with bloodborne viruses (hepatitis B, hepatitis C and HIV). https://www.gov.uk/government/publications/bbvs-in-healthcare-workers-health-clearance-and-management (accessed 28 July 2022).

Walker, J.T., Jhutty, A.J., and Parks, S. (2014, 2014). *Investigation of healthcare-acquired infections associated with Pseudomonas aeruginosa biofilms in taps in neonatal units in Northern Ireland*. Journal of Hospital Infection 86: 16–23.

Weston, D. (2013). Fundamentals of Infection Prevention and Control – Theory and Practice, 2e. Oxford: Wiley Blackwell.

Wilson, J.A., Loveday, H.P., Hoffman, P.N., and Pratt, R.J. (2007). *Uniform: an evidence review of the microbiological significance of uniforms and uniform policy in the prevention and control of healthcare-associated infections. Report to the Department of Health (England)*. Journal of Hospital Infection 66 (4): 301–306.

World Health Organization (WHO) (2009). *Guidelines on hand hygiene in health care: first global patient safety challenge, clean care is safe care*. http://whqlibdoc.who.int/publications/2009/9789241597906_eng.pdf (accessed 27 June 2022).

World Health Organization (WHO) (2011a). *Report on the burden of endemic health care-associated infection worldwide*. https://apps.who.int/iris/bitstream/handle/10665/80135/9789241501507_eng.pdf (accessed 27 June 2022).

World Health Organization (WHO) (2011b). *Antimicrobial resistance: no action today, no cure tomorrow*. https://www.who.int/director-general/speeches/detail/antimicrobial-resistance-no-action-today-no-cure-tomorrow (accessed 27 June 2022).

World Health Organization (WHO) (2021). *Antimicrobial Resistance*. https://www.who.int/news-room/fact-sheets/detail/antimicrobial-resistance (accessed 28 July 2022).

Wright, S.N., Gerry, J.S., Busowski, M.T. et al. (2012). *Gordonia bronchialis sternal wound infection in 3 patients following open heart surgery: intraoperative transmission from a healthcare worker*. Infection Control and Hospital Epidemiology 33: 1238–1241.

Further reading

Chief Medical Officer (CMO) (2002) Getting Ahead of the Curve: A Strategy for Infectious Diseases (Including Other Aspects of Health Protection). London, Department of Health

Davies S (2013) The Drugs Don't Work – A Global Threat. London: Penguin

Loveday, H.P., Wilson, J.A., Pratt, R.J., Golsorkhi, M., Tingle, A., Bak, A., Browne, J., Prieto, J., Wilcox, M. (2014) *Epic 3: National Evidence-Based Guidelines for preventing healthcare-associated infections in NHS hospitals in England*. Journal of Hospital Infection 86 S1 S1–S70

NHS England and NHS Improvement (2022) National infection prevention and control manual for England. https://www.england.nhs.uk/wp-content/uploads/2022/04/C1636-national-ipc-manual-for-england-v2.pdf (accessed 28 July 2022).

National Institute for Clinical Excellence (NICE) (2019). Surgical site infections: prevention and treatment. https://www.nice.org.uk/guidance/ng125 (accessed 28 July 2022).

National Institute for Clinical Excellence (NICE) (2012) Prevention and control of healthcare-associated infections in primary and community care. https://www.nice.org.uk/Guidance/CG139 (accessed 27 June 2022).

Royal College of Nursing (2017). Essential practice for infection prevention and control. https://www.rcn.org.uk/professional-development/publications/pub-005940 (accessed 28 July 2022).

Chapter 14

Intravenous and intra-arterial access and infusions

Anne Ho[1], Hannah Barron[2], and Lorna O'Rourke[3]

[1]RN (Child), BSc (hons) Child Health: Central venous Access CNS, Great Ormond Street Hospital, London, UK

[2]RN (Child); Senior Staff Nurse, PICU, GOSH

[3]BSc (hons), RN (Adult), RN (Child); Sister, NICU, GOSH

Chapter contents

Introduction	250
Aseptic nontouch technique (ANTT®) for intravenous therapy	250
Visual infusion phlebitis (VIP)	260
Types of central venous access devices (CVADs)	268
CVAD dressings	269
Common CVAD complications	280
Safety aspects for staff and families	287
Neonatal longlines (PICCs): Nursing management	294
Arterial lines	298
References	306
Further reading	309

Procedure guidelines

14.1	ANTT® for intravenous therapy	251
14.2	General principles: cannulation	255
14.3	Planning and preparation for peripheral venous cannulation	256
14.4	Peripheral venous cannulation	256
14.5	Cannula dressing	259
14.6	Flushing the peripheral venous cannula	261
14.7	Administration of a bolus medication via a peripheral cannula	262
14.8	Administration of an infused medication via a peripheral cannula	263
14.9	Blood sampling from a peripheral cannula	265
14.10	Removal of a peripheral cannula	267
14.11	CVAD: CVAD dressing	271
14.12	CVAD: changing the needle-free access device	272
14.13	Accessing CVADs: flushing	272
14.14	Accessing CVADs: administration of a medication bolus	273
14.15	Accessing CVADs: administration of a medication infusion via a syringe pump	274
14.16	Accessing CVADs: administration of a medication infusion via a volumetric pump	275
14.17	Accessing an implanted port	277
14.18	De-Accessing an implanted port	279
14.19	Assessing a CVAD for occlusions	283
14.20	Instillation of alteplase into a CVAD	284
14.21	Immediate care of a PICC or Hickman® with a fracture, hole, or split	287
14.22	Action required with a pulled-out PICC or Hickman®	287
14.23	Repair of a single lumen Groshong® NXT ClearVue® PICC	288
14.24	Repair of a Broviac® or Hickman®	290
14.25	Removal of a noncuffed PICC stitched in situ	293
14.26	Neonatal longline dressing change	296
14.27	Neonatal longlines: nursing care (general)	297
14.28	Removal of neonatal longlines	298
14.29	Intra-arterial lines: preparation of child and family	298
14.30	Insertion of an intra-arterial line	299
14.31	Preparation: system setup (intra-arterial infusion)	301
14.32	Maintenance: calibration	301
14.33	Maintenance: maintaining patency	302
14.34	Maintenance: observations	302
14.35	Blood sampling (arterial)	303
14.36	Troubleshooting: dampened trace	304
14.37	Troubleshooting: abnormal readings	305
14.38	Troubleshooting: puncture site bleeding	305
14.39	Troubleshooting: circulation compromise	305
14.40	Troubleshooting: no waveform	305
14.41	Removal of arterial cannula	306

The Great Ormond Street Hospital Manual of Children and Young People's Nursing Practices, Second Edition. Edited by Elizabeth Anne Bruce, Janet Williss, and Faith Gibson.
© 2023 John Wiley & Sons Ltd. Published 2023 by John Wiley & Sons Ltd.

Introduction

Intravenous (IV) and intra-arterial (IA) access is a common component of medical care, facilitating blood sampling and the administration of medication, fluids, and parenteral nutrition.

This chapter describes the insertion and management of vascular access devices (VADs) commonly used with children and young people (CYPs), including peripheral venous catheters (cannulas), peripherally inserted central catheters (PICCs), skin tunnelled cuffed central venous catheters (e.g. Broviac®/Hickman®) and subcutaneously implanted ports (e.g. Port-a-cath®). The insertion and management of arterial lines and neonatal longlines is also described in this chapter. Some guidance regarding the administration of medication via these lines is also included. For further information regarding the administration of medicines see Chapter 8: Administration of Systemic Anti-cancer Treatments, Chapter 12: Immunisations, and Chapter 17: Administration of Medicines. The use of epidural, nurse-controlled, and patient-controlled analgesia (PCA) is covered in Chapter 24: Pain Management.

The choice of VAD for the CYP will depend on the type of medication or therapy required, duration of treatment, family lifestyle, and the age of the CYP (Kaye et al. 2000). Early assessment of venous access needs can facilitate insertion of the right VAD and help reduce/prevent discomfort and repeated venepunctures (Bowe-Geddes and Nichols 2005). Play therapy is an important aspect of the preparation for procedures and needs to be an integral part of hospital care for the CYP. For more information see Chapter 27: Play as a Therapeutic Tool.

Aseptic nontouch technique (ANTT®) for intravenous therapy

Aseptic nontouch technique (ANTT®) is the standard aseptic technique used in the UK (Rowley and Clare 2011). The purpose of ANTT® is to minimise the introduction of micro-organisms, which can occur during preparation and administration of IV therapy. Fundamental principles pertaining to infection prevention and control must be followed, including effective hand hygiene, and the use of alcohol-based solutions for decontamination with adequate cleaning and natural evaporation of the alcohol. If alcohol-based products are not allowed to dry naturally then the antibacterial properties of the agent will be ineffective, placing the patient at risk of developing an infection (Rowley et al. 2010; Centers for Disease Control and Prevention (CDC) 2011; RCN 2016). For more information on hand hygiene see Chapter 13: Infection Prevention and Control.

Standard ANTT® is principles-based, clearly defined and focusses on the essential elements required for all IV therapy, regardless of intravenous device, administration route or clinical condition (Rowley et al. 2010).

The underlying principles of ANTT® are the protection of 'key parts' and 'key sites,' i.e. equipment that come into direct contact with the patient and therefore have the potential to transmit microorganisms, and the parts of equipment that come into direct contact with the infusate. Identifying and protecting key parts and key sites is paramount (see Table 14.1). For tips on maintaining ANTT®, see Table 14.2.

Gloves

Gloves should be used with discretion when performing infusion-related procedures. To prevent gloves being worn unnecessarily, it is important that healthcare workers are able to differentiate between specific clinical situations when gloves should be worn (e.g. when there is a risk of exposure to blood or body fluids) and those when their use is not required (e.g. when taking a blood pressure). The use of gloves in situations when their use is not recommended represents a waste of resources without necessarily leading to a reduction of cross-transmission and may also result in missed opportunities for hand hygiene (WHO, 2009). The use of nonsterile or sterile gloves will depend on the procedure being undertaken, contact with susceptible sites or clinical devices, the risks involved, and the local organisational policies and procedures in place (Loveday et al. 2014).

Where gloves are required, it is important that well-fitting gloves are selected. They should be neither too small, with the potential to be punctured by wearer's fingernails, nor too large, as they may impede manual dexterity (RCN 2016).

Table 14.1 Examples of key parts and key sites (not an exhaustive list)

- Syringe tip
- Needle – both the needle tip and the needle hub
- Needle-free access device on catheter lumen
- IV infusion lines – several key parts, such as fluid bag spikes, all bungs/caps/three-way taps, infusion ports, the end of the infusion line which connects to the patient
- Extension tubing (both the end that attaches to the IV administration set and the point where tubing connects to the patient)
- The hub of the CVAD/VAD
- The tip of the implanted port needle and the hub end
- Dressings – the parts of dressings that come into direct contact with skin
- Sponge sections of 2% chlorhexidine/70% alcohol applicators (e.g. ChloraPrep™)
- Sterile gauze – the centre of the sterile gauze squares (used for dressing changes)
- Rubber tops of vials containing medications, etc.
- Ends of bungs used to protect syringe tips
- Inner packaging where the syringe is positioned

Table 14.2 Tips for maintaining ANTT®

- Remember that the tray is not sterile – do not drop your equipment into your tray.
- Ensure other equipment in the tray does not come into contact with key parts (e.g. syringe caps, blood bottles rolling around tray, extension tubing being placed on top of equipment/key parts).
- Use plastic trays and always clean the tray prior to use. Do not use paper trays for IV preparations.
- Gloves are not a replacement for hand hygiene, staff must decontaminate their hands before donning and after removing gloves.
- Due to hand contamination that occurs when collecting equipment and touching cupboard handles, hand hygiene must be performed after this part of the process has been completed.
- Take care when inserting the needle into vials/ampoules not to touch the outer sides.
- Take care not to contaminate syringe tips when placing into and removing from syringe packet.

Cleaning trays

Correct decontamination of trays is another essential component of ANTT® (see Table 14.2). Before use, the IV tray should be decontaminated with a sanitising wipe and allowed to dry. After use, the IV tray should be decontaminated with a sanitising wipe and left to dry. Alternatively, the trays can be washed with hot water and liquid (dishwashing) detergent (Hibiscrub® or any other liquid hand soap are not suitable for this purpose) and dried immediately with a paper towel.

Accessing venous access devices

When applying ANTT® to intravenous therapy procedures, the actions required are the same for accessing peripheral, midline or central venous access devices (CVADs). It is essential that all staff accessing VADs are fully trained and competent to undertake these procedures.

Procedure guideline 14.1 ANTT® for intravenous therapy

Statement	Rationale
14.1.A The highlighted steps below should be adhered to at the start of all procedures:	
1 To prepare for the procedure: a) Put on a plastic apron if required. b) Perform hand hygiene. c) Collect plastic tray. d) Wipe tray with a sanitising wipe immediately prior to use. e) Clean all surfaces of the tray internally, then externally. f) Once cleaned, allow the tray to dry naturally.	1 a) As part of standard precautions. b) To minimise the risk of infection.
2 Collect all necessary equipment, diluents, medications, etc. Calculate all dosages and dilutions. Write/print all labels.	2 To ensure the procedure can be undertaken efficiently.
3 Perform hand hygiene.	3 To minimise the risk of infection and prevent any cross-contamination when collecting equipment.
4 Open equipment by carefully peeling back packaging.	
5 Connect all needles to syringes and draw up and prepare all medications. Ensure all key parts remain uncontaminated. If at any time you think you may have come into contact with any key part, dispose of it and use a new piece.	5 Using potentially contaminated equipment can lead to an increased risk of infection.
6 When all equipment/medication has been prepared, remove all needles from syringes and leave in syringe packet.	6 To prevent any risk of airborne or key part contamination.
7 On entry to the room/bed space, perform hand hygiene.	
8 Take the tray to the CYP. Undertake the appropriate identity checks.	8 To ensure you have the right CYP.
9 Locate the VAD to be used and if applicable, identify the lumen to be used. Check the VAD and site for any problems.	
10 Clean the needle-free access device attached to the end of the VAD with a 2% chlorhexidine/70% alcohol wipe for 15 seconds using friction. Allow to dry naturally for 30 seconds, visibly checking that it is dry.	10 To ensure adequate cleaning and enable the product to work effectively.
11 Carefully remove the syringe from the packet, taking care not to contaminate the syringe tip. Insert syringe(s) into the needle-free access device of the VAD and administer medications as prescribed.	11 To maintain sterility of key parts.
12 When all medications have been administered, rebandage, and tuck away the CYP's VAD.	12 To prevent accidental dislodgement or damage to the VAD.
14.1.B The highlighted steps below should be adhered to at the end of all procedures:	
1 To complete the procedure: Dispose of all waste/used equipment appropriately. Dispose of any sharps in a sharps container.	1 To ensure clinical waste is disposed of according to hospital policy.
2 Clean the plastic tray with a chlorhexidine based sanitising wipe and allow to dry naturally. or Wash with liquid detergent and dry immediately. Store in an appropriate and dry location.	2 To ensure appropriate cleaning of tray and reduce risk of cross contamination.
3 Perform hand hygiene.	3 To prevent cross-contamination.
4 Record all care in the CYP's health care record.	4 To maintain accurate records.

Safe sharps

Sharps injuries are one of the most common risks to healthcare workers. The 2010 EU directive, along with the Health and Safety Regulations (European Union 2010; Health and Safety Executive 2013) aim to achieve a safer working environment to prevent injuries with all medical sharps by requiring employers to promote the use of sharps safety devices and safe use and disposal of medical sharps.

In reality it will be difficult, if not impossible, to remove all sharps from the healthcare setting (RCN 2013), so the focus is on reducing the use of sharps where practical, or alternatively to introduce products with sharps safety mechanisms and implement controls that will minimise the risk of needlestick/sharps injuries. Within the field of IV therapy, these include the use of blunt needles for vials, sterile plastic quills for drawing up from ampoules, and cannulas and needles with safety mechanisms. In the following procedures, where the use of sharps is listed, the aim is that safe sharps (incorporating protection mechanisms) will be used to protect the healthcare worker from sharps-related injuries.

Disinfection of needle-free access devices and catheter hubs

Current recommendations are to use wipes containing 2% chlorhexidine in 70% isopropyl alcohol to clean the hubs of venous access devices and the needle-free devices for between 15 and 30 seconds with friction, and allow to dry prior to use, with the aim of reducing catheter-related bloodstream infections (Soothill et al. 2009; CDC 2011; National Institute for Health and Care Excellence [NICE] 2012; Loveday 2014). Proper disinfection of the IV connector is crucial in preventing bacterial contamination of the intraluminal fluid pathway (Macklin 2010). Studies by Kaler and Chinn (2007) and Smith et al. (2012) showed that prolonged contact with the alcohol wipe and the use of friction were effective in disinfecting needle-free devices. Individually packaged wipes impregnated with 2% chlorhexidine in 70% isopropyl alcohol are easily available and should be used.

Flushing VADs

This section covers:

- Volumes of flushes and heparinisation
- Flushing techniques
- Syringe size

Volumes of flushes and heparinisation of VADs/CVADs

Routine flushing with 0.9% sodium chloride or another compatible solution is performed at established intervals to promote and maintain patency and prevent the mixing of incompatible medications and solutions (RCN 2016). Heparinised sodium chloride is commonly used to maintain patency when the CVAD is not in use (Hadaway 2006a; Richardson 2007; Dougherty and Lister 2015).

Low-dose heparin flushes are frequently used to fill the lumens of CVADs between use with the aim of preventing thrombus formation and prolonging the duration of catheter patency. However, the efficacy of this practice is unproven (Bishop et al. 2007; Loveday et al. 2014). A review of the evidence regarding heparin flushes indicated that the benefits of this practice are unclear and inconclusive (Goossens 2015). A rapid response report from the National Patient Safety Agency (NPSA) advised organisations to review local policies to minimise the use of heparin flush solutions for all VADs due to risks associated with heparin flush use (NPSA 2008). It is not known whether withdrawing heparin from use in maintaining patency of VADs and CVADs will lead to an increase in occlusion rates.

When flushing CVADs, the internal volume of the catheter differs depending on the type and size of catheter (Dougherty 2006). Many long-term CVADs will have been cut in theatre to fit each individual CYP; therefore the internal volume of the catheters will be less than the stated catheter priming volume. The volume of the flush solution should be equal to at least twice the volume of the catheter and add-on devices (RCN 2016). For recommended flush volumes, see Table 14.3.

Table 14.3 Flush volumes and heparinisation of VADs

The flush volume tables below are a guide. The CYP's size and clinical condition will influence the clinician's clinical judgement regarding the volume of flush to use.		
Peripheral venous cannula		
Flushing volumes for peripheral venous cannula		
Action	**Volume**	**Solution**
To assess patency preaccess	1–2 ml	Sodium chloride 0.9%
In between/after IV medication	1–2 ml	Sodium chloride 0.9% or dextrose 5%
To lock the catheter	1–2 ml 0.5 ml	Sodium chloride 0.9% heparinised saline 10 units per ml if used (Klenner et al. 2003)
To flush after blood sampling	2 ml	Sodium chloride 0.9%
PICC – valved: 3 Fr, 4 Fr (single) and 5 Fr (dual)		
Flushing volumes for PICC – valved: 3 Fr, 4 R (single) and 5 Fr (dual)		
Action	**Volume**	**Solution**
To assess patency preaccess	1–2 ml	Sodium chloride 0.9%
In between/after IV medication	2 ml	Sodium chloride 0.9% or dextrose 5%
To lock the catheter – weekly	3 ml	Sodium chloride 0.9%
To flush after blood sampling	3 ml	Sodium chloride 0.9%
PICC open-ended/nonvalved		
Flushing volumes for PICC – open-ended 3 Fr (single) and 4 Fr (double)		
Action	**Volume**	**Solution**
To assess patency preaccess	1–2 ml	Sodium chloride 0.9%
In between/after IV medication	2 ml	Sodium chloride 0.9% or dextrose 5%
Frequently accessed catheters (three times daily or more), after each use as a lock	1–2 ml	Sodium chloride 0.9%

Table 14.3 Flush volumes and heparinisation of VADs (continued)

Action	Volume	Solution
Infrequently accessed catheters (once or twice daily), after each use as a lock	1–2 ml 2 ml	Sodium chloride 0.9% Heparinised saline 10 units per ml
To lock the catheter – weekly	2 ml	Heparinised saline 10 units per ml
To flush after blood sampling	3 ml	Sodium chloride 0.9%

Skin tunnelled central venous catheter (CVC): 2.7 Fr, 4.2 Fr, 6.6 Fr (single lumen) 5 Fr (double lumen)

Flushing volumes for skin tunnelled CVC: 2.7 Fr, 4.2 Fr, 6.6 Fr (single lumen), 5 Fr (double lumen)

Action	Volume	Solution
To assess patency preaccess	1–2 ml	Sodium chloride 0.9%
In between/after IV medication	1–2 ml	Sodium chloride 0.9% or dextrose 5%
Frequently accessed catheters (three times daily or more), after each use as a lock	1–2 ml	Sodium chloride 0.9%
Infrequently accessed catheters (once or twice daily), after each use as a lock	1–2 ml 1.5 ml	Sodium chloride 0.9% Heparinised saline 10 units per ml
To lock the catheter – weekly	1.5 ml	Heparin sodium 10 units per ml
To flush after blood sampling	2–3 ml	Sodium chloride 0.9%

Skin tunnelled CVC: 9.6 Fr (single lumen), 7 Fr, 9 Fr, 10 Fr and 12 Fr (dual lumen)

Flushing volumes for skin tunnelled CVCs: 9.6 Fr (single lumen), 7 Fr, 9 Fr, 10 Fr and 12 Fr (dual lumen)

Action	Volume	Solution
To assess patency pre access	2–4 ml	Sodium chloride 0.9%
In between/after IV medication	2–4 ml	Sodium chloride 0.9% or Dextrose 5%
Frequently accessed catheters (three times daily or more) after each use as a lock	2–4 ml	Sodium chloride 0.9%
Infrequently accessed catheters (once or twice daily), after each use as a lock	2–4 ml 2.5 ml	Sodium chloride 0.9% Heparinised saline 10 units per ml
To lock the catheter – weekly	2.5 ml	Heparinised saline 10 units per ml
To flush after blood sampling	5–10 ml	Sodium chloride 0.9%

Subcutaneous implanted port (large)

Flushing volumes for implanted port large

Action	Volume	Solution
To assess patency pre access	2–3 ml	Sodium chloride 0.9%
In between/after IV medication	2–3 ml	Sodium chloride 0.9% or dextrose 5%
Frequently accessed catheters (three times daily or more), after each use as a lock	2–3 ml	Sodium chloride 0.9%
Infrequently accessed catheters (once or twice daily), after each use as a lock	2–3 ml 2.5 ml	Sodium chloride 0.9% Heparinised saline 10 units per ml
Deaccessing the port – weekly	2.5 ml	Heparinised saline 10 units per ml
Deaccessing the port – monthly	2.5 ml	Heparinised saline 100 units per ml
To flush after blood sampling	5 ml	Sodium chloride 0.9%

Actual catheter priming volumes: port = 0.6 ml, catheter = 0.6 ml – Total 1.2 ml

Subcutaneous implanted port (low profile)

Flushing volumes for implanted port low profile

Action	Volume	Solution
To assess patency pre access	1–2 ml	Sodium chloride 0.9%
In between/after IV medication	1–2 ml	Sodium chloride 0.9% or dextrose 5%
Frequently accessed catheters (three times daily or more) after each use as a lock	1–2 ml	Sodium chloride 0.9%
Infrequently accessed catheters (once or twice daily), after each use as a lock	1–2 ml 2 ml	Sodium chloride 0.9% Heparinised saline 10 units per ml
Deaccessing the port – weekly	2 ml	Heparinised saline 10 units per ml*

(continued)

Table 14.3 Flush volumes and heparinisation of VADs *(continued)*

Deaccessing the port – monthly	2 ml	Heparinised saline 100 units per ml
To flush after blood sampling	3 ml	Sodium chloride 0.9%
Actual catheter priming volumes: Port = 0.2 ml, catheter = 0.6 ml – Total 0.8 ml (Bishop et al. 2007; Frey 2007; Hagle 2007; Bravery 2008).		

Haemodialysis/apheresis CVCs (long and short term)

Flushing volumes for haemodialysis/apheresis CVCs (long and short term)

Action	Volume	Solution
To lock after each access or weekly	Equivalent to the catheter/priming volume usually found writing on the catheter or clamp.	Heparin sodium 1000 units per ml
To access the catheter before use	Withdraw 1–2 ml blood/heparin and discard. Then flush with 2–5 ml of sodium chloride 0.9%. This must be performed prior to every access/intervention	N/a
To flush in between drugs	3–5 ml	Sodium chloride 0.9% or Dextrose 5%
To flush after haemodialysis/extracorporeal procedures	2–5 ml	Sodium chloride 0.9%
To flush after blood sampling	5 ml	Sodium chloride 0.9%

Note: Before using the catheter the indwelling heparin must be aspirated from the catheter and lumen(s) and flushed with 0.9% sodium chloride. This is to prevent systemic heparinisation and to remove any clots present

Short-term nontunnelled CVC

Flushing volumes for short-term nontunnelled CVC

Action	Volume	Solution
To assess patency pre access	1–3 ml	Sodium chloride 0.9%
In between/after IV medication	1–3 ml	Sodium chloride 0.9%
Frequently accessed catheters (four times daily or more) after each use as a lock	1–3 ml	Sodium chloride 0.9%
Infrequently accessed catheters (one to three times daily) after each use as a lock	1–3 ml 1 ml	Sodium chloride 0.9% Heparinised saline 10 units per ml
To lock the catheter – weekly	1 ml	Heparinised saline 10 units per ml
To flush after blood sampling	3–5 ml	Sodium chloride 0.9%

Flushing techniques
Actual flushing techniques impact on the patency of CVADs. There are two main methods of flushing used; the turbulent or pulsatile flush, and positive pressure (Dougherty 2006; Hadaway 2006b; Dougherty and Lister 2015; RCN 2016).

Turbulent/pulsatile flush
This method is used to clear the catheter of blood or drugs that adhere to the catheters internal inner surface. It utilises a pulsating, push-pause, turbulent flush, allowing turbulent flow to remove any medication or blood residue from the internal lumen of the catheter and minimising the risk of occlusion (Moureau 2000, Dougherty and Lamb 2008). When first accessing the CVAD, gentle pressure must be used initially to assess the patency of the catheter. Then, firmly pulsate 1 ml of the flush solution at a time into the catheter, so creating turbulent flow within the lumen (Dougherty and Lamb 2008).

This technique is based on the concept of laminar and turbulent fluid flow. Laminar fluid flows in undisturbed layers, with the fastest current in the centre of the lumen. Turbulent flow moves in swirls and eddies. Therefore, in theory, turbulent flow removes blood/debris attached to the catheter wall and thus reduces the risk of catheter lumen occlusion (Hadaway 2006b).

Positive pressure flushing
Use of positive pressure when flushing off a CVAD helps maintain catheter patency (Goodwin and Carlson 1993; Dougherty and Lister 2015; RCN 2016). The use of positive pressure helps to prevent a vacuum forming after completion of the flush and prevents blood being sucked (refluxing) back into the catheter, reducing catheter occlusion. The technique involves clamping the catheter while instilling the last part of the flush, so that 0.5–1 ml of solution is left in the syringe, immediately after which the pressure is released on the syringe.

For tunnelled, cuffed central venous catheters (e.g. Hickman®), venous ports, and open-ended/nonvalved PICCs, positive pressure is achieved by closing the clamp while flushing in the heparin. For valved PICCs, flush the PICC while removing the luer-slip syringe from the needle-free access device.

This technique is not needed if a positive-displacement or positive-pressure needle-free access device is being used (Richardson 2007). Always follow the manufacturers' instructions, as different techniques may be required.

Syringe size
Before use, the CVAD must be checked for patency using a 10 ml or larger syringe to flush the CVAD (Bishop et al. 2007; Dougherty

and Lister 2015). Syringe size has a significant impact on the risk of catheter damage, the basic principle being that when flushing a device, smaller syringes generate higher internal pressures with very little force compared with larger syringes (Hadaway 2006b; Douglas et al. 2009). Therefore, using a 10 ml syringe helps to prevent excessive pressure being exerted on the vein and CVAD (Todd 1998). If force is applied to the syringe plunger when resistance is felt, this can result in high pressure within the catheter, which may rupture. 10 ml syringes or larger should be used when first accessing/flushing any CVAD. Catheter fracture/rupture can be internal or external. An internal break can result in possible catheter emboli. Smaller size syringes can be used for medication administration, to ensure dose accuracy, once catheter patency has first been established using a 10 ml syringe (Hadaway 1998).

Smaller syringes can exceed 25 pounds per square inch (psi) which can cause venous damage and catheter rupture. For example, exerting normal pressure on a 10 ml syringe produces 11 psi, on a 3 ml syringe, 29 psi, and a 1 ml syringe produces >100 psi. CVADs can burst when pressures above 25–40 psi are applied (Bard Access Systems 2016). The reverse applies when aspirating the catheter. Small syringes exert less negative pressure when withdrawing blood samples from CVADs (Macklin 1999; Registered Nurses Association of Ontario (RNAO) 2005). If difficulty is experienced withdrawing blood from a CVAD, switching to a 5 ml syringe or smaller may help (Macklin 1999).

Peripheral venous catheters

Peripheral venous cannulas are the most commonly used VADs. Cannulation is a procedure commonly performed on CYPs in hospital. Cannulas provide short-term IV access for the infusion of fluids, medications, blood products, and blood sampling.

An intravenous cannula is a plastic flexible catheter with a needle stylet that can be inserted into a peripheral vein (Weller 2005). There are a variety of sizes/gauges (G) of cannulas. The size selection should depend on the size of the CYP and their veins, along with the medication(s) and volumes required to be administered. For example, a 24G cannula is suitable for neonates, while a 22G cannula is commonly used for young children.

Cannulation in CYPs can be difficult due to vein size, adherance, and the number of previous cannulation attempts. Recommendations from the CDC (2011) specify that the replacement of peripheral catheters in children should only occur when clinically indicated (Keogh 2013). Care must be taken to monitor the cannula site for signs of infection, phlebitis, infiltration and extravasation.

While the insertion of a cannula is a routine event for health care practitioners (HCP), many CYPs and their families associate cannulation with serious illness. Cannulation can be both traumatic and painful for the CYP (Humphrey et al. 1992;) as well as stressful for the family. It is essential that pain and anxiety are minimised through preparation, explanation, and the use of drug and nondrug interventions during cannulation. For more information see Chapter 27: Play as a Therapeutic Tool, and Chapter 24: Pain Management.

Procedure guideline 14.2 General principles: cannulation

Statement	Rationale
1 Take time to plan the procedure and review any previous cannulation experiences for the CYP. Ensure appropriate play/other preparation is undertaken.	1 To maximise the chance of a successful procedure and aid compliance by the CYP.
2 The HCP should record and evaluate the procedure in the CYP's health record. In addition, the date, time, size of cannula, and site should be recorded.	2 To ensure that the CYP's health record is comprehensive.
3 If the first attempt at cannulation is unsuccessful, it is considered good practice that the same HCP should have no more than one further attempt.	
4 If this attempt is unsuccessful, a more experienced colleague should be asked to perform the procedure.	4 Repeated attempts by the same healthcare professional will damage both their self-confidence and the confidence of the CYP and family in their ability and skill.
5 In the event that repeated attempts (maximum of two attempts) by various healthcare professionals are unsuccessful, the team should consider and discuss with the CYP and family: • The relative importance and urgency of the procedure. • The reasons why a cannula is required. • The staff that may be able to help, e.g. senior colleagues, anaesthetists. • Equipment and products that may make the procedure easier, e.g. different types of cannula, use of a light source. • The need to preserve veins for future use. • Alternative methods of venous access, e.g. longlines and PICC. • The ability of the CYP to tolerate further attempts and interventions. • Alternative therapies not requiring venous access.	5 Repeated attempts at cannulation are stressful for all involved (McGowan 2014).
6 If after consideration and discussion it is concluded that further attempts will be made, the CYP and family should have a break if possible.	6 This will allow the CYP to regain their composure.

Procedure guideline 14.3 Planning and preparation for peripheral venous cannulation

Statement	Rationale
Planning and preparation: CYP and family	
1 Obtain verbal consent for the procedure from the CYP and family (Department of Health [DH] 2009).	1 To obtain agreement to the cannulation.
2 Explain the entire procedure to the CYP and family, giving information appropriate to the CYP's age and developmental understanding.	2 To ensure that the CYP and family understand the reason for the procedure.
3 Provide play preparation.	3 To prepare the CYP and reduce anxiety.
4 Consider which hand the CYP favours and avoid using if possible. However, do not make promises to use sites that are not accessible.	4 To promote a trusting relationship and keep dominant hand free for the CYP to use if possible.
5 Consult the CYP and family on their preferred choice of pain relief. If a local anaesthetic for topical application is used, ensure that it remains in situ for the appropriate time.	5 To minimise pain (Association of Paediatric Anaesthetists of Great Britain and Ireland (APAGBI) 2012). For more information see Chapter 24: Pain Management.
6 Always check for previous allergic reactions.	
7 Apply the topical local anaesthetic cream, if used, to two or more suitable venous sites and leave in situ for the recommended time to prevent any adverse reactions.	7 To allow the topical anaesthetic cream time to take effect. More than one site is selected to allow choice during cannulation and in case a second access site is required.
8 Use an adhesive dressing to cover the topical anaesthetic cream. Alternatively, Clingfilm can be wrapped around the cream if preferred.	8 Sterile polyurethane dressings are the method of choice for securing any local anaesthetic creams (Needham and Strehle 2008). Using cling film avoids the discomfort of removing the dressing later.
Planning and preparation – equipment and environment	
9 Use a clinical room if possible. Avoid using the CYP's own bed-space or room.	9 To ensure the CYP's bed space remains a safe haven (Bruce 2009).
Planning and preparation: Site assessment	
10 Limbs and venous sites should be inspected.	10 To select the most appropriate site and the best veins to use.
11 Avoid selecting veins adjacent to joints if possible. The veins should be straight and feel soft and bouncy when lightly pressed. Avoid veins that are sclerosed, fibrosed, or hard. A suitable vein will be palpable or visible, of good width and length, with a brisk refill capacity. Straight, nontortuous veins, without valves, are preferable.	11 To decrease the risk of extravasation and phlebitis (Paquette et al. 2011).
Preparation and preparation: Staff roles	
12 Seek the assistance of a colleague to hold the CYP's limb, assist with the securing of the device, and to provide distraction if appropriate.	12 The assistance of a colleague will help to maximise the chance of a successful insertion procedure.
13 Allow the parents to be as involved as they wish, but also give them the option of being absent if they prefer (Gilboy and Hollywood 2009).	13 To assist with holding and distraction and provide emotional support.
14 All HCPs involved should be aware of the level of restrictive physical intervention and therapeutic holding that will be required for the individual CYP. This should have been agreed in advance.	14 For more information on therapeutic holding, see Chapter 19: Moving and Handling.

Procedure guideline 14.4 Peripheral venous cannulation

Statement	Rationale
Prepare for the procedure as per Procedure Guideline 14.1.A.	
1 Gather equipment: • Sterile 2% chlorhexidine/70% isopropyl alcohol applicator (e.g. ChloraPrep™) in the appropriate size • Cannulas (appropriate size) • Needle-free access device • T-extension • 0.9% sodium chloride drawn up in a 10ml syringe • Wound closure strips • Semipermeable dressing • Cotton wool or gauze • Bandage • Single-use splint if required • Single-use tourniquet	1 To ensure the procedure can be performed efficiently.

Procedure guideline 14.4 Peripheral venous cannulation *(continued)*

Statement	Rationale
2 Place yourself in a comfortable position, sitting facing the CYP.	
3 Remove the local anaesthetic cream, if used, and wipe dry with a tissue or gauze.	
4 If appropriate, confirm with the CYP that the cream has caused numbness of the skin effectively.	4 To reassure them that the pain of the procedure will be reduced.
5 Apply an appropriate size tourniquet 7–8 cm above the intended vein to allow compression.	5 To facilitate filling of the vein and enhance visualisation.
6 Do not occlude arterial supply to the limb (indications of occluded arterial supply include loss of colour, compromised pulse, and pain). Loosen and remove the tourniquet immediately if this occurs.	6 To differentiate veins from arteries (arteries pulsate) and to locate valves.
7 Lightly tap the vein or instruct the CYP to clench or pump the fist.	7 To encourage further venous filling.
8 Palpate the intended vein by placing one or two fingers over the vein and pressing lightly.	
9 Perform hand hygiene.	
10 Disinfect the skin at the site at which you intend to insert the needle, with 2% chlorhexidine gluconate/70% isopropyl alcohol applicator, (e.g. ChloraPrep™) using firm back and forth and left to right strokes for 30 seconds. Discard ChloraPrep™ away from equipment in tray.	10 To clean and disinfect the skin, and prevent introduction of infection.
11 Allow the site to completely dry.	11 To ensure the required contact time of the skin disinfectant.
12 Do not repalpate the vein once the skin has been cleaned.	12 To prevent recontaminating the skin.
13 Select the appropriate size cannula to ensure the correct flow rates required for the procedure.	13 Ideally the smallest gauge of cannula should be selected for the prescribed therapy to prevent damage to the vessel intima (inner lining), and ensure adequate blood flow around the cannula to reduce the risk of phlebitis.
14 Stabilise the vein by gently stretching the skin over the vein and maintaining the support throughout the insertion of the cannula.	13 To ensure easy penetration of the skin with the cannula and to immobilise and anchor the vein.
15 With the bevel up, at the sharpest part of the needle, insert the cannula through the skin at an angle of between 10 and 45°, depending on the depth of the vein to be entered (Weinstein 2007).	15 **To ensure easy penetration of the skin with the cannula needle at the sharpest point.**
16 On entering the vein, a first flashback of blood is seen in the chamber of the stylet.	16 This is known as primary flashback. It may be accompanied by a giving way sensation, felt by the HCP as a result of resistance from the vein wall as the cannula enters the lumen of the vein.
17 Decrease the angle of the cannula so that it is now resting on the skin and withdraw the stylet slightly: a second flashback of blood, known as secondary flashback, will be observed along the shaft of the cannula.	
18 Maintain skin traction while the device is advanced. Slowly advance the cannula without advancing the stylet until it is fully inserted.	18 There are various documented techniques for this; floating, two-handed, one-step and pushing off the stylet. See Tables 14.4a and 14.4b.
19 Release the tourniquet.	19 **To restore the usual venous blood flow.**
20 Taking care to hold the cannula in position, remove the stylet while applying digital pressure just above the cannula entry site with one finger.	
21 Place the stylet safely away from other equipment in the tray, ensuring it is not allowed to contaminate clean, unused materials.	21 To reduce the risk of an accidental needle stick injury and minimise the risk of infection.
22 Continuing to protect the cannula, connect a T-extension using ANTT® and flush with 1–2 ml of 0.9% sodium chloride, using a 10 ml syringe.	22 To ensure the cannula is correctly inserted, ensure patency, and prevent clotting.
23 Flush using a pulsating push pause technique to create turbulent flow, followed by a smooth flush during which the clamp the T-extension is closed (positive pressure).	23 To prevent occlusion and blood back flow into the T-extension.
24 Remove the syringe and apply a needle-free access device (e.g. MicroClave®) to the end of the T-extension.	
25 Secure the cannula as per the dressing procedure.	
26 Complete the procedure as per Procedure Guideline 14.1.B.	
27 Document cannula insertion. The HCP should record and evaluate the procedure in the CYP's health records, ensuring that the date and time, number of attempts, size of the cannula, and site are recorded.	27 To maintain accurate records.

The Great Ormond Street Hospital Manual of Children and Young People's Nursing Practices

Table 14.4a Approaching the vein

How to approach a vein

1 Approaching the vein from the top:

Insert the cannula at a 15–25° angle depending on the vein depth. Take care not to insert it too far into the lumen or it may penetrate the back wall.

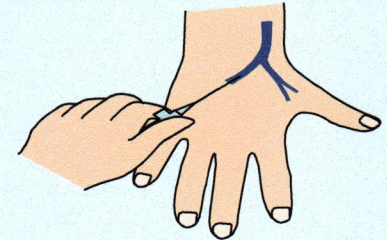

2 Approaching the vein from the side:

Position the cannula tip adjacent to the vein aimed toward it. This method, which is preferred if you have injected a local anaesthetic, prevents piercing the vein's back wall.

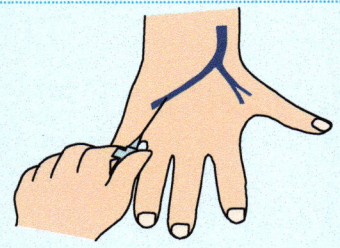

3 Approaching below a bifurcation:

A bifurcated vein looks like an inverted 'V'. It may be easier to cannulate than a single vein because it is more stable and less likely to roll. Insert the cannula about 1cm below the bifurcation, then tunnel it into the vein at the inverted 'V'. This approach prevents you from entering the vein at too steep an angle, reducing trauma to the vein wall on insertion. You are also less likely to pierce the vein's opposite wall.

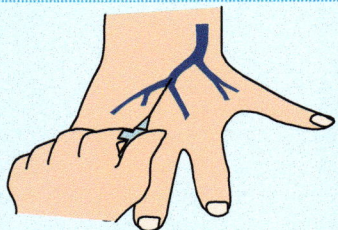

4 Approaching a vein that is palpable but only visible for a short segment:

This technique may help you to cannulate a vein that extends into the deep tissues where you cannot see or feel it. Insert the cannula about 1cm in front of the vein's visible segment, and then tunnel the cannula through the tissue to enter the vein. Tunnelling may reduce trauma to the vein wall on insertion.

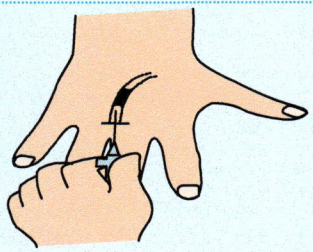

Table 14.4b Advancing the cannula

Advancing the cannula: four options

1 Floating the cannula into the vein

With this method you will remove the stylet before fully advancing the cannula. It is a good technique to use if you are inexperienced – you will be less likely to puncture the vein's opposite wall because you will advance the cannula only after you see adequate blood return (secondary flashback). Also, the fluid flow helps to float the cannula into place.

Perform venepuncture and advance the cannula about one third to a half of its length into the vein or when you observe primary flashback in the hub.

Place a sterile gauze or cotton wool under the catheter hub to catch any blood that escapes when you remove the stylet.

Release the tourniquet and remove the stylet.

Attach the tube and start the IV infusion at a slow rate.

Use one hand to maintain vein stretch while advancing the cannula with the other hand.

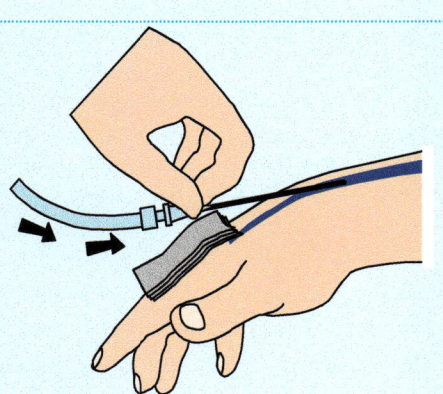

Chapter 14 Intravenous and intra-arterial access and infusions

Table 14.4b Advancing the cannula *(continued)*

Advancing the cannula: four options

2 The two-handed technique

Many practitioners use this technique because the stylet partially obstructs the cannula as it is advanced. This method reduces blood spillage.

- Insert the cannula into the vein approximately half its length or until primary flashback is visible in the hub.
- With one hand hold the hub of the cannula while retracting the stylet about halfway with the other hand.
- While maintaining vein stretch, advance the cannula until it is inserted fully.
- Remove tourniquet. If the vein is small leave the tourniquet tied to increase vein size during cannula advancement.
- Remove the stylet and attach the IV tubing or flush with 1–2 ml of 0.9% normal saline and attach the T-connector.

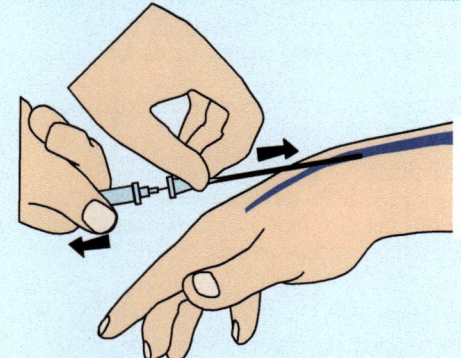

3 One-step technique

You might choose this method if you are experienced in venepuncture and the vein you are accessing is straight, even and superficial. An experienced, skilful practitioner can place the cannula in the vein lumen with one deft motion without injuring the vein.

- In one step, enter the skin and advance the cannula into the vein completely up to the hub.
- Remove the stylet and attach the IV tubing or T-connector.

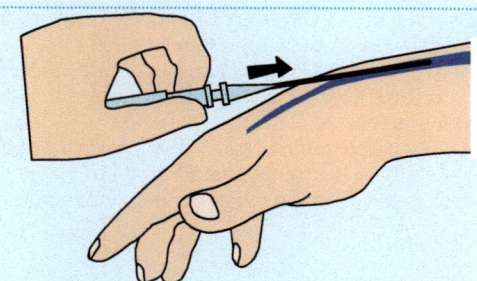

4 Pushing the cannula off the stylet

This technique is recommended for cannulae with a raised lip on the hub, e.g. quik-cath®.

- Advance the cannula halfway into the vein.
- Pressing your forefinger or thumb against the hub's lip, slide the cannula forward, so it moves off the stylet and into the vein.
- Discard the stylet, remove the tourniquet, and attach the IV tubing or T-connector.

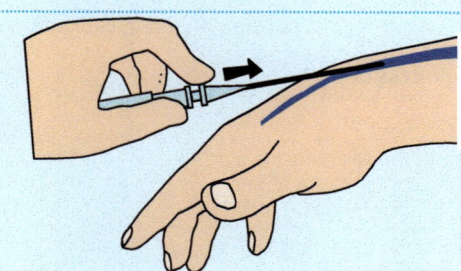

Procedure guideline 14.5 Cannula dressing

The dressing on the cannula should be changed only if it is likely to become ineffective in securing the cannula or there is water under the dressing. Take care not to dislodge the cannula when removing the dressing.

Statement	Rationale
1 The cannula can be secured using a sterile clear hand polyurethane dressing, such as: • Opsite® • IV3000® • Tegaderm IV®	1 Helps reduce the risk of dislodgment, mechanical phlebitis, and reduce the risk of infection. Clear dressings facilitate easy observation of the cannula insertion site.
2 Taking care to hold the cannula in position, apply wound closure strips (e.g. SteriStrips®) and a ported hand dressing after.	
3 Do not use opaque tapes or elastic adhesive plaster.	3 Risk of cross-contamination and lack of site visualisation.
4 Apply an appropriate size splint if necessary and bandage the entire area, leaving a small visible window at the cannula exit site.	4 To be able to visualise the exit site for signs of infection, phlebitis, and infiltration/extravasation. Bandaging the area around cannula helps to minimise dislodgement.
5 The fingers and toes should remain visible.	5 To facilitate checks of the CYP's circulation.
6 Complete the procedure as per Procedure Guide 14.1.B.	

Visual infusion phlebitis (VIP)

Peripheral catheter related phlebitis is the inflammation of the tunica intima of the vein and results from chemical, infective, or mechanical irritation (Macklin 2003; Lavery and Ingram 2006). Infusion phlebitis is defined as the acute inflammation of the vein directly linked to the presence of an intravenous access device.

The three most common causes of irritation are:

Chemical
- Properties of fluids or medications related to their pH or osmolarity. Children may be at increased risk of chemical phlebitis due to their smaller veins.

Mechanical
- Irritant cannula material, length or gauge.
- An inexperienced HCP lacking the skill of cannula insertion.
- Poor site placement of the cannula.
- Poor fixation of the cannula, allowing movement, such as rubbing against the vessel wall (Macklin 2003).
- Activity of the CYP or manipulation of the cannula, which may contribute to the development of phlebitis, e.g. a cannula in the foot of a mobile CYP.
- A larger-size cannula used, resulting in limited blood flow around the cannula (Higginson and Parry 2011).
- Prolonged duration of the cannula without review.

Infective
- Contamination by microscopic particles, which may be transferred to the CYP by infusion fluids and drugs (Higginson and Parry 2011).

Infective phlebitis if left untreated can lead to systemic sepsis.

Prevention of phlebitis and the visual infusion phlebitis (VIP) score (Table 14.5)

The aim of cannula care is to reduce the incidence of peripheral intravenous cannula infection and phlebitis. The use of the Visual Infusion Phlebitis (VIP) score supports a standardised approach when checking cannula sites (RCN 2016). To minimise the risk of phlebitis:

- Avoid using veins in areas over joints and splint if possible.
- Select veins with ample blood volume when infusing irritant substances.
- Securely anchor the cannula and replace loose or contaminated dressings.
- Inspect the cannula site frequently.
- Remove the cannula at the first sign of discomfort and inflammation (score of two or above on VIP scale) (Jackson 1998; RCN 2016).

All children with an IV access device in situ must have the site inspected at least once every shift for signs of infusion phlebitis using the VIP score (LaRue and Peterson 2011). Where CYPs are

Table 14.5 Visual infusion phlebitis (VIP) score

Appearance	Score	Action	Stage
IV site appears healthy:	0	Observe cannula site.	No signs of phlebitis
One of the following is evident: • Slight pain near IV site • Slight redness near IV site	1	Caution: Observe cannula site	First signs of potential phlebitis
Two of the following are evident: • Pain at IV site • Erythema • Swelling	2	Resite cannula.	Medium stage of phlebitis
All of the following signs are evident: • Pain along path of the cannula • Erythema • Induration or a palpable venous cord less than 5cm above the IV site	3	Resite cannula.	Advanced stage of phlebitis
All of the following signs are evident and extensive: • Pain along the path of the cannula • Erythema • Induration or a palpable venous cord more than 5cm above the IV site	4	Resite cannula, consider treatment.	Advanced stage of phlebitis or start of thrombophlebitis
All of the following signs are evident and extensive: • Pain along the path of the cannula • Erythema • Induration • Palpable venous cord • Pyrexia	5	Resite cannula, consider treatment.	Advanced stage of thrombophlebitis

Source: Jackson (1998) and RCN (2016)

receiving continuous intravenous fluids/medication, the VIP score should be documented hourly on the fluid balance chart for the duration of the infusion, when bolus medications are being administered, and when any other IV input occurs (RCN 2016). The VIP score and action taken, if any, should be documented in the CYP's health record (Nursing and Midwifery Council [NMC] 2015).

The VIP score is based around a traffic light design (see http://www.vipscore.net/wp-content/uploads/2012/04/002-IV3000-A4-score-and-vein-card.pdf).

Procedure guideline 14.6 Flushing the peripheral venous cannula

If the cannula is being accessed regularly (at least every eight hours) for the administration of medication or for blood sampling, no further flushing is required. In the event of infrequent access, the following regime should be followed with 8–12 hourly flushes using 0.9% sodium chloride (Goode et al. 1991; Kleiber et al. 1993; Gyr et al. 1995). The use of heparin is no more effective than 0.9% sodium chloride in prolonging cannula patency (Arnts et al. 2011; Cook et al. 2011); however some hospitals do still opt to use heparin.

Statement	Rationale
1 Prepare for the procedure as per Procedure Guideline 14.1.A.	
2 Gather equipment; this may include: • 10ml syringe • Needle • 0.9% sodium chloride for injection • 2% chlorhexidine in 70% isopropyl alcohol wipe	
3 Decontaminate hands with alcohol gel.	3 To adhere to the hand hygiene policy.
4 Open equipment by carefully peeling back packaging. If at any time there is a suspicion that a piece of equipment may have become contaminated, dispose of it immediately, and use a new piece.	4 Using potentially contamination equipment can lead to the risk of infection.
5 Connect the needle to the syringe. Draw up 0.9% sodium chloride, taking care that the needle does not touch the outside of any vials/ampoules. Ensure all key parts remain uncontaminated.	
6 When all equipment/medication has been prepared, remove all needles from syringes and leave in syringe packet.	6 To adhere to ANTT® and prevent any key part contamination.
7 Remove the bandage from over the cannula.	7 To facilitate easy observation of the cannula exit site during the procedure.
8 Assess the entry site using the visual infusion phlebitis (VIP) score.	
9 Perform hand hygiene.	
10 Clean the cannula's needle-free access device with the 2% chlorhexidine in 70% isopropyl alcohol wipe for 15 seconds using friction and allow to dry naturally for 30 seconds. Visibly check that the device is dry.	10 To ensure adequate cleaning of the device and enable the product to work effectively.
11 Unclamp the T-extension and slowly flush the cannula with 1–2 ml of 0.9% sodium chloride.	11 To check device patency and minimise discomfort. Studies suggest that 1–2 ml is sufficient (Goode et al. 1991; Gyr et al. 1995; RCN 2016).
12 Ask the CYP to report any pain or discomfort experienced and, while flushing, observe the cannula entry site and surrounding area for any sign of swelling, phlebitis, or infiltration.	12 To assess for any problems.
13 If there are no problems. Clamp the T-extension, while still flushing, to create positive pressure.	13 To prevent blood backflow into the cannula and T-extension causing occlusion.
14 If resistance is so strong that it is either not possible or very difficult to flush the cannula, check for kinks in the tubing, especially under the clamp. Consider replacing the T-extension (especially if there is blood visible), having first primed it with 0.9% sodium chloride, and repeat the process above.	14 The clamp can leave stress points on the plastic tubing, resulting in kinking of the tubing. The T-extension may be blocked due to blood backflow or other occlusion.
15 If it is not possible to flush the cannula using the techniques described it must be removed (see Procedure Guideline 14.10).	
16 If there are no problems with the cannula, ensure the splint is still in the correct position and rebandage the area over the cannula.	16 To immobilise the limb, preventing movement that may cause occlusion, phlebitis, and infiltration/extravasation.
17 Complete the procedure as per Procedure Guideline 14.1.B.	
18 Record the VIP score, as described below, in the CYP's health record and document any important information, e.g. relative ease of flushing, or any pain experienced.	18 To maintain accurate records.

Procedure guideline 14.7 Administration of a bolus medication via a peripheral cannula

Statement	Rationale
Prepare for the procedure as per Procedure Guideline 14.1.A.	
1 Gather equipment, this may include: • 10ml syringes • Other sizes of syringes for dose accuracy • Needles to draw up the required solutions • Medication(s) and appropriate diluents to prepare, if required • 0.9% sodium chloride for injection/5% dextrose or appropriate fluid depending on medication compatibility • Required amount and strength of heparin as needed • 2% chlorhexidine in 70% isopropyl alcohol wipe plus extra for cleaning the top/rubber bung of any vial	1 To ensure the procedure is undertaken efficiently and prevent later contamination of gloves.
2 Work out any medication calculations, collect medication vials or preprepared medication syringes. Write out/print any medication labels that may be needed and research any relevant information required.	
3 Perform hand hygiene.	3 To reduce possible hand contamination from collecting equipment.
4 Open equipment by carefully peeling back packaging.	
5 Connect the needles to the syringes, as required and draw up the first solution, taking care that the needle does not touch the outside of any vials/ampoules.	5 To prevent key part contamination.
6 Using the same technique detailed above, draw up all medication(s), flushes, heparin, and diluents required for the procedure. Prepare all medications as per guidelines.	
7 When all equipment/medication has been prepared, remove all needles from syringes and leave in syringe packet.	7 To adhere to ANTT® and minimise the risk of key part contamination.
8 Label syringes.	8 To help reduce medication errors (NPSA 2007).
9 Check the medication(s) to be administered against the CYP's prescription.	9 To adhere to the hospital medication administration policy.
10 When all medication(s), flushes, etc., have been prepared, take the tray and prescription to the CYP.	
11 Check the CYP's identification against the details on the prescription.	11 To correctly identify patient and minimise the risk of medication errors (NMC 2015).
12 Inspect the cannula entry site for any sign of phlebitis or infection using the VIP score.	12 To assess for any problems.
13 Perform hand hygiene. Clean the cannula's needle-free access device with the 2% chlorhexidine in 70% isopropyl alcohol wipe for 15 seconds using friction and allow to dry naturally for 30 seconds. Visibly check that the device is dry.	13 To ensure adequate cleaning of the device/bung and enable the product to work effectively.
14 Unclamp the T-extension and slowly flush the cannula with 1–2ml of 0.9% sodium chloride.	
15 Ask the CYP to report any pain or discomfort experienced and, while flushing, observe the cannula entry site and surrounding area for any sign of swelling, phlebitis or infiltration.	
16 If a vesicant medication is being administered, 0.5ml of blood should be aspirated from the cannula prior to administration. Administer any vesicant medicine first if several medications are to be administered.	16 To reduce the risk of extravasation (Hadaway 2007).
17 If there are no problems, remove the syringe containing the flush and insert the syringe containing the medication. Administer the medication over the required time period, observing the CYP and cannula site at all times. If there are problems flushing the cannula, follow Procedure Guideline 14.6.	
18 Following the procedure above, administer all required medications, ensuring adequate flushing between each of the medications to prevent medication incompatibilities.	
19 Attach the flush syringe to the needle-free access device and gently instil the first part of the flush followed by the turbulent flushing technique.	19 To clear the cannula of any medication/blood residue and minimise the risk of subsequent CVAD occlusion.

Chapter 14 Intravenous and intra-arterial access and infusions

Procedure guideline 14.7 Administration of a bolus medication via a peripheral cannula *(continued)*

Statement	Rationale
20 Clamp the T-extension, while still flushing, to create positive pressure.	20 To prevent blood backflow into the cannula and T-extension causing occlusion.
21 Ensure the splint is still in the correct position and rebandage the cannula.	
22 The CYP's fingers and toes should remain visible.	22 To facilitate checks of their circulation.
23 Complete the procedure as per Procedure Guideline 14.1.B.	
24 Record the VIP score as described below in the CYP's health record and document any important information, e.g. relative ease of flushing, any pain experienced. Record any medicines administered.	24 To maintain accurate records.

Procedure guideline 14.8 Administration of an infused medication via a peripheral cannula

Administration of any infusions via a peripheral cannula will require the use an infusion pump. The type of pump will depend on the volume of the infusate: Hydration fluids will require infusion via a volumetric pump, while medications ≤ 50 ml in volume can be administered with a syringe pump. Medications > 50 ml may require administration via a burette infusion set through a volumetric pump and those > 150 ml will be added to a bag of compatible IV fluids and administered through an infusion set and a volumetric set.

Statement	Rationale
Prepare for the procedure as per Procedure Guideline 14.1.A.	
1 Gather equipment, this may include: • 10 ml syringes • Other sizes of syringes for dose accuracy • Needles to draw up the required solutions • Medication(s) and appropriate diluents to prepare, if required • 0.9% sodium chloride for injection/5% dextrose or appropriate fluid depending on medication compatibility • 2% chlorhexidine in 70% isopropyl alcohol wipe, plus extra for cleaning the top rubber bung of any vial • Infusion set (buretted or nonburetted) • Bag of compatible fluid for medication or hydration fluid required	1 To ensure the procedure is undertaken efficiently.
2 Calculate any medication and look up relevant information. Collect medication vials or preprepared medication. Write out any medication labels.	
3 Perform hand hygiene.	3 To minimise the risk of hand contamination from collecting equipment.
4 Open equipment by carefully peeling back packaging. If at any time a piece of equipment may have become contaminated, dispose of it immediately and use a new piece.	4 Using potentially contaminated equipment will increase the risk of infection.
5 Connect the needles to the syringes, as required, and draw up the first solution, taking care that the needle does not touch the outside of any vials/ampoules.	
6 Using the same technique detailed above, draw up all medication(s), flushes, and diluents required for the procedure. Prepare all medications as per guidelines.	
7 When all equipment/medication has been prepared, remove all needles from syringes and leave in syringe packet.	7 To adhere to ANTT® and minimise risk of key part contamination.
8 Label syringes.	8 To help reduce medication errors (NPSA 2007).
9 Open the required infusion administration set and close all roller clamps to the off position.	
10 Check the medications/fluid bags as per medication policy. Open the required bag of infusion fluid and check the bag to ensure it contains no visible precipitate, leaks or damage to bag. Twist off the connector at the bottom of the fluid bag to reveal the connection port.	
11 Remove the plastic cover over the spike on the infusion set, taking care not to touch the spike. Taking care not to touch any part of the spike, hold the bung of the fluid bag in one hand and the bottom of the spike on the infusion set in the other. Insert the spike into the connection port on the infusion bag using a twisting motion. Ensure the spike is inserted fully.	

(continued)

Procedure guideline 14.8 Administration of an infused medication via a peripheral cannula *(continued)*

Statement	Rationale
12 Hang the fluid bag which is now connected to the infusion administration set onto a stand.	
If using a nonburetted set: 13 Gently squeeze the drip chamber to allow fluid into it, filling the chamber halfway.	
14 Slowly open the roller clamp until the fluid begins to move down the infusion set.	
15 Prime the infusion set until fluid is seen at the end of the line and then close the roller clamp off.	
If using a buretted set: 16 Open the roller clamp between the fluid bag and the buretted set and fill the burette with the required amount of fluid to prime the line. Close the roller clamp.	
17 Gently squeeze the drip chamber to allow fluid into it, filling the chamber approximately halfway. Prime the infusion set until fluid is seen at the end of the line and then close off the roller clamp.	
18 If a medication is to be infused: Connect the syringe containing the medication to the needle-free connector on the top of the burette (clean device first if it may have been contaminated during handling). Push the medication into the burette until the syringe is empty	
19 Remove syringe from needle-free access device and dispose.	
20 Gently shake the burette to ensure drug and fluid mix thoroughly.	
21 If large amounts of fluid are contained within the burette, close the white clamp on the top of the burette to prevent fluid leaking out when shaken. Remember to open this clamp once mixing is complete as it acts as an air inlet.	
22 Attach a medication-added label to the burette with all appropriate details.	22 To help reduce medication errors (NPSA 2007).
23 Set the appropriate settings on the infusion pump, including pressure limits, volume to be infused, and rate.	
24 **If using a 50ml syringe:** Prepare all medications as per IV/pharmacy guidelines. Use a luer-lock syringe for administering the infusion.	
25 Open the required infusion administration set (i.e. long extension) and connect the needle-free access device. Then connect the luer-lock syringe with the medication to the needle-free access device.	
26 Prime the infusion set until fluid is seen at the end of the set and then close the slide clamp to off.	
27 Attach a medication-added label to the syringe with all required details.	27 To help reduce medication errors (NPSA 2007).
28 Check any medication(s) to be administered against the prescription.	28 To minimise the risk of medication errors (NMC 2015).
29 When all medication(s), flushes, etc., have been prepared, take tray and prescription to the CYP.	
30 Check the CYP's identification against the details on the prescription to correctly identify the patient.	30 To adhere to the hospital medication administration policy and minimise the risk of medication errors.
31 Remove the bandage from over the cannula.	
32 Inspect entry of the cannula for any sign of phlebitis or infection using the VIP score.	
33 Perform hand hygiene.	
34 Clean the cannula's needle-free access device with the 2% chlorhexidine in 70% isopropyl alcohol; wipe for 15 seconds using friction and allow to dry naturally for 30 seconds. Visibly check that the device is dry.	34 To ensure adequate cleaning of the device and enable the product to work effectively.
35 Unclamp the T-extension and slowly flush the cannula with 1–2ml of 0.9% sodium chloride.	35 To check the patency of the device.
36 If a vesicant medication is being administered, 0.5ml of blood should be aspirated from the cannula prior to administration.	36 To reduce the risk of extravasation.
37 Ask the CYP to report any pain or discomfort experienced and, while flushing, observe the cannula entry site and surrounding area for any sign of swelling, phlebitis, or infiltration.	

Procedure guideline 14.8 Administration of an infused medication via a peripheral cannula *(continued)*

Statement	Rationale
38 If there are no problems, remove the syringe containing the flush and connect the infusion set. If there are problems with flushing the cannula, then follow the guidelines in Procedure Guideline 14.6.	
39 Attach the infusion line to the extension tubing. Open the clamp. Commence infusion as prescribed, ensuring rates, pressure limits, and volumes to be infused limits are set.	
40 Ensure that the splint is still in the correct position and rebandage the area over the cannula, leaving a small window over the cannula site.	40 The window will allow visualisation of the cannula site to allow for observation for phlebitis and infiltration/extravasation.
41 The CYP's fingers and toes should remain visible.	41 To facilitate checks of the CYP's circulation.
42 When infusing a medication, it is essential that a flush is infused using the pump. The rate of the flush must remain the same as the medication. • For burettes, add a compatible diluent of 20 ml via the needle-free access device at the top of the burette (remember to clean the device first). • For nonburettes, change the infusion bag to a bag of compatible fluid at the spike attachment. Set a 'volume to be infused' for 20 ml. • For syringe administration, remove the medication syringe and attach another luer-lock syringe containing 5 ml of compatible fluid. The 'flush' MUST be labelled to prevent extra flushes or lack of flush.	42 To ensure all of the medication in the infusion tubing is administered.
43 When the flush has finished, attach the flush syringe to the needle-free access device and gently instil the first part of the flush, followed by the turbulent flushing technique.	43 To clear the cannula of any medication/blood residue and minimise the risk of future VAD occlusion
44 Clamp the T-extension, while still flushing, to create positive pressure.	44 To prevent blood backflow into the cannula and T-extension causing occlusion.
45 Ensure the splint is still in the correct position and rebandage the area over the cannula.	
46 The CYP's fingers and toes should remain visible.	46 To facilitate checks of the site and circulation
47 Complete the procedure as per Procedure Guideline 14.1.B.	
48 Record the VIP score, as described below, and document in the CYP's health record	48 To maintain an accurate record.

Procedure guideline 14.9 Blood sampling from a peripheral cannula

Principles of Blood Sampling from a Cannula

It may be appropriate to insert a cannula specifically for the purposes of blood sampling if this is likely to be more convenient, as taking blood samples from an existing peripheral cannula reduces the trauma of venepuncture for the CYP and family. Always insert as large a cannula as possible when it is to be used for blood sampling. Generally, smaller cannulae are unsuitable as they do not allow easy sampling of blood and can become occluded during the procedure (Danek and Norris 1992). However, some tests cannot be performed on blood sampled from a peripheral cannula; examples include:

- Blood glucose monitoring when the cannula has been used for the administration of a glucose solution, as dextrose adheres to the lining of the cannula, resulting in inaccurate results.
- Measurement of antibiotic levels when the cannula has been used to administer the antibiotic, as it can adhere to the lining of the cannula, resulting in inaccurate levels.
- Blood cultures; these should only be taken from a newly inserted cannula to prevent contamination.

Safety systems are available for staff, including vacuum blood collection systems. These closed systems reduce the risk of the healthcare practitioner coming into contact with blood (Dougherty and Lamb 2008).

Procedure Guideline

Statement	Rationale
1 Ensure adherence to laboratory guidelines for taking and sending samples.	1 To ensure an accurate result is obtained: Some tests must be undertaken within a specified time or delivered to the laboratory under certain conditions.

(continued)

The Great Ormond Street Hospital Manual of Children and Young People's Nursing Practices

Procedure guideline 14.9 Blood sampling from a peripheral cannula *(continued)*

Statement	Rationale
Prepare for the procedure as per Procedure Guideline 14.1.A.	
2 Gather equipment; this may include: • 10 ml syringes • 2 and 5 ml syringes • Needle • 0.9% sodium chloride for injection • 2% chlorhexidine in 70% isopropyl alcohol wipe • S-Monovette® blood bottle(s) • S-Monovette system adaptors (multiadapter and membrane adapter) • Sterile sealed caps • Non sterile gloves	
3 Perform hand hygiene.	3 To reduce possible hand contamination from collecting equipment.
4 Open equipment by carefully peeling back packaging. If at any time there is a suspicion that a piece of equipment may have become contaminated, dispose of it immediately, and use a new piece.	4 Using potentially contaminated equipment can increase the risk of infection.
5 Connect the needle to the syringe. Draw up 0.9% sodium chloride, taking care that the needle does not touch the outside of any vials/ampoules. Ensure all key parts remain uncontaminated. Carefully peel open the membrane adapter and connect to the hub of an empty syringe. Peel back the paper cover on the S-Monovette multiadapter and place in tray with the plastic packaging acting as a holder. When all equipment has been prepared, remove all needles from syringes and leave in syringe packet.	5 To adhere to ANTT® and minimise the risk of airborne or key part contamination.
6 Take tray and blood request forms to the CYP. Check the CYP's name band against the details on the blood request form to correctly identify patient.	6 To ensure that blood sample is obtained from the correct patient.
7 Keep the cannula splinted if it is positioned adjacent to a join.	7 To prevent the cannula from bending, as this can cause occlusion, phlebitis, or extravasation.
8 Remove the bandage from over the cannula. Thoroughly inspect the site of entry of the cannula for any sign of phlebitis or infection. Assess the entry site using the visual infusion phlebitis (VIP) score.	8 So that the entry site may be observed throughout the procedure.
9 Apply an appropriately sized tourniquet, 7–8 cm, above the cannula but not so tightly as to occlude arterial supply.	9 To assist filling of the vein, improving blood flow from the cannula.
10 Perform hand hygiene	
11 Clean the cannula's needle-free access device with the 2% chlorhexidine in 70% isopropyl alcohol wipe for 15 seconds using friction and allow to dry naturally for 30 seconds. Visibly check that the device is dry.	11 To minimise the risk of infection.
12 Unclamp the T-extension and **either:** Connect the S-Monovette multiadapter to the needle-free access device on the CVAD and attach the empty 10 ml syringe with the membrane adapter to the multiadapter. Then withdraw 1 ml of blood. Remove the waste syringe and collect the required samples directly into the appropriate bottles using the vacuum method.	12 A closed system reduces the risk of contamination and splash injuries.

Or:

13 Using a 2 or 5 ml syringe, withdraw 1 ml of blood and discard. Then using the other 2 or 5 ml syringe, slowly withdraw the required quantity of blood. Transfer the required quantities of blood from the syringe to the appropriate Monovette® blood bottle(s). Please note the correct order of draw for Monovette blood bottles, if required:	13 To withdraw the flush within the cannula and haemodilute samples.
14 Release the tourniquet.	14 To restore usual venous blood flow.
15 Slowly flush the cannula with 1 ml of 0.9% sodium chloride, and then flush using the pulsing technique.	
16 Ask the CYP to report any pain or discomfort experienced and, while flushing, observe the cannula entry site and surrounding area for any sign of swelling, phlebitis or infiltration.	16 To assess for any problems.

Procedure guideline 14.9 Blood sampling from a peripheral cannula *(continued)*

Statement	Rationale
17 If there are no problems, clamp the T-extension while still flushing to create positive pressure.	17 To prevent blood backflow into the cannula and T-extension causing occlusion.
18 Ensure the splint is still in the correct position and rebandage the area over the cannula, leaving a window for site assessment.	18 To immobilise the limb and minimise the risk of occlusion, phlebitis and infiltration/extravasation.
19 The CYP's fingers and toes should remain visible. Label blood samples.	19 To facilitate checks of the circulation.
20 Complete the procedure as per Procedure Guideline 14.1.B.	
21 Record the VIP score (see Table 14.5), blood collected and tests performed in the CYP's health record and document any important information, e.g. relative ease of flushing, any pain experienced.	21 To ensure that the CYP's health record is comprehensive and to provide information to other practitioners who may collect samples from the cannula later.

Procedure guideline 14.10 Removal of a peripheral cannula

1 Reasons for removal of the cannula:

   1 Intravenous access no longer required (ensure this is correct before removing).
   2 The cannula may no longer be functioning effectively.
   3 The cannula may be causing excessive discomfort.
   4 The VIP score is two or above.
   5 Infiltration and extravasation.

Statement	Rationale
2 Prepare for procedure as per Procedure Guideline 14.1.A	
3 Collect the equipment required for the procedure; this may include: • Packet of sterile gauze or cotton wool balls • Medical adhesive tape • Plaster as needed	3 To ensure the procedure is undertaken efficiently and prevent later contamination of gloves.
4 Remove the bandage and splint. Inspect the exit site and assess for phlebitis or infection, utilising the VIP scoring system.	
5 Perform hand hygiene.	5 As part of standard precautions.
6 Put on well-fitting nonsterile gloves.	6 Close fitting gloves improve dexterity.
7 Carefully remove the old dressing, holding the cannula in place.	
8 Hold a piece of sterile gauze over the exit site without applying any pressure.	8 Pressure should not be applied until the cannula has been fully removed or it will cause the tube to be dragged out of the vein causing pain and venous damage.
9 Slowly withdraw the cannula, maintaining a neutral angle with the skin.	
10 Immediately apply gentle digital pressure to the exit site for several minutes until haemostasis is achieved.	10 To absorb any blood that escapes and to prevent the formation of a haematoma.
11 Examine the cannula and place it carefully into a tray.	11 To ensure that no cannula parts remain in the vein.
12 After 2–3 minutes, lift the gauze and inspect the exit site to check that bleeding has ceased. Reapply digital pressure if further bleeding is observed.	12 To achieve haemostasis.
13 If blood/dirt is present in the area, clean the area.	13 The exit puncture site is a potential entry point for infection.
14 Apply a plaster directly over the exit site. If there is further bleeding from the exit site, a folded square of gauze can be secured with medical adhesive tape.	
15 If the CYP prefers, they may choose only sterile gauze and tape without a plaster. The plaster/gauze and tape should remain in situ for at least a few hours.	15 To minimise the risk of infection.
16 Dispose of the cannula in a sharps container.	16 To minimise the risk of a sharps injury.
17 Document the procedure, date of removal, duration of cannula, VIP score, and action taken in the CYP's health records.	17 To maintain accurate records.

Types of central venous access devices (CVADs)

A long-term CVAD is a catheter that is inserted into the central venous system with the internal tip sitting in the superior/inferior vena cava (IVC) or right atrium (Dougherty and Lister 2015; RCN 2016). They can have single or multiple lumens.

The types of long-term CVADs commonly used include:

- PICCs: There are two types of PICCs used, which may have one or two separate lumens, open-ended/nonvalved, i.e. Cook® PICC with clamps, or valved, i.e. Groshong NXT ClearVue™ PICC – Tunnelled Noncuffed CVCs.
- Skin tunnelled cuffed central venous catheters (commonly referred to as Hickman® or Broviac®): These devices may have one, two, or three separate lumens and a tissue ingrowth cuff.
- Subcutaneous implanted ports: These are commonly referred to as ports, port-a-cath, or Bardport®).

The usual sites for insertion of tunnelled CVCs are the subclavian vein or the internal/external jugular vein. However, where access to the upper veins is difficult or unsuitable, the femoral vein can be used and the catheter threaded into the IVC (Josephson 2004). CYPs usually require a general anaesthetic for the placement of CVADs.

Peripherally inserted central catheter (PICC)

PICCs are central catheters and should not be confused with peripherally inserted catheters (PICs), i.e. long lines or midlines. The two are different in terms of the length of time the device can be used, the types of medication that can be administered, and where the tip of the catheter is placed.

A PICC is a thin catheter (ranging between 2 and 8 Fr) that is generally inserted in one of the veins in the upper arm above the antecubital fossa so as to not impede arm movement or affect the administration of IVs. It is threaded through to the lower third of the superior vena cava (SVC)/proximal right atrium. PICCs can be held in place with either a securement device or sutures and can be used as any other CVAD.

In babies, due to their small peripheral vein size, these CVCs may be tunnelled under the skin along the same principles as a Hickman®, but since this is no longer a peripheral insertion, the CVC is referred to as a tunnelled noncuffed CVC. Care of this device is very similar.

In CYPs, PICCs are commonly inserted by interventional radiologists, clinical nurse specialists, and radiographers, or by surgical teams. PICCs can be placed under general or local anaesthetic.

PICCs were originally designed for short-term use, but are increasingly being inserted as the first option for longer-term CVAD access (Abedin and Kapoor 2008). The PICC provides a less invasive, minimal risk alternative to other CVADs. PICCs are an option for a CYP who needs mid to long-term access, for example, where they require IV medication for four weeks or more, have poor peripheral access, or their condition temporarily prohibits the insertion of the tunnelled CVAD.

There are a number of companies that manufacture PICCs, with two main types available, both offering devices with one or two separate lumens:

- Open-ended/nonvalved, i.e. Cook PICC.
- Valved, i.e. Groshong NXT ClearVue™ PICC, Vaxcel® PICCs with PASV® valve technology.

Open-ended/nonvalved PICCs will have clamps in situ and may require a heparin lock when not in use and more frequent flushing.

Valved PICCs have an internal Groshong® valve and a closed catheter tip. This is a three-way pressure sensitive valve that allows infusions, blood aspiration and when not in use, remains closed to restrict the backflow of blood into the catheter (Bard Access Systems 2015, 2016).

Power-injectable PICCs are also used within child healthcare. These can withstand higher flow rates and can be used to deliver rapid contrast injections (Klees 2011).

Skin tunnelled cuffed central venous catheters (Hickman®)

A skin tunnelled cuffed central venous catheter is made of a radiopaque medical-grade silicone or polyurethane, that has a tissue ingrowth cuff for fixation of the catheter in the subcutaneous tunnel when tissue grows into the cuff area. The catheter is inserted in the chest region and tunnelled under the skin, usually into the jugular vein, where it accesses the venous system and is threaded to the lower third of the SVC or the proximal right atrium. A stitch is often placed at the exit site to provide a temporary hold until the cuff is secure. The stitch can also be removed, if required after four to –six weeks when the cuff has had chance to bond.

As the CVC is tunnelled, the distance between the vein entry site and the exit site on the chest reduces the risk of infection (Dougherty 2000). The tissue ingrowth cuff works to secure the catheter, but may also help as a barrier to microbes.

Hickmans are frequently placed by interventional radiologists, clinical nurse specialists, and radiographers. Surgical teams also place Hickmans under a general anaesthetic in child healthcare.

Historically, the brand name of Hickman® has always been used to refer to all different brands of skin tunnelled cuffed CVCs: Broviac/Hickman/Leonard® are all produced by Bard Access Systems, but other companies produce similar CVCs which need to be cared for in the same way. Due to the common usage of this brand name by healthcare professionals around the UK, the term 'Hickman' will be used to refer to all versions of this device within this chapter.

Subcutaneous/totally implanted port (Port)

Implanted ports are commonly referred to as ports, port-a-cath®, Bardport (Port).

A subcutaneous or totally implanted port consists of a reservoir or chamber with a self-sealing septum (the portal) which is attached to a catheter. The reservoir is implanted in a pocket formed under the skin in the subcutaneous tissue, commonly in the chest region (they can also be implanted in the arm, if required). The catheter runs in a tunnel under the skin and accesses the jugular vein, from where it is threaded into the lower third of the SVC or the proximal right atrium. Since it is completely internal, it is not visible externally, apart from a bump under the skin.

Access to the port reservoir is via a dedicated port (Huber) needle, which is a noncoring gripper needle. Standard hypodermic needles and other needles cannot be used to access the port as they are not 'noncoring', and will therefore remove a piece of the silicon septum, leaving a hole. The port can be accessed approximately 1000 times according to manufacturer guidelines, and can be used over many years. Once accessed, the port needle can stay for seven days or longer, depending on the CYP's diagnosis and treatment. The port needle should be changed every seven days, especially in the immunosuppressed CYP.

Both the port reservoir and the catheter are available in a variety of sizes to accommodate all ages of CYPs. Dual chamber ports are also available for CYPs who require two lumens for therapy.

CVAD dressings

Maintaining the dressing site is important to reduce the risk of infection (Rickard et al. 2002) and to minimise the risk of CVAD dislodgement, fracture, or accidental removal. Daily checks of the CVAD dressing and exit site need to be undertaken to observe for signs of infection and to ensure that the dressing remains in situ and is effective in securing the CVAD.

The first choice for a CVAD dressing is a sterile semipermeable transparent dressing, e.g. IV3000™ (O'Grady et al. 2011; Loveday et al. 2014; RCN 2016). This provides a sterile barrier, which is permeable to water vapour from the skin, and reduces the growth of local microflora. It also reliably secures the CVAD and port needle, permits continuous visual inspection of the catheter site, allows patients to bathe and shower without saturating the dressing, and requires less frequent changes than standard gauze dressings. Gauze-based dressings are not waterproof, require frequent changing in order to inspect the catheter site, and are rarely useful in patients with long-term CVADs.

The dressing must be changed if it becomes wet, soiled, or loose. CYPs and their families must be shown how to protect the CVAD and site during showers and baths to prevent any water from getting under the dressing. Moisture under dressings not only allows bacteria to flourish, but also provides a medium for transit over the skin and down the catheter tract (Macklin 2010).

CVAD dressings need to be changed the day after insertion if there is any blood left underneath the dressing, to reduce the risk of infection (RCN 2016). After this, CVAD dressings are changed weekly, unless the exit site has bled, oozed, or the dressing is not secure.

Other dressings

Self-adhesive island nonwoven dressings, e.g. Mepore®, need to be used where there is oozing from the exit site to absorb any exudate. Remnant exudate around the site increases the risk of infection (RCN 2016). The dressing needs to be changed daily if exudate is present and the exit site reviewed. The dressing can be left for 48 hours if there is no ooze. When the oozing has resolved, it is recommended that transparent, semipermeable dressings are used as soon as possible (Loveday et al. 2014).

If an allergy to any dressing is suspected or for sensitive skin or those with mild reactions, a barrier film in the form of a foam applicator (not a spray), such as Cavilon™, may be used to protect the skin prior to dressing application.

A soft silicone adherent dressing (e.g. Mepitel® film, Mepiform®, or Mepilex® BorderLite) can be used as an alternative if the CYP has an allergy to the above dressings. The adhesive is silicon-based and less likely to cause reactions/irritation. These dressings also peel off easily, causing less trauma to the CYP's skin. Dermatology or a Tissue Viability team may need be contacted for advice.

Antimicrobial dressings

Antimicrobial dressings such as BioPatch® can be considered for use in CYPs to provide antimicrobial activity at the catheter exit site (Loveday et al. 2014). Biopatch® is a polyurethane foam disc impregnated with chlorhexidine gluconate (CHG). It is effective against a variety of gram-positive and gram-negative bacteria. The device provides a steady release of CHG around the insertion site over a seven day period. Biopatch has been shown to reduce the rate of central line infections by up to 69% (Timsett et al. 2009). At GOSH, all CVADs should have a Biopatch applied at insertion of the device. Biopatch should be used on all short-term and temporary CVADs for the duration of the time that they are inserted.

Tunnelled and cuffed CVADs (e.g. permanent Hickman®) should have Biopatch applied for the first eight weeks from insertion. CYPs who are colonised with MRSA and have tunnelled and cuffed CVAD's in situ should have Biopatch applied for the duration of the time the line is in situ. Biopatch is not used with subcutaneous implanted ports (e.g. Port-a-cath) or neonatal longlines at GOSH.

Skin cleaning

The CVAD exit site should be cleaned with a single patient use application of alcoholic chlorhexidine-based cleaning solution, preferably 2% CHG in 70% isopropyl alcohol (Loveday et al. 2014; RCN 2016). Alcohol-based cleaning solutions have demonstrated good activity against bacteria, viruses, and most fungi. 2% CHG in 70% isopropyl alcohol should not be used on the skin of preterm infants under 35 weeks gestational age. It can be used with caution in children under two months of age. However, if there is any evidence of skin reaction in this age group, discontinue its use and consider alternative antiseptic solutions, such as 0.5% CHG in 70% denatured ethanol B or Povidone-iodine 10% (Bravery 2008).

Catheter securement

The purpose of the dressing is to keep the exit site clean and dry and to stabilise the catheter (Macklin 2010). Securement prevents migration of the catheter in or out of the entry site, which in turn reduces infective and thrombotic risk (Maki et al. 2000). In addition, it is important that the weight of multiple lines for infusions are supported so that tension is not applied to the catheter. Hickmans and other CVADs need the external length of the catheter securing so that it cannot be tugged (Macklin 2010).

There are a variety of options to help secure a CVAD, including dressing technique, sutures, and devices that function as a securement device. Current evidence suggests that either sutures or sutureless fixation devices are recommended (Yamamoto et al. 2002; Graf et al. 2006).

Dressing technique

For multiple lumen CVADs, the bifurcation must be effectively secured under the dressing, while the smaller French single and multilumen CVADs require the thinner section of the catheter to be secured well within the dressing to minimise the risk of catheter fracture. The addition of a loop, S-shape, or curve with the catheter, which is secured under the dressing, (Figure 14.1) also minimises the risk of CVAD dislodgement.

The catheter leg(s) are thicker and heavier than the section of the catheter exiting the body, so can dislodge the loop out or, with the smaller French lines, expose the thinner section of the catheter.

Statlock® PICC and dialysis stabilisation device

The Statlock device is a post and door design that houses the wings of PICC (Figure 14.2) or the bifurcation of the double lumen Hickman® (Statlock® Dialysis version) (Figure 14.3) and adheres securely to the skin. Statlocks are changed weekly with dressing changes.

SecurAcath

The SecurAcath is a subcutaneous catheter securement system which can be placed alongside indwelling catheters in order to prevent migration (Hughes 2014). It can remain in place until the PICC is removed.

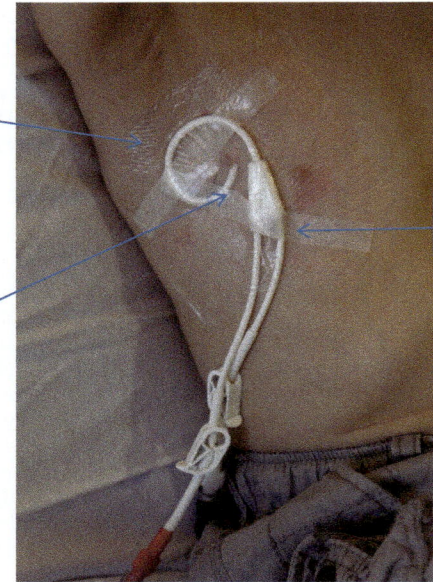

Figure 14.1 Recommended CVAD dressing securement.

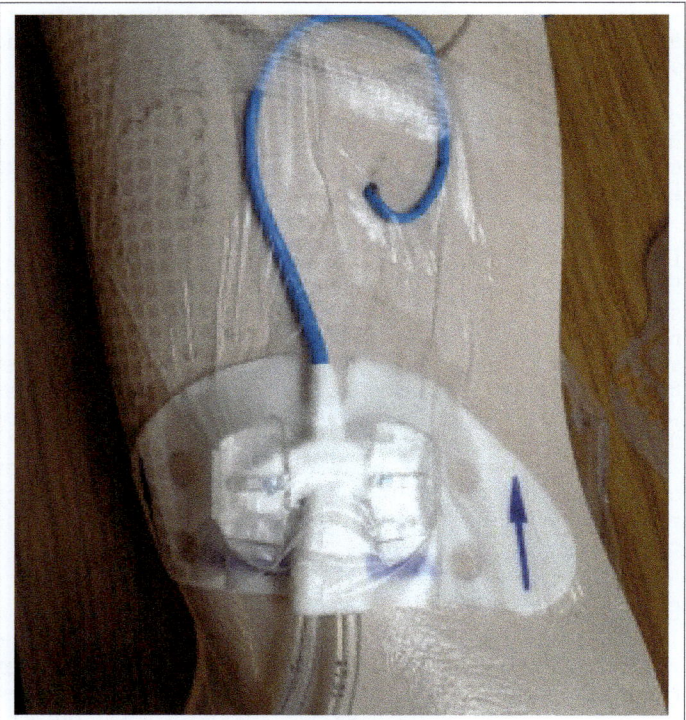

Figure 14.2 Statlock® PICC stabilisation device. Statlock is a registered trademark of C.R. Bard Inc. or an affiliate.

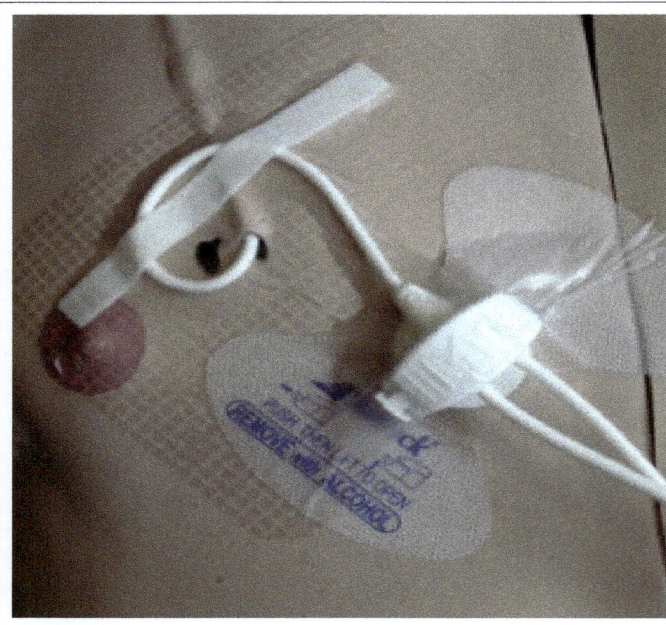

Figure 14.3 Statlock double-lumen CVAD stabilisation device.

Procedure guideline 14.11 CVAD: CVAD dressing

Assess the CVAD site prior to preparing for dressing so that the correct equipment can be prepared and to minimise any delays that can distress the CYP.

Statement	Rationale
Prepare for the procedure as per Procedure Guideline 14.1.A.	
1 Gather equipment; this may include: • New dressing • Sterile wound closure strips, if required • 3 ml 2% chlorhexidine/70% isopropyl alcohol applicator (e.g. ChloraPrep™) • Spare pair of nonsterile well-fitting gloves, as required • Pack(s) of sterile gauze and sodium chloride sachet(s) if blood/debris is present under dressing • Receptacle for collecting discarded equipment at bedside	1 To ensure the procedure is undertaken efficiently.
2 Disinfect hands using alcohol gel.	2 To reduce possible hand contamination from collecting equipment.
3 Peel off paper section of the 3 ml applicator and leave sitting in plastic packaging until just before use.	
4 Open the dressing and take out of packaging, placing it in the precleaned plastic tray. Leave protective backing on the dressing.	
5 Open wound closure strips, leaving the protective backing on, and place paper side down into plastic tray on top of dressing.	
6 Prepare CYP for the dressing change; remove any clothing/net vests, etc.	6 To allow easy access to the site.
7 Put on gloves at this point if there is any blood present.	
8 Remove old dressing, being particularly careful around the exit site not to pull CVAD.	8 To minimise discomfort or catheter dislodgement.
9 After the dressing has been removed:	
10 Perform hand hygiene and put on nonsterile gloves if there is blood present.	10 To minimise cross-contamination.
11 Additional skin cleaning may be required if there is blood/ooze present. Any blood/ooze adherent to the skin and catheter must be first removed, using sodium chloride 0.9% and sterile gauze, before disinfecting the skin with 2% chlorhexidine/70% isopropyl alcohol.	11 To ensure adequate cleaning of the site and enable the product to work effectively.
12 Remove the 3 ml applicator from the packaging. Pinch the wings to 'pop' the enclosed ampoule to release the solution. Hold sponge-side down to allow liquid to drain into the sponge applicator.	
13 Firmly press the applicator against the exit site for 10 seconds and then apply the 2% chlorhexidine/70% isopropyl alcohol, using firm repeated up and down strokes, then back and forth strokes for another 20–30 seconds. Remember to clean the skin around and up to the catheter exit site.	13 To clean and disinfect the skin and prevent the introduction of infection.
14 Discard applicator away from clean equipment in tray.	14 To prevent contamination of other equipment.
15 Allow the skin to dry naturally. Do not dry the skin with sterile gauze.	15 Drying is needed to allow the required contact time of the disinfectant and to help prevent dermatitis.
16 Loop or curve/S-shape the catheter onto the chest/arm and secure with the wound closure strips if required. Ensure they do not cover the exit site.	16 To maintain visibility.
17 Take off protective cover of the dressing and place dressing over the catheter, ensuring it covers the exit site and the reinforced section of the catheter.	17 To help prevent the loop being dislodged and minimising the risk of breakage, dislodgement, or preventable early dressing changes.
18 Press down the dressing, ensuring that there are minimal air pockets present.	18 Good dressing adherence allows the skin to breathe and moisture to disperse, while air pockets can trap moisture.
19 Once completed, tuck away the CYP's CVAD.	19 To minimise risk of breakage or dislodgement.
20 Complete the procedure as per Procedure Guideline 14.1.B.	
21 Document dressing change in the CVAD record.	21 To maintain accurate records.

The Great Ormond Street Hospital Manual of Children and Young People's Nursing Practices

Procedure guideline 14.12 CVAD: changing the needle-free access device

Statement	Rationale
Prepare for the procedure as per Procedure Guideline 14.1.A.	
1 Gather equipment; this may include: • Needle-free access device(s) • 2% chlorhexidine in 70% isopropyl alcohol wipe	1 To ensure the procedure is taken efficiently
2 Each separate lumen will require its own set of equipment.	2 Reusing the same equipment for a different lumen can lead to cross-contamination.
3 Perform hand hygiene.	3 To prevent cross-contamination from collecting equipment.
4 Open the needle-free access device by removing the paper backing but placing the connector into the tray still contained in its plastic wrapping.	
5 Place 2% chlorhexidine in 70% isopropyl alcohol wipe into plastic tray on one side away from the clean equipment.	5 To prevent contamination of key parts.
6 Take the plastic tray containing equipment to the CYP.	
7 Locate the CVAD and visibly ensure any clamps are closed.	7 To minimise the risk of haemorrhage or air embolism, which occurs if clamp is left open and the needle-free access device is removed.
8 Perform hand hygiene.	
9 Remove old device.	
10 Clean the CVAD hub with the 2% chlorhexidine in 70% isopropyl alcohol wipe firmly for 15 seconds using friction and allow to dry naturally for 30 seconds. Visibly check that the device is dry.	10 To ensure adequate cleaning of the device/bung and enable the product to work effectively.
11 Remove the cover over the needle-free access device, taking care not to contaminate the key part. Connect the device to the hub of the CVAD.	
12 Once completed, tuck away the CYP's CVAD.	12 To minimise risk of breakage or dislodgement.
Complete the procedure as per Procedure Guideline 14.1.B.	
13 Document device change in the CVAD record.	13 To maintain accurate records.

Procedure guideline 14.13 Accessing CVADs: flushing

Statement	Rationale
Prepare for the procedure as per Procedure Guideline 14.1.A.	
1 Gather equipment: • 10ml syringes • Needles to draw up the required solutions • 0.9% sodium chloride for injection • Ampoule(s) of heparin, if required • 2% chlorhexidine in 70% isopropyl alcohol wipe	1 To ensure the procedure is undertaken efficiently.
2 NB: For multilumen CVADs, individual sets of the above equipment will be needed for each lumen.	2 To reduce the risk of cross-contamination.
3 Perform hand hygiene.	3 To reduce possible hand contamination from collecting equipment.
4 Open equipment by carefully peeling back packaging. If at any time there is a suspicion that a piece of equipment may have become contaminated, dispose of it immediately and use a new piece.	
5 Connect the needles to the syringes, as required. Draw up 0.9% sodium chloride and heparin, as required. Ensure all key parts remain uncontaminated.	5 To adhere to ANTT®.
6 Locate the CVAD to be used and if applicable, identify the lumen to be used. Check the CVAD catheter and exit site for any problems.	
7 Perform hand hygiene.	
8 Clean the CVADs needle-free access device with the 2% chlorhexidine in 70% isopropyl alcohol wipe for 15 seconds using friction and allow to dry naturally for 30 seconds. Visibly check that the device is dry.	8 To ensure adequate cleaning of the device and enable the product to work effectively.

Chapter 14 Intravenous and intra-arterial access and infusions

Procedure guideline 14.13 Accessing CVADs: flushing *(continued)*

Statement	Rationale
a) Attach the syringe of 0.9% sodium chloride to the needle-free access device. b) Open the clamp and gently instil the first part of the flush. c) If patent, follow with turbulent flushes.	b) To check device patency. To minimise the risk of accidental catheter rupture from increased flushing pressure. c) To clear the CVAD of any blood residue and minimise the risk of subsequent CVAD occlusion.
9 Administer heparin, if required. Whichever solution is used for the final flush, positive pressure must be used when flushing off the CVAD. For CVCs, ports, and open-ended PICCs, positive pressure is achieved by closing the clamp while flushing. For valved PICCs, continue to flush the PICC while removing the luer-slip syringe from the needle-free access device.	9 Positive pressure helps to prevent blood refluxing back into the catheter which can result in occlusion.
10 Once completed, tuck away the CYP's CVAD.	10 To minimise risk of breakage or dislodgement.
11 Complete the procedure as per Procedure Guideline 14.1.B.	
12 Document procedure in care record.	12 To maintain accurate records.

Procedure guideline 14.14 Accessing CVADs: administration of a medication bolus

Alternate lumens on multilumen devices should be used for antimicrobials.

Statement	Rationale
Prepare for the procedure as per Procedure Guideline 14.1.A.	
1 Gather equipment; this may include: • 10 ml syringes • Other sizes of syringes for dose accuracy • Needles to draw up the required solutions • Medication(s) and appropriate diluents to prepare if required • 0.9% sodium chloride for injection/5% dextrose or appropriate fluid depending on medication compatibility • Required amount and strength of heparin as needed • 2% chlorhexidine in 70% isopropyl alcohol wipe plus extra for cleaning the top/rubber bung of any vial Work out any medication calculations, collect medication vials or preprepared medication syringe from CIVAS/satellite. Write out any medication labels that may be needed and research any relevant information, as required.	1 To ensure the procedure is undertaken efficiently.
2 Perform hand hygiene.	2 To reduce possible hand contamination from collecting equipment.
3 Open equipment by carefully peeling back packaging. If at any time there is a suspicion that a piece of equipment may have become contaminated, dispose of it immediately and use a new piece.	3 Using potentially contamination equipment can lead to the risk of infection.
4 Check the medication(s) to be administered against the prescription.	4 To ensure the correct medication/s and dose/s are prepared.
5 Connect the needles to the syringes, as required, and draw up the first solution, taking care that the needle does not touch the outside of any vials/ampoules.	5 To prevent key part contamination.
6 Using the same technique detailed above, draw up all medication(s), flushes and diluents required for the procedure. Prepare all medications as per pharmacy guidelines.	
7 When all equipment/medication has been prepared, remove all needles from syringes and leave in syringe packet.	7 To adhere to ANTT® and minimise risk of key part contamination.
8 Label syringes as you prepare each medicine.	8 To reduce medication errors (NPSA 2007).
9 When all medication(s), flushes, etc., have been prepared, take tray and prescription to the CYP.	
10 Check the CYP's identification against the details on the prescription to correctly identify the patient.	10 To ensure that the drug is being given to the correct CYP.
11 Locate the CVAD to be used and if applicable, identify the lumen to be used. Check the CVAD catheter and exit site for any problems.	

(continued)

Procedure guideline 14.14 Accessing CVADs: administration of a medication bolus *(continued)*

Statement	Rationale
12 Perform hand hygiene.	
13 Clean the needle-free access device with the 2% chlorhexidine in 70% isopropyl alcohol wipe firmly for 15 seconds using friction and allow to dry naturally for 30 seconds. Visibly check that the device is dry.	13 To ensure adequate cleaning of the device/bung and enable the product to work effectively.
14 For ports and vesicant medications, 1–2 ml of blood return must be established prior to administration.	14 To reduce the risk of extravasation (Hadaway 2007).
15 Insert 10 ml syringe of 0.9% sodium chloride or compatible diluent into the needle-free access device. Open the clamp of the CVAD if present and inject flush into the CVAD to ascertain its patency, taking care to gently instil the first part of the flush.	15 To check device patency and minimise the risk of accidental catheter rupture from increased flushing pressure.
16 When the patency of the device has been established, remove the syringe containing the flush and insert the syringe containing the medication. Administer the medication over the required time, observing the patient and CVAD throughout.	16 To ensure safe administration of the medication and to observe for any side effects.
17 Following the procedure above, administer all required medications, ensuring adequate flushing between each one.	17 To prevent mixing of incompatible medications.
18 Attach the flush syringe to the needle-free access device and gently instil the first part of the flush, followed by the turbulent flushing technique.	18 To clear the CVAD of any medication residue and minimise the risk of subsequent CVAD occlusion.
19 Administer heparin, if required. Whichever solution is used for the final flush, positive pressure must be used when flushing off the CVAD.	19 To minimise the risk of CVAD occlusion. To prevent blood refluxing into the catheter and resulting in CVAD occlusion.19
20 Once completed, tuck away the CYP's CVAD.	20 To prevent accidental dislodgement or damage to the CVAD.
Complete the procedure as per Procedure Guideline 14.1.B.	
21 Complete prescription/administration documentation.	21 To maintain accurate records.

Procedure guideline 14.15 Accessing CVADs: administration of a medication infusion via a syringe pump

Statement	Rationale
Prepare for the procedure as per Procedure Guideline 14.1.A.	
1 Collect the equipment required for the procedure, this may include: • 10 ml syringes • Luer-lock syringe for syringe pump • Other sizes of syringes for dose accuracy • Needles to draw up the required solutions • Medication(s) and appropriate diluents to prepare, if required • 0.9% sodium chloride for injection, 5% dextrose, or other appropriate fluid, depending on medication compatibility • Sterile syringe caps • Ampoules of heparin, if required • 2% chlorhexidine in 70% isopropyl alcohol wipe plus extra for cleaning the top rubber bung of any vials • Infusion set-long extension set • Needle-free access device (e.g. MicroClave®) • Compatible fluid for diluting medication, if required	1 To ensure the procedure is taken efficiently and prevent later contamination.
2 Work out any medication calculations and infusion rates, collect medication vials or prepared medication syringe from CIVAS. Write/print any medication labels required and research any relevant data.	2 To minimise the risk of medication errors.
3 Perform hand hygiene.	3 To prevent any cross-contamination after collecting equipment.
4 Open equipment by carefully peeling back packaging.	
5 Connect the needles to the syringes, as required and draw up the first solution, taking care that the needle does not touch the outside of any vials/ampoules.	5 Using potentially contaminated equipment can lead to an increased risk of infection.
6 Check the medication/s to be administered against the prescription.	6 To ensure the correct medication/s and dose/s are prepared.

Procedure guideline 14.15 Accessing CVADs: administration of a medication infusion via a syringe pump *(continued)*

Statement	Rationale
7 Using the same technique detailed above: Draw up all medication(s), flushes, heparin, and diluents required for the procedure. Prepare all medications as per IV/pharmacy guidelines. Use a luer-lock syringe for administering the infusion.	7 Use of a luer-lock syringe prevents accidental disconnection, which could cause inaccurate administration of medication.
8 Open the required infusion administration set and connect the needle-free access device. Then connect the luer-lock syringe to the needle-free access device.	8 Using a needle-free access device reduces the risk of contamination and air embolism with syringe changes.
9 Prime the infusion set until fluid is seen at the end of the set and then close the slide clamp.	
10 Attach a medication-added label to the syringe with all required details.	10 To minimise the risk of medication errors (NPSA 2007).
11 When all equipment/medication has been prepared, remove all needles from syringes and cover syringe tips with a sterile cap.	11 To prevent any risk of airborne contamination or key part contamination.
12 Take the tray/prescription to the CYP.	
13 Check the CYP's identification band against the details on the prescription to correctly identify patient.	13 To ensure that the drug is given to the correct CYP.
14 Locate the CVAD to be used and, if applicable, identify the lumen to be used. Check the CVAD catheter and exit site for any problems.	
15 Perform hand hygiene.	
16 Clean the end of the needle-free access device with the 2% chlorhexidine in 70% isopropyl alcohol wipe for 15 seconds using friction and allow to dry naturally for 30 seconds. Visibly check that the device is dry.	16 To ensure adequate cleaning of the device/bung and enable the product to work effectively.
17 For ports and vesicant medications, 1–2 ml of blood return must be established prior to administration.	17 To minimise the risk of extravasation (Hadaway 2007).
18 Insert 10 ml syringe of 0.9% sodium chloride or compatible diluent into needle-free access device. Open the clamp of the device and gently flush into the CVAD.	18 To ascertain CVAD patency.
19 Attach infusion set to the CVAD's needle-free access device. Open clamp. Commence infusion as prescribed, ensuring rates and pressure limits are set.	
20 After infusing a drug, it is essential that when the syringe empties it is flushed using a compatible diluent at the same rate. Use a luer-lock syringe for administering all flushes. The 'flush' syringe must be labelled to prevent potential extra unnecessary flushes or lack of.	
21 When the infusion is completed, disconnect the infusion set from the CVAD. Attach the flush syringe to the needle-free access device and gently instil the first part of the flush followed by the turbulent flushing technique. Administer heparin, if required. Whichever solution is used for the final flush, Positive pressure must be used when flushing off the CVAD.	21 To maintain catheter patency.
22 Once completed, tuck away the CYP's CVAD.	22 To prevent accidental dislodgement or damage to the CVAD.
23 Complete the procedure as per Procedure Guideline 14.1.B.	
24 Complete prescription/ administration documentation.	24 To maintain accurate records.

Procedure guideline 14.16 Accessing CVADs: administration of a medication infusion via a volumetric pump

Statement	Rationale
Prepare for the procedure as per Procedure Guideline 14.1.A.	
1 Gather equipment; this may include: • 10 ml syringe(s) • Other sizes of syringes for dose accuracy • Needles to draw up the required solutions • Medication(s) and appropriate diluent to prepare, if required • 0.9% sodium chloride for injection/5% dextrose or appropriate fluid depending on medication compatibility • Ampoule of heparin, if required • 2% chlorhexidine in 70% isopropyl alcohol wipe plus extra for cleaning the top/rubber bung of any vials • Infusion set (buretted or nonburetted) • Bag of compatible fluid for medication or hydration fluid required	1 To ensure the procedure is undertaken efficiently.

(continued)

The Great Ormond Street Hospital Manual of Children and Young People's Nursing Practices

Procedure guideline 14.16 Accessing CVADs: administration of a medication infusion via a volumetric pump *(continued)*

Statement	Rationale
2 Work out any medication calculations and infusion rates, collect medication vials or preprepared medication syringes from CIVAS/satellite. Write/print out any medication labels that may be needed and research any relevant information, as required.	2 To minimise the risk of drug errors.
3 Perform hand hygiene.	3 To reduce possible hand contamination from collecting equipment.
4 Open equipment by carefully peeling back packaging. If at any time a piece of equipment may have become contaminated, dispose of it immediately and use a new piece.	
5 Check the medication/s to be administered against the prescription.	5 To ensure the correct medication/s and dose/s are administered.
6 Connect the needles to the syringes, as required, and draw up the first solution, taking care that the needle does not touch the outside of any vials/ampoules.	6 To prevent contamination of any key parts.
7 Using the same technique detailed above: Draw up all medication(s), flushes, heparin, and diluents required for the procedure. Prepare all medications as per pharmacy guidelines.	
8 When all equipment/medication has been prepared, remove all needles from syringes and leave in syringe packet.	8 To adhere to ANTT® and minimise the risk of key part contamination.
9 Open the required infusion administration set and close all roller clamps to the off position.	
10 Check the medications/fluid bags as per medication policy. Open the required bag of infusion fluid and check the bag to ensure it contains no visible precipitate, leaks, or damage to bag. Twist off the connector at the bottom of the fluid bag to reveal the connection port.	10 To minimise drug errors and adhere to the hospital medication administration policy.
11 Remove the plastic cover over the spike on the infusion set, taking care not to touch the spike. Holding the bung of the fluid bag in one hand and the bottom of the spike on the infusion set in the other, insert the spike into the connection port on the infusion bag using a twisting motion, taking care not to touch any part of the spike. Ensure the spike is inserted fully into the fluid bag.	11 To prevent contamination of both key parts and the bag of infusion fluid.
12 Hang the fluid bag which is now connected to the infusion administration set onto a stand.	
13 If using a nonburetted set: Gently squeeze the drip chamber to allow fluid into it, filling the chamber halfway. Prime the infusion set until fluid is seen at the end of the line and then close the roller clamp.	13 To prevent air embolism.
14 If using a buretted set: Open the roller clamp between the fluid bag and the buretted set and fill the burette with the required amount of fluid to prime the line. Close the roller clamp. Gently squeeze the drip chamber to allow fluid into it, filling the chamber approximately halfway. Prime the infusion set until fluid is seen at the end of the line and then close off the roller clamp.	14 To prevent air embolism.
15 If a medication is to be infused, connect the syringe containing the medication to the needle-free connector on the top of the burette (clean device first if it may have been contaminated during handling). Push the medication into the burette until the syringe is empty.	
16 Remove syringe from needle-free access device and dispose.	
17 Gently shake the burette to ensure drug and fluid mix thoroughly.	
18 If there is a large amount of fluid in the burette, close the white clamp on the top of the burette to facilitate effective mixing. Remember to open this clamp after as it acts as an air inlet.	
19 Attach a medication-added label to the burette with all appropriate details.	
20 When all medication(s), flushes, etc., have been prepared, take tray and prescription to the CYP.	
21 Check the CYP's identification against the details on the prescription.	21 To correctly identify patient.
22 Locate the CVAD and if applicable, identify the lumen to be used.	22 Alternating lumens on multilumen devices should be used for antimicrobial dosing to cover all lumens for infection.

Chapter 14 Intravenous and intra-arterial access and infusions

Procedure guideline 14.16 Accessing CVADs: administration of a medication infusion via a volumetric pump *(continued)*

Statement	Rationale
23 Perform hand hygiene.	
24 Clean the end of the needle-free access device with the 2% chlorhexidine in 70% isopropyl alcohol; wipe for 15 seconds using friction, and allow to dry naturally for 30 seconds. Visibly check device is dry.	24 To ensure adequate cleaning of the device/bung and enable the product to work effectively.
25 For ports and vesicant medications, 1–2 ml of blood return must be established prior to administration. Insert 10 ml syringe of 0.9% sodium chloride or compatible diluent into needle-free access device. Open any clamps on the CVAD and inject the flush gently into the CVAD to ascertain its patency.	25 To reduce the risk of extravasation (Hadaway 2007.) To check device patency and to minimise the risk of accidental catheter rupture from increased flushing pressure.
26 Attach infusion line to extension tubing. Open clamp. Commence infusion as prescribed, ensuring rates, pressure limits, and volume to be infused limits are set.	
27 After infusing a drug, 'flush' or clear the empty burette and line with at least 18 ml of a compatible fluid (e.g. 0.9% sodium chloride). The rate of the flush should remain the same as the drug infusion.	27 To clear the CVAD of any medication/blood residue and minimise the risk of subsequent CVAD occlusion.
28 The flush MUST be labelled on the burette.	28 To prevent extra or no flush being infused and reduce medication errors (NPSA 2007).
29 When the infusion is complete, disconnect the infusion set from the CVAD.	
30 Attach the flush syringe to the needle-free access device and gently instil the first part of the flush followed by the turbulent flushing technique.	30 To minimise the risk of CVAD occlusion.
31 Administer heparin, if required.	
32 Whichever solution is used for the final flush, positive pressure must be used when flushing off the CVAD.	32 To prevent blood refluxing into the catheter and resulting in CVAD occlusion.
33 Once completed, tuck away the CYP's CVAD.	33 To minimise risk of breakage or dislodgement.
34 Complete the procedure as per Procedure Guideline 14.1.B.	
35 Complete prescription/administration documentation.	35 To maintain accurate records.

Procedure guideline 14.17 Accessing an implanted port

Statement	Rationale
1 Apply a local anaesthetic cream if the CYP wishes, according to prescription or patient group direction. Allow for the cream to take effect.	1 To reduce any discomfort caused by the port needle puncturing the skin over the port.
2 Prepare for the procedure as per Procedure Guideline 14.1.A.	
3 Gather equipment; this may include: • 10 ml syringes • Needles to draw up the required solutions • 0.9% sodium chloride for injection • Ampoule(s) of heparin • 2% chlorhexidine in 70% isopropyl alcohol wipe • Dressing (preferably a sterile transparent semipermeable dressing) • Sterile wound closure strips (e.g. Steri-Strips®) • One packet of sterile gauze (5 × 5 cm) • 2% chlorhexidine in 70% isopropyl alcohol applicator (e.g. ChloraPrep™ (3 ml) • Port access needle • Needle-free access device (e.g. MicroClave®) Two trays may be required if there is a risk of key contamination with all the equipment required.	3 To ensure the procedure is undertaken efficiently.
4 Perform hand hygiene.	4 To reduce possible hand contamination from collecting equipment.
5 Open equipment by carefully peeling back packaging. If at any time a piece of equipment may have become contaminated, dispose of it immediately and use a new piece.	

(continued)

The Great Ormond Street Hospital Manual of Children and Young People's Nursing Practices

Procedure guideline 14.17 Accessing an implanted port *(continued)*

Statement	Rationale
6 Connect the needles to the syringes, as required. Draw up the 0.9% sodium chloride and heparin, as required. Ensure all key parts remain uncontaminated.	
7 When all equipment/medication has been prepared, remove all needles from syringes and leave in syringe packet.	7 To adhere to ANTT® and minimise the risk of key part contamination.
8 Connect the needle-free access device to the port needle hub. Prime the Port needle with 0.9% sodium chloride and close the clamp.	
9 Carefully open the packs of sterile gauze without touching and leave gauze on the unlabelled side of the paper. Place into tray with the paper-side down acting as a holder for the sterile gauze.	
10 Open the dressing and take out of packaging, placing it inside plastic tray. Leave protective backing on the dressing.	
11 Open the wound closure strips, leave protective backing on and place into plastic tray.	
12 Peel off paper section of the ChloraPrep applicator and leave sitting in packaging until just before use.	
13 Go to the CYP and ensure easy access to the port site. Remove any clothing that may contaminate the port site once cleaned.	
14 Remove the dressing. If using a local anaesthetic cream; wipe off any excess cream.	
15 Locate port and identify the septum if port is implanted deep with the subcutaneous tissues.	
16 Perform hand hygiene.	
17 Put on gloves.	17 To minimise contamination.
18 Pinch the wings of the ChloraPrep applicator to 'pop' the enclosed ampoule and release the solution. Hold lollipop-side down to allow liquid to drain into the sponge applicator.	
19 Firmly press the applicator against the port chamber site for 10 seconds and then apply the ChloraPrep using firm repeated up and down, then back and forth strokes for 20–30 seconds over the port site.	19 To ensure adequate cleaning of the site.
20 Discard ChloraPrep away from equipment in tray.	
21 Allow the skin to dry naturally. Do not dry the skin with sterile gauze.	21 To enable the product to work effectively.
22 Pick up the port needle and remove the needle guard.	
23 Locate and firmly secure the sides/top and bottom of the port firmly between your finger and thumb.	23 To stabilise the port and prevent movement with port needle insertion.
24 Take care not to touch the skin surface over the port.	24 To prevent contaminating the skin over the port prior to port needle access.
25 Insert the needle at a 90°/perpendicular angle through the septum until the internal base/backplate of the port is felt.	
26 The port needle can be secured to the chest first, if required. See point 32 for principles on securing the port needle.	
27 Clean the needle-free access device with the 2% chlorhexidine in 70% isopropyl alcohol wipe for 15 seconds using friction and allow to dry naturally for 30 seconds. Visibly check that the device is dry.	
28 Connect an empty syringe to the needle-free access device.	
29 Withdraw approximately 1–2 ml of fluid/blood from the Port. If blood sampling is required, refer to appropriate section.	29 To check patency and port needle position.
30 Insert the 10 ml syringe of 0.9% sodium chloride into the needle-free access device. Open the clamp of the port needle and gently instil the first part of the flush into the port. If patent, follow with turbulent flushes as described. If the port patency is in doubt, check needle position.	30 To check device patency and minimise the risk of accidental catheter rupture from increased flushing pressure. To clear the CVAD of any blood residue and minimise the risk of subsequent CVAD occlusion.
31 Use positive pressure when flushing off the port as described previously. The port may need to be heparinised according to the guidelines.	31 To prevent blood refluxing into the catheter and resulting in CVAD occlusion.

Procedure guideline 14.17 Accessing an implanted port (continued)

Statement	Rationale
32 Secure the port needle to the port using gauze and wound closure strips, as required. a) Take care not to obscure the upper half of the port site. b) Do not overpad the port needle with gauze (it is better to underpad). Put a small S-curve in the tubing and apply a transparent semipermeable dressing over the port needle and tubing without covering the clamp.	a) To allow visibility to monitor the port site for signs of infection or extravasation. b) Overpadding will cause needle dislodgement and impede fluid flow.
33 Complete the procedure as per Procedure Guideline 14.1.B.	
34 Document procedure and needle size used in the CVAD record.	34 To maintain accurate records.

Procedure guideline 14.18 De-Accessing an implanted port

Statement	Rationale
1 Depending on the type of port needle, two people may be recommended for deaccessing a port, one to flush the port and the other to secure/stabilise the port, while the port needle is withdrawn. Where there is only one person available, the port can be flushed and clamped prior to withdrawing the port needle otherwise a parent, the young person, or a family member may be able to help flush while the health care professional stabilises the port and withdraws the port needle.	1 To support the port during port needle removal and prevent possible trauma.
2 Prepare for the procedure as per Procedure Guideline 14.1.A.	
3 Gather equipment; this may include • 10 ml syringes • Needles to draw up the required solutions • 0.9% sodium chloride for injection • Required amount and strength of heparin • 2% chlorhexidine in 70% isopropyl alcohol wipe • Small plaster, if required	
4 Perform hand hygiene.	4 To reduce possible hand contamination from collecting equipment.
5 Open equipment by carefully peeling back packaging. If at any time there is a suspicion that a piece of equipment may have become contaminated, dispose of it immediately and use a new piece.	
6 Connect the needles to the syringes, as required. Draw up the 0.9% sodium chloride and heparin, as required.	
7 When all equipment/medication has been prepared, remove all needles from syringes and leave in syringe packet.	7 To adhere to ANTT® and minimise the risk of key part contamination.
8 Perform hand hygiene	
9 Clean the needle-free access device with the 2% chlorhexidine in 70% isopropyl alcohol wipe for 15 seconds using friction and allow to dry naturally for 30 seconds. Visibly check that the device is dry.	9 To ensure adequate cleaning of the device and enable the product to work effectively.
10 Insert 10 ml syringe of 0.9% sodium chloride into the needle-free device. Open the clamp of the port needle and attach the flush syringe to the needle-free access device and gently instil the first part of the flush followed by the turbulent flushing technique. NOTE: If the port patency is in doubt, do not force fluid and seek advice.	10 To check device patency and minimise the risk of accidental catheter rupture from increased flushing pressure. To clear the CVAD of any blood residue and minimise the risk of subsequent CVAD occlusion.
11 Carefully peel dressings completely away from the skin. Locate and firmly secure the sides/top and bottom of the port firmly between your finger and thumb.	11 To avoid dislodging the port needle. Reassess the port needle position and reflush with 0.9% sodium chloride if the Port needle may have been dislodged.
12 Reclean the needle-free access device.	12 To adhere to ANTT® and reduce the risk of infection.
13 Attach the syringe of heparin syringe. Inject the heparin and maintain positive pressure by asking a second person to firmly secure/hold down the port, while withdrawing the port needle.	13 To prevent blood refluxing into the catheter and resulting in CVAD occlusion. To support the port during port needle removal and prevent possible trauma.
14 Dispose of any sharps in a sharps container.	14 To reduce the risk of needle stick injury.
15 Use a small plaster/gauze and tape to cover needle site, if required.	
16 Complete the procedure as per Procedure Guideline 14.1.B.	
17 Document procedure in CVAD record chart.	17 To maintain accurate records.

Common CVAD complications

Athale et al. (2012) estimate that 40–46% of CVADs develop complications. The most common complications are infection, mechanical, thrombotic and nonthrombotic occlusion, migration/malpositions, fractures, and dislodgement /accidental removal.

Infection

Infection is the most common CVAD-related problem. Overall, the organisms most frequently responsible for catheter-related blood stream infections (CRBSIs) are coagulase-negative staphylococci, *Staphylococcus aureus*, enterococci, *Escherichia coli*, Klebsiella species, and Candida species (Abad and Safdar 2012). Colonisation of the CVAD may be extra or intra luminal.

Once an infection is suspected, blood culture specimens should be taken from all lumens of a CVAD to avoid any missed infections. Antimicrobial treatment must be administered through alternating lumens to treat any infection in all lumens and prevent seeding of infection from one lumen to another. Extra luminal infections will need swabs sent for microscopy, culture, and sensitivity.

Management of CRBSIs relies on systemic antimicrobial treatment or catheter removal, depending on the organism/s and the clinical condition of the CYP. Catheter salvage strategies, such as antibiotic lock therapy, are also used where appropriate as an adjunct to systemic therapy.

Adherence to strict guidelines for line care is essential to avoid bloodstream infection, along with close monitoring for signs of intravascular infection and/or exit site infection, such as fever, sepsis, local site redness, swelling, oozing (pus or blood) or pain.

Flushing problems

When a catheter is totally patent, the internal pressure will not increase during flushing (Hadaway 1998). Excessive force must never be used when flushing any device. Should this occur, stop flushing the CVAD immediately, assess for the following, and seek assistance from a more experience colleague if needed:

- Resistance is felt (never flush against resistance due to the risk of catheter damage).
- The CYP reports pain.
- Inability to inject flush (never force fluid into the catheter).
- Swelling is observed from inside the catheter (i.e. bulging/ballooning).
- Swelling is observed along the skin tunnel, around the chest site, or in the neck area.
- Leakage of fluid from the catheter or exit site.

Occlusions

Occluded catheters compromise patient care and require skilled nursing interventions to restore catheter patency. Adherence to recommended maintenance and flushing techniques reduces the risk of catheter occlusions (Holt et al. 2010). Untreated CVAD occlusions increase the risk of CRBSIs.

Catheter occlusion can manifest as a withdrawal, partial or total occlusion, and can occur due to a range of factors. See Table 14.6 for types of CVAD occlusions and the possible causes and Table 14.7 for the management of these.

The cause of any occlusion should be ascertained; mechanical, thrombotic or nonthrombotic. The experienced HCP should be able to spot the subtle warning signs of catheter occlusion/malfunction. Withdrawal and partial occlusions are easier to treat effectively than total occlusions, so early assessment and prompt treatment increase treatment success and results in minimal delay to patient care.

Mechanical occlusions

Mechanical occlusions obstruct free flow through a CVAD. These include kinking of the catheter, clamps being left in a closed position while attempting to flush the CVAD, catheter adherence under the clamp when left in the same position for long periods, and tip malposition against a vessel wall. Tip malposition against a vessel is more common with distal tip positioning high in the SVC, and is more prevalent with left-sided insertion.

For most mechanical occlusions, the occlusion can be resolved on reassessment of the CVAD and any connected infusion tubing for kinks or closed clamps or removal/change of the needle-free access device.

Thrombotic occlusion

A normal functioning CVAD should flush easily with free-flowing blood return. Catheter occlusion is a common complication in paediatric patients (Hovda Davis 2013) and is commonly associated with CVADs after an infection.

Any device inserted into the vascular system increases the risk of thrombus formation, either in the vessel or in the catheter. Fibrin build-up, a natural consequence of catheter placement, contributes to thrombus formation. Fibrin can develop into a sheath that may either completely encase the catheter or build up on a catheter without completely enclosing it (in this scenario, a small piece of fibrin referred to as a fibrin tail hangs off the catheter tip). In both cases, infusions will still be possible, but the sheath or tail will occlude the internal catheter tip during aspiration and prevent withdrawal of blood from the catheter. This is known as a withdrawal occlusion.

Intraluminal thrombi can form inside the CVAD lumen and can result in partial or complete occlusion. This can be due to inadequate CVAD flushing resulting in blood refluxing back into the

Table 14.6 Types of CVAD occlusions

	Withdrawal	Partial	Total
Definition	CVAD flushes easily, but no blood present on aspiration, or difficulty in free aspiration of blood.	Able to flush CVAD, but stiff to flush (extra pressure used on flushing).	Unable to flush or withdraw from CVAD.
Possible causes	• Fibrin sheath or tail/thrombus • Catheter tip against the vein wall • Catheter malposition/migration	• Intraluminal thrombus partially occluding the catheter • Extra luminal thrombus – still attached to catheter • Partial medication/lipid precipitates • Incorrect position of port needle • Kink in catheter • Suture constriction	• Intraluminal thrombus • Extra luminal thrombus – still attached to catheter • Medication/lipid precipitates • Incorrect position of port needle • Severe kink in catheter • Mechanical obstruction

Table 14.7 Occlusion troubleshooting guide

	Try with all CVADs	**With PICCs include**	**With Hickmans include**	**With implanted ports include**
Withdrawal occlusion	• Access without needle-free access device. • Try flushing 20 ml 0.9% sodium chloride. • Ask the CYP to look up and away from the CVAD (especially for CYPs with very chunky necks). • Change CYP's position.	• Check catheter for kinks under and outside of dressing.	• Check catheter for kinks under and outside of dressing. • Check for internal catheter adhesion under clamp(s).	• Check port needle is correctly inside port chamber and not against inner/outer wall of chamber. • Check for overpadding of port needle causing dislodgement. **If needle position is correct, do not remove as routine.**
Total occlusion	• Access without needle-free access device. • Try gently flushing 10 ml 0.9% sodium chloride.	• Check for kinks in catheter. • Check for catheter twisting at catheter hub junction.	• Check for catheter twisting at catheter hub junction for smaller French catheter. • Check for internal catheter adherence under clamp(s).	• Check port needle not sitting inside the silicon septum.
Mechanical occlusion	Check that clamps are open.	• Check for kinks in catheter. • Check for catheter twisting at catheter hub junction.	• Check for catheter twisting at catheter hub junction for smaller French catheter. • Check for internal catheter adherence under clamp(s).	

Withdrawal occlusions can progress to a total occlusion if left untreated, so prompt treatment is required. It is not acceptable practice to leave a withdrawal occlusion untreated in one lumen while continuing to use the other lumen (Kerner et al. 2006).

catheter or blood clotting within the catheter during blood sampling.

Within child health, any suspected thrombotic occlusion should be treated with the instillation of a thrombolytic agent (Baskin et al. 2009). This is an effective noninvasive method of clearing thrombotic occlusions in CVADs and has a catheter clearance rate of 80–90% after one or two doses (Baskin et al. 2009). Alteplase and urokinase are commonly used in CYPs. Alteplase is currently used at GOSH and hence urokinase is not discussed here – please refer to local guidelines.

Alteplase

Alteplase is a recombinant tissue type plasminogen activator. It acts as a thrombolytic by activating plasminogen to form plasmin, which degrades fibrin and breaks up thrombi. The most frequent adverse reaction associated with all thrombolytics is bleeding. Alteplase should be used with caution in CYPs with a higher risk of bleeding. It is instilled into the occluded CVAD and left for a set period of time to allow the fibrinolytic effect to take place.

Alteplase dosing for CVAD occlusion in young children tends to depend on the volume of the affected catheter. 110% of the catheter fill volume is administered to account for intraluminal thrombus and the fibrin sheath/tail on the internal catheter (Anderson et al. 2013). However, accurate dosing of Alteplase in paediatrics is difficult because of customisation of catheter length, resulting in variability of intraluminal volume. Most trusts have a standardised dosing schedule based on catheter sizes (Doellman 2011). For further information, see Table 14.8.

If repeated thrombotic therapy fails to alleviate the CVAD withdrawal occlusion, then refer for radiographic imaging to check for catheter tip malposition or a contrast study, i.e. linogram to check for extensive fibrin formation, will be necessary (Doellman 2011). Treatment for extensive/persistent fibrin sheath/tail/flap usually involves removal of the CVAD. Other options include fibrin sheath stripping, but fibrin sheaths usually redevelop after stripping (Steiger 2006) or administering an infusion of low-dose Alteplase over two to four hours, but again, the fibrin tail may redevelop.

With total occlusions, the complete dose of thrombolytic needs to be instilled inside the catheter. The aim is to seep the thrombolytic around the thrombus by very gently stretching the catheter around the thrombus. There is a high risk of the catheter ballooning or bursting if too much pressure is applied, especially if the occlusion has been left for a long period of time and the thrombus has solidified inside the catheter. Experienced HCPs need to either undertake this task or supervise any less experienced colleagues. Radiographic imaging (X-ray) and contrast studies (linogram) offer no diagnostic benefit with total occlusions as the internal lumen is not visible or accessible to offer any rationale for the occlusion, so the exposure to radiation is not justified.

Nonthrombotic occlusions

Medication related nonthrombotic occlusions occur when medication crystallisation and precipitation when the pH of a solution varies too much from the medication's normal stability range. Lipid occlusions also occur and are more prevalent with silicone catheters, as lipid emulsion adheres to silicone.

To determine whether the partial or total occlusion is result of medication precipitate or lipid deposit, the compatibility of the medications recently administered must be reviewed (Doellman 2011). In addition, lipid debris can sometimes be seen at the catheter hub, or medication precipitation can be seen during attempts to flush or aspirate the CVAD. If the medication history leads to a suspected medication-related occlusion, treatment involves adding a solution that brings the pH back to the normal range, which may liquefy the drug and dissolve the precipitate. For crystallised medications with a normally high pH, such as phenytoin sodium, sodium bicarbonate can be infused to raise the pH, which may cause the medication to revert to its liquid state. With naturally low pH solutions, such as vancomycin, hydrochloric acid

Table 14.8 Alteplase doses

Alteplase administration volumes for the management of withdrawal/total occlusion	
Alteplase (Actilyse Cathflo®) is available as 2 mg vials.	
Central venous access device	Alteplase Dose
PICC 3 Fr 4 Fr 5 Fr	0.5 mg (0.5 ml) 0.5 mg (0.5 ml) 0.5 mg (0.5 ml) down each required lumen
Single lumen CVC (Broviac®) 2.7 Fr/4.2 Fr/6.6 Fr	0.5 mg (0.5 ml)
Single lumen CVC (Hickman®) 9.6 Fr	1 mg (1 ml)
Dual lumen CVC (Hickman®) 7 Fr/9 Fr/10 Fr	1 mg (1 ml) down each required lumen
Triple lumen CVC (Hickman®) 10 Fr/12 Fr	1 mg (1 ml) down each required lumen
Implantable port: Mini port Low profile (small) Large/standard	0.7 mg (0.7 ml) 1 mg (1 ml) 1.5 mg (1.5 ml)
Central venous access (temporary) for extracorporeal therapies (Gamcath®/Vascath®) catheter Various sizes	The amount instilled must be the equivalent of the volume of the dead space of the catheter The priming volumes for the catheter are printed on the catheter or clamps itself and in the insertion leaflet
Central venous access (permanent/cuffed) for extracorporeal therapies (Kimal/Gambro/Tyco/Permcath®) catheter Various sizes	The amount instilled must be the equivalent of the volume of the dead space of the catheter The priming volumes for the catheter are printed on the catheter or clamps itself and in the insertion leaflet

Source: Boehringer Ingelheim Limited (2021)

can be used to dissolve a precipitate occlusion. To dissolve lipid occlusions, 70% ethyl alcohol is used.

Ethanol, sodium bicarbonate, and hydrochloric acid administration may also include risks and side effects, so use of these medications for CVAD occlusions needs to be assessed carefully. They should only be administered by HCPs expert in treating CVAD occlusions, and follow trust protocols, with appropriate monitoring, to reduce the risk of harm to the CYP.

Catheter migration/malposition

CVAD migration/malposition occurs when the internal catheter migrates out of its insertion placement site to another location, usually within the venous system, but into an undesired vein, such as the opposite brachiocephalic (Savader and Trerotola 2000). This can result from the external catheter being pulled, from forceful flushing, from changes in intrathoracic pressure occurring during forceful coughing or vomiting, and from physical activity. Migration can also occur spontaneously for no apparent reason.

The malpositioned CVAD can lead to difficulty in blood aspiration, thrombophlebitis, or other serious complications. For example, tip positioning in the distal right atrium or in the right ventricle can lead to arrhythmia. Some signs and symptoms of malposition may include difficulty with aspiration or infusion, increased external catheter length or exposure of the Dacron cuff, leaking of fluid at exit site, or complaints of gurgling/clicking sound in the ear. There may also be no obvious signs of malposition.

If migration/malposition is suspected, the CYP will require an X-ray to verify the catheter tip position. Once malposition is confirmed, the CVAD position will need to be corrected if possible. Depending on the tip position, this might be by saline injection, length readjustment or repositioning if feasible – externally migrated CVADs cannot be readvanced due to the risk of infection (Savader and Trerotola 2000; Burn et al. 2013) – or ultimately, the device will need to be replaced.

Catheter fracture/rupture

All CVADs can split, develop holes, rupture or fracture, both internally and externally. Internal damage will require complete CVAD removal. With implanted ports, where there is external damage to the port needle, the needle will just need to be deaccessed and the port reaccessed with a new port needle.

If a Hickman®/PICC or similar device is damaged, immediate action is required to ensure the CYP's safety. See Procedure Guideline 14.21.

CVAD dislodgement/accidental removal

In order to minimise the risk of dislodgement/accidental removal the CVAD needs to be checked at least daily, to ensure that the dressing is secure and there is a loop/curve firmly secured underneath the dressing. If the catheter is completely pulled out immediate action is required to ensure the CYP's safety. See Procedure Guideline 14.22.

Chapter 14 Intravenous and intra-arterial access and infusions

Procedure guideline 14.19 Assessing a CVAD for occlusions

Statement	Rationale
Prepare for the procedure as per Procedure Guideline 14.1.A.	
1 Gather equipment; this may include: • 10 ml luer-lock syringes • 20 ml syringe **for withdrawal occlusions only** • Needle • 0.9% sodium chloride for injection • 2% chlorhexidine in 70% isopropyl alcohol wipes • Needle-free access device • Sterile closed caps NB: For multilumen CVADs, individual sets of the above equipment will be needed for each lumen to reduce the risk of cross-contamination.	1 To ensure the procedure is undertaken efficiently.
2 Perform hand hygiene.	
3 Open equipment by carefully peeling back packaging. If at any time you think you may have come into contact with any key part, dispose of it immediately and use a new piece.	3 Using potentially contamination equipment can lead to the risk of infection.
4 Connect the needles to the syringes, as required. Draw up 0.9% sodium chloride in a 10 ml syringe. Include a 20 ml syringe filled with 0.9% sodium chloride if a withdrawal occlusion is suspected. Ensure all key parts remain uncontaminated. Open an empty 10 ml syringe as well.	
5 When all equipment/medication has been prepared, remove all needles from syringes and leave in syringe packet.	5 To adhere to ANTT® and minimise the risk of key part contamination.
6 Open the needle-free access device, but leave in plastic covering at the side of the tray away from key parts.	6 To minimise cross-contamination.
7 Put on gloves, locate the CVAD to be used, and identify the lumen to be assessed. Check the CVAD catheter and exit site for any problems.	7 As part of standard precautions.
8 Check that the CVAD clamp is closed and remove the needle-free access device and any add-on devices.	8 To assess the CVAD without any add-on devices that may be contributing to the occlusion.
9 Perform hand hygiene.	
10 Clean the CVAD's hub with the 2% chlorhexidine in 70% isopropyl alcohol; wipe for 15 seconds using friction and allow to dry naturally for 30 seconds. Visibly check the hub is dry.	10 To ensure adequate cleaning of the device and enable the product to work effectively.
11 Attach the empty syringe and attempt to withdraw blood. Remove syringe.	
12 N.B. Remember to clamp the CVAD between syringe changes	12 To prevent blood loss or air embolism.
13 Attach the 10 ml syringe of 0.9% sodium chloride to the hub, open the clamp, and gently try to instil the first part of the flush to check the patency of the CVAD. Do not apply excessive pressure.	13 To check device patency. To minimise the risk of accidental catheter rupture from increased flushing pressure.
14 **If CVAD flushes easily, but does not aspirate**, then use the 20 ml of sodium chloride to give a firm turbulent flush, and then try aspirating blood again. If still unable to aspirate, then refer to procedure for instillation of Alteplase (withdrawal occlusion). **If CVAD can be flushed, but extra pressure needs to be applied**, then refer to procedure for instillation of Alteplase (partial occlusion). **If CVAD cannot be flushed or aspirated,** then refer to procedure for instillation of Alteplase (total occlusion).	
15 **If CVAD flushes and aspirates easily**, then clean off any blood on the CVAD's hub with the 2% chlorhexidine in 70% isopropyl alcohol; wipe for 15 seconds using friction and allow to dry naturally for 30 seconds. Visibly check the hub is dry, then follow the rest of the procedure guidelines for flushing a CVAD.	15 To remove any blood present from accessing the CVAD without a needle-free access device. To complete the procedure and maintain patency of the CVAD.
16 Replace needle-free access device on CVAD.	
17 Once completed, tuck away the CYP's CVAD.	17 To minimise risk of breakage or dislodgement.
18 Complete the procedure as per Procedure Guideline 14.1.B.	
19 Document procedure in care record.	19 To maintain accurate records.

The Great Ormond Street Hospital Manual of Children and Young People's Nursing Practices

Procedure guideline 14.20 Instillation of alteplase into a CVAD

This procedure describes how to use alteplase as the thrombolytic (see also Figure 14.4). However, the same principles of assessment and administration can be used for urokinase following the manufacturer's, pharmacy, or prescription guidelines for the appropriate dilution and dose.

There are three methods to instil alteplase into a CVAD: The single syringe method; the two syringe method; and the three-way tap method. The procedure below uses the single syringe method.

Statement	Rationale
Prepare for the procedure as per Procedure Guideline 14.1.A.	
1 Collect the equipment required for the procedure; this may include: • 10 ml syringes • 2.5 or 3 ml syringe • Needles to draw up the required solutions • Vial of alteplase • Vial of sterile water for injection • 0.9% sodium chloride for injection • 2% chlorhexidine in 70% isopropyl alcohol wipes	1 To ensure the procedure is undertaken efficiently and prevent later contamination.
2 Write label including the date and time that the alteplase is instilled and the time it can be removed.	2 To minimise the risk of drug errors.
3 Review any medication side effects and check that the correct dose is prescribed.	3 To confirm alteplase dose.
4 For a 2 mg vial of alteplase, 2.2 ml of water for injection is added; Alteplase has a **final concentration of 1 mg/ml.**	4 See medicinal product information leaflet (Boerhringer Ingelheim Limited 2018).

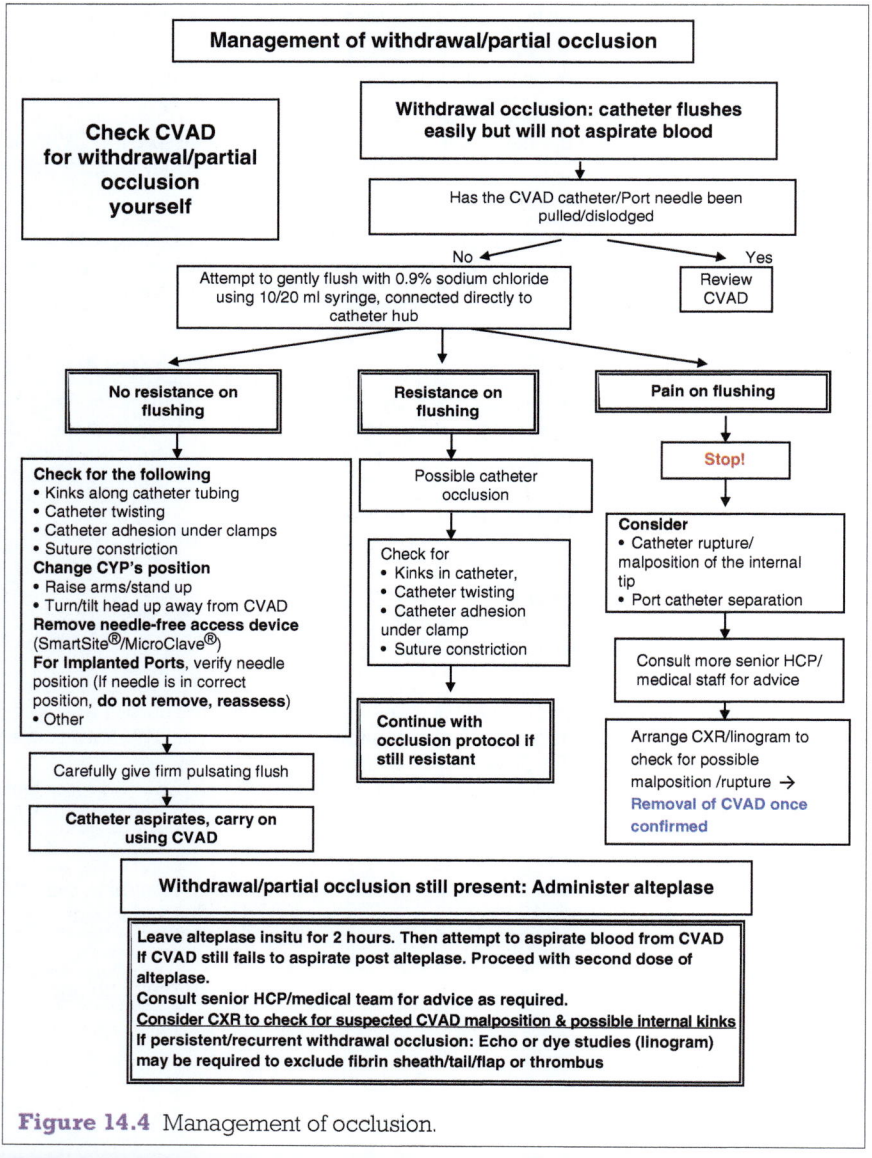

Figure 14.4 Management of occlusion.

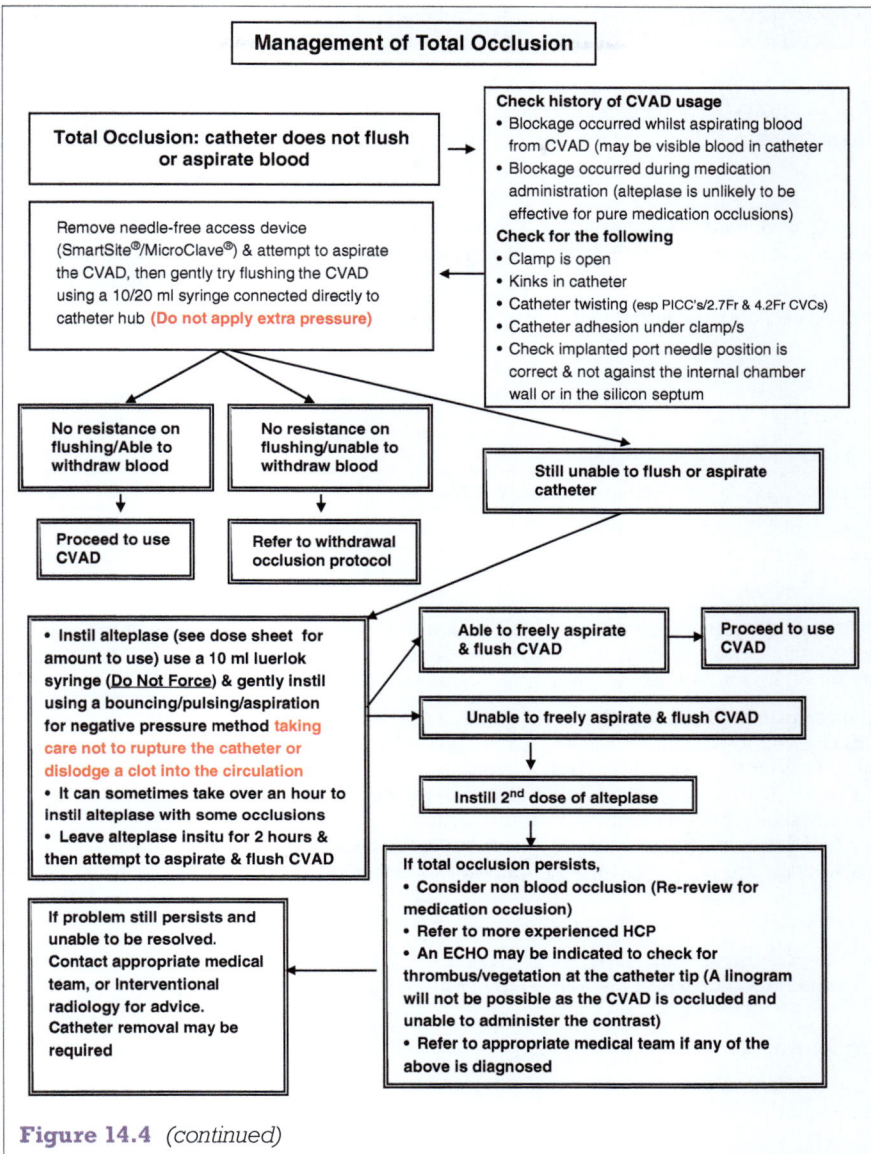

Figure 14.4 *(continued)*

Procedure guideline 14.20 Instillation of alteplase into a CVAD *(continued)*	
Statement	**Rationale**
5 Perform hand hygiene.	5 To reduce possible hand contamination from collecting equipment.
6 Open equipment by carefully peeling back packaging. If at any time there is a suspicion that a piece of equipment may have become contaminated, dispose of it immediately and use a new piece.	
7 Clean the top of the alteplase vial with a 2%chlorhexidine/70%isopropyl alcohol wipe.	7 To prevent contamination of the vial contents.
8 Check the medication(s) to be administered against the CYP's prescription. Also check that the alteplase volume is correct for the type and size of catheter.	8 To ensure that the correct dose is administered for the size of the CVAD.
9 Connect the needles to the syringes, as required and draw up 2.2 ml of the water for injection, taking care that the needle does not touch the outside of any vials.	
10 Add the water for injection to the 2 mg alteplase vial. Gently shake to dissolve the powder and when completely dissolved, draw up the required dose of Alteplase in the 10 ml luer-lock syringe.	10 10 ml syringes exert less pressure on flushing. Luer-lock syringes ensure that the syringe does not accidently become disconnected during administration.

(continued)

Procedure guideline 14.20 Instillation of alteplase into a CVAD *(continued)*

Statement	Rationale
11 If you are unsure whether the CVAD lumen currently contains anything other 0.9% sodium chloride, then draw up a 0.9% sodium chloride flush.	11 To prevent alteplase incompatibility with any other medications that may be left in the CVAD lumen leading to increased catheter occlusion.
12 Cover all exposed syringe tips with sterile sealed caps, taking care not to contaminate key parts when placing them on and removing prior to use.	12 To adhere to ANTT®. To prevent any risk of airborne or key part contamination.
13 Open an additional sterile sealed cap, leaving it in the plastic packaging at the side of the tray.	
14 Label syringes.	14 To help reduce medication errors (NPSA 2007).
15 Take tray and prescription to the CYP.	
16 Perform hand hygiene on entry to the room/bed space.	
17 Check the CYPs identification against the details on the prescription.	17 To correctly identify the patient.
18 Locate the CVAD to be used and if applicable, identify the lumen to be used. Check the CVAD catheter and exit site for any problems.	
19 Visibly check any CVAD clamps are closed.	
20 Remove the needle-free access device and clean the CVAD hub with the 2% chlorhexidine in 70% isopropyl alcohol wipe firmly for 15 seconds using friction and allow to dry naturally for 30 seconds. Visibly check that the hub is dry.	20 To ensure adequate cleaning of the hub and enable the product to work effectively.
21 **If withdrawal/partial occlusion:** Flush with the 10ml syringe of 0.9% sodium chloride as needed. Then instil the dose of alteplase, observing for any pain/discomfort or bulging/ballooning/leaking in the catheter. **If total occlusion:** Attach the 10ml syringe containing the dose of alteplase and gently using negative pressure and no positive pressure, instil the complete dose of alteplase. Use a mainly aspirating/negative pressure method for instilling the alteplase, taking care not to rupture the catheter or dislodge a clot into the circulation. It can sometimes take over 30 minutes or longer to instil alteplase with total occlusions.	
22 Cover the hub with the sterile sealed cap and place the label with the alteplase details on the CVAD leg.	22 To prevent accidental access before the alteplase has had time to take effect.
23 Leave the alteplase in situ for 2 hours.	23 To allow sufficient time for the alteplase to be effective.
24 After the 2 hours: Prepare another tray containing an empty 10ml syringe, a 10ml syringe containing 10ml of 0.9% sodium chloride, 2% chlorhexidine in 70% isopropyl alcohol wipes and a needle-free access device.	
25 Confirm CVAD clamp is still closed and remove the label and cap on the CVAD hub.	
26 Perform hand hygiene.	
27 Clean the CVAD hub with the 2% chlorhexidine in 70% isopropyl alcohol; wipe firmly for 15 seconds using friction and allow to dry naturally for 30 seconds. Visibly check that the hub is dry.	27 To ensure adequate cleaning of the hub and enable the product to work effectively.
28 Using the empty 10ml syringe, attempt to aspirate the CVAD, and withdraw 2ml of blood. Whether the CVAD aspirates freely or not, connect the 0.9% sodium chloride. Open the clamp of the CVAD if present and very gently using minimal pressure flush the CVAD.	28 To attempt to remove the alteplase from the CVAD. To ascertain the CVAD patency.
29 If able to freely flush the CVAD without any pressure, use the turbulent flushing technique followed by positive pressure to complete the flush.	29 To prevent any further occlusion.
30 If unable to flush the CVAD or extra pressure is required to flush the CVAD, follow procedure for a second dose of alteplase.	
31 If CVAD flushing freely, attach the needle-free access device to the CVAD hub. Clean hub as per procedure if blood is visible on hub.	
32 Once completed, tuck away the CYP's CVAD.	32 To prevent accidental dislodgement or damage to the CVAD.
33 Complete the procedure as per Procedure Guideline 14.1.B.	
34 Complete prescription/administration documentation.	34 To maintain accurate records.

Safety aspects for staff and families

Prior to the CYP leaving the ward area or being discharged from hospital, CVAD safety must be taught to them (if appropriate) and their family. This is essential to maintain the safety of a CVAD outside the ward environment and ensure that the family can deal with any situation that may arise. It includes:

- Advice and teaching regarding daily care of the CVAD.
- What to do if the dressing becomes dirty/wet or is peeling off.
- How to check for signs of infection.
- What to do if the PICC/CVC/Hickman® is pulled out.
- What to do if there is a hole/split or break in the PICC/CVC/Hickman®.

Safety pack contents and information leaflets

A CVAD safety pack and safety information should be given to the family to reinforce the safety issues they have been taught.

Other safety measures

Extra security for the CVAD can be achieved by adopting one of the following:

- Wearing a vest/armband made out of elastic net retention bandage (e.g. Surgifix®) or similar product.
- Wearing cropped vests with elastic edging.
- Attaching pockets using Velcro or sewn into place on the inside of vests/T-shirts to tuck the ends of the catheter into.
- Wearing bags with ties to hold the distal end of the CVC. Often referred to as Hickman®/wriggly bags (NB: The CYP must not sleep with the tape/ribbon around their necks).
- Ensuring any CVC tubing is tucked away and not allowed to hang down outside clothing.

Ensure that the above are changed regularly or washed.
Do not tuck catheters into nappies due to the risk of contamination

Procedure guideline 14.21 Immediate Care of a PICC or Hickman® with a fracture, hole, or split

Statement	Rationale
1 Gather the required equipment: • Nonsterile gloves • Pack sterile gauze • 2 small 6 × 7 cm semipermeable dressings • 2 plastic clamps • 1 roll of medical tape	
2 Perform hand hygiene and put on gloves.	
3 Take a plastic clamp from the safety pack and clamp Hickman®/PICC catheter ABOVE the hole, ensuring that the section of the clamp used to clamp seals the catheter effectively.	3 To seal the catheter and stop any bleeding.
4 You may need to peel off some of the dressing over the CVAD.	4 To get access to the catheter for clamping.
5 Take the second plastic clamp and one piece of gauze. Fold the gauze in half and then place around the catheter above the first clamp. Clamp the second clamp over this piece of gauze, then move the first clamp and reclamp over the gauze.	5 Backup, in case one of the clamps falls off. A layer of gauze is usually placed between the clamp and the catheter as plastic or metal clamps can potentially cause stress points which can result in further catheter damage.
6 Open the small clear occlusive dressing and place this over the hole or around the breakage (do not put any gauze underneath).	6 To reduce the risk of further infection.
7 Take a piece of medical tape and secure the Hickman®/PICC to the CYP's chest.	7 To prevent pulling on as the Hickman®/PICC with the clamps on will be heavy.
8 Arrange for the CYP to have the Hickman®/PICC repaired.	8 For the required IV therapy to continue.
9 Document in the CYP's healthcare record and complete incident form.	

Procedure guideline 14.22 Action required with a pulled-out PICC or Hickman®

Statement	Rationale
1 Gather the required equipment: • Gloves • Pack sterile gauze • 2 small semipermeable plastic dressings	
2 Perform hand hygiene and put on gloves.	2 As part of standard precautions.
3 Immediately apply firm pressure for five minutes to the: • Neck site for Hickman® or tunnelled noncuffed CVCs (there will be the small scar site on the neck from the CVAD insertion). • Arm area for PICCs, i.e. where it exited the arm.	3 To stop any bleeding from the vein.
4 After 5 minutes observe the neck site/arm site closely for any swelling or blood; if you see any blood, continue to apply pressure.	4 To confirm haemostasis has been achieved.

(continued)

Procedure guideline 14.22 Action required with a pulled-out PICC or Hickman® *(continued)*

Statement	Rationale
5 After the bleeding has stopped, open the small clear dressing and apply it over the exit site (on the chest for Hickmans® and on the arm for PICCs).	5 To seal the hole and prevent air embolism.
6 Continue to monitor for any further bleeding.	6 Risk of bleeding restarting.
7 Check the Hickman®/PICC to confirm that the catheter is intact and has been completely removed.	7 Risk of catheter embolus if segment retained internally.
8 Arrange for a new CVAD to be inserted, if required.	8 To continue with IV treatment, as required.
9 Document in the CYP's healthcare record and complete clinical incident form.	

CVAD repair

Catheter damage can occur with any CVAD, sometimes due to defective products but more often from improper care, such as improper securement or excessive use of pressure when flushing the device. Damage can occur as a result of contact with sharp objects, such as scissors or teeth, or catheter fracture when the CVAD is pulled or entangled in the sides of pushchairs/car doors. Once a catheter has been damaged, it is contaminated and there is a risk of infection to the CYP.

Externally damaged catheters can be repaired rather than replaced.

PICC repair

The ability to repair a PICC will depend on the type and brand as not all brands of PICCs have repair kits. Where there is no repair kit, the PICC will need to be removed and a new PICC inserted if still required. Where PICC repair kits are available, the catheter repair must be done by an experienced healthcare professional, using only the repair kit provided by the PICC manufacturer.

The following PICC repair procedure refers to the repair of a Bard single-lumen Groshong NXT ClearVue PICC. A minimum of 5 cm undamaged catheter below the exit site is essential when repairing any PICC line. The Bard dual-lumen PICCs require 'red' and 'white' lumens to be repaired separately with a different connector. They cannot be repaired if the break is above the bifurcation (i.e. at the blue catheter).

Sterile gloves are used alongside the ANTT® to reduce the already high risk of line infection following the fracture (Gordon and Gardiner 2013).

Procedure guideline 14.23 Repair of a single lumen Groshong® NXT ClearVue® PICC

Statement	Rationale
1 Prepare for the procedure as per Procedure Guideline 14.1.A.	
2 Clean a (metal) trolley using a sanitising wipe working from top to bottom. Let the trolley dry completely.	2 To prevent cross-infection.
3 Gather equipment, to include: • Correct size repair kit • 0.5% or 2% Chlorhexidine in 70% denatured ethanol • Blue plastic clamps • Two packs of sterile gauze swabs • Sterile scissors • Dressing pack or field • Well-fitting sterile gloves • 10 ml luerslip syringes ×2 • Needle • 10 ml vial of 0.9% sodium chloride • Blood culture bottles • 3 ml 2%chlorhexidine/70% isopropyl alcohol sterile applicators (e.g. ChloraPrep®) • Wound closure strips • Large clear dressing • Needle-free access device	3 To ensure the procedure is undertaken efficiently.
4 Perform hand hygiene.	
5 Open out the sterile field or dressing pack and drop the required equipment onto the field without touching any of the sterile equipment. Pour the Chlorhexidine in 70% denatured ethanol on the gauze swabs.	
6 The syringes and flushes required for accessing the PICC can be prepared in the already cleaned IV tray.	
7 Remove CYP's clothing if necessary.	7 To allow easy access to the PICC and prevent contamination of the area with clothing.
8 Remove the dressing and reposition the clamp on the catheter, as required, leaving at least 3 cm of catheter to work with.	
9 Get a colleague to hold the clamp and prevent any pulling of the PICC.	9 To minimise discomfort for the CYP and reduce the risk of dislodgement.

Procedure guideline 14.23 Repair of a single lumen Groshong® NXT ClearVue® PICC (continued)

Statement	Rationale
10 Perform hygienic hand wash.	10 To minimise cross-infection.
11 Put on the well-fitting **sterile** gloves.	11 Well-fitting gloves improve dexterity.
12 Get your colleague to hold up the catheter while you place the sterile field underneath.	12 To ensure the area under the repair is clean.
13 Taking a piece of the gauze, lift up the end of the PICC.	13 To minimise contamination of sterile gloves.
14 Clean the broken segment of the catheter or where you intend to cut the PICC with the chlorhexidine-soaked gauze firmly for 30 seconds. Repeat twice more with a new piece of soaked gauze.	14 To minimise any further risk of infection from contamination (Gordon and Gardiner 2013).
15 Allow time for the solution to dry completely.	15 To allow the chlorhexidine to work effectively and minimise any further risk of infection.
16 Once dry, using the sterile scissors, cut the PICC catheter cleanly and straight above the damaged portion.	
17 Reclean the end of the PICC three times with the chlorhexidine-soaked gauze and allow to air dry completely.	
18 Slide the smaller oversleeve part of the repair and advance it over the cut end of the catheter, feeding in the narrow side first. If resistance is felt while advancing the oversleeve, gently twist back and forth while feeding in the catheter.	
19 The oversleeve should slide over the catheter and 2–3 cm of the catheter should protrude at the end.	
20 Gently insert the metal stent of the connector repair into the PICC catheter, pushing it up so the blue catheter end meets the hub. The catheter should lie flat on the stent without any kinks or ruching.	20 To enable a neat join with the catheter and stent. Kinks/ruching will occlude the internal catheter and impede fluid flow.
21 Slide the oversleeve part to the winged portion and align the 'grooves' between the 'wings'. Push together until a locking sensation is felt. This will ensure that the two pieces are fully engaged.	
22 Very gently, stretch the catheter at the hub slightly.	22 To ensure there are no gathers under the oversleeve.
23 Attach the 10 ml syringe and aspirate blood for culture. You may have to flush with a very small amount of 0.9% sodium chloride if the PICC does not bleed back initially.	23 The risk of infection will have increased with a hole/break in the catheter.
24 Flush gently with 0.9% sodium chloride.	
25 If blood is present at the hub, clean with a 2% chlorhexidine in 70% isopropyl alcohol wipe firmly for 15 seconds using friction and allow to dry naturally for 30 seconds. Visibly check that the device is dry.	25 There is a risk of infection if blood is left present.
26 Attach the needle-free access device.	26 To provide a closed system.
27 Attach the flush syringe to the needle-free access device and gently instil the first part of the flush followed by the turbulent flushing technique.	27 To check patency and confirm intact PICC catheter.
28 Use positive pressure when flushing off the valved PICC; flush the PICC while removing the luer-slip syringe from the needle-free access device.	28 To minimise the risk of blood refluxing into the lumen of the catheter and resulting in catheter occlusion.
29 Follow CVAD dressing procedure to secure the repaired PICC.	29 To secure the PICC and help prevent any further holes/breaks.
30 Once completed, tuck away the CYP's CVAD	30 To minimise risk of breakage or dislodgement.
31 Complete the procedure as per Procedure Guideline 14.1.B.	
32 Document in the CYP's healthcare record.	32 To maintain accurate records.

Hickman® repair

Externally damaged Hickman® or similar catheters can be repaired rather than replaced. A minimum of 5 cm undamaged catheter below the exit site is essential when repairing any Hickman® type catheter. Repair kit availability will depend on the type and brand. A few CVADs do not have repair kits. In these cases, or where the catheter cannot be repaired due to insufficient length, the catheter will need to be removed and a new CVAD inserted if still required.

There are various types of repairs that can be performed, depending on the fracture/hole position, leg repairs available, as well as the complete catheter segment. The correct size/French repair must be used.

Some CVADs have identifying features that allow easy identification of the catheter size. For single lumen Hickmans, where the device size is not written on the line, or if the printed wording on the catheter has worn away with time, check the medical/operation notes for the correct size. Multi lumen catheters often have the identifying features written on the bifurcation. Leg repairs are colour coded with Hickman® legs being red, white or blue. The Hickman® leg repairs are generic for all their multiple lumen/legs.

Sterile gloves are used alongside the ANTT® to reduce the already high risk of infection following the catheter fracture (Gordon and Gardiner 2013).

The procedure guidelines below refer to the repair of a Bard Hickman®, but the principles can be followed for all glue related CVAD repairs, including other brands of CVCs, such as Cook medical or Vygon®. The catheter repair must be done by an experienced healthcare professional, using only the repair kit provided by that specific CVAD manufacturer. If there are any queries about the type or brand of CVAD, then the medical team that placed it must be contacted for clarification.

Procedure guideline 14.24 Repair of a Broviac® or Hickman®

Statement	Rationale
Prepare for the procedure as per Procedure Guideline 14.1.A.	
1 Clean a (metal) trolley using a sanitising wipe working from top to bottom. Let the trolley dry completely.	1 To prevent cross-infection.
2 Collect the equipment required for the procedure, this may include: • Well-fitting sterile gloves • One sterile dressing pack or two sterile fields • Packs of sterile gauze • Appropriate number of 10ml luerlock syringes needed for blood cultures, flushing and heparin. For example, a double lumen repair would require six syringes whereas a leg repair would only require three. • Appropriate number of needles • Vial/s of 0.9% sodium chloride • Vial/s of heparin 10 units in 1ml • Two packs of large wound closure strips • One 2ml syringe plunger • One pair of sterile scissors • Three 10cm by 12cm clear dressings • 0.5%/2% chlorhexidine in 70% denatured ethanol • A 3ml 2% chlorhexidine/70% isopropyl alcohol applicator • Needle-free access device • Repair kit specific to the catheter that is to be repaired • Plastic clamp • Sanitising wipes – 2% chlorhexidine/70% isopropyl alcohol individual wipes • Blood culture bottle(s)	2 To ensure the procedure is undertaken efficiently
3 Perform hand hygiene.	3 To reduce possible hand contamination from collecting equipment.
4 If you have no assistant, open out sterile field/dressing pack onto the trolley, taking care not to touch the sterile area (use the corners of the field).	
5 Peel open the packs of gauze and drop onto the sterile field.	
6 Open the required number of 10ml syringes and then the 2ml syringe.	
7 Open the needles, needle-free access device/s, large wound closure strips, Large transparent dressings, sterile field, sterile scissors and ChloraPrep.	
8 Remove the repair kit from the box. Double check it is the correct size. Remove outer plastic packaging and drop sealed inner box onto sterile field. Each repair kit is supplied in a double sterile package.	8 To check correct size kit is used and to save wasting incorrect equipment.
9 NOTE: Do not touch the contents on the trolley/sterile field until you are wearing the sterile gloves.	9 To maintain the sterile equipment on the trolley.
10 Perform hand hygiene.	
11 Put on the sterile gloves and ensure that they fit well).	11 To improve manual dexterity; repairing any CVC requires good dexterity.
12 Arrange your equipment in a systematic way:	
13 Place the needles on the syringes.	
14 Get a colleague to open the 0.9 sodium chloride vial. Draw up the 0.9% sodium chloride without touching the outside of the vial.	
15 Using the same technique, draw up 3ml of the heparin.	
16 Dispose of all needles in sharps container.	16 To prevent sharps injuries.
17 Remove the outer barrel of the 2ml syringe; you will only need the plunger.	17 To use as a splint and support the repair join.
18 Separate 3 layers of gauze into a separate pile. Place away from the main stack of gauze.	18 To place under the syringe plunger.

Chapter 14 Intravenous and intra-arterial access and infusions

Procedure guideline 14.24 Repair of a Broviac® or Hickman® *(continued)*

Statement	Rationale
19 Get a colleague to pour the chlorhexidine/70% denatured ethanol solution onto the large pile of gauze only, allowing the solution to soak through to the bottom.	19 For catheter cleaning.
20 Peel off the paper packaging of the repair kit, taking extra care not the drop the atraumatic needle.	20 The needle is packaged at the side of the box, so can be dropped easily when peeling off the paper.
21 Carefully manipulate the plastic sleeve up toward the metal stent, leaving a 1 cm gap. Do not pull too firmly/quickly as the sleeve may slide past the tip of the catheter and be difficult to retract back.	
22 Without touching the line, ensure that the clamps on the repair are closed.	22 To prevent blood backflow when the repair is fixed.
23 <u>DO NOT</u> prime the repair with 0.9% sodium chloride.	23 The glue will not adhere if the catheter/stent is wet.
24 Pull out the plunger from the syringe in the repair kit and squeeze the adhesive into the syringe; approximately 1–1.5 ml. Push back in the plunger. Attach the atraumatic needle and prime with the adhesive.	
25 <u>Colleague</u> Prepare the CYP, removing any clothing that may contaminate the line repair area.	
26 Remove the CVC dressing, as required to get to the repair site.	
27 Moving one clamp at a time, reposition both clamps further up the catheter, ensuring there is a layer of gauze between the clamp and the catheter (be aware that this will make the catheter very heavy and may tug on the CYP's skin, so make provision to support the catheter and clamps).	27 To prevent the clamps marking the catheter. To prevent the CVC tugging and causing pain or dislodgement.
28 Peel off any dressing covering the break or cut.	
29 You can now take over supporting the line/clamps during the repair.	29 To prevent the line tugging and causing pain or dislodgement.
30 <u>Repairer</u> Get your colleague to hold up the catheter while you place the sterile field underneath.	30 To have a clean area under the repair.
31 Decide the best place to cut the catheter considering the amount of room needed for future repairs and the length of the catheter post the repair. There must be at least 5 cm of intact catheter to be able to easily perform the repair (if unsure, seek advice).	31 Any previous repair must be cut off. A repair must **not** be added onto a preexisting repair.
32 Using one piece of the sterile gauze to hold the catheter, take a second piece of chlorhexidine soaked gauze to firmly clean the catheter where it will be cut (NB: Clean at least 4 cm above and over the selected cut site).	32 To prevent contamination of the sterile gloves.
33 Firmly clean this site at least 3 times for 30 seconds each time.	33 To prevent contamination of the site when cut (Gordon and Gardiner 2013).
34 Allow to air dry and visibly check that the catheter is completely dry.	
35 Holding onto the catheter with your fingers, taking care not to stretch it, carefully cut, ensuring the cut is as straight as possible. Also inspect the catheter to ensure that both inner and outer tubing are in alignment.	35 To enable a neat join with the catheter and stent.
36 The catheter can be trimmed if necessary to ensure the join is straight.	
37 Re-clean the end at least three times again, ensuring that any dried blood in the catheter is removed.	37 To minimise any further risk of infection from contamination.
38 Allow time for the cleaned catheter to completely air dry	38 To allow the chlorhexidine to work effectively and minimise any further risk of infection. The glue will not adhere/set if the catheter is wet.
39 Take the repair and insert the stent into the cut section, ensuring the inner tubing is not pushed up. Do not push the ends together fully at this time; leave a 2 mm gap.	39 Pushing up the inner lining means that the seal will not be intact and it will leak at the join.
40 With double and triple lumens, ensure that the correct sized stent is inserted into the corresponding hole.	40 Multi lumen catheters can have different diameters/stents within each lumen. Incorrect use will lead to weak joins/leakage.
41 Place a line of glue all the way around the join and push the two ends of the spliced segments of the catheter until they are flush together. Do not allow the repair and existing catheter to overlap or bulge up.	41 Positioning the repair in the centre correctly with no gaps at the repair site means that the repair will be better supported during use.

(continued)

Procedure guideline 14.24 Repair of a Broviac® or Hickman® (continued)

Statement	Rationale
42 Carefully slide the plastic sleeve up the catheter until the repair site is in the centre of the sleeve. The sleeve needs to be slid up the line: Avoid pulling the catheter from below as this will pull the repair apart. If needed, small amount of glue can be applied underneath the plastic sleeve at both ends to help the sleeve slide up.	
43 When the repair is centred, fill the sleeve with glue from both ends, starting by inserting the atraumatic needle up to where the two catheter sections join, and slowly retract the needle as the glue is gently squeezed in. When inserting the needle, ensure it is pointed against the sleeve and not the catheter. The sleeve needs to be completely filled with glue with no air bubbles. Take care not to overfill the sleeve.	43 To minimise air bubbles under the plastic stent. To prevent puncturing a hole in the catheter. Overfilling could cause the repair to be pushed apart.
44 Wipe off any excess glue from outside the plastic sleeve.	
45 Take the 2 ml syringe plunger and secure it to the plastic sleeve with the wound closure strips, ensuring that the plunger top is furthest away from the exit site. Do not place them over the repair site.	45 To provide support while the glue is setting. To allow clear visualisation of the repair site in case of any fluid/blood leaking out during use.
46 Carefully remove the clamps.	46 To prevent pulling.
47 Clean the skin with 2% chlorhexidine/70% isopropyl alcohol applicator and allow to dry.	47 To ensure adequate cleaning of the site and enable the product to work effectively.
48 Place a loop or 'S' in the catheter.	48 To support the catheter repair in case of accidental pulls.
49 Place a piece of dry gauze underneath the plunger end only and secure the plunger to the skin at each end with wound closure strips.	49 To prevent the plunger causing a pressure sore and allow clear visualisation of the repair site in case of any fluid/blood leaking out during use.
50 Use wound closure strips to secure the rest of the catheter in a loop/curve/S-shape onto the chest. Ensure they do not cover the exit site.	
51 Apply dressings, ensuring all parts of the catheter are secured up to the catheter clamps and the repair/plunger is completely sealed under the dressings.	51 To provide extra support while the glue is setting over the next 48 hours.
52 Access the repaired lumen(s) using ANTT®:	
53 Aspirate the lumen(s) first to obtain blood cultures. If unable to aspirate, try gently flushing with a small amount of 0.9% sodium chloride.	53 The risk of infection will have increased with a hole/break in the catheter.
54 Always observe the repair site when aspirating or flushing the catheter. Do not use any pressure when flushing the catheter(s) as this will push the repair apart or cause the 0.9% sodium chloride to leak out from the repair and flush away the glue.	54 To observe for signs of leakage.
55 If you are able, gently flush the catheter and lock it with the heparin 10 units in 1 ml.	
56 If you are unable to flush or aspirate the catheter, leave for at 4 hours and try again. You may need to gently instil Alteplase or similar thrombolytic at this point.	56 This time allows the glue to be initially set. Very minimal pressure must be used, otherwise the repair site can be pushed apart and/or the glue will be flushed out.
57 Place needle-free access device(s) on the ends of the lumens.	
58 Once completed, tuck away the CYP's CVAD.	58 To minimise risk of breakage or dislodgement.
59 Complete the procedure as per Procedure Guideline 14.1.B.	
60 Document the repair in the CYP's healthcare record. Inform any required parties, i.e. community teams, of the care required.	60 To maintain accurate documentation. Effective communication means that the repair will not be used incorrectly.

Remember:
- The Hickman® can be used for boluses after at least 1 hour and for infusions after at least 4 hours, allowing the glue to initially set, but ideally leave for at least 12 hours where feasible.
- The glue will take at least 48 hours to fully set.
- The plunger can be removed after 48 hours and the Hickman® cleaned and redressed as usual.

CVAD removal

Any CVAD should be removed when no longer indicated (Macklin 2010; O'Grady et al. 2011; Loveday et al. 2014). Noncuffed CVADs can be removed on the ward by competent healthcare professionals (Drewitt 2009), while cuffed CVADs and implanted devices should be removed within an interventional radiology or theatre environment.

PICC removal

When assessing whether to remove a PICC, it is important to consider how it is secured. PICCs may be secured with equipment that can be easily removed on the ward, e.g. sutures, a StatLock®, or via other methods, such as an internal cuff or devices such as a SecurAcath. With an internal cuff, local policy much be adhered to and the risks assessed as to whether these PICCs are removed with surgical support, to prevent internal catheter fracture during removal. If using a SecurAcath, knowledge of removal of these devices is vital to prevent complications (Hughes 2014).

Removal of noncuffed PICCs or tunnelled noncuffed CVCs is usually a straightforward procedure. The person removing the catheter must have knowledge of potential complications and be competent to safely remove these devices.

The same principles of removing a noncuffed PICC can be applied to removal of tunnelled noncuffed CVCs, short-term CVCs and temporary dialysis/apheresis catheters.

Potential complications may include
Bleeding

The CYP's platelet count and clotting history should be assessed to minimise any risk of prolonged bleeding. A platelet count ≥ 50 is advised to aid haemostasis (Kaye et al. 2000).

Correct digital pressure needs to be applied at the venous entry site. In PICCs, this will commonly be placed in the upper arm. For tunnelled noncuffed CVCs this will be at the neck (jugular) site and not the chest exit site. Short-term CVCs and temporary dialysis/apheresis catheters will be at the neck (jugular) or groin (femoral) site.

Venous spasm

Venous spasm can occur during removal, as the movement of the catheter through valves and curves can stimulate the smooth muscles in the tunica media to contract (Wall and Kierstead 1995).

If venous spasm occurs during PICC removal, i.e. resistance is felt, stop immediately. Tips to resolve the spasm include:

- Pausing the procedure for a few minutes (Braswell 2011).
- Gentle pulling; this may overcome the venous spasm, however, aggressive pulling can result in internal catheter fracture.
- Covering the PICC site with a dressing and placing a warm compress on the arm and waiting 10–20 minutes may relieve the spasm and allow safe removal of the PICC.

Persistent venous spasm may require referral to interventional radiology for removal.

Temporarily stuck PICC

In some cases, if the CYP is anxious, they may hold their breath; continually catch their breath while crying, or become tense while the PICC is being removed. This will cause them to tighten/clamp around the catheter, resulting in the PICC being resistant when being pulled. In this situation, temporarily stop the procedure and get the CYP to try and relax. Continue when they have relaxed sufficiently for you to pull out part or the rest of the catheter without any resistance. It is important that this is not confused with venous spasm and to remember that gentle pulling is used to prevent catheter fracture.

Thrombosis

A thrombus can form at the tip of the catheter or outside of the catheter on the vein wall. Signs include decreased catheter flow rates, resistance on flushing or aspiration, and swelling in the neck, forearm, and hand. PICC removal should not be undertaken unless this has been confirmed with the clinical team and the size/location of the thrombus has been confirmed by a venogram or ECHO.

Vagal reactions

Vagal reactions can be caused by emotional stress and worry about the procedure. Signs include pallor, cold sweats, nausea, sinus bradycardia, and hypotension leading to dizziness and fainting. If any of these symptoms occurs, stop the procedure and apply cold compresses to the neck and forehead of the CYP and keep them supine on the bed/cot. If there are any signs that the CYP is likely to be anxious, involvement of the play specialist and/or planned distraction techniques are essential before starting the procedure.

PICC catheter fracture (external or internal)

- External fracture: Hold onto the catheter immediately. It is still possible to remove the rest of the catheter. Continue the removal procedure, taking care not to cause any further fractures. If removal is not possible, apply a clamp or similar, to stop the catheter migrating into venous system, and cover the exit site with an occlusive dressing. Refer to a senior colleague or interventional radiology for advice and treatment.
- Internal fracture: This is a clinical emergency for catheter embolism. Place the CYP in the left lateral Trendelenburg position and administer oxygen. Immediate referral to interventional radiology is required for catheter removal. Signs and symptoms of a catheter embolism will include shortness of breath, pallor, tachycardia (rapid weak pulse), hypotension, chest pain, anxiety, and loss of consciousness (Simcock 2001).

Procedure guideline 14.25 Removal of a noncuffed PICC stitched in situ

Unless a PICC is being removed due to a suspected PICC infection, there is usually no indication to send off the tip for cultures for end of treatment removal. If the PICC is being removed due to a suspected infection, however, the tip should be sent for microscopy, culture, and sensitivity (MC&S)

Statement	Rationale
Prepare for the procedure as per Procedure Guideline 14.1 A.	
1 Gather equipment; this may include: • Two packs of sterile gauze swabs • Sterile stitch cutter • Sterile, well fitting gloves • Clear occlusive dressing	1 To ensure the procedure is undertaken efficiently and prevent later contamination of gloves.

(continued)

Procedure guideline 14.25 Removal of a noncuffed PICC stitched in situ *(continued)*

Statement	Rationale
2 If infection is suspected, to send the PICC tip for bacterial culture, gather additional equipment required: • 3 ml 2% chlorhexidine/70% isopropyl applicator • Sterile scissors • Specimen pot	
3 Perform hand hygiene.	3 To reduce possible hand contamination from collecting equipment.
4 Open out the sterile field or dressing pack and drop the required equipment onto the field without touching any of the sterile equipment. Pour the 0.5% Chlorhexidine in 70% denatured ethanol on the gauze swabs.	
5 Remove CYP's clothing, if necessary.	5 To allow easy access to the PICC for removal.
6 Ensure the CYP is lying supine on the bed/cot with the arm extended, as required, and clothing removed as needed.	6 To facilitate easy access in case of complications.
7 Remove dressing over the PICC.	
8 Perform hand hygiene.	8 To decontaminate hands from dressing removal.
9 Put on the well-fitting **sterile** gloves.	9 Close fitting gloves improve dexterity.
10 To send the PICC tip for bacterial culture: Pinch the 2% chlorhexidine/70%isopropyl alcohol applicator wings to 'pop' the enclosed ampoule to release the solution. Hold lollipop/sponge-side down to allow liquid to drain into the sponge applicator. a) Firmly press the applicator against the exit site for 10 seconds and then apply the ChlorPrep using firm, repeated up and down, then back and forth strokes for another 20–30 seconds around the area. b) Allow the skin to dry naturally. Do not dry the skin with sterile gauze.	a) To ensure adequate cleaning of the site and enable the product to work effectively. b) Allowing any cleaning solution to dry is vital for disinfection to be effective.
11 Using the stitch cutter, remove the two sutures securing the wings to the skin. Ensure the stitches are completely removed from the skin.	
12 Slowly start to gently pull out the PICC, then release, and use a hand-over-hand method, continue to gently remove the PICC, holding onto the catheter section as it exits the skin, and taking care not to stretch the catheter.	12 This technique allows greater control and reduces the risk of the PICC catheter snapping as minimal pressure is used.
13 As soon as the PICC is removed, press on the exit site and apply sufficient firm digital pressure for 5 minutes.	13 To achieve haemostasis.
14 To send the PICC tip for bacterial culture, try to minimise the PICC tip from touching the skin on removal. • Hang the tip of the PICC over the open specimen pot. • Get a colleague to cut the PICC with the sterile scissors, allowing the cut tip to drop into the pot without anyone touching the section to be sent.	14 To prevent skin flora contamination. To prevent any contamination from external sources.
15 After five minutes, gently lift the pad and check for any further bleeding. Reapply pad and digital pressure if subsequent bleeding is observed.	
16 Once haemostasis has been achieved, apply the small occlusive dressing to the site.	16 To allow review of the site for any signs of bleeding or infection.
17 Inspect the PICC to ensure the whole catheter is intact.	17 To ensure the whole catheter has been removed due to risk of catheter embolism.
18 Complete the procedure as per Procedure Guideline 14.1.B	
19 Document PICC removal in the CYP's healthcare record.	19 To maintain accurate records.

Neonatal longlines (PICCs); nursing management

This section describes the management and ongoing care of neonatal longlines or peripherally inserted central venous catheters (PICCs). For information regarding the care and management of all other central venous catheters, please see the previous sections in this chapter.

Introduction

A longline is a type of central venous line, which is a peripherally inserted central venous catheter (PICC), commonly used in neonates for central vascular access. They are inserted peripherally, via an upper or lower limb vein, and then threaded/tunnelled to the SVC if an upper limb vein is used (e.g. brachial or cephalic veins), or to the IVC if inserted via a lower limb vein (e.g. femoral or saphenous vein) (Lloreda-García et al. 2016). They are used in neonates due to the small lumen size of the catheter and can remain in situ for four to six weeks, making them ideal for long-term use.

Key points
There are specific key points to highlight regarding the care of neonatal longlines that differ from the care of other CVADs. This is due to the small lumen size of the catheters (Size 1–2 Fr).

When using these longlines:

- Never administer bolus fluids through the longline.
- Never administer blood products through the longline.
- Never aspirate from the longline.
- Always use a 10 ml luerlock syringe when accessing the longline.
- Always have an infusion of minimum 0.5 ml/hr running through the longline.

Duration of use should be discussed with the consultant on an individual basis, but typically, they can remain in situ for four to six weeks.

Confirmation of longline position
Confirmation of longline position can only be undertaken by performing a chest X-ray. As these longlines cannot be aspirated, checking for blood return is NOT a means of assessing longline position before use (Soe 2007).

The Department of Health (UK) (DH 2001) recommend that the line tip is placed OUTSIDE the heart, either in the superior (SVC) or inferior (IVC) vena cava, to avoid risks of cardiac tamponade. Cardiac tamponade can pose serious health risks and may result in death (Lloreda-García et al. 2016). This may occur if the position of the longline is intra-atrial. The position can only be confirmed by the medical team or specifically trained nurse practitioners. If the longline is in the incorrect position, the medical team or nurse practitioner team can pull it back by 1–2 cm. However, position complications will frequently require removal or replacement of the longline (Sharpe 2014; Lloreda-García et al. 2016).

Longline pressures
Due to the small lumen size, these longlines can run at extremely high pressures of between 100 and 300 mmhg, and it is important not to assume that the longline is blocked.

Types of longline used at GOSH
There are various types of longlines (PICC) used for neonates at GOSH. These are:

- Vygon Premicath (size 1 Fr)
- Vygon Nutriline PICC Line (size 2 Fr)
- Vygon Epicutaneo-Cava-Catheter (size 2 Fr)

The Vygon premicath Size 1 Fr, is specifically designed for patients who require the smallest size catheter available, typically babies less than 1 kg in weight. This catheter is made of polyurethane.

The Vygon Nutriline PICC Line, (size 2 Fr): is also a polyurethane catheter, but with a larger diameter.

Advantages of polyurethane include:
- Easier catheter placement
- Higher pressure tolerance and burst strengths
- Greater flow rates achieved over silicone catheters

Disadvantages of polyurethane include:
- Greater risk of vessel irritation
- Greater risk of perforation

The Vygon Epicutaneo-Cava-Catheter is a size 2 Fr silicone catheter typically used for those >1 kg.

Advantages of silicone include:
- Soft lumen, therefore less trauma and irritation caused to vessel
- Greater resistance to cracking or snapping of catheters

Disadvantages of silicone include:
- Higher difficulty of insertion
- Lower pressure tolerance and burst strengths
- Higher incidence of catheters blocking

(Corzine and Willett 2010).

Risks and complications
The presence of a neonatal longline has risks, which include:

- Vascular compromise
- Pleural and pericardial effusion
- Cardiac tamponade
- Occlusion/obstruction of the vessel
- Thrombosis
- Catheter-related sepsis
- Tip migration
- Leakage and breakage

Ongoing care and maintenance of longlines to maintain patency and reduce the risk of complications
As per manufacturers guidelines, due to the small lumen sizes of these longlines (size 1 Fr and size 2 Fr) there are essential aspects of care which must be undertaken to reduce the risks of complications, e.g. line occlusion, bursting, and snapping of the catheters.

Essential instructions for use
- **Never administer bolus fluids through the catheter:**
  - This may result in the catheter bursting due to the low pressure tolerance and burst strengths of the longline.
- **Never administer blood products through the catheter:**
  - Due to the small lumen size, blood products may clot and occlude the longline.
- **Never aspirate from the catheter:**
  - Due to the soft lumen, this may result in trauma or vessel irritation.
- **Always ensure an infusion of a minimum 0.5 ml/hr running through the longline:**
  - To reduce the risk of the longline occluding. This can be via a syringe pump or infusion pump.

N.B. Longlines may be flushed when assessing for patency if occlusion suspected. These longlines are stiff to flush and this can often be mistaken for the longline being blocked. If flushing the longline, no more than 1 ml volume should be used and a 10 ml luerlock syringe must be used to ensure that the optimal pressure is achieved.

(Petit and Wyckoff 2007)

Accessing the Longline
Principles of asepsis must be adhered to whenever the longline is accessed to administer a medication or to change and existing infusion. An ANTT® must be used. Refer to the Procedure Guideline 14.1 ANTT® for Intravenous Therapy for more information.

Prior to accessing the longline, adequate decontamination of the hub as per CVAD clinical guideline is essential. 2% chlorhexidine in 70% isopropyl alcohol wipes should be used to clean the hubs of venous access devices and the needle-free access devices for 30 seconds with friction and then allow hub to dry for a further 30 seconds to let alcohol sufficiently evaporate. Infusions may then be connected.

NB: As these longlines cannot be aspirated, checking for blood return is NOT a means of assessing longline position before use. This can be undertaken only by chest X-ray.

Dressing Changes

Longline/PICC exit site dressings provide a protective barrier for the catheter entrance site. An effective dressing will minimise the risk of longline migration, leakage, breakage, and CRBSIs (Gustafon 2010).

These longlines have low infection rates and low risks of complications, so it is recommended that dressing changes are not performed routinely, but only changed 'as required' (Sharpe and Pettit 2013). The need to change a dressing should be determined by visually assessing the site and identifying whether the line or skin integrity is at risk.

Indications for dressing change include:

- The dressing integrity appears affected or is lifting.
- If the hub or any part of the entrance site of the longline has become exposed.
- If the loop has become uncoiled or is pulling and the longline position may be compromised.
- If the longline or skin is visibly dirty or oozing blood/serous fluid where it is affecting the dressing integrity.
- If it appears to have any signs of infection, such as redness, swelling, purulent ooze.

The site must be regularly assessed for signs of:

- Redness
- Swelling
- Oozing
- Phlebitis
- Tracking

The assessment should be recorded in the CYP's healthcare record. Equipment needed for dressing change:

- New dressing (e.g. IV3000)
- Aprons and gloves
- ChloraPrep applicator
- Adhesive remover wipes (e.g. Appeel®)
- Sterile wound closure strips (e.g. Steri-Strips)
- Pack of sterile gauze
- 0.9% sodium chloride

Procedure guideline 14.26 Neonatal longline dressing change

Statement	Rationale
1 Ensure safe environment before approaching the patient, and plan suitable time for dressing change.	1 To minimise adverse effects and to enable clustering of cares to reduce handling of the baby.
2 Prepare for the procedure as per Procedure Guideline 14.1.A	
3 A two-nurse technique should be used; one to perform the dressing change and one to assist.	3 To allocate roles for each nurse to reduce the risk of infection and accidental longline displacement during the dressing change.
4 Gather equipment: • New dressing (e.g.IV3000) • Aprons and gloves • Sterile 2% chlorhexadine gluconate/70% isopropyl alcohol (ChloraPrep) applicator • Adhesive remover wipes (e.g. AppeelR) • Sterile wound closure strips (e.g. Steri-Strips) • Pack of sterile gauze • 0.9% sodium chloride	4 To ensure the procedure can be performed safely.
5 Both nurses must don aprons and perform hand hygiene.	5 To minimise the risk of infection.
6 The assisting nurse should clean and prepare the surface of trolley being used for procedure using sanitising wipes and allowing this to dry. Hand hygiene should again be performed.	6 To reduce the risk of catheter related blood stream infection or sepsis and to ensure aseptic environment.
7 Aseptic nontouch technique must be used at all times (see section titled Aseptic Nontouch Technique (ANTT®) for Intravenous Therapy). Gloves should be applied.	7 To ensure aseptic environment.
8 Adhesive remover wipes (e.g. Appeel) should be used to loosen the adhesive from the old dressing. The old dressing should be removed very carefully, while holding the stabilising wing on the catheter. It should be peeled from the outside toward the insertion site.	8 To protect skin integrity and prevent catheter dislodgement, or breakage of the longline.
9 Remove the old steristrips.	
10 The insertion site should be closely observed and specific position of length of insertion noted, oozing, or for signs of infection.	10 To prevent movement of catheter position or identify is this occurs.
11 The site should be cleaned using a 2% Chlorhexidine gluconate 70% isopropyl alcohol applicator (e.g. ChloraPrep™) in up and down motions beginning from the insertion site and moving outwards.	11 This prevents movement of microorganisms toward the insertion site. Chlorhexidine is recommended by manufacturers. ChloraPrep™ is not licenced for use on infants below the age of two months but has been approved locally as the product of choice for skin decontamination on all children with intact skin including those below 32 weeks gestation and less than 2 weeks of life.
12 For babies < 30 weeks gestation chlorhexidine 0.5% alcohol free topical solution should be used for skin prep.	12 To minimise the risk of chemical skin burns.

Procedure guideline 14.26 Neonatal longline dressing change (continued)

Statement	Rationale
13 The skin must be allowed to dry for a minimum of 30 seconds.	13 Asepsis is much more effective if the skin is adequately dry post cleaning.
14 Proceed to loop or coil the longline and place on surface of skin.	14 To give allowance for unintended movement or pulling of the line.
15 A small square of sterile gauze or duoderm® should be placed under the stabilisation hub.	15 To protect skin integrity.
16 Place a wound closure strip (e.g. Steri-strip®) over loop and entrance site and place another strip over the stabilisation hub (see Figure 14.5).	16 To secure loop to skin and to secure stabilisation hub.
17 Visually assess site by observing the markings on the longline and ensure skin integrity remains intact.	17 To ensure line has not been dislodged and skin is intact.
18 Cover the longline, including all of the thin segment and the stabilisation wing with a semipermeable transparent dressing (e.g. IV 3000®/Tegaderm®), being careful not to encircle the limb (see Figure 14.5).	18 To secure line to prevent migration, dislodgement and breaking. A clear dressing is used to allow for constant revaluation of the insertion site. Encircling the limb with a dressing may compromise perfusion.
19 Document dressing change and observation of site in healthcare record.	19 To maintain accurate records and ensure effective communication.
20 Complete the procedure as per Procedure Guideline 14.1.B	

Source: Hill et al. (2010), Sharpe (2014) and Ullman et al. (2015).

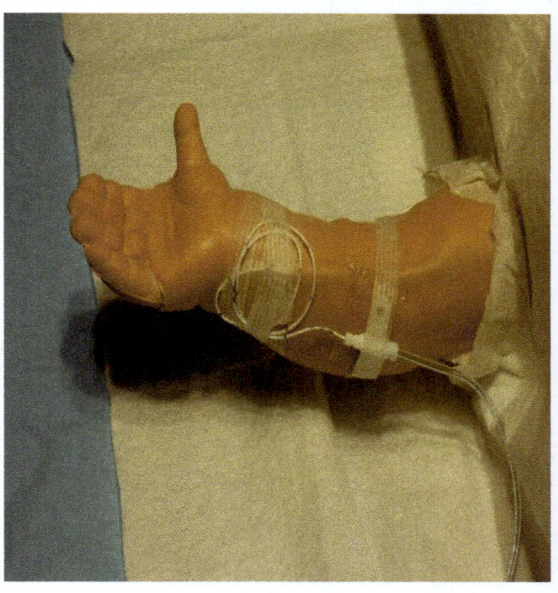

Figure 14.5 Securing a neonatal longline. *Source:* Courtesy of Dr Rashmi Gandhi, Neonatal Consultant, King's College Hospital.

Procedure guideline 14.27 Neonatal longlines: nursing care (general)

Statement	Rationale
1 **Documentation:** All longline (PICC) care should be documented.	1 To ensure clear and accurate records (NMC 2015).
2 Regular observations and routine assessments should be clearly and concisely documented in the healthcare record to include: • Longline type and date of insertion • Size of longline inserted • Length of longline inserted • Visual infusion phlebitis (VIP) score • Dressing information including time and date last changed • Observation of entry site at each dressing change	
3 Catheter Breakage: A broken catheter must be removed and replaced.	3 These longlines cannot be repaired.

Procedure guideline 14.28 Removal of neonatal longlines

Statement	Rationale
4 Removal of longlines must be discussed with the consultant and removed by a health care professional who is trained and competent to do so.	4 To minimise complications: These longlines pose a high risk of breaking or snapping.
5 The catheter should be removed in small stages, approx. 1 cm at a time, with pauses in between. Steady and gentle traction should be used, starting at the insertion site. The process should take approx. 60 seconds.	5 To reduce the risk of pulling and stretching the longline, putting it at risk of breaking. Pulling the longline at 1 cm intervals and pausing intermittently will allow the longline to recoil if it's been stretched.
6 No pressure should be applied at insertion site when removing the longline (Vygon 2012).	6 This increases the risk of spasm, thrombosis or occlusion, making it more difficult to remove the longline.

Arterial lines

An arterial line is an invasive cannula inserted into an artery. It is used for continuous accurate monitoring of blood pressure, frequent blood sampling, especially for arterial blood gas analysis, in theatre, intensive and high-dependency care settings, as well as during interhospital transfers. It is normally sited in the radial, femoral, or axillary artery using percutaneous puncture. The umbilical artery may be used in newborns, but the care and management of these are not covered in these guidelines.

The use of heparin to maintain the patency of arterial lines is a topic of extensive discussion. While studies in adults suggest it offers no advantages over 0.9% sodium chloride further research in paediatrics is required (NPSA 2008a, b; Dixon and Crawford 2012; Robertson-Malt et al. 2014). At GOSH, patency of the arterial cannula is maintained with an infusion of 0.9% sodium chloride, and 1 unit of heparin per ml (BNF 2021; Robertson-Malt et al. 2014). Heparin can be omitted in patients with severe bleeding disorders and 0.45% sodium chloride can be used in patients with high serum sodium and neonates, (NPSA 2008a). Drugs and hypertonic solutions must never be given via an arterial line as these can cause severe tissue necrosis in high concentrations (Cardinal et al. 2000; NPSA 2008a,b; Woodrow 2009). Arterial lines must therefore be clearly labelled and the cannula site needs to be exposed and continually monitored. The CYP should never be left unattended, as any bleeding or disconnection must be quickly identified.

The arterial line is connected to a transducer and haemodynamic monitor. The transducer converts the arterial pulsatile oscillations into kinetic energy, which is displayed as an electrical waveform on the monitor, (Esper and Pinsky 2014). Arterial waveform analysis can provide valuable diagnostic information as well as the absolute systolic and diastolic pressure (Hazinski 2013; Esper and Pinsky 2014). The blood pressure recordings may be correlated with noninvasive blood pressure recording, as required or according to local policy. However, invasive monitoring is normally more accurate, especially in the critically ill and will produce readings 5–10 mmHg higher than noninvasive measurements (Woodrow 2009).

All those involved in the siting and management of arterial cannula must be trained and competent in the techniques involved.

Procedure guideline 14.29 Intra-arterial lines: preparation of child and family

Statement	Rationale
1 a) Explanation and preparation to the CYP and family should be included as part of the whole preoperative preparation. b) In emergency situations explanations may need to be repeated after the initial resuscitation process. The CYP is often anaesthetised or heavily sedated during insertion, but if not, some restraint or therapeutic holding may be necessary; for more information see Chapter 19: Moving and Handling.	1 a) To ensure they understand the reason for the procedure and can give informed consent. b) Effective preparation demonstrates a means of promoting coping behaviours and reducing stress levels (Twycross et al. 2014).
2 Explain the procedure to the CYP and family, avoiding medical jargon, including the following: • That a cannula is necessary • The reason for the cannula • What it entails • The potential risk of the cannula • The length of time it is likely to be in situ	2 To comfort a conscious CYP, minimise distress and optimise treatment outcomes, (Jaaniste et al. 2007). To provide a safe environment. Well-informed parents are more likely to stay calm and support their CYP (APAGBI 2012; Royal College of Anaethetists (RCoA) 2022).
3 The parents/carers may be present but they should be given the option of leaving if they prefer. The practitioner inserting the cannula must be comfortable and willing to perform the procedure in the parents'/carers' presence.	3 Being present with their CYP through a difficult procedure should be negotiated.
4 Appropriate methods of distraction may be required for the semiconscious CYP.	4 To prevent the CYP's whole attention being centred on the invasive procedure (APAGBI 2012; RCoA 2022).

Procedure guideline 14.30 Insertion of an intra-arterial line

Statement	Rationale
1 Only a suitably trained and competent practitioner should undertake arterial cannulation.	1 To ensure the procedure is carried out safely and correctly.
2 Prepare for the procedure as per Procedure Guideline 14.1.A. An ANTT® should be employed throughout the procedure. Standard precautions must be adhered to. An apron, gloves and eye protection should be worn.	2 To minimise the risk of infection (DH 2007; Rowley and Clare 2011; NICE 2012; Loveday et al. 2014).
3 Prepare the following equipment on a clean surface or tray: • Dressing pack • 0.9% sodium chloride for injection • 2 ml syringes • 5 ml syringe • 21 G needles • cannula, appropriate gauge • short low compliance extension tubing • Three-way tap • 2% Chlorhexidine in 70% isopropyl alcohol applicator (e.g. ChloraPrep™) • Lidocaine 1% • Skin closure strips • Transparent dressing • Disposable splint	3 To ensure equipment is readily available and reduce risk of infection (Garretson 2005; O'Grady et al. 2011; Loveday et al. 2014).
4 Select the most appropriate artery to cannulate; in children the radial artery is preferred, but femoral or axillary arteries may be used. Ultrasound guidance can be used where possible.	4 There is a reduced risk of infection compared with femoral access (Garretson 2005; Danckers et al. 2022). Collateral blood supplied to hand by the ulnar artery. To prevent multiple attempts at cannulation (Aouad-Maroun et al 2016).
5 The brachial artery is not recommended if other sites are available and the ulnar or posterior tibial vessels are not used.	5 The brachial artery is difficult to immobilise with risk of nerve damage, (Dixon and Crawford 2012). Cannulation of the ipsilateral radial or dorsalis pedis may result in the development of digital ischaemia (Woodrow 2009).
6 Arterial cannulae are usually sited in sedated or anaesthetised CYPs, however if an arterial line is being considered in an awake CYP intravenous analgesia and sedation may be required, including infiltration of the area with lidocaine 1% (Advanced Life Support Group 2016).	6 To reduce pain and fear and to ensure the patient remains still. Topical anaesthesia may be ineffective for arterial puncture and administration of local analgesia can be painful (APAGBI 2012; Danckers et al. 2022; RCoA 2022).
7 Perform an Allen's test before using the radial artery to check that an ulnar artery is present and patent: • Occlude both arteries at the wrist. • Release the pressure on the ulnar artery. • Observe the circulation returning to the hand, i.e. that it will flush pink. If this does not happen, do not proceed with a radial puncture on that side.	7 To ensure an adequate circulation is maintained (Perrin and MacLeod 2013; Advanced Life Support Group 2016). There are some discussions around the use of an Allen's test but it is still recommended in paediatrics.
8 Seek the assistance of a colleague with the securing of the line and to position the CYP as follows: • Radial artery: Hyperextend and restrain the wrist over a small roll. • Femoral artery: Elevate buttocks with a small roll. • Axillary artery: Arm abducted to 90 degrees with the hand near the ear or above the head. Place rolled up towel under the chest to rotate the axilla upwards. Consider ultrasound guidance with cannulation.	8 To provide better access and maximise the success of the procedure (Ishii et al. 2013; Aouad-Maroun et al 2016).
9 Identify the vessel by palpation.	9 To ensure it is suitable and can be found.
10 Perform hand hygiene.	10–13 To minimise the risk of infection.
11 Put on protective clothing including sterile gloves and eye protection.	
12 Establish a sterile field around the chosen cannulation site.	
13 Disinfect the skin at intended cannulation site with the 2% chlorhexidine and 70% isopropyl alcohol applicator (e.g. ChloraPrep™), using firm repeated up and down and then back and forth strokes for at least 30 seconds and allow to dry for 30 seconds.	
14 a) **Unless the CYP is anaesthetised or a neonate, infiltrate the skin with a very small volume of 1% lidocaine. This is not required in the anaesthetised CYP and is contra-indicated in neonates.** b) **Topical anaesthesia can be used safely in premature neonates from 28 weeks gestation.**	14 To minimise pain. b) Lidocaine can cause cardiac arrhythmias in neonates (APAGBI 2012).

(continued)

Procedure guideline 14.30 Insertion of an intra-arterial line *(continued)*

Statement	Rationale
15 Examine the cannula for faults and attach a 2 ml syringe.	15 To ensure it will meet its purpose.
16 Gently stretch the skin over the artery.	16 To immobilise the vein.
17 Break the skin with a sterile lancet or 21 G needle.	17 For ease of cannula insertion; an inadequate skin nick may cause significant resistance.
18 Insert the cannula through the skin parallel to the vessel at an approach angle of 45° and advance it slowly.	
19 If the vessel is not entered, pull back slowly as an artery may be transfixed. If so advance after flashback of blood. If not pull back the skin and redirect, so that the needle does not become blocked thus preventing adequate flashback.	
20 When the artery is punctured, blood will be seen to pulsate in the syringe.	
21 Collect the required amount of blood in the syringe for analysis.	
22 Decrease the angle of the cannula so that it is resting on the skin and withdraw the stylet slightly.	
23 A second flashback of blood will be observed up the shaft of the cannula, blood may rush back or be easily aspirated.	
24 Slowly advance the cannula over the needle and into the artery.	24 To ensure the cannula is correctly inserted and patent.
25 If the artery is entered but the catheter cannot be fully advanced, a guide wire, (e.g. Cook™ positive placement wire or a kimal™ guide wire) (size 0.18 for a 22 G cannula) may help.	
26 Never re-advance the needle into the cannula.	26 There is a risk of puncturing the cannula and embolising the tip.
27 During attempted arterial cannulation sluggish backflow indicates either inadvertent venous cannulation or para-arterial placement, i.e. a haematoma.	
28 Press firmly on the artery to occlude the blood flow, keep the cannula in position and withdraw the stylet.	
29 Continuing to protect the cannula, connect a 5 ml syringe and flush with 0.9% sodium chloride.	29 To prevent clotting and to check the patency of the line.
30 Check the site for swelling and skin blanching.	30 To ensure prompt detection of extravasation.
31 Occlude the artery, remove the syringe and attach low compliance tubing primed with heparinised 0.9% sodium chloride.	31 To avoid blood loss from the cannula.
32 Taking care at all times to protect the cannula, apply 2 × 1 cm skin closures, e.g. Steri-strips, a sterile occlusive transparent dressing. Some additional secure strapping of the tubing may be required to ensure adequate fixation while maintaining good site visualisation.	32 To facilitate observation of the cannula site and reduce the risk of infection (Woodrow 2009; Hazinski 2013).
33 If required, apply an appropriate sized splint, ensuring the cannula remains visible for regular inspection. Radial lines should be splinted with the wrist extended.	33 To prevent movement, which may cause extravasation, phlebitis or cannula damage (Hazinski 2013).
34 Attach the arterial line set to the transducer and monitor.	
35 Calibrate the transducer following the manufacturer's instructions (see maintenance: calibration).	35 To ensure accurate monitoring of blood pressure.
36 Observe arterial trace on the monitor for appropriate waveform.	
37 Set appropriate alarm limits on the monitor.	37 To maintain patient safety.
38 Complete the procedure as per Procedure Guideline 14.1.B.	
39 Dispose of all used equipment correctly according to local disposal of used sharps policy.	39 To minimise risk of sharps injury.
40 Perform hand hygiene	40 To minimise risk of cross-infection.
41 Document cannulation in the CYP's healthcare records.	41 To maintain an accurate record.
42 Following this procedure, time should be taken to give comfort and positive feedback to the aware CYP and the parents/carers.	42 To reassure them and acknowledge the parents/carers contribution.

Procedure guideline 14.31 Preparation: system setup (inter-arterial infusion)

Statement	Rationale
1 There are two delivery methods of intra-arterial infusion available, which provide different levels of accuracy of fluid administration (Hazinski 2013). a) An optimal system that uses a syringe pump with a variable pressure alarm. b) A nonoptimal system that uses a high-pressure bag with manual pressure gauge; this does not allow for accurate documentation of fluid administered each hour (Hazinski 2013).	1 To maintain catheter patency. a) To be used when small volumes and/or very accurate fluid intake is required, e.g. neonates, infants less than 10kg, and intensive care patients. b) To be used where a moderately accurate record of fluid administration is sufficient, e.g. peri-operative procedures and children 10kg and over.
2 The following equipment should be gathered: a) Haemodynamic monitoring system (monitor) b) Arterial line set c) Heparinised 0.9% sodium chloride d) Transducer e) Pressure bag or syringe pump, dispensing pin, and 50ml syringe f) Clean tray	2 To set up the system: a) An alarm monitor for prompt detection of occlusion and for blood pressure monitoring is required. b) To maintain patency (BNF 2021).
3 Check the arterial pressure monitoring system for any faults or loose connections.	3 To avoid accidental disconnection.
4 Using aseptic nontouch technique (ANTT®), prime the system thoroughly with heparinised 0.9% sodium chloride or the prescribed approved fluid. Ensure that: a) Air is thoroughly removed. b) All connections are well secured. c) All ports are primed. d) The system is clearly labelled. e) Complete appropriate safety checks on prescribed fluid and patient.	4 To prevent air embolism and minimise errors. a) To prepare the line b) Air in low compliant tubing, or loose connections can cause a dampened waveform, leading to inaccurate pressure readings.

Procedure guideline 14.32 Maintenance: calibration

Statement	Rationale
1 The transducer must be calibrated following the insertion of an arterial line, at the beginning of a shift, when the CYP's position is changed, or when an intra-arterial line has been accessed.	1 To ensure the haemodynamic measurements are accurate. A change in position or any intervention with the monitoring system may affect the accuracy of measurements (Hazinski 2013; Esper and Pinsky 2014; Chambers et al 2019).
2 For calibration the transducer must be level with the right atrium.	2 To ensure accurate measurement of intra-arterial pressures (Garretson 2005; Hazinski 2013).
3 Using the mid-clavicle as a guide, locate the fourth intercostal space and follow this space across the chest wall to the mid-axillary line. This is called the phlebostatic axis (Hazinski 2013).	3 To landmark the right atrium (Hazinski 2013).
4 The CYP can be either lying flat or their head elevated by not more than 45°.	4 The right atrium and the phlebostatic axis remain constant up to a 45° (Perrin and MacLeod 2017).
5 Level the transducer at the phlebostatic axis.	5 To obtain and accurate invasive pressure measurement, (Perrin and MacLeod 2017).
6 Silence alarms.	6 To prevent occlusion or pressure alarms.
7 Turn the three-way tap off to the CYP.	7 To isolate the transducer for calibration.
8 Turn the three-way tap on to the atmosphere (air).	8 To calibrate to atmospheric pressure.
9 Press the zero key on the monitor. When the monitor indicates that the process is complete close the three-way tap to the atmosphere and open the three-way tap to the CYP.	9 To calibrate to atmospheric pressure.
10 Select a suitable waveform scale on the monitor.	10 To provide a clear arterial pressure trace.
11 Select correct monitor label.	11 To identify which pressure is being monitored.
12 Select appropriate upper and lower alarm limits for the CYP's age and condition.	12 To alert the practitioner to any significant changes.

Procedure guideline 14.33 Maintenance: maintaining patency

Statement	Rationale
1 A continuous intravascular pressurised infusion should be maintained through the cannula.	1 To keep the cannula patent. To reduce risk of backflow into the monitoring system (Hazinski 2013).
2 Intermittent irrigation is not recommended.	2 To reduce the risk of obstruction, clotting and loss of access, (Woodrow 2009).
3 Heparinised 0.9% sodium chloride or an approved fluid should be prescribed and continually infused.	3 The debate regarding the most appropriate solution to maintain arterial patency is ongoing; current practice at GOSH supports the use of heparinised saline to maintain patency of arterial lines, (Robertson-Malt et al. 2014).
4 Heparin may be omitted especially in patients with severe bleeding disorders.	4 To reduce risk of haemorrhage and contamination of blood samples (Anand 2008; Del Cotillo et al. 2008; Leslie et al. 2013; Robertson-Malt et al. 2014).

Procedure guideline 14.34 Maintenance: observations

Statement	Rationale
1 Check the monitor is set to display the arterial pressure trace and numerical values.	1 To ensure accurate and continuous monitoring of the arterial blood pressure.
2 Check for a normal waveform, which should have a sharp peak systole upstroke, a clear dicrotic notch and a definite end diastole (Hazinski 2013 Esper and Pinsky 2014; Chambers et al, 2019).	2 To ensure accurate and continuous monitoring of the arterial blood pressure.
3 Record volume of fluid administered via the line each hour on the CYP's fluid balance chart.	3 To maintain accurate records.
4 a) The cannula site must be exposed and observed by a competent practitioner. b) The patient must not be left unattended.	4 a) To check for adequate blood supply. b) To reduce the risk of cannula dislodgement or loss of patency and to reduce risk of blood loss due to disconnection.
5 Any abnormalities must be reported to medical staff immediately.	5 The cannula may need to be replaced.
6 The circulation of the cannulated limb should be continuously monitored for signs of the following: Cyanosis, decreased pulse, blanching, cool extremities, sluggish capillary refill or bleeding.	6 To detect reduced circulation distal to the cannula site, arterial spasm or clot formation (Garretson 2005; Woodrow 2009; Hazinski 2013; Perrin and MacLeod 2017).
7 The cannula must be removed if the circulation is compromised.	7 To maintain circulation to the limb (Dixon and Crawford 2012).
8 Observe for signs of cannula displacement including swelling, bleeding, lack of a normal arterial waveform, fluid leakage, blanching, or pain or discomfort.	8 To maintain patient safety and comfort (Dixon and Crawford 2012, Jevon et al. 2012).
9 Observe the tissues around the cannula for signs of infection, including pain, redness, pus, temperature change, and swelling.	9 For prompt recognition and management of signs of infection, (Jevon et al. 2012).
10 Observe for bleeding around cannula due to cannula movement within the vessel (a normal arterial waveform will be displayed on the monitor).	10 For prompt recognition of complications.
11 Ensure cannula is secure, immobilised with a splint if necessary, and that the site is visible at all times.	11 To prevent dislodgement and maintain cannula.
12 If necessary, clean the site and re-secure the dressing when bleeding has stopped.	12 To minimise risk of infection and prevent risk of retained cannula (NPSA 2008a).
13 Accidental removal of the arterial cannula will require the immediate application of pressure to the site for 5–15 minutes or until bleeding has stopped. The site should be covered with a sterile pressure dressing until bleeding has stopped (Burns and Chulay 2014).	13 To prevent blood loss.
14 The administration set and tubing must be checked for unsecure connections and kinks in the tubing.	14 To ensure there are no loose connections, avoid line occlusion and ensure that accurate pressure readings are displayed (Esper and Pinsky, 2014).

Procedure guideline 14.34 Maintenance: observations (continued)

Statement	Rationale
15 Perform hourly assessment of the continuous infusion and for normal pressures within the infusion device.	15 The pressure bag may deflate.
16 Monitor the general condition of the CYP; any pyrexia should be investigated and acted on according to local policy.	16 To detect signs of cannula related infection; antibiotics may be required (Garretson 2005; Burns and Chulay Burns and chulay, (2014)).
17 The cannula should be re-sited when clinically indicated, e.g. signs of inflammation, pyrexia, or positive blood cultures.	17 Micro-organisms in the cannula may have been flushed into the circulation.
18 The transducer system and prescribed fluid should be changed every 72 hours to prevent bacterial growth (Burns and Chulay 2014). If an optimal system that uses a syringe pump is being used the prescribed fluid should be changed every 24 hours.	18 To reduce the risk of infection (Burns and Chulay 2014).
19 All observations must be recorded in the CYP's healthcare records.	19 To maintain an accurate record.

Procedure guideline 14.35 Blood sampling (arterial)

Statement	Rationale
1 Prepare the CYP and family by explaining: • That a blood sample is required. • What the procedure will entail. • The implications of any results. • When the results will be available.	1 To ensure they understand the reason for the procedure and can give informed consent, (De Lourdes et al. 2003; APAGBI 2012; NMC 2015; RCoA 2022).
2 The CYP may require play or distraction during the procedure.	2 To minimise anxiety (Jaaniste et al. 2007; APAGBI 2012; Hazinski 2013; Twycross et al. 2014).
Prepare for the procedure as per Procedure Guideline 14.1.A	
3 Depending on the blood tests required, gather suitable equipment, for example: • Clean plastic tray • Blood bottles • 1 × 2–5 ml syringe (for dead space) • 1 × 2–10 ml syringe for blood samples required • Wipes impregnated with 2% chlorhexidine in 70% alcohol sterile hubcap • Syringe cap • Protective paper sheet or towel • Nonsterile gloves	3 To minimise infection risk (NICE 2012; Loveday et al. 2014).
4 Prepare working surface, perform hand hygiene.	4 To minimise infection risk.
5 Standard precautions must be adopted when blood sampling from an arterial line including gloves, eye protection and an apron should be worn (Rowley and Clare 2011; Loveday et al. 2014).	5 To minimise infection risk and risk of cross infection (Rowley and Clare 2011; Loveday et al. 2014).
6 An aseptic nontouch technique should be used.	6 To minimise infection risk.
7 If it is difficult to obtain blood, seek assistance from a doctor or an experienced practitioner.	7 To avoid artery damage or occlusion.
8 Apply non sterile gloves.	8 To adhere to ANTT® and minimise the risk on infection
9 Stop infusion line, clamp pressure bag and silence alarms.	9 To prevent occlusion or pressure alarms. A continuing alarm disturbs patients and others (Xie et al. 2009).
10 Remove cap from sampling port and clean hub for 15 seconds with 2% chlorhexidine in 70% isopropyl alcohol wipe and allow to dry naturally.	10 To ensure adequate cleaning of the device minimising risk of infection.
11 Connect a 2–5 ml syringe.	
12 Open the three-way tap to CYP and syringe and withdraw a minimum of 3 ml dead space.	12 To clear the system of heparin, old blood and small emboli (Woodrow 2009).
13 Turn the three-way tap off to hub/ CYP /infusion.	
14 Remove the syringe and place on a clean tray.	

(continued)

The Great Ormond Street Hospital Manual of Children and Young People's Nursing Practices

Procedure guideline 14.35 Blood sampling (arterial) *(continued)*

Statement	Rationale
15 Reaccess the device using a 2–10ml syringe or Monovette™ system.	15 To enable sample to be taken.
16 Open three-way tap to CYP and syringe.	
17 Withdraw required quantity of blood.	
18 Turn the three-way tap off to the hub and remove syringe containing blood sample and place cap on the sample.	18 To prevent backflow of blood, movement of infusion fluid, and minimise blood loss (Hazinski 2013).
19 Replace dead space fluid slowly, if free of blood clots or debris. Leave syringe in hub.	19 To reduce risk of arterial spasm or irritation and may result in retrograde arterial flow. To minimise unnecessary blood loss and iatrogenic anaemia (Andrews and Waterman 2008; Hazinski 2013).
20 Turn off the three-way tap to the CYP and open to syringe and infusion press purge and release flow limiting valve to clear hub.	20 To prevent blood collection in hub.
21 Turn three-way tap off to hub and open to infusion and CYP.	
22 Close hub and cover with a sterile hub.	
23 Flush the line from the infusion device to clear any blood.	23 Blood left in a line could cause a dampened trace with lower blood pressure readings and occlude the cannula (Hazinski 2013; Esper and Pinsky 2014; Chambers et al, 2019).
24 Observe site for any blanching.	24 Can be present with excessive pressure used to flush the line however can indicate early recognition of compromise to the limb (Dixon and Crawford 2012).
25 Ensure infusion is turned on and unclamped.	
26 Switch all alarms back on.	
27 Observe monitor for normal trace.	
28 Ensure arterial line is secure.	28 To maintain cannula patency and reduce risk of dislodgment.
29 Complete the Procedure as per Procedure Guideline 14.1.B.	
30 Perform bedside blood analysis tests and/or send samples for laboratory analysis.	
31 Remove PPE and perform hand hygiene.	31 To reduce risk of infection.
32 Record blood samples taken in the CYP's healthcare records.	32 To maintain an accurate record.

Procedure guideline 14.36 Troubleshooting: dampened trace

Statement	Rationale
1 Assess and report changes in the CYP's cardiovascular status, including pulse check, ECG waveform, pulse oximetry, and noninvasive blood pressure.	1 To monitor for inadequate or absent cardiac output (pulseless electrical activity) or low blood pressure requiring treatment.
2 Check arterial line site, connections and infusion flow rate.	2 To prevent backflow of blood into line caused by the CYPs arterial pressure exceeding the flush pressure (Hazinski 2013).
3 Check appropriate arterial scale is in use on monitor.	
4 Check arterial line set for clots, air, and back-flow of blood and change entire system if necessary.	4 To prevent dampened trace and ensure accurate pressure readings (Esper and Pinsky, 2014).
5 Check that blood can easily be aspirated at access port.	5 Occlusion may be due to a blood clot (Burns and Chulay 2014).
6 Attempt to aspirate any clot, using a 2ml syringe.	6 To clear line occlusion.
7 Do not forcefully flush the catheter if resistance is high.	7 This may traumatise vessel, release clot, and damage local blood circulation.
8 Redress cannula site; check for kinks or poor positioning of the cannula.	8 To clear line occlusion.
9 Reposition the CYP and/or their cannulated limb.	9 To clear line occlusion if catheter tip is resting against vessel wall (Hazinski 2013).

Chapter 14 Intravenous and intra-arterial access and infusions

Procedure guideline 14.37 Troubleshooting: abnormal readings

Statement	Rationale
1 Abnormally high or low readings must be investigated promptly and any change in the CYP's condition reported immediately to medical staff.	1 Patient safety is paramount.
2 Assess the CYP's cardiovascular status, including pulse check, ECG waveform, pulse oximetry and noninvasive blood pressure	2 To determine whether there is a monitoring problem or a real change in the CYP's condition: Changes in arterial waveform frequently reflect pathological changes in the CYP's condition that require urgent medical treatment, for example, hypovolaemia, cardiac compromise, sudden hypotension or hypertension (Garretson 2005; Jevon et al. 2012).
3 Observe trace for arterial swing (Hazinski 2013).	3 Artificial elevation of peak systolic pressure trace may be noted.
4 Position transducer level with the right atrium, using the mid-axilla as a guide (please see maintenance: calibration for land marking guide).	4 To ensure accurate measurements.
5 Ensure low compliance tubing of minimal length is used.	5 To minimise distortion and ensure accurate measurements.
6 Recalibrate transducer.	6 Ensure accurate calibration and measurements.

Procedure guideline 14.38 Troubleshooting: puncture site bleeding

Statement	Rationale
1 If bleeding occurs at the puncture site apply firm pressure for 5–15 minutes (Burns and Chulay 2014).	1 To stop bleeding
2 Ensure catheter is securely strapped and the limb is immobilised.	2 To minimise catheter and limb movement.
3 Check circulation to cannulated limb.	3 To ensure adequate blood supply to effected limb.

Procedure guideline 14.39 Troubleshooting: circulation compromise

Statement	Rationale
1 If circulation is compromised distal to the puncture site decreased pulse, blanching, cyanosis, or cool skin may be seen.	1 This may be due to artery spasm (Jevon et al. 2012).
2 Using a gentle irrigation technique maintain a continuous flush and ensure extremity is kept warm.	2 To promote vasodilation (Jevon et al. 2012).
3 Check extremity for signs of adequate circulation. The cannula must be removed if there is sustained blanching to the limb, distal to the cannula site.	3 To maintain circulation to the limb, (Jevon et al. 2012).

Procedure guideline 14.40 Troubleshooting: no waveform

Statement	Rationale
1 If there is no waveform visible on the monitor, assess and report changes in the CYP's cardiovascular status, including pulse check, pulse oximetry, and ECG waveform.	1 To ensure patient safety.
2 Perform noninvasive blood pressure monitoring to ensure it is not due to a change in the CYP's clinical condition.	
3 Check the system is correctly set up and attached with all three-way taps open to CYP (Garretson 2005).	
4 Flush arterial catheter with 0.9% sodium chloride	4 To ensure patency of arterial cannula
5 Check appropriate arterial scale is in use on the monitor.	
6 Ensure monitor display settings are correctly set.	
7 Try an alternative transducer and module.	7 To determine if equipment is faulty.
8 Consult a biomedical engineer.	8 To determine if equipment is faulty and initiate repair.

Procedure guideline 14.41 Removal of arterial cannula

Statement	Rationale
1 The arterial line should be removed when: • Limb circulation is compromised. • The cannula is misplaced. • It is no longer required for monitoring or frequent blood sampling. • There are signs of infection (Burns and Chulay 2014).	1 To minimise risks associated with arterial cannula.
2 Check for normal blood coagulation levels.	2 To avoid prolonged bleeding from site following cannula removal.
3 CYPs with severe clotting disorders may require an infusion of depleted clotting factors (e.g. Octaplas) immediately prior to arterial cannula removal.	3 To avoid prolonged bleeding from site following cannula removal.
4 Inform the CYP and family of the following: • Why the arterial line needs to be removed. • What this entails. • Prepare the CYP using distraction techniques.	4 To ensure they understand the reason for the procedure and can give informed consent, promoting coping behaviours and reducing stress levels (De Lourdes et al. 2003; Jaaniste et al. 2007; APAGBI 2012; Twycross et al. 2014; NMC 2015; RCoA 2022).
5 Standard precautions must be adopted including nonsterile gloves, eye protection, and an apron.	5 To minimise infection risks (Loveday et al. 2014).
Prepare for the procedure as per procedure Guideline 14.1.A.	
6 Use an ANTT® throughout.	6 To minimise infection risks (Rowley and Clare 2011; NICE 2012).
7 Gather the following equipment: • Clean tray • Nonsterile gloves • Eye protection • Sterile gauze • Surgical tape • Small sterile plaster (if required)	
8 Perform hand hygiene and put on apron, eye protection and nonsterile gloves.	8 To maintain standard precautions (Loveday et al. 2014).
9 Loosen all dressings.	
10 Withdraw line from artery.	
11 Using sterile gauze immediately apply firm pressure for up to 5 minutes or until bleeding has stopped.	11 To stop the bleeding and reduce risk of haematoma formation.
12 Apply a sterile plaster or pressure dressing over the site.	12 To protect site and minimise blood loss (Burns and Chulay 2014).
13 Complete the procedure as per Procedure Guideline 14.1.B.	
14 Dispose of all used equipment according to the local trust waste management policy.	14 To meet health and safety standards.
15 Perform hand hygiene.	15 To minimise infection risks.
16 Observe site frequently for signs of rebleeding and the extremity should be checked for circulatory compromise including pulse check, cyanosis, sluggish capillary refill time and temperature for a few hours following removal (Burns and Chulay 2010).	16 To detect further bleeding. To detect deceased circulation from clot formation (Burns and Chulay 2014; Garretson 2005; Hazinski 2013; Perrin and MacLeod 2013; Woodrow 2009).
16 Record the procedure in the CYP's healthcare records.	16 To maintain accurate records.

References

Abad, C.L. and Safdar, N. (2012). Catheter-related bloodstream infections. *Pharmacy Practice News: Education Review*: 11–18.

Abedin, S. and Kapoor, G. (2008). Peripherally inserted central catheters are a good option for prolonged venous access in children with cancer. *Pediatric Blood & Cancer* 51 (2): 251–255.

Advanced Life Support Group (2016). *Advanced Paediatric Life Support*, A Practical Approach to Emergencies 6e. London: BMJ Books.

Anand, K. (2008). Heparinised saline or normal saline? *The Journal of Perioperative Practice* 18 (10): 440.

Anderson, D.M., Pesaturo, K.A., Casavant, J., and Ramsey, E.Z. (2013). Alteplase for the treatment of catheter occlusion in pediatric patients. *The Annals of Pharmacotherapy* 47: 405–410.

Andrews, T. and Waterman, H. (2008). What factors influence blood gas sampling patterns? *Nursing in Critical Care* 13 (3): 132–137.

Aouad-Maroun M, Raphael CK, Sayyid SK, Farah F, Akl EA (2016). Ultrasound-guided arterial cannulation for paediatrics. Cochrane Database of Systematic Reviews 2016, Issue 9. Art. No.: CD011364. DOI: 10.1002/14651858.CD011364.pub2.

Arnts, I.J.J., Heijnen, J.A., Wilburs, H.T.M. et al. (2011). Effectiveness of heparin solution versus normal saline in maintaining patency of intravenous locks in neonates: a double blind randomised controlled study. *Journal of Advanced Nursing* 67 (12): 2677–2685.

Association of Paediatric Anaesthetists of Great Britain and Ireland (APAGBI) (2012). Good practice in postoperative and procedural pain management. 2. *Pediatric Anesthesia* 22 (1): 1–79.

Athale, U.H., Sicilianao, S., Cheng, J. et al. (2012). Central venous line dysfunction is an independent predictor of poor survival in children with cancer. *Journal of Pediatric Hematology/Oncology* 34 (3): 188–193.

Bard Access Systems (2015). Nursing procedure manual. Groshong® central venous catheter. https://www.bd.com/assets/documents/pdh/initial/BAW0738860-Groshong-CVC-IFU.pdf (accessed 18 July 2022).

Bard Access Systems (2016). Nursing procedure manual. Hickman®, Leonard®, and Broviac® central venous catheters. https://www.bd.com/assets/documents/pdh/initial/BPV-CVCA-1115-0002v-1.1-Hickman-Leonard-Broviac-Nursing-Procedure-Manual.pdf (accessed 18 July 2022).

Baskin, J.L., Pui, C., Reiss, U. et al. (2009). Management of occlusion and thrombosis associated with long-term indwelling central venous catheters. *Lancet* 374 (9684): 159–169.

Bishop, L., Dougherty, L., Bodenham, A. et al. (2007). Guidelines on the insertion and management of central venous access devices in adults. *International Journal of Laboratory Hematology* 29 (4): 261–278.

Boehringer Ingelheim Limited (2021). Actilyse Cathflo 2mg. Electronic medicines compendium.® www.medicines.org.uk/emc/medicine/24604/SPC/Actilyse+Cathflo+2+mg (accessed 18 July 2022).

Bowe-Geddes, L.A. and Nichols, H.A. (2005). An overview of peripherally inserted central catheters. *Topics in Advanced Practice Nursing e-journal*. 5 (3).

Bravery, K. (2008). Paediatric intravenous therapy in practice. In: *Intravenous Therapy in Nursing Practice* (eds. L. Dougherty and J. Lamb). Oxford: Blackwell Publishing.

Bravo, K. and Cochran, G. (2016). Nursing strategies to increase medication safety in inpatient settings. *Journal of Nursing Care Quality* 31 (4): 335–341.

British Medical Association and Royal Pharmaceutical Society of Great Britain (2021). *British National Formulary for Children*. London: BMJ Group.

Bruce, E. (2009). Chapter 10. Management of Painful Procedures. In: *Managing Pain in Children: A Clinical Guide* (eds. A. Twycross, S.J. Dowden and E. Bruce). Wiley-Blackwell.

Burn, J., Monzon, L., Kashef, E., and Moser, S. (2013). Malfunctioning central venous catheters. *CardioVascular and Interventional Radiology* 36 (S278).

Burns, S.M. and Chulay, M. (2014). *AACN Essentials of Critical Care Nursing*, 3e. New York: McGraw Hill.

Cardinal, P., Allan, J., Pham, B. et al. (2000). The effects of sodium citrate in arterial catheters on acid base and electrolyte measurements. *Critical Care Medicine* 28 (5): 1388–1392.

Centers for Disease Control and Prevention (CDC) (2011). Guidelines for the prevention of intravascular catheter-related infections. https://www.cdc.gov/infectioncontrol/guidelines/bsi/index.html (accessed 18 July 2022).

Chambers D, Huang C, Mathhews G, (2019) Section 3, Cardiovascular Physiology, Basic physiology for Anaethetists: Cambridge university press, Pages 111–188.

Cook, L., Bellini, S., and Cusson, R.M. (2011). Heparinized saline vs normal saline for maintenance of intravenous access in neonates: an evidence-based practice change. *Advanced Neonatal Care* 11 (3): 208–215.

Corzine, M. and Willett, L.D. (2010). Neonatal PICC: one Unit's six year experience with limiting catheter complications. *Neonatal Network* 29 (3): 161–173.

Danckers, M., Fried, E.D., Windle, M.L., and Rowe, V.L. (2022) Arterial blood gas sampling, *Medscape online article*. http://emedicine.medscape.com/article/1902703-overview (accessed 23 September 2022).

Danek, G.D. and Norris, E.M. (1992). Pediatric IV catheters; efficacy of saline flush. *Pediatric Nursing* 18 (2): 111–113.

De Lourdes, L.M., Larcher, V., and Kerz, R. (2003). Informed consent/assent in children. Statement of the ethics working group of the confederation of European specialists in paediatrics (CESP). *European Journal of Paediatrics* 162 (9): 629–633.

Del Cotillo, M., Grane, N., Llavore, M., and Quintana, S. (2008). Heparinised solution vs saline solution in the maintenance of arterial catheters: a double blind randomised clinical trial. *Intensive Care Medicine* 34: 339–343.

Department of Health (DH) (2001). *Review of Four Neonatal Deaths Due to Cardiac Tamponade Associated with the Presence of a Central Venous Catheter: Recommendations and Department of Health Response*. London: DH.

Department of Health (DH) (2007). *Saving Lives: Reducing Infection, Delivering Clean and Safe Care: Taking Blood Cultures, a Summary of Best Practice*. London: Department of Health.

Department of Health (DH) (2009). *Reference Guide to Consent for Examination and Treatment*, 2e. London: Department of Health.

Dixon, M. and Crawford, D. (2012). *Paediatric Intensive Care Nursing*. Oxford: Wiley Blackwell.

DoellmanA, D. (2011). Prevention, assessment and treatment of central venous catheter occlusions in neonatal and young pediatric patients. *Journal of Infusion Nursing* 34 (4): 251–258.

Dougherty, L. (2000). Central venous access devices. *Nursing Standard* 14 (43): 45–50.

Dougherty, L. (2006). *Central Venous Access Devices: Care and Management*. Oxford: Blackwell Publishing.

Dougherty, L. and Lamb, J. (2008). *Intravenous Therapy in Nursing Practice*, 2e. Oxford: Blackwell Publishing.

Dougherty, L. and Lister, S. (eds.) (2015). Chapter 14: vascular access devices: insertion and management. In: *The Royal Marsden Hospital Manual of Clinical Nursing Procedures*, 9e. Chichester: Wiley Blackwell Publishing.

Douglas, L., Aspin, A., Jimmeson, N., and Lawrance, V. (2009). Central venous access devices: review of practice. *Paediatric Nursing* 21 (5): 19–22.

Drewitt, S. (2009). Removal of central venous access. In: *Central Venous Catheters* (eds. H. Hamilton and A.R. Bodenham). Wiley.

Esper, S A., Pinsky M R. (2014) Arterial waveform analysis, Best practice and research clinical anesthesiology, volume 28, pages 363–380.

European Union (EU) (2010). Council directive 2010/32/EU of May 2010 implementing the framework agreement on prevention from sharps injuries in the hospital and healthcare sector concluded by HOSPEEM and EPSU. *Official Journal of the European Union* 53: 66–72.

Frey, A.M. (2007). Pediatric intravenous therapy. In: *Plumer's Principles and Practice of Intravenous Therapy* (ed. S.M. Weinstein). Philadelphia: Lippincott Williams and Wilkins.

Garretson, S. (2005). Haemodynamic monitoring: arterial catheters. *Nursing Standard* 19 (31): 55–64.

Gilboy, S. and Hollywood, E. (2009). Helping to alleviate pain for children having venepuncture. *Paediatric Nursing* 21 (8): 14–19.

Goode, C.J., Titler, M., Rakel, B. et al. (1991). A meta-analysis of effects of heparin flush and saline flush: quality and cost implications. *Nursing Research* 40 (6): 324–330.

Goodwin, M.L. and Carlson, I. (1993). The peripherally inserted central catheter: a retrospective look at three years of insertions. *Journal of Intravenous Nursing* 16 (2): 92–103.

Goossens, GA. (2015). Flushing and Locking of Venous Catheters: Available Evidence and Evidence Deficit. *Nurs Res Pract.* 2015;2015:985686. doi:10.1155/2015/985686 (accessed 18 July 2022).

Gordon, S. and Gardiner, S. (2013). Central line infections in repaired catheters: a retrospective review. *The Journal of the Association for Vascular Access*. 18 (3): 164–166.

Graf, J.M., Newman, C.D., and McPherson, M.L. (2006). Sutured securement of peripherally inserted central catheters yields fewer complications in pediatric patients. *Journal of Parenteral and Enteral Nutrition* 30 (6): 532–535.

Gustafon, R. (2010). Best practices for the care and maintenance of argyle™ neonatal peripherally inserted central catheters. *Covidien*: 1–15.

Gyr, P., Burroughs, T., Smith, K. et al. (1995). Double blind comparison of heparin and saline flush solutions in maintenance of peripheral infusion devices. *Paediatric Nursing* 21 (4): 383–389. 366.

Hadaway, L.C. (1998). Major thrombotic and non-thrombotic complications. Loss of patency. *Journal of Intravenous Nursing* 21 (5S): 143–160.

Hadaway, L. (2006a). Heparin locking for central venous catheters. *The Journal of the Association for Vascular Access* 11: 224–231.

Hadaway, L. (2006b). Technology of flushing vascular access devices. *Journal of Infusion Nursing* 29 (3): 129–145.

Hadaway, L. (2007). Infiltration and extravasation, preventing a complication of IV catheterization. *American Journal of Nursing* 107 (8): 64–72.

Hagle, M. (2007). Central venous access. In: *Plumer's Principles and Practice of Intravenous Therapy* (ed. S.M. Weinstein). Philadephia: Lippincott Williams and Wilkins.

Hazinski, M.F. (2013). *Nursing Care of the Critically Ill Child*, 3e. Elsevier Mosby: St Louis.

Health and Safety Executive (2013). Health and Safety (Sharp Instruments in Healthcare) Regulations 2013. Guidance for employers and employees. HSE information sheet. Health Services Information Sheet 7. https://www.hse.gov.uk/pubns/hsis7.htm (accessed 18 July 2022).

Higginson, R. and Parry, A. (2011). Phlebitis: treatment, care and prevention. *Nursing Times* 107 (36): 18–21.

Hignett, R. and Stephens, R. (2006). Radial arterial lines. *British Journal of Hospital Medicine* 67 (5): m3–m4.

Hill, M.L., Baldwin, L., Slaughter, J.C. et al. (2010). A silver alginate coated dressing to reduce peripherally inserted central catheter (PICC) infections in NICU patients: a pilot randomized control trial. *Journal of Perinatology* 30: 469–473.

Holt, D.M., Lewis, C., Klimpel, K. et al. (2010). The effects of focused nursing education on 3F Groshong™ PICC occlusion rates: the experience of one tertiary pediatric care facility. *Journal of the Association for Vascular Access* 15 (4): 213–221.

Hovda Davis, M. (2013). Pediatric central venous catheter management: a review of current practice. *Journal of the Association for Vascular Access* 18 (2): 93–98.

Hughes, M.E. (2014). Reducing PICC migrations and improving patient outcomes. *British Journal of Nursing*. IV Therapy supplement 23 (2): S12–S18.

Humphrey, G.B., Boo, C.M., van Linden van den Heuvell, G.F., and van de Wiel, H.B. (1992). The occurrence of high levels of accurate behavioural distress in children and adolescents undergoing routine venepunctures. *Pediatrics* 90 (1): 87–91.

Ishii, S., Shime, N., Shibasaki, M., and Sawa, T. (2013). Ultrasound-guided radial artery catheterisation in infants and young children. *Paediatric Critical Care Medicine* 14 (5): 471–473.

Jaaniste, T., Hayes, B., and Von Baeyer, C. (2007). Providing children with information about forthcoming medical procedures: a review and synthesis. *Clinical Psychology* 14 (2): 124–143.

Jackson, A. (1998). Infection control: a battle in vein infusion phlebitis. *Nursing Times* 94 (4): 68–71.

Jevon, P., Ewens, B., and Pooni, J.S. (2012). *Monitoring the Critically Ill Patient*, 3e. Oxford: Wiley Blackwell.

Josephson, D.L. (2004). *Intravenous Infusion Therapy for Nurses: Principles and Practice*, 2e. New York: Delmar Learning.

Kaler, W. and Chinn (2007). Successful disinfection of needle-free mechanical access ports: a matter of time and friction. *Journal of the Association of Vascular Access* 12: 203–205.

Kaye, R., Sane, S.S., and Towbin, R.B. (2000). Pediatric intervention: an update-part 2. *Journal of Vascular and Interventional Radiology* 11: 807–822.

Keogh, S. (2013). New research: change peripheral intravenous catheters as clinically indicated, not routinely. *Journal of the Association for Vascular Access* 18 (3): 153–154.

Kerner, J., Garcia-Careaga, M., Fisher, A., and Poole, R.L. (2006). Treatment of catheter occlusion in pediatric patients. *Journal of Parenteral and Enteral Nutrition* 30 (1): S73–S81.

Klees, S.J. (2011). The ideal use of the power injectable peripherally inserted central catheter in the pediatric population. *Journal of the Association for Vascular Access* 16 (2): 86–93.

Kleiber, C., Hanrahan, K., Fagan, C.L., and Zittergruen, M.A. (1993). Heparin vs. saline for peripheral i.v. locks in children. *Pediatric Nursing* 19 (4): 405–409.

Klenner, A.F., Fusch, C., Rakow, I. et al. (2003). Benefit and risk of heparin for maintaining peripheral venous catheters in neonates: a placebo-controlled trial. *The Journal of Pediatrics* 143 (6): 741–745.

LaRue, G.D. and Peterson, M. (2011). The impact of dilution on intravenous therapy. *Journal of Infusion Nursing* 34 (2): 55–60.

Lavery, I. and Ingram, P. (2006). Prevention of infection in peripheral intravenous devices. *Nursing Standard* 20 (49): 49–56. quiz 57.

Leslie, R.A., Gouldson, S., Habib, N. et al. (2013). Management of arterial lines and blood sampling in intensive care: a threat to patient safety. *Anaesthesia* 68: 1114–1119.

Lloreda-García, J.M., Lorente-Nicolás, A., Bermejo-Costa, F., and Fernández-Fructuoso, J.R. (2016). Catheter tip position and risk of mechanical complications in a neonatal unit. *Anales de Pediatría* 85 (2): 77–85.

Loveday, H.P., Wilson, J.A., Pratt, R.J. et al. (2014). Epic 3: national evidence-based guidelines for preventing healthcare-associated infections in NHS hospitals in England. *Journal of Hospital Infection* 86 (supplement 1): S1–S70.

Macklin, D. (1999). What's physics got to do with it? *Journal of Vascular Access Devices* 4: 7–11.

Macklin, D. (2003). Phlebitis, a painful complication of peripheral IV catheterization that may be prevented. *American Journal of Nursing* 103 (2): 55–60.

Macklin, D. (2010). Catheter management. *Seminars in Oncology Nursing* 26 (2): 113–120.

Maki, D.G., Mermel, L.A., Kluger, D., Narans, L., Knasinki, V., Parenteau, S., and Covington, P. (2000). The efficacy of a chlorhexidine-impregnated sponge (Biopatch) for the prevention of intravascular catheter related infection – a prospective randomized controlled multi center study. Abstract. Fortieth Interscience Conference on Antimicrobial Agents and Chemotherapy. https://www.epistemonikos.org/documents/b5e036312e5d4f772cb87dd4bb774e989936f248/ (accessed 18 July 2022).

McGowan, D. (2014). Peripheral intravenous cannulation: managing distress and anxiety. *British Journal of Nursing* 23 (Suppl 19): S4–S9.

Moureau, N. (2000). Training for turbulence. *Journal of Vascular Access Devices* 5 (4): 2.

National Institute for Health and Care Excellence (2012). *Infection: Prevention and Control of Healthcare-Associated Infections in Primary and Community Care*. London: National Institute for Health and Clinical Excellence.

National Patient Safety Agency (NPSA) (2007). Patient Safety Alert 20: Promoting safer use of injectable medicines. https://healthcareea.vctms.co.uk/assets/content/9652/4759/content/injectable.pdf (accessed 18 July 2022).

National Patient Safety Agency (NPSA) (2008). Rapid Response Report NPSA/2008/RRR002. Risks with intravenous heparin flush solutions. https://www.patientsafetysolutions.com/docs/May_2008_UK_NPSA_Alert_on_Heparin_Flushes.htm (accessed 23 September 2022).

National Patient safety Agency (NPSA) (2008a). Rapid response report NPSA/2008/RRR006 Problems with infusions and sampling from arterial lines, London NPSA. https://www.patientsafetysolutions.com/docs/August_19_2008_Arterial_Line_Issues.htm (accessed 18 July 2022).

National Patient Safety Agency (NPSA) (2008b). Supporting information for Rapid Response Report NPSA/2008/RRR006, London, NPSA.

Needham, R. and Strehle, E.M. (2008). Evaluation of dressings used with local anaesthetic creams and for peripheral venouscannulation. *Paediatric Nursing* 20 (8): 34–36.

Nursing and Midwifery Council (NMC) (2015). *The Code: Professional standards of practice and behaviours for nurses, midwives and nursing associates*. London: NMC https://www.nmc.org.uk/standards/code/ (accessed 18 June 2022).

O'Grady, N.P., Alexander, M., Dellinger, E.P. et al. (2011). CDC- guidelines for the prevention of intravascular catheter-related infections. *Morbidity and Mortality Weekly Report* 51: 1–26.

Paquette, V., McGloin, R., Northway, T. et al. (2011). *The Canadian Journal of Hospital Pharmacy* 64 (5): 340–345.

Perrin, K.O. and MacLeod, C.E. (2013). *Understanding the Essentials of Critical Care Nursing*, 2e. New Jersey: Pearson.

Petit, J. and Wyckoff, M.M. (2007). *Peripherally Inserted Central Catheters*, 2e. Guidelines for Practice.

Registered Nurses Association of Ontario (RNAO) (2005). Care and maintenance to reduce vascular access complication. https://bpgmobile.rnao.ca/category/guidelines/care-and-maintenance-reduce-vascular-access-complications (accessed 18 July 2022).

Richardson, D.K. (2007). Vascular access nursing. Practice, standards of care, and strategies to prevent infection: a review of flushing solutions and injection caps. *Journal of the Association of Vascular Access* 12: 74–84.

Rickard, C.M., Wallis, S.C., Courtney, M. et al. (2002). Intravascular administration sets are accurate and in appropriate condition after 7 days of continuous use: an in vitro; study. *Journal of Advanced Nursing* 37 (4): 330–337.

Robertson-Malt, S., Malt, G.N., Farquhar, V., and Greer, W. (2014). *Heparin Versus Normal Saline for Patency of Arterial Lines, the Cochrane Collaboration ®, Issue 5*. Wiley.

Rowley, S. and Clare, S. (2011). ANTT: a standard approach to aseptic technique. *Nursing Times* 107 (36): 12–14.

Rowley, S., Clare, S., Macqueen, S., and Molyneux, R. (2010). ANTT v2: an updated practice framework for aseptic technique. *British Journal of Nursing* 19 (5).

Royal College of Nursing (RCN) (2013). *Sharps Safety: RCN Guidance to Support the Implementation of the Health and Safety (Sharp Instruments in Healthcare Regulations)*. London: RCN.

Royal College of Nursing (RCN) (2016). *Standards for Infusion Therapy*, 4e. London: RCN https://www.rcn.org.uk/clinical-topics/Infection-prevention-and-control/Standards-for-infusion-therapy (accessed 18 July 2022).

Royal College of Anaethetists (RCoA) (2022). Guidelines for the Provision of Anaesthetic Services. Chapter 10: Guidelines for the Provision of Paediatric Anaesthesia Services 2022. https://www.rcoa.ac.uk/gpas/chapter-10 (accessed 23 September 2022).

Savader, S.J. and Trerotola, S.O. (2000). *Venous Interventional Radiology with Clinical Perspectives*, 2e. Thieme: New York.

Sharpe, E. (2014). Neonatal peripherally inserted central catheter practices and their association with demographics, training and radiographic monitoring. *Results from a National Survey. Advances in Neonatal Care* 14 (5): 329–335.

Sharpe, E. and Pettit, J. (2013). A National Survey of neonatal peripherally inserted central catheter (PICC) practices. *Advances in Neonatal Care* 13 (1): 55–74.

Simcock, L. (2001). Complications of CVCs and their nursing management. *Nursing Times* 97 (20): 36–39.

Smith, J.S., Irwin, G., Viney, M. et al. (2012). Optimal disinfection times for needle-free intravenous connectors. *Journal of the Association of Vascular Access* 17 (3): 137–143.

Soe, A. (2007). Central venous catheterisation in newborn infants. *Infants* 3 (5): 172–175.

Soothill, J., Bravery, K., Ho, A. et al. (2009). A fall in bloodstream infections followed a change to 2% chlorhexidine in 70% isopropanol for catheter connection antisepsis: a pediatric single centre before/after study on a hemopoietic stem cell transplant ward. *American Journal of Infection Control* 37 (8): 626–630.

Steiger, E. (2006). Dysfunction and thrombotic complications of vascular access devices. *Journal of Parenteral and Enteral Nutrition* 30 (1): S70–S72.

Timsett, J., Schwebel, C., Bouadma, L. et al. (2009). Chlorohexidine impregnated sponges and less frequent dressing changes for prevention of catheter related infections in critically ill adults- a randomised control trial. *JAMA* 301 (12): 1231–1241.

Todd, J. (1998). Peripherally inserted central catheters (PICC). *Professional Nurse* 13 (5): 297–302.

Twycross, A., Reid, K., and Tuterra, D. (2014). Management of painful procedures. In: *Managing Pain in Children a Clinical Guide for Nurses and Healthcare Professionals*, 2e (eds. A. Twycross, S. Dowden and J. Stinson). Oxford: Wiley Blackwell.

Ullman, A., Cooke, M., and Rickard, C. (2015). Examining the role of securement and dressing products to prevent central venous access device failure: a narrative review. *JAVA* 20 (2): 99–110.

Vygon (2012). *Neonatal & Paediatric Catheters*. Specialist Products for Newborns & Young Children.

Wall, J.L. and Kierstead, V.L. (1995). Peripherally inserted central catheters: resistance to removal: a rare complication. *Journal of Intravenous Nursing* 18 (5): 251–254.

Weinstein, S.M. (2007). *Plumer's Principles and Practices of Intravenous Therapy*, 8e. Philadelphia: Lippincott Williams and Wilkins.

Weller, B.F. (ed.) (2005). *Bailliere's Nurse's Dictionary for Nurses and Health Care Workers*, 24e. Edinburgh: Elsevier.

Woodrow, P. (2009). Arterial catheters: promoting safe clinical practice. *Nursing Standard* 24 (4): 35–40.

Xie, H., Kang, J., and Mills, G.H. (2009). Clinical review: the impact of noise on patients sleep and effectiveness of noise reduction strategies in intensive care units. *Critical Care* 13 (2): 208.

Yamamoto, A.J., Solomon, J.A., Soulen, M.C. et al. (2002). Sutureless securement device reduces complications of peripherally inserted central venous catheters. *Journal of Vascular and Interventional Radiology* 13 (1): 77–81.

Further reading

Adlard, K. (2008). Examining the push-pull method of blood sampling from central venous access devices. *Journal of Pediatric Oncology Nursing* 25 (4): 200–207.

Arrowsmith, J. and Campbell, C. (2000). A comparison of local anaesthetics for venepuncture. *Archives of Disease in Childhood* 82 (4): 309–310.

Baker, R.B., Summer, S.S., Lawrence, M. et al. (2013). Determining optimal waste volume from an intravenous catheter. *Journal of Infusion Nursing* 36 (2): 92–96.

Biccard, B. (2001). EMLA-1hr is not enough for venous cannulation. *Anaesthesia* 56 (10): 1027–1028.

Bravery, K. and Hannan, J. (1997). The use of long-term central venous access devices in children. *Paediatric Nursing* 9 (10): 29–37.

Bregenzer, T. (1998). Is routine replacement of peripheral intravenous catheters necessary? *Archives of Internal Medicine* 158: 151–156.

Brenner, M. (2007). Child restraint in the acute setting of pediatric nursing: an extraordinary stressful event. *Issues in Comprehensive Pediatric Nursing* 31 (1–2): 29–37.

Brown-Smith, J.K., Stoner, M.H., and Barley, Z.A. (1990). Tunnelled catheter thrombosis: factors related to incidence. *Oncology Nurses Forum* 17 (4): 543–549.

Camara, D. (2001). Minimising risks associated with peripherally inserted central catheters in the NICU. *MCN. The American Journal of Maternal/Child Nursing* 26 (1): 17–22.

Capka, M.B., Carey, S., Marks, D. et al. (1993). Nursing observations of central venous catheters: the effect on patient outcome. In: *The Best of Critical Care Nursing* (eds. C.E. Guzetta, T. Ahrens and D. Fontaine). St Louis: Mosby.

Chiang, V.W. and Baskin, M.N. (2000). Uses and complications of central venous catheters inserted in a pediatric emergency department. *Pediatric Emergency Care* 16 (4): 230–232.

Claar, R., Walker, L., and Smith, C. (2002). The influence of appraisals in understanding children's experiences with medical procedures. *Journal of Paediatric Psychology* 27 (7): 553–563.

Clarke, S. and Radford, M. (1986). Topical anaesthesia for venepuncture. *Archives of Disease in Childhood* 61: 1132–1134.

Cohen, L.L. (2008). Behavioural approaches to anxiety and pain management for pediatric venous access. *Pediatrics* 122 (Supplement 3): S134–S139.

Cohen, L.L., Bernard, R.S., Greco, L.A., and McClellan, C.B. (2002). A child focused intervention for coping with procedural pain: are parent and nurse coaches necessary? *Journal of Pediatric Psychology* 27 (8): 747–757.

Cole, M., Price, L., Parry, A. et al. (2006). A study to determine the minimum volume of blood necessary to be discarded from a central venous catheter before a valid sample is obtained in children with cancer. *Pediatric Blood & Cancer* 48: 687–695.

Conn, C. (1993). The importance of syringe size when using an implanted vascular access device. *Journal of Vascular Access Networks* 3: 11–18.

Davies, S. (1998). The role of nurses in intravenous cannulation. *Nursing Standard* 12 (17): 43–46.

Department of Health (DH) (2003). *Getting the Right Start; NSF for Children. Emerging Findings*. London: Department of Health.

Department of Health (DH) (2010). *Advanced Level Nursing: A Position Statement*. London: Department of Health.

Dougherty, L. (1996). Intravenous cannulation. *Nursing Standard* 11 (2): 47–51.

Dougherty, L. (2008). Peripheral cannulation. *Nursing Standard* 22 (52): 49–56.

Dougherty, L. and Lamb, J. (eds.) (1999). *Intravenous Therapy in Nursing Practice*. London: Churchill Livingstone.

Dunn, D. and Lennihan, S. (1987). The case for saline flush. *American Journal of Nursing* 6: 689–699.

Flynn, S. (1999). Administering intravenous antibiotics at home. *Professional Nurse* 14 (6): 399–402.

Franklin, L. (1998). Skin cleansing and infection control in peripheral venepuncture and cannulation. *Paediatric Nursing* 10 (9): 33–34.

Frey, A.M. (1995). Pediatric peripherally inserted central catheter program report: a summary of 4,496 catheter days. *Journal of Intravenous Nursing* 18 (6): 280–291.

Frey, A. (1998). Success rate for peripheral IV insertion in a children's hospital. *Journal of Intravenous Nursing* 21 (3): 160–165.

Frey, A.M. (1999). PICC complications in neonates and children. *Journal of Vascular Access Devices* Spring: 17–26.

Frey, A.M. (2003). Drawing blood samples from vascular access devices: evidence-based practice. *Journal of Infusion Nursing* 26 (5): 285–293.

Fuhrman, B.P. and Zimmerman, J.J. (1998). *Paediatric Critical Care*, 2e. St Louis: Mosby.

Gabriel, J. (1996a). Care and Management of Peripherally Inserted Central Catheters. *British Journal of Nursing* 5 (10): 594–599.

Gabriel, J. (1996b). Peripherally inserted central catheters: expanding UK Nurses' practice. *British Journal of Nursing* 5 (2): 71–74.

Gabriel, J. (1997). Fibrin sheaths in vascular access devices. *Nursing Times* 93 (10): 56–57.

Gabriel, J. (2001). PICC securement: Minimising potential complications. *Nursing Standard* 15 (43): 42–44.

Goodwin, M. and Carlson, I. (1993). The peripherally inserted central venous catheter. *British Journal of Intensive Care* 12 (4): 96–97.

Hadaway, L. (1998). Catheter connection. *Journal of Vascular Access Devices* 3 (3): 129–145.

Haslam, D. (1969). Age and perception of pain. *Psychological Science* 15: 86–87.

Hecker, J. (1988). Improved technique in IV therapy. *Nursing Times* 84 (34): 28–33.

Henderson, N. (1997). Central venous lines. *Nursing Standard* 11: 49–56.

Hijazi, O.M., Cheyney, J.J., Guzzetta, P.C. Jr., and Toro-Figueroa, L.O. (1997). Venous access and catheters. In: *Essentials of Pediatric Intensive Care (Vol 2)*, 2e (eds. D.L. Levin and F.C. Morriss). New York: Churchill Livingstone.

Hindley, M. (1997). Reducing exit site infections and the risk of accidental removal of Hickman lines in children within the first month post insertion. *Journal of Cancer Nursing* 1 (1): 54–55.

Holcombe, B.J., Forloines-Lynn, S., and Garmhausen, L.W. (1992). Restoring patency of long-term central venous access devices. *Journal of Intravenous Nursing* 15 (1): 36–41.

Howie, S. (2011). Blood sample volumes in child health research: review of safe limits. *Bulletin of the World Health Organization* 89 (1): 46–53.

Intravenous Nurses Society (1990). Intravenous nursing standards of practice. *Journal of Intravenous Nursing* 13: S1–S98.

Infusion Nurses Society (2011). Infusion nursing standards of practice. *Journal of Infusion Nursing* 34: S1–S109.

James, L., Bledsdoe, L., and Hadaway, L.C. (1993). A retrospective look at tip location and complications of peripherally inserted central catheter lines. *Journal of Intravenous Nursing* 16 (12): 104–109.

Keller, C.A. (1994). Methods of drawing blood samples through central venous catheters in pediatric patients undergoing bone marrow transplant: results of a national survey. *Oncology Nursing Forum* 21 (5): 879–884.

Kolk, A., Hoof, R., and Fiedeldij, D.M. (1999). Preparing children for venepuncture. *Child: Care, Health and Development* 26 (3): 251–260.

Kumar, R. and Russell, H. (1995). Parental presence during procedures: a survey of attitudes amongst paediatricians. *Journal of the Royal Society of Medicine* 88: 508–510.

Lai, K. (1998). Safety of prolonged peripheral cannula and IV tubing use from 72 hours to 96 hours. *American Journal of Infection Control* 26 (1): 56–70.

Lamb, J. (1995). Peripheral IV therapy. *Nursing Standard* 9 (30): 32–35.

Livesley, J. (1993). Reducing the risks: management of paediatric intravenous therapy. *Child Health* 1 (2): 68–71.

MacGeorge, L., Steeves, L., and Steeves, R.H. (1988). Comparison of the mixing and reinfusion methods of drawing blood from a Hickman catheter. *Oncology Nursing Forum* 15 (3): 335–338.

Macklin, D. (2000). Removing a PICC. *American Journal of Nursing* 100 (1): 52–54.

Magnusson, S. (1996). Oh, for a little humanity. *British Medical Journal* 313: 1601–1603.

Maki, D. and Ringer, M. (1991). Risk factors for infusion-related phlebitis with small peripheral venous catheters. *Annals of Medicine* 114: 845–854.

Maki, D. (1976). Preventing infection in intravenous therapy. *Hospital Practice* April: 104.

Maki, D., Ringer, M., and Alvarado, C.J. (1991). Prospective randomised trial of povidone iodine, alcohol and chlorhexidine for prevention of infection associated with central venous and arterial lines. *Lancet* 338: 339–343.

Marcoux, C., Fisher, S., and Wong, D. (1990). Central venous access devices in children. *Pediatric Nursing* 16 (2): 123–133.

Marx, M. (1995). The management of the difficult peripherally inserted central venous catheter line removal. *Journal of Intravenous Nursing* 18 (5): 243–249.

Mayo, D.J. and Pearson, D.C. (1995). Chemotherapy extravasation: a consequence of fibrin sheath formation around venous access devices. *Oncology Nursing Forum* 22 (4): 675–680.

McCann, B. (2003). Securing peripheral cannulae: evaluation of a new dressing. *Paediatric Nursing* 15 (5): 23–26.

Miall, L.S., Das, A., Brownlee, K., and Conway, S.P. (2001). Peripherally inserted central catheters in children with cystic fibrosis. Eight cases of difficult removal. *Journal of Infusion Nursing* 24 (5): 297–300.

Millam, D.A. (1992). Starting IVs how to develop your venepuncture expertise. *Nursing* September: 33–46.

Murdoch, L. and Bingham, R. (1990). Venous cannulation in infants and small children. *British Journal of Hospital Medicine* 44 (6): 405–407.

Needham, R. and Strehle, E.M. (2008). Evaluation of dressings used with local anesthetic cream and for peripheral venous cannulation. *Paediatric Nursing* 20 (8): 34–36.

Nelson, D.B. and Garland, J.S. (1987). The natural history of Teflon catheter-associated phlebitis in children. *American Journal of Diseases of Children* 141 (10): 1090–1092.

Oldham, P. (1991). A sticky situation: microbiological study of adhesive tape used to secure IV cannulae. *Professional Nurse* 6: 268–269.

Orr, F. (1999). The role of the paediatric nurse in promoting paediatric right to consent. *Journal of Clinical Nursing* 8 (1): 291–298.

Pearch, J. (2005). Restraining children for clinical procedures. *Paediatric Nursing* 17 (7): 36–38.

Perdue, M. (1995). Intravenous complications. In: *Intravenous Therapy Clinical Principles and Practice* (eds. J. Terry, L. Bararanowski, R. Lonsway and C. Hedrick). Philadelphia: W.B. Saunders.

Perucca, R. and Micek, J. (1993). Treatment of infusion related phlebitis: review and nursing protocol. *Journal of Intravenous Nursing* 16 (5): 282–286.

Phelps, S. and Helms, R. (1987). Risk factors affecting infiltration of peripheral venous lines in infants. *The Journal of Pediatrics* 111: 384–389.

Pierce, C., Wade, A., and Mok, Q. (2000). Heparin bonded central venous lines reduce thrombotic and infective complications in critically ill children. *Intensive Care Medicine* 26: 967–972.

Polderman, K.H. and Girbes, A.R.J. (2002). Central venous catheter use part 1. Mechanical complications. *Intensive Care Medicine* 28: 1–17.

Power, K. (1997). Legal and ethical implications of consent to nursing procedures. *British Journal of Nursing* 6 (15): 885–888.

Reed, T. and Philips, S. (1996). Management of central venous catheter occlusions and repairs. *Journal of Intravenous Nursing* 19 (6): 289–294.

Richardson, D. and Brusco, P. (1993). Vascular access devices: management of common complications. *Journal of Intravenous Nursing* 16 (5): 44–49.

Rowley, S. (2001). Aseptic non-touch technique. *Nursing Times* 97 (7): 6–8.

Royal College of Nursing (RCN) (1995). *Leukaemia and Bone Marrow Transplant Forum. Skin Tunnelled Catheters Guidelines for Care*. London: RCN.

Royal College of Nursing RCN (2010). *Restrictive Physical Intervention and Therapeutic Holding for Children and Young People*. London: RCN.

Rumsey, K.A. and Richardson, D.K. (1995). Management of infection and occlusion associated with vascular devices. *Seminars in Oncology Nursing* 11 (3): 174–183.

Ryder, M.A. (1993). Peripherally inserted central venous catheters. *Nursing Clinics of North America* 28 (4): P937–P971.

Turner, T. (1989). Catalogue of disaster. *Nursing Times* 89 (49): 19.

Van Cleve, L., Johnson, L., and Pothier, P. (1996). Pain responses of hospitalised infants and children to venepuncture and intravenous cannulation. *Journal of Pediatric Nursing* 11 (3): 161–168.

World Health Organization (WHO) (2009). Guidelines on hand hygiene in health care: first global patient safety challenge, clean care is safe care. https://www.who.int/publications/i/item/9789241597906 (accessed 18 July 2022).

Wiener, E. (1998). Venous access in pediatric patients. *Journal of Intravenous Nursing* 21 (5s): 122–133.

Woodrow, P. (2002). Central venous catheters and central venous pressure. *Nursing Standard* 16 (45–52): 54.

Zempsky, W.T. (2008). Pharmacologic approaches for reducing venous access pain in children. *Pediatrics* 122: S140–S153.

Chapter 15

Investigations

Barbara Brekle[1], Annabel Linger[2], Di Robertshaw[3], and Melanie Hiorns[4]

[1] RN (Child), BSc (Hons); Deputy Lead Nurse, Infection Prevention and Control, Great Ormond Street Hospital, London, UK
[2] RN (Child), Dip HEd Nursing Sciences, BSc (Hons) Child Health Nursing, ENB 405 & 998; Lead Sister, NICU, GOSH
[3] RN (Adult), RN (Child), RNT, BSc (Hons) Child Health, Dip N (Paediatrics), Dip Nursing Education; Practice Educator, Cardiac Unit, GOSH
[4] FRCR, FRCP; Clinical Director International and Private Patients and Consultant Radiologist, GOSH

Chapter contents

Introduction	314
Collection of microbiological specimens	314
Ward-based investigations	331
Radiological investigations	346
References	353

Procedure guidelines

15.1 Taking a blood culture	315	
15.2 Capillary blood sampling	317	
15.3 Collecting a sample of chest drain fluid	320	
15.4 Collecting fungal samples	321	
15.5 Collecting gastric samples	321	
15.6 Collecting a nasopharyngeal aspirate	322	
15.7 Collecting sputum samples	322	
15.8 Collecting a stool (faecal) specimen	323	
15.9 Taking a cough swab	323	
15.10 Taking an ear swab	324	
15.11 Taking an eye swab	324	
15.12 Collecting nose swabs	325	
15.13 Taking an oral fluid (saliva) swab	325	
15.14 Collecting pernasal swabs	326
15.15 Taking skin (screening) swabs	326
15.16 Taking throat swabs	326
15.17 Taking a vulval swab for the investigation of simple vaginal discharges	327
15.18 Taking a wound swab	328
15.19 Collecting a urine specimen	328
15.20 Collecting vesicular fluids	330
15.21 Blood glucose monitoring	332
15.22 Three-lead continuous ECG monitoring	335
15.23 Performing a 12-lead ECG	337
15.24 Measuring glomerular filtration rate	339
15.25 Care of the CYP during a radiological investigation	347

The Great Ormond Street Hospital Manual of Children and Young People's Nursing Practices, Second Edition. Edited by Elizabeth Anne Bruce, Janet Williss, and Faith Gibson.
© 2023 John Wiley & Sons Ltd. Published 2023 by John Wiley & Sons Ltd.

Introduction

This chapter covers a wide range of investigations which are carried out by health care professionals on the ward and in radiology. Many children and young people (CYPs) undergo investigations while in hospital. These range from minimally invasive to high risk and/or invasive investigations, but most will cause the CYP to worry, or experience a degree of anxiety around what is to be expected. Parents/carers will also worry; therefore, as with all nursing practices, preparation is essential. Preparation is underpinned by knowledge of the reason for, process, and outcome of the investigation. Throughout this chapter the practical considerations that will underpin family preparation are addressed. The first section covers the collection of microbiological specimens, section two considers ward-based investigations, and the chapter concludes with the preparation for and care of CYPs during radiological Investigations. This chapter should be read in conjunction with Chapter 27: Play as a Therapeutic Tool, which provides detailed information regarding preparing CYPs for procedures through play. For pulse oximetry and monitoring of vital signs, see Chapter 1: Assessment, and for the care of CYPs undergoing liver, skin, or renal biopsies and bone marrow aspirate or trephine, see Chapter 3: Biopsies. For more information regarding blood sampling see Chapter 14: Intravenous and Intra-arterial Access and Infusions Obtaining a sampling of cerebrospinal fluid (CSF) is covered in Chapter 21: Neurological Care.

Collection of microbiological specimens

Microbiological and virological laboratory testing of specimens has a key role in the management of CYPs with infections. Accurate and rapid identification of significant microorganisms is vital for guiding optimal antimicrobial therapy and improving outcomes from infections and infectious diseases. Laboratory diagnosis is also essential for effective infection prevention and control in both the hospital and community settings, as well as providing valuable epidemiological data. In addition, accurate diagnosis reduces the overprescribing of antimicrobial agents and contributes significantly to reductions in the emergence and spread of antimicrobial resistance (Public Health England 2015).

Clinicians have the responsibility of using the correct procedure during the collection and safe transportation of samples to the laboratory. The validity of test results largely depends on good practice in the 'pretest' stage and it is essential that documentation is accurate and comprehensive (Higgins 1994). Microbiological tests are not as standardised as some other laboratory tests; the ways in which a sample is processed and the results are interpreted depend significantly on the information provided with the specimen. Contamination of samples, especially those from normally sterile sites such as blood or cerebrospinal fluid (CSF), can lead to misleading results, inappropriate antibiotic usage, unnecessary laboratory work, and potential delay in effective treatment for the CYP. Prolonged periods of storage at ambient temperatures and delay in transporting specimens to the laboratory may increase the number of contaminants present. It is therefore essential that every effort should be made to avoid these problems.

Rationale for specimen collection

Specimen collection is undertaken when laboratory investigation is required for the examination of material, e.g. blood, body fluid, tissue, or faeces to aid diagnosis.

Preparation

Laboratory request forms can be either:

- Printed through an electronic patient information management or similar system. The available labels on the form should be used to label the specimen the form was generated for. These are usually bar-coded to aid the audit trail.
- Handwritten on the appropriate laboratory request form.

All specimens must be clearly labelled to identify their source. Specimen containers should not be prelabelled as this may increase the risk of errors. The specimen should be labelled next to the CYP at the time the sample is taken. The laboratory request form must be checked against the wristband or other suitable identification of the CYP to positively identify them and avoid mislabelling specimens.

A laboratory request form with the following information must accompany the specimen. This aids interpretation of results and reduces the risk of errors. It should include:

a Name, date of birth, ward/department, and hospital/NHS number.
b Type of specimen and the site from which it was obtained (where necessary).
c Date and time collected.
d Diagnosis or suspected diagnosis with history, such as returning from abroad (specify country) with diarrhoea and vomiting, rash, pyrexia, catheters in situ or invasive devices used, or surgical details regarding postoperative wound infection.
e Any antimicrobial drug(s) given.
f Consultant's name.
g Cost code (if applicable).
h Name/bleep number of the clinician who ordered the investigation, as it may be necessary to telephone preliminary results and discuss treatment before the result is authorised.

- Always explain the procedure to the CYP and parent/carer and the reasons for taking the specimen. Separate permission must be obtained from the CYP and parent/carer if specimens are sought for research purposes; they have a right to refuse without any obligation (Royal College of Paediatrics and Child Health Ethics Advisory Committee 2000).
- Hands should be cleaned before and after specimen collection. Standard precautions should be applied and the appropriate personal protective equipment (PPE) worn when collecting or handling specimens to protect the healthcare worker (HCW) from exposure to blood and/or body fluids (Loveday et al. 2014).
- If an infection is suspected, e.g. when a CYP has respiratory symptoms or loose stools, the appropriate isolation precautions should be applied, even before the results of the specimen are available. The isolation precautions should be based on the symptoms the CYP is presenting with. Once the result of the specimen is available, the need and type of the isolation precautions can be reassessed. For more information on hand hygiene, see Chapter 13: Infection Prevention and Control.
- When collecting certain specimens, e.g. catheter urines and CSF, every effort should be made to minimise the risk of infecting the CYP. An appropriate aseptic or aseptic nontouch technique (ANTT) should be used.
- All pathological specimens must be treated as potentially infectious and local written laboratory protocols should be followed for the safe handling and transportation of specimens (Health and Safety Executive (HSE) 2003). Specimens should be collected in sterile containers with tight-fitting lids to avoid contamination and spillage. All specimen containers must be transported in a double-sided, self-sealing polythene bag with one compartment containing the laboratory request form and the other the specimen.
- In CYPs suspected of suffering from hazard group 3 or 4 pathogens, e.g. Middle East respiratory syndrome (MERS), severe acute respiratory syndrome (SARS), or viral haemorrhagic fevers (HSE Advisory Committee on Dangerous Pathogens 2021), the Infection Prevention and Control Team or Consultant in Communicable Diseases Control (CCDC) must be consulted before any specimens are taken (HSE 2003).
- Ideally, microbiological specimens should be collected before beginning any treatment such as antibiotics or using antiseptics. However, in the case of serious sepsis, treatment must not be delayed.

- When collecting a pus specimen, as much material as possible should be obtained, as this increases the chance of isolating microorganisms that may be difficult to grow or are minimal in number, e.g. tuberculosis.

Transport medium is used to preserve microorganisms during transportation:

- Charcoal medium improves the isolation of bacteria by neutralising toxic substances such as naturally occurring fatty acids found on the skin.

For virology specimens a viral transport medium should be used, as many viruses do not survive well outside the body.

Transport to the laboratory

- Specimens are generally delivered to the laboratories by hospital porters, via a pneumatic tube delivery system, by CYPs/parents (if from the community), or by post.
- Specimens sent by post must be packed and sent according to UN3373 regulations (United Nations Economic Commission for Europe 2020). The laboratory will have the relevant equipment for packaging. It is imperative that the regulations are followed, as the sender may be liable (with a financial penalty) for any spillage that may occur.
- Spillage kits must be available for cleaning and decontamination of any spillages of blood and/or body fluids. The manufacturer's instructions must be followed (HSE 2021).

Equipment

This will vary according to the specimen required, but must include:

- Disposable gloves
- Additional PPE where applicable (e.g. apron/gown, mask/respirator, goggles/visor)
- Tray
- Sterile container for the specimen with (if required) appropriate transport medium
- Laboratory request form
- Polythene transportation bag
- Biohazard label, if required

Blood samples

Blood sampling should be performed using the ANTT by an HCW trained and competent in the procedure (Loveday et al. 2014). As there are many different microbiological and virological blood tests, the clinician should seek information as to the appropriate laboratory containers required for specific tests and the amount of blood required. PPE should be worn as appropriate. The 'Broken Needle Technique' (breaking the hub of the needle to obtain blood from small infants) poses an additional risk of injury to the CYP and user and must NOT be used.

Analysis of antibiotic levels

The relationship between drug dose, drug concentration in biological fluid, and the individual CYP's metabolic process must be understood for interpreting results. The results may be affected by the route of administration, age of the CYP and disease process, such as liver and renal disease. The analysis involves testing levels in blood serum or plasma in direct relationship to drug administration:

- For timing of sampling for antibiotic concentrations, see local antibiotic policy.
- Record on the laboratory form the name of the drug, dose, and mode of administration, the time the drug is given, and whether the sample is a peak, trough, or random level.
- Trough levels are taken immediately prior to the time a drug is due; peak levels are taken one hour after the bolus or infusion has been administered.
- Blood for antibiotic assay should preferably be taken from a venepuncture, heel/finger-prick or arterial line; it should not be taken through the same catheter that has been used to give the antibiotic at any time. Some antibiotics bind to plastic and the drug may release intermittently, giving false results.

Blood culture

Detection of microorganisms by culture of blood is essential in the diagnosis of bloodstream infections, including infective endocarditis, infections presenting as pyrexia of unknown origin, prosthetic material infections, and intravenous catheter infections. Blood cultures may also detect bacteraemia associated with primary infections such as pneumonia and septic arthritis. Accurate positive results provide valuable information to guide optimal antibiotic therapy early on, which can improve the outcome from these conditions (NHS England 2022). Contaminated blood cultures can, however, cause considerable diagnostic confusion and lead to unnecessary or suboptimal antimicrobial therapy. This can be prevented by careful collection of the blood using the ANTT (Rowley and Clare 2011). The specimen should preferably be taken during pyrexial episodes, as more bacteria may be present at that time. Blood cultures should only be taken when there is a clinical need to do so in response to a deteriorating clinical picture and any of the following clinical signs suggestive of sepsis:

- Abnormalities in heart rate, core temperature, or leucocyte count
- Presence of rigours or chills
- Other focal signs of infection, such as pneumonia, septic arthritis, meningism, urinary tract infection, pyelonephritis, and acute abdominal pathology.

Procedure guideline 15.1 Taking a blood culture

Statement	Rationale
1 Perform hand hygiene and put on gloves and apron.	1 To comply with standard precautions.
2 Use an aerobic and an anaerobic blood culture bottle. Remove the plastic caps, wipe the bung with a 2% chlorhexidine in 70% alcohol wipe for 15 seconds, then allow to dry prior to inoculation.	2 To ensure sterility and prevent contamination.
3 Prior to the venepuncture, soap and water should be used to clean any visibly soiled skin. The skin must then be decontaminated with a 2% chlorhexidine in 70% alcohol applicator and allowed to dry. After decontamination the vein should not be repalpated (even with a gloved hand).	3 To prevent contamination.

(continued)

Procedure guideline 15.1 Taking a blood culture (continued)

Statement	Rationale
4 After withdrawing the blood, remove and safely discard the needle. Insert the blood into the blood culture bottle with a new sterile needle.	4 To prevent contamination of skin organisms on the needle used to withdraw the blood.
5 The anaerobic blood culture bottle should be inoculated first and the aerobic culture bottle second.	5 To prevent oxygen trapped in the syringe being transferred to the anaerobic bottle.
6 The volume of blood is the most critical factor in the detection of blood stream infections. Place up to 4 ml in the aerobic bottle (priority) and up to 10 ml in the anaerobic bottle. For neonates 1–2 ml of blood is recommended (Kellogg et al. 2000). However, the sensitivity of neonatal blood cultures is increased if more blood is cultured.	6 This optimises the identification of the microorganism if present.
7 Inoculation of the blood into the blood culture bottles should be performed first before inserting blood into other specimen bottles.	7 Many other blood bottles are not sterile and accidental contamination may occur.
8 Where available, a closed system should be used to inoculate blood culture bottles.	8 To prevent needle stick injuries.
9 Discard used needles into a sharps container.	9 To dispose of equipment safely.
10 After completion of the procedure, remove apron and gloves and perform hand hygiene.	10 To comply with standard precautions.
11 In CYPs with suspected central venous line sepsis, blood for culture may be taken from a peripheral vein stab and also from the appropriate intravascular lines.	11 If the same microorganism is identified from both sites, this indicates line colonisation or infection.
12 Blood cultures should only be taken from newly inserted peripheral cannulae and only if it is not possible to obtain the blood sample for culture through a separate venepuncture. Strict asepsis must be maintained.	12 Peripheral cannulae that have been in situ for some time are likely to be contaminated with skin organisms, increasing the risk of contamination of the blood culture.
13 Label blood culture bottles and place together with the laboratory form in the polythene transportation bag.	13 To ensure correct process and safe transport to the laboratory.
14 Document date and time when the blood culture was taken in the CYP's records.	14 To maintain accurate records.

Capillary blood sampling

A heel prick or finger puncture (see Table 15.1) is a useful and simple way of collecting a blood sample. It involves puncturing the cutaneous layer of the skin in a highly vascular area and can be used to monitor; blood sugar levels (see Procedure Guideline 15.20: Blood Glucose Monitoring), drug levels, blood gases, full blood counts, urea and electrolytes, bilirubin levels, and newborn bloodspot screening tests, see Chapter 20: Neonatal Care. Capillary blood sampling should NOT be used to obtain samples for blood cultures or coagulation studies, as it will not provide accurate results. Although this is a simple procedure, complications can arise, including pain; collapsed veins if the tibial artery is lacerated from puncturing the medial aspect of the heel; osteomyelitis of the heel bone (calcaneus) (Lilien et al. 1976, cited by WHO 2010); nerve damage if the fingers of neonates are punctured; haematoma and loss of access to the venous branch used; scarring; and localised or generalised necrosis from repeated procedures (WHO 2010). These problems can be avoided by using a good technique. Good quality sampling not only minimises complications but ensures accuracy of results, reduces unnecessary repeat samples and delays in obtaining results, and minimises distress to the CYP.

Table 15.1 Selecting an appropriate site for blood sampling. *Source:* From WHO (2010) WHO guidelines on drawing blood: best practices in phlebotomy. © 2010 World health organization

Condition	Heel-prick	Finger-prick
Age	Birth to about 6 months	Over 6 months
Weight	From 3 to 10 kg, approximately	Greater than 10 kg
Placement of lancet	On the medial or lateral plantar surface	On the side of the ball of the finger perpendicular to the lines of the fingerprint
Recommended finger	Not applicable	Second and third fingers (i.e. middle and ring fingers); avoid the thumb and index finger because of calluses, and avoid the little finger because the tissue is thin

(WHO 2010)

Procedure guideline 15.2 Capillary blood sampling

15.2.1 Preparation

Statement	Rationale
1 Ensure the CYP and family are informed of the following: • That a blood sample will be needed • What this will involve • Aftercare following obtaining the sample. A full explanation should be given to the parents and the CYP should be appropriately prepared with consideration of their age, level of understanding, anxiety, and past experiences.	1 To increase co-operation and understanding and minimise anxiety.
2 Gather the following equipment: a) Gloves and aprons b) Cotton wool or gauze c) Capillary tube and/or blood bottle d) Tenderfoot® or other age/size appropriate automated incision device (see point 3 below) e) Clean tray to hold equipment f) Sharps disposal box	2 To prepare for the procedure a) To minimise the risk of contamination d) To minimise pain and bruising, obtain the sample more quickly and reduce the risk of accidental injury from manual lancets f) To safely dispose of lancet device and capillary tubes.
3 Select an appropriate device: Choose an appropriately sized and age-appropriate automated incision device. For a neonate and baby less than six months this will normally be a heel-prick device (see Table 15.2); for a child over six months a finger-prick is recommended.	3 There is some evidence that an arch-shaped incision device (e.g. Tenderfoot® heel incision device) causes less trauma to the tissue, is more effective in providing a good quality sample, and reduces the number of heel punctures per sample, the time taken to complete the sample, bruising, and the need to repeat the sample (Glenesk et al. 2006; Shepherd et al. 2006).
4 a) The recommended depth for a finger-prick is: • Age six months to eight years: ≤ 1.5mm; • Age over eight years: ≤ 2.4mm. b) Too much compression should be avoided. c) Manual lancets must not be used.	4 a) To minimise trauma. b) This may cause a deeper puncture than is needed to get good flow (WHO 2010). c) To minimise pain and tissue damage (Cavanagh and Coppinger 2009).
5 Prepare the CYP and family/carer: Comfort measures and the use of sucrose are recommended to reduce the pain and discomfort caused to the patient during the blood sampling process. For neonates, an assessment of the baby's ability to tolerate handling must be made prior to obtaining the sample.	5 To minimise pain and discomfort during the blood sampling process (Association of Paediatric Anaesthetists of Great Britain and Ireland (APAGBI) 2012; Frank and Gilbert 2003; Yilmaz and Arikan 2011).
6 Select an appropriate site for blood sampling (see Figure 15.1): a) For full-term and preterm neonates, the external and internal limits of the calcaneus (the sides of the heels) are the preferred puncture sites (Public Health England 2016). b) For neonates who have had repeated heel punctures, the whole plantar surface may also be used. The use of the plantar surface should be limited to rare occasions and if in doubt, speak to the nurse in charge/an experienced nurse before undertaking. c) When using the whole planter surface, an automated incision device with a penetrative depth of no more than 1mm is recommended (Public Health England 2016). d) The back of the heel (posterior curvature) should be avoided as the device may puncture the bone. e) The site chosen for sampling should continually be rotated and be free from previous injury. f) Document skin integrity in the health care record. g) The procedure should be avoided on poorly perfused, oedematous, inflamed or swollen tissue, and localised areas of infection. h) Capillary blood sampling should never be taken from the fingers of a neonate. i) Please see Figure 15.1 for recommended sites for neonatal capillary blood sampling.	6. To ensure an effective procedure and cause minimal trauma. a) To reduce the risk of calcaneal puncture, which may lead to calcaneal osteomyelitis. b) To reduce the soft tissue damage and pain from repeated heel punctures in the same area. c) To reduce the risk of calcaneal puncture that may lead to calcaneal osteomyelitis. To reduce the soft tissue damage and pain from repeated heel punctures in the same area. e) To reduce the soft tissue damage and pain from repeated heel punctures in the same area. To minimise the risk of further trauma. g) To minimise the risk of contamination of the sample. To ensure a viable sample. To minimise the risk of infection. h) To avoid nerve damage.

(continued)

Table 15.2 Suggested size of Tenderfoot to use, according to weight/age

Device	Depth	Case Colour	Indications
Tenderfoot Preemie®	0.65 mm	White	Low birth weight 1000–2500 g
Tenderfoot Newborn®	0.85 mm	Pink and Blue	Low birth weight 1000–2500 g

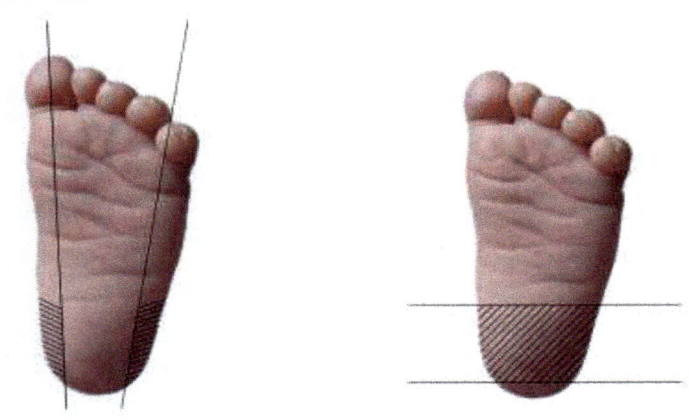

Figure 15.1 Recommended sites for capillary sampling. *Source:* Public Health England (2016)

Procedure guideline 15.2 Capillary blood sampling *(continued)*

15.2.2 Obtaining the sample

Statement	Rationale
1 Confirm the CYP's identity.	1 To ensure that the sample is collected from the correct CYP.
2 Perform a social handwash.	2, 3. To minimise the risk of infection.
3 Don apron and gloves.	
4 Place equipment in a convenient position.	4 To ensure a smooth and seamless procedure
5 To obtain the sample: a) Ensure that the CYP is in a safe and secure position. b) Clean the intended puncture site by washing with plain water using gauze/cotton wool. Do not heat the water. c) Soap and alcohol impregnated wipes should not be used. d) Allow the area to dry. e) Ensure the finger/heel is warm but additional prewarming is not required. f) Soft paraffin solutions such as Vaseline® should not be used.	5. a) To assist procedure and reduce pain/discomfort. b) To minimise the risk of infection. To prevent contamination of the sample. c) Soap or detergent can irritate the skin. Alcohol is drying and has been associated with chemical burns in premature infants (Lund et al. 2001; Reynolds et al. 2005) and can cause injury to delicate or healing tissue (Lund et al. 2001). d) Test results may be affected if the skin is not allowed to dry properly. e) To avoid the risk of scalding/burns (Hassan and Shah 2005; Public Health England 2016). To increase blood flow to the area. To aid collection. f) Soft paraffin solutions such as Vaseline increase the risk of infection, can alter blood results, and clog equipment.
6 For a finger-prick: Hold the finger that has been selected for puncture between your thumb and index finger with the palm of the CYP's hand facing up.	6 To produce a steady grip and minimise movement.
7 For a heel prick, hold the baby's heel with the nondominant hand with a moderately firm grip (Figure 15.2a). The forefinger is placed at the arch of the foot and the thumb below the puncture site at the ankle. Use other fingers to steady the baby's leg.	7 To keep the dominant hand free for the procedure. To produce a steady grip and minimise movement.
8 To perform the procedure: a) Place the automated incision device against the finger/heel in accordance with the manufacturer's instructions. Do not use undue pressure/compression of the device against the skin (Figure 15.2b). b) Depress button to activate the device to puncture the skin in a steady and intentional manner. After triggering, immediately remove the device from the finger/heel (Figure 15.2c).	a) Excessive pressure/compression from a heel stick device when placed against the skin can significantly increase the depth of the puncture.

Procedure guideline 15.2 Capillary blood sampling *(continued)*

Statement	Rationale
c) There is no need to discard the first drop of blood.	c) This can be used if the area has been cleaned thoroughly (Public Health England 2016).
d) While maintaining grip, hold the finger/heel so that blood is allowed to hang downwards.	d) To increase blood flow to the area and aid collection.
e) Gently but firmly compress the finger/heel to form a large droplet of blood.	e) Steady compression aids collection.
f) Do not squeeze the finger/foot in an attempt to increase blood flow.	f) Squeezing can cause haemolysis and potentially inaccurate results. It can also cause pain, bruising and soft tissue damage.
g) Hold the capillary tube or blood bottle to the blood droplet and touch (Figure 15.2d).	g, h, i) To obtain an adequate blood sample.
h) Momentarily release pressure to collect subsequent blood then reapply pressure, allowing the blood to flow.	
i) Continue until sufficient blood has been obtained.	
j) If blood flow ceases, wipe the area firmly with gauze and gently massage the foot, avoiding squeezing to try to promote blood flow. If there is no blood flow, a second puncture may be necessary – this should be performed on a different part of the same foot or on the other foot.	j) To ensure a viable sample.

15.2.3 Completing the procedure

Once the sample has been obtained:	
1 Wipe excess blood from the heel and apply gentle pressure to the site with gauze (Figure 15.2e).	1 To stop bleeding and protect the wound.
2 Maintain pressure until bleeding has stopped. Apply gauze and hypoallergenic tape to the site if required. Do not use Elastoplast®.	2 To prevent bruising. Certain adhesive tapes can damage fragile skin and cause infection.
3 The baby/child should be left comfortable.	
4 Waste should be disposed of according to local policy.	
5 Staff involved should wash their hands.	
6 The sample should be sent for analysis as soon as possible.	6 To promote effectiveness of testing.

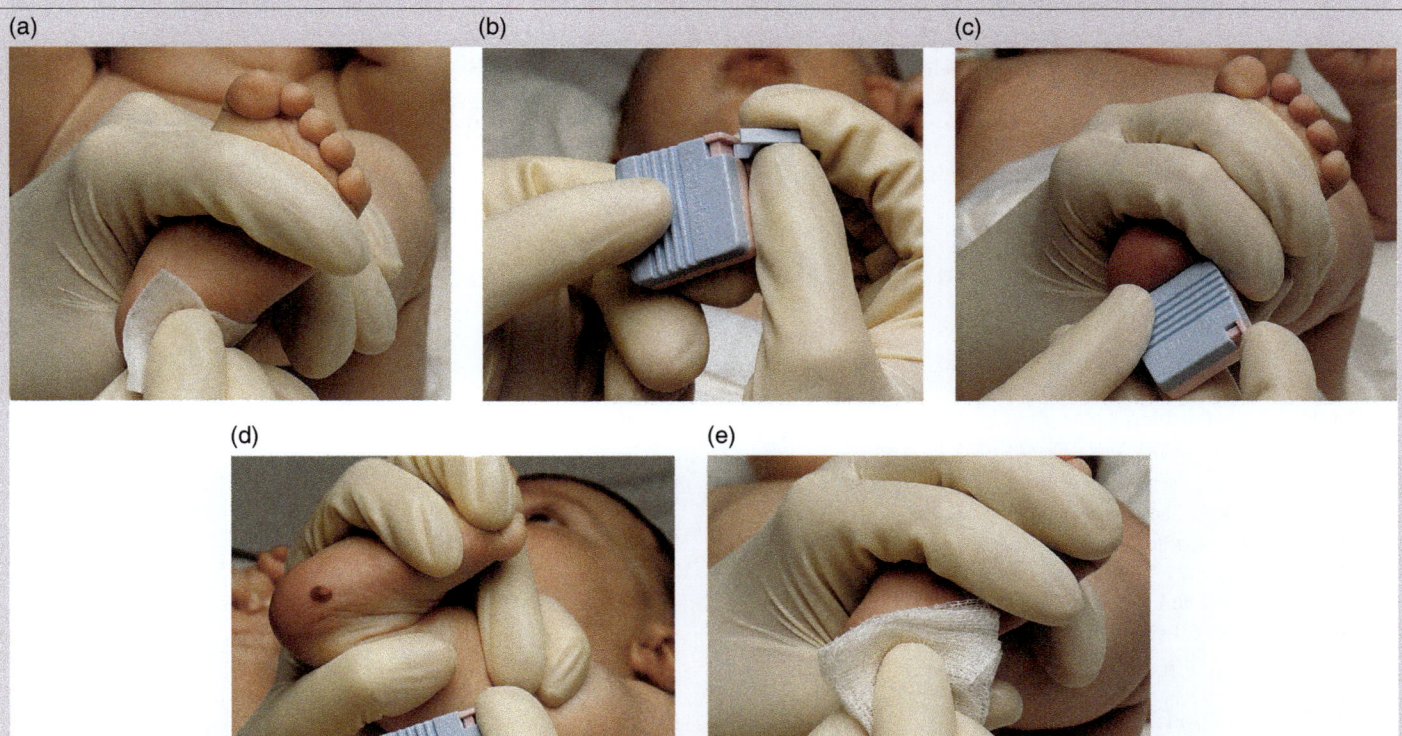

Figure 15.2 Obtaining a capillary sample from a heel using a Tenderfoot Heel Incision Device. *Source:* International Technidyne Corporation.

Biopsy Material

Specimens such as skin, muscle, kidney, liver, jejunal tissue, or brain biopsies are generally obtained by medical staff under either general or local anaesthetic, depending on the site. A sterile technique is required for all procedures. Biopsy specimens, especially if small, or when requesting multiple tests, must be discussed with the relevant laboratory personnel in order to:

- Ensure that the most appropriate specimen and laboratory tests are undertaken. If the specimen is small, it may be necessary to limit the range of tests.
- Check whether the specimen is to be fixed in formalin. Formalin **must not be used** if the specimen is for microbiological investigation. In many cases, histopathological, microbiological, and virological analysis will be required and it is critical that separate specimens are sent for these purposes so that they are processed and transported appropriately.

For more information see Chapter 3: Biopsies.

Cerebrospinal fluid (CSF)

CSF is usually obtained via a lumbar puncture performed by medical staff. Sampling of CSF is essential for the accurate diagnosis of infectious meningitis and may aid in the diagnosis of encephalitis. A sterile technique is required, as there is a risk of introducing infection during the procedure. Specimens of CSF should be dispatched to the laboratory immediately. Out of office hours it is essential that the on-call laboratory staff are contacted when the sample is being transported. It is important not to store the specimen in a refrigerator as this may cause the cells to deteriorate or lyse, giving rise to misleading results. It is common practice to send three separate collection tubes of CSF when investigating for evidence of subarachnoid haemorrhage, as the initial part of the sample may be contaminated with blood from outside the subarachnoid space. If this is performed, it is important to label the tubes as such and specifically request counts on the first and third samples. It is also important to remember that a CSF glucose level (sent separately to chemical pathology) can only be accurately interpreted in conjunction with a simultaneous plasma glucose level. For more information regarding obtaining a sample of CSF see Chapter 21: Neurological Care.

Chest Drain Fluid Collection

Samples of chest drain fluid can be taken directly from the drainage tubing to be tested for the presence of infection markers, white blood cells, and chyle.

Fungal Samples (Hair, Nail, and Skin)

These samples may be required for the investigation of suspected fungal infections.

Gastric Washings (Lavage)

Infants and young children are generally not able to expectorate enough sputum for laboratory analysis. It may therefore be necessary to obtain swallowed sputum through gastric washings (lavage), particularly to aid the diagnosis of pulmonary *Mycobacterium tuberculosis*. The detection of alcohol acid fast bacilli (AAFB) is not adequate alone for diagnosis of *Mycobacterium tuberculosis* as other environmental AAFBs may be present. Culture of the organism is always performed and may take between 6 and 12 weeks to confirm diagnosis. Three consecutive early morning specimens should be obtained. There are usually only small numbers of microorganisms present, so as much material as possible should be obtained. Sterile water must be used for the gastric lavage, as AAFB are often found in tap water.

NB: Performing this procedure may cause the CYP to cough, which can expose the HCW to pathogens. It is therefore essential that appropriate respiratory protection and eyewear is worn when performing this procedure.

Nasopharyngeal Aspirate (NPA)

A nasopharyngeal aspirate (NPA) is required for the diagnosis of viral respiratory infections such as influenza, parainfluenza, metapneumovirus, and respiratory syncytial virus (RSV). It is also the preferred type of specimen for the diagnosis of *Bordetella pertussis* infections by polymerase chain reaction (PCR) and culture.

Procedure guideline 15.3 Collecting a sample of chest drain fluid

Statement	Rationale
1 Wash hands and perform aseptic nontouch technique (ANTT) to prepare the following equipment: • Small dressing pack • Appropriate cleaning solution (such as chlorhexidine gluconate 0.5%, in 70% alcohol) • Nonsterile gloves • Syringe and needle • Chest drain clamps • Specimen pot(s) • Specimen form.	
2 Clamp drainage tubing below fluid level.	2 To obtain the specimen and avoid secondary infection.
3 Perform hand hygiene and put on apron and gloves.	3 To comply with standard precautions.
4 Clean tubing with chlorhexidine gluconate 0.5% in 70% alcohol wipe and allow to dry.	
5 Insert a green needle and aspirate fluid using a 10 ml syringe.	
6 Dispose of used sharps safely in line with local guidelines.	
7 Remove clamp. Tube is self-sealing.	
8 A specimen can also be taken from the back of the drainage unit, which does not require a needle. a) Follow ANTT and PPE and clean the site with chlorhexidine gluconate 0.5% in 70% alcohol wipe. b) Attach a syringe directly onto the specimen access point at the back of the drain.	
9 Ensure the specimen is correctly labelled.	9 To ensure that analysis is carried out correctly.
10 Ensure amount removed is documented.	10 To maintain an accurate fluid balance.

Procedure guideline 15.4 Collecting fungal samples

Statement	Rationale
1 Special containers for the collection of dermatological material for mycological investigations may be obtained from the laboratory.	1 These containers aid the visibility of the material against a dark background under the microscope.
2 Perform hand hygiene and put on apron and gloves.	2 To comply with standard precautions.
3 Hair: Samples of infected hair should be removed by plucking the hair with forceps or gloves.	3 The root of the hair is infected, not the shaft.
4 Nail: Samples of the whole thickness of the nail or deep scrapings should be obtained.	4 To enable as much infected material as possible to be obtained to increase the chances of identification.
5 Skin: The skin should be cleaned with an alcohol swab. Obtain epidermal scales scraped from the active edge or roof of a lesion.	5 To prevent secondary infection.
6 Label specimen and put with the laboratory form in the polythene transport bag.	6 To ensure correct process and safe transport to the laboratory.
7 Remove apron and gloves and perform hand hygiene.	7 To comply with standard precautions.
8 Document date and time when the specimen was taken in the CYP's records.	8 To maintain accurate records.

Procedure guideline 15.5 Collecting gastric samples

Statement	Rationale
1 Fast the CYP for at least six hours overnight or as long as possible.	1 Feeds may not be sterile and environmental AAFB found normally in substances, such as water, will confuse results.
2 Put on an apron, respirator, and goggles or visor.	2 To comply with standard precautions.
3 Perform hand hygiene and put on gloves.	3 To comply with standard precautions.
4 Pass a nasogastric tube.	4 To obtain the gastric washings.
5 Aspirate the stomach contents and place in a plain sterile container.	5 The fasted stomach contents may contain sputum with AAFB.
6 a) Instil at least 30 ml of sterile water down the tube to obtain as much stomach content as possible. b) The medical condition and age of the CYP must be taken into consideration.	6 a) To increase the amount of material to be tested. b) In preterm or young infants the amount of the water to be instilled may have to be reduced.
7 Aspirate the contents back and place in the same container.	7 To increase the amount of material to be examined.
8 Remove the tube if it is no longer required.	
9 Label specimen and put together with the laboratory form in a polythene transport bag.	9 To ensure correct process and safe transport to the laboratory.
10 Remove PPE and perform hand hygiene.	10 To comply with standard precautions.
11 Document date and time when the specimen was taken in the CYP's records.	11 To maintain accurate records.

NB: Performing an NPA may generate either droplets, aerosols or both, which can expose HCWs to these pathogens. It is therefore essential that appropriate respiratory protection and eyewear is worn when performing this procedure.

Sputum samples
Sputum cultures have been shown to accurately reflect lower airway secretions (Hoppe et al. 2015). For CYPs who produce and are able to expectorate sputum, this proves to be a more accurate method of microbiological sampling, and therefore improves identification of respiratory pathogens (Equi et al. 2001). This may be required for microbiological diagnosis of pneumonia, as well as acute tracheitis, and bronchitis. It is routinely used for CYPs with chronic and often progressive suppurative lung diseases such as cystic fibrosis and primary ciliary dyskinesia. However, samples contaminated with oropharyngeal secretions and saliva are difficult to interpret and can be misleading.

NB: Obtaining a sputum specimen may generate either droplets, aerosols or both, which can expose the HCW to pathogens. It is therefore essential that appropriate respiratory protection and eyewear is worn when performing this procedure.

Stool (Faeces) specimen
In CYPs, stool specimens are frequently collected to identify bacteria, viruses, or parasites that cause diarrhoea. Other reasons may be to assess gastrointestinal function, or to check for occult blood.

Swabs: Cough swab
Early recognition and eradication of respiratory pathogens may delay disease progression in CYPs with cystic fibrosis and other conditions that cause progressive suppurative lung disease (Koch and Hoiby 2000). Cough swabs are a sampling method used for the identification of respiratory pathogens with CYPs who do not produce or expectorate sputum. Antibiotic therapy can then be directed accordingly.

Procedure guideline 15.6 Collecting a nasopharyngeal aspirate

Statement	Rationale
1 Put on an apron, respirator and goggles or visor.	1 To comply with standard precautions.
2 Perform hand hygiene and put on gloves.	2 To comply with standard precautions.
3 Attach a mucus trap to the suction system and the appropriately sized catheter, leaving the wrapper on the suction catheter.	3 This maximises the material for analysis and prevents contamination.
4 Turn on the suction and adjust the pressure.	4 To obtain the material for analysis.
5 Using a clean glove technique and without applying suction, remove the catheter from the wrapper. Gently insert the catheter into the nose, directed posteriorly and towards the opening of the external ear. NB: The depth of insertion necessary to reach the posterior pharynx is equivalent to the distance between the anterior naris and external opening of the ear. When resistance is felt the posterior nasopharynx has been reached.	5 To prevent contamination of the specimen or injury to the nasopharynx.
6 a) Apply suction and slowly withdraw the catheter using a rotating movement. The mucus trap should be kept upright. b) The catheter should remain in the nasopharynx for no longer than 10 seconds.	6 a) To obtain the material. b) To minimise discomfort or hypoxia.
7 If necessary, rinse the catheter with a small volume of sterile 0.9% sodium chloride to ensure adequate specimen volume.	7 To obtain any material left in the tubing.
8 Disconnect suction and seal mucus trap, either with tubing or the attached lid.	8 To safely send the sputum trap to the laboratory and avoid contamination.
9 Label specimen and put together with the laboratory form in a polythene transport bag.	9 To ensure correct process and safe transport to the laboratory.
10 Remove PPE and perform hand hygiene.	10 To comply with standard precautions.
11 Document date and time when the specimen was taken in the CYP's records.	11 To maintain accurate records.

Procedure guideline 15.7 Collecting sputum samples

Statement	Rationale
1 Put on an apron, respirator and goggles or visor.	1 To comply with standard precautions.
2 Perform hand hygiene and put on gloves.	2 To comply with standard precautions.
3 Encourage the CYP to cough (especially after sleep) and expectorate into a plain sterile container. Alternatively, a sample may be obtained from a nasopharyngeal, oropharyngeal, or tracheal suction using a sputum trap.	3 To obtain a suitable sample.
4 Chest physiotherapy may be performed and/or a saline nebuliser given (normal of 0.9% sodium chloride or hypertonic of 3% or 7%) prior to the sample being taken. NB: If hypertonic saline is to be used it must be prescribed, along with a bronchodilator, and the CYP must be monitored with oxygen saturation, spirometry, and auscultation. This should be done by an appropriately qualified professional, such as physiotherapist or specialist nurse.	4 This may help facilitate expectoration.
5 Ensure the material obtained is sputum and not saliva.	5 The cells in the sputum are required for analysis.
6 Label specimen and put together with the laboratory form in a polythene transport bag.	6 To ensure correct process and safe transport to the laboratory.
7 Remove PPE and perform hand hygiene.	7 To comply with standard precautions.
8 Document date and time when the specimen was taken in the CYP's records.	8 To maintain accurate records.

Procedure guideline 15.8 Collecting a stool (faecal) specimen

Statement	Rationale
1 Perform hand hygiene and put on apron and gloves.	1 To comply with standard precautions.
2 a) Continent CYPs should be asked to urinate first, flush the toilet, and then defecate into a bed pan that is placed on the toilet. b) In nappy-wearing children a urine bag can be applied.	2 To prevent contamination of the stool with urine.
3 The specimen can be obtained from a nappy, clean potty, or bed pan that is placed on the toilet.	3 The specimen does not need to be sterile.
4 Using the scoop attached to the inside of the lid of the specimen container, place faecal material into the stool specimen container.	4 To prevent contamination of the outside of the container.
5 Where diarrhoea is present, a small piece of nonabsorbent material lining the nappy can be used to obtain a suitable specimen.	5 To prevent faeces soaking into the nappy.
6 Examine the sample for consistency, odour, or blood and record observations.	6 To monitor any changes.
7 If segments of tapeworm are seen, send to the laboratory. a) For the identification of *Enterobius vermicularis* (threadworm/pinworm) material should be obtained first thing in the morning on awakening by using a clear adhesive tape slide. b) Place the sticky side of a strip of adhesive clear tape briefly over the anal region to obtain the material, remove and stick the clear adhesive tape smoothly onto a glass slide.	7 Tapeworm segments can vary from the size of rice grains to a ribbon shape, 1 inch long. a) Threadworms lay their ova on the perianal skin at night and will therefore not be seen in a faecal specimen. b) The worms and/or ova can then be identified under the microscope.
8 Where acute amoebic dysentery is suspected, the specimen of stool must be freshly dispatched to the laboratory.	8 The parasite causing amoebic dysentery exists in a free-living motile form and in the form of nonmotile cysts. Both forms are characteristic in their fresh state, but the motile form cannot be identified when dead. 'Hot faeces' should be discussed with the laboratory prior to collection to ensure they are processed immediately.
9 Label specimen and put together with the laboratory form in a polythene transport bag.	9 To ensure correct process and safe transport to the laboratory.
10 Remove gloves and apron and perform hand hygiene.	10 To comply with standard precautions.
11 Document date and time when the specimen was taken in the CYP's records.	11 To maintain accurate records.
12 NB: A faecal specimen is more suitable than a rectal swab.	12 A stool specimen is likely to contain more microorganisms than a rectal swab. However, rectal swabs may be taken from neonates before the first stool is passed.

Procedure guideline 15.9 Taking a cough swab

Statement	Rationale
1 Put on apron, respirator, and goggles/visor.	1 To comply with standard precautions, as the CYP may cough and infectious material poses a risk to the healthcare worker.
2 Perform hand hygiene and put on gloves.	2 To comply with standard precautions.
3 Place a cotton-tipped swab in, but not touching, the posterior pharynx.	3 To enable accurate sampling.
4 Ask the CYP to cough or stimulate a cough, holding the swab in position.	4 To obtain the sample.
5 Remove the swab without touching the oropharynx and place into transport medium.	5 To send the swab to the laboratory and preserve the sample.
6 Label the specimen and place together with the laboratory form in the polythene transportation bag.	6 To ensure correct process and safe transport to the laboratory.
7 Remove PPE and perform hand hygiene.	7 To minimise the risk of infection.
8 Document date and time when the specimen was taken in the CYP's records.	8 To maintain accurate records.

Swabs: Ear Swabs

Procedure guideline 15.10 Taking an ear swab

Statement	Rationale
1 Perform hand hygiene and put on apron and gloves.	1 To comply with standard precautions.
2 Place a sterile swab into the outer ear and gently rotate to collect the secretions.	2 This material is required to identify any microorganisms.
3 If there is purulent discharge this should be sampled.	3 To obtain an adequate specimen.
4 For deeper ear swabbing a speculum may be used.	4 Only experienced medical staff should undertake this procedure as damage to the tympanic membrane may occur.
5 Place the swab in a specimen container with transport medium.	5 To preserve the growth of any microorganisms.
6 Label the specimen and put together with the laboratory form in the polythene transport bag.	6 To ensure correct process and safe transport to the laboratory.
7 Remove gloves and apron and perform hand hygiene.	7 To comply with standard precautions.
8 Document date and time when the specimen was taken in the CYP's records.	8 To maintain accurate records.
9 NB: No antibiotics or other therapeutic agents should have been applied in the aural region for about three hours prior to sampling the area.	9 Local antibiotics may inhibit the growth of microorganisms.

Swabs: Eye Swabs

Procedure guideline 15.11 Taking an eye swab

Statement	Rationale
1 Perform hand hygiene and put on apron and gloves.	1 To comply with standard precautions.
2 Where possible ask the CYP to look upwards and gently pull down the lower lid or gently part the eyelids.	2 To expose the area to be swabbed.
3 Use a sterile cotton wool swab and gently roll the swab over the conjunctival sac inside the lower lid. Hold the swab parallel to the cornea.	3 This avoids injury if the CYP moves.
4 Place the swab in a specimen container with transport medium.	4 To preserve the growth of microorganisms.
5 For viral investigation follow same as above, but place in viral transport medium.	5 To preserve any viral material.
6 Label specimen and put together with the laboratory form in the polythene transport bag.	6 To ensure correct process and safe transport to the laboratory.
7 Remove gloves and apron and perform hand hygiene.	7 To comply with standard precautions.
8 Document date and time when the specimen was taken in the CYP's records.	8 To maintain accurate records.
9 For suspected *Chlamydia trachomatis* infection obtain a special chlamydia sampling kit from the laboratory:	
a) Perform hand hygiene and put on apron and gloves.	a) To comply with standard precautions
b) Clean the eye first with sterile normal saline.	b) To obtain a clear view of the conjunctiva.
c) Using the swab, part the eyelids and gently rub the conjunctival sac of the lower lid.	c) To obtain epithelial cells.
d) Place the swab in the transport medium provided.	d) To preserve the growth of microorganisms.
e) Label specimen and put together with the laboratory form in the polythene transport bag.	e) To ensure correct process and safe transport to the laboratory.
f) Remove gloves and apron and perform hand hygiene	f) To comply with standard precautions.
g) Document date and time when the specimen was taken in the CYP's records.	g) To maintain accurate records.

Swabs: Nose Swabs

Procedure guideline 15.12 Collecting nose swabs

Statement	Rationale
1 Perform hand hygiene and put on apron and gloves.	1 To comply with standard precautions.
2 Moisten the swab with sterile 0.9% saline solution beforehand.	2 This enhances the collection of material and alleviates discomfort.
3 Insert the swab into the anterior nares and direct it up into the tip of the nose and gently rotate.	3 Both nares should be swabbed using the same swab to obtain adequate material.
4 Place in specimen container with transport medium.	4 To preserve any microorganisms.
5 For viral investigation follow same as above, but place in viral transport medium.	5 To preserve any viral material.
6 The outside of the nostrils may be rubbed after the procedure to alleviate the unpleasant sensation of swabbing.	6 This procedure may stimulate sneezing.
7 Label specimen and put together with the laboratory form in the polythene transport bag.	7 To ensure correct process and safe transport to the laboratory.
8 After the procedure remove gloves and apron and perform hand hygiene.	8 To comply with standard precautions.
9 Document date and time when the specimen was taken in the CYP's records.	9 To maintain accurate records.

Swabs: Oral fluid (Saliva) swab

This test is used to confirm suspected cases of measles, mumps and rubella.

NB: Ideally the sample should be taken as soon as possible after onset of the first symptoms.

Swabs: Pernasal swabs

This investigation is most commonly used to diagnose whooping cough (*Bordetella pertussis*). Specimens for PCR can be taken at any age if there is a clinical diagnosis. If acute infection is suspected, the pernasal swab can also be cultured, but must be taken to the laboratory immediately after collection.

A NPA is the preferred type of specimen for the diagnosis of *Bordetella pertussis*. Pernasal swabs may be sent, but only special thin wire swabs for pernasal specimen collection are used. The HCW must be proficient in obtaining a pernasal swab and must ensure that suction, oxygen, and resuscitation equipment are easily available, as the procedure may induce paroxysmal coughing and/or vomiting. The CYP should be held securely during the procedure and be observed carefully during and immediately after the procedure.

NB: Performing this procedure may generate droplets and/or aerosols, which can expose HCWs to this pathogen. It is therefore essential that appropriate PPE (gloves, apron, respirator, and goggles/visor) is worn when performing this procedure.

Swabs: Skin (Screening) swabs

These swabs are generally taken to comply with hospital admission screening protocols for *meticillin-resistant Staphylococcus aureus* (MRSA) or on the advice of the infection prevention and control team. The purpose of the screening is to detect those individuals with asymptomatic MRSA carriage or colonisation, as they represent the most important reservoir of MRSA in healthcare facilities (Grundmann et al. 2006).

As part of the routine admission screen each CYP should have a nose and throat swab taken in the 30 days prior to admission or within the first 24 hours of admission and then at least every 30 days during admission (Coia et al. 2006; DH 2014). In addition, any skin lesions and sites of indwelling devices (e.g. tracheostomy or gastrostomy) should be swabbed. In neonates the umbilicus should be swabbed. CYPs already known to be colonised with MRSA should have a full MRSA screen (nose, throat, hairline, axillae, groyne/perineum, any skin lesions and sites of indwelling devices) taken on admission. In CYPs with *Epidermolysis bullosa* taking a nose and throat swab may cause mucosal damage and should therefore be avoided. However, these CYPs should still be screened on nonmucosal sites such as hairline, axillae, groyne, and sites of indwelling devices (if applicable).

For the screening of nose and throat, refer to Procedure Guidelines 15.12 and 15.16.

Procedure guideline 15.13 Taking an oral fluid (saliva) swab

Statement	Rationale
1 Special oral fluid test kits may be obtained from the laboratory.	1 This kit includes a sponge swab which will aid the collection of adequate material.
2 Perform hand hygiene and put on apron and gloves.	2 To comply with standard precautions.
3 Place the CYP in a position with a good light source.	3 This will ensure maximum visibility of the area to be swabbed.
4 Ask the CYP to open the mouth wide and say 'aahh'.	4 This will ensure maximum visibility of the area to be swabbed.
5 Remove pink sponge swab from the clear tube and swab the area between the cheek and gum by rubbing the pink sponge swab all along the gums and teeth (if present) for one to two minutes.	5 To obtain adequate material.

(continued)

Procedure guideline 15.13 Taking an oral fluid (saliva) swab *(continued)*

Statement	Rationale
6 Replace pink swab in the clear tube, attach label, and put together with the laboratory form in the polythene transport bag.	6 To ensure correct process and safe transport to the laboratory.
7 Remove apron and gloves and perform hand hygiene.	7 To comply with standard precautions.
8 Document date and time when the specimen was taken in the CYP's records.	8 To maintain accurate records.

Procedure guideline 15.14 Collecting pernasal swabs

Statement	Rationale
1 Put on apron, respirator and goggles or visor.	1 To comply with standard precautions.
2 Perform hand hygiene and put on gloves.	2 To comply with standard precautions.
3 Place the CYP in a position with a good light source.	3 This facilitates better observation of the CYP.
4 Use a special pernasal swab (dry, thin cotton-tipped wire swab in a plain dry tube).	4 This minimises trauma to the nasal tissue.
5 Holding the head upwards, pass the swab along the floor of the nasal cavity to the posterior wall of the nasopharynx.	5 This is where the *Bordetella pertussis* bacterium commonly resides.
6 Gently rotate and withdraw the swab and place in its container, dispatch immediately to the laboratory.	6 This ensures maximum chance of growth of the organism.
7 For PCR tests, the sample should be taken in the same way and delivered immediately to the microbiology laboratory.	7 Do not put the sample in charcoal medium as this inhibits PCR.
8 Label specimen and put together with the laboratory form in the polythene transport bag.	8 To ensure correct process and safe transport to the laboratory.
9 Remove PPE and perform hand hygiene.	9 To comply with standard precautions.
10 Document date and time when the specimen was taken in the CYP's records.	10 To maintain accurate records.

Procedure guideline 15.15 Taking skin (screening) swabs

Statement	Rationale
1 Perform hand hygiene and put on apron and gloves.	1 To comply with standard precautions.
2 As skin is usually dry, moisten the swab with sterile 0.9% saline solution beforehand.	2 This enhances the collection of material (Perry 2007).
3 Rotate the moistened swab gently but firmly over the area to be swabbed.	3 To obtain adequate material.
4 Place in specimen container with transport medium.	4 To preserve any microorganisms.
5 Label specimen and put together with the laboratory form in the polythene transport bag.	5 To ensure correct process and safe transport to the laboratory.
6 After the procedure remove apron and gloves and perform hand hygiene.	6 To comply with standard precautions.
7 Document date and time when the specimen was taken in the CYP's records.	7 To maintain accurate records.

Procedure guideline 15.16 Taking throat swabs

Statement	Rationale
1 Perform hand hygiene and put on apron and gloves.	1 To comply with standard precautions.
2 Place the CYP in a position with a good light source.	2 This will ensure maximum visibility of the tonsillar bed.
3 Either depress the tongue with a spatula or ask the CYP to say 'aahh'. Quickly but gently rub the swab over the tonsillar fossa (tonsillar bed) or area where there is exudate or a lesion.	3 The procedure is likely to cause gagging and the tongue will move to the roof of the mouth. This can prevent accurate sampling.

Procedure guideline 15.16 Taking throat swabs (continued)

Statement	Rationale
4 Care should be taken that the swab does not come into contact with the tongue or oral mucosa on removal.	4 To prevent contamination of the swab with oral bacterial flora.
5 Place the sample into transport medium or, if for viral investigation, place into viral transport medium.	5 To preserve the microorganisms.
6 Label specimen and put together with the laboratory form in the polythene transport bag.	6 To ensure correct process and safe transport to the laboratory.
7 Remove gloves and apron and perform hand hygiene.	7 To comply with standard precautions.
8 Document date and time when the specimen was taken in the CYP's records.	8 To maintain accurate records.

Procedure guideline 15.17 Taking a vulval swab for the investigation of simple vaginal discharge

Statement	Rationale
1 Perform hand hygiene and put on apron and gloves.	1 To comply with standard precautions.
2 The girl should lie on an examination couch with her legs in a froglike position.	2 To ensure the CYP is comfortable and to allow good visibility.
3 Gently separate and retract the labia.	3 To allow visualisation of the external genitalia.
4 Swab the posterior fourchette without inserting the swab into the vagina.	4 Discharge often pools in the posterior fourchette.
5 • In older girls a routine charcoal swab can be used. • In very young girls a dry, thin, cotton-tipped wire swab can be used (same as for pernasal swabs).	5 To minimise discomfort.
6 Label specimen and put together with the laboratory form in the polythene transport bag.	6 To ensure correct process and safe transport to the laboratory.
7 Remove gloves and apron and perform hand hygiene.	7 To comply with standard precautions.
8 Document date and time when the specimen was taken in the CYP's records.	8 To maintain accurate records.

In case of suspected or actual sexual abuse:

- Prior to any examination being undertaken, the named safeguarding doctor must be contacted for advice and support.
- The named safeguarding doctor will advise on the appropriate investigations, as well as the appropriateness of a forensic procedure.
- **Do not clean the area** (unless clinically indicated), as identification of semen or sexually transmitted diseases may be required for evidence.
- Local safeguarding protocols must be adhered to.

Swabs: Vaginal/vulval swabs

Taking a vaginal or vulval swab is a sensitive procedure and the medical context, as well as the potential sexual activity of the girl need to be considered to decide if a swab is clinically indicated.

The procedure should be explained to the girl and the parents/carers. It should be done, if preferred, by a female HCW, proficient in the procedure and usually in the presence of a parent/carer in a relaxed and private space. In some circumstances, young girls should be given the choice whether or not they would like to have a parent or carer present.

Swabs: Wound swabs

Interpretation of results must be in conjunction with clinical signs. In the absence of clinical signs of infection, wound swabs will provide little, if any, useful information, and simply reflects colonisation (Gilchrist 1996).

Urine Samples

Bedside urine testing for the presence of blood, protein, and other analytes is usually undertaken with reagent strips, the results of which indicate that further laboratory investigation is required (Cook 1995).

Most urine samples sent to the microbiology laboratory are for bacteriological investigation. The same collection techniques also apply to samples sent for virological investigation.

Urine samples should be dispatched to the laboratory as soon as possible and no more than 4 hours if kept at room temperature or up to 24 hours if kept at 4°C to avoid overgrowth of organisms and misleading results (Griffiths 1995).

All methods used to collect urine samples can result in contamination with bacteria from outside the bladder. This can lead to an inaccurate diagnosis, involve unnecessary treatment, or require a sample to be repeated, which has implications for patient care and cost effectiveness (Lewis 1998).

Prior to collection of the specimen normal social hygiene, such as washing the genitalia with soap and water and drying thoroughly, is considered sufficient to minimise contamination from the skin. Assess the clinical and psychosocial needs of the CYP as to whether cleaning the genitalia is necessary. The HCW must be sensitive to the cultural issues surrounding touching intimate parts of the body.

The most popular noninvasive method to obtain a urine specimen is the midstream or 'clean catch' specimen. National Institute for Health and Care Excellence (NICE) (2007) defines this method as the gold standard. However, obtaining a midstream or 'clean catch' specimen in precontinent babies, nontoilet trained toddlers, or incontinent CYPs can be challenging.

Urine collection pads or urine collection bags are often used but are more susceptible to contamination due to close contact with the ano-genital area. NICE (2007) suggests urine collection pads as the next best option to 'clean catch' specimen. When using urine collection pads, manufacturer's instructions should be followed. Cotton-wool balls, gauze, or sanitary pads should not be used (NICE 2007).

Collection of urine by a supra-pubic aspirate should only be considered when a clean and accurate sample is required, as this is a painful and invasive procedure. Ultrasound guidance should be used to indicate the presence of urine in the bladder before a supra-pubic aspirate is attempted (NICE 2007).

Vesicular fluid sample for herpes polymerase chain reaction (PCR)

This test may be necessary to confirm a suspected diagnosis of *herpes simplex* or *varicella zoster* (chickenpox or shingles). Vesicle fluid may be collected into a syringe or onto a swab and placed in viral transport medium for testing by PCR.

Procedure guideline 15.18 Taking a wound swab

Statement	Rationale
1 Obtain the specimen prior to any dressing or cleaning procedure of the wound.	1 This will maximise the material obtained and prevent killing of the organism by the use of antiseptics.
2 Perform hand hygiene and put on apron and gloves.	2 To comply with standard precautions.
3 a) Use a sterile swab and gently rotate on the area to collect exudate from the wound and place into transport medium. b) Where there is pus, collect as much as possible in a sterile syringe or sterile container (do not use a swab) and send to the laboratory.	3 a) To obtain the material for analysis. b) Pure pus may contain a concentration of micro-organisms and maximise analysis of the material.
4 For detection of *Mycobacterium tuberculosis*, pus collected neat into a pot or tissue biopsy is preferred; however, a calcium alginate swab can be used.	4 The alginate swab gradually dissolves, maximising the isolation of the microorganism as the number of microorganisms is usually small.
5 Label specimen and put together with the laboratory form in the polythene transport bag.	5 To ensure correct process and safe transport to the laboratory.
6 Remove gloves and apron perform hand hygiene.	6 To comply with standard precautions.
7 Document date and time when the specimen was taken in the CYP's records.	7 To maintain accurate records.

Procedure guideline 15.19 Collecting a urine specimen

15.19.1 Collecting a midstream or 'clean catch' urine specimen

Statement	Rationale
1 Perform hand hygiene and put on apron and gloves.	1 To comply with standard precautions.
2 Ensure that the CYP's genitalia have been washed with soap and water and dried thoroughly. Ask them to wash their hands with soap and water.	2 To prevent contamination of the specimen.
3 **In the female**, encourage separation of the labia while passing urine. **In the male,** encourage retraction of the prepuce, if appropriate while passing urine.	3 To prevent contamination of the specimen while passing urine.
4 Ask the CYP to void a small amount of urine into the toilet first.	4 To avoid meatal contamination of the specimen.
5 Then ask the CYP to urinate 10–20ml directly into the specimen container.	5 To decrease the possibility of contaminating the specimen.
6 Instruct the CYP that the remaining urine can be passed into the toilet.	6 To empty the bladder.
7 Place the lid securely on the specimen container. Wipe the outside of the container with a sanitising wipe and place container in polythene transport bag together with the laboratory form.	7 To avoid leakage and contamination and ensure safe transport to the laboratory.
8 Assist the CYP with handwashing if required.	8 To promote personal hygiene.
9 Remove apron and gloves and perform hand hygiene.	9 To comply with standard precautions.
10 Document date and time when the specimen was taken in the CYP's records.	10 To maintain accurate records.

Procedure guideline 15.19 Collecting a urine specimen *(continued)*

15.19.2 Collecting a urine specimen using a urine collection pad

Statement	Rationale
1 Perform hand hygiene and put on apron and gloves.	1 To comply with standard precautions.
2 Remove nappy and clean the perineum or prepuce of the infant with soap and water. Do not apply any creams.	2 To prevent contamination of the specimen.
3 Place the urine collection pad across vulva or penis in a lengthwise fashion. Remove the adhesive backing from the pad and secure to a clean nappy.	3 To obtain the specimen.
4 Change urine collection pad every 30–45 minutes and also when the child has passed stool.	4 To reduce the risk of contamination with skin or faecal flora.
5 Once the child has passed urine remove the nappy with the urine collection pad in it.	5 To obtain the specimen.
6 <ul><li>Lay the pad down wet side up on an appropriate clean surface.</li><li>Take a sterile 5 ml syringe and place the tip on the pad.</li><li>Extract urine by pulling the plunger.</li><li>Repeat until required amount of urine is obtained.</li><li>Empty syringe into a sterile container.</li></ul>	6 To obtain the specimen.
7 Dispose of urine collection pad, syringe and nappy in the appropriate waste bin.	7 To comply with standard precautions.
8 Label specimen and put together with the laboratory form in a polythene transport bag.	8 To ensure correct process and safe transport to the laboratory.
9 Remove gloves and apron and perform hand hygiene.	9 To comply with standard precautions.
10 Document date and time when the specimen was taken in the CYP's records.	10 To maintain accurate records.

15.19.3 Collecting a urine specimen using a urine collection bag

Statement	Rationale
1 Select the correct size sterile urine bag.	1 To avoid leakage or contamination with faeces.
2 Perform hand hygiene and put on apron and gloves.	2 To comply with standard precautions.
3 Remove nappy and clean the perineum or prepuce of the infant with soap and water.	3 To prevent contamination of the specimen.
4 Dry area thoroughly. Do not apply any creams.	4 To ensure that the bag will adhere to skin.
5 Remove the protective backing from the bag, then:<ul><li>**For the female**, place the bag over the vulva, starting from the perineum and working upward, pressing the adhesive to perineum and symphysis.</li><li>**For the male**, insert penis and scrotum into the opening of the bag and press adhesive to perineum and symphysis.</li></ul>	5 To avoid leakage and contamination from faeces.
6 Cut a hole in the nappy and pull the urine bag through the opening.	6 To be able to observe when urine has been passed.
7 Once the child has passed urine, perform hand hygiene, put on apron and gloves and remove the bag.	7 To obtain the specimen.
8 Hold the bag over a sterile urine specimen container and cut off the tip of the bottom corner of the bag with a sterile pair of scissors. Empty the urine into the container.	8 To reduce transmission of microorganisms.
9 After the procedure wash the child's genitalia and put on clean nappy.	9 To prevent soreness of the skin.
10 Label specimen and put together with the laboratory form in a polythene transport bag.	10 To ensure correct process and safe transport to the laboratory.
11 Remove gloves and apron and perform hand hygiene.	11 To comply with standard precautions.
12 Document date and time when the specimen was taken in the CYP's records.	12 To maintain accurate records.

(continued)

Procedure guideline 15.19 Collecting a urine specimen *(continued)*

15.19.4 Urine specimen taken from a urinary catheter: The sample is collected from the self-sealing bung of the urinary drainage tubing in a CYP who is already catheterised (Loveday et al. 2014; NICE 2015).

Statement	Rationale
1 Perform hand hygiene and put on apron and gloves	1 To comply with standard precautions
2 Using an aseptic nontouch technique, clean the catheter sampling site with 2% chlorhexidine in 70% alcohol wipe for 15 seconds and allow to dry.	2 To decontaminate the sampling site.
3 Collect the urine using sterile equipment appropriate to access port, i.e. either by using a sterile syringe and needle and inserting the needle into the bung at an angle of 45° degrees or by using a needleless system.	3 This will minimise penetration of the wall of the tubing and subsequent needle-stick injury.
4 Gently withdraw the urine into the syringe.	4 To diminish any pressure on the bladder and obtain the specimen.
5 Remove the needle and syringe, wipe the area with a 2% chlorhexidine in 70% alcohol wipe for 15 seconds and allow to dry.	5 To prevent contamination. The rubber bung will self-seal.
6 Place the urine in a sterile specimen container.	6 To obtain the specimen.
7 Discard the needle and syringe into a sharps container.	7 To dispose of equipment safely.
8 Label specimen and put together with the laboratory form in a polythene transport bag.	8 To ensure correct process and safe transport to the laboratory.
9 Remove gloves and apron and perform hand hygiene.	9 To comply with standard precautions.
10 Document date and time when the specimen was taken in the CYP's records.	10 To maintain accurate records.
11 NB: The closed drainage system must not be disconnected (DH 2001).	11 To prevent microorganisms being introduced.
12 NB: The urine sample must not be taken from the urinary drainage bag.	12 The sample may be contaminated, which will give a false result.

Procedure guideline 15.20 Collecting vesicular fluid

Statement	Rationale
1 Explain to the CYP and parent/carer that the procedure is usually pain free.	1 The needle only penetrates the vesicle, not the skin.
2 Obtain a sterile syringe and needle, sterile swab, and viral transport medium.	2 To obtain the specimen and avoid secondary infection.
3 Perform hand hygiene and put on apron and gloves.	3 To comply with standard precautions.
4 a) Pierce the top of the vesicle with the sterile needle and if there is sufficient fluid draw up the exudate into a syringe. Keep the needle flush to the skin. b) Draw up some viral transport medium into the syringe and flush the medium plus vesicle fluid back into the bottle of viral transport medium. c) If fluid is easy to collect the vesicle may be punctured with the sterile needle and fluid collected on a dry swab, which is then placed in the viral transport medium.	4 a) To prevent accidental stabbing if the CYP moves. b) This maximises the material to be analysed.
5 Discard the needle and syringe in a sharps bin.	5 To dispose of equipment safely.
6 Place a sterile dressing over the vesicle until dry.	6 To avoid leakage of infected material and prevent secondary infection.
7 Label specimen and put together with the laboratory form in a polythene transport bag.	7 To ensure correct process and safe transport to the laboratory.
8 Remove gloves and apron and perform hand hygiene.	8 To comply with standard precautions.
9 Document date and time when the specimen was taken in the CYP's records.	9 To maintain accurate records.
10 NB: If the vesicle is already ruptured and moist or dry, a positive diagnosis may be reached from a dry swab that has been vigorously rubbed over the dry vesicle and then placed in viral transport medium.	

Ward-based investigations

Blood glucose monitoring

Staff performing blood glucose monitoring should be trained in both the theoretical and practical aspects, including the use of the glucose measuring device and instruction of quality control. Without the appropriate knowledge and skill staff may obtain inaccurate or misleading results, which can lead to incorrect management and adversely affect the CYP. A normal blood glucose level is between approximately 4–7 mmol/l (Gilbert 2009; Hanas 2007). Different parameters will be indicated for specific clinical conditions, e.g. congenital hyperinsulinism (Hussain et al. 2007) and should be specified in local protocols. Staff should report blood glucose levels in mmol/l rather than describing the level as high or low.

Standard Monitoring

Blood glucose monitoring should commence within one hour of starting (intravenous) IV dextrose of 10% or higher. For neonates, this applies to ANY concentration of dextrose including 5% and blood glucose must continue to be measured four hourly if within normal range of 4–7 mmol/l and more frequently if outside this range (National Patient Safety Agency (NPSA) 2010).

In exceptional circumstances the clinician responsible for the CYP's care may decide that an individualised clinical management plan is required. The rationale for this, together with the detailed clinical management plan, must be documented in the CYP's health care record and reviewed daily.

When changing the IV glucose concentration or the rate of administration, blood glucose monitoring should also occur within one hour of the changes (NPSA 2010).

If a CYP continues to be symptomatic of either hypo or hyperglycaemia and has normal blood glucose levels (4–7 mmol/l), despite appropriate interventions, a true glucose sample should be sent to the laboratory as directed by an experienced nurse or doctor.

All blood glucose samples should be taken from a capillary or artery, not from a venous line, to prevent contamination from the intravenous glucose solution (Gilbert 2009).

With very small neonates it is not always possible to take a capillary sample due to the skin integrity and size of the baby. A consultant should be responsible for deciding whether a capillary sample is to be taken, or if the sample can be taken from a line. If the decision is to take the blood glucose sample from a line this must be documented in the healthcare record.

Any sample from a central line which is recorded 'out of range' must then result in a capillary sample being taken.

At handover for neonates receiving a glucose infusion, the most recent blood glucose level must be checked to ensure it is within acceptable limits in accordance with the clinical management plan (NPSA 2010).

Blood glucose monitoring is necessary for CYPs who are:

- Receiving intravenous or subcutaneous insulin for dose adjustment.
- Receiving medication that can alter blood glucose levels, e.g. octreotide, diazoxide.
- Receiving intravenous glucose solutions; this includes parenteral nutrition.
- Nil by mouth for four hours without intravenous fluids
- Nil by mouth and receiving only intravenous fluids for more than 12 hours.
- Commencing parenteral nutrition and during 'wind down' of cyclical parenteral nutrition until stable.
- Diagnosed with some endocrine and metabolic conditions, e.g. hyperinsulinism and glycogen storage disease.
- Having blood glucose levels outside of normal parameters 4–7 mmol/l or parameters as specified by local policy and medical instruction specific to CYP's condition.
- Postoperatively as per local guidelines, i.e. procedure specific.
- Presenting with seizures and/or unexplained loss of consciousness.
- Commencing steroid therapy.
- Following a ketogenic diet.

Neonatal risk factors include:

- Intrauterine growth retardation
- Prematurity
- Infants of insulin-dependent diabetic mothers
- Hypoxic ischaemic encephalopathy
- Hypothermia
- Polycythaemia
- Haemolytic disease of the newborn
- Other syndromes, e.g. Beckwith-Weidermann
- Metabolic metabolism disorders, e.g. galactosaemia, glycogen storage disease

Medical teams responsible for individual CYPs MUST write a clear, daily plan in the healthcare record to specify what blood glucose range is expected for these CYPs, as well as a step-by-step plan to follow if the blood glucose is outside of these specified ranges. CYPs with hyperinsulinism should not have blood glucose levels of less than 3.5 mmol/l without intervention, as they are unable to produce alternative fuel sources such as ketones, and are therefore at high risk of brain damage (Hussain et al. 2007). A lower level of 3.0 mmol/l may be accepted for CYPs with other conditions before intervention (Chowdhury 2015), but the named consultant for the CYP must direct this.

If the blood glucose level is outside of the parameters 4–7 mmol/l, or if the CYP is displaying symptoms of hypo- or hyperglycaemia (see Table 15.3), contact an experienced nurse or doctor for advice.

Contraindications associated with extra-laboratory blood glucose measurement

Staff performing capillary blood glucose monitoring should be aware that:

- Haematocrit values should be between 10 and 65%.
- Intravenous (IV) infusion of ascorbic acid; this will cause overestimation of results.
- Lipaemic samples (triglycerides) in excess of 20.3 mmol/l may produce elevated results.
- In impaired peripheral circulation; collection of capillary blood is not advised as the results might not be a true reflection of the physiological blood glucose level. This may apply in the following circumstances:
  - Severe dehydration as a result of diabetic ketoacidosis
  - Hyperglycaemic hyperosmolar nonketotic syndrome
  - Hypotension
  - Shock
  - Decompensated heart failure NYHA Class IV
  - Peripheral arterial occlusive disease
- Blood concentrations of Galactose >0.83 mmol/l will cause overestimation of blood glucose results (normally galactose is <0.28 mmol/l). CYPs with a known or suspected diagnosis of galactosaemia must be monitored using laboratory glucose results only.

(Medicine and Healthcare products Regulatory Agency 2021)

Table 15.3 Symptoms of hypo- and hyperglycaemia

Hypoglycaemia	Hyperglycaemia
pallor	increased thirst
lethargy	increased urine output
clammy skin	irritability
irritability	abdominal pain
seizures	weight loss

The Great Ormond Street Hospital Manual of Children and Young People's Nursing Practices

Procedure guideline 15.21 Blood glucose monitoring

15.21.1 Preparation

Statement	Rationale
1 Inform the CYP and family of the following: • That the monitoring of blood glucose is necessary. • The reason for monitoring. • The implications of the result. • What it entails • The proposed duration of the procedure.	1 To obtain informed consent. To aid efficiency. To promote safety. To promote involvement and enable partnership in care.
2 Age appropriate play, distraction, and other coping techniques should be employed.	2 To minimise distress and promote concordance – for more information see Chapter 27: Play as a Therapeutic Tool.
3 Standard or isolation precautions must be adhered to.	3 To minimise the risk of cross infection.
4 If the CYP has an arterial line, this can be used for blood sampling. If not, recommended puncture sites vary with age: a) For neonates, follow the guideline for blood sampling from a neonatal capillary. b) Under one year, use the side of the heel. c) Over one year, use the side of a fingertip or toe; avoid thumb and index finger.	c) To avoid affecting the pincer grip and fine motor skills.
5 The back of the heel and tips of fingers should be avoided (Jain and Rutter 1999; Jain et al. 2001).	5 To prevent damage to underlying structures (Jain and Rutter 1999; Jain et al. 2001; Naughten 2005).
6 The chosen puncture site should be continually rotated.	6 Continued use of the same puncture site can cause pain and the development of calluses (Naughten 2005).
7 Excessive squeezing should be avoided.	7 To prevent pain and tissue damage (Naughten 2005).
8 White soft paraffin and alcohol impregnated wipes must not be used to prepare the CYP's skin.	8 Alcohol toughens the skin when used frequently. Alcohol and white soft paraffin can interfere with strip and meter analysis and may give incorrect results.
9 Age-appropriate lancing devices should be used to avoid tissue damage; these would include puncture devices as supplied by the Trust. A guillotine device should not be used for standard blood glucose monitoring as this can cause pain and tissue damage.	9 To prevent pain and tissue and damage (Jain and Rutter 1999; Jain et al. 2001; Naughten 2005).

15.21.2 Quality control (QC) testing of the glucose meter

1 Quality control (QC) testing of the Glucose Meter must be performed every 24 hours.	1, 2. To meet the manufacturer's recommendations. To exclude meter error and incorrect results.
2 QC testing must also be performed when: • The meter is dropped. • Unexplained blood glucose levels contradict the clinical appearance of CYP. • Using a new batch of test strips.	

15.21.3 Obtaining the sample

1 Gather the following equipment: a) Glucose meter. b) Test strips (in date and with lid on). c) Nonsterile gloves and an apron. d) Nonsterile gauze – avoid use of cotton wool. e) Sharps bin. f) A retractable puncture device as supplied by the Trust.	1 a) To ensure that the procedure can be carried out in a timely manner. b) Out-of-date strips and exposing test strips to moisture may give incorrect results. c) To minimise the risk of infection d) Cotton wool fibres can interfere with strip and meter analysis and may give incorrect results. e) To promote safety and prevent needle stick injury. f) To promote safety and prevent needle stick injury. To achieve optimum depth of penetration.
2 To obtain the measurement: a) Ensure site is clean and free from glucose contamination. b) Perform hand hygiene. c) Put on nonsterile gloves and apron. d) Prepare meter **immediately** before sampling. e) Puncture the skin using a retractable lancet device, or take the sample from an arterial line.	2 a) To prevent incorrect test results. b) To minimise the risk of cross infection. c) To minimise the risk of cross infection. d) To facilitate analysis. e) To obtain blood sample.

Procedure guideline 15.21 Blood glucose monitoring *(continued)*

Statement	Rationale
f) Wipe away first drop of blood (unless using an arterial line or the site has been washed and dried).	f) To reduce the risk of contamination and ensure circulating blood is measured (Hortensius et al. 2011).
g) Gently squeeze or massage area to create a teardrop size of blood.	g) To encourage blood flow to the site.
h) Place the edge of the strip to the drop of blood. The test area will draw in the blood sample. Ensure yellow window on strip is completely filled with blood.	h) To obtain accurate and reliable results.
i) Apply nonsterile gauze to the puncture site and apply pressure.	i) To ensure that the bleeding has stopped and CYP is comfortable.
j) Wait for result to be displayed on meter.	j) To maintain accurate records.
k) Read off result. If the monitor reads 'LO' or 'HI', check sampling techniques **immediately** and call for senior help.	k) To initiate appropriate intervention and management. Both situations are potential medical emergencies.
l) Dispose of used equipment according to local policy and perform a hygienic handwash.	l) To minimise risk of cross infection.
m) If the result is out of range, inform an experienced nurse or doctor of the result and commence interventions as directed.	m) To initiate appropriate intervention and management.
n) Record the results in the health care records. Inform the CYP/family of the result and explain the implications.	n) To promote involvement and enable partnership in care.
3 After the procedure: a) Clean the glucometer as per manufacturer's guidelines. A damp cloth will usually suffice. Surface wipes can be used but ensure that any excess residue is removed. The meter should be cleaned after every use. b) Do not immerse in water c) Do not attempt to clean the optics or inside the meter.	3 a) To minimise the risk of cross infection b), c) To prevent equipment damage.

Chemical Pathology must be contacted if the glucometer has malfunctioned and additional support or equipment is required.

NB: Patient's own meters and lancet devices may be used by the CYP or parent to gain practice in the technique of blood glucose monitoring or promote involvement, but Trust meters must also be used as they are quality controlled and can be deemed accurate.

Electrocardiograph (ECG) monitoring (3-Lead and 12-Lead Diagnostic)
What is an ECG?
The ECG is a graphical representation of the flow of electrical activity within the heart (Figure 15.3) recorded from the surface of the body. The graph is displayed as voltage change on the y axis against time on the x axis; see Figure 15.4 (Park and Guntheroth 2006).

Why is the ECG used?
The ECG is used to clinically assess the cardiac electrical activity and conduction pathways within the heart. Arrhythmias, damage to the heart, and some structural abnormalities can also be assessed (Hampton 2013). The ECG does not provide information regarding the heart's mechanical performance as a pump and cannot be used to assess blood pressure or cardiac output.

What Should the ECG Look Like?

PQRST is the international nomenclature assigned to identify the different components of the ECG.

P wave: Represents atrial depolarisation, conduction of the electrical impulse originating from the Sino-atrial (SA) node and spreading across the atrium, causing atrial contraction. Atrial repolarisation cannot be seen on the ECG as it is masked by the QRS depolarisation (Marieb 2014).

PR interval: Represents the time taken for the electrical impulse to be conducted through the atrium and the atrio-ventricular (AV) node.

QRS: Represents ventricular depolarisation, the electrical impulse is conducted through the Bundle of His, the right and left bundle branches to the Purkinje fibres. This results in ventricular contraction (systole) and ejection of blood from the ventricles.

T wave: Represents ventricular repolarisation (diastole) and refilling of blood in the ventricles. This is the period when the ventricular cells are recovering, ready to be depolarised again (Park and Guntheroth 2006).

Electrodes and leads
The 'electrode' is the means of connecting the CYP to the electrical ECG equipment. An electrode comprises of a lead connected to a metal strip or wire that is in contact with a conducting substance. This may be a wet electrolyte gel surrounded by a dry adhesive (hypoallergenic) or a dry conductive adhesive pad positioned on the skin (Coviello 2016). A variety of sizes are available; infant, child, and adult, so that the most appropriate electrode may be selected to prevent distortion of the ECG trace (Hazinski 2012).

The term 'lead' has two slightly different meanings:

i An insulated electrical wire that attaches each electrode to the ECG machine. Each lead is specifically labelled/colour coded with the position to which it should be attached.
ii Gives rise to the nomenclature given to describe the different electrical views obtained using different electrodes, e.g. Lead I is the electrical activity recorded between the right and left arm electrodes

(Hampton 2013).

The Great Ormond Street Hospital Manual of Children and Young People's Nursing Practices

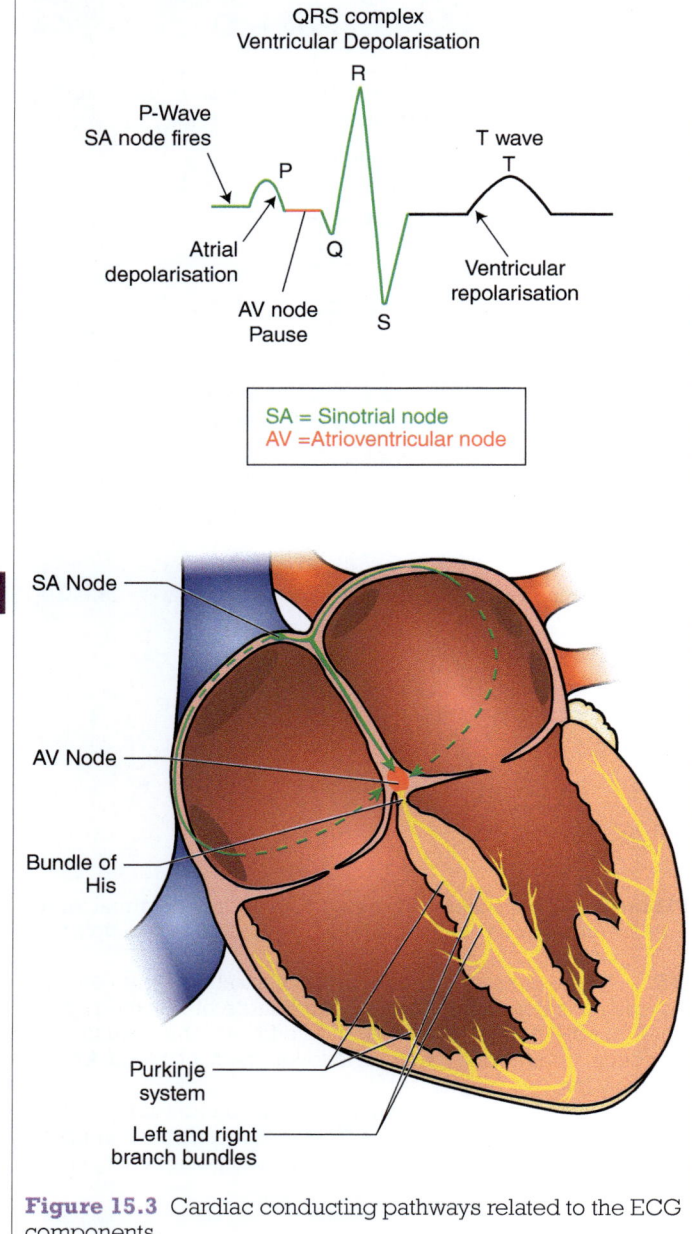

Figure 15.3 Cardiac conducting pathways related to the ECG components.

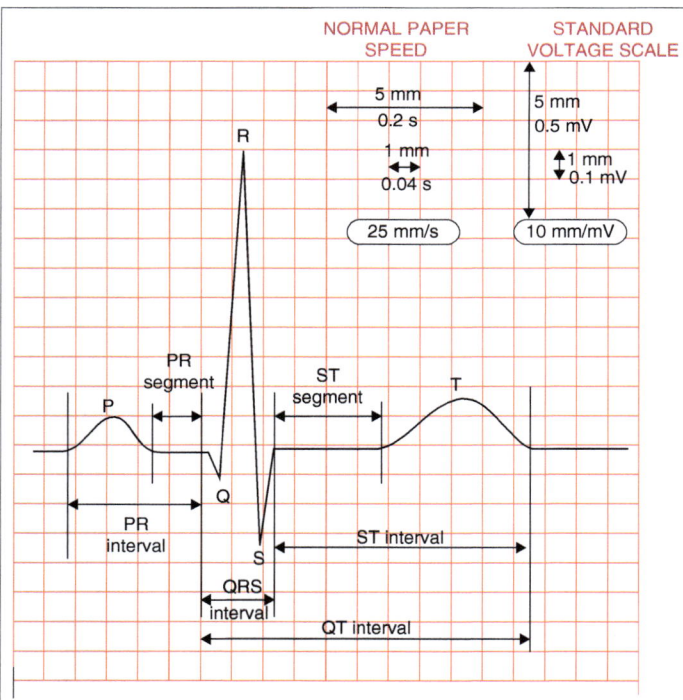

Figure 15.4 The normal ECG Waveform. Source: Adapted from Davey (2013) ECG at a Glance.

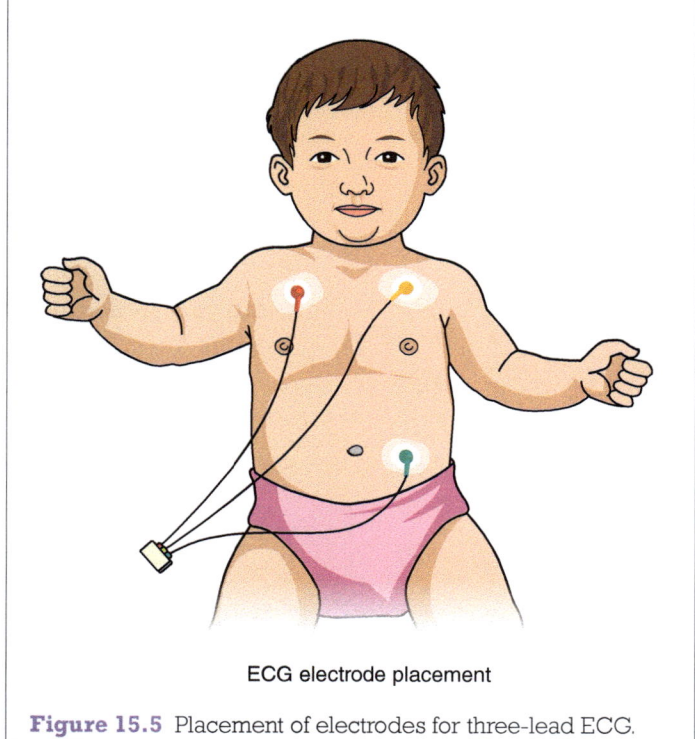

Figure 15.5 Placement of electrodes for three-lead ECG.

For three-lead ECG monitoring on a bedside or portable monitor the three electrodes are placed on the skin in a 'triangular' arrangement around the heart. Placement is normally to the right arm/upper chest (red), left arm/upper chest (yellow) and left leg/left abdominal wall (green) (Figure 15.5). This gives the different electrical views: Lead I, Lead II, and Lead III if selected on the monitor.

For a 12-lead formal ECG, a standard ECG recording machine is required but only 10 leads and electrodes are utilised. Using these 10 leads, 12 electrical 'views' can automatically be taken by the machine – Leads I, II, III, aVR, aVL, aVF and the chest leads V1–V6 (Figure 15.8).

Three-lead ECG monitoring

This may be used to continuously monitor the heart rate and rhythm of a CYP accurately in the clinical environment and to enable timely interventions and management.

The ECG may be used to:

- Give a baseline of heart rate and rhythm prior to an intervention or drug administration.
- Assess the effectiveness of a drug treatment or intervention.
- Alert to a deteriorating condition, reveal a rhythm disturbances or adverse haemodynamic events.
- Contribute to patient assessment; changes in the ECG can indicate underlying medical conditions (Hazinski 2012).

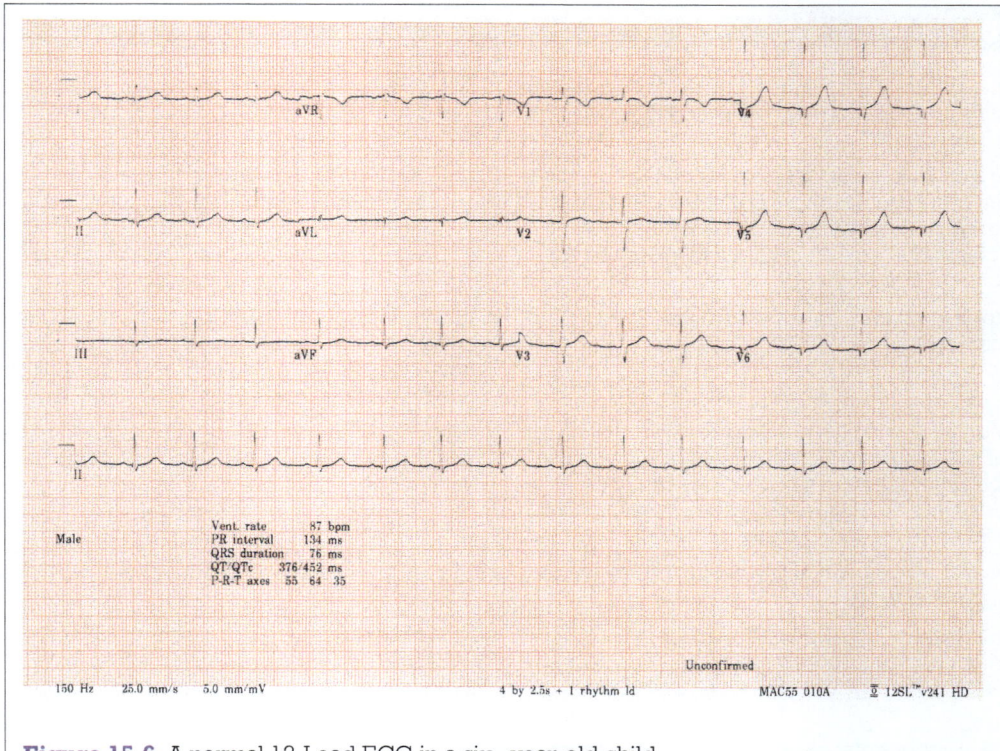

Figure 15.6 A normal 12-Lead ECG in a six –year-old child.

CYPs who require continuous ECG monitoring should be cared for in an environment where their ECG may be monitored continuously by physical presence of a nurse nearby or via remote telemetry observation of the CYP by appropriate nursing/medical/technical staff with good communications to the multidisciplinary team.

If changes to electrical cardiac activity are not anticipated but the CYP's situation requires monitoring, then consideration may be given to using pulse oximetry rather than monitoring ECG (see Chapter 1: Assessment) as the CYP/family may find this less concerning and disturbing. Pulse oximetry monitoring may give a more rapid alert to changes in heart rate, oxygenation and pulsatile flow than changes on the ECG monitoring (Tremper 1992).

Equipment
ECG Electrodes

- Self-adhesive pregelled electrodes.
- Age, size, and machine specific.
- ECG leads to attach to monitor.
- ECG monitor: All users should have had the appropriate training in the use of the device and the correct technique (Royal College of Nursing [RCN] 2013).
- Razor for hirsute CYPs.

Procedure guideline 15.22 Three-lead continuous ECG monitoring

Statement	Rationale
1 If safe/appropriate time to do so, provide information about this monitoring and why it is required.	To ensure the CYP or carer can give informed consent.
2 Ensure the CYP and parents/carers receive appropriate information and are aware of the risks and benefits of the procedure.	To obtain verbal consent (Green and Huby 2010).
3 Inspect the skin condition. Consider shaving the electrode placement areas if necessary. If the skin is soiled, sweaty, or greasy, consider washing and wiping the area dry before electrode placement.	To ensure good electrode contact and electrical conduction to minimise artefacts (Green and Huby 2010). Skin sweat, oils, or dead cells may inhibit conduction (Horrox 2002, Coviello 2016).
4 a) Apply electrodes to right arm/upper chest, left arm/upper chest, and left side of abdomen, below the heart (as shown in Figure 15.5), or upper left leg, and according to the manufacturer's guidelines, which are usually illustrated on the machine. b) Avoid bony prominences, dressings, wounds, sore skin, and other attachments.	a) To ensure the trace is accurate. b) The electrode gel is an irritant and may damage the skin integrity if already sore/inflamed.
5 Attach leads to electrodes ensuring the colours are in the correct place. Ensure the leads are not pressing or pulling on skin, and are not in a position to become easily tangled with other pieces of equipment/clothing etc.	To protect skin and lead integrity, maintenance of monitoring, and ensure a good trace (RCN 2013).

(continued)

Procedure guideline 15.22 Three-lead continuous ECG monitoring *(continued)*

Statement	Rationale
6 Connect to monitor with the correct colour coding connections and switch on.	To establish an acceptable monitoring trace.
7 a) Lead II is the standard monitoring lead. If trace is not clear (showing artefact), consider moving electrodes to different positions (American Heart Association 2006). b) Ensure that electrodes are firmly attached to skin by gently pressing on them.	7 a) Lead II is usually the most positive upright ECG trace as the direction of electrical flow is towards the positive monitoring electrode. b) To ensure good conduction through the skin.
8 The ECG monitoring will only be accurate if the CYP is relatively quiet and still.	8 Infants and children are likely to be more mobile and less cooperative when attached to the ECG monitoring. Movement will cause the ECG trace to show artefacts from muscle tremors and movement and create a difficult trace to interpret (Hazinski 2012).
9 Set age and condition appropriate alarms on the monitor and check functionality. Observe, record and analyse changes in the ECG or if concerned, assess all vital signs and seek advice from a proficient colleague who has age-related skill in ECG interpretation (Park and Guntheroth 2006).	9 To ensure early detection and recording of changes in heart rate, rhythm, and CYP status (Green and Huby 2010; RCN 2013).
10 Check that the CYP's name band and labelling on the monitor correlate at every shift change.	10 To ensure that the observations are recorded for the correct CYP
11 Change electrodes and skin position if in situ for over 24 hours, or if detached from skin. Skin should be assessed regularly and at each electrode change.	11 To prevent damage to the skin and promote good skin integrity (RCN 2013). There is a risk of skin damage, a reaction to the gel or burns if left too long especially the vulnerable neonate (Hazinski 2012).
12 If the trace appears suboptimal consider changing electrodes as the gel may have become dry and fail to conduct.	12 To ensure good trace and good skin contact (Green and Huby 2010).
13 If removing adhesive electrodes consider using adhesive remover.	13 To prevent damage to the skin and minimise stress and discomfort for the CYP.
14 Before discontinuing ECG monitoring discuss this with the family and CYP and explain why this is now appropriate.	14 To reduce anxiety and reassure the family that their child will still be assessed frequently by the staff.
15 When discontinuing ECG monitoring, remove the electrodes, using adhesive remover if appropriate, and wash the skin.	15 To assess skin condition and ensure good skin integrity (Hazinski 2012).
16 Ensure leads are cleaned according to local policy and coiled, ready for the next CYP	16 To ensure good infection control standards and protect integrity of the wires (Green and Huby 2010; RCN 2013)

12-Lead ECG

A 12-Lead ECG is a 'snapshot' in time of the electrical activity within the heart. This is depicted in graphical form, voltage change on the y axis against time on the x axis (see Figure 15.6).

The individual leads each give a different electrical 'view' of the heart, and it is possible to diagnose structural abnormalities or rhythm abnormalities by analysing an ECG thoroughly. Taking an accurate 12-Lead ECG is important to allow this analysis to be clinically significant (Hampton 2013).

12-Lead ECG's may be performed by any competent member of a multidisciplinary team – allied health professionals, healthcare assistants, nurses, and medical staff – however, they should be analysed only by someone trained in age-related ECG analysis (Sharieff and Rao 2006).

Equipment

- ECG machine with 10* lead attachments: All users should have had the appropriate training in the use of the device and the correct technique (RCN 2013).
- ECG electrodes specific to the machine connect to the ECG leads. These electrodes are usually small tags, with a thin metal layer over a layer of adhesive conducting gel.

*Only 10 leads and electrodes are utilized, giving 12 electrical 'views'.

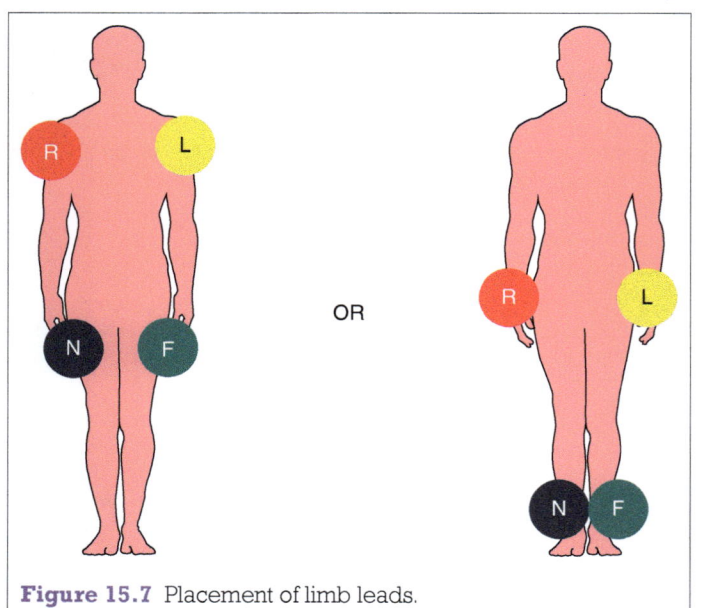

Figure 15.7 Placement of limb leads.

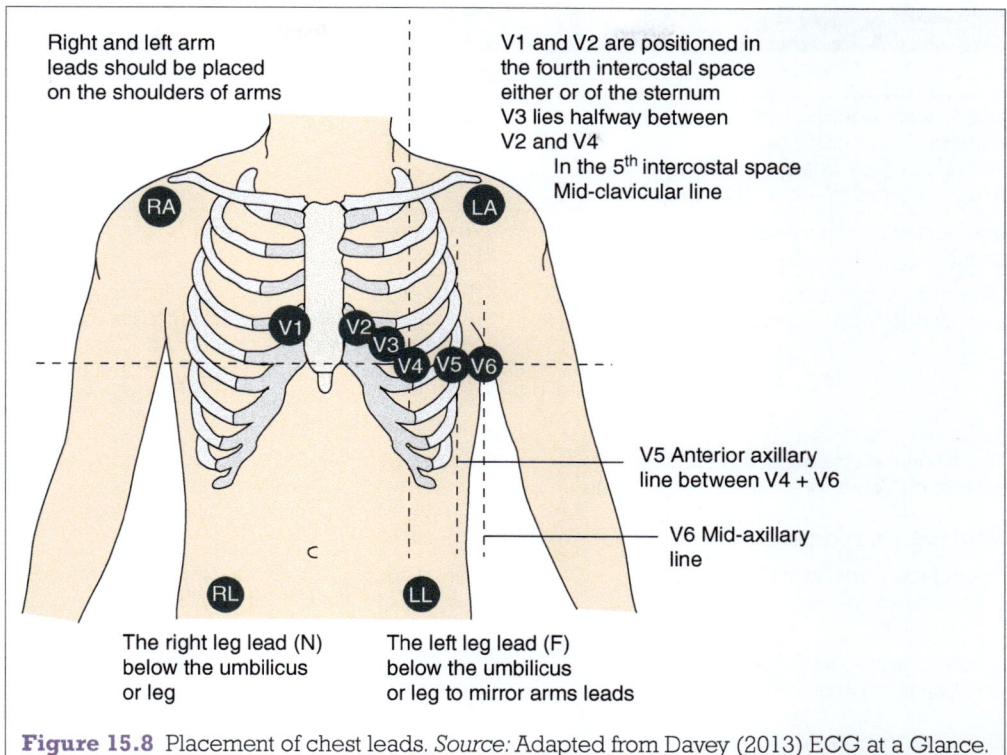

Figure 15.8 Placement of chest leads. *Source:* Adapted from Davey (2013) ECG at a Glance.

Procedure guideline 15.23 Performing a 12-lead ECG

Statement	Rationale
1 Explain the 12-lead ECG to the CYP and carer, including steps for the procedure and what information will be gathered. It is not possible to perform this procedure without removal of clothing/underwear covering the chest. Adolescent girls should be given the option of a female technician or chaperone to maintain dignity and modesty (Nursing and Midwifery Council (NMC) 2018).	1 To ensure informed consent and consideration of appropriate personnel present at procedure.
2 Ensure the CYP and parents/carers receive appropriate information and are aware of the risks and benefits of the procedure.	2 To gain verbal consent for the investigation (Green and Huby 2010).
3 Ensure skin is clean and dry. Consider washing if necessary to remove oils and creams. If CYP is particularly 'hairy' consider shaving.	3 To ensure good electrode contact and conduction (Green and Huby 2010).
4 Apply the electrodes to prepared skin in the correct position, ensuring privacy and dignity to the CYP. Electrodes must not be touching each other. **Limb Leads** (see Figure 15.7) N – right ankle/lower leg R – Right wrist/lower arm L – Left wrist/lower arm F – Left ankle/lower leg **Chest leads** (see Figure 15.8) V1 – 4th intercostal space – right of sternum. V2 – 4th intercostal space – left of sternum. V3 – Between V2 and V4. V4 – Placed 5th intercostal space in the mid-clavicular line. V5 – 5th intercostal space, between V4 and V6. V6 – Mid-axillary line, 5th intercostal space. (Coviello 2016; Wren 2012) NB: Smaller electrodes are available for infants and young children if necessary. If not available, adult electrodes may be cut in half longitudinally, if not contraindicated by the manufacturer.	4 To ensure that the trace is correct, without interference or artefacts. Incorrect placement can affect the resulting ECG. This is an international standard, to ensure consistent interpretation. NB: It is important to ensure that electrodes are placed equidistant on the wrists/ankles where possible, positioning of the limb leads affects the R-wave voltage. This may provide inaccurate information, which may be detrimental in the management of a CYP, particularly post heart transplant (American Heart Association 2006).

(continued)

Procedure guideline 15.23 Performing a 12-lead ECG (continued)

Statement	Rationale
5 Turn on machine and input required data. Ensure details are correct with CYP's name band or through a verbal check with the parent present. Ensure voltage, speed and filters are correct (normally 10.0 mm/mV and 25.0 mm/s, 150hZ).	5 These are international standards for ECG recording (Wren 2012).
6 Connect the named/coded leads to each corresponding electrode. This must be correct.	6 To ensure an accurate trace.
7 Ensure CYP is still and settled; consider using sucrose (under three months of age) or distraction techniques.	7 ECG recording in young or distressed CYPs requires patience. Infants and children are likely to be more mobile and less cooperative with the procedure (Cook and Langton 2009). Movement will cause the ECG machine to pick up muscle tremors and movement artefact and create a difficult trace to interpret (Hazinski 2012).
8 When rhythm is stable on the screen, press the correct print button for ECG to print out. Then press for a rhythm strip if required. Do not press 'Copy' (depending on manufacturer's instructions).	8 To print out the 12-lead ECG tracing. A rhythm strip is helpful if rhythm abnormalities are present. 'Copy' may print a previous electronically stored ECG if the CYP's details have not been inserted correctly (NHS England 2014).
9 Check print-out for artefacts (American Heart Association 2006), correct CYP details, and repeat ECG if required.	9 To ensure all aspects of the recording are correct and meet the international standard (Coviello 2016).
10 Analyse ECG or show to proficient colleague who has age-related skill in ECG interpretation (Park and Guntheroth 2006). Record arrhythmias/abnormalities observed. Ensure the ECG is filed in the CYP's record or transferred/stored electronically as per local policy.	10 To detect irregularities that may need immediate attention and maintain a record of changes observed (Coviello 2016; RCN 2013).
11 Remove ECG electrodes ensuring privacy and dignity. Advise who will inform CYP and family of results. Clean and dry the electrode areas if required	11 To ensure that the CYP is left clean and with dignity intact.
12 Ensure leads are cleaned according to local policy and coiled, ready for the next CYP.	12 Ensure good infection control standards and protect integrity of the wires (Green and Huby 2010).

Glomerular filtration rate

The glomerular filtration rate (GFR) refers to the rate of renal clearance of a substance from the plasma compartment. Clearance is assumed to be due to the glomerular filtration of the solute. The GFR is measured in ml per minute, i.e. the volume the kidneys can filter per unit of time. Measuring the GFR using the clearance of an exogenous compound (such as iohexol) is a useful way to determine how well the kidneys are working. If the concentration of iohexol in the blood is measured at two points, it is easy to calculate the rate of elimination (KE). However, this does not give a particularly good estimate of kidney function as it does not identify how widely distributed the substance is. In order to calculate the clearance (ml/min), we need to know the volume that iohexol is distributed in, to make sense of our measurements of concentration. This volume of distribution (VD) is a theoretical volume calculated from the dose divided by the concentration at the instant the dose is given (C0). Iohexol elimination follows a mono-exponential decay. From this, C0 can be calculated by drawing a graph of ln (serum iohexol concentration) versus time. If two or more concentrations are measured at different times a straight line joining the points and bisecting the concentration axis (where time = 0) allows C0 to be estimated and VD calculated. The clearance can then be calculated using the VD, and KE. For the calculation to be accurate, the following parameters must be accurately measured:

1. Dose (this is used to calculate VD).
2. Dose and sampling times (used to calculate C0 – errors here will affect VD).
3. Serum iohexol concentrations (used to calculate C0 – errors here will affect VD).

In order to compare GFR values they are routinely standardised to body size. This is because larger individuals need to have higher clearances in order to eliminate compounds at the same rate. Generally, larger people have a higher VD and as discussed above KE = CL/VD. GFR measurements are therefore 'corrected' to $1.73\,m^2$, a typical adult body surface area (and better measure of size than weight alone), which is calculated from the height and weight. It is for this reason that height and weight must be accurately be recorded on the day of GFR testing.

A normal corrected GFR is: $80–120\,ml/min/1.73\,m^2$ (after one year of age). For the purposes of these guidelines, the following definitions will be used:

Mild renal impairment	$70–80\,ml/min/1.73\,m^2$
Moderate renal impairment	$50–70\,ml/min/1.73\,m^2$
Severe renal impairment	$<50\,ml/min/1.73\,m^2$
Hyperfiltration	$>120\,ml/min/1.73\,m^2$

The GFR test is primarily used to monitor CYPs with normal renal function or mild to moderate impairment. It is less useful for those with severe impairment as blood samples have to be taken later and other tests are used to build a more complete picture of renal function.

Plasma creatinine concentration increases with age due to growth; therefore, a formula relating creatinine and height has been advocated as a rough estimate of GFR, e.g.:

GFR = height in cms × 33 / plasma creatinine concentration.

In routine clinical practice, the GFR is inferred from the plasma creatinine concentration using this formula. It is assumed that a normal creatinine concentration indicates normal glomerular function. This may not apply in some CYPs, hence the need for a more accurate GFR test. The measurement of GFR is based on the determination of the clearance of a marker, either endogenous (e.g. urea, creatinine) or exogenous (e.g. iohexol, inulin). This assumption may be invalid in CYPs who are malnourished, whose dietary protein is severely restricted, whose growth is poor, or who have reduced muscle mass. In these CYPs, GFR is formally determined by the iohexol method.

Various methods have been used to assess GFR. In the UK the single injection slope clearance method has been adopted as the most practical. The test assumes that after intravenous injection, the marker is instantaneously mixed throughout the plasma compartment and only excreted by glomerular filtration. This method has been established for many years and is widely used (Chantler et al. 1969; Counahan et al. 1976). Iohexol, a nonradioactive substance, replaced chromium-51-EDTA, a radioactive isotop, in 2007. Three 1 ml blood samples are usually taken; the first before the iohexol injection, and then at three and four hours. A further sample is taken at six hours if expected GFR < 40 ml/min (Nilsson-Ehle 2001). An accurate result is calculated by measuring the quantity of the marker remaining in the circulating blood at these times.

The advantages of this method are:

- It is established, safe, and cost effective.
- It is reliable, and iohexol is not radioactive.
- It involves a small dose of marker, which is safe to use in a ward environment, provided this guideline is followed.
- It uses much smaller blood samples than the chromium EDTA method.
- Samples can be stored without loss of accuracy.
- There is a sensitive, reproducible assay for iohexol in clinical biochemistry.
- A wider range of staff can perform the test than with the chromium EDTA method. Basic IV training plus iohexol-specific training will be required.

The disadvantages of this method are:

- As with other GFR test methods, it is most useful for detecting mild to moderate renal impairment and is less accurate at 'normal,' 'hyperfiltration,' and 'severe' GFR values.
- The test has to be booked in advance and preferably performed in working hours.

Procedure guideline 15.24 Measuring glomerular filtration rate

Statement	Rationale
1 An aseptic nontouch technique (ANTT) should be employed throughout the procedure, whether it is performed peripherally or utilising a central venous access device (CVAD).	1 To prevent cross infection.
2 A GFR test may be required for CYPs with: • Reduced renal function. • Urological abnormalities. • Following extensive renal surgery. • Those taking nephrotoxic drugs. • Prior to treatment with certain types of cytotoxic chemotherapy. • As part of a research study where there is a clear need to accurately define renal function.	2 To monitor any deterioration in renal function.
3 GFR is contraindicated in: a) Ascites or generalised oedema, e.g. relapse of nephrotic syndrome. b) Manifest thyrotoxicosis. c) Previous severe reaction to iohexol or iodine products. d) Severely compromised venous access e) Presence of external drain, e.g. an external ventricular drain or chest drain. f) Fasted/dehydrated individuals: The CYP should have had their usual fluid intake during the previous 24 hours and for the duration of the test. g) Hyper-hydrated individuals (e.g. those undergoing hyper-hydration for certain types of chemotherapy). h) CYPs due to receive radioiodine therapy in the next week. i) CYPs who have eaten a heavy meal including large protein load or large caffeine intake (> 1 cup of tea/coffee) on the morning of, or during the test.	3 a) The test is likely to fail due to abnormal distribution of the marker. b) Free iodine may be liberated which is taken up by the thyroid gland. c) There is an increased risk of anaphylaxis. d) There is an increased risk of extravasation and likelihood that adequate postinjection samples will not be available. e) This is likely to lead to abnormal losses of the marker. f) Dehydration may lead to deranged electrolytes, which could cause an inaccurate result. Iohexol may rarely precipitate acute renal failure in dehydrated individuals. g) Hyperhydration may affect the distribution of iohexol, and therefore the result of the test. h) To prevent avid uptake of any free iodine from iohexol 'blocking' the uptake of the radioiodine by the thyroid gland. GFR should be postponed until after therapy. i) Protein and caffeine may affect the measured GFR.
4 The CYP's temperature must be recorded prior to commencement of the test. The test should be rescheduled in the event of pyrexia (> 38°C). Confirm with the appropriate team prior to cancelling the test.	4 Pyrexia may cause a false result due to insensible loss.

(continued)

Procedure guideline 15.24 Measuring glomerular filtration rate *(continued)*

Statement	Rationale
5 GFR should be performed with caution in the following CYPs: a) Those with a hospital visit due to asthma in the past two years, asthma requiring regular inhaled corticosteroids, allergies to other foods/drugs, and severe hay fever requiring regular antihistamines. These CYPs should be closely monitored for 15 minutes after injection of iohexol, and if the dose was given through a cannula, it should be left in situ at least until the end of the observation period. b) Infants (under one year) require special consideration. c) Those taking metformin (e.g. Type 2 diabetes, polycystic ovary syndrome): This group should be assessed individually by the consultant requesting the test. d) CYPs taking amiodarone (e.g. cardiac problems such as arrhythmias). This group should be individually assessed; they should be referred back to the referring consultant for a risk/benefit assessment. e) CYPs with phaeochromocytoma were considered at risk, but this is no longer a contraindication.	5 a) This group are at increased risk of anaphylaxis. NB: There is a small chance of allergic-type reactions in all CYPs; they should remain on the ward for at least 15 minutes after iohexol administration. b) Renal function matures during the first year of life so the test result may be less useful in this age group. Venous access may be difficult in very young children. c) There is a theoretical risk of developing lactic acidosis if metformin is given after iohexol treatment (Thomson Healthcare Inc. 2006). d) Concurrent administration of iohexol and amiodarone can prolong QT-interval (Goernig et al. 2004). The risk is probably small as the dose of iohexol used for GFR measurement is low. However, the benefit of obtaining an accurate GFR must be weighed against the risk of ventricular arrhythmia. e) Iohexol does not cause significant changes in plasma catecholamine levels in CYPs with phaeochromocytomas (Mukherjee et al. 1997).
Pregnancy and breastfeeding	
1 Adolescent/menstruating girls, generally 10 years or older, should be asked if there is a possibility of their being pregnant. If they suspect, or know they are pregnant, the benefit of obtaining an accurate GFR must be weighed against the risk to the developing foetus.	1 Iohexol is classified as risk category B, i.e. there is no known teratogenicity in animals. No human teratogenicity has been seen, but there is an absence of clinical trial data to support this (Thomson Healthcare Inc. 2006). There may be a risk to the developing foetus with iohexol exposure, but it is probably small compared with many other medicinal products.
2 Adolescent mothers who are breastfeeding could be advised to avoid doing so for 24 hours after the test.	2 Iohexol is excreted in small amounts into breast milk. Iohexol is poorly absorbed from the gastrointestinal tract so there is minimal risk to the infant; cautious mothers may wish to avoid breastfeeding for 24 hours after the test.
3 Staff must exercise caution in dealing with this sensitive situation.	3 To maintain confidentiality, privacy, and dignity and offer appropriate advice, support, and counselling.
Training	
1 GFR must only be performed by a healthcare professional (HCP) who has been trained and assessed as competent.	1 To ensure practice safe and effective (General Medical Council 2013; NMC 2018).
Preparation of CYP and family	
1 Explain the procedure, including the reason for the GFR. Information must be given according to the CYP's age and developmental understanding. A factsheet is available for families (https://www.gosh.nhs.uk/teenagers/tests-and-treatments/glomerular-filtration-rate-gfr-test/).	1 To ensure that the family understands the reason for the procedure and are psychologically prepared. Well-informed parents are more likely to stay calm and will be in a position to support their child (Frederick 1991).
2 Explain the following: • What is a GFR test? • How long will it take? • Why do they need the test? • Why do need the test? • Are there any side effects? • Are there any alternatives? • What happens before the test, what does it involve, and what happens between blood samples? • What happens afterwards and when the CYP returns home?	2 To ensure that informed consent is obtained and to allow the family to develop coping strategies.
3 If a CVAD is not being used a topical anaesthetic should be offered and/or applied to two potential vein sites **on separate limbs**, prior to commencing the test. Alternatively, the CYP may choose a local anaesthetic spray that should be applied according to product instructions.	3 To minimise pain and distress (APAGBI 2012).
4 Provide play preparation if appropriate, involving the play specialist if possible.	4 To provide explanation in a nonthreatening manner, and give the CYP the opportunity to express fears in a familiar environment (Broome 1990; Lansdown 1993).

Procedure guideline 15.24 Measuring glomerular filtration rate *(continued)*

Statement	Rationale
5 Consider involvement of a clinical psychologist if appropriate, particularly if previous procedures have been stressful for the CYP or if he/she is known to have, or exhibits signs of, anticipatory anxiety and distress.	5 To minimise fear and distress and increase the likelihood of successful cannulation (Claar et al. 2002; Duff 2003).
6 Prepare appropriate methods of distraction for the CYP to use during the procedure itself. Attempt to discover from the CYP and family what techniques are most likely to consume his attention; e.g. pop-up or musical books, blowing bubbles, and guided imagery.	6 To prevent the CYP's whole attention being centred on the invasive procedure. These techniques can help to distract and relax the CYP (Heiney 1991; Langley 1999). For more information see Chapter 27: Play as a Therapeutic Tool.
7 Check that the CYP has had their normal fluid intake over the previous 24 hours.	7 Dehydration may lead to deranged electrolytes, which could cause an inaccurate result. Iohexol may precipitate acute renal failure in dehydrated individuals.
8 Measure and record the CYP's weight and height accurately before commencing the procedure (see Chapter 11: Assessment).	8 An accurate height and weight are essential to enable accurate calculation of the dose and to correction of the result based on surface area.
9 Take a full drug history and list all medicines taken in the last week in the healthcare record, including over-the-counter medicines.	9 Some drug metabolites may interfere with the assay (Nilsson-Ehle 2001). These can be corrected for using the 'predose' sample but it is important to alert biochemistry to any potential interactions.
10 Check that the CYP has not had any iohexol administered within the last 72 hours, i.e. radiological test with contrast. If the CYP has had a radiological test or scan involving an injection within the previous 72 hours, check with the radiology department who performed the imaging if iohexol was used.	10 Any radiological test or scan involving the injection of contrast is likely to have used iohexol, which will affect parameters used to calculate the GFR.
11 If the CYP is currently taking metformin, take advice from the consultant who ordered the test or if unavailable, a member of the renal team responsible for GFR measurement.	11 There is a risk of developing lactic acidosis if metformin is given after iohexol treatment.
12 If the CYP is currently taking amiodarone, take advice from the consultant who ordered the test or if unavailable, a member of the renal team responsible for GFR measurement.	12 There is a risk of iohexol causing a prolonged QT-interval in CYPs taking amiodarone.
13 Ascertain whether the CYP suffers from asthma.	13 CYPs with bronchial asthma may be at increased risk of allergic-type reactions (Morcos 2005).
14 Ascertain whether they have any allergies.	14 To ensure that the CYP has had no previous allergic reaction to iohexol or other contrast media containing iodine.
15 If the CYP/family report an allergy to latex, ward staff should initiate the relevant policy (iodine/products) and alert medical staff.	15 To minimise the risk of anaphylaxis.
16 The CYP must be wearing an identity bracelet or have photographic ID.	16 To ensure correct identification of the CYP and to prevent critical incidents
17 Tea, coffee, fizzy drinks, ice cream, chocolate, and a heavy or protein-rich meal are best avoided for the duration of the test. Bananas should be avoided pretest but can be eaten during. If the CYP has had a small intake of any of the above proceed with the test and note on the GFR Record Form.	17 Some foods, e.g. protein load and/or caffeine, stimulate the kidneys, causing a false result.

Preparation of equipment, iohexol, and the environment

1 Print out the request forms for GFR test.	1, 2a) To ensure samples and test data are attributed to the correct CYP.
2 Check and record the following: a) The CYP's name, hospital number, date of birth, gender, ward. b) Body weight and height.	b) The dose will be calculated using a recent measurement of weight.
3 Check that there is sufficient iohexol 300 to perform the required number of GFRs.	3 To ensure there is sufficient iohexol available for the test to proceed.
4 NB: The vials are for single use only. Multiple doses may be drawn from the vial on a single occasion. Opened vials containing iohexol should be disposed of according to local waste policy.	4 While iohexol is a relatively stable compound, dosing accuracy is crucial, so new vials should be used wherever possible. This also reduces the risk of microbial contamination.
5 The iohexol should, wherever possible, be administered before midday, so that samples can be delivered to chemical pathology by 4:30 p.m.	5 To ensure that blood sampling can be completed with the same staff members, giving continuity of care and arriving at chemical pathology during main working hours.
6 Prepare PPE (gloves and apron).	6 To prevent cross infection.

(continued)

Procedure guideline 15.24 Measuring glomerular filtration rate *(continued)*

Statement	Rationale
7 Gloves should be of a comfortable fit, but tight to the skin, particularly at the fingertips.	7 To allow easier palpation of the vein and manual dexterity in handling equipment.
8 Prepare the equipment: • Clean plastic tray. • Apron. • Nonsterile gloves (latex free if required). • Syringes: 2 x 5 ml, or 1 x 5 ml and 1 x 2 ml, depending on the dose to be administered. • Blue or green butterfly needle or appropriate cannula for venepuncture. • Blue needle for drawing up the iohexol. • Green needle for drawing up the 0.9% sodium chloride. • 5 ml 0.9% sodium chloride. • Latex-free filter (if required) • 2% chlorhexidine gluconate /70% isopropyl alcohol solution applicator (see antiseptic skin preparation – first line use of 2% chlorhexidine/70% isopropyl alcohol for vascular line insertion for further information) • Sterile gauze • Plaster spot dressing • Sharps disposal box.	8 To ensure the smooth and efficient running of the procedure.
9 Perform a social hand wash and put on PPE.	9 To prevent cross infection.
10 Draw up 5 ml of 0.9% sodium chloride; label the syringe.	10 For flushing the cannula. Labelling minimises the risk of drug errors.
11 Take a vial of Iohexol 300 and calculate dose according to the following ranges. This should be checked by two registered staff and written on the GFR Record Form. The dose should also be prescribed as per Trust policy.	11 To ensure an appropriate dose for the CYP's size. To ensure that the correct dose is given to the correct CYP. To prevent medication errors.
Weight <40 kg > = 40 kg	**Iohexol 300 dose (ml)** 2 ml 5 ml
12 Draw up the iohexol in an appropriate sized syringe and have this checked by a trained member of staff.	12 Using the correct sized syringe improves the accuracy of the dose.
13 Discard the blue needle once the iohexol has been drawn up and label the syringe.	13 To minimise drug errors.

Performing the test using peripheral venous access

Statement	Rationale
1 An aseptic nontouch technique (ANTT) and standard precautions must be used throughout the procedure.	1 To minimise the risk of cross infection.
2 Position the CYP on a chair, treatment couch, or on a parent/carer's lap.	2 To minimise the trauma of the procedure.
3 Whenever possible, allow the CYP to select their chosen position. Ensure that this will be comfortable for the CYP, parents and HCPs for the duration of the procedure. Consider moving and handling risks.	3 To maximise the chance of a successful procedure and to aid compliance by the CYP (RCN 2019). For more information see Chapter 19: Moving and Handling.
4 Perform hand hygiene, put on PPE and ensure that all HCPs assisting are similarly attired.	4 To prevent cross infection.
5 Place yourself in a comfortable position, sitting facing the CYP and family.	5 Good eye contact should be maintained to aid compliance with the procedure.
6 Check the CYP's name, date of birth, hospital number and allergies against the prescription datasheet.	6 To prevent medication error.
7 Remove the local anaesthetic cream if used and wipe dry with a tissue or gauze. If an occlusive transparent dressing was used, remove by stretching parallel with the skin.	7 This breaks the glue, causing less irritation and pain.
8 Confirm with the CYP, if appropriate, that the cream has caused numbness of the skin effectively.	8 To reassure the CYP that the pain of the procedure will be minimised.
9 Apply an appropriate size tourniquet 5–8 cm above the chosen vein but not so tight to occlude arterial supply. Indications of occluded arterial supply include loss of colour, compromised pulse, and pain.	9 To facilitate filling of the vein, enhance visualisation and to allow the assisting nurse to have his/her hands free for other tasks (Millam 1992).
10 Lightly tap the vein or instruct the CYP to clench or pump the fist.	10 To encourage further venous filling

Procedure guideline 15.24 Measuring glomerular filtration rate *(continued)*

Statement	Rationale
11 Palpate the chosen vein.	11 To ensure that it can still be found and is still considered suitable. To ascertain the calibre and direction of the vein.
12 Cleanse the skin at the intended needle insertion site, working outwards, with a 2% chlorhexidine gluconate/70% isopropyl alcohol solution for at least 30 seconds.	12 To clean the skin and prevent introduction of infection (Franklin 1998).
13 Do not fan, blow-dry, or otherwise attempt to accelerate the drying process. Do not re-palpate the vein once the skin has been sterilised.	13 To prevent re-contaminating the skin (Millam 1992).
14 Apply local anaesthetic spray if this is the preferred pain management strategy. This should not be used in children aged under five years.	14 To minimise pain during venepuncture/cannulation. To adhere to product recommendations.
15 Advise the CYP that venepuncture will now occur.	15 To allow the CYP/family to initiate planned coping strategies and to confirm implied consent.
16 a) Using the butterfly needle or cannula, access one of the prepared venous sites. b) If any routine blood tests are required, this is a good time to take them. c) Collect a **predose sample** (0.5–1 ml) in a white serum bottle and label this as "predose sample". d) Flush with 1–2ml of sodium chloride. e) Remove the syringe with 0.9% sodium chloride and attach the iohexol syringe.	16 c) To ensure no iohexol is present before the test and to correct for any substances that may affect the assay. d) To check patency of the vein.
17 Administer the iohexol over 20–30 seconds. **Note down the time to the nearest minute that the iohexol is administered on the GFR Record Form.**	17 To ensure the GFR can be accurately calculated.
18 Detach the iohexol syringe once administered and reattach the 0.9% sodium chloride syringe. Flush the remaining 0.9% sodium chloride through the butterfly or cannula.	18 To ensure the whole dose is administered.
19 Continuously observe the butterfly/cannula site for blanching and any other adverse local reaction.	19 To monitor for infiltration.
20 In the event of iohexol infiltration into the surrounding tissue, stop administration immediately. a) If the infiltration occurs while administering the initial 0.9% sodium chloride flush, repeat venepuncture and attempt to administer the iohexol. b) If infiltration occurs while administering the iohexol the test should be abandoned. c) If infiltration of iohexol occurs, this must be documented in the health record and the test will be abandoned.	20 To minimise the risk of tissue damage. b) Infiltration is a major cause of inaccurate results, as the whole dose will not enter the circulation. c) Iohexol is nontoxic but nevertheless accurate record keeping should be maintained
21 Hold a piece of sterile gauze over the exit site but do not apply pressure. Slowly withdraw the butterfly needle/cannula, maintaining a neutral angle with the CYP's skin.	21 Pressure should not be applied until the needle has been fully removed or it will cause the needle to be dragged out of the vein, causing pain and venous damage.
22 Immediately apply gentle digital pressure to the exit site for three to four minutes.	22 To absorb any blood that escapes and to prevent the formation of a haematoma.
23 Place the used equipment carefully into the tray.	23 To prevent possible inoculation injury.
24 a) Lift the soiled gauze and inspect the exit site. b) **DO NOT** wipe the exit site with the gauze.	24 a) To check that bleeding has ceased. b) This could reactivate bleeding by dislodging the thrombus.
25 Once the bleeding has ceased apply the spot plaster.	25 To prevent infection of the puncture site.
26 a) Record the time the iohexol injection was administered accurately, using the same watch/clock throughout, to the nearest minute. Note which clock/watch was used and use the same one to record blood sampling times. b) Also note which limb was used.	26 a) To facilitate accurate calculation of the GFR and to determine the sites and times for the subsequent blood samples to be collected. To ensure accurate record keeping. b) Blood sampling should ideally be taken from an alternate limb.
27 Dispose of used equipment and sharps according to local policy, remove protective clothing, and perform a social hand wash.	27 To prevent inoculation injury and minimise the risk of cross infection.
28 If the procedure is abandoned for any reason dispose of any iohexol as for other IV drugs; empty vials may be disposed in a sharps bin, partially full vials should be returned to pharmacy.	28 To facilitate safe disposal.

(continued)

Procedure guideline 15.24 Measuring glomerular filtration rate *(continued)*

Statement	Rationale
Performing the test using a central venous access device (CVAD)	
1 If the CYP has a double lumen CVAD, the iohexol may be given through one lumen and the blood samples taken from the other lumen.	1 To ensure that the same lumen is not used for both functions
2 Accurate recording of which lumen was used for which function is vital. There is space for this on the GFR Record Form.	2, 3 To ensure an accurate result
3 If the CYP has a single lumen CVAD, PICC, or implantable port, the iohexol may be given through a butterfly needle and the blood samples collected through the CVAD, or the iohexol given through the CVAD and the blood samples collected peripherally. In either of these events the procedure for performing the test remains as described above.	
Positive reinforcement and reward	
1 Time should be taken to give positive feedback to the CYP for tolerating the invasive procedure.	1 To pass control back to the CYP.
2 The parents should also be given positive feedback for their valuable contribution.	2 To acknowledge the value of their involvement, teach mastery of the event, and equip them with coping strategies for future occasions.
3 If a story or game has been used for distraction purposes, allow the CYP to complete the activity.	3 To conclude the procedure with a positive outcome and maintain/improve compliance for subsequent blood sampling. Any reward, however small, will help the CYP to feel a sense of achievement and control.
Subsequent blood sampling	
1 When collecting the subsequent blood samples, all HCPs involved must: • Use an aseptic nontouch technique (ANTT). • Wear PPE. • Perform a social handwash before and after the procedure. • Dispose of all waste and sharps in accordance with local policy.	1 To minimise the risk of cross infection
2 It is important that there is a delay of three hours between administration of iohexol and the second blood sample and an hour's delay before the third blood sample. (T = 0 hrs, T = 3 hrs, and T = 4 hrs).	2 To ensure the iohexol level will have dropped sufficiently to accurately measure the line slope.
3 Take 1 ml of blood at 180 and 240 minutes post injection, from either a new butterfly or cannula (preferably inserted into an alternative limb from which the iohexol was administered), a finger-prick, the indwelling central line (if the CYP has one and provided iohexol was not administered via this), or an alternate lumen of a multiple lumen central line to the one used to administer iohexol. If the first sample is delayed, e.g. at 200 minutes, take the second sample 60 minutes later.	3 Sampling from the same limb as that used for administration of the iohexol may give a false result.
4 If the expected GFR is less than 40 ml/min, a further sample at 360 minutes (six hours) post injection is required. The requesting doctor should state whether this is the case.	4 Elimination of the marker is slower in these CYPs.
5 In some circumstances it may be appropriate to take blood samples using a finger-prick (see capillary blood sampling guideline). An absolute minimum of 0.5 ml of blood is required.	5 Finger pricks may be preferred to cannulation where venous access is difficult.
6 **It is very important to accurately record on the GFR Record Form the exact times at which samples are taken, to the nearest minute, from the same clock/watch.**	6 Accurate time keeping is imperative to calculate an accurate result.
7 Place the blood sample in a white serum bottle and label accurately with the CYP's details and the date and **time of sampling to the nearest minute**. Place in a clear specimen bag. All blood samples, request form and the GFR Record Form should be packaged together and sent to the biochemistry by chute or by porter collection on completion of the test. Additional name labels should also be included which should be on the request form. Where possible they should arrive in chemical pathology by 4:30 p.m.	
8 The HCP performing the procedure must sign and date the GFR Record Form upon completion of the test.	8 To maintain an accurate record and ensure that laboratory staff know who to contact in the event of a query.
9 Serum will be separated promptly and stored until the assay is performed.	9 To ensure that the samples are collected and processed in the right way at the right time.

Pregnancy testing

There is evidence which indicates that some treatments, such as surgery and radiological examinations, carry the risk of spontaneous abortion and interuterine growth retardation. In order to reduce the risks to any unborn child all females of childbearing age must be assessed for the possibility of pregnancy prior to a surgical or interventional procedure under general anaesthetic (GA). The possibility of pregnancy should be considered in all females (age 12 and over) before surgery and exposure to radiation, as these pose risks to the mother and foetus. Routine pregnancy checking is NOT required for every radiology or MRI procedure (Department of Health and Social Care (DHSC) 2018). The need to determine pregnancy status depends on the risk presented by the GA/ procedure on the foetus. If pregnancy is confirmed, the risks and benefits of the procedure can be discussed with the young person and/or parents as appropriate. Surgery may be postponed or anaesthetic and surgical approaches modified if necessary. In emergency situations, confirmation of pregnancy should not delay treatment and should be judged within clinical assessment of risk. Obtaining pregnancy status of all females of 12 years of age and over undergoing surgical or interventional procedures under GA needs to be undertaken in a consistent, sensitive, and confidential manner. In some instances, both the law and/or child protection guidelines may have to be considered a priority and the HCP's duty of confidentiality to the young person may be overridden. Additionally, pregnancy testing may be required as part of the routine investigations for CYPs presenting with certain conditions or where there is suspicion of sexual abuse.

When to assess for pregnancy

Assessment for the possibility of pregnancy must be approached sensitively and in a simple and clear manner. The pregnancy test result is confidential. Young women should be reassured that staff will respect their right to confidentiality. The only exception to this is where staff think that the health, safety, or welfare of the young woman (or another person) is at risk. If staff plan to share the test result with anyone other than a healthcare professional (e.g. Social Work Team, or the police) they must first explain to the young woman why they need to share the test result and support the young woman to talk about this.

A pregnancy test should be performed on all young women aged 12 or over:

- Prior to undergoing a surgical interventional procedure under GA.
- Before X-ray examinations in which the primary beam will irradiate the lower abdomen or pelvis.
- Before receiving medicines known to be teratogenic: The young person should receive counselling regarding pregnancy and sexual health prior to the commencement of treatment. Evidence of this discussion should be documented. Pregnancy testing will then be considered.

In emergency situations, priority is given to any lifesaving care which the young woman may require. The Royal College of Paediatrics and Child Health (RCPCH) has information to support clinicians (RCPCH 2012). Information sheets are available (GOSH 2019).

Requesting a pregnancy test

Information should be provided to the young woman. This should include:

- The risks associated with performing a surgical or interventional procedure under GA or giving a high risk medicine on a pregnant female.
- How a pregnancy test is performed.
- How the young woman will receive the results.
- What will happen after receiving the results.

Young women under 16 years

If the young woman is under 16 years old and is Gillick competent, she can give consent for the test for herself. A young person under 16 years old is Gillick competent if she has sufficient intellectual maturity, emotional maturity, and understanding of the nature of test to provide consent to the pregnancy testing. If she is not Gillick competent, someone with parental responsibility may be asked to agree on her behalf. If there are any concerns regarding the competency of a young woman under the age of 16 years the legal services team should be contacted for advice during office hours.

Young women aged 16 years and over

If the young woman is 16 years old or over, staff must assume that she has mental capacity and is, therefore, able to consent to the pregnancy test for herself. If there are doubts about the young woman's capacity the clinician must assess her capacity to give consent herself by considering whether she has an impairment of, or a disturbance in the functioning of the mind or brain that causes her to be unable to make the decision about pregnancy testing at the material time. A young woman of 16 years or over is not able to make a decision if they are not able to: understand the relevant information; retain the relevant information long enough to make a decision; use or weigh up that information as part of the decision-making process; or communicate her decision by some means. If she lacks capacity, she is not able to give consent fherself, and someone with parental responsibility may be asked to agree on her behalf. If there are any concerns regarding the mental capacity of a young woman of 16 years or over, contact the legal services team during office hours.

When requesting a urine sample the young woman's privacy, dignity, and confidentiality must be respected and the procedure should be approached sensitively and in a simple and clear manner. All efforts should be made to ensure the young woman is comfortable and able to answer questions truthfully. This should be done without the parent(s)/guardian(s) present. The most suitable time for this may be when measuring and weighing the young woman. For young women with communication difficulties, every attempt must be made to overcome these, e.g. using an interpreting service and/or sign language, and it should not be assumed that because a young woman has a physical or learning disability they are unable to consent for themselves. The questions should be asked as part of the preassessment check list. Prior to any questioning, explain that these particular questions, although sensitive, are asked routinely of all females of this age group. It is important that these questions are worded in a nonaccusatory manner and that they are presented as part of a group of standard preoperative safety checks.

Refusal of a pregnancy test

In the event that either the young woman or the person with parental responsibility refuses the test, the surgeon, medical doctor, or radiographer will decide if the procedure can continue. The social work service will need to be informed of the refusal if the young woman is either under 16 or is over 16 but lacks mental capacity.

Obtaining the information regarding possibility of pregnancy prior to the procedure

A sample of urine will be collected, and the testing carried out on admission, not at a preadmission clinic. If the procedure is rescheduled the test must be repeated, even if a previous test has been negative during the same admission period.

Test results

The result should be clearly, but discreetly, noted in the health records and where applicable by recording urine HCG +ve or urine HCG −ve on the preop checklist and affixing the printed sticker. All results (positive and negative) should be given to young women by an appropriate clinician confidentially, on the day that the test is performed, and documented in the health records. Parents must not be present when the young woman is given the result unless the young woman specifically wants them to be present. Parents will not routinely be told the result of the test and should be discouraged from asking staff for the result. They should be encouraged to help staff to respect their daughter's confidentiality. It may be necessary to reassure parents that sometimes procedures are cancelled or delayed at short notice and that if this happens they should not assume that it has anything to do with the result of their daughter's pregnancy test. If the young woman wants staff to share the result of the test with her parent(s) without her being present, they can do so.

If the pregnancy test is negative, treatment may then be undertaken. If the young woman wants to tell someone this result they may want help from staff to do so. However, if the young woman does not want to share the negative result, staff must not do so.

If the pregnancy test is positive, the surgical, radiological, or medical team will decide if the procedure should continue or be delayed. The rules for who needs to be told of a positive pregnancy test result vary, depending on the young woman's age and mental capacity. The young woman should be reassured that staff will support her, whatever her age. If any young woman is found to be pregnant, discuss the benefits with her of confiding in either her parent/guardian(s), in another trusted member of her family, or in a service that can provide support for her.

If the young woman is **under 16** and pregnant:

- The surgical, radiological or medical team will decide if the procedure should continue or be delayed. This should be explained to the young woman.
- Staff must inform the Social Work Service.
- If staff want to tell the parent(s) about the result, they must talk to the young woman first, and consider her confidentiality.
- If the young woman would like to tell her parent(s) or anyone else about the result, and they want help from staff in telling them, this can be arranged.

If the young woman is **16 or over** and pregnant:

- The surgical, radiological, or medical team will decide if the procedure should continue or be delayed. This should be explained to the young woman.
- If the young woman has capacity, it will be her decision when (or if) she tells her parent(s) the result of the pregnancy test. If the young woman would like help in telling her parent(s) or anyone else, this can be arranged.
- If the young woman lacks mental capacity, staff must inform the Social Work Service. If staff want to inform the parent(s) of the result, they must talk to the young woman first, and consider her confidentiality.

If a young woman (of any age) feels that she will be at risk of physical danger if her parent(s) were informed of a positive pregnancy test result, this must be discussed in line with the Trust's safeguarding policy and a referral made to social service before she is discharged. If any young woman is found to be pregnant, she should be advised that informing her GP would provide the best opportunity for continuity of care on an informed basis. Even if the young woman does not want the Trust to share this information with the GP, it may be necessary to do so.

Radiological investigations

This section provides an overview of the specialties within radiology and the examinations or procedures performed. Guidelines are provided which will enable the nurse to:

- Prepare CYPs for a radiological procedures
- Assist in maintaining safety throughout the procedure
- Ensure the CYP's safe recovery and return to the ward

Introduction to radiological investigations

The aim of this section is to help nurses understand their role in preparing CYPs for and assisting the radiologist to perform radiological investigations in CYPs. Some radiology departments have a designated radiology nurse experienced in all aspects of the department's work and the procedures that occur. When this facility is not available the role will often fall to the ward nurse who accompanies the CYP to the radiology department. It is frequently the case that the most optimal imaging is achieved when the nurse caring for the CYP remains with them to support them, facilitate holding, provide advice on the CYP's condition, and build on previously established nurse–patient or parent/carer rapport. The role of the accompanying nurse therefore is to support the CYP and their family, act as the patient's advocate, and assist with the preparation of the CYP and carer, based on a thorough assessment of the CYP and knowledge of the examination required. The nurse may also be involved in the preparation of equipment prior to the examination and assist the radiographer in ensuring that the CYP remains in the correct position.

Any test can make a CYP or parent/carer apprehensive, so reassurance that most tests are not painful or uncomfortable, if asked, is critical to avoid difficult or lengthy procedures due to an uncooperative or frightened CYP. It is really important to avoid negative suggestions to the CYP such as 'barium does not taste nice'; instead, say 'you will need to drink a plain drink and we can add your favourite flavour to it if you like.' Parents/carers may also inadvertently give negative messages without realising it; for example, repeatedly saying 'it will not hurt' introduce the idea that it might when this may never have occurred to the CYP previously. It is therefore important that HCWs have the knowledge to support the CYP and family through these commonly performed procedures.

Whether the CYP is an inpatient or daycase, preparation using toys to demonstrate the test can help. Parents/carers can be given information and encouraged to do this at home prior to admission. The radiology department should have a space that is decorated in a suitable way for CYPs, with toys and more grown-up activities to distract them before and during the test. The X-ray room is a controlled environment where CYPs can feel they have no choice about whether the procedure is performed. It may be helpful for the CYP to take a favourite toy or storybook, tablet, music, or video with them to the X-ray department to distract them. Small rewards such as stickers or certificates should be available to help to make it a positive experience and reduce anxiety for any subsequent visits. For more information see Chapter 27: Play as a Therapeutic Tool.

The X-ray room should be kept warm to avoid cooling of the CYP. Some clothing can be left in place, depending on the type of X-ray examination, and the nurse should check with the radiographer to determine what is allowed. It is more common to remove any clothes with metal poppers or zippers beforehand.

For inpatients, the stability of the CYP's condition must be assessed before considering a move to the radiography department. The use of portable X-ray machines within intensive care units is well established and should be considered for all CYPs when transferring them to the department is difficult, poses an infection risk, or is likely to cause further deterioration in an already unwell child. The risks and benefits of moving the CYP versus performing a portable X-ray should always be considered.

Wall-mounted oxygen, suction, and monitoring equipment should be available in every radiology room. Resuscitation equipment for all ages of CYP must be present within the department and trained personnel available.

Many tests in the radiology department use X-rays, which involve the use of ionising radiation. Within diagnostic radiology these are generally of an ultra-low or very low dose. We are all exposed to background radiation all our lives and a CYP's chest X-ray is typically the equivalent of one day of background radiation, i.e. the CYP is one day 'older' in radiation terms, which is negligible. Other tests, such as computed tomography (CT) use a higher dose, and are only performed after careful clinical consideration by the referring doctor and the radiologist; nevertheless, the diagnostic benefit for the CYP usually far outweighs any potential risk from the radiation.

Factors to note
- The need for radiological information that can aid in clinical diagnosis or treatment must be balanced against the potential hazards of the exposure to radiation.
- It is a legal requirement that tests involving ionising radiation can only be requested by a doctor or other specially trained health professional, such as a nurse practitioner (DHSC 2018).
- The X-ray examination is clinically directed by the radiologist or trained physicist.
- The radiographer normally directs and is responsible for the examination.

Chapter 15 Investigations

- All X-rays hold a potential risk.
- It is important to remember that although the risk to the individual CYP is minimal it is a general philosophy that the dose to the general public from medical use of ionising radiation should be reduced.
- The net gain outweighs the risk, i.e. CYP undergoing frequent X-ray examinations.
- Before any investigations are performed on any CYP, the principles laid down in the regulations must be adhered to (DHSC 2018).
- The radiographer will ask all female patients over the age of 12 requiring X-rays of the abdomen, pelvis, or spine whether they have started their periods and if there is a chance they could be pregnant. They may also then ask the date of their last period in order to meet legal requirements (DHSC 2018).
- Nurses should act as an advocate for the CYP to ensure there is no possibility of pregnancy in girls over 12 years of age.
- Nurses or mothers who are pregnant should not assist with X-ray examinations in order to protect their unborn foetus.

Preparation

Adequate preparation and explanation is important to ensure successful examinations for CYPs within the radiology department, particularly if they may need to stay still for a long period of time, or may experience some discomfort during the procedure. Preparation of both the CYP and their parent/carer is essential to minimise anxiety and support a smooth procedure. Where procedures are long and lengthy, for example in MRI, there are distraction aides such as DVD's; alternatively, sedation or a GA may be required. For more information regarding preparation and distraction see Chapter 27: Play as a Therapeutic Tool.

Restraint or immobilisation is a common dilemma in radiology when CYPs are unwilling or unable to remain still during a procedure. Restraining CYPs should be a last resort (RCN 2019). Immobilisation techniques such as Velcro straps and sandbags, are useful aides in radiology departments. Verbal consent should always be sought from the CYP/parent/carer prior to any examination, and any restrictive physical intervention or therapeutic holding should be discussed and agreed ahead of the procedure.

Procedure guideline 15.25 Care of the CYP during a radiological investigation

General preparation for all radiological investigations

Statement	Rationale
1 Ensure that the test or procedure is necessary and has been requested by a doctor or other authorised HCW.	1 To minimise exposure to ionising radiation and ensure that the procedure is justified and is the best imaging modality for the clinical question.
2 All request forms should state the diagnosis, examination required, the reason for the request, and any additional information relevant, such as infectious status or relevant medical history.	2 To ensure that the correct procedure is performed and to minimise risk.
3 Where possible the CYP should come to the department for their examination.	3 Optimal imaging for diagnosis is best achieved in the department.
4 Some imaging may be performed on the ward if the CYP is: • Deteriorating • On intensive care • Immune suppressed with reverse barrier nursing • Highly infectious	4 To ensure the safety of the CYP and others.
5 Ensure that the CYP is suitably dressed for the procedure. a) Remove any clothing with metal zips, poppers, or wires that will be within the field of examination. Orthopaedic back braces must also be removed if possible. b) For interventional radiological procedures, the CYP should wear a hospital gown.	5 a) These can cause artefacts and alter image quality or obstruct the area of examination.
6 Inform the CYP/carer of the need to lie still and agree on any holding restraints if these need to be used.	6 To plan for a smooth procedure and determine whether sedation or GA may be required.
7 For any female over the age of 12, consider the need for a pregnancy test.	7 To minimise the risk to the foetus.
8 Provide information regarding the procedure and obtain consent.	
9 Ensure CYP is nil by mouth as required (2, 4, 6 rule – see Chapter 26: Perioperative Care).	9 To minimise the risk of aspiration.
10 Use hoists as appropriate (see Chapter 19: Moving and Handling).	10 To provide a safe environment for both the CYP and staff.

Preparation of CYP and Family

1 The CYP and parents/carers should have been given a full explanation of why the imaging is being undertaken and details of the procedure, equipment, and processes involved prior to arriving in X-ray. This must include any activity expected of the CYP, e.g. drinking medication, holding their breath, and procedures such as cannulation or catheterisation.	1 To fully inform and prepare the family and increase concordance during imaging.

(continued)

Procedure guideline 15.25 Care of the CYP during a radiological investigation *(continued)*

Statement	Rationale
2 An assessment and care plan are recommended prior to complex procedures.	2 To ensure correct management of the CYP and minimise the effects of any pain or distress.
3 Books and leaflets written for CYPs can help explain the type of equipment that will be used and the procedures involved. There are some very good inexpensive publications available, which can be adapted to the needs of the individual department.	3 These provide a simple explanation of the process during the procedures. To minimise fear; X-ray machines, for example, are large and may need to be moved around the CYP during the procedure, which may be frightening.
4 Check that the name, date of birth, and hospital number of the CYP are correct. Inpatients must have a name band or alternative ID with them.	4 To ensure that the correct procedure is performed on the correct patient.
5 Girls who have passed the menarche should be asked in private if they might be pregnant.	5 X-rays can cause harm to an unborn foetus.
6 If medications or intravenous contrast media are likely to be administered the CYP should be weighed prior to the test.	6 To enable the correct doses of drugs and contrast media to be given.
7 Accompanying adult(s) should be aware that they may be required to immobilise the CYP by gently holding. They should be both comfortable with this and not pregnant, as this would prevent their involvement.	7 To ensure a smooth procedure with minimal delays and minimal risk.

Other factors requiring consideration

Privacy

1 Privacy is an important aspect of any procedure. All CYPs should have their investigation in private and only the people necessary for the procedure should remain in the X-ray room.	1 To maintain the privacy and dignity of the CYP and parent/carer and reduce the general exposure of individuals to radiation.

Protection

2 Any person assisting with an X-ray examination must wear the lead covering apron and thyroid collar provided. Local protection for the CYP may be required, e.g. pelvic/gonad protection. When X-rays are being taken on the ward using portable equipment a safe zone should be established, ensuring that no unnecessary personnel are present in the area and that those who are required are wearing protective clothing.	2 To minimise radiation dose.

Positioning

3 The radiographer will assist the nurse/parent/carer to position the CYP correctly.	3 To get the best exposure the first time, so minimising radiation exposure for everyone. The correct positioning of the CYP and the maintenance of the position during the X-ray examination is one of the most important aspects of the procedure.

Restraint

4 It is the nurse's role, as the child and family's advocate, to ensure that the CYP is not restrained unnecessarily or for any great length of time and that appropriate explanation and reassurance is given.	4 To comply with national restraint guidelines (RCN 2019).

Special Needs

5 In the case of a CYP who is a wheelchair user or physically disabled it is advisable to ask the carer how to move the CYP. It may not be possible to obtain particular X-rays on some physically disabled CYPs, due to their inability to move or maintain a particular position. Those CYPs with a learning disability may need additional time, a quieter environment and other reasonable adjustments to be made.	5 To ensure a smooth procedure and avoid harm to the CYP, parent/carer, or nurse. To comply with local lifting and handling policies.

Praise and reward

6 At the end of any X-ray examination the CYP must be praised for their cooperation and if appropriate, a bravery certificate or sticker can be awarded.	6 To provide positive feedback and reassurance to the CYP.

Environment and physical safety

Many examination areas within radiology departments are deemed to be 'controlled environments' and these will be denoted by clear warning signs outside the room/scanner. Entering any clinical room should be done with caution, and only after checking for warning signs. This is to ensure the safety of both staff and the CYP, particularly within MRI where there is a strong magnetic field, or in areas where ionising radiation is being used (X-rays, CT scanners, interventional radiology, and nuclear medicine). It is also important to respect the privacy and dignity of the CYP during these examinations.

Checking pregnancy status

For most diagnostic radiological examinations, exposure to ionising radiation poses little risk to the unborn foetus. However, pregnancy status should be sought from all females who are of 'child-bearing potential,' and this is generally accepted to be all females over 12 years old. Asking pregnancy status questions can sometimes pose difficulties within a paediatric hospital if family members are present when the question is asked, and can cause offence; discretion and privacy should be sought. The usual way to do this is to tell the female CYP that everyone is asked this and it is a legal obligation to ask (this helps remove any suggestion that the question is specific to them) and then to ask the CYP using the words 'is there is any chance that you might be pregnant'. If they answer with a definite 'no' the examination goes ahead. If there is any uncertainty whatsoever they are then asked when their last period was. If the period is overdue (i.e. more than 28 days prior) consideration will be given to postponing the examination, after discussion with the radiologist and/or clinician. For more information see the "Pregnancy Testing" section above.

Types of radiological investigations
General X-ray

General or plain film X-ray is the most common examination occurring in any radiology department and is noninvasive. Very low levels of ionising radiation are used to take a 2D X-ray image to look at the anatomy in any part of the body, including bone, lung, or soft tissue. It can be taken in the Anterior/Posterior (AP) (i.e. front to back) or lateral (i.e. sideways) plane, depending on which part of the body needs to be examined. Most commonly an examination involves one image of the chest, abdomen, or pelvis and two images of any part of the limbs or spine. When suspecting nonaccidental injury a skeletal survey is taken, which involves multiple X-ray images of the whole body in both planes (often around 20 X-rays or more).

Fluoroscopy

Fluoroscopy uses ionising radiation at a typical X-ray pulse rate of three images per second, giving a real-time moving 2D picture that is viewed instantly on the monitor and then saved. These images then create a dynamic study similar to a real-time video and can be saved as single images or as a series. This type of examination is particularly useful when the radiologist needs to see how something actually happens, e.g. how the CYP swallows, how the gut is working or what happens to the urinary tract during micturition. Two broad types of contrast agents are used; water-soluble contrast agents (iodine based), which are clear and look like water, but show on X-rays; and barium-based contrast agents, which are white and also show on X-rays. These agents work in completely different ways:

Water-soluble contrast:	Typically used for intravascular examinations, urology examinations, if there is a risk of aspiration, and when bowel perforation is suspected.
Barium:	Typically used when investigating the gastrointestinal tract, observing swallowing or gastric emptying and anatomy, or bowel 'follow-through' examinations. Barium is an inert, white, 'chalky' agent. It passes undigested through the gastrointestinal tract and can take up to three days to clear. To make barium palatable it can be mixed with flavouring or food, depending on the procedure. Barium is NEVER used intravenously.

Air can also be used as an agent and its use will be explained later. Some examinations in fluoroscopy can carry a clinical risk. Emergency equipment and the appropriate level of medical or nursing support must be available as the condition of the CYP dictates. The following is a brief description of the types of examinations most commonly performed in fluoroscopy and the preparation required.

Upper gastrointestinal series

An upper gastrointestinal (GI) series (previously called barium/contrast swallow and barium/contrast meal), examines the gut from the pharynx to the first loop of jejunum. Barium (or water-soluble contrast medium) is given orally and observed as it transits the upper GI tract. Several images will be acquired by the radiologist with the CYP in various positions on the table. It is usually performed supine in CYPs, but erect in adults. The most common indications in CYP include looking for structural anatomical abnormalities such as malrotation and to observe for gastro-oesophageal reflux. The examination takes approximately 15 minutes.

Dysphagia swallow using videofluoroscopy

Dysphagia swallow with videofluoroscopy is used to assess swallowing safety and coordination and is usually performed by the radiologist or radiographer in conjunction with a speech and language therapist. The CYP is usually seated (or placed in a specially formed seat like a car seat) and offered a variety of consistencies from fluids through to solids mixed with barium. Swallowing is then observed with fluoroscopy and simultaneously recorded on videotape or DVD. The test usually takes 15 minutes.

Barium follow-through

A barium follow-through examines the gut from the pharynx to the caecum. Its main purpose is to examine the small intestine, as this cannot be reached by endoscopy. Like an upper GI series barium, it is usually given orally, but may also be administered by nasogastric, nasojejunal, or gastrostomy tube. A series of images will be acquired at intervals during the study. The CYP does not have to stay in the X-ray room all the time but will be brought in intermittently to monitor the progress of the barium. The most common indication is to look for anatomy before or after surgery. The test usually takes between 45 minutes and 3 hours, depending on how long the barium takes to transit the small bowel. Barium follow-through is increasingly being replaced by MRI of the bowel and may soon be obsolete for most indications.

Tube oesophagram

This is a specialist test that is less commonly performed, but is used to assess for a fistula between the trachea and the oesophagus.

Contrast enema

A contrast enema is used to examine the large bowel from the rectum to the caecum. The most common indication in CYPs is in unexplained chronic constipation or following surgery to the lower GI tract. The CYP will need to lie on the couch and will be asked to turn on their side while the radiologist passes a thin soft plastic catheter a few centimetres into the rectum. Water soluble contrast is then given through the catheter. The radiologist follows its progress under X-ray screening until it reaches the appendix and the whole of the colon has been visualised. This may involve turning the CYP onto their side, back and so on. The radiologist will take a limited series of X-ray images. The test normally takes about 30 minutes.

Air enema

This is a specialist, but important procedure used to treat an intussusception. The diagnosis of intussusception is usually made by ultrasound and an air enema is only performed once the diagnosis has been made. A catheter is placed into the rectum and air is introduced at a continuous pressure under fluoroscopic guidance to push back (reduce) the intussuscepted bowel. This procedure may take up to 30 minutes. The main complication is perforation of the bowel. An air enema is contraindicated if a perforation is already present, or if the CYP has not been adequately fluid resuscitated before the procedure.

Micturating cystourethrogram

A micturating (or voiding) cystourethrogram (MCUG/VCUG) examines the bladder and urethra and may provide information about the ureters and upper urinary tract if there is reflux of contrast. A catheter is passed into the bladder, usually via the urethra, although a suprapubic catheter can be used if it is already in place, and water-soluble contrast is instilled. Images of the bladder are taken, and images of the urethra are acquired when the CYP micturates. The most common indications for an MCUG include looking for anatomical abnormalities of the lower urinary tract (such as posterior urethral valves in boys) and to look for ureteric reflux if other abnormalities have already been identified on ultrasound.

Linogram

A linogram involves injecting intravenous contrast through a central venous access line, often a 'Hickman' line, under fluoroscopy to check its position and integrity. Most commonly this is performed if there have been problems with injecting or aspiration through the line. The test takes 15 minutes.

Ultrasound

Ultrasound is an excellent imaging modality to examine parts of the body comprising soft tissue, e.g. liver, kidney, thyroid, testes, breast, musculoskeletal structures, and fluid containing structures such as the bladder, gall bladder, or vessels. It is less useful in examining structures that contain gas, such as the bowel. Ultrasound uses sound waves that are of high frequency and cannot generally be heard by the human ear. A transducer (probe) is used to both send and receive the returning ultrasound signal, and this is then converted to an image on the screen. The CYP cannot feel the ultrasound waves and therefore this examination causes little or no discomfort, other than when positioning the CYP or use of the probe on an already painful area.

Ultrasound gel is used to ensure good contact between the probe and the skin, which may tickle a little. For many ultrasound examinations no preparation is necessary. However, examination of the bladder and/or pelvis requires that the bladder is full and examination of the biliary tree (as part of an abdominal scan) requires that the CYP is fasted. After the scan, the gel is wiped off and the CYP is free to go.

Nuclear medicine

In most hospitals 'nuclear medicine' is part of the Radiology Department. Virtually every nuclear medicine examination involves the CYP having a radioisotope injected via a butterfly needle or a cannula. Central intravenous lines cannot be used, as the injection (isotope) can become attached to the inside of the lines. For specialist tests of the bowel the radioisotope is sometimes taken orally, mixed with food.

Every radioisotope injection is specific to the individual CYP, as it is calculated for their weight and the type of examination. It is prepared the day before the procedure in a specialist laboratory and it is essential that it is given before the radioactivity decays. The 'decaying' process means that the energy of the isotope is constantly decreasing, and consequently the images become poorer in quality. If a CYP is late for their appointment their isotope may have decayed beyond the level required for a reliable image and the appointment will have to be cancelled; timing is crucial.

Specific 'labels' are attached to isotopes, e.g. technetium, allowing it to be specifically taken up by one type of organ or cell type.

After the injection, the gamma camera (scanner) detects the gamma rays being emitted from the isotope. The amount of radiation used for these diagnostic tests is very small and there are no side effects, but the CYP may need to use a separate toilet in the department directly after the scan, as the urine may have low levels of decaying radioactivity. These scans require the CYP to lie still for a period of time and, depending on age and/or ability, can be performed while awake, sedated, or if needed, under a GA.

Table 15.4 Types of radiological isotopic scans

Procedure	Purpose	Special considerations
Bone Scan	Assesses for infection, fractures, or areas of overactive bone – such as in metastatic cancer.	An isotope (technetium) is injected 2–3 hours before the scan commences. Preparation involves ensuring CYP is well hydrated to get a good result.
Direct Isotope Cystogram (DIC)	Looking for vesico ureteric reflux on bladder emptying	A small catheter is inserted into the urethra and an isotope is injected into the bladder. A course of oral antibiotics should be started five days prior to study and if already on antibiotics, the dose should be doubled (as for an MCUG, which also requires catheter placement).
DMSA and MAG3 scans	DMSA examines structure, location, and function of the kidneys. MAG3 looks for delay or obstruction to drainage from the kidneys.	Both involve injecting isotopes into a vein. It can take up to two hours before the isotope is present in the kidneys to perform the scan.
Gall bladder (HIDA) scan	Examines size, structure, function, and location of liver and gall bladder.	

Table 15.4 Types of radiological isotopic scans (continued)

Procedure	Purpose	Special considerations
Labelled white cell scan	Looks for areas of infection or inflammation.	Involves taking a blood sample, which is mixed with an isotope and injected into a vein three hours later. The isotope attaches itself to the white cells in the blood. The scan follows as it circulates throughout the body; if infection or inflammation is present, it will collect in those areas.
Lung (VQ) scans	Assesses lung function.	This is done by injecting an isotope into a vein, which shows the blood supply to the lungs. The CYP breathes in a gas isotope, showing how well oxygen passes into the lungs.
Meckel's scan	Assesses for the presence of a Meckel's diverticulum.	Involves injecting an isotope that is taken up by ectopic stomach or pancreas cells in the mucosa of the Meckel's diverticulum in the distal ileum.
MIBG scan	Looks for abnormal cell types associated with certain tumours.	Injection of radioisotope into a vein.
Perchlorate discharge test	Detects abnormal tissues of neurogenic origin, e.g. neuroblastoma.	Both involve injecting an iodine-based radioisotope. NB: CYPs who have previously had iodine-based reactions to seafood or medicines containing iodine are not suitable for this examination.
Thyroid/parathyroid scans	Assesses thyroid function.	
SPECT scan	Assesses brain activity in CYPs with epilepsy.	CYPs must be monitored closely as their anti-seizure medicines are stopped to deliberately evoke a seizure. Once seizing, the radioisotope is injected and the scan commenced. These CYPs also have further radioisotope scans when not seizing.
DEXA scan	Assesses bone density	

Computer tomography

A computer tomography (CT) scan is an X-ray procedure that combines many X-ray images with the aid of a computer to generate cross-sectional images (like 'slices') and if needed, 3D images of the internal structures of the body. A CT scan is used to define normal and abnormal structures in the body and/or to assist in procedures by helping to guide the placement of instruments, as in biopsies. Compared with standard X-rays, the images are much more detailed and can be viewed in multiple planes. The scanner consists of a large doughnut-shaped structure containing an X-ray tube and special image detectors, which rotate around the CYP, who lies on the scanner bed. The detectors send signals to a computer for processing and a cross-sectional image or 'slice' is displayed on a monitor/computer screen.

Contrast material may be given either orally or intravenously to highlight certain structures. CT is a low-risk (but relatively high X-ray dose) procedure, the most common problem being an adverse reaction to intravenous contrast media, which is iodine-based. Care should be taken with CYPs who have a positive history of allergy, asthma, or untoward reactions to iodinated contrast media.

While the scan is in progress the CYP needs to be very still, as the scanner takes very fine slices through the body. The actual scan is so quick (typically 15 seconds) that even very young children can usually comply. Occasionally it has to be done under GA. Metal objects cause artefacts on the images, so clothes with metal fastenings need to be removed prior to the scan.

Magnetic resonance imaging (MRI)

Magnetic resonance imaging (MRI) is a way of looking inside the body without using X-rays. MRI can produce two- or three-dimensional images using a very large magnet, radio waves, and a computer. The MRI scanner is a large tube, big enough for the patient to lie down inside it, which is why it is sometimes referred to as a tunnel. The magnetic fields used are not known to be harmful, which means that the CYP can have someone with them in the room, sitting right beside the scanner. MRI is used for diagnosis and monitoring disease, giving detailed information on bone, organ, soft tissue, tendon, ligament, or muscle structures, including the heart, brain, and blood vessels. It is increasingly used for examinations of the urinary tract (MRU) and the bowel (MRE).

There is no specific preparation required for an MRI scan, but everyone entering the magnetic area will be checked for metallic objects, which may not be taken into the room, as they can damage the magnet or the CYP if they become projectile. No-one with a pacemaker, aneurysm clip, or other metalware may enter the scan room. Often it is necessary to inject a small amount of contrast, which does not contain iodine, into the arm. Allergic reactions are therefore rare.

The CYP can wear what they like during the scan, as long as the clothes do not have zips or other metal parts, so do not have to undress. The CYP must keep very still during the scan, as one movement can spoil all the images, unlike X-rays. It can be good to practice this in advance, as the CYP who cannot cope with this will usually need a GA. A favourite toy can be taken in with the CYP, if there is no metal in it. There is a lot of helpful information available on the internet for parents/carers to help prepare their child (GOSH 2016).

Once the scan starts, the machine starts to make a whirring and thumping noise, which can get very loud, and this continues throughout the scan. The CYP can talk to the radiographer while in the magnet and is given a bell to press should they wish to stop the procedure. No special care is required following a scan, provided the CYP has not received a GA or sedation. The CYP can have someone with them throughout the entire examination, which can take between 20 and 60 minutes.

Interventional radiology (IR)

IR uses image-guided techniques; ultrasound, fluoroscopy (X-rays) and occasionally CT, which are minimally invasive, to diagnose and/or treat certain conditions as an alternative to surgery (see Table 15.5). These procedures are generally less costly and less traumatic for the CYP as they have quicker recovery times due to the smaller incisions required and shorter stays in hospital.

IR procedures are mostly performed under GA but can be undertaken while the CYP is awake if they are able to cooperate. They can also be undertaken with sedation or Entonox (see Chapter 24: Pain Management). For care of the anaesthetised CYP, see Chapter 26: Perioperative Care.

Consent needs to be obtained for all procedures to ensure that the CYP and their parent/carer receive the appropriate information and are aware of the benefits and risks of the examination.

Some procedures require preoperative blood tests to be taken and reviewed prior to the examination. Any concerning results, particularly relating to coagulation, should be discussed with a haematologist to determine whether it is safe to proceed with the procedure. IR techniques are minimally invasive and involve less risk, both at the time of the procedure and in preservation of veins for future access, and should be utilised for all elective procedures.

Table 15.5 Procedures performed in interventional radiology

Type of procedure	Description and nursing considerations
Central venous line placement	This is the placement of a soft flexible plastic tube (catheter) into a centrally located vein using vascular interventional techniques. The most commonly placed lines include PICC (peripherally inserted central catheter), Hickman® lines (single and double lumens), Port-a-Caths, VasCaths, and Perm Caths). Depending on the type of central venous access required, the procedure can either be carried out under local or GA. For a PICC line or femoral vascath in older/co-operative CYPs, local anaesthetic, with or without sedation, is sufficient. However, for tunnelled catheter insertions such as a Hickman catheter®, which requires a large amount of cooperation, a general anaesthetic is usually needed. The line is ready for use as soon as the procedure is finished.
Airway procedures	Diagnostic procedures involve injecting a small amount of contrast into the airways under fluoroscopy and then observing the trachea and bronchi while the CYP is under GA. A **bronchogram** can identify malacia (softening), stenosis (narrowing), and other abnormalities of the trachea and smaller airways. A **bronchoscopy** involves passing a scope into the airways and directly visualising the trachea and bronchi for physical abnormalities such as granulation tissue, foreign body, and structural abnormalities. If a diagnosis is made, a ballooning or stenting procedure may be performed.
Gastrointestinal interventions	This includes insertion of new gastrostomy tubes, gastrostomy or gastrojejunal tube maintenance, oesophageal, or other GI dilatations. Those having a gastrostomy for the first time will need to ingest barium before the procedure, which can be taken up to 12 hours prior to the procedure. The barium coats the inside of the large bowel, which then makes it visible on X-ray, reducing the risk of bowel perforation. **Oesophageal dilatation** is the most common procedure undertaken within the GI tract and involves inserting balloon catheters over guide wires under fluoroscopy and inflating at the point of the narrowing or stricture.
Arterial/venous procedures	This typically involves the insertion of a sheath (outer tubing), usually into a femoral artery, but other vessels can also be used. Catheters and wires are then passed through the sheath and positioned in the vessels/area being investigated. Diagnosis involves injecting contrast into the vessel to assess pathology under fluoroscopy. Contrast doses must be monitored due to the potential for toxicity when high concentrations are used. Procedures include **angioplasty, stenting, embolisation,** and **thrombolysis**. **Nursing considerations:** The administration of oral or IV fluids postprocedure assists with flushing the contrast from the system. Postprocedure care includes bed rest and close neurovascular monitoring of the leg or arm where the sheath has been placed. This is because the sheath has been impeding normal blood flow to that particular limb. It is not uncommon for the limb to be a little cooler than the other, but this should improve within the period of monitoring as specified by the interventional radiologist, typically 6–12 hours. For CYPs who have had neuro-interventional procedures, neuro-observations need to be carried out; see Chapter 21: Neurological Care.
Sclerotherapy and lasering	**Sclerotherapy** of venous or lymphatic malformations involves inserting needles into the malformation and injecting an agent with the intention of shrinking or sclerosing the malformation. This may require a number of staged treatments. Endovascular laser treatment (EVLT) is performed in CYPs who have atypically large veins that become sluggish and lose the ability to return blood back to the heart, resulting in an enlarged affected limb. **Nursing considerations:** If the malformation is on a limb then a pressure bandage is applied for a few days postprocedure to assist with ongoing sclerosing effect. These procedures are often performed as day cases. Hypervascular lesions in areas such as the tongue or on the face require close monitoring, as it is not uncommon for swelling to occur. CYPs undergoing orbital sclerotherapy require a night in hospital postprocedure due to the risks associated with swelling and proptosis, where the eyeball is pushed forward and vision may be compromised. If **laser treatment** is given, local laser safety rules must be followed; these include making sure the room is safe, with doors locked during lasering, windows blacked out, shiny surfaces covered, eye protection for the CYP and staff when laser is in use, and fire safety precautions available. A specific register records the CYP's details, vessel, length of time, and wattage of laser and the personnel present in the room.

Table 15.5 Procedures performed in interventional radiology (continued)

Type of procedure	Description and nursing considerations
Renal biopsy and tumour biopsy	**Renal biopsy** is undertaken to identify a specific disease process in the kidney (or transplant kidney). The kidney is visualised using ultrasound guidance. Local anaesthetic is given to the chosen area of the kidney. The specialist biopsy needle has a sharp cutting edge that slices and removes tiny samples of the kidney tissue. **Tumour biopsies** are performed in much the same way, depending on where the tumour is. **Nursing considerations:** In older CYPs this procedure is successfully performed with sedation or Entonox; otherwise a GA is needed. As there is a small risk of postoperative bleeding it is imperative that clotting results are obtained prior to the procedure and the operator is informed if the CYP is currently on aspirin. Postoperative observations are essential to ensure early detection of complications such as bleeding. For more information regarding Biopsies see Chapter 3.
Other interventional radiology procedures	**Aspirations and drain insertions** of fluid collections or abscesses anywhere in the body with the use of ultrasound predominately or X-ray/CT for difficult lesions. This can be performed under GA or on the awake CYP if cooperative. **Nephrology and urology interventions:** These include nephrostomy tube insertions for the nonfunctioning or obstructed kidney, ureteric dilatation and stenting, antegrade pyelogram, which assesses the calyces and ureter by directly injecting contrast under ultrasound guidance, and using X-rays and percutaneous nephrolithotomy (PCNL); ultrasound guided insertion of an endoscope, to remove or crush kidney stones. **Ultrasound or X-ray guided injections** of steroids into joints and/or tendon sheaths can be performed for CYPs with idiopathic juvenile arthritis. Ultrasound guided needle placement can also be used to inject botulinum into salivary glands to reduce saliva production in a CYP with a difficult or unsafe swallow.

References

American Heart Association (2006). *ECG Basics*. American Heart Association: Dallas.

Association of Paediatric Anaesthetists of Great Britain and Ireland (APAGBI) (2012). Good practice in postoperative and procedural pain management. *Pediatric Anesthesia* 22 (1): 1–79.

Broome, M.E. (1990). Preparation of children for painful procedures. *Pediatric Nursing* 16 (6): 537–541.

Chowdhury, T.A. (2015). Hypoglycaemia (low blood sugar) in diabetes. netdoctor (e-pub). www.netdoctor.co.uk/conditions/diabetes/a834/hypoglycaemia-low-blood-sugar-in-diabetes (accessed 23 August 2022).

Cavanagh, C. and Coppinger, C. (2009). Newborn blood spot sampling. *Infant* 5 (3): 83–86.

Chantler, C., Garnett, E.S., Parsons, V., and Veall, N. (1969). Glomerular filtration rate measurement in man by the single injection methods using 51Cr-EDTA. *Clinical Science* 37 (1): 169–180.

Claar, R.L., Walker, L.S., and Smith, C.A. (2002). The influence of appraisals in understanding children's experiences with medical procedures. *Journal of Pediatric Psychology* 27 (7): 553–563.

Coia, J.E., Duckworth, G.J., Edwards, D.I. et al. (2006). Joint working Party of the British Society of antimicrobial chemotherapy; hospital infection society; Infection Control Nurses Association. Guidelines for the control and prevention of meticillin-resistant Staphylococcus aureus (MRSA) in healthcare facilities. *The Journal of Hospital Infection* 63 (Suppl 1): S1–S44.

Cook, R. (1995). Urinalysis. *Nursing Standard*, CE Article 343 9 (28): 32–37.

Cook, K. and Langton, H. (eds.) (2009). *Cardiothoracic Care for Children and Young People – A Multidisciplinary Approach*. Chichester: Wiley-Blackwell.

Counahan, R., Chantler, C., Ghazali, S. et al. (1976). Estimation of glomerular filtration rate from plasma creatinine concentration in children. *Archives of Disease in ChildhoodArch Dis Child* 51 (11): 875–878.

Coviello, J.S. (ed.) (2016). *ECG Interpretation: Made Incredibly Easy*, 5e. Ambler, PA Lippincott: Williams and Wilkins.

Davey, P. (2013). *ECG at a Glance*. Chichester, UK: Wiley.

Department of Health (DH) (2001). Guidelines for preventing infections associated with the insertion and maintenance of short-term indwelling urethral catheters in acute care. The EPIC project: developing National Evidence-based Guidelines for preventing healthcare associated infections. *Journal of Hospital Infection*: 47 (S3–S4), 39–46.

Department of Health and Social Care (DHSC) (2018) Guidance to the Ionising Radiation (Medical Exposure) Regulations 2017 (IRMER). https://www.gov.uk/government/publications/ionising-radiation-medical-exposure-regulations-2017-guidance (accessed 23 August 2022).

Department of Health Expert Advisory Committee on Antimicrobial Resistance and Healthcare Associated Infection (ARHAI) (2014). Implementation of modified admission MRSA screening guidance for NHS. https://assets.publishing.service.gov.uk/government/uploads/system/uploads/attachment_data/file/345144/Implementation_of_modified_admission_MRSA_screening_guidance_for_NHS.pdf (accessed 23 August 2022).

Duff, A. (2003). Incorporating psychological approaches into routine paediatric venepuncture. *Archives of Diseases in Childhood* 88: 931–997.

Equi, A., Pike, S., Davies, J., and Bush, A. (2001). Use of cough swabs in a cystic fibrosis clinic. *Archives of Disease in Childhood* 85: 438–439.

Frank, L. and Gilbert, R. (2003). Reducing the pain during blood sampling in infants. *Clinical Evidence* 9: 419–435.

Franklin, L. (1998). Skin cleansing and infection control in peripheral venepuncture and cannulation. *Paediatric Nursing* 10 (9): 33–34.

Frederick, V. (1991) Paediatric IV therapy: soothing the patient). *RN* 54 (12): 40–42.

General Medical Council (2013). Good Medical Practice. https://www.gmc-uk.org/ethical-guidance/ethical-guidance-for-doctors/good-medical-practice (accessed 23 August 2022).

Gilbert, C. (2009). Investigation and management of congenital hyperinsulinism. *British Journal of Nursing* 18 (20): 1256–1260.

Gilchrist, B. (1996). Wound infection – sampling bacterial flora: a review of the literature. *Journal of Wound Care* 5 (8): 386–388.

Glenesk, A., Shepherd, A., and Niven, C. (2006). Blood spot testing: comparing techniques and automated devices. *British Journal of Midwifery* 14 (2): 96–99.

Goernig, M., Kirmeier, T., Krack, A. et al. (2004). Iohexol contrast medium induces QT prolongation in amiodarone patients. *British Journal of Clinical Pharmacology* 58 (1): 96–98.

Great Ormond Street Hospital (GOSH) (2016) Your child is having an MRI scan without sedation or general anaesthetic. https://www.gosh.nhs.uk/conditions-and-treatments/procedures-and-treatments/your-child-having-mri-scan-without-sedation-or-general-anaesthetic/ (accessed 23 August 2022).

Great Ormond Street Hospital (GOSH) (2019) Routine pregnancy testing before treatment. https://www.gosh.nhs.uk/conditions-and-treatments/procedures-and-treatments/routine-pregnancy-testing-treatment/ (accessed 23 August 2022).

Green, M. and Huby, K. (2010). Cardiovascular system, chapter. 9. In: *Clinical Skills in Children's Nursing* (eds. I. Coyne, F. Neill and F. Timmins). Oxford: Oxford University Press.

Griffiths, C. (1995). Microbiological examination in urinary tract infection. *Nursing Times* 91 (11): 33–35.

Grundmann, H., Aires-de-Sousa, M., Boyce, J., and Tiemersma, E. (2006). Emergence and resurgence of meticillin-resistant Staphylococcus aureus as a public health threat. *Lancet* 368: 874–885.

Hampton, J.R. (2013). *The ECG Made Easy*, 8e. Edinburgh, Churchill Livingstone: Elsevier.

Hanas, R. (2007). *Type 1 Diabetes in Children, Adolescents and Young Adults*, 3e. London: Class Publishing.

Hassan, Z. and Shah, M. (2005). Scald injury from the Guthrie test: should the heel be warmed? *Archives of Disease in Childhood - Fetal and Neonatal Edition* 90 (6): F533–F534.

Hazinski, M.F. (2012). *Nursing Care of the Critically ill Child*. St. Louis: Mosby.

Health and Safety Executive (HSE) (2003). Safe Working and the Prevention of Infection in clinical Laboratories and Similar Facilities. https://www.hse.gov.uk/pubns/clinical-laboratories.pdf (accessed 23 August 2022).

Health and Safety Executive (HSE) (2021). Blood-borne viruses. https://www.hse.gov.uk/biosafety/blood-borne-viruses/index.htm (accessed 23 August 2022).

Health and Safety Executive (HSE) (2021). The Approved List of biological agents. (4th Ed.). Advisory Committee on Dangerous Pathogens. https://www.hse.gov.uk/pubns/misc208.pdf (accessed 23 August 2022).

Heiney, S.P. (1991). Helping children through painful procedures. *The American Journal of Nursing* 91 (11): 20–24.

Higgins, C. (1994). An introduction to the examination of specimens. *Nursing Times* 90 (47): 29–32.

Hoppe, J.E., Towler, E.E., Wagner, B.D. et al. (2015). Sputum induction improves detection of pathogens in children with cystic fibrosis. *Pediatric Pulmonology* 50 (7): 638–646.

Horrox, F. (2002). *Manual of Neonatal and Paediatric Heart Disease*. London: Whurr.

Hortensius, J., Slingerland, R.J., Kleefstra, N. et al. (2011). Self-monitoring of blood glucose: the use of the first or the second drop of blood. *Diabetes Care* 34 (3): 556–560.

Hussain, K., Blackenstein, O., De Lonlay, P., and Christessen, H.T. (2007). Hyperinsulinaemic hypoglycaemia: biochemical bias and the importance of maintaining normoglycaemia during management. *Archive of Diseases in Childhood* 92 (7): 568–570.

Jain, A. and Rutter, N. (1999). Ultrasound study of heel to calcaneum depth in neonates. *Archives of Disease in Childhood-Fetal and Neonatal Edition* 80 (3): F243–F245.

Jain, A., Rutter, N., and Ratnayaka, M. (2001). Topical amethocaine gel for pain relief on heel prick blood sampling: a randomised double blind controlled trial. *Archives of Disease in Childhood* 84: 56–59.

Kellogg, J.A., Manzella, J.P., and Bankert, D.A. (2000). Frequency of low-level bacteraemia in children from birth to fifteen years of age. *Journal of Clinical Microbiology* 38 (6): 2181–2185.

Koch, C. and Hoiby, N. (2000). Diagnosis and treatment of cystic fibrosis. *Respiration* 67: 239–247.

Langley, P. (1999). Guided imagery: a review of effectiveness in the care of children. *Paediatric Nursing* 11 (3): 18–21.

Lansdown, R. (1993). Managing pain in children. Playing monsters and dragons. *Nursing Standard* 7 (25 Suppl): 11.

Lewis, J. (1998). Clean-catch versus urine collection pads: a prospective trial. *Paediatric Nursing* 10 (1): 15–16.

Lilien, L.D., Harris, V.J., Ramamurthy, R.S., and Pildes, R.S. (1976). Neonatal osteomyelitis of the calcaneus: complication of heel puncture. *Journal of Pediatrics* 88 (3): 478–480. Cited in World Health Organisation (WHO) (2010) WHO guidelines on drawing blood: best practices in phlebotomy. p41–45.

Loveday, H.P., Wilson, J.A., Pratt, R.J., Golsorkhi, M., Tingle, A., Bak, A., Browne, J., Prieto, J., Wilcox, M. (2014). Epic 3: national evidence-based guidelines for preventing healthcare-associated infections in NHS hospitals in England. Journal of Hospital Infection, 86S1: S1–S70. https://www.his.org.uk/media/1185/epic3_national_evidence-based_guidelines_for_preventing_hcai_in_nhse.pdf (accessed 23 August 2022).

Lund, C.H., Osborne, J.W., Kuller, J. et al. (2001). Neonatal skin care: clinical outcomes of the AWHONN/NANN evidence-based clinical practice guideline. *Journal of Obstetric, Gynecologic, and Neonatal Nursing* 30 (1): 41–51.

Marieb, E. (2014). *Essentials of Human Anatomy and Physiology*, 10e. International, San Francisco: Benjamin Cummings/Pearson Imprint.

Medicine and Healthcare products Regulatory Agency (2021) Management and use of IVD point of care test devices. https://www.gov.uk/government/publications/in-vitro-diagnostic-point-of-care-test-devices/management-and-use-of-ivd-point-of-care-test-devices (accessed 23 August 2022).

Millam, D.A. (1992). Starting i.v.s: how to develop your venepuncture expertise. *Nursing* 22 (9): 33–46.

Morcos, S.K. (2005). Review article: Acute serious and fatal reactions to contrast media: our current understanding. *The British Journal of Radiology* 78 (932): 686–693.

Mukherjee, J.J., Peppercorn, P.D., Reznek, R.H. et al. (1997). Pheochromocytoma: effect of nonionic contrast medium in CT on circulating catecholamine levels. *Radiology* 202 (1): 227–231.

National Health Service (NHS England) (2014). Risk of associating ECG records with wrong patients, National Patient Safety Alert NHS/PSA/W/2014/003. https://www.england.nhs.uk/2014/03/risk-associating-ecg-records-wrong-patients/ (accessed 23 August 2022).

National Health Service (NHS) England (2022). Improving the blood culture pathway - Executive summary. https://www.england.nhs.uk/wp-content/uploads/2022/06/B0686-improving-the-blood-culture-pathway--executive-summary.pdf (accessed 23 August 2022).

National Institute for Health and Care Excellence (NICE) (2015). Healthcare associated infections: prevention and control in primary and community care. Long-term use of urinary catheters. Clinical Guideline CG139. (Updated 2017). https://www.nice.org.uk/guidance/cg139/ifp/chapter/Your-care (accessed 23 August 2022).

National Institute for Health and Care Excellence (2007). Urinary tract infection in under 16's: diagnosis and management. Clinical guideline (CG54) (Updated 2018). https://www.nice.org.uk/Guidance/CG54 (accessed 23 August 2022).

National Patient Safety Agency (NPSA) (2010). Rapid Response Report NPSA/2010/RRR015: Prevention of over infusion of intravenous fluid and medicines in neonates. https://www.networks.nhs.uk/nhs-networks/staffordshire-shropshire-and-black-country-newborn/documents/1264_RRR_Prevention_of_over_infusion__FINAL.pdf (accessed 23 August 2022).

Naughten, F. (2005). The heel prick: how efficient is common practice? *RCM Midwives* 8 (3): 112–114.

Nilsson-Ehle, P. (2001). Iohexol clearance for the determination of glomerular filtration rate: 15 years' experience in clinical practice. *Electronic Journal of the International Federation of Clinical Chemistry* 13 (2): 48–52.

Nursing and Midwifery Council (2018). *The Code: Professional Standards of Practice and Behaviour for Nurses, Midwives and Nursing Associates*. London: Nursing and Midwifery Council. https://www.nmc.org.uk/standards/code/ (accessed 23 August 2022).

Park, M.K. and Guntheroth, W.G. (2006). *How to Read Pediatric ECGs*, 4e. Philadelphia: Mosby, Elsevier.

Perry, C. (2007). *Infection Prevention and Control*. Oxford: Blackwell Publishing.

Public Health England (2015). Start smart – then focus. Antimicrobial stewardship toolkit for English hospitals. Updated March 2015 https://www.gov.uk/government/publications/antimicrobial-stewardship-start-smart-then-focus (accessed 23 August 2022).

Public Health England (2016). *Guidelines for Newborn Blood Spot Sampling*. London: Public Health England Publications PHE publications gateway number: 2015750. (Updated 2021). https://www.gov.uk/government/publications/newborn-blood-spot-screening-sampling-guidelines (accessed 23 August 2022).

Reynolds, P.R., Banerjee, S., and Meek, J.H. (2005). Alcohol burns in extremely low birthweight infants. Archive of disease in childhood. *Fetal & Neonatal Edition* 90 (1): F10.

Rowley, S. and Clare, S. (2011). ANTT: an essential tool for effective blood culture collection. *British Journal of Nursing* 20 (14).

Royal College of Nursing (RCN) (2013). *Standards for Assessing, Measuring and Monitoring Vital Signs in Infants, Children and Young People London*. Royal College of Nursing.

Royal College of Nursing (RCN) (2019). Restrictive physical interventions and clinical holding of children and young people – guidance for nursing staff. London. https://www.rcn.org.uk/professional-development/publications/pub-007746 (accessed 23 August 2022).

Royal College of Paediatrics and Child Health (2012). Pre-procedure pregnancy checking for under 16s: guidance for clinicians. https://www.rcpch.ac.uk/resources/pre-procedure-pregnancy-checking-under-16s-guidance-clinicians (accessed 23 August 2022).

Royal College of Paediatrics and Child Health Ethics Advisory Committee (2000). Guidelines for the ethical conduct of medical research involving children. *Archives of Disease in Childhood* 82: 177–182.

Sharieff, G.Q. and Rao, S.O. (2006). The pediatric ECG. *Emergency Clinics of North America* 24: 195–208.

Shepherd, A.J., Glenesk, A., Niven, C., and Mackenzie, J. (2006). A Scottish study of heel-prick blood sampling in newborn babies. *Midwifery* 22 (2): 158–168.

Thomson Healthcare INC (2006). Iohexol in DRUGDEX drug evaluations. *Micromedex Healthcare Series* 128.

Tremper, K.K. (1992). Noninvasive monitoring of oxygenation and ventilation-40 years in development. *Western Journal of Medicine* 156: 662–663.

United Nations Economic Commission for Europe (UNECE) (2020). Agreement concerning the International Carriage of Dangerous Goods by Road. https://unece.org/transport/publications/agreement-concerning-international-carriage-dangerous-goods-road-adr-2021 (accessed 23 August 2022).

Wren, C. (2012). *Concise Guide to Pediatric Arrhythmias*. Chichester: Wiley-Blackwell.

Yilmaz, F. and Arikan, D. (2011). The effects of various interventions to newborns on pain and duration of crying. *Journal of Clinical Nursing* 20 (7–8): 1008–1017.

Chapter 16

Learning (intellectual) disabilities

Jim Blair

RNLD, CNLD, DipSW, MA, BSc, BA, MSDipHE, PGDipHE, Formerly Consultant Nurse Learning (Intellectual) Disabilities, Great Ormond Street Hospital, London, UK

Chapter contents

Introduction	358
Principles underpinning practice	358
Families as allies	358
What is a learning (intellectual) disability?	358
The need for change in services and practice	359
Challenges health professionals face when working with people with learning (intellectual) disabilities	359
See the person and understand behaviour that challenges	359
Diagnostic overshadowing	360
Positive behaviour support reducing the use of restrictive practices	361
Becoming an adult: All change	361
Making decisions: Consent to treatment	361
Health needs and the transition	362
Getting care right in practice	362
Reasonable care adjustments	362
Hospital passport	362
Protocols to improve care outcomes	362
The learning (intellectual) disability protocol for preparation for theatre and recovery	364
Getting communication right	364
Pictures say more than words	364
Books beyond words	364
Tips to getting it right	364
Conclusion	365
Useful websites	365
References	365

The Great Ormond Street Hospital Manual of Children and Young People's Nursing Practices, Second Edition. Edited by Elizabeth Anne Bruce, Janet Williss, and Faith Gibson.
© 2023 John Wiley & Sons Ltd. Published 2023 by John Wiley & Sons Ltd.

Introduction

For children and young people (CYPs) with learning disabilities, coming into hospital can seem like a whirlpool of white noise and bright lights, where the route to travel along is not clear. This often makes them very agitated, anxious, distressed, and frightened, which in turn makes their behaviour become more difficult for clinicians to interpret. Health professionals may experience higher levels of anxiety and uncertainty regarding how to assess, treat, and ensure that safe, reasonable care is provided for CYPs with a learning disability. The purpose of this chapter is to assist health professionals to 'get it right'; providing information regarding solutions such as the hospital passport, reasonable adjustments, and alerts used in primary care, hospitals, emergency departments, and other specialist health services.

In 2015, there were about 1.1 million people with learning disabilities in England, including 160 000 CYPs aged under 17 (Public Health England 2016). These individuals and their families often require additional adjustments to their care and in the way things are communicated to them, so that they can understand what is happening when in contact with health services. Parents/carers with a learning (intellectual) disability may need to have their ability to consent to treatment for their child assessed in accordance with the Mental Capacity Act. This issue is highlighted within this chapter in relation to assessing a person's capacity. The practical solutions highlighted in this chapter can be adapted and adopted to aid any CYP, with or without disabilities, or with autism, mental health issues, or other specific health requirements.

A core element flowing through this chapter is that everybody's life has worth and each human being has abilities that need to be acknowledged and celebrated for what they are. Health professionals often struggle to accept or interpret what a person is saying to them or to change their (the professionals) communication methods to enhance understanding of the person's needs. As a result, health needs may not be adequately met. It is also common for professionals to misinterpret a person's behaviour as being part of their disability, rather than exploring a health reason for a behaviour change (Gates and Barr 2009).

Positive values, attitudes, and principles are integral to good service planning, delivery, and outcomes, since these form the bedrock of care and should be infused within the behaviour of every person who provides a service within a health setting.

Principles underpinning practice

A central principle that should underpin practice is the active understanding that parents/carers and CYPs with learning disabilities are experts by their lived experience. In order to get care right, it is essential that they are fully engaged in the planning, design, delivery, and teaching of staff in how to provide services that effectively meet required needs in a tailored way. These principles can apply to any healthcare worker (HCW) or patient interaction, but are particularly important for those with learning disabilities and are outlined below:

1. **Value driven:** CYPs can contribute to their care.
2. **Positive communication:** Increase the use of positive terminology and place an emphasis on appropriate communication.
3. **Appreciate the interaction:** Between the individual and their environment; understand the CYP's life experiences and how they express themselves.
4. **Increase independence:** While acknowledging the stage or age of a CYP, it is important to focus on developing their independence.
5. **Promote emotional literacy:** Ensure that CYPs have opportunities to express themselves and help and support them to understand their own feelings.
6. **Create a positive environment:** Create a welcoming setting – It is important to acknowledge each CYP's individuality, culture, and life experience so that they are valued and important members of the hospital community.
7. **Focus on individual support:** Each person is an individual and will respond to being positively addressed by their name and by having their individual needs considered, rather than merely those of a group.
8. **Work toward achievable goals:** Set goals that motivate and are achievable within a timescale that is reasonable for that CYP and for the service they are using. HCWs need to see those who use their services as allies to work with and alongside to ensure improvements are continually made where needed.

Families as allies

When caring for CYPs with learning disabilities, positive engagement with the family is essential. Parents and families are at times labelled as being difficult, which is often highly inappropriate. Families of CYPs with learning (intellectual) disabilities face multiple daily challenges and very difficult situations that can often feel like a 24-hour struggle with a system that pays lip service to valuing their expertise in loving and supporting their CYP. All staff must remember that parents and families are constantly their best allies in ensuring safe, effective, timely care and outcomes for their children, who often have complex multiple needs.

What is a learning (intellectual) disability?

The Department of Health (DH) (2001) defines a learning disability as; *'A significantly reduced ability to understand new or complex information, to learn new skills (impaired intelligence) with: a reduced ability to cope independently (impaired social functioning) which started before adulthood, with a lasting effect on development'* (DH 2001, p. 14).

Having a learning (intellectual) disability can also affect a person's behaviour, particularly if they struggle to communicate or get their needs and wishes met in more conventional ways.

There are three core criteria that must be met for the term learning (*intellectual*) *disability* to apply:

- Significant impairment of intellectual function.
- Significant impairment of adaptive and or social function (ability to cope on a day-to-day basis with the demands of his/her environment and the expectations of age and culture).
- Age of onset before adulthood.

How do you know if someone has a learning (intellectual) disability?

If they:

- Have been diagnosed as having a learning disability by an appropriately qualified health professional, e.g. paediatrician, psychiatrist, clinical psychologist.
- Have an IQ lower than 70.

This will mean they are likely to:

- Be unable to read, write, interpret, and process new information to the expected level for their age.
- Find recalling information very difficult.
- Find it hard to maintain their own self-care.
- Need significant assistance to carry out their daily lives.

What is *not* a learning (intellectual) disability?

- The development of cognitive, adaptive, or social impairments after 18 years of age.
- Acquired brain inquiry after the age of 18.
- Complex medical conditions that affect intellectual and social/adaptive functioning, e.g. dementia.
- Specific learning difficulties: e.g. literacy or numeracy problems, dyslexia, or delayed language and speech development.
- Dyspraxia – developmental coordination disorder.
- Attention deficit disorder.
- Attention deficit hyperactive disorder.
- Asperger's syndrome.
- Challenging behaviour.
- Physical impairment.
- Sensory impairment.

The label 'learning difficulties' is frequently used in educational settings to portray people with specific learning problems, but this does not denote that a person has a learning disability as defined here.

When giving families a diagnosis, always be mindful that it is life changing and future altering information, which is neither good nor bad, as you do not know how the person in front of you will take the news. It is important to be aware of how they may react and be in a position to link them into organisations and support structures that may be able to assist them in their coming to terms with their changing circumstances (Ainsworth and Blair 2018).

The need for change in services and practice

The past 10 years has witnessed a number of episodes in the United Kingdom where care has been very poor for people with learning disabilities and the services they receive unequal to those members of society without a learning (intellectual) disability. In 2012 Mencap published 'Death by Indifference: 74 Deaths and Counting'; which is a stark reminder of the effect healthcare inequalities continue to have on people with learning disabilities. Mencap (2012) highlighted constant failings, such as ignoring vital advice from families and an inability of staff to meet basic care needs. Diagnostic overshadowing has led to untimely deaths. In 2013 the Confidential Inquiry into the Premature Deaths of People with Learning Disabilities (CIPOLD) found the most common reasons for deaths being viewed as premature were delays or problems with diagnosis or treatment and difficulties identifying needs and providing appropriate care in response to altering needs (Heslop et al. 2013). In addition, CIPOLD highlighted that a lack of reasonable adjustments to facilitate healthcare of people with learning disabilities, particularly when accessing clinics for appointments and investigations, was a contributory factor in a number of the deaths they investigated. Key issues arising from this in relation to clinical risk is the lack of coordination of care across sectors and between the varying disease pathways and service providers, and the single episodic nature of care provision (Heslop et al. 2013). A lack of clarity between services can lead to fragmented pictures of a person and their quality of life, which may cloud clinical decision making. This is a core component behind the work that is being undertaken within GOSH and discussed within this chapter.

Challenges health professionals face when working with people with learning (intellectual) disabilities

CYPs and adults with learning disabilities may present with a range of difficulties, including:

- Expressing their needs and communicating their choices.
- Comprehending their diagnosis, treatment options, or the services available to them.
- Interpreting the consequences that their decisions can have on their health status.
- Adapting to a hospital environment and what is expected of them within hospital.
- Behaving in unpredictable ways and in a manner that would be considered unusual for CYPs without a learning (intellectual) disability.

Each of these will prove problematic for HCWs seeking to engage with and care for the these CYPs and their families. It is vital that all health professionals effectively engage with and involve the CYP with learning (intellectual) disabilities and their families/carers to identify how they can best interact, understand and support them while they are under their care. This chapter offers some suggestions for such engagement.

See the person and understand behaviour that challenges

It is essential to explore behind every behaviour change or increase in existing behaviour, whether or not there is a health cause. Challenging behaviour is a term that is frequently used and has many interpretations. It was coined to remove the many other problematic terms that placed the person as 'difficult'. Challenging behaviour focuses on the understanding; 'this person presents us with a challenge in how to support him/her' as opposed to 'this person is being difficult'. As with many terms, challenging behaviour has been misused to mean 'this person has challenging behaviour'. A return to the original meaning is necessary and advocated for by the Challenging Behaviour Foundation (https://www.challengingbehaviour.org.uk/).

A helpful and widely accepted definition is:

Behaviour can be described as challenging when it is of such an intensity, frequency, or duration as to threaten the quality of life and/or the physical safety of the individual or others and it is likely to lead to responses that are restrictive, aversive, or result in exclusion.
(Royal College of Psychiatrists, British Psychological Society, Royal College of Speech and Language Therapists 2007, p. 14)

Many challenging behaviours are effective methods for a person with a learning (intellectual) disability to control what is going on around them and to express what is happening to them. Numerous unmet health needs are often behind the behaviours, and these need to be considered when exploring why someone is behaving in a certain way.

Behaviours might include:

- Hurting others (e.g. hair pulling, hitting, head-butting).
- Self-injury (e.g. head banging, eye poking, hand biting).
- Destructive behaviours (e.g. throwing things, breaking furniture, tearing things up).
- Eating inedible objects (e.g. cigarette butts, pen lids, bedding).
- Other behaviours (e.g. spitting, smearing, repetitive rocking, stripping off clothes, running away).

(From the Challenging Behaviour Foundation http://www.challengingbehaviour.org.uk/about-us/about-challenging-behaviour/what-is-challenging-behaviour.html)

The CYP who presents with such behaviours is not difficult; the challenge is for HCWs to explore what is happening for, to, and with the individual, especially if there is a health issue behind the behaviour, pain, distress, and / or anxiety. Yet commonly health professionals put challenging behaviours down to the person's disability without finding out more about why the person is doing this. This is known as diagnostic overshadowing.

Diagnostic overshadowing

The term *diagnostic overshadowing* refers to a very significant problem when health professionals see the disability and not the person and attribute existing or new behaviours to the learning disability, rather than exploring what health problems may lie behind them (Gates and Barr 2009). This can lead to a delay in investigating and treating a person in an effective and timely manner, which can lead to poor health outcomes and in some cases result in avoidable deaths (Heslop et al. 2013). It is always essential to see beyond a diagnosis and explore a health reason behind any new behaviours or increase in existing behaviour, especially if the individual has a severe learning disability with limited verbal language (Blair 2017a, b).

A key way to reduce the likelihood of diagnostic overshadowing from occurring is to use tools such as the DisDAT tool (Northumberland Tyne and Wear NHS Trust and St. Oswald's Hospice 2006).

Assessing pain and distress – disability distress assessment tool (DisDAT)

Being able to clearly identify when someone is in distress or pain can be difficult to assess. The DisDAT tool was created in Northgate Hospital by a combined learning disability and palliative care team to assess distress in people with severe communication difficulties.

Distress signs and behaviours are not always linked to a specific cause and every CYP has their own repertoire of behaviours and distress signs. The DisDAT tool is useful in identifying distress accurately and carers find it easy to use.

How the DisDAT tool can be used

The DisDAT tool can be used to create a baseline profile of a person and will then serve as an aid to HCWs' understanding of the person when they meet. The tool illustrates how a person behaves when they are content or distressed and involves the following aspects; the person's appearance: vocal signs, habits and mannerisms, postures and observations, known triggers of distress, skin appearance, speech, facial signs, jaw movements, appearance of eyes, and ability to communicate.

To use the tool:

- Observe the individual when content and when distressed – document this on the inside pages of DisDAT. Anyone who cares for the patient can do this.
- Observe the context in which distress is occurring.
- Identify possible causes of distress. Use the clinical decision distress checklist on the back page of DisDAT to help you.
- Use the monitoring sheets if the cause is not obvious. Sometimes the cause of distress only becomes clear by monitoring daily (or even hourly for 24 hours) to show a pattern of distress.
- Pick whichever set of monitoring sheets make most sense to the situation you are in.
- Treat or manage the likeliest cause of the distress.
- Monitor the distress: if necessary, use the monitoring sheets to see how the distress changes over time.
- What then? If the distress resolves, the process stops. If not, you start an intervention for the second possible cause of distress.
- The goal is a reduction in the number or severity of distress signs and behaviours.

https://www.stoswaldsuk.org/how-we-help/we-educate/education/resources/disability-distress-assessment-tool-disdat/

What is behind the change in or new behaviour?

Gaining a clearer picture of new or unusual behaviour is essential. Table 16.1 illustrates the types of issues and concerns that should be considered; this can greatly enhance understanding and subsequent action.

One pain tool that has been validated to assess pain in CYPs with learning and communication difficulties is the revised FLACC (Malviya et al. 2006), which can be used alongside other tools (see Chapter 24: Pain Management). It is always important to understand that someone may present pain in unusual ways, such as curling up into a foetal position, becoming increasingly quiet and withdrawn, and not engaging in activities they usually enjoy. It is important to notice these behaviours and recognise them as possible signs of pain and treat accordingly. In the following example, Lauretta illustrates how her four-year-old, learning-disabled, autistic son, Otito, appears to express pain in 'atypical' ways. Here she discusses experiences with Otito when he was in hospital with pancreatitis (Blair et al. 2017a).

Table 16.1 Possible causes of changes in behaviour

Behaviour/Characteristics	Possible causes to consider
• Repeated rapidly?	• Pleuritic pain (in time with breathing) • Colic (comes and goes every few minutes) • Repetitive movement due to boredom or fear
• Associated with breathing?	• Infection, chronic obstructive pulmonary disease (COPD), pleural effusion, tumour
• Worsened or precipitated by movement?	• Movement-related pains
• Related to eating?	• Food refusal through illness, fear, or depression • Food refusal because of swallowing problems • Upper GI problems (oral hygiene, peptic ulcer, dyspepsia) or abdominal problems
• Related to a specific situation?	• Frightening or painful situations
• Associated with vomiting?	• Causes of nausea and vomiting
• Associated with elimination (urine or faecal)?	• Urinary problems (infection, retention) • GI problems (diarrhoea, constipation)
• Present in a normally comfortable position or situation?	• Anxiety, depression, pain at rest (e.g. colic, neuralgia), infection, nausea

Source: Northumberland Tyne and Wear NHS Trust and St. Oswald's Hospice (2006).

"The pain charts recorded higher scores for pain based on normal responses. For example, screaming, being irritable, and displaying active movements, especially kicking to show pain was ranked highly. They could not justify the need to give the level of pain relief I was requesting since the pain scores they charted did not support my claim. However, given his status as a severely autistic child with learning disabilities it was really not far-fetched. As time went by my son became very withdrawn. While what the health professionals saw was more of a quiet boy, what I saw was less of my child and more of a chronic patient. To them his quietness was only a confirmation that he was after all unwell.

The new pain document accommodated my son's unique responses to pain. Things that were previously being overlooked (like being quiet, curling up in a foetal position, not moving around, staying in corners, grinding his teeth, closing his eyes even while awake, interacting less with people or toys, etc.) were not only taken into account but in fact given higher scores using the new pain score sheet. It helped the doctors understand my son better. By using this new pain score sheet they could also justify the need for a higher level of pain relief (something that was also an important requirement for dispensing them)" (Blair et al. 2017a).

A person may present with behaviour that is challenging due to their being in pain. About 50% of people with a learning (intellectual) disability and challenging behaviour are subject to physical interventions such as restraint (see Chapter 19: Moving and Handling). Positive behavioural approaches can be helpful in reducing restrictive practices. For more information see the British Institute of Learning Disabilities website (http://www.bild.org.uk/our-services/positive-behaviour-support).

Positive behaviour support reducing the use of restrictive practices

Positive behaviour support (PBS) approaches are established as the preferred method when working with people with learning disabilities of all ages who demonstrate behaviours described as challenging. A key aspect to PBS is that of assisting an individual to develop personal relationships, improve their health, become more active within their lives and communities, and to develop personally. PBS plans should be written following detailed assessments; aspects that the individual finds challenging are then highlighted and addressed. A variety of techniques that aid distraction, diversion, and at times disengagement, can be incorporated into the plan. These should be used by carers/staff when a person starts to become anxious, aroused, or distressed (DH 2014). There are also quality of life improvements for the individual, both as an intervention and as an outcome measure. This way of thinking inherently concerns itself with reducing restrictive practices which do not just involve restraint but also any practices that limit freedom of choice (http://www.bild.org.uk/our-services/positive-behaviour-support).

Improving care reducing restrictive practices
The following are key examples of practices that reduce the need for restrictions in caring for CYPs with learning disabilities:

- 'Staff must not deliberately restrain people in a way that impacts on their airway, breathing, or circulation, such as face down restraint on any surface, not just on the floor.
- If restrictive intervention is used it must not include the deliberate application of pain.
- If a restrictive intervention has to be used, it must always represent the least restrictive option to meet the immediate need.
- Staff must not use seclusion other than for people detained under the Mental Health Act 1983.
- People who use services, families, and carers must be involved in planning, reviewing, and evaluating all aspects of care and support.
- Individualised support plans, incorporating behaviour support plans, must be implemented for all people who use services who are known to be at risk of being exposed to restrictive interventions'.

(*Source:* DH 2014, p. 10)

Becoming an adult: All change

Throughout life, transitions take place; possibly the most difficult and challenging changes for families and young people with learning (intellectual) disabilities are those experienced when becoming an adult and moving from children's to adults' services. Entering the world of adult services happens at around the age of 18 but planning should begin around 13 years of age. Every parent wants their child to have a fulfilling life as an adult, but the future may seem uncertain to a young person after the familiarity of local children's health services and hospitals (The Foundation for People with Learning Disabilities 2014). A further factor is the feeling that families are no longer in control or able to consent on behalf of their child, and this can enhance the feelings of anxiety that are frequently experienced during this tumultuous period.

Making decisions: Consent to treatment

From the age of 16 (or younger if assessed as Gillick competent), a young person has the right to provide consent to their own treatment. If they are unable to do so, this is done by the parent, carer or other person with parental responsibility. It is important to remember that parents may have a learning disability themselves and may lack the capacity to consent on behalf of their child, or understand what is happening to them. At such times, the Mental Capacity Act applies, and an assessment of their capacity should be undertaken in accordance with the Act (HM Government 2005).

It is essential to remember that each decision is time, location, and decision specific. Just because a person may lack capacity at one time about one particular decision, it does not mean that they lack capacity in other areas or aspects of their life (Blair 2013). A variety of communication methods, such as signs, photos, videos, music, and "books beyond words" (www.booksbeyondwords.co.uk), should be used to and ascertain a clearer picture of a person's understanding. These tools will assist health professionals to get care right. For further information on consent see section 7 in the Introduction of this book.

If the capacity of an individual over the age of 18 is in question, clinicians need to carry out a four-point capacity test.

Is the person able to:

- Understand the information relevant to the decision?
- Retain the information long enough to make the decision?
- Use or weigh up the information?
- Communicate their decision?

If the person lacks capacity the HCW must:

- Consider delaying the decision if the person may regain capacity.
- Act in the best interests of the person.
- Consider holding a Best Interest meeting under the Mental Capacity Act (HM Government 2005).
- Always use the less restrictive option.
- Encourage participation in the decision.

- Consult all relevant people.
- If the person has no relatives consider a referral to the Independent Mental Capacity Advocate Service (IMCA).

Health needs and the transition

A young person's health needs are a central factor within the transition to adulthood. As with other areas, such as social care and education, there needs to be a health transition plan to support them, and this should link in with other plans that they are being supported to make during the transition stage. Until the age of 18 the young person with learning (intellectual) disabilities is likely to be under the care of a community paediatrician or child development team, who coordinates care. Once the young person becomes 18, this ceases and it can be difficult to find a health professional who will continue to coordinate care, although the GP will provide some continuity, often in partnership with the Community Learning Disability Nurses from the local Community Learning Disability Team. GPs are currently expected to undertake annual health checks on adults with learning disabilities who are known to social services; this is being extended to young people from the age of 14. These are essential in ensuring that people with learning (intellectual) disabilities have their health and well-being needs identified and a plan of how to address them activated to enhance their health outcomes (Figure 16.1).

Getting care right in practice

This section examines how services can organise their systems, structures, and working practices to embed improvements in care provision, including making reasonable adjustments and the use of the hospital passport (see Figure 16.1). Areas to focus on include:

- **Beware of missing serious illness:** Do not ignore medical symptoms by seeing them as part of the person's disability. ACT QUICKLY.
- **Find the best way to communicate:** With the person, their families, carers, and friends. Not everyone speaks – use photos, signs, symbols, and pictures alongside speech.
- **Read and act on the hospital passport:** It provides vital information about a person's needs.
- **Make reasonable care adjustments:** To minimise waiting; adapting the environment, e.g. dimmer switches to reduce impact of bright lights, quieter place to be seen.
- **Clinical alerts – Making sure adjustments can be made:** Identifying those with a learning (intellectual) disability in advance of them coming to hospital is essential; this will ensure that their needs are identified and a plan of care can be developed. This will enable staff to get it right for them and improve their experience and health outcomes. In addition, reports can be generated that enable the hospital to identify patients a learning (intellectual) disability and enables them to audit whether adjustments to care were effectively in place.

Reasonable care adjustments

Reasonable adjustments to care are a legal requirement under the Equality Act (HM Government 2010) and must be provided to ensure equal treatment for all. Equal treatment does not mean treatment should be the same, but necessary additions need to be in place to ensure that everyone is able to access the services they need. For example, all staff should offer people with learning (intellectual) disabilities:

- The first or last appointment when attending an outpatient appointment.
- A double appointment, so there is more time to enable participation in the consultation.
- A hospital passport to facilitate communication.
- Accessible information by using a communication book, photographs, signs, symbols, and jargon-free language.
- Changes to the environment, e.g. altering lighting, seeking quieter places, calmer waiting/clinic areas.
- Involve the CYPs and their families/ carers in the decision making process around care, treatment, and discharge home.

A TEACH approach to implementing reasonable adjustments is helpful, as first created by the Hertfordshire Community Learning Disability Team:

T = Time: Take time to work with the person.
E = Environment: Alter the environment, e.g. quieter areas, reducing lighting and waiting.
A = Attitude: Have a positive solution focus.
C = Communication: How does the person communicate; share the information with colleagues.
H = Help: What help is needed for the person and for colleagues to get care right.

Hospital passports play a core role in ensuring safe effective care that is tailored to the individual can be delivered in a timely manner. These along with other examples such as the creation of specific focused protocols should ensure better outcomes and experiences for all involved.

Hospital passport

Hospital passports (also called health passports, my health) play a core role in ensuring safe, effective care that is tailored to the individual can be delivered in a timely manner. They contain vital information that will enhance the quality of health interactions, diagnosis, and outcomes. They are completed by the person or their family prior to admission or attendance at a clinic and can greatly enhance the outcome and the proposed plan for treatment because of the depth of detail contained within them (see Figure 16.1). However, they do require health professionals to know about them and to ask for them of every person who has a learning disability.

A great many other individuals with a range of disabilities and health conditions can benefit from the use of a hospital passport, since they enable health professionals to know and understand the person behind the health problem. Passports can come in a variety of formats, such as video or photographs, however, there is no one that fits all. They may be called health passports, my health and a variety of other names, but they all provide vital information that will enhance the quality of health interactions, diagnosis, and outcomes.

Protocols to improve care outcomes

Protocols can provide clear structural guidance for staff to help them traverse difficult or challenging situations in a clear, easy manner. They should be created from learning from past experiences, trialled, and formerly agreed on. In general, protocols should be applicable to all, but there are times when they necessarily need to be specific to certain individuals to reduce clinical risk and ensure safety. One such example is in operation at Great Ormond Street Hospital to improve perioperative care, which is described below (see also Figure 16.2).

Chapter 16 Learning (intellectual) disabilities

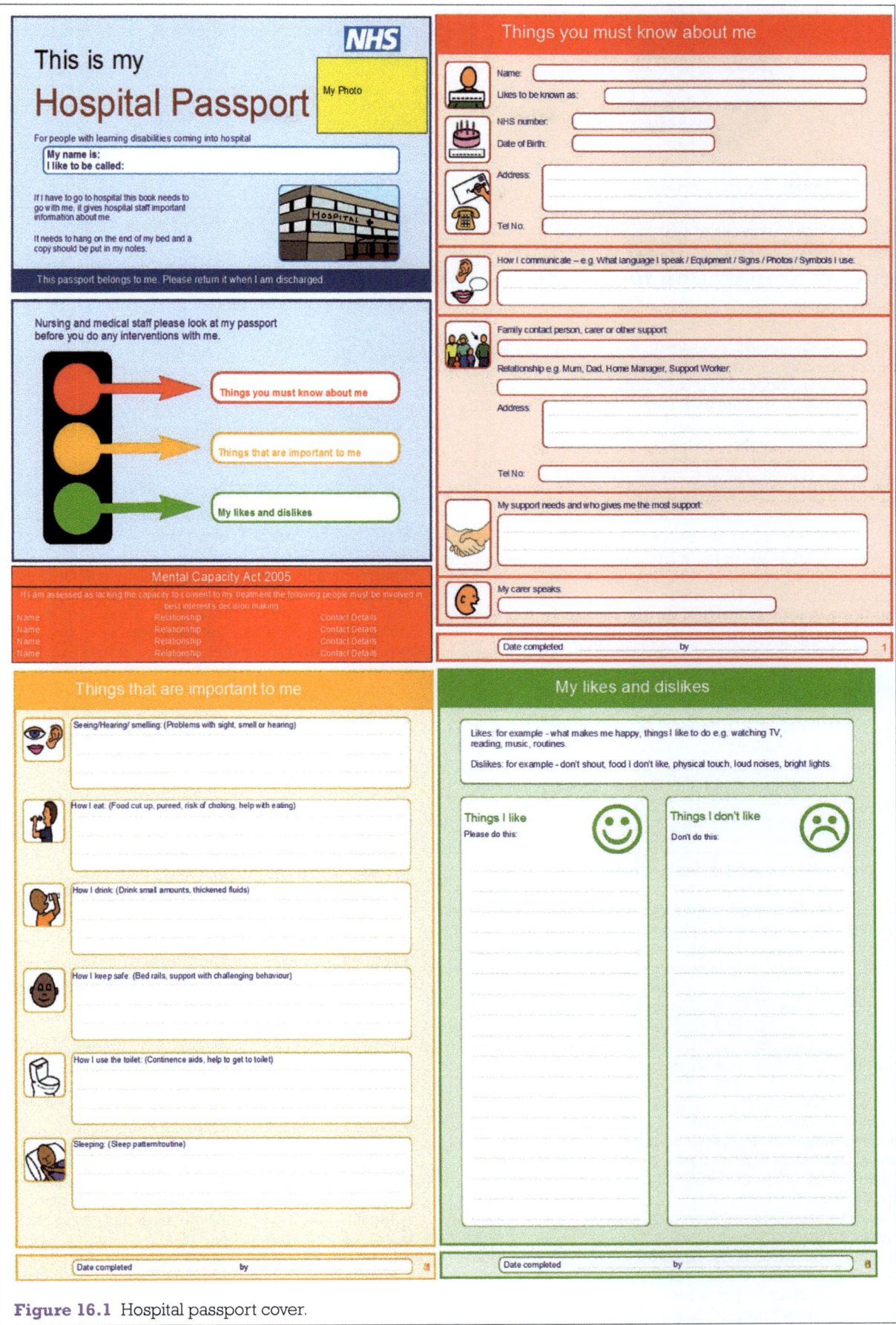

Figure 16.1 Hospital passport cover.

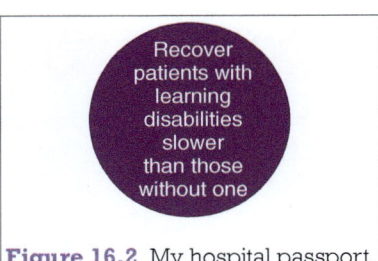

Figure 16.2 My hospital passport.

The learning (intellectual) disability protocol for preparation for theatre and recovery

This protocol was developed in order to improve the experience, safety, and outcomes for CYPs with learning (intellectual) disabilities and their families. It provides a clear structure to ensure the safest and best outcome for the patient and their families as well as the staff.

- Discuss the patient's needs with them and their family/carers.
- Use 'comforters' to relax the patient during pre op and in recovery.
- Document and handover to colleagues.
- Lower levels of noise and light.
- Place the patient in a quiet area within recovery.
- Ensure parents/carers are present and involved.
- Gradually recover observing how the patient is progressing and ensuring pain has been reviewed.

If the patient is still disturbed or distressed in Recovery, please then consider:

a Call an anaesthetist to use sedation to induce a relaxed, sleepier state.
b Increase levels of sedation as required.

The brevity and clarity of this protocol is ensuring it's efficacy in reducing difficult and challenging, as well as distressing situations, which can lead to unsafe practice with poor outcomes. For more information about the impact of the theatre protocol see (Blair et al. 2017d).

Getting communication right

Words and being able to read are key parts of communication, yet not everyone uses these as methods of communicating with or interpreting the world around them. It is vital that health professionals think differently and act creatively when seeking to communicate and interact with CYPs with learning (intellectual) disabilities and their families/carers. The key to successful communication is to always involve the CYP directly in their care as well as involving their families/carers. Getting communication right is not easy and what works with one person will not necessarily work with all.

Modify your language
- Keep language short and simple.
- Say what you mean and mean what you say.
- Avoid or explain irony, sarcasm, jokes, metaphors.
- Be positive – avoid 'no' and 'don't' and say what you want, not what you don't want.
- Say your name first.
- Speak in the correct order.
- Give time for processing of information.
- Be explicit – avoid inferred and implied concepts.
- Use concrete, not abstract concepts.
- Look for and interpret nonverbal communication and be aware of your own.
- Listen to and involve the family/carers.
- Take more time; this will save time in the long run as key information will be acquired.
- Be aware that the ability to talk does not mean someone understands.
- Rely less on body language and intonation and more on visual information.
- Jargon-free language.

Pictures say more than words

Be creative, communicate differently, and be guided by the individual with a learning (intellectual) disability and those who know them well. Consider using:

- Photographs
- Pictures
- Signs
- Drawings
- Symbols
- Music
- Videos

Books beyond words

Communicating as fully as possible with a disabled CYP can sometimes seem quite daunting. Books Beyond Words are stories told in pictures that help the reader, including readers who understand pictures better than words, to explore a situation or experience and share their understanding with you, the observer, or supporter.

Books Beyond Words stories have no words in them, so they work well regardless of the language spoken by the CYP or supporter. They include stories about going into hospital and a range of investigations as well as some specific conditions such as epilepsy, diabetes, and heart problems. Go to www.booksbeyondwords.co.uk.

Tips to getting it right

- People with learning (intellectual) disabilities, their families, and carers are likely to be exhausted, scared, and worried – slow down what you are doing.
- Be relaxed, calm, clear, kind.
- Use jargon-free words.
- Working collaboratively with the person, their family, and carers ensures the outcomes are better.

Every person is an individual and unique. Each interaction and contact has to count. Health professionals do need to think differently and act creatively together with the CYP with a learning disability and their families. In order to get care right, health professionals need to:

Dedicate time to being with the person with a learning disability and their families to tune into their lived experiences.
Take a whole person approach, not just looking at the diagnosis.
Tap into how the person with a learning disability communicates, interacts, and usually is.
Listen to parents and other people who love the CYP.
Invest time and energy, not just for the moment, but for the future as well.
Pick up on what is and is not said and avoid hurrying the interaction (Blair et al. 2016).

Conclusion

Small changes lead to big changes. This chapter has highlighted the need and shown from examples how HCWs and services need to think differently and act creatively to meet the requirements of CYPs with learning (intellectual) disabilities and their families. The central message is to look, listen, engage, value, and act on what people with learning (intellectual) disabilities and their families have to share in order to ensure effective, safe, and lawful health outcomes can happen.

Individuals with learning (intellectual) disabilities and their families are the experts and it is vital that they are involved in planning, designing, and evaluating services, as well as educating health professionals about their needs in order for services to improve and for better lives to prevail. If services get it right for people with learning (intellectual) disabilities, it will be very much better for all.

Useful websites

https://www.bild.org.uk
British Institute of Learning Disabilities services help develop the organisations who provide services, and the people who give support.

https://www.booksbeyondwords.co.uk
Stories in pictures to help people with learning and communication disabilities explore and understand their own experiences.

https://www.challengingbehaviour.org.uk
Charity for people with severe learning disabilities whose behaviour challenges.

https://www.easyhealth.org.uk
Accessible health information.

https://www.gosh.nhs.uk/your-hospital-visit/before-you-come-gosh/if-your-child-has-additional-needs/children-and-young-people-learning-disabilities/
Information for CYPs with learning disabilities, families, and staff on what is provided at GOSH.

www.intellectualdisability.info
Health information for health professionals about people with learning disabilities.

https://www.learningdisabilities.org.uk
Foundation for People with Learning Disabilities provides information about issues affecting the lives of people with learning disabilities, publications, workshops, conferences, and funds research and service.

https://www.mencap.org.uk/gettingitright
Getting it right when treating people with a learning disability.

References

Ainsworth, V. and Blair, J. (2018). *Ten rules for delivering a diagnosis of autism or intellectual disabilities in a way that ensures lasting emotional damage . . . and maybe what to do about it*. Pavilion Publishing.

Blair, J. (2013). Everybody's life has worth – getting it right in hospital for people with an intellectual disability and reducing clinical risks. *Clinical Risk* 19: 58–63.

Blair, J. (2017a). Diagnostic overshadowing: see beyond the diagnosis. *British Journal of Family Medicine* 17: 34–35.

Blair, J. (2017b). What you see isn't all there is . . . Understanding people with learning disabilities and health issues. Care Talk, 62 (June 17): 12.

Blair, J., Bush, M., Goleniowska, H. et al. (2016). Through our eyes: what parents want for their children from health professionals.' Chapter 18. In: *Supporting the Physical Health Needs of People with Learning Disabilities* (eds. S. Hardy, E. Chaplin and P. Woodward), 197–212. Pavilion Press.

Blair, J., Anthony, T., Gunther, I. et al. (2017d). A protocol for the preparation of patients for theatre and recovery. *Learning Disability Practice* 20 (2): 22–26.

Blair, J., Busk, M., Hawtrey-Woore, S. et al. (2017c). Refocusing: what you see isn't all there is – getting healthcare right in hospitals for autistic and learning disabled people. In: *Autism and Intellectual Disability in Adults*, vol. 2 (eds. D. Milton and N. Martin). Pavilion Publishing. https://www.herts.ac.uk/intellectualdisability/how-to-guides/articles/refocusing-what-you-see-isnt-all-there-is-getting-healthcare-right-in-hospitals-for-autistic-and-learning-disabled-people (accessed 13 August 2022).

Department of Health (DH) (2001). *Valuing people*. London: HMSO.

Department of Health (DH) (2014). Positive and Proactive Care: reducing the need for restrictive interventions. London: HMSO. https://assets.publishing.service.gov.uk/government/uploads/system/uploads/attachment_data/file/300293/JRA_DoH_Guidance_on_RP_web_accessible.pdf (accessed 13 August 2022).

The Foundation for People with Learning Disabilities (2014) Children and young people with complex health needs: a one-stop booklet for families. https://www.learningdisabilities.org.uk/cy/node/2000 (accessed 13 August 2022).

Gates, B. and Barr, O. (2009). *Learning and Intellectual Disability Nursing*. Oxford: Oxford University Press.

Heslop, P., Blair, P., Fleming, P., Houghton, M., Marriott, A., & Russ, L. (2013). Confidential enquiry into premature deaths of people with learning disabilities (CIPOLD). Bristol University, Norah Fry Research Centre. https://www.bristol.ac.uk/cipold/ (accessed 13 August 2022).

HM Government (2010). Equality Act 2010. https://www.legislation.gov.uk/ukpga/2010/15/contents (accessed 13 August 2022).

HM Government (2005). Mental Capacity Act 2005. www.legislation.gov.uk/ukpga/2005/9/contents (accessed 13 August 2022).

Malviya, S., Vopel-Lewis, T.B., Merkel, S., and Tait, A.R. (2006). The revised FLACC observational pain tool: improved reliability and validity for pain assessment in children with cognitive impairment. *Pediatric Anesthesia* 16: 258–265.

Mencap (2012). *Death by Indifference: 74 Deaths and Counting*. London: Mencap.

Northumberland Tyne & Wear NHS Trust and St. Oswald's Hospice (2006). DisDAT Disability Distress Assessment Tool. https://www.stoswaldsuk.org/how-we-help/we-educate/education/resources/disability-distress-assessment-tool-disdat/ (accessed 13 August 2022).

Public Health England (2016). Learning Disabilities Observatory People with learning disabilities in England 2015: Main report. https://www.gov.uk/government/publications/people-with-learning-disabilities-in-england-2015 (accessed 13 August 2022).

Royal College of Psychiatrists, British Psychological Society, Royal College of Speech and Language Therapists (2007). *Challenging behaviour – a unified approach*. Clinical and service guidelines for supporting people with learning disabilities who are at risk of receiving abusive or restrictive practices, p.14. https://www.rcpsych.ac.uk/improving-care/campaigning-for-better-mental-health-policy/college-reports/2005-07-college-reports (accessed 13 August 2022).

# Chapter 17

Administration of medicines

Jacqueline Robinson-Rouse[1], Mandy Matthews[2], Emily Baker[3], and Bhumik Patel[4]

[1]RN (Child), BSc (Hon), MSc, Formerly Lead Nurse, Nursing Workforce, Great Ormond Street Hospital, London, UK
[2]RN (Adult), RN (Child), PGDip in Learning and Teaching for Professional Practice, Formerly Head of International Practice Development, GOSH
[3]Dip (He) Nursing Child Branch, BSc (Hons) Children's Cancer Nursing, MA Practice Education, Senior Clinical Research Nurse Haematology/Oncology, GOSH
[4]MPharm, MSc, PGCert; Senior Specialist Pharmacist in Paediatric Palliative Care, GOSH

Chapter contents

Section 1: General principles	368
Introduction	368
Child development considerations	370
Checking the medicine prescription	370
Drug calculations	370
Section 2: Routes of administration	371
Oral	371
Enteral via a tube or device	372
Buccal	372
Sublingual	373
Intranasal	374
Inhalation	374
Rectal	375
Intradermal (ID), subcutaneous (SC), and intramuscular (IM)	376
Intradermal	377
Subcutaneous	377
Intramuscular	378
Intravenous	380
Intraosseous	380
Intrathecal	380
Epidural	381
Transdermal (skin patches)	381
References	402

Procedure guidelines

17.1 Oral medication administration	384
17.2 Enteral tube administration	384
17.3 Buccal and sublingual administration	386
17.4 Intranasal administration	387
17.5 Inhalation administration	388
17.6 Rectal administration	390
17.7 Preparation of medication for injections using an aseptic nontouch technique	392
17.8 Intradermal (ID) administration	393
17.9 Subcutaneous (SC) administration	394
17.10 Intramuscular (IM) administration	396
17.11 Intraosseous administration	398
17.12 Intrathecal administration	398
17.13 Skin patch administration	402

Principles table

17.1 General guidelines	382

The Great Ormond Street Hospital Manual of Children and Young People's Nursing Practices, Second Edition. Edited by Elizabeth Anne Bruce, Janet Williss, and Faith Gibson.
© 2023 John Wiley & Sons Ltd. Published 2023 by John Wiley & Sons Ltd.

Section 1: General principles

Introduction

A key component of many healthcare treatments for children and young people (CYPs) involves the prescription and administration of pharmaceutical products. Medication administration in contemporary healthcare is a dynamic and complex process. Professional competencies, theoretical knowledge, critical reflection, use of advanced technologies and the ability to engage CYPs in participation are required by the registered practitioner to ensure medication is administered safely.

Administration of medication is part of everyday nursing practice and there is potential for error every time this occurs. Medication administration errors are among the most common errors reported in healthcare environments, the consequences of which can be serious or even fatal (NHS England (2022b). NHS England (formerly NHS Improvement) also issues specific alerts and guidance promoting the safe use of medicines, to rapidly provide guidance to healthcare systems on preventing potential incidents that may lead to harm or death (NHS England 2022a). NPSA issued several specific alerts and guidance promoting the safe use of medicines between 2007 and 2012. These included guidance promoting the safety of oral and injectable medicines (NPSA 2007a, b), reducing risks associated with the administration of heparin (NPSA 2008), oxygen (NPSA 2009), loading doses (NPSA 2010a), insulin (NPSA 2010b; NHS Improvement 2018), and buccal midazolam (MHRA 2014), as well as safety alerts and guidance regarding the safe use of equipment and intravenous (IV) fluids involved in medicine administration (NPSA 2010c, 2011a, b, c). Monthly reports of 'never events' are now made available on the NHS England website as part of their commitment to be open and transparent about patient safety incident reporting (NHS England 2022).

Nurses, in line with all registered practitioners, are professionally responsible for their actions and must ensure that they act in the best interests of the patient at all times (NMC 2015). When administering medicines, nurses must exercise their professional judgement and apply their knowledge and skill in the given situation (NMC 2015). The nurse is accountable for their actions and omissions in administering medication, delegating or assisting, or overseeing any self-administration of medication. A registrant is responsible for ensuring that the patient, carer, or care assistant is competent to carry out the task and apply the appropriate level of supervision. The registrant may delegate an unregistered practitioner or student nurse to assist the patient in the ingestion or application of the medicinal product (RCN 2020).

It is important that nurses/registered practitioners understand the law that governs the prescription, supply, and administration of medicines, as well as having an understanding of the classification and licencing of medicine for human use for medicinal purposes, which within the UK allows appropriate practitioners to supply and administer medication. The legislation covering the sale, use, and production of medicines includes the Human Medicines Regulations (2012), and the Medicines and Healthcare Products Regulatory Agency (MHRA); the national body responsible for regulating medicines and medical devices in the UK (MHRA 2022).

Medicines are classified into three categories; prescription-only medicine (POM), general sale medicine (GSL)/over-the-counter (OTC), and pharmacy-only medicine (P). Some medicines are subject to further specific controls through the Misuse of Drug Act (1971), Misuse of Drugs Regulations (MDR) 2001), and Psychoactive Substances Act (Her Majesty's Stationery Office [HMSO] 2016), which regulates possession, supply, and manufacture of controlled drugs (CDs), to prevent the nonmedical use of certain drugs. The Controlled Drugs Regulations (Department of Health [DH] 2013) classify CDs into five schedules; each represents a different level of control for the management and storage of medicines by professionals. The nurse should be familiar with these regulations and other relevant guidance, including the Health Act (2006) and NICE guidelines (2016).

Prior to the administration of a medicine, nurses must be aware of the legal considerations around the manufacturing, marketing authorisations (previously termed licences), labelling, and prescribing of medicines to CYPs. All medicines used for CYPs must be tested to stringent standards and specifically licenced for this use. However, some medicines used to treat children's healthcare conditions are unlicensed. This may be due to the challenges around testing medications with children; manufacturers may have not included children in the clinical trials, so cannot include them on the licence, or because they are used to treat extremely rare conditions. The complexities in prescribing and administering 'off licence' and 'off label' (licenced medicines for unlicensed use) is addressed in the British National Formulary for Children (BNFC) (2022). Medicines tend to be labelled using nonproprietary (generic) drug names, unless there is a clinical or legal reason why brand switching isn't allowable (BNFC 2022). Since 1992, nonmedical prescribing has been allowed in the UK and development and changes in legislation over the past 25 years have enabled the progression toward independent prescribing for nurses, pharmacists, and a range of allied health professionals. This practice continues to expand, with steadily increasing numbers of nonmedical prescribers and the recent evolution of undergraduate nonmedical healthcare prescribing education programmes (Cope et al. 2016). Currently, an approved accredited nurse prescribing course needs to be undertaken, and once this has been obtained the qualification must be registered with the NMC in order to practice as a nurse prescriber (NMC 2019).

There are two main types of nurse prescribers (NMC 2019; RCN 2022):

- **Community Practitioner Nurse Prescribers:**
  Nurses working in the community who are qualified to prescribe only from the Nurse Prescribers Formulary, which includes appliances, dressings, pharmacy, and general sales list and 13 prescription-only medications.
- **Nurse Independent Prescribers:**
  This course covers both independent and supplementary prescribing. An independent prescriber can prescribe any medicine within the BNF, unlicensed medicines, and all controlled drugs in schedules 2 to −5, as long as it is within their competency to do so. Supplementary nurse prescribers can prescribe in partnership with an independent prescriber within an agreed clinical management plan and with the patient/ carer's permission.

Registered practitioners must only supply and administer medicinal products in accordance with one or more of the following processes (Royal Pharmaceutical Society (RPS) 2021):

- Patient specific direction (PSD).
- Patient medicines administration chart (may be called medicines administration record or MAR).
- Patient group direction (PGD).
- Medicines Act exemption.
- Standing order.
- Homely remedy protocol.
- Prescription forms.

Patient group/specific directions

The main two types of patient directions:

- **Patient Specific Direction (PSD)** is a written instruction from an independent prescriber to supply or administer a medicine to a named patient. A PSD may be used to administer medicines to several named patients, e.g. on a clinic list. It is a direct instruction and uses the prescriber's assessment of need. Anyone competent to do so may supply and administer the medicine

- **Patient Group Direction (PGD)** is a written instruction for the supply or administration of a named medicine to a specific group of patients who may not be individually identified before presenting for treatment (RPS and RCN 2019). They must only be used by individually named registered practitioners and use the registered practitioner's assessment of need without referral to a prescriber. The instruction is agreed on and signed by a senior doctor and pharmacist and includes the following information:
  - The name of the health professional who can supply or administer the medicine.
  - The condition(s) included.
  - A description of those patients who should not be treated under the direction.
  - A description of circumstances where referral to another professional should be made.
  - The description, dosage, and strength of the medicines and the method of administration.

The legislation currently permits nurses to administer or supply medicines under a PGD (MHRA 2014, updated 2017).

Medications are available in a variety of preparations for administration via multiple routes. The choice of prescribed route can depend on a number of factors, including the availability and cost of the medication, the condition being treated, the required speed of onset of action of the medication, and the CYP's tolerance to the route of administration.

Medicines should only be given to CYPs when they are necessary and, in all cases, the potential benefit of administering the medicine should be considered in relation to the risk involved. It is important that CYPs are involved in decisions about treatment options and taking medication when able and are encouraged to take responsibility for using them correctly (BNFC 2022). Parents/carers should be encouraged to participate in the administration of medication to their child where appropriate. Many CYPs are also able to self-administer. The degree of involvement will depend on age, level of understanding, and personal circumstances.

Nurses must follow correct procedures in order to administer medication safely to CYPs. Alongside professional standards and legislation, organisations need to have clear policies in place to support practitioners with prescribing, storage, ordering, administration, and disposal of medicines.

Interruptions and distractions during the medicine checking and administration process, poor medicine calculation skills, inadequate training, and noncompliance with policies are all associated with medication errors (Alsulami et al. 2014; Bennett et al. 2010, Ofosu and Jarrett 2015; Raban and Westbrook 2014; Westbrook et al. 2010).

There are a variety of methods and checking processes recommended to ensure the safe administration of medication to patients; these include adhering to the 6 Rs of medicine administration and utilising effective independent checking processes. Some medicines require two registered professionals to check, others can be administered by one professional.

The six principles, the 6 Rights (6Rs) NICE (2018) provides a useful checklist to ensure that:

the	**r**ight medication is administered
to the	**r**ight patient
in the	**r**ight dose
via the	**r**ight route
at the	**r**ight time
with the	**r**ight to decline

Independent check of medicines

The nurse is responsible for checking any medicine that they are going to administer. They are responsible for checking and resolving any queries they have about the prescription or the administration of the medicine with the prescriber, reference source, or pharmacist prior to the administration of the medicine. The person giving the medicine may request any checks that they feel they require. A second registered practitioner may be required to check the preparation and/or administration of a medicine to reduce the risk of any errors that may have been made or missed by the person who is to administer the medicine. (NMC 2015). Any check made by a second person must be made independently of the first person, i.e. the practitioners check the medicine separately from each other and do not verbalise their checks to each other. The use of an independent second check is considered to be more effective at detecting errors (Institute of Healthcare Improvement (IHI) 2022) because it reduces the risk of confirmation bias, when individuals see what they expect to see or select out something that is familiar to them (Baldwin and Walsh 2014). This method of second checking is endorsed by the IHI (2022) and the British Committee for Standards in Haematology (Davidson 2014; British Society for Haematology 2022), and has been adopted as policy at GOSH.

Timeliness of medicine administration

The administration of medication at the right time is important in providing quality care to CYPs. Delays and omissions of medicines can result in harm to patients. National Institute for Health and Care Excellence (NICE) (2022), and NHS England (2022) recommend the use of 'red flag events', which warn when nurses in charge of shifts must act immediately to ensure they have enough staff to meet the needs of patients on that ward. These 'red flag events' include patients not being provided with basic care such as pain relief, unplanned omissions in providing patient medications, and delays of more than 30 minutes in providing pain relief.

Documentation

Following administration of any medicine the correct documentation must be completed. This is essential to ensure that there is a record of the medicine administered, a reason documented if this was not administered, and this also reduces the risk of a repeat dose being given.

Patient self-administration

CYPs are often discharged home on prescribed medication regimens and there are obvious benefits while in hospital to adjusting the responsibility to self/carer administration with professional support prior to discharge. For those CYPs or carers who wish to participate in the administration of medication, the responsibility and professional duty of the practitioner does not diminish and it is the responsibility of the registered nurse to educate, train, and assess the CYP or carer's competence in carrying out the task. Once competence is achieved, the practitioner should ensure the ongoing provision of support and regular reviews of competence (NMC 2018). Organisational policies to support medicine administration by patients and carers should be in place within hospitals. It should also be acknowledged that in some instances, CYPs/carers may wish to take a break from the responsibility of self-administration, and this should be negotiated with them as appropriate.

Child development considerations

Developmentally, infants and CYPs are going through a process of physical, metabolic, and psychological change. This section briefly describes some of the principles based on developmental age that need to be taken into account when administering medicines to CYPs. It goes on to outline the various routes of medicine administration, the benefits and contraindications for each route, and provides guidance in the safe practice of administering medication to CYPs.

Administering medication to CYPs can be facilitated by considering some general basic principles:

- Be confident and firm.
- Approach the procedure, CYP, and family with a positive attitude.
- Be honest and understanding.
- Empower the CYP to have some control (where appropriate).
- Encourage involvement in decision making.
- Use language appropriate to the level the CYP understands.
- Explain, if appropriate, what they will smell, taste, feel, see, and hear.
- Listen to all involved.
- Explain the benefits of taking the medication.

Infants (1–12 months)
At this stage of development, the infant is usually developing basic trust and needs to have a parent or carer near.

- Use sensory measures, i.e. touching of skin, talking softly.
- Provide comfort, i.e. a cuddle before, during, and after administering the medication.
- If the infant has a familiar/favourite blanket or toy, have it nearby for comfort.
- Encourage parental/carer involvement.

Toddlers (1–3 years)
At this stage of development, the toddler is developing their use of language slowly and remains very clearly attached to the parent/carer.

- Use a calm and confident approach and encourage the child to express their feelings.
- Use basic language that they will understand to explain what is going to happen, using toys/dolls, etc. and encourage them to role-play with their own toys.
- Give one instruction at a time, e.g. 'sit down.'
- Prepare the child shortly or immediately before the administration.

Pre-schoolers (3–5 years)
By this stage the child has usually further developed the ability to communicate.

- Give simple explanations so the child understands what is going to happen and does not perceive it to be a punishment.
- Use a positive approach and statements/reinforcement, e.g. that they are good *at* taking the medicine, not that they are good *for* taking the medicine.
- Allow the child some control by asking them to choose which method of administration they would prefer (if a choice is available) or where and how they would like to position themselves.

School-age (6–12 years)
At this stage of development the child is self-aware and has an awareness of the environment, etc. around them. They have some understanding of illness and treatments.

- Explain what is happening using teaching dolls, models, diagrams, drawings, etc.
- Involve the child in the decision making and allow time to answer questions.
- Prepare in advance of administration and suggest ways of maintaining control, e.g. counting.

Young people
- Young people value their independence and increasingly want to make their own decisions while secure in the knowledge that help or support is available if needed.
- Encourage and support them to take responsibility for their own treatment and make decisions as appropriate.

Checking the medicine prescription

There are some key requirements for any prescription: The drug name must be written in capitals, in full, and using the generic name. The route of administration must be clearly identified, the quantity of medicine required written in full (e.g. micrograms/milligrams) and it must be signed and dated by an independent prescriber.

Dose calculation in CYPs' medicine is usually based on either body weight in mg/kg (most commonly used due to simplicity and ease of calculation); or body surface area in mg/m^2 for which both accurate body weight and height are required.

NB: Body surface area is calculated on the CYP's ideal weight and will require adjustment for those whose weight falls outside this. Doses must also be modified in infants weighing **less than 10 kg** and care taken not to exceed the maximum safe daily dose in young people at the upper end of the spectrum, see body surface area calculator (BNFC 2022).

Guidance for safe practice in paediatric drug calculation:

- Ensure all dosages are reviewed regularly as the CYP grows.
- Check in an approved formulary whether the dose prescribed or stated is in terms of a single dose (mg/kg/dose, mg/m2/dose) or total daily dose (TDD). If TDD is used, this should be divided by the number of times the drug is to be administered.
- Displacement volumes must be accounted for when reconstituting freeze-dried injections. If not, this will result in significant dosing errors when drugs have large displacement volumes or small doses are administered.
- The calculated dose should not normally exceed the maximum recommended dose for an adult. e.g. If dose is 8 mg/kg (maximum dose 300 mg), then a CYP who weighs 40 kg should receive 300 mg rather than 320 mg (BNFC 2022).
- The use of decimal points when writing prescriptions should be discouraged, e.g. "100 micrograms" should be written instead of "0.1 milligram. This is to reduce the risk of decimal point errors in medicine prescribing and/or in calculation prior to administration being made. These types of errors are not infrequent, and result in a 10-fold difference in dosage for the CYP, which could be fatal.
- Always consider the presentation of drug, strength and form to encourage compliance and ease of administration for the CYP and parent/carer.

Drug calculations

The drug formula is:

$$\frac{\text{Dose required}}{\text{Present standard quantity of drug}} \times \text{Present quantity of liquid in which standard quantity of drug is dissolved} = \text{Correct dosage to be given}$$

In other words:

$$\frac{\text{What you want}}{\text{What you have}} \times \text{What it is in (dilution)} = \text{Correct dosage to be given}$$

For example:
A child is prescribed 90 mg of paracetamol and the medication supplied is 120 mg of paracetamol in 5 ml:

$$\frac{90}{120} \times \frac{5}{1} = 3.75 \text{ml}$$

Section 2: Routes of administration

Oral

The oral route is the most common route of administration for medicines in CYPs; this is for several reasons:

- It is generally associated with less pain and anxiety compared to other routes, e.g. injections.
- It is often cheaper than other preparations, e.g. IV medication.
- It usually requires less equipment to administer and can therefore be less time-consuming.
- There is a slower absorption of medication compared to other routes (e.g. IV) allowing more time to react should adverse reactions occur.

Medication administered orally passes through the gastrointestinal tract, with absorption usually through the small intestine, and it is then transported to the liver via the portal vein. After the medication has been metabolised by enzymes in the liver it enters the circulatory system, usually for systemic effect (Anderson and Saneto 2012). However, some oral medication can have a local effect, e.g. oral antacids which reduce the acidity of stomach contents, while stimulant laxatives increase intestinal motility (McKay and Walters 2013).

Considerations
The following should be taken into consideration when administering medicines orally:

- Refer to an approved medication formulary for information about the medicine, e.g. BNFC (2022).
- Ensure the CYP has a gag reflex present and the ability to maintain their airway in the presence of fluid.
- If the CYP is critically ill, gastric absorption of the medication may be slow and erratic.
- The therapeutic effect of some oral medications can be inhibited by the presence of food/milk, e.g. Ampicillin (BNFC 2022).
- Some oral medications, such as nonsteroidal anti-inflammatory drugs, can irritate the gastrointestinal lining. Taking these oral medications during or after consuming food or milk may prevent or partially reduce the irritation.
- Unless contra-indicated, administer oral medication to a baby prior to a feed to reduce the risk of loss of medication with any postfeed vomiting.
- Refer to the responsible practitioner if the CYP is nil by mouth, e.g. preoperative fasting. In some circumstances the CYP may still need to take the medication orally, while in others an alternative route of administration may need to be prescribed. NB: The dose of medication may differ depending on the route of administration.

Preparations
- The therapeutic dose of oral medication may vary depending on its preparation, e.g. 92 mg phenytoin suspension is equivalent to 100 mg tablet (BNF for Children 2022).
- The therapeutic duration of effect of oral medication may also vary depending on its preparation, e.g. modified release.
- Some IV preparations are suitable for oral administration. ALWAYS refer to the manufacturer's guidelines and liaise with pharmacy before administering.
- Some oral suspensions can taste extremely unpleasant.
- Some suspensions have a high sugar content and can cause dental caries with prolonged use; consider sugar-free formulations, if available.
- Crushing tablets or opening capsules generally renders the medication unlicensed for use, is not covered by the product licence, and may alter its therapeutic properties. Crushing a tablet will cause the drug to be released more quickly than desired.
- Some tablets are not suitable for crushing, as the coating prevents the release and absorption of the drug until it reaches the small intestine, e.g. enteric-coated tablets.
- It is good practice to avoid crushing or dissolving tablets or capsules; however, if it is necessary, care should be taken in order to deliver as safe and accurate a dose as possible. This should include pharmacist advice and referring to manufacturer's guidelines.
- Do not break tablets in half in order to administer half the dose unless they are scored.
- The mixing of medicines for administration should be avoided whenever possible. It must only be done when clinically appropriate and to meet the needs of the patient (MHRA 2014a; DH 2010).
- Unused medicines should always be disposed of in a pharmaceutical waste bin and never flushed down a sink.

Equipment
- Protective clothing should be worn when handling some medications, e.g. cytotoxic medication; see Chapter 8: Administration of Systemic Anticancer Treatments and Chapter 13: Infection Prevention and Control.
- Developmental level and understanding of the CYP can influence the method of administration and form of oral medication used, e.g. oral syringe or spoon, suspension, or tablet.
- Only use syringes that are labelled for oral/enteral use. These cannot be connected to IV catheters or ports, which reduces the risk of the administration of oral medications via the IV route, which can be fatal (NPSA 2007a). The UK standard is to use purple syringes to differentiate between oral syringes and those used for other routes.
- Medicines to be given in a clinical setting by either the oral or enteral route must be measured and administered using a single-use disposable medicine measure, a specific oral/enteral syringe, cup, spoon, or dropper provided specifically for that medicine and to be single patient use only.
- If crushing tablets, a glass or porcelain mortar must be used, as marble and granite may retain some of the medicine, resulting in the CYP not receiving the prescribed dose. The pestle must also be made of glass or porcelain and should have not have a wooden handle. Wooden handles are difficult to clean and may pose an infection risk. Any residual medicine must be wiped out of the mortar with a paper towel and then disposed of in a pharmaceutical waste bin. The pestle and mortar should be cleaned with water and dishwashing detergent after each use, dried, and stored in a dry location. Tablet crushers should not be used in a hospital setting as they are difficult to clean.
- Tablet splitters can be used in a home setting for single patient use; they must be cleaned with water and dishwashing detergent after each use, dried, and stored in a dry location.

Contraindications	Cautions
• Unconscious CYP • Absent gag reflex • Inability to swallow • Vomiting	• Gastrointestinal tract trauma/illness/malabsorption • Post gastrointestinal surgery • Nil by mouth, e.g. preoperative fasting • Nausea

Enteral via a tube or device

Administration of medication via feeding tubes placed either in the stomach or small intestine can provide a systemic or local effect similar to oral administration, depending on the position of the tube. There are numerous types of enteral tubes and different reasons why CYPs may require them. For more information see Chapter 22: Nutrition and Feeding.

The benefits of enteral tube administration of medication include:

- An alternative route of administration for CYPs who are unable to take oral medications.
- Slower absorption of medication compared to some other routes (e.g. IV), allowing more time to react should adverse reactions occur.

Considerations

- The administration of medication via oral and enteral tube differs depending on the type and location of the tube.
- It is essential that the nurse administering a medicine via an enteral tube is familiar with the type of tube being used and, importantly, whether it requires aspiration or flushing prior to administering medications.
- Some medications are not suitable for enteral administration.
- Most medications are not licenced for enteral administration (Santos et al. 2012).
- Medicines may be given via a nasogastric tube without the absorption of the medicine being affected. However, the therapeutic effect of some medications can be inhibited by the presence of enteral feeds, e.g. phenytoin (Barker et al. 2012).
- Medicines must not be administered via a tube that by-passes the stomach, e.g. a nasojejunal tube, without reference to the prescribing guideline or the advice of a pharmacist. This is because the absorption of the medicine may be affected.
- Medications should not be added to enteral feeds because of the increased risk of tube blockage (Williams 2008).
- Administration of crushed tablets or viscous suspensions should be avoided as they could block enteral tubes. If a crushed tablet must be used, this should be in liaison with a pharmacist, and be dissolved in an appropriate solution.
- Suspension medication with a high sorbital content or osmolarity can cause bloating, stomach cramps, and diarrhoea (White and Bradnam 2015).
- Medication should not be administered to CYPs who have enteral tubes on free drainage unless the drainage can be stopped for an appropriate amount of time following administration of the medication.
- CYPs requiring complete aspiration of stomach contents should not have medication administered prior to the procedure.
- In the critically ill CYP, gastric absorption of medication may be slow and erratic.
- Sterile water is recommended for flushing enteral tubes in hospitals. Cooled boiled water or tap water is used in the community setting for CYPs over the age of one year – always refer to local policies (Guidelines and Audit Implementation Network [GAIN] 2015).
- The volume of medication and flush administered should be monitored and recorded, especially in CYPs who are fluid restricted or who require large amounts of medication.
- A 20 or 50 ml syringe is recommended for flushing enteral devices, as this minimises the pressure delivered and reduces the risk of damage to the enteral device (GAIN 2015; NICE 2012). In neonates a 5 ml syringe should be used (Knox and Davie 2009).

Equipment

In most healthcare settings, medicines given by the enteral route must be measured and administered using a single patient use disposable medicine measure, or a specific oral/enteral syringe, provided specifically for that medicine. In the home setting, syringes may be washed in fresh soapy water and reused for the same CYP (Medicines for Children 2014).

An oral/enteral syringe must be used to administer the medication. Syringes for injection must never be used to administer oral/enteral medicines and feeds (NPSA 2007a; NHS Improvement 2018).

It is widely documented in the literature that the smaller the syringe used to administer a liquid via an enteral tube, the higher the risk of tube rupture (Perry et al. 2014; Reising and Neal 2005; White and Bradnam 2015). However, there is little agreement over the safe size of syringe that should be used, with syringes ranging from 10–60 ml being recommended. In practice, aspiration and flushing should be undertaken with nothing smaller than a 20 ml syringe. Administration of medication on the other hand is often undertaken using a smaller syringe to ensure accuracy of measurement of the medication. Syringes and containers of enteral medicines must be labelled to ensure that the medicine can be identified if there is a problem.

Contraindications	Cautions
• Enteral tube that must remain on continuous free drainage • Vomiting	• Nil by mouth, e.g. preoperative fasting • Post-gastrointestinal tract surgery • Gastrointestinal malabsorption/trauma/illness/obstruction

Buccal

Buccal administration can be used for medicines with either a local or systemic effect. It involves administering medication between the facial cheek and upper or lower gum for absorption through the buccal mucous membranes (tissues which line the mouth) (Figure 17.1). The medication diffuses through the oral mucosa and enters directly into the bloodstream, thereby avoiding the gastrointestinal system.

Advantages of this route of administration include:

- Rapid absorption and onset due to higher bioavailability of the drug. As the drug enters the systemic circulation directly, without having to pass through the gastrointestinal system, it is protected from degradation due to pH and enzymes (Narang and Sharma 2011).
- Faster onset of action compared to the oral route (Narang and Sharma 2011).
- Due to its rapid action and onset it is widely used in urgent/emergency situations, e.g. to administer midazolam for seizure management.
- Fast dissolution without the need for water or chewing (Narang and Sharma 2011).
- An alternative route of administration for some medications when there is no IV access.

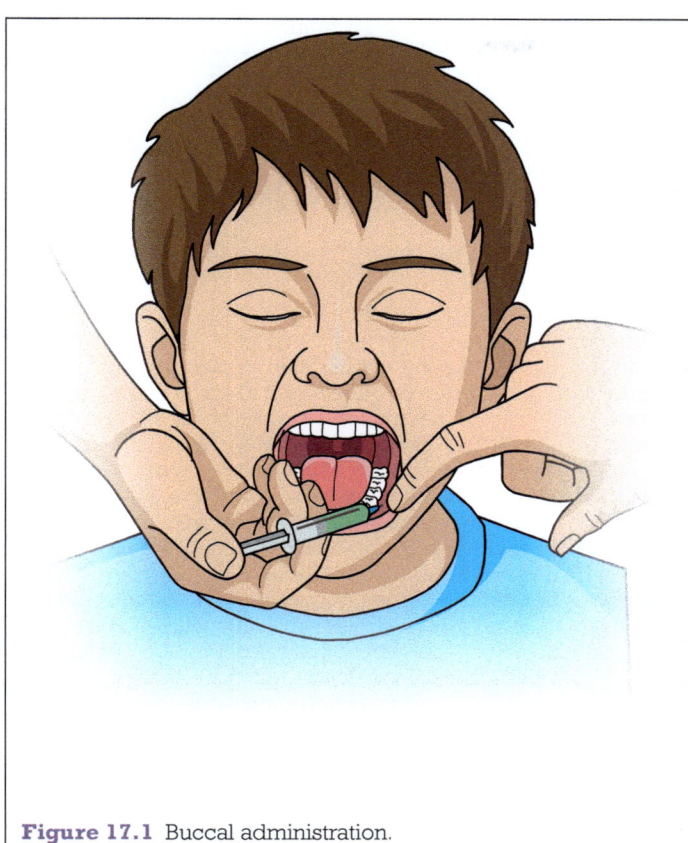

Figure 17.1 Buccal administration.

- May have better compliance with some CYPs compared to oral ingested tablets (Narang and Sharma 2011).
- Generally associated with less pain and anxiety compared with other routes.

Considerations

- The MHRA (2014) recommends that Trusts develop a written protocol for the use of buccal midazolam, ensuring that the dose is always prescribed in mg. and ml. and is only administered using oral syringes that are not compatible with IV or other parenteral devices.
- Buccal and sublingual forms of medication and administration are different and should not be confused.
- There is currently limited availability of medication suitable for buccal administration.
- The therapeutic dose and duration of effect of buccal medication may be different than with other routes of administration. It has a faster onset of action compared to the oral route and has a longer acting duration than sublingual (Narang and Sharma 2011).
- The tablet form (soluble or effervescent) of buccal medication is only suitable for CYPs who understand that the tablet should be allowed to dissolve and not chewed or swallowed and needs to be retained in the cheek and left to dissolve (BNFC 2022).
- Large volumes of medication may not be suitable for buccal administration.
- Liquid form of buccal medication should be carefully administered in small amounts to reduce the risk of swallowing or aspirating the medication.
- Eating, drinking, cleaning of teeth, rinsing the mouth, and talking must be temporarily restricted; see manufacturer's guidance.
- Smoking should be discouraged, as it decreases the absorption of medication due to vasoconstriction (Narang and Sharma 2011).
- Refer to manufacturer's guidelines and liaise with pharmacy regarding the use of IV preparations of medication; some may be suitable for buccal administration but can taste unpleasant.
- Unpleasant taste may affect the CYP's compliance with administration of the medication.
- Prolonged or repeated administration could potentially cause deterioration in the buccal cavity and tooth discoloration or decay.

> **Contraindications and cautions**
>
> There currently does not appear to be any readily available documented contraindications or cautions for buccal administration of medication. The following conditions should be discussed with the responsible prescriber prior to administration of buccal medication:
>
> - Oral trauma
> - Postoperative maxillo-facial surgery
> - Buccal mucous membrane abrasions, lesions, or infections
> - Tooth discolouration or decay

Sublingual

Sublingual (under the tongue) medication is only administered for systemic effect and involves administering medication into the space under the CYP's tongue for absorption through the sublingual mucous membranes into the systemic circulation (Narang and Sharma 2011). Medicines administered by this route include cardiovascular drugs, e.g.; antianginal, antihypertensives, and analgesics e.g.; morphine, steroids, and antiemetics.

Benefits of this route are;

- Higher bioavailability of a drug results in rapid absorption and onset. As the drug enters the systemic circulation directly, without having to pass through the gastrointestinal system, it is protected from degradation due to pH and enzymes (Narang and Sharma 2011).
- Faster onset of action compared to the less permeable buccal area and oral routes and has a shorter duration of effect (Narang and Sharma 2011).
- Due to its rapid action and onset it is widely used in emergency situations.
- Fast dissolution without the need for water or chewing (Narang and Sharma 2011).
- An alternative route of administration for some medications when there is no IV access.
- Better compliance in CYPs than the oral route (Narang and Sharma 2011).
- It is generally associated with less pain and anxiety and considered less invasive than other routes, particularly the IM and rectal routes.

Considerations

- Buccal and sublingual forms of medication and administration are different and should not be confused.
- There is limited availability of medication suitable for sublingual administration.
- The therapeutic dose and duration of effect of sublingual medication may be different from other routes of administration; it has a faster onset, but a shorter duration of effect compared to buccal and oral routes (Narang and Sharma 2011).
- Tablet form (soluble or effervescent) of sublingual medication is only suitable for CYPs who understand that the tablet should be allowed to dissolve and must not be chewed or swallowed.
- Liquid form (drops or spray) of sublingual medication should be carefully administered. The sublingual dosages are convenient for CYPs with dysphagia (difficulty in swallowing) (Narang and Sharma 2011).
- Eating, drinking, and talking can be temporarily restricted.

- Smoking should be discouraged, as it decreases the absorption of medication due to vasoconstriction (Narang and Sharma 2011).
- Refer to manufacturer's guidelines and liaise with the pharmacy regarding the use of IV preparations of medication, some of which may be suitable for sublingual administration.
- Unpleasant tasting medications, particularly IV preparations, may affect the CYP's compliance with administration of the medication.
- Prolonged or repeated administration could potentially cause deterioration in the sublingual cavity and tooth discolouration or decay.

Contra-indications and cautions

There are currently no readily available documented contraindications or cautions for sublingual administration of medication. However, it is suggested that the following conditions should be discussed with the responsible prescriber prior to administration of sublingual medication:

- Oral trauma
- Postoperative maxillo-facial surgery
- Tooth discolouration or decay
- Sublingual abrasions or lesions

Intranasal

Intranasal medication is used for both local and systemic effect; the medication can be rapidly absorbed through the large mucous membranes in the nasal cavities. Antihistamines, decongestives, corticosteroids, and antibiotic medications are administered for local effect, while analgesia, sedatives, hormones, and vaccines are administered via the intranasal route for systemic effect (Bitter et al. 2011; Grassin-Delyle et al. 2012).

Benefits

- Higher bioavailability of a drug results in a rapid absorption and onset through the thin vascularised mucosa in the nasal cavity, which allows the drug to enter directly into the systemic circulation and avoids gastrointestinal destruction and hepatic first-pass metabolism (destruction of drugs by liver enzymes) (Bitter et al. 2011 and Grassin-Delyle et al. 2012).
- Faster absorption and onset of action compared with the oral and IM routes. This route is used in emergency situations e.g. where immediate, rapid analgesia is required and no IV access is available, e.g. following a fracture, burn, or soft tissue injury (Bitter et al. 2011; Grassin-Delyle et al. 2012).
- An alternative route of administration for some medications as it is easily accessible when IM and IV access are either inappropriate or difficult (Hadley et al. 2010).
- Better compliance with CYPs because generally it is associated with less pain and anxiety compared with other routes such as IM injections.
- Less invasive than some other routes of administration, e.g. rectal route (Bitter et al. 2011).

Considerations

- Medications suitable for this route are generally potent, as the volume that can be sprayed into the nasal cavity is limited.
- Nasal administration can be associated with a high variability in the amount of drug absorbed.
- Unpleasant smell/taste may affect the CYP's compliance with administration of the medication.
- May sting or cause an unpleasant sensation during administration.
- Prolonged or repeated administration may be less suitable due to the harmful long-term effects on the nasal mucosa (epithelium) (Fransén 2008).

Cautions and contraindications

- Nasal trauma/fractures
- Postoperative nasal surgery
- Mucus obstructing the nasal passage
- Nasal infection, blood or discharge
- Epistaxis

Inhalation

This method is used to deliver fine particles of medication directly into the respiratory tract by nebulisation or aerosolisation. These routes of administration are primarily used to achieve local effects in the respiratory tract (although some medications will also have a systemic response) and are most commonly used in the treatment of respiratory tract conditions, e.g. acute asthma, cystic fibrosis. The aim of inhalation therapy is to reverse or prevent airway inflammation and constriction to control symptoms and maximise respiratory flow (British Thoracic Society and Scottish Intercollegiate Network (BTS/SIGN) 2019 and NICE (2002). Nebulisation is achieved by the passage of air or oxygen (if required) through a solution of medication to form a fine spray, e.g. sodium chloride, antibiotics, or bronchodilators. Medication for aerosolisation is prepared in an inert diluent, either in the form of solution or powder (inhalers). A measured amount is passed through a valve under pressure, which delivers the medication to the patient in a very fine spray in a controlled dose and particle size, e.g. bronchodilators or steroids. With this method, although a minimal amount of medication is administered, the concentration at the site is high. This usually achieves effective and rapid control of symptoms without the side effects associated with other systemic routes of administration, e.g. IV, of the same medication. This route is most commonly used to treat acute and chronic asthma.

Benefits

- Delivers the medication directly to where it is required.
- Usually achieves control of symptoms with fewer systemic side effects than other routes, for example IV.

Nebuliser

- The nebuliser solution for administration may need to be further diluted according to manufacturer's recommendations and requires an air or oxygen (if required) flow of between 6 and -8 litres per minute in order to produce adequate droplet formation (Boe et al. 2001).
- Some nebuliser types are more suitable for specific drugs and only connectors specifically modified to connect nebulisers to ventilator tubing must be used.
- The air or oxygen can be delivered via a cylinder, piped gas supply, or a compressor.
- The use of oxygen instead of air is dependent on the CYP's condition and must be prescribed if required.
- An appropriately sized mask or mouthpiece attached to the nebuliser pot should be used. If neither of these attachments is used the dose of medication administered to the CYP can be significantly reduced, as the medication can escape into the surrounding atmosphere.
- Ideally a facemask should be avoided when administering steroids to minimise steroid application to the skin and eyes (Boe et al. 2001). If unavoidable, ensure that the CYP's face is cleaned or wiped with water following administration.

Aerosoliser (inhalers)

There are a variety of different inhaler devices on the market that offer different features, each with its own advantages and disadvantages. The selection of a suitable device for the administration of inhalation medication for a CYP depends on the complexity of their treatment, including previous history of their condition. It also depends on their:

- Age (fine and motor skills and understanding)
- Respiratory function
- Lifestyle – portability, convenience, stigma
- Adherence to treatment
- Inhaler technique

There are three main types of inhaler devices:

- Press and breathe pressurised metered dose inhalers (pMDIs)
- Breath-actuated pressurised metered dose aerosol inhalers (breath activated pMDIs)
- Dry powder inhalers (DPIs) (NICE 2002)

pMDIs: The user presses down on the metal container held in a plastic cover (actuation), which releases the medication in a pressurised metered dose and simultaneously breathes in. This method requires actuation-inhalation coordination (NICE 2002; BTS/SIGN 2019).

Breath activated pMDIs: These remove the need for coordination of actuation and inhalation by delivering a pressurised aerosol metered dose of medication which is automatically activated by the user inhaling through the mouthpiece. However, the sound and sensation of the automatic actuation may cause adherence issues, as they differ from other devices (NICE 2002; BTS/SIGN 2019).

DPIs: Another breath-activated inhaler; a dose of micronised medication in an inert powder is delivered as the user inhales. Like the breath-activated inhaler, actuation-inhalation coordination is not required. However, some CYPs may find it difficult to exert a high enough inspiration to enable an effective dose delivery. This may also present a problem for CYPS in acute respiratory distress. There are a variety of DPI devices available and some find one device easier to use than another (NICE 2002; BTS/SIGN 2019).

Spacers: There are currently two general types of spacer systems available; these attach directly to the pMDIs, which resolves some of the problems associated with these inhalers.

- Detachable chambers (small, medium, or large volume) – this type is attached to the press and breathe pMDIs mouthpiece. The spacer acts as a holding chamber for the aerosol and medication, which allows the CYP to take in the medication over several breaths. As this type has a valve system, it is imperative that the correct inhalation technique is taught (NICE 2002; BTS/SIGN 2019).
- Small-volume extended mouthpiece spacers – these provide an increased distance between the point of release of the medication and the oropharyngeal area. This type of spacer can be used with press and breathe and breath-actuated pMDIs (NICE 2002; BTS/SIGN 2019).

Detachable plastic chamber spacers are prone to developing a buildup of static, which can cause adhesion of the medication to the chamber walls, and reduce medication delivery. It is important to follow manufacturer's guidelines; careful washing and thorough drying of the device at appropriate intervals can reduce this problem (NICE 2002; BTS/SIGN 2019).

For children under 5 years, a pMDI should be used with a spacer device with a facemask attached if required. With the correct technique, this is considered as good as a nebuliser in treating mild to moderate asthmatic attacks. If this is not effective nebulisation should be considered for this age group. A DPI could also be considered. The selection of the type of device should be governed by the specific need and the child and/or their parent/carer's adherence to the treatment regimen (BTS/SIGN 2019).

The education and training of the parent/carer is also important in this age group, as this can influence their child's adherence to and the effectiveness of the inhalation treatment.

If requiring daily corticosteroid therapy, a suitable spacer device is recommended, in order to achieve maximum benefit of the preventive therapy and minimise potential systemic absorption.

NICE (2002) and BTS/SIGN (2019) recommendations on inhaler device selection for 5 to 15 year-olds with asthma include individual training on the use of specific inhaler device/devices as a key influence on the effective delivery of inhalation therapy. Regular monitoring and review (at least annually) of inhaler technique are used to assess the continued effectiveness, adherence to therapy, and suitability of inhaler type, which may change with increasing age and the CYPs condition or preference.

Establishing the history of the CYP's condition and the therapeutic interventions they have undergone may also influence what type of inhalation therapy to administer, if required.

Contra-indications

- Airway obstruction
- A depressed level of consciousness (unless ventilated)

Cautions

- Oral/maxillary-facial surgery.
- Artificial airways.
- Severely compromised airways, e.g. acute inflammation of the airway – croup, epiglottitis.
- Flexion and hyperextension of the neck.
- History of ingestion or inhalation of a foreign body or volatile chemical.
- Congenital malformations or trauma of the head, neck, or chest.
- Recent history of general anaesthesia or sedation.
- Generalised muscle weakness, e.g. Guillain–Barré syndrome.

Rectal

Rectal medications are available in two main forms, suppositories and enemas, which can deliver medicine that has a systemic or local effect, e.g. anti-inflammatory medication can provide local effect for ulcerative colitis (Rang et al. 2003), while other medications such as analgesia, antibiotics, and anticonvulsants provide a systemic effect.

Suppositories are solid forms of medication that dissolve through the rectal mucosa at body temperature. Enemas are medication solutions used for rectal administration. There are two main types of enema; medicated enemas, which are absorbed through the rectal mucosa, and cleansing enemas, used for evacuation of the large intestine. A foam enema is a medicine that is mixed into a foam, which is sprayed into the rectum, and a liquid enema is a medicine that is mixed into a liquid, which is squeezed into the rectum (Medicines for Children 2014).

This section will focus on the administration of suppositories and medicated enemas. For information regarding cleansing enemas see Chapter 5: Bowel Care.

The benefits of rectal administration of medication include:

- An alternative route of administration for some medications if the CYP either cannot have the oral form of medication and/or there is no IV access.
- It is generally associated with less pain compared with other routes such as injections.

Considerations
- There is a limited range of medication type and strength available in rectal form.
- Suppositories should not be cut in half, as there is no guarantee of the dosing accuracy (Perry et al. 2014).
- If a smaller dose of an enema is prescribed than is available, the volume should be measured and not estimated.
- Medicated enemas provide more rapid absorption than suppositories.
- The therapeutic dose of rectal medication may be different than other routes of administration, e.g. a higher dose of diazepam is required to be prescribed when administered rectally instead of intravenously for the treatment of seizures (BNFC 2022).

- The presence of faeces in the large intestine can delay or inhibit absorption of medication.
- For many CYPs, using the rectal route can be a very distressing experience.
- Suppositories should be inserted rounded end first to minimise trauma during insertion (Perry et al. 2014).
- Many parents are unfamiliar and/or uncomfortable with the use of the rectal route for their child. Some cultural and religious beliefs may oppose the CYP and family to rectal administration of medication.
- Rectal administration of medications should be avoided if there is a history of child abuse.
- The CYP's privacy and dignity should be maintained at all times.
- It is recommended that a chaperone is present during administration of a rectal medication.
- The rectal route should only be used in the treatment of constipation if oral laxatives do not work, and then only if the CYP and family consent (NICE 2010).
- Colostomies may be used but must be well established, not newly formed, and a rectal stump may also be used if there is a good blood supply (Higgins 2007).

Contra-indications

- Diarrhoea
- Certain bowel conditions, e.g. imperforate anus
- During the postoperative period following certain types of bowel or pelvic surgery, e.g. Duhamel pull through
- Peri-anal injury, e.g. abrasions and lesions
- Blood clotting disorders such as thrombocytopenia
- New formed colostomy
- Rectal stump with poor blood supply

Caution

Discuss administration of rectal medication with the responsible doctor if the CYP:

- Has a rectal stump
- Has any history of bowel, cardiac, or haematological disorder
- Is constipated (NB: Not a caution for laxative suppositories)
- Has a cardiac arrhythmia
- Is immunosuppressed; the risks of infection/trauma/bleeding due to the vulnerable mucosal membrane in the rectum mean this method of administration is contraindicated (Selwood 2008)

Intradermal (ID), subcutaneous (SC), and intramuscular (IM)

Injections via the ID, SC and IM routes are used less frequently in CYPs due to the availability of alternative techniques, such as epidural infusions and IV patient- and nurse-controlled analgesia (see Chapter 24: Pain Management). However, there are some circumstances where injections are unavoidable; this may be because:

- The CYP is unable to take the medication via any other route.
- The medicine is not available to be given via an alternative route.
- The medicine is not as effective when administered by another route (Ford et al. 2010).

This section will focus on administration of medication via intradermal (ID), subcutaneous (SC) and intramuscular (IM) routes. For IV administration, see Chapter 14: Intravenous and Intra-arterial Access. For injection routes and techniques, refer to the Royal College of Paediatricians and Child Health (RCPCH) guidelines (2002). Using evidence-based practice will reduce discomfort and complications for CYPs receiving injections (Clancy and Furyk 2012; Greenway 2014; Hunter 2008).

Considerations

- ID, SC, and IM administration methods are different and should not be confused.
- Medication for injection is usually supplied either as a sterile solution or freeze-dried powder as the stability of the medication is often limited once dissolved.
- Consider involving the play specialist for play therapy and/or distraction therapy.
- If the CYP needs to be held this should be in accordance with the local restraint and therapeutic holding policies.
- Unless contraindicated, consider applying a prescribed local anaesthetic cream, cold/spray, or using a cold pack to numb the site prior to the injection.
- Administration of cold medication may be more painful. Refer to manufacturer's guidelines and pharmacy to see if refrigerated medication can be allowed to warm to room temperature before use.
- Administration of large volumes of medication is more painful. Refer to pharmacy regarding available strengths of medication.
- The choice of needle size for the different routes, ages, and the size of the CYP need to be assessed on an individual basis. It is not only the length of the needle that is important to consider, but also the gauge (width) of the needle and the viscosity of the medication.
- For many CYPs, using the ID, SC, and IM route can be a very distressing experience.

There are many differences of opinion regarding skin cleansing prior to administering injections (Pratt et al. 2005). The World Health Organisation (WHO) (2010) and the DH (2017) do not recommend the use of alcohol swabs if the skin is visibly clean. The RCPCH (2002) say that formal skin disinfection is not necessary prior to immunisation. For the immunocompromised CYP, however, it is recommended that a sterile 70% alcohol impregnated swab is used prior to an IM injection and then allowed to dry for 30 seconds before the injection is given (Dougherty et al. 2015). Prior to IM injections, skin disinfection with a sterile 70% alcohol swab (e.g. Steret®) is recommended. This must be allowed to dry before injection.

Where the CYP is not immunocompromised and has no skin infections, the practitioner administering the injection should ensure that the skin is visibly clean and is, if required, washed with soap and water prior to the administration of an injection.

Skin disinfection with an alcohol swab is not necessary prior to ID, SC or IM injection, irrespective of the CYP's immune status.

All ID, SC and IM medications should be prepared for administration using an aseptic nontouch technique (see Chapter 14: Intravenous and Intra-arterial Access).

General equipment required for ID, SC, and IM injections includes:

- Prescription
- Medication formulary
- Manufacturer's drug information
- Medication
- Clean plastic medication tray
- Syringe
- Needle(s)
- Sterile 70% isopropyl alcohol impregnated wipe for skin preparation (if required for IM injection)
- Nonsterile gauze
- Apron

Cautions and contraindications

- CYPs with a bleeding disorder (e.g. haemophilia) should always have the need for a SC, ID, or IM injection discussed with their haematology team before any injections are given.
- Injury or infection at injection site.
- Factors which may affect the absorption from the site (i.e. shock, poor tissue perfusion).

Intradermal

Intradermal (ID) injections allow the injection of a medicine into the dermis of the skin. This is the outer most layer of the skin, found underneath the skin, just beneath the epidermis. This route of administration is usually used for either anaesthetising the skin prior to an invasive procedure, or to test for allergies or tuberculosis. The BCG vaccination is also given via the ID route. Although not often used in children, there are also ID implants, which are inserted using a minor surgical procedure into dermal pockets in order to release medication, e.g. hormones over several months or a year.

Benefits
- Provides a local effect
- Lower risk of infection than with IV administration
- Lower risk of accidentally injecting a blood vessel compared with IM injection

Considerations
- In order to reduce the pain of the procedure only small volumes should be injected via the ID route, i.e. less than 0.5 ml (Brown 2015).
- Care should be taken when measuring the amount of medicine in the syringe, as the measurements are very small.
- The use of an alcohol skin swab is not recommended if the skin is clean.
- Resistance may be felt and a small wheal may form where the medication is injected into the skin (Public Health England (PHE) 2013).
- The most common site for ID testing is the inner forearm due to its hairlessness. If it is not possible to use this site the upper back under the scapula can be used, or if necessary one of the SC sites (Love 2006).
- An injection site must be free from lesions, rashes, moles, hair or scars (Lynn 2011).
- Practitioners should ensure they are competent to administer an ID injection, as the angle and needle length are different to other injections.
- For allergy testing, there is the risk of the test being invalid if not injected correctly (Perry et al. 2014).
- If testing for allergens, the area on the skin should be labelled, in order to monitor the allergic response.

Note: When allergen testing, ensure emergency equipment, including anaphylaxis management drugs, is readily available. For further information see Chapter 2: Allergy and Anaphylaxis.

Subcutaneous

Subcutaneous (SC) injections allow the injection of a medicine into SC tissue/fat under the skin, i.e. the layer of connective and adipose tissue located between the skin dermis and muscle fascia. SC medication can be administered as either a bolus or an infusion and delivers either a local or systemic effect. The most common sites of administration in CYPs are the lateral upper arm, anterior thigh, and lower abdomen (see Figure 17.2a). Medicines given subcutaneously include growth hormone, insulin and epinephrine. This route can also be used to provide a continuous infusion where parental administration is required but there is no IV access.
Benefits of SC administration of medication include:

- Lower risk of infection than with IV administration
- Lower risk of accidental injection into a blood vessel compared with IM injection
- Longer duration of effect than IM and IV medication
- Some medicines are more effective when injected subcutaneously

Considerations
- There are a range of devices used for administration including standard needles and syringes, prefilled syringes, auto injector and pen devices and SC cannula.
- Some medications, e.g. insulin, are prescribed in units and must always be prescribed in units and administered in syringes measured in the same units (NPSA 2010b; NHS Improvement 2018).
- SC injections can be painful; there are various ways the pain can be reduced including:
  - Avoiding nerve endings; most CYPs find some areas of the thigh less painful than the abdomen.
  - How the needle is inserted; the needle is cut at 45° angle so should be inserted with angle facing upwards-see Figure 17.2b.
  - Rotation of injection sites.
- Suitable areas are those with a substantial amount of fat below the skin, such as the thigh, buttocks, and abdomen.
- Sites of administration should be rotated to reduce the risk of fibrosis of SC tissue and the development fatty lumps (liphypertrophy), which could influence the absorption of medication.
- Accidental IM administration of SC medication could result in faster absorption of medication with a shorter duration of effect.
- The size of syringe should be determined by the volume of medication. Due to the ability of the SC layer to accommodate infusion of fluid there is no evidence base for a maximum bolus volume.
- If regular SC injections are required consider administration via a SC cannula. This can be left in situ for several days to minimise trauma.

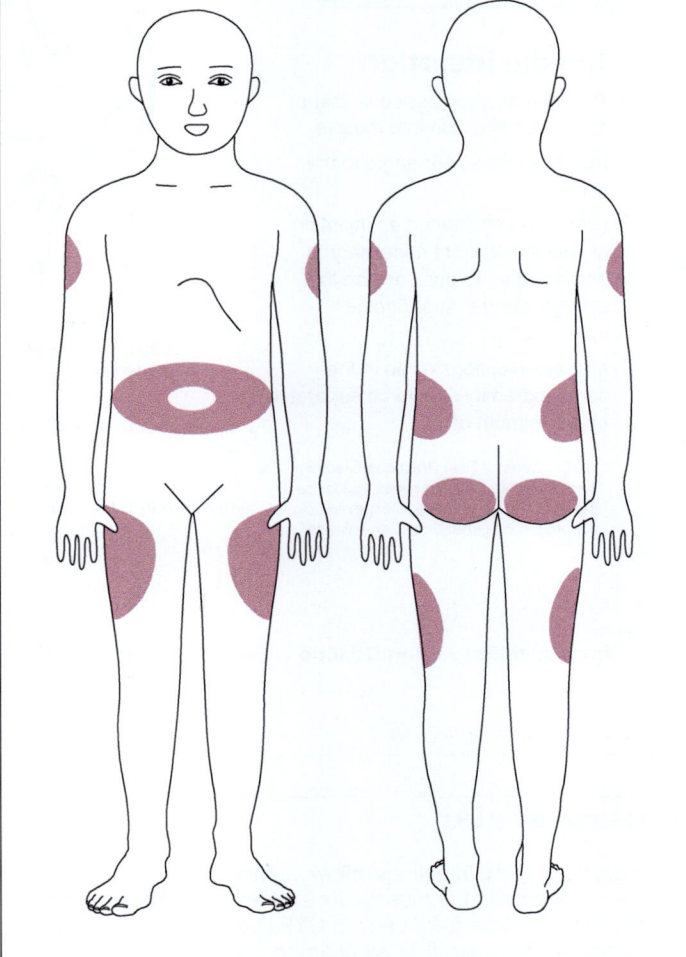

Figure 17.2a Sites of subcutaneous (SC) administration.

The Great Ormond Street Hospital Manual of Children and Young People's Nursing Practices

Administration by the Subcutaneous (Subcut) Route

Administer these vaccines via Subcut route

- Measles, mumps, and rubella (MMR)
- Varicella (VAR)
- Zoster, live (ZVL)

Administer inactivated polio (IPV) and pneumococcal polysaccharide (PPSV23) vaccines either IM or Subcut.

PATIENT AGE	INJECTION SITE	NEEDLE SIZE
Birth to 12 months	Fatty tissue overlying the anterolateral thigh muscle	5/8" (23–25 gauge)
12 months and older	Fatty tissue overlying the anterolateral thigh muscle or fatty tissue over triceps	5/8" (23–25 gauge)

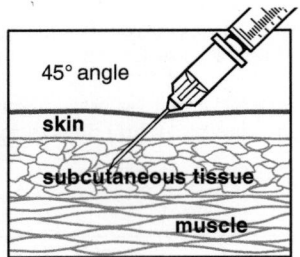

Needle insertion

Pinch up on subcutaneous tissue to prevent injection into muscle.

Insert needle at 45° angle to the skin.

(Before administering an injection of vaccine, it is not necessary to aspirate, i.e., to pull back on the syringe plunger after needle insertion.*)

Multiple injections given in the same extremity should be separated by a minimum of 1".

*CDC. "General Best Practices Guidelines for Immunization: Best Practices Guidance of the ACIP" at https://www.cdc.gov/vaccines/hcp/acip-recs/general-recs/downloads/

Subcutaneous (Subcut) injection site for infants

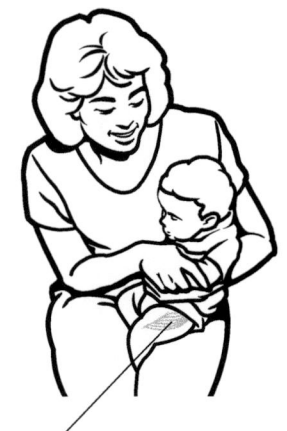

Subcut injection site (shaded area)

Insert needle at a 45° angle into fatty tissue of the anterolateral thigh. Make sure you pinch up on subcutaneous tissue to prevent injection into the muscle.

Subcutaneous (Subcut) injection site for children (after the 1st birthday) and adults

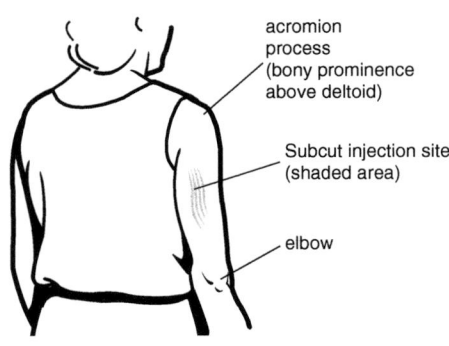

Insert needle at a 45° angle into the fatty tissue overlying the triceps muscle. Make sure you pinch up on the subcutaneous tissue to prevent injection into the muscle.

Immunization Action Coalition • Saint Paul, Minnesota • 651-647-9009 • www.immunize.org • www.vaccineinformation.org

www.immunize.org/catg.d/p2020.pdf • Item #P2020 (1/18)

Figure 17.2b (continued)

Intramuscular

Intramuscular (IM) injections allow a medicated solution to be injected directly into the muscle fibre underneath the SC layer. The IM route is used less frequently in CYPs because many are fearful of injections. However, it is sometimes used, either because the medication is currently not available in a form suitable for administration by any other route, e.g. Hepatitis B vaccination, or because local reaction occurs with SC administration.

There are two main sites used for the administration of IM injections in children (Figure 17.3):

- The **deltoid muscle** is the preferred site for IM and deep SC injections in larger children. It is suitable for small volume injections such as immunizations, but not for repeated use or large volumes. It should be used with caution in children under three years old (Hemsworth 2000).
- The **vastus lateralis** is the preferred site for IM and deep SC injections in infants under one year and children up to three

Administration by the Intramuscular (IM) Route

Administer these vaccines via IM route

- Diphtheria-tetanus-pertussis (DTaP, Tdap)
- Diphtheria-tetanus (DT, Td)
- *Haemophilus influenzae* type b (Hib)
- Hepatitis A (HepA)
- Hepatitis B (HepB)
- Human papillomavirus (HPV)
- Inactivated influenza (IIV)
- Meningococcal serogroups A,C,W,Y (MenACWY)
- Meningococcal serogroup B (MenB)
- Pneumococcal conjugate (PCV13)
- Zoster, recombinant (RZV)

Administer inactivated polio (IPV) and pneumococcal polysaccharide (PPSV23) vaccines either IM or subcutaneously (Subcut).

PATIENT AGE	INJECTION SITE	NEEDLE SIZE
Newborn (0–28 days)	Anterolateral thigh muscle	⅝"* (22–25 gauge)
Infant (1–12 mos)	Anterolateral thigh muscle	1" (22–25 gauge)
Toddler (1–2 years)	Anterolateral thigh muscle	1–1¼" (22–25 gauge)
Toddler (1–2 years)	Alternate site: Deltoid muscle of arm if muscle mass is adequate	⅝*–1" (22–25 gauge)
Children (3–10 years)	Deltoid muscle (upper arm)	⅝*–1" (22–25 gauge)
Children (3–10 years)	Alternate site: Anterolateral thigh muscle	1–1¼" (22–25 gauge)
Children and adults (11 years and older)	Deltoid muscle (upper arm)	⅝†–1" (22–25 gauge)
Children and adults (11 years and older)	Alternate site: Anterolateral thigh muscle	1–1½" (22–25 gauge)

* A ⅝" needle usually is adequate for neonates (first 28 days of life), preterm infants, and children ages 1 through 18 years if the skin is stretched flat between the thumb and forefinger and the needle is inserted at a 90° angle to the skin.

† A ⅝" needle may be used in patients weighing less than 130 lbs (<60 kg) for IM injection in the deltoid muscle only if the skin is stretched flat between the thumb and forefinger and the needle is inserted at a 90° angle to the skin; a 1" needle is sufficient in patients weighing 130–152 lbs (60–70 kg); a 1–1½" needle is recommended in women weighing 153–200 lbs (70–90 kg) and men weighing 153–260 lbs (70–118 kg); a 1½" needle is recommended in women weighing more than 200 lbs (91 kg) or men weighing more than 260 lbs (118 kg).

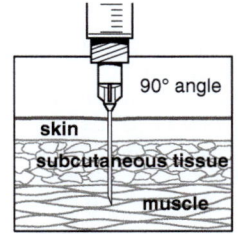

Needle insertion

Use a needle long enough to reach deep into the muscle.

Insert needle at a 90° angle to the skin with a quick thrust.

(Before administering an injection of vaccine, it is not necessary to aspirate, i.e., to pull back on the syringe plunger after needle insertion¶.)

Multiple injections given in the same extremity should be separated by a minimum of 1", if possible.

¶ CDC. "General Best Practices Guidelines for Immunization: Best Practices Guidance of the ACIP" at https://www.cdc.gov/vaccines/hcp/acip-recs/general-recs/downloads/general-recs.pdf

Intramuscular (IM) injection site for infants and toddlers

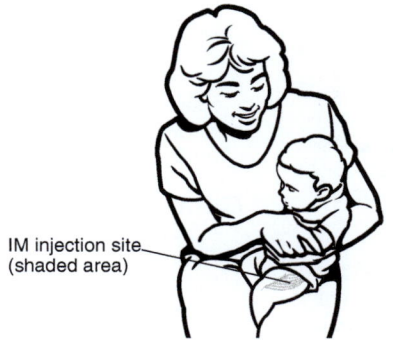

Insert needle at a 90° angle into the anterolateral thigh muscle.

Intramuscular (IM) injection site for children and adults

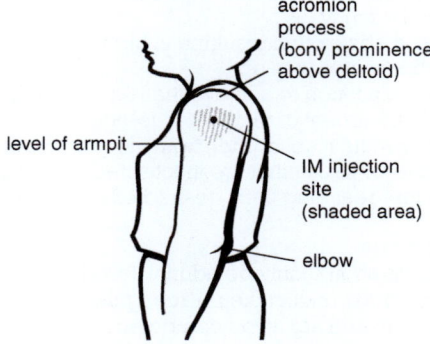

Give in the central and thickest portion of the deltoid muscle – above the level of the armpit and approximately 2–3 fingerbreadths (~2") below the acromion process. See the diagram. To avoid causing an injury, do not inject too high (near the acromion process) or too low.

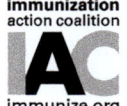

immunization action coalition

Saint Paul, Minnesota • 651-647-9009 • www.immunize.org • www.vaccineinformation.org

Technical content reviewed by the Centers for Disease Control and Prevention

Figure 17.3 Sites of intramuscular (IM) injections.

---

years old (Cook and Murtagh 2005; World Health Organization 2010).

The benefits of IM administration of medications include:

- Reduced risk of local reaction compared with SC and IV administration.
- Faster absorption in an emergency situation (such as anaphylaxis).
- Alternative route for some medications when there is no IV access, e.g. administration of IM antibiotics for suspected meningitis by the GP.

Considerations

- Awareness of potential complications such as haematoma, abscess, fibrosis or necrosis of the muscle, and nerve injury.
- The age, size and condition of the CYP and the volume and viscosity of medication should determine the choice of muscle to be used for the injection.

- Care should be taken to avoid the dorso-gluteal area in young children as this muscle is not well developed until they are walking.
- Sites of administration should be rotated to reduce the risk of fibrosis of IM tissue developing which could influence the absorption of medication.
- Accidental SC administration of IM medication could result in slower absorption of the medication with a longer duration of effect.
- The size of syringe should be determined by the volume of medication. The maximum volume of an IM injection should ideally not exceed 2 ml (Aronson 2008), as larger volumes cause more pain and influence the absorption of medication.

Intravenous

Intravenous (IV) administration of medication involves the administration of medication directly into a vein for systemic action. It can be given by bolus injection, intermittent infusion, or continuous infusion, depending on the type of medication prescribed and the condition of the CYP. There are different types of intravascular access devices including peripheral and central percutaneous intravenous catheters; nontunnelled and tunnelled central venous catheters, and implanted ports. Guidelines for the administration of IV medications are not provided in this chapter; see Chapter 14: Intravenous and Intra-arterial Access Infusions.

The benefits of IV medication include:

- Reduced use of needles once access is established.
- Rapid onset of action of medication, which is particularly important in an emergency.
- More effective absorption resulting in higher plasma levels compared to other routes, e.g. oral.
- Titration of medication to achieve the required response, e.g. IV insulin in the treatment of diabetic keto-acidosis.
- An alternative route if absorption from the gut is poor or variable.
- An alternative for drugs that are inactivated in the stomach or by the liver before reaching their desired effect in the circulation.

Considerations

- IV medications should only be administered by registered practitioners who have undertaken a recognised period of training and assessment and achieved competence. Refer to local policy for details.
- An aseptic nontouch technique should be adhered too, to reduce the risk of infection.
- Awareness of potential complications and their management is required, including phlebitis, infiltration, extravasation, fluid overload, air embolism, and anaphylaxis. For more information see Chapter 14: Intravenous and Intra-arterial Access.
- Certain IV medications require monitoring of plasma concentration levels.
- Some medications may not be suitable for administration via peripheral catheters due to their pH or osmolarity, due to the high risk of infusion related complications. Always check local guidelines and liaise with the pharmacist if unsure.
- Medications should not be added to blood transfusions, parenteral nutrition, alkaline or strong acidic solutions.
- If a CYP is receiving parenteral nutrition and there is a need to intermittently interrupt this to allow for administration of IV medication, this should be planned with the dietitian and pharmacist.
- Refer to local policy for guidance on changing IV infusion giving sets, as this may be affected by the type of medication and the length of time over which it is administered.

Intraosseous

The administration of medications via the intraosseous (IO) route, involves inserting a cannula or needle into the medullary cavity of a long bone, passing through the skin, periosteum and cortex of the bone. This route is usually reserved for emergency situations where rapid access to the central circulation is urgently required and access via more conventional routes have failed or cannot be achieved quickly. It has all the advantages of central venous access and can be rapidly and easily achieved (Advanced Life Support Group 2011; Resuscitation Council (UK) 2011). The proximal and distal tibia and distal femur are the most commonly used sites in CYPs. For more information see Chapter 30: Resuscitation.

Benefits

- The medullary cavity does not collapse in the presence of hypovolaemia or circulatory failure. It acts like a rigid vein, making it an ideal site in a situation where vascular access is urgently required (e.g. clinical shock or cardiac arrest).
- Rapid onset of medication action.
- The IO route has become the route of choice when the CYP has no other central access in situ in a clinical emergency situation (Resuscitation Council UK 2011).
- All resuscitation fluids, drugs and blood products can be given via the IO route
- It can be used in any situation where there is no or inadequate IV access and IV access is difficult or has failed and there is an immediate or urgent need for IV fluids and/or IV medication.
- Insertion of the IO needle is quick and easy.

Considerations

- Medications and fluids can only be delivered as a manual bolus.
- This is a vascular route of administration and therefore medications should only be administered via this route by medical staff or registered practitioners who have undergone a recognised period of training and assessment and achieved competence. Refer to local policy for details.
- An aseptic nontouch technique must be used to minimise the risk of infection.
- Knowledge and awareness of potential complications and their early detection and management is essential.

Complications

- Infection
- Extravasation
- Subperiosteal infusion
- Embolism
- Compartment syndrome
- Fracture
- Skin necrosis
- Pain on use
- Dislodgement
- Skin necrosis

Contraindications

- Coagulopathies, e.g. haemophilia
- Fractures in the target bone
- Previous orthopaedic surgery near the insertion site
- Previous IO insertion in the target bone within the preceding 48 hours
- Infection at the insertion site
- Loss of skin integrity
- Osteogenesis imperfecta (if using a Cooks needle only)
- Osteoporosis (if using a Cooks needle only)

Intrathecal

Intrathecal administration allows medication to be administered directly into the cerebrospinal fluid in either the subdural or subarachnoid space between the arachnoid and pia mater, e.g. via a lumbar puncture or directly into the ventricles (intraventricular), e.g. via a reservoir or an external ventricular drainage system. It can only be administered by injection or infusion through a shunt reservoir, an intraventricular reservoir, a drainage system or a lumbar puncture (Lindsay et al. 2010). This route is only used for specific intrathecal medications such as spinal anaesthesia, antispasmodics, antibiotic therapy, specific cytotoxic therapies and X-ray or contrast media containing those substances that do not penetrate the blood–brain barrier (Dougherty et al. 2015). Only medication specially prepared for the intrathecal route should be used. For more information on intrathecal administration see Chapter 8: Administration of Systemic Anticancer Treatments (SACT).

Benefits
- Allows direct administration of medication to the central nervous system (CNS) of medication that is either normally excluded by the blood–brain barrier or that cross the blood–brain barrier in very limited amounts (Dougherty et al. 2015).

Considerations
- Intrathecal medication must only be administered by medical staff/practitioners who have undergone specific training and been assessed as competent (DH 2011).
- The storage, preparation, dispensing, supply and administration of intrathecal medication must always be separate from medication intended for IV administration.
- Check the CYP's treatment protocol and determine stage of treatment.
- If administrating intrathecal antibiotics, ensure the antibiotic level in the cerebrospinal fluid has been checked prior to administration, as the medication dose may need to be altered to maintain therapeutic drug levels (Arnell et al. 2007).
- Establish the CYP's neurological status prior to administration, so any alteration in their neurological condition during and post administration can be detected early.
- Refer to local prescription guidelines, usually the medication and route of administration 'intrathecal' should be clearly written in full on the chart.

All equipment used to obtain lumbar puncture samples and administer intrathecal medications must not be able to connect with IV Luer connectors (NPSA 2011b).

Intrathecal cytotoxic medication must only be administered by medical staff/practitioners who have undergone specific training, been assessed as competent and registered to administer intrathecal cytotoxic medication. Refer to the specific national and local guidelines that exist in relation to administration of cytotoxic intrathecal medication (DH 2011).

Intrathecal cytotoxic medication should be prescribed on specifically designed intrathecal chemotherapy prescriptions. For more information see Chapter 8: Administration of Systemic Anticancer Treatments (SACT).

Cautions and contra-indications
- Alteration of intracranial pressure
- Infection
- Haemorrhage
- Shock
- Fatality (if incorrect medication is administered)

Epidural

The epidural route is indicated for relief of moderate to severe pain that is likely to be difficult to control via an alternative route. The range of medicines that can be administered into the epidural space is limited. Administration of medicine via the epidural route should only be performed by registered professionals who have undergone specific training and are competent in this area of practice. Organisations should have clear local guidelines for staff. Medicines administered via this route have direct access to the brain without having to pass the blood–brain barrier. They should be formulated for epidural use and not contain preservatives, as these can cause neurotoxicity.

Benefits
- Allows direct administration of medication to the CNS (Patel 2006).
- Can provide more effective analgesia than the IV route
- Reduces opiate requirement if the epidural block is effective.
- Useful as part of a multimodal approach to pain management in CYPs (Saul et al. 2016).

Considerations
- Each patient should be assessed on an individual basis to ensure that the potential benefits outweigh the risks.
- Insertion of an epidural catheter should be performed by a consultant anaesthetist with experience of performing this technique in CYPs, or an anaesthetic registrar under supervision.

Contra-indications
- Local or generalised sepsis
- Coagulation disorders
- Anticoagulation therapy
- Some diseases of the CNS
- Spinal deformity

Epidural medicines can be given as a bolus or as a continuous infusion. For more information on epidural analgesia, see Chapter 24: Pain Management.

Transdermal (skin patches)

These provide an alternative route for the administration of medication through the skin into the bloodstream to produce a systemic effect. Skin patches are reservoirs of medicine contained within thin pads with an adhesive backing, which enables them to be applied directly to the skin. The medicine within the patch diffuses slowly through the skin into the bloodstream. It usually provides a controlled release of medication through either a porous membrane covering the reservoir or body heat melting thin layers of medication embedded in the adhesive patch. Although the skin is normally impermeable to substances, solutions are used to increase the skins permeability and allow specific drugs to pass through the skin to the interstitial fluid and hence the bloodstream. There are five main types of transdermal patch; single, multi-layer, reservoir, matrix, and vapour patches.

Benefits
- The continual slow release of the drug and its absorption into the skin provide more consistent blood levels and effect over time, e.g. analgesia.
- Alternative route of administration for CYPs who are unable to take, tolerate or absorb medicines via the enteral route.
- A noninvasive and pain-free route of administration (Delgado-Charro and Guy 2014).
- A discreet way to administer medicine.

Considerations
- There is currently limited availability of medications suitable for transdermal administration.
- The therapeutic dose of medication within the skin patch may be different to that administered by other routes; for example, the oral medication dose is usually higher to allow for the malabsorption and metabolism of the drug.
- Only small portions of transdermal patches may be required for CYPs: Although some patches can be cut for partial administration, cutting others destroys the release of the medication (Lee and Phillips 2002) and could result in inaccurate dose administration.

The Great Ormond Street Hospital Manual of Children and Young People's Nursing Practices

- Do not remove the patch from its protective pouch or remove the protective backing until just before applying it.
- Do not put a patch on straight after a bath or shower; allow the skin to cool down first to reduce the possibility of increased absorption through the skin.
- Do not use moisturiser, creams, or powder on the skin prior to application, as this may stop the patch from sticking properly.
- The patch should be applied to clean, dry, hairless skin on the upper arm, or hip.
- Avoid placing the patch under tight clothing or around the waistband area.
- Ensure that the patch is not placed near the genital / nappy area to avoid contamination as this may irritate the skin and affect absorption of the drug.
- Young children have a tendency to remove patches; cover with clothing so that the patch is out of sight.
- Some patches need to be removed before swimming, showering, or bathing; check the manufacturer's information sheet before applying.
- Assess the skin under the patch every time a patch is changed to be certain that the site is not irritated.
- Change the site every time a new patch is applied to reduce the possibility of irritation to the skin.
- Dispose of the used patch carefully as it will still contain some active medicine. Fold the patch so it sticks to itself prior to disposal (MHRA 2014b).

Contra-indications

- Broken, burned, cut, oily or irritated skin
- Epidermolysis bullosa

Caution

- Eczema or other skin conditions
- Previous surgery near the insertion site
- Infection near site
- Sensitive skin.

Principles table 17.1 General guidelines

The following sections of this chapter provide details for the administration of medications via the different routes referred to earlier in this chapter. For each route there are several general principles that should be followed, the reader must be familiar with and adhere to the following principles in each situation.

Principle	Rationale
1 Refer to local policy for administration of medications.	1 To adhere to local policy.
2 Avoid distractions while dispensing and administering medications.	2 To reduce the risk of medication error.
3 Never administer medication you have not checked yourself.	3 To reduce the risk of medication error.
4 Obtain equipment needed for the procedure. For all procedures you will need: • Prescription • Medication formulary • Manufacturer's drug information (if required) • Medication • Device for administration • Diluent (if required) • Personal protective equipment (PPE) (if required)	4 To be adequately prepared for dispensing and administering medication.
5 Check the expiry date of all equipment, e.g. syringes.	5 To reduce the risk of harm to the CYP.
6 Refer to local guidelines on writing prescriptions. Check that the prescription is clear and correctly written.	6 To adhere to local policy and national guidance. To reduce the risk of medication error. To reduce the risk of harm to the CYP.
7 Check that the medication is required and has not already been given.	7 To prevent a medication error.
8 Check that the CYP does not have any known allergy or contra-indication to the prescribed medication. If they do, do not give the medication and inform the responsible prescriber immediately.	8 To reduce the risk of medication error and harm to the CYP. To enable the responsible prescriber to make a decision about the CYP's treatment.
9 Check in an approved medication formulary that the dose, route and frequency of the prescribed medication are accurate and ensure that they have been verified by a pharmacist (where necessary).	9 To reduce the risk of medication error and harm to the CYP.
10 If more than one medication is prescribed, check with the prescriber or pharmacist that they are compatible.	10 To reduce the risk of medication error and harm to the CYP. To enable the responsible prescriber to make a decision about the CYP's treatment.
11 Remove the medication from the box/holding the canister and check the name, dose and expiry date of the medication's actual container, e.g. ampoule or canister/inhaler, bottle label.	11 To reduce the risk of a medication error and to ensure that the medication has not been placed in the incorrect box and that the medication is the correct strength.

Principles table 17.1 General guidelines *(continued)*

Principle	Rationale
12 Perform hand hygiene and don appropriate PPE as required.	12 To comply with standard precautions.
13 Dispense the medication according to the CYP's prescription and local policy. **Remember the 6Rs** • Right medicine • Right patient • Right dose • Right route • Right time • Right documentation	13 To reduce the risk of a medication error.
14 Take the medication directly to CYP for administration.	14 To prevent tampering of medication. To prevent misuse of medication by others.
15 Do not attempt to administer medication while the CYP is distressed.	15 To promote the development of a trusting relationship. To reduce the risk of aspiration of medication.
16 Identify if the CYP has any previous experience in taking medication and, if so, what the experience was like.	16 To facilitate the provision of an appropriate explanation of the administration of the medication.
17 a) Explain to the parent/carer and CYP, using age and developmentally appropriate language, what medication is due and why. b) Negotiate roles for the administration of the medication with the CYP and parent/carer.	17 a) To allow them to ask questions and discuss any concerns. b) To work in partnership with the family and obtain informed consent.
18 Check that the name, date of birth and hospital number on the prescription corresponds with the details on the CYP's identification band.	18 To ensure the correct CYP receives the correct medication.
19 Where possible allow the CYP choice and control in the procedure, e.g. they could choose to administer the medicine themselves or with assistance from their parent/carer or nurse. Be firm but fair.	19 Involvement of the CYP and family in decision making can help reduce anxiety and facilitate successful administration of medication.
20 Allow time for the CYP to take the medication.	20 Rushing the CYP could increase feelings of anxiety, which could result in them refusing administration of the medication.
21 Provide positive reinforcement as appropriate during and following administration of medication.	21 To encourage the CYP to take the medication.
22 Assist the CYP in repositioning (if required) to promote comfort following the administration of the medication.	22 To maintain comfort.
23 a) Inform the responsible prescriber if the CYP refuses or is unable to take the medication. b) Document in the appropriate area on the medication chart.	23 a) To maintain safety and enable the responsible prescriber to make a decision regarding the CYP's treatment. b) To maintain accurate records.
24 a) Discard any unused medication in a pharmaceutical waste bin or according to local waste management policy. b) Unused medications should not be flushed down a sink.	24 a) To prevent the misuse of unused medication b) To prevent contamination of water and the environment.
25 Dispose of equipment according to local waste management policy.	25 To minimise the risk of harm.
26 Remove PPE (if worn) and perform hand hygiene.	26 To comply with standard precautions.
27 Record the administration of the medication on the prescription chart/medicine administration system immediately after this has been completed.	27 To maintain an accurate record of medication administered. To reduce the risk of medication being administered twice.
28 Observe, report, and document any reaction or abnormality.	28 To enable the responsible doctor to make a decision about the CYP's treatment, and to maintain accurate records.
29 Observe for and report any adverse effects of the medication immediately to the nurse in charge and responsible prescriber.	29 To facilitate early detection and action of any adverse effects of medication.

Procedure guideline 17.1 Oral medication administration

Statement	Rationale
1 Check the medication supplied is suitable for oral administration.	1 To reduce the risk of error and harm to the CYP.
2 a) Negotiate with the parent/carer and CYP who will be administering the medication (self-administration where possible and agreed) and whether to mix medications with food/drinks. b) The potential benefits and risks of covert administration of medication in fluid or food should be considered carefully by the nurse and parent/carer and be avoided wherever possible.	2 Covert administration of medication should be avoided as this increases mistrust. To reduce the risk of the CYP becoming fearful of medication being hidden in food or drinks.
3 If a choice is available, identify the CYP's preference for the form of oral medication, e.g. suspension or tablet, and the type of device to be used for administration.	3 To promote the development of a trusting relationship between the CYP, parent/carer and nurse. This also facilitates partnership working with the CYP and parent/carer.
4 Gather equipment as in Section 17.1.4 and additionally: • A spoon, cup, dropper, oral syringe, or pot and tablet cutter as appropriate.	4 To ensure that you are adequately prepared for the procedure.
5 Perform hand hygiene and dispense medication into the appropriate device without directly touching the medication with your hands. Shake the bottle before opening (if required).	5 To comply with standard precautions. To ensure liquid suspension is mixed before administration.
6 a) Sit the CYP upright or hold a baby in their usual feeding position if possible. b) Do not force the medication device into the CYP's mouth. c) The oral syringe/spoon can be inserted into the side of the mouth between the cheek and the gum, or alternatively the syringe/spoon placed onto the tip of the tongue. d) Gently squirt or tip in a small amount and administer slowly.	6 a) To prevent choking and promote safe ingestion. b) To prevent oral trauma and the development of a trusting relationship. c–d) To aid safe administration and prevent choking.
7 a) Ensure the medication is administered slowly. b) Gently stroking the cheek or under the chin may encourage a baby's sucking and swallowing reflexes. c) A medicine spoon can be used to retrieve any medicine spilt on the chin.	7 a) To promote safe ingestion of medication. b) To reduce the risk of the CYP spitting out the medication and to reduce the risk of aspiration of medication. c) To reduce the risk of spillage of medication.
8 Unless contraindicated, offer the CYP a drink or ice cube in-between and after ingestion of medication.	8 To promote ingestion of medication.
9 Dispose of waste following local policy.	9 To dispose of equipment safely.
10 Perform hand hygiene.	10 To comply with standard precautions.
11 Record medication administered.	11 To meet local and legal requirements.

Procedure guideline 17.2 Enteral tube administration

Statement	Rationale
1 Check that the medication supplied is suitable for enteral administration. Refer to the manufacturer's guidelines and liaise with the pharmacist.	1 To reduce the risk of error and harm to the CYP. To promote safe administration of medication. Some medications are not suitable for enteral administration. The dose of medication may differ from other routes of administration.
2 Gather equipment as in Section 17.1.4 and additionally: • Enteral syringe for administration. • Water for flushing. • CE marked universal indicator.	2 To ensure that you are adequately prepared for the procedure.
3 Liaise with dietitian if necessary, to manage the timing of medicine administration and fluid volumes; e.g. the feed regimen may need to be altered to allow for sufficient gaps for administration of incompatible medications. In the patient who is fluid restricted, the volume/type of feed may need altering to allow for the volume of medications and flushes administered.	3 To facilitate adequate hydration and nutrition.
4 a) Perform hand hygiene and prepare the medication using an aseptic nontouch technique, without directly touching it with your hands. b) Use only enteral syringes to draw up medication.	4 a) To comply with standard precautions. b) To prevent the risk of incorrect administration via another route.

Procedure guideline 17.2 Enteral tube administration *(continued)*

Statement	Rationale
5 If the medication is viscous, liaise with the pharmacist regarding alternative preparations of the medication or dissolving the suspension further with sterile water. Also consider flushing the tube with water halfway through administering the medication. NB: Caution should be taken when administering to a CYP who is on restricted fluids.	5 To reduce the risk of enteral tube blockage.
6 Record volume of medication and flush on the CYP's fluid balance chart. The size of the flush is dependent on the size of the CYP, length of the tube and any fluid restrictions.	6 To maintain accurate fluid balance chart.
7 **Orogastric/nasogastric tube:** a) Check the tube is in the correct position prior to medicine administration by placing a small amount of aspirate on CE marked universal pH indicator paper. If unable to obtain aspirate for testing, use alternative method of testing in accordance with local protocol. b) **Use a syringe of 20 ml or greater in size to aspirate the tube.** c) Once the position has been confirmed, flush the tube with 5–10 ml of sterile water. d) Administer the medication slowly. e) Stop administering the medication if aspiration is suspected and inform the nurse in charge/responsible prescriber. f) Flush the tube with 5–10 ml of sterile water between medications. g) Flush the tube with a turbulent flush with 5–10 ml of sterile water after administration of medications.	7 a) To check position of tube and promote safe administration of medication (for more information see Chapter 22: Nutrition and Feeding). b) **Smaller syringes create high intraluminal pressures and can cause damage to the tube** (White and Bradnam 2015). c) To ensure the tube is clear for administration of medication and to reduce the risk of tube blockage. d) To reduce the risk of aspiration of medication. e) To promote early detection and prompt action of complications. f) To reduce the risk of tube blockage. g) To reduce the risk of medication remaining in the tube resulting in the CYP not receiving the full dose of the medication at the prescribed time.
8 **Nasoduodenal/nasojejunal tube:** a) Liaise with the pharmacist as many medicines are not suitable for nasoduodenal/nasojejunal administration. b) Check the tube is in the correct position prior to feeding by confirming the length of tube left outside of the body against the length documented from insertion in the patient's notes (see Chapter 22: Nutrition and Feeding). If uncertain of position, use alternative method of testing in accordance with hospital protocol. c) Flush the tube with a turbulent flush with 3–5 ml of sterile water (1–2 ml for neonates). d) Administer the medication slowly. e) Stop administering the medication if aspiration is suspected and inform the nurse in charge/responsible prescriber. f) Flush the tube with 3–5 ml of sterile water between medications (1–2 ml for neonates). g) Flush the tube with 3–5 ml (1–2 ml for neonates) of sterile water after administration of medications.	8 a) To promote safe administration of medication. b) To reduce the risk of a medical error and harm to the CYP. c) To ensure the tube is clear for administration of medication and to reduce the risk of tube blockage. d) To reduce the risk of aspiration of medication. e) To promote early detection and prompt action of the complications. f) To reduce the risk of tube blockage. g) To reduce the risk of medication remaining in the tube resulting in the CYP not receiving an accurate dose of medication at prescribed time and to reduce the risk of tube blockage.
9 **Gastrostomy:** a) Using a syringe size no smaller than 20 ml, flush the tube with 5–10 ml sterile water. b) Administer the medication slowly. c) Stop administering the medication if CYP appears in discomfort or becomes distressed and inform the nurse in charge/responsible prescriber. d) Flush the tube with 5–10 ml of sterile water between medications. e) Flush the tube with 10–20 ml of sterile water after administration of medications.	9 a) To ensure the tube is clear for administration of medication, and to reduce the risk of tube blockage. b) To reduce the risk of aspiration of medication. c) To promote early detection and prompt action of complications. d) To reduce the risk of tube blockage. e) To reduce the risk of medication remaining in the tube resulting in the CYP not receiving an accurate dose of medication at prescribed time and to reduce the risk of tube blockage.

(continued)

Procedure guideline 17.2 Enteral tube administration *(continued)*

Statement	Rationale
10 **Jejunostomy:** a) Liaise with the ward pharmacist, as many medicines are **not** suitable for jejunostomy administration. b) Using a syringe no smaller than 20 ml, flush the tube with 5–10– ml of sterile water. c) Administer the medication slowly. d) Stop administering the medication if patient appears in discomfort or becomes distressed and inform the nurse in charge/responsible prescriber. e) Flush the tube with 5–10– ml of sterile water between medications,. f) Flush the tube with 5–10 ml of sterile water after administration of medications.	10 a) To promote safe administration of medication and to reduce the risk of a medical error. To reduce the risk of harm to the CYP. b) To ensure the tube is clear for administration of medication and to reduce the risk of tube blockage. c) To promote the safe administration of medication and to reduce the risk of aspiration of medication. d) To promote early detection and prompt action of the complications. e) To reduce the risk of tube blockage and ensure that the CYP receives the whole dose. f) To reduce the risk of tube blockage.
11 Dispose of waste according to local policy.	11 To dispose of equipment safely.
12 Perform hand hygiene.	12 To comply with standard precautions.
13 Record medication administered.	13 To meet local and legal requirements.

Procedure guideline 17.3 Buccal and sublingual administration

Statement	Rationale
1 a) Check the medication supplied is suitable for buccal or sublingual administration. b) Gather equipment as in Section 17.1.4 and additionally: • Oral syringe (for liquid form of medication)	1 a) To reduce the risk of medical error and harm to the CYP. b) To prepare for the procedure.
2 Perform hand hygiene and draw up a suspension medication into an appropriate size syringe, e.g. a 1 ml syringe calibrated with 0.1 ml increments for doses less than 1 ml, or use prefilled oral syringes.	2 To facilitate accurate measurement and administration of medication.
3 If a tablet form of medication is being used, dispense the tablet into a medicine pot or spoon without touching it.	3 To reduce the risk of cross-infection. In addition, contact with skin could initiate breakdown of the medication.
4 Allow time for the CYP to take the medication.	4 Rushing the CYP could increase feelings of anxiety, which could result in the CYP refusing administration of the medication.
5 Advise the CYP not to swallow the medication.	5 To promote safe administration and absorption of the medication.
6 Check the condition of the CYP's buccal or sublingual area (depending on the route of administration prescribed). Refer to the responsible prescriber if abrasions or lesions are observed.	6 To reduce the risk of harm to the CYP. To enable the responsible prescriber to make a decision about the child/young person's treatment.
7 Do not force the syringe containing the liquid preparation of medication into the CYP's mouth.	7 To reduce the risk of oral trauma, as well as to promote a trusting relationship.
8 **Buccal administration:** • Slowly administer small amounts of liquid medication between the CYP's facial cheek and upper or lower gum. • Administer half of the medication on each side of the mouth (see Figure 17.1). • If a tablet form is being used, place the tablet in between the CYP's facial cheek and lower gum.	8 To promote successful absorption of the medication and minimise the risk of it being swallowed, aspirated or spat out.
9 **Sublingual administration:** Place the tablet preparation or slowly administer small amounts of the liquid medication into the space under the CYP's tongue (Figure 17.4).	9 To reduce the risk of spillage of the medication. To promote safe absorption of the medication.
10 Ensure the CYP does not have any oral fluid or food until all the medication has been absorbed.	10 To promote successful absorption of the medication.
11 Dispose of waste according to local policy.	11 To dispose of equipment safely.
12 Perform hand hygiene.	12 To comply with standard precautions.
13 Record medication administered.	13 To meet local and legal requirements.

Procedure guideline 17.4 Intranasal administration

Statement	Rationale
1 Check the medication supplied is suitable for nasal administration.	1 To reduce the risk of medical error and to reduce the risk of harm to the CYP.
2 Check the condition of the CYP's nostrils. Refer to the responsible prescriber if any abrasions, lesions, or other contraindications are observed.	2 To reduce the risk of harm to the CYP and enable the responsible prescriber to make a decision regarding treatment.
3 If appropriate ask the CYP to gently blow their nose to clear any congestion.	3 To promote safe administration of the medication.
4 Perform hand hygiene.	4 To comply with standard precautions
5 **Intranasal spray** a) Intranasal medication in spray form should be labelled with the CYP's name and hospital number and for individual use only. b) Ensure the spray nozzle is primed before use. c) Assist the CYP as necessary in repositioning for administration of medication. Unless contraindicated by their condition or treatment, the CYP should be assisted to sit or stand upright with their head upright or neck hyperextended. d) Do not force the nozzle into the CYP's nostrils. e) Block one nostril and insert the spray nozzle gently into the opposite nostril (just inside at the midline) and administer one spray. If more than one spray is prescribed both nostrils should be used. If appropriate ask the CYP to gently inhale the medication into the nostril as the spray is squeezed. f) Refer to manufacturer's guidelines regarding cleaning the spray nozzle.	5 a) To reduce the risk of cross-infection. b) To promote safe administration of the medication. c) To promote comfort and reduce the risk of leakage of the medication. d) To reduce the risk of nasal trauma and facilitate safe administration of intranasal medication. e) Touching the external nares could stimulate sneezing. f) To reduce the risk of infection.
6 **Intranasal dropper** a) Intranasal medication in dropper form should be labelled with the CYP's name and hospital number and for individual use only. b) Assist the CYP as necessary in repositioning for administration of medication. Unless contraindicated by their condition or treatment, the CYP should be assisted to either lie supine with the neck hyperextended or sit with their back tilted backwards and neck hyperextended. A pillow can be placed behind the CYP's neck to assist with positioning and comfort. c) Do not force the dropper into the CYP's nostrils. The dropper should be positioned at the midline entry of the nostril and the rubber top of the dropper squeezed to administer one drop into the nostril. If more than one drop is prescribed, both nostrils should be used.	6 a) To reduce the risk of cross-infection and to promote safe administration of the medication. b) To promote comfort and reduce the risk of leakage of the medication. c) To reduce the risk of nasal trauma and to promote safe intranasal administration of medication. d) Touching the external nares could stimulate sneezing.
7 **Intranasal medication via syringe** a) Draw up the suspension medication into an appropriate size syringe. b) Assist the CYP as necessary in repositioning for administration of medication. Unless contraindicated by their condition or treatment, the CYP should be assisted to either lie supine with the neck hyperextended or sit with their back tilted backwards and neck hyperextended. A pillow can be placed behind the CYP's neck to assist with positioning and comfort. c) Do not force the syringe into the CYP's nostrils. d) Gently insert the tip of the syringe at the midline of the nostril and administer small amounts of the medication slowly. Administer half of the medication into each nostril.	7 a) To facilitate accurate measurement and administration of medication and to promote safe administration of the medication. b) To promote comfort and reduce the risk of leakage of the medication. c) To reduce the risk of nasal trauma. d) To promote safe intranasal absorption of medication and reduce the risk of leakage to the medication. e) Touching the external nares could stimulate sneezing.
8 **Encourage the CYP not to blow their nose until all the medication has been absorbed.**	8 To promote safe intranasal absorption of medication and to reduce the risk of leakage of the medication.

(continued)

Procedure guideline 17.4 Intranasal administration (continued)

Statement	Rationale
9 a) **Use gauze or tissue to wipe any observed leakage following administration of medication and** b) **Inform the responsible prescriber.** c) **Document the incident in the appropriate area on the medication chart.**	9 a) To maintain the CYP's safety. b) To enable the responsible prescriber to make a decision regarding treatment. c) To maintain accurate records.
10 Dispose of waste according to policy.	10 To safely dispose of equipment.
11 Perform hand hygiene.	11 To comply with standard precautions.
12 Record medication administered.	12 To meet local and legal requirements.

Procedure guideline 17.5 Inhalation administration

Statement	Rationale
1 Check the medication supplied is suitable for inhalation administration.	1 To reduce the risk of error and harm to the CYP.
2 a) Assess the CYP's respiratory function, e.g. respiratory rate and effort, skin colour etc., prior to the administration of the medication. b) Gather equipment as in Section 17.1.4 and additionally: • Inhaler with spacer and mask (if required) OR • nebuliser pot and mask or mouthpiece.	2 a) To enable monitoring of medication effects on condition. b) To prepare for the procedure.
3 Perform hand hygiene.	3 To comply with standard precautions.
4 **Nebuliser** a) Dispense the correct amount of nebuliser solution into the nebuliser pot. Further dilute to the volume recommended by the manufacturers. b) Assist the CYP as necessary in repositioning for administration of medication. Unless contraindicated by their condition or treatment, they should be assisted to sit upright with their head forward. c) Connect the nebuliser to either the mask or mouthpiece and then to the tubing. Connect the tubing (connected to the nebuliser pot) to the gas supply or compressor. d) Place the mouthpiece in the CYP's mouth, ensuring that they form a seal around the mouthpiece, or place the mask gently over the CYP's mouth and nose. The nebuliser pot should remain vertical/upright throughout the nebulisation. e) Turn the air or oxygen (if prescribed) flow to 8–10 l/min. f) Encourage the CYP to breathe in and out slowly and gently, if appropriate for their age and development. g) Tap the nebuliser pot gently occasionally during administration until all the solution has evaporated. h) Observe and document the CYP's condition during and after the administration of medication. i) When administration is complete, the CYP should rinse their mouth. j) After administration, either discard the nebuliser pot or dismantle and wash it according to manufacturer's guidelines, allow to dry, and store for the same CYP's use only.	4 a) To ensure effective delivery of the medication. b) To increase lung capacity and maximise absorption of the medication. c) To promote safe administration of the medication. d) To promote absorption of the medication. e) To promote the safe delivery of the medication. f) To promote absorption of the medication. g) To ensure the large droplets are shaken down and the medication is delivered. h) To monitor the effectiveness of the treatment. i) To reduce systemic absorption of the medication. j) To reduce the risk of infection.

Procedure guideline 17.5 Inhalation administration *(continued)*

Statement	Rationale
5 **Inhaler with small volume extended mouthpiece spacer (baby or toddler under 5 years old)** a) Position the baby or toddler lying supine. b) Attach the appropriate size mask to the spacer mouthpiece, if required. c) Remove the protective cap from the inhaler device, shake the inhaler thoroughly and insert into the back of spacer. d) Place the mouthpiece of the spacer in the child's mouth and ensure they seal their lips around the mouthpiece, or position the mask gently over the baby/toddler's nose and mouth and form a seal. e) Encourage the child to breathe in and out slowly and gently, if appropriate for their age and development. A whistling sound may be heard if they breathe too quickly. However, this sound may not be heard if using a small volume extended mouthpiece with a mask. When this is established, actuate the medication inhaler once, with your free hand. f) Hold the spacer in position, while the child takes several breaths. Then remove it from their mouth. g) Wait for 30 seconds, before administering a second dose. If this is required, repeat points d–f. h) When administration is complete, rinse the child's mouth.	5 a) To promote the safe delivery of the medication. b) To promote absorption of the medication. c) To promote the safe delivery of the medication. d) To promote absorption of the medication. e) To promote the safe delivery of the medication, to promote absorption of the medication. f) To promote the absorption of the medication and increase lung capacity. g) To promote the safe delivery of the medication. h) To reduce systematic absorption of the medication.
6 **Inhaler with small volume extended mouthpiece spacer (CYPs 5–15 years old)** a) Assist the CYP as necessary in repositioning for administration of medication. Unless contraindicated by their condition or treatment, they should be assisted to sit or stand upright. b) Attach the appropriate size mask to the spacer mouthpiece, if required. c) Remove the protective cap from the inhaler device. Shake the inhaler thoroughly and insert it into the back of the spacer. Place the mouthpiece of the spacer in the CYP's mouth and ensure they seal their lips around the mouthpiece, or position the mask gently over the CYP's nose and mouth and form a seal. Actuate the medication inhaler once, to release a dose of medication. d) Encourage the CYP to take a slow deep breath in. A whistling sound may be heard if they breathe too quickly. However, this sound may not be heard if using a small volume extended mouthpiece with a mask. Encourage the CYP to hold their breath for about 10 seconds, then breathe out through the mouthpiece and to breathe in again but not to actuate the inhaler and release another dose of medication. Then remove the mouthpiece from the CYP's mouth and ask them to breathe out. Wait for a few seconds, before administering a second dose if required, repeat points c and d. e) When administration is complete, ask the CYP to rinse their mouth.	6 a) To promote the safe delivery of the medication. b) To promote absorption of the medication. c) To promote absorption of the medication. d) To reduce systemic absorption of the medication and promote the absorption of the medication and increase lung capacity. e) To reduce systemic absorption of the medication.

(continued)

Procedure guideline 17.5 Inhalation administration *(continued)*

Statement	Rationale

7 **Pressurised metered dose inhaler (pMDIs)**
   a) When not using spacers, inhaler devices should be labelled with the CYP's name and hospital number and be for individual use only.
   b) Assist the CYP as necessary in repositioning for administration of medication. Unless contraindicated by their condition or treatment, they should be assisted to sit or stand upright. Remove the protective cap from the inhaler device. Shake the inhaler thoroughly. Ask the CYP to breathe out. Then place the mouthpiece of the inhaler in their mouth and ensure they seal their lips around the mouthpiece. Encourage them to take a slow deep breath in, simultaneously pressing the inhaler once, on inhalation. Then hold their breath for about 5–10 seconds.
   c) Remove the device from their mouth and ask them to breathe out.
   d) Wait for a few seconds, prior to administering a second dose if required then repeat points b and c.
   e) When administration is complete, ask the CYP to rinse their mouth.
	7
	   a) To promote the safe delivery of the medication.
	
	   b) To promote the safe delivery of the medication and promote absorption of the medication.
	
	   c) To reduce systemic absorption of the medication.
	
	   d) To promote the absorption of the medication and increase lung capacity.
	   e) To reduce systematic absorption of the medication.

8 **Breath-actuated pressurised metered dose inhaler or dry powder inhalers (DPIs)**
   a) When not using spacers, inhaler devices should be labelled with the CYP's name and hospital number and for individual use only.
   b) Assist the CYP as necessary in repositioning for administration of medication. Unless contraindicated by their condition or treatment, they should be assisted to sit or stand upright. Remove protective cap from the inhaler device. Shake the inhaler thoroughly or preload the dry powder inhaler. Ask the CYP to breathe out. Place the mouthpiece of the inhaler in their mouth and ensure they seal their lips around the mouthpiece.
   c) Encourage them to take a sharp, deep breath in; to hold their breath for about 5–10 seconds; then, remove the device from their mouth and breathe out.
   d) Wait for a few seconds, prior to administering a second dose, and if this is required; repeat points a and b.
   e) When administration is complete, ask the CYP to rinse their mouth.
	8
	
	   a) To promote the safe delivery of the medication.
	
	   b) To promote safe delivery of the medication.
	
	   c) To promote absorption of the medication.
	
	   d) To promote absorption of the medication.
	
	   e) To reduce systemic absorption of the medication.

9 Dispose of waste according to local policy.	9 To prevent cross infection.
10 Perform hand hygiene.	10 To comply with standard precautions.
11 Record medication administered.	11 To meet local and legal requirements.

Procedure guideline 17.6 Rectal administration

Statement	Rationale

1 a) Check that the medication supplied is suitable for rectal administration.
   b) Gather equipment as in Section 17.1.4 and additionally:
     • Water-soluble lubricant or warm water
     • Incontinence pad
	1 a) To reduce the risk of medical error.
	
	   b) To prepare for the procedure.

2 Advise the CYP to open their bowels if necessary and appropriate prior to administration of rectal medication.	2 To reduce the risk of expulsion and promote absorption of rectal medication.
3 Perform hand hygiene and apply nonsterile gloves and apron.	3 To comply with standard precautions.

Procedure guideline 17.6 Rectal administration *(continued)*

Statement	Rationale
4 Assist the CYP as necessary in repositioning for administration of the medication. Unless contraindicated by condition or treatment, ask the CYP to lie on their left side with their left leg in a flexed position. Babies can also be positioned supine with their legs elevated and flexed. The CYP can be in any of the following positions: • Squatting down • Lying on one side with one leg straight and the other bent • Standing up with one leg raised	4 To promote safe administration of the medication. To ensure smooth insertion of suppository or enema. To reduce risk of harm to the CYP.
5 Check the condition of the perianal area. Do not administer the medication if abrasions, lesions, or any abnormality are observed. Inform the responsible doctor immediately.	5 To reduce the risk of harm to the CYP.
6 **Suppositories** a) Remove the suppository from its plastic cover and unless contraindicated, lubricate the pointed end of the suppository with a water-soluble lubricant or warm water. Gently lift the CYP's right buttock and insert suppository, pointed end first, fully into the rectum against the rectum wall, using the index finger. Alternatively, support the CYP with self-administration. b) Where possible, gently hold buttocks together after insertion, c) Unless being given to relieve constipation, encourage the CYP not to have a bowel action for as long as they feel comfortable.	a) To facilitate insertion of the suppository. b) To reduce the risk of expulsion of the suppository. c) To allow time for absorption of the suppository. The onset of action for a suppository depends on the time it takes to dissolve, which can be 3–50 minutes depending on its ingredients.
7 **Suppositories via a ileostomy and colostomy** Suppositories can be inserted into a well-established colostomy or a rectal stump with a good blood supply, using the same principles as above.	7 To use appropriate route of administration.
8 **Medicated enemas** a) Position an incontinence pad underneath the CYP. b) Remove the lid of the enema tube and, if necessary, lubricate the nozzle with either water-soluble lubricant or warm water. NB: Refer to manufacturer's guidelines as some enemas are now designed with prelubricated nozzles. c) Lift the CYP's right buttock and gently insert the nozzle of the enema into the rectum. d) Gently squeeze the contents of the enema into the rectum, maintaining pressure on the enema until it is removed from the rectum. e) Hold the CYP's buttocks together for a few minutes. f) Where possible encourage the CYP not to have a bowel action for as long as feels comfortable.	8 a) To minimise the risk of disruption due to the CYP spillage of the enema or leakage of bowel contents onto bed linen. b) To facilitate insertion. d) To prevent backflow of the contents of the enema. e)-f) To reduce the risk of expulsion and allow time for absorption of the enema. For management of constipation, see Chapter 5: Bowel Care.
9 Provide positive reinforcement as appropriate during and following administration of the medication.	9 To encourage the CYP to take the medication.
10 Utilise distraction techniques such as asking the CYP to whistle / blow if they are CYP clenching their buttocks.	10 To facilitate administration of rectal medication. The procedure will be more comfortable if the CYP is relaxed.
11 Dispose of waste according to local policy.	11 To dispose of equipment safely.
12 Perform hand hygiene.	12 To comply with standard precautions.
13 Record medication administered.	13 To meet local and legal requirements.

The Great Ormond Street Hospital Manual of Children and Young People's Nursing Practices

Procedure guideline 17.7 Preparation of medication for injections using an aseptic nontouch technique

Statement	Rationale
1 **Medicated solution in a glass vial** a) Perform hand hygiene. b) Tap the top of the vial gently to move any medication into the lower part of the vial. c) Cover the top of the vial with the inside of a sterile alcohol wipe package and break open the vial on the premarked line. d) Inspect the medicated solution for any glass fragments or signs of contamination. Discard if any signs are observed and start the procedure again. e) Insert the filter needle or needle size 23 G attached to the syringe into the vial and withdraw the prescribed amount of medication with the vial held tilted upside down, keeping the tip of the needle below the level of the medication. f) With caution recap the needle after removal from the vial. g) Hold the syringe in a vertical position and tap the syringe gently to expel the air bubbles. h) Remove the needle and attach an appropriate size needle depending on the route of administration. Syringes are calibrated to give the correct volume of medication accounting for the medication that remains in the hub of the syringe and needle after administration.	1 a) To comply with standard precautions. b) To facilitate collection of medication. c) To reduce the risk of glass injury. d) To reduce the risk of harm to the CYP. e) To reduce the risk of contamination of medication with shards of glass after opening the vial. f) To reduce the risk of needle-stick injury. g) To ensure the correct amount of medication is administered. h) To reduce the risk of harm and accidental tracking of medication.
2 **Freeze dried medication in a rubber-topped vial** a) Perform hand hygiene and don chemotherapy gloves if drawing up cytotoxic drugs. b) Remove the metal/plastic cap and clean the rubber bung on the top of the vial using a 70% isopropyl alcohol wipe for at least 15 seconds and allow to dry. c) Do not touch the rubber bung after cleaning it. d) Refer to manufacturer's and pharmacy guidelines for the type and volume of diluents suitable for dissolving the freeze-dried medication. e) Draw up the appropriate volume of diluent with a filter needle or needle size 23 G and syringe. f) Insert the needle into the rubber top of the vial and inject the required volume of diluent slowly into the vial. g) Allow the freeze-dried medication to disperse completely in the solution. h) Check the dissolved medication for any signs of contamination, e.g. cloudiness. If any signs of contamination are observed discard and start the procedure again. i) Using the same syringe and needle as used for diluting, withdraw all the medication with the vial held tilted upside down, keeping the tip of the needle below the level of the medication. j) Recap the needle after removal from the vial. k) Hold the syringe in a vertical position and tap the syringe gently to expel the air bubbles. l) Discard (according to local waste management policy), any additional medication from the syringe in a pharmaceutical waste bin, leaving the prescribed amount of medication in the syringe. m) Remove the needle and attach an appropriately sized new needle, depending on the route of administration.	2 a) To comply with standard precautions. b) To reduce the risk of cross-infection. c) To reduce the risk of cross-infection. d) To account for displacement volumes when reconstituting the medication so that the correct dose is administered. e) To reduce the risk of contamination with particles of rubber through the rubber bung on the vial. f) Fast injection of the diluent can create bubbles in the vial. g) To ensure the correct dose of medication is administered. h) To reduce the risk of harm to the CYP. i) To ensure the medication is in the correct volume of solution. j) To reduce the risk of needle-stick injury. k) To reduce the risk of harm to the CYP and ensure the correct amount of medication is administered. l) To ensure the correct amount of medication is administered. m) Syringes are calibrated to give the correct volume of medication accounting for the medication that remains in the hub of the syringe and needle after administration, to reduce the risk of tracking of medication during administration.
3 After the procedure: a) Dispose of waste according to local policy. b) Perform hand hygiene. c) Record medication administered.	 a) To dispose of equipment safely. b) To comply with standard precautions c) To meet local and legal requirements.

Procedure guideline 17.8 Intradermal (ID) administration

Statement	Rationale
1 Check the medication supplied is suitable for ID administration.	1 To reduce the risk of medication error.
2 Prepare and administer medication using aseptic nontouch technique.	2 To reduce the risk of cross-infection.
3 Perform hand hygiene and don PPE.	3 To comply with standard precautions.
4 a) Prepare the medications for injection (see procedure guideline 17.7). b) Check the medication supplied is suitable for ID administration: Volume should be 0.5 ml or less.	4 a) To ensure safe preparation of the medication. b) To reduce the risk of medication error.
5 If not using a prefilled syringe, draw up medication using a 1 ml syringe calibrated in 0.01 ml increments,. a) You will need to use a 26 G 10 mm needle for administration (PHE 2013).	5 To ensure the correct amount of medication is administered, and to reduce the risk of medical error. a) To ensure the medication is delivered to the intradermal layer.
6 If air bubbles are present in the syringe, tap the syringe gently with your hand and expel the air bubbles.	6 To ensure the correct amount of medication is administered, and to reduce the risk of harm to the CYP.
7 Utilise distraction techniques with the assistance of parent/carer or play specialist as appropriate.	7 To reduce fear (Dahlquist et al 2002).
8 Identify an appropriate site for administration of the medication. Do not use an area that feels tender, hard, or lumpy if the CYP is having regular ID injections.	8 To reduce the risk of a fibrous area developing and to promote effective absorption of the medication.
9 Check the site is clean.	9 To reduce risk of infection.
10 Choose the site; ensure the skin is not highly pigmented, or keratinised, or covered with hair, i.e. median inner forearm area or between the scapulae. Avoid moles, lesions and scars.	10 To promote effective absorption of the medication.
11 Stretch the skin taut between thumb and forefinger with the nondominant hand.	11 Making the skin taut makes needle entry smoother
12 With the other hand insert the needle into the skin with the bevel up, at a 10–15° angle (almost parallel with the surface) to the depth of 2–5 mm just under the epidermis.	12 To avoid the risk of accidental subcutaneous administration of medication.
13 When administering the medication, a raised blanched bleb (blister or large vesicle) or small wheal may form around the injection site.	13 This is a sign of correct administration of the medication.
14 Administer the medication according to manufacturer's guidelines.	14 To administer the medication correctly and prevent a medication error.
15 Do not massage the site following administration of medication.	15 Massaging the site could cause additional discomfort.
16 Do not resheath the needle after administration of the medication.	16 To reduce the risk of needle-stick injury.
17 Dispose of sharps and other equipment according to trust waste management policy.	17 To reduce the risk of needle-stick injury and to dispose of equipment safely.
18 Check injection site and surrounding area.	18 To observe site for any signs of inflammatory reaction and taken appropriate action if required.
19 Perform hand hygiene.	19 To comply with standard precautions.
20 Record medication administered. a) This may include site of administration. b) Observe, report and document any local reaction or abnormality at the site of injection.	20 To meet local and legal requirements. a) To enable monitoring for signs of reaction. b) To facilitate early detection of and prompt action to manage any complications.

Procedure guideline 17.9 Subcutaneous (SC) administration

Statement	Rationale
1 Check the medication supplied is suitable for SC administration.	1 To reduce the risk of medication error.
2 Perform hand hygiene and don PPE.	2 To comply with standard precautions.
3 Prepare and administer medication using aseptic nontouch technique.	3 To reduce the risk of cross infection.
4 Refer to preparation of medications for injections (see procedure guideline 17.7).	4 Safe preparation of medication.
5 Remove the needle used for preparation of medication and attach an appropriate size needle. a) Needle length and gauge will depend on the size of the CYP: 23G (blue) or 25G (orange), length 16mm, or insulin needle (Shin and Kim 2006).	5 Syringes are calibrated to give the correct volume of medication accounting for the medication that remains in the hub of the syringe and needle after administration. a) The needle needs to be long enough to deliver the medication to the SC tissue without penetrating the intramuscular layer.
6 Utilise distraction techniques with the assistance of parent/carer and/or play specialist as appropriate.	6 Distraction could help reduce any feelings of anxiety the CYP experiences.
7 Identify an appropriate site for administration of the medication. For daily injections, ensure rotation of injection sites (see Figure 17.2a). Do not use an area that feels tender, hard, or lumpy. Ensure injection sites are rotated if the CYP is having regular SC injections or cannulas.	7 To reduce the risk of SC fibrosis. To promote effective absorption of medication.
8 **When using a needle and syringe** a) Check the site is clean. b) Gently bunch up a small area of skin and SC tissue; aspiration is not necessary. Insert the needle with the cut angle facing upwards at 90° when using a short insulin needle, but at 45° if the needle length is greater than 8mm or if the CYP does not have much SC tissue (Annersten and Willman 2005) - see Figure 17.5. The needle entry should be quick. Push the plunger on the syringe slowly and smoothly to administer the medication. c) Release the grip on the skin and SC tissue and withdraw the needle quickly. d) Do not massage the site following administration of medication. e) Use gauze to apply gentle pressure if the injection site bleeds. f) Do not resheath the needle after administration of the medication. g) Dispose of sharps in a sharps bin and equipment according to local waste management policy. Perform hand hygiene. h) Document administration of medicine. This may include the site of administration. i) Observe, report, and document any local reaction or abnormality at the site of administration.	8 a) To reduce risk of infection. b) To reduce the risk of accidental IM administration of medication. To reduce the risk of pain from the needle insertion. c) To reduce the risk of accidental administration of IV medication. d) To reduce the risk of haematoma formation and additional discomfort. e) To reduce the risk of leakage of the medication. f) To reduce the risk of needle-stick injury. g) To dispose of equipment safely and comply with standard precautions. h) To follow local and legal requirements. i) To facilitate early detection of and prompt action to manage any complications. To maintain accurate records.
9 **Inserting a SC cannula** a) Check that the medication supplied is suitable for administration via SC cannula. Check the packaging is intact and expiry date is valid before removing the SC cannula from its packaging. b) Check the site is clean. Consider cleansing the site for administration of medication with a sterile alcohol impregnated wipe using a circular movement, moving from inwards out for 30 seconds and allow to dry. c) Gently bunch up a small area of skin and SC tissue with the nondominant hand. Holding the cannula between the forefinger and thumb of the dominant hand insert the full length of the needle at a 45° angle, bevel upwards. d) Holding the SC cannula in position, release the bunched-up skin and SC tissue and slowly remove the needle from the cannula. e) Secure the SC cannula with a nonocclusive adhesive dressing.	9 a) To reduce the risk of medical error. b) To minimise the risk of infection. c) To reduce the risk of accidental IM administration of medication. d) To reduce the risk of harm to the CYP. e) To facilitate observation of cannula site

Chapter 17 Administration of medicines

Procedure guideline 17.9 Subcutaneous (SC) administration *(continued)*

Statement	Rationale

10 **Administering medication via a SC cannula**
Insert the needle attached to the syringe of medication into the SC cannula bung and slowly inject the medication into the cannula.
  a) Remove the needle and syringe from the cannula bung after the medication has been administered.
  b) Document date of insertion of SC cannula and refer to manufacturer's guidelines regarding length of time the SC cannula can remain in situ.
	
	a) To ensure accurate record keeping and minimise the risk of infection.
	b) To reduce the risk of harm to the CYP.

11 Observe, report, and document any local reaction or abnormality at the site of SC cannulation.
  The SC cannula should be removed/replaced if any of the following are observed:
  • Redness
  • Pain
  • Swelling
  • Fibrosis
  • Leakage.
	11 To facilitate the early detection of and prompt action to manage any complications.

12 Place sharps in a sharps bin and dispose of all waste according to local policy.	12 To dispose of equipment safely.
13 Perform hand hygiene.	13 To comply with standard precautions.
14 Record medication administered.	14 To meet local and legal requirements.

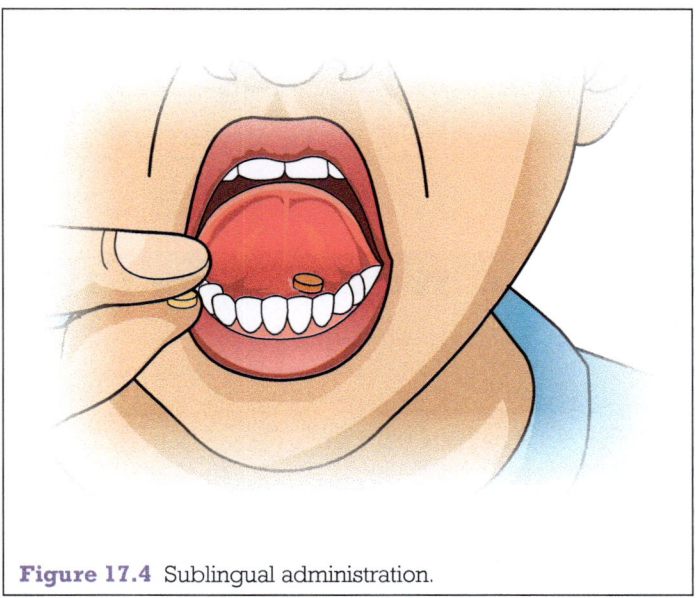

Figure 17.4 Sublingual administration.

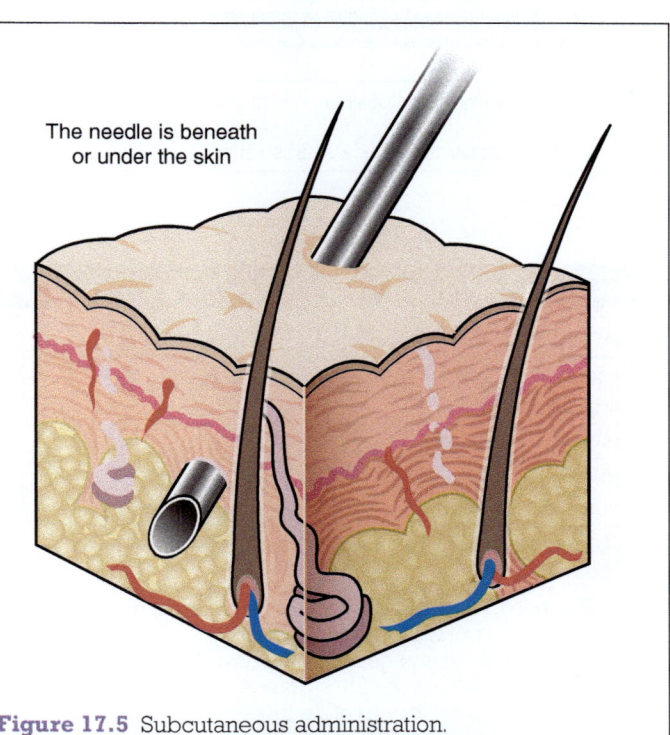

Figure 17.5 Subcutaneous administration.

How to Administer Intramuscular (IM) Injections

Patient age	Site	Needle size	Needle insertion
Infants (birth to 12 mos. of age)	Vastus lateralis muscle in anterolateral aspect of middle or upper thigh	7/8" to 1" needle, 23–25 gauge	Use a needle long enough to reach deep into the muscle. Insert needle at an 80–90° angle to the skin with a quick thrust. There are no data to document the necessity of aspiration." Multiple injections given in the same extremity should be separated by a minimum of 1". *American Academy of Pediatrics 2000 Red Rock Respect of the Committee on Infectious Disease: p.18.
Young children (12 to 36 mos, of age)	Vastus lateralis muscle preferred until deltoid muscle has developed adequate mass	7/8" to 1" needle, 23–25 gauge	
Older children (>36 mos. of age) and adults	Thickest portion of deltoid muscle—above level of armpit and below acromion	1" to 1" needle, 23–25 gauge	

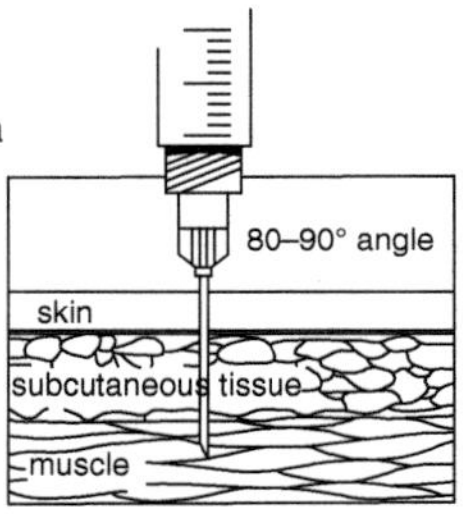

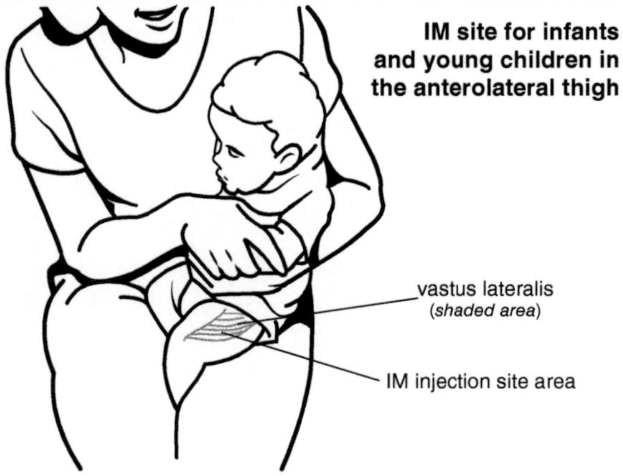

IM site for infants and young children in the anterolateral thigh

Insert needle at an 80–90° angle into vastus lateralis muscle in the anerolateral aspect of middle or upper thigh.

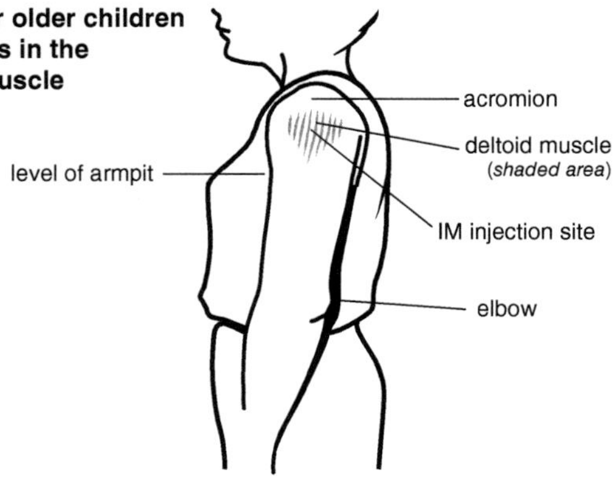

IM site for older children and adults in the deltoid muscle

Insert needle at an 80–90° angle into densest portion of deltoid muscle—above the level of armpit and below the acromion.

Adapted by the Immunization Action Coalition courtesy of the Microsoft Department of Health

Immunization Action Coalition • 1573 Selby Aye,. Ste. 234 • St.Paul. MN 55104 • (651) 647-9009 • www.immunize.org • admin@immunize.org

Figure 17.6 Intramuscular administration.

Procedure guideline 17.10 Intramuscular (IM) administration

Statement	Rationale
1 Check the medication supplied is suitable for IM administration.	1 To reduce the risk of medical error and harm to the CYP.
2 Perform hand hygiene and don PPE.	2 To comply with standard precautions.
3 Prepare and administer medication using an aseptic nontouch technique.	3 To minimise the risk of infection.
4 Refer to preparation of medications for injections (see Procedure Guideline 17.7).	4 For safe preparation of medication.
5 a) Remove the needle used for preparation of medication and attach an appropriate size needle. b) Needle length and gauge will depend on the size of the CYP: A 23 G(blue) or 25 G(orange), length 25 mm (short 25G available for premature infants).	5 a) Syringes are calibrated to give the correct volume of medication accounting for the medication that remains in the hub of the syringe and needle after administration. b) The needle must be long enough to deliver the medication to the IM layer.
6 Utilise distraction techniques with the assistance of parent/carer and/or play specialist as appropriate.	6 To reduce any feelings of anxiety the CYP experiences (Dahlquist et al 2002).
7 Identify an appropriate site for administration of the medication (See Figure 17.6). Do not use an area that feels tender, hard or lumpy. Ensure injection sites are rotated if the CYP is having regular IM injections.	7 To promote effective absorption of medication. To reduce the risk of muscle fibrosis.

Procedure guideline 17.10 Intramuscular (IM) administration *(continued)*

Statement	Rationale
8 Unless administering a vaccine, cleanse the skin with a sterile alcohol impregnated wipe, using a circular movement, from the centre outwards for 30 seconds and allow to dry. A sterile 70% alcohol swab (e.g. Steret®) is recommended. Allow to dry before the injection. **There is more than one technique for administering IM injections – they are described here.**	8 To reduce the risk of infection.
9 **Skin stretch technique** Stretch the skin between the forefinger and thumb of one hand and, using the other hand, insert the needle in a dartlike motion at a 90°angle and then release the stretch on the skin (DH 2013).	9 To reduce the risk of accidental SC administration of medication in obese CYPs.
10 **Pinch up technique** Gently pinch up a small area of skin, SC tissue, and muscle and insert the needle in a dart like motion at a 90° angle and then release the pinched-up skin.	10 To maximise access to muscle and reduce the risk of hitting bone in CYPs with wasted muscle.
11 **Z-track technique** Push the skin down and then pull the skin taut in one direction. Then insert the needle in a dartlike motion at a 90° angle and keep the pull on the skin until the needle is ready for removal from the site (Dougherty et al. 2015). This technique requires the co-operation of the CYP and is not advised for immunisations.	11 To reduce the risk of medication leaking into SC tissue. To reduce the risk of some medications staining the skin, e.g. iron. This technique has been shown to reduce pain (Barron and Hollywood 2010).
12 Unless administering a vaccine, aspirate with the syringe and observe for the presence of blood. If no blood is observed, administer the medication, pushing the plunger slowly and smoothly. NB: If blood is observed, do **not** administer the medication; remove and dispose of the needle, syringe, and medication and start the procedure again. For immunisations there is no need to aspirate (DH 2013).	12 To reduce the risk of accidental IV administration of medication.
13 Depress the syringe plunger at a rate of 10 seconds per ml of medication (Mitchell and Whitney (2001). For immunisations, a rapid injection is recommended (Taddio et al. 2009). Wait 10 seconds following administration of medicine before removing the needle from the site of administration. NB: If using the Z-track technique, release the pull on the skin after removal of the needle.	13 To allow time for the medication to disperse and reduce the risk of leakage of the medication.
14 Do not massage the site following administration of the medication.	14 Massaging the site could cause additional discomfort.
15 Use gauze to apply gentle pressure if the injection site bleeds.	15 To reduce the risk of haematoma formation.
16 Dispose of sharps in a sharps bin and dispose of waste according to local policy.	16 To dispose of equipment safely.
17 Perform hand hygiene.	17 To comply with standard precautions.
18 a) Record medication administered. This may include the site of administration. b) Observe and report any local reaction or abnormality at the site of administration.	18 a) To meet local and legal requirements. b) To facilitate early detection of and prompt action to manage any complications.

Procedure guideline 17.11 Intraosseous administration

Statement	Rationale
1 Check the medication supplied is suitable for IO administration (these are the same medications that are deemed suitable for central IV administration).	1 To reduce the risk of medication error.
2 Check the medication(s) including dosage as per local policy.	2 To prevent medication error.
3 Gather equipment as in Section 17.1.4 and additionally: • Powered device needle drill (EZ-IO) and appropriately sized needle or manual IO needle • Plastic medication tray • Alcohol based skin preparation fluid – 2% chlorhexidine/70% isopropyl alcohol applicator (e.g. Chloraprep®) • Sterile gloves • Apron • Syringes • Sterile 3-way tap with extension tubing • 0.9% Sodium Chloride for injection	
4 Perform hand hygiene and put on gloves and apron.	4 To comply with standard precautions.
5 Prepare the medication(s) as per local policy and manufacturer's guidelines. Use an ANNT throughout.	5 To minimise risk of infection and prevent medication error.
6 Following insertion of the IO needle, (see chapter 30) attach a previously primed three-way tap (with 0.9% sodium chloride) and flush the cannula with 2–3 ml 0.9% sodium chloride for injection.	6 To confirm correct placement and to ensure patency of cannula.
7 Administer appropriate medications/fluids as prescribed.	7 To comply with treatment plan.
8 Ensure appropriate volume of 0.9% sodium chloride for injection is used to flush after and/or between each medication.	8 To ensure full dosage of medication is delivered. To ensure no drug interactions.
9 Ensure three-way tap is turned to 'off' position or fluid infusion is continued as prescribed following administration of medication.	9 To maintain patient safety, minimise infection risks, to adhere to the prescribed treatment plan.
10 Dispose of sharps in a sharps bin and all equipment used as per local waste management policy.	10 To dispose of equipment safely
11 Remove PPE and perform hand hygiene.	11 To comply with standard precautions.
12 Record medication administered.	12 To meet local and legal requirements.

Procedure guideline 17.12 Intrathecal administration

Statement	Rationale
1 **Intrathecal medication must only be administered by medical or nursing staff who have undergone training and been assessed as competent to administer medication via this route.**	1 To adhere to policy introduced following fatal errors in administration (DH 2011).
Gather equipment as in Section 17.1.4 and additionally: • Treatment protocol • Patient's medical records with current dated treatment protocol • Intrathecal medication • 0.9% sodium chloride for injection • Clean plastic medication tray • Sterile field • Sterile dressing pack (if required) • Sterile alcohol impregnated wipes • 1 × 1 or 2 ml syringe • 2 × 10–30 ml syringe • Needles (if required) • Small noncoring butterfly 23 or 25 G or lumbar puncture needle (specifically designed needle that will not connect with IV syringes) (NPSA 2011b) • Three-way tap (if required) • Sterile gauze and tape (if required) • Alcohol based skin preparation fluid – 2% chlorhexidine/70% isopropyl alcohol applicator (Killeen et al. 2012) • Transparent film dressing spray, e.g.: Op-site® spray or similar • Sterile gloves and gown • Apron, visor	

Chapter 17 Administration of medicines

Procedure guideline 17.12 Intrathecal administration *(continued)*

Statement	Rationale
2 Check that the medication supplied is suitable for intrathecal administration.	2 To reduce the risk of medical error.
3 Check the CYP's treatment protocol and determine stage of treatment, e.g. the level of the medication in the cerebrospinal fluid (antibiotic assay, if applicable).	3 The medication level in cerebrospinal fluid directly influences whether the medication dose may need to be altered to maintain therapeutic levels.
4 Refer to the manufacturer's guidelines and liaise with the ward pharmacist regarding the administration of the intrathecal medication.	4 The presence of some medications inhibits the effects of other medications.
5 **External ventricular drainage system**	5
a) Check CYP's treatment protocol and determine stage of treatment.	a) To ensure that the medication is due according to treatment protocol.
b) Close clamps on the drainage system as near to the injection port as possible.	b) To prevent the drug entering drainage system.
c) Put on an apron and visor and perform a surgical hand wash then put on a sterile gown and sterile gloves.	c) To reduce the risk of infection and to comply with standard precautions
d) Check medication according to local policy.	d) To prevent a medication error.
e) Prepare the medication using an aseptic technique.	e) To minimise risk of infection.
f) Remove stopcock protection box and clean injection port/needle free access device on the drainage system with 2% chlorhexidine in 70% isopropyl alcohol; wipe for 30 seconds using friction and allow to dry naturally.	f) To minimise the risk of infection.
g) Insert a 10 ml syringe and slowly withdraw 4 ml of CSF, remove syringe and discard.	g) To check free flow of CSF and patency of the drainage system.
h) Insert syringe containing medication and administer according to manufacturer's guidelines. Remove syringe.	h) To ensure safe administration of the medication.
i) Insert syringe containing 0.9% sodium chloride into catheter opening and gently flush catheter with 4 mls 0.9% sodium chloride. Remove syringe and replace stopcock protection box.	i) To ensure safe administration and absorption of the medication.
j) Keep the drainage system clamped for 1 hour ONLY after administration.	j) To ensure absorption of the medication.
6 **Intracerebroventricular access device (reservoir)**	6
a) To be administered with local anaesthesia, e.g. EMLA or Ametop gel, if required.	a) To minimise pain and anxiety.
b) Check CYP's treatment protocol and determine stage of treatment.	b) To ensure that medication is due according to treatment protocol.
c) Put on an apron and perform a surgical hand wash, then don personal protective clothing, i.e. visor according to local policy and sterile gloves.	c) To reduce the risk of infection and comply with standard precautions.
d) Check medication according to local policy.	d) To prevent medication error.
e) Position CYP comfortably on parent/carer's lap or lying down.	e) To facilitate the procedure.
f) Assist the practitioner (doctor/nurse) to locate the reservoir by slightly depressing the dome several times.	f) To facilitate the procedure.
g) Clean the site using 3 × 3 ml ChloraPrep® applicators. Gently press the applicator against the skin and then apply the antiseptic using firm repeated up and down, then back and forth strokes for 30 seconds over the device site and allow to dry completely	g) To minimise the risk of infection.
h) Using a small noncoring butterfly needle (25 G) or a Gripper needle connected to a three-way tap, access the reservoir, collect 1 ml of waste CSF, and discard. Collect required volume of CSF for laboratory testing (if required).	h) To check free flow of CSF and patency of the reservoir, and to send CSF to laboratory for analysis if required.

(continued)

Procedure guideline 17.12 Intrathecal administration *(continued)*

Statement	Rationale
i) Connect syringe containing medication to butterfly needle/Gripper needle extension puncture and inject slowly. Compress and release the dome after all medication has been given. If infusing a medication, secure the needle as required, using steristips/posey/surgifix or similar material, while ensuring that the entry site is visible throughout the infusion.	i) To facilitate safe, effective administration of the medication.
j) Remove the needle and syringe or syringe when the administration is complete.	j) To maintain the safety of the CYP
k) Spray with Op-site spray and apply pressure with a gauze pad. If CSF continues to leak, apply a small dressing with gauze and tape. This must be removed within 24 hours post procedure.	k) To prevent leakage of CSF and to reduce risk of infection.

7 **Administration of intrathecal chemotherapy via a lumbar puncture**

a) To be administered with a general anaesthesia, local anaesthesia, and/or Entonox, in a designated area.	a) To minimise pain and anxiety, in line with the national guidelines (DH 2011)
b) If a general anaesthesia or Entonox is to be administered, an appropriately trained person must be present to administer this. The CYP must be fasted according to hospital policy.	b) To ensure patient safety and minimise the risk of aspiration of stomach contents while under anaesthetic.
c) Check the CYP's treatment protocol and determine stage of treatment.	c) To ensure that medication is due according to treatment protocol.
d) Check CYP's full blood count (on preop check list) • Minimum platelet count of $50 \times 10\ 9/l$. • Ensure coagulation factors are normal. If patient has a known clotting abnormality or if there is any doubt. Ensure that a recent coagulation result is also available.	d) To ensure the safety of the CYP and minimise the risk of bleeding.
e) Check the CYP's consent form, prescription chart, and name band.	e) To adhere to local policy.
f) The doctor must collect the intrathecal chemotherapy from the designated fridge and complete the relevant documentation.	f) To confirm that the chemotherapy has been collected from a designated area and to minimise the risk of errors in line with national policy (DH 2011).
g) Put on an apron and visor and perform a surgical handwash, then don a sterile gown and sterile gloves.	g) To reduce the risk of infection, comply with standard precautions, and protect from cytotoxic spillage in line with current local policy.
h) The doctor administering the medication must check the intrathecal chemotherapy according to local policy with a nurse who is chemotherapy competent (DH 2011).	h) To minimise the risk of errors and adhere to national policy.
i) Once the CYP is anaesthetised/inhaling Entonox they should be monitored according to local policy. This should include monitoring of oxygen saturations and observing the following: i) Respiratory rate and pattern ii) Heart rate iii) Colour iv) Airway v) Conscious level	i) To maintain patient safety and to promote safe administration of medication. For more information on the use of Entonox see Chapter 24: Pain Management. i) To monitor effect on cardio-respiratory systems. iv) To determine need for suction or atropine. v) To determine need for further anaesthetic agent.
j) Position the CYP on their side with head flexed onto chest and knees drawn up (Dougherty and Lister 2011).	j) To facilitate procedure.
k) Open a sterile dressing pack and pour out some alcohol based skin preparation fluid:– 2% chlorhexidine/70% isopropyl alcohol (e.g. Chloraprep).	k-m) To minimise the risk of infection.
l) Open intrathecal chemotherapy drugs by cutting open plastic sealed pack.	
m) Prepare skin and clean site.	
n) Insert a lumbar puncture needle and collect 20 drops of cerebrospinal fluid (CSF) for Laboratory testing as required.	n) To facilitate procedure.

Procedure guideline 17.12 Intrathecal administration (continued)

Statement	Rationale
o) Connect syringe containing chemotherapy to lumbar puncture needle and inject slowly.	o) To facilitate the safe, effective administration of the medicine.
p) Remove the needle and syringe or syringe when the administration is complete.	p) To maintain the safety of the CYP.
q) Spray with Op-site spray and apply pressure with gauze pad. If CSF continues to leak apply a small dressing with gauze and tape. This dressing must be removed within 24 hours post the procedure or as soon as the leak has stopped.	q) To prevent leakage of CSF and chemotherapy, to reduce risk of infection.
p) Send CSF to laboratory for cytospin.	r) For diagnostic testing.
8 Administration of chemotherapy via an intraventricular access device (Ommaya reservoir)	**8**
a) To be administered with local anaesthesia (Emla or Ametop gel) in a designated area (DH 2011).	a) To minimise pain and anxiety (DH 2011).
b) Check the CYP's treatment protocol and determine stage of treatment.	b) To ensure that the medication is due according to treatment protocol.
c) Check the CYP's full blood count (on preop check list): • Minimum platelet count of 50 × 10 9/l. • Ensure that coagulation factors are normal. If the CYP has a known clotting abnormality or if there is any doubt, ensure that a recent coagulation result is also available.	c) To ensure the safety of the CYP and minimise the risk of bleeding.
d) Check the CYP's prescription chart and name band.	d) To ensure that the right drug is being given to the right CYP (RCN 2020).
e) The doctor must collect the intrathecal chemotherapy from the designated fridge complete the relevant documentation.	e) To confirm that the chemotherapy has been collected from a designated area, to minimise risk, and adhere to national policy (DH 2011).
f) Put on apron and visor and perform a surgical hand wash, then don a sterile gown and sterile gloves.	f) To reduce the risk of infection and protect from chemotherapy spillage and contamination.
g) The doctor administering the medication must check the intrathecal chemotherapy according to local policy and with a nurse who is chemotherapy competent (DH 2011).	g) To minimise risk in line with national policy.
h) Position the CYP comfortably on the parent/carer's lap or ask them to lie down.	h) To facilitate procedure.
i) Open sterile dressing pack and pour out some alcohol based skin preparation fluid – 2% chlorhexidine/70% isopropyl alcohol	i) To minimise the risk of infection.
j) Open intrathecal chemotherapy drugs by cutting open plastic sealed pack.	j) To minimise the risk of infection.
k) Locate the reservoir by slightly depressing the dome several times. Prepare skin and clean the site.	k) To check free flow of CSF and patency of the reservoir. To minimise the risk of infection.
l) Use a small noncoring butterfly needle 25 G connected to a three-way tap, access the reservoir and collect a small amount of CSF.	l) To send to the laboratory for cytospin to look for leukaemic cells.
m) Connect syringe containing chemotherapy to butterfly needle extension puncture and inject slowly. Compress and release the dome after all medication is given.	m) To facilitate medication administration.
n) Remove the needle and syringe or syringe when the administration is complete.	n) To disperse the drug and promote safe administration of the medication.
o) Spray with Op-site spray and apply pressure with gauze pad. If CSF continues to leak apply a small dressing with gauze and tape. This dressing must be removed within 24 hours post the procedure or as soon as the leak has stopped.	o) To facilitate dispersal of the medication, to prevent leakage of CSF and chemotherapy, to reduce risk of infection.
p) Dispose of sharps in a sharps bin and all equipment used as per local waste management policy.	p) To dispose of equipment safely.
q) Remove PPE and perform hand hygiene.	q) To comiply with standard precautions.
r) Record medicine administration.	r) To meet local and legal requirements.

Procedure guideline 17.13 Skin patch administration

Statement	Rationale
1 Expose the area of skin where the patch will be applied as specified in the manufacturer's drug information instructions. Always apply over the trunk or major muscle, not on distal extremities. Use a patch of skin that is free from hair, lesions, scars and pigmentation.	1 To prepare for administration and ensure that the patch is applied to the right location on the body. To ensure best absorption.
2 If the skin needs cleaning use **clear water only; no soap or alcohol wipes**. Ensure that the area is completely dry before applying the patch.	2 Soap or alcohol may affect the absorption of the medication.
3 Perform hand hygiene and don PPE if required.	3 To comply with standard precautions and reduce risk of absorbing medication.
4 Carefully remove the patch from its pouch, taking care not to tear the patch. Do not use scissors when removing the patch from its pouch.	4 To ensure the patch remains intact and to avoid damaging the patch.
5 Peel off the protective strip exposing the adhesive surface. Do not touch the sticky surface of the patch.	5 To reduce the risk of interfering with the medication dose.
6 Immediately place the adhesive side against the skin.	6 To reduce the exposure of the medication to the air.
7 Press the patch firmly, for about 10–20 seconds, with the palm of your hand. Ensure that the edges adhere to the skin. Run your finger around the edge of the patch once applied to checked that it is sealed properly	7 To ensure that the patch is completely sealed to the skin and that no air or water can get in.
8 Observe for and report immediately to the nurse in charge and responsible prescriber any adverse effects of the medication.	8 To facilitate early detection of any adverse effects of the medication.
9 Dispose of waste according to local policy.	9 To dispose of equipment safely.
10 Perform hand hygiene.	10 To comply with standard precautions
11 Record medication administered.	11 To meet local and legal requirements.

References

Advanced Life Support Group (2011). *Advanced Paediatric Life Support. The Practical Approach*, 5e. London: BMJ Publishing Group.

Alsulami, Z., Choonara, I., and Conroy, S. (2014). Nurse's knowledge about the double checking process for medicine administration. *Nursing Children and Young People* 26 (9): 21–25.

Anderson, G.D. and Saneto, R.P. (2012). Current oral and non-oral routes of anti-epileptic drug delivery. *Advanced Drug Delivery Reviews* 64: 911–918.

Annersten, M. and Wilmann, A. (2005). Performing subcutaneous injections: a literature review. *Worldviews on Evidence-Based Nursing* 2 (3): 122–130.

Arnell, K., Enblad, P., Wester, T., and Sjolin, J. (2007). Treatment of cerebrospinal fluid shunt infections in children using systemic and intraventricular antibiotic therapy in combination with externalization of the ventricular catheter: efficacy in 34 consecutively treated infections. *Journal of Neurosurgery* 107 (3 Suppl): 213–219.

Aronson, J.K. (2008). Routes of drug administration: uses and adverse effects. Part 1: Intramuscular and subcutaneous injection. Adverse Drug Reaction Bulletin, No 253.

Baldwin, K. and Walsh, V. (2014). Independent double-checks for high-alert medications: essential practice. *Nursing* 44 (4): 65–67.

Barker, C., Nunn, A.J., and Turner, S. (2012). Paediatrics. In: *Clinical Pharmacy and Therapeutics* (eds. R. Walker and C. Whittlesea), 132–148. Edinburgh: Churchill Livingstone.

Barron, C. and Hollywood, E. (2010). Drug administration. In: *Clinical Skills in Children's Nursing* (eds. I. Coyne, F. Neill and F. Timmins), 147–181. Oxford: Oxford University Press.

Bennett, J., Dawoud, D., Maben, J. (2010).Effects of interruptions to nurses during medication administration. Nursing Management 16(9): 22–23. https://www.researchgate.net/profile/Jill-Maben/publication/41908581_Effects_of_interruptions_to_nurses_during_medication_administration/links/54d4a8120cf2970e4e6364d4/Effects-of-interruptions-to-nurses-during-medication-administration.pdf (accessed 16 September 2022).

Bitter, C., Suter-Zimmermann, K., and Surber, C. (2011). Nasal drug delivery in humans. *Current Problems in Dermatology* 40: 20–35.

Boe, J., Dennis, J.H., O'Driscoll, B.R. et al. (2001). European Respiratory Society guidelines on the use of nebulizers. *European Respiratory Journal* 18 (1): 228–242.

British Society for Haematology (2017). Administration of blood components. Section 14.3. One or two person checks. p. 35. https://b-s-h.org.uk/guidelines/guidelines/administration-of-blood-components/ (accessed 16 September 2022).

British National Formulary for Children (BNFC) (2022). British Medical Association, Royal Pharmaceutical Society, the Royal College of Paediatrics and Child Health, and the Neonatal and Paediatric Pharmacists Group. London. https://about.medicinescomplete.com/publication/british-national-formulary-for-children/ (accessed 05 July 2022).

British Thoracic Society and Scottish Intercollegiate Network (BTS/SIGN) (2019). British guideline on the management of asthma. https://www.brit-thoracic.org.uk/quality-improvement/guidelines/asthma/ (accessed 16 September 2022).

Brown, T.L. (2015). Pediatric Variations of Nursing Interventions. In: *Wong's Nursing Care of Infants and Children*, 10e (eds. M.J. Hockenberry and D. Wilson), 575–632. Missouri: Elsevier.

Clancy, M. and Furyk, J. (2012). Paediatric intramuscular injections for developing world settings: a review of the literature for best practices. *Journal of Transcultural Nursing* 23 (4): 406–409.

Cook, I.F. and Murtagh, J. (2005). Optimal technique for intramuscular injection of infants and toddlers: a randomised trial. *Medical Journal of Australia* 183 (2): 60.

Cope, L.C., Abuzour, A.S., and Tully, M.P. (2016). Nonmedical prescribing: where are we now? *Therapeutic Advances in Drug Safety Journal* 7 (4): 165–172.

Dahlquist, L.M., Busby, S.M, Slifer, et al. (2002). Distraction for children of different ages who undergo repeated needle sticks. *Journal of Pediatric Oncology Nursing* 19 (1): 22–34.

Delgado-Charro, M.B. and Guy, R.H. (2014). Effective use of transdermal drug delivery in children. *Advanced Drug Delivery Reviews* 73: 63–82.

Department of Health/Royal Pharmaceutical Society (2007). Safer management of controlled drugs. A guide to good practice in secondary care (England). Gateway 8157.

Department of Health (DH) (2010). Mixing of medicines prior to administration in clinical practice: medical and non-medical prescribing. https://www.gov.uk/government/publications/mixing-of-medicines-prior-to-administration-in-clinical-practice-medical-and-non-medical-prescribing (accessed 16 September 2022).

Department of Health (DH) (2011). Health Circular: HSC 2008/001 Updated national guidance on the safe administration of intrathecal chemotherapy. https://webarchive.nationalarchives.gov.uk/ukgwa/20130104235816mp_/http://www.dh.gov.uk/prod_consum_dh/groups/dh_digitalassets/documents/digitalasset/dh_086844.pdf (accessed 16 September 2022).

Department of Health (DH) (2013). Controlled drugs (supervision of management of use) regulations 2013. https://assets.publishing.service.gov.uk/government/uploads/system/uploads/attachment_data/file/214915/15-02-2013-controlled-drugs-regulation-information.pdf (accessed 16 September 2022).

Department of Health (DH) (2013). Immunisation against Infectious Diseases (The Green Book) https://www.gov.uk/government/collections/immunisation-against-infectious-disease-the-green-book (accessed 16 September 2022).

Dougherty, L., Lister, S., and West-Oram A (2015). *The Royal Marsden Hospital Manual of Clinical Nursing Procedures*, 9e. Sussex: Wiley.

Ford, L., Maddox, C., Moore, E., and Sales, R. (2010). The safe management of medicines for children. In: *Practices in Children's Nursing: Guidelines for Community and Hospital*, 3e (eds. E. Trigg and T.A. Mohammed), 417–445. Edinburgh: Churchill Livingstone.

Fransén, N. (2008). Studies on a novel powder formulation for nasal drug delivery. DIVA. https://www.diva-portal.org/smash/get/diva2:172562/FULLTEXT01.pdf (accessed 16 September 2022).

Guidelines and Audit Implementation Network (GAIN (2015). Guidelines for caring for an infant, child, or young person who requires enteral feeding. Guidelines and Audit Implementation Network. https://www.rqia.org.uk/RQIA/files/4f/4f08bb34-7955-49ea-adf1-9de807d3da66.pdf (accessed 16 September 2022).

Grassin-Delyle, S., Buenestado, A., Naline, E. et al. (2012). Intranasal drug delivery: an efficient and non-invasive route for systemic administration: focus on opioids. *Pharmacology and Therapeutics* 134 (3): 366–379.

Greenway, K. (2014). Rituals in nursing: intramuscular injection. *Journal of Clinical Nursing* 23 (23–24): 3583–3588.

Hadley, G., Maconochie, and Jackson, A. (2010). A survey of intranasal medication use in the paediatric emergency setting in England and Wales. *Emergency Medicine Journal* 27: 553–554.

Health Act (2006). Health Act 2006, c28. https://www.legislation.gov.uk/ukpga/2006/28/contents (accessed 16 September 2022).

Hemsworth, S. (2000). Intramuscular (IM) injection technique. *Pediatric Nursing* 12 (9): 17–20.

Her Majesty's Stationery Office (HMSO) (2016). Psychoactive Substances Act 2016. The Stationery Office, London. https://www.legislation.gov.uk/ukpga/2016/2/contents/enacted (accessed 5 November 2018).

Higgins, D. (2007). Bowel care. Part 6: administration of a suppository. *Nursing Times* 103 (47): 26–27.

Hollis, R. (2002). Accidental intrathecal administration of chemotherapy agents. *Cancer Nursing Practice* 1 (1): 8–9.

Human Medicines Regulations (2012). Statutory Instruments No. 1916. The Human Medicines Regulations. www.legislation.gov.uk/uksi/2012/1916/pdfs/uksi_20121916_en.pdf (accessed 16 September 2022).

Hunter, J. (2008). Intramuscular injection techniques. *Nursing Standard* 22 (24): 35–40.

Institute for Healthcare Improvement (2022). Conduct independent double checks on the unit. http://www.ihi.org/resources/Pages/Changes/ConductIndependentDoubleChecksonUnit.aspx (accessed 16 September 2022).

Killeen, T., Kamat, A., Walsh, D. et al. (2012). Severe adhesive arachnoiditis resulting in progressive paraplegia following obstetric spinal anaesthesia; a case report and review. *Anaesthesia Journal of Association of Great Britain and Ireland* 67 (12): 1386–1394.

Knox, T. and Davie, J. (2009). Nasogastric tube feeding-which syringe size produces lower pressure and is safest to use? *Nursing Times* 105 (27): 24–26.

Lee, M., and Phillips, J. (2002). Transdermal patches: High risk for error? Drugs Topic (April 1): 54–55.

Lindsay, K.W., Bone, I., and Fuller, G. (2010). *Neurology and Neurosurgery Illustrated*, 5e. London: Churchill Livingstone Elsevier.

Love, G.H. (2006). Clinical Do's and Don'ts, administering an intradermal injection. *Nursing* 36 (6): 20.

Lynn, P. (2011). *Fundamentals of Nursing: The Art and Science of Nursing Care*. Philadelphia: Lippincott Williams & Wilkins.

McKay, G. and Walters, M. (2013). *Clinical Pharmacology and Therapeutics*, 9e. London: Wiley-Blackwell.

Medicines and Healthcare Products Regulatory Agency (MHRA) (2014a). Medical and non-medical prescribing: mixing medicines in clinical practice. https://www.gov.uk/drug-safety-update/medical-and-non-medical-prescribing-mixing-medicines-in-clinical-practice (accessed 16 September 2022).

Medicines and Healthcare Products Regulatory Agency (MHRA) (2014b). Fentanyl skin patches: importance of safe use and disposal https://assets.publishing.service.gov.uk/media/54730808e5274a1301000046/con437440.pdf (accessed 16 September 2022).

Medicines and Healthcare Products Regulatory Agency (MHRA) (2014, updated 2017). Patient group directions: who can use them. Medicines & Healthcare Products Regulatory Agency: London. https://www.gov.uk/government/publications/patient-group-directions-pgds (accessed 16 September 2022).

Medicines and Healthcare Products Regulatory Agency (MHRA). (2022). Medicines & Healthcare Products Regulatory Agency: London. https://www.gov.uk/government/organisations/medicines-and-healthcare-products-regulatory-agency (accessed 16 September 2022).

Medicines for Children (2014). How to give medicines: rectal medicines. Medicines for Children, London. https://www.medicinesforchildren.org.uk/advice-guides/giving-medicines/how-to-give-medicines-rectal-medicines/ (accessed 16 September 2022).

MHRA (2014). Buccal Midazolam (Buccolam ▼): new authorised medicine for paediatric use. https://www.gov.uk/drug-safety-update/buccal-midazolam-buccolam-new-authorised-medicine-for-paediatric-use (last accessed 16 September 2022).

Misuse of Drugs Act (1971). The Stationery Office, London. https://www.legislation.gov.uk/ukpga/1971/38/contents (accessed 16 September 2022).

Misuse of Drugs Regulations (2001). The Stationery Office, London www.legislation.gov.uk/uksi/2001/3998/contents/made (accessed 16 September 2022).

Mitchell, J.R. and Whitney, F.W. (2001). The effect of injection speed on the perception of intramuscular injection pain: a clinical update. *American Association of Occupational Health Nurses Journal* 49 (6): 286–292.

Narang, N. and Sharma, J. (2011). Sublingual mucosa as a route for systemic drug delivery. *International Journal of Pharmacy and Pharmaceutical Sciences* 3 (Suppl 2): 18–22.

NHS England (2022). Never Events data. https://www.england.nhs.uk/patient-safety/never-events-data/ (accessed 16 September 2022).

National Institute for Health and Care Excellence (NICE) (2002). Inhaler devices for routine treatment of chronic asthma in older children (aged 5–15 years). London. National Institute for Health and Clinical Excellence. www.nice.org.uk/guidance/ta38 (accessed 16 September 2022).

National Institute for Health and Care Excellence (NICE) (2010). Constipation in children and young people: diagnosis and management. NICE Guidelines (CG99). www.nice.org.uk/Guidance/CG99 (accessed 16 September 2022).

National Institute for Health and Care Excellence (NICE)) (2012). Infection: prevention and control of healthcare-associated infection in primary and community care. NICE Clinical guideline 139. London: National Institute for Health and Clinical Excellence. www.nice.org.uk/guidance/cg139 (accessed 16 September 2022).

National Institute for Health and Care Excellence (NICE) (2014). Safe staffing for nursing in adult inpatient wards in acute hospitals NICE guidelines [SG1]. https://www.nice.org.uk/guidance/sg1 (accessed 16 September 2022).

National Institute for Health and Care Excellence (NICE) (2016). Controlled drugs: safe use and management. NICE guideline [NG46]. https://www.nice.org.uk/guidance/ng46 (accessed 20 September 2021).

National Institute for Health and Care Excellence (NICE) (2018). Discussing and planning medicines support. https://www.nice.org.uk/about/nice-communities/social-care/quick-guides/discussing-and-planning-medicines-support (accessed 01 November 2022).

National Patient Safety Agency (NPSA) (2007a). Patient safety alert; Promoting safer measurement and administration of liquid medicines via oral and other enteral routes. https://webarchive.nationalarchives.gov.uk/ukgwa/20170906191124/http://www.nrls.npsa.nhs.uk/alerts/?entryid45=59808&cord=DESC&p=3 (accessed 16 September 2022).

National Patient Safety Agency (NPSA) (2007b). Promoting the safer use of injectable medicines. Patient Safety Alert 20. p 2, https://webarchive.nationalarchives.gov.uk/ukgwa/20180501173536/http://www.nrls.npsa.nhs.uk/resources/search-by-audience/hospital-doctor/?entryid45=59812&p=3 (accessed 16 September 2022).

National Patient Safety Agency (NPSA) (2008). Risks with intravenous heparin flush solutions. Patient Safety Alert 002. https://europepmc.org/article/HIR/287902 (accessed 16 September 2022).

National Patient Safety Agency (NPSA) (2009). Oxygen safety in hospitals: Rapid Response Report NPSA/2009/RRR006. September. https://www.england.nhs.uk/wp-content/uploads/2019/12/Patient_Safety_Alert_-_Reducing_the_risk_of_oxygen_tubing_being_connected_to_a_bDUb2KY (accessed 16 September 2022).

National Patient Safety Agency (NPSA). (2010a). Preventing fatalities from medication loading doses: Rapid Response Report NPSA/2010/RRR018. https://webarchive.nationalarchives.gov.uk/ukgwa/20171030132005/http://www.nrls.npsa.nhs.uk/resources/patient-safety-topics/medication-safety/?entryid45=92305&p=1 (accessed 16 September 2022).

National Patient Safety Agency (NPSA). (2010b). Safer administration of insulin: Rapid Response Report NPSA/2010/RRR013 June. https://webarchive.nationalarchives.gov.uk/ukgwa/20180501172252/http://www.nrls.npsa.nhs.uk/resources/collections/10-for-2010/?entryid45=74287&p=2 (accessed 16 September 2022).

National Patient Safety Agency (NPSA). (2010c). Prevention of over infusion of intravenous fluid and medicines in neonates: Rapid Response Report NPSA/2010/RRR015. August. https://webarchive.nationalarchives.gov.uk/ukgwa/20171030140238/http://www.nrls.npsa.nhs.uk/resources/clinical-specialty/medicine/?entryid45=75519&p=4 (accessed 16 September 2022).

National Patient Safety Agency (NPSA), (2011a). Multiple use of single use injectable medicines: Signal. March. https://webarchive.nationalarchives.gov.uk/ukgwa/20170906173951/http://www.nrls.npsa.nhs.uk/resources/type/signals/?entryid45=130185&p=1 (accessed 16 September 2022).

National Patient Safety Agency (NPSA) (2011b). Safer spinal (intrathecal), epidural and regional devices – Part A. https://webarchive.nationalarchives.gov.uk/ukgwa/20171030130405/http://www.nrls.npsa.nhs.uk/resources/patient-safety-topics/medical-device-equipment/?entryid45=94529 (accessed 16 September 2022).

NHS England (2014). Safer staffing: a guide to care contact time. NHS England. Leeds. https://www.england.nhs.uk/wp-content/uploads/2014/11/safer-staffing-guide-care-contact-time.pdf (accessed 16 September 2022).

NHS England (2022a). Our national patient safety alerts. https://www.england.nhs.uk/patient-safety/patient-safety-alerts/ (16 September 2022).

NHS England (2022b). Never Events data. NHS Improvement: London. https://www.england.nhs.uk/patient-safety/never-events-data/ (accessed 16 September 2022).

Nursing and Midwifery Council (NMC) (2015). *The Code. Professional Standards of Practice and Behaviour for Nurses, Midwives and Nursing Associates.* https://www.nmc.org.uk/standards/code/ (accessed 22 September 2022).

Nursing and Midwifery Council (NMC) (2018). Future nurse: Standards of proficiency for registered nurses. https://www.nmc.org.uk/globalassets/sitedocuments/standards-of-proficiency/nurses/future-nurse-proficiencies.pdf (accessed 01 November 2022).

Nursing and Midwifery Council (NMC) (2019). Standards for prescribers. https://www.nmc.org.uk/standards/standards-for-post-registration/standards-for-prescribers/ (accessed 16 September 2022).

Ofosu, R. and Jarrett, P. (2015). Reducing nurse medicine administration errors. *Nursing Times* 111 (20): 12–14.

Patel, D. (2006). Epidural analgesia for children. *Continuing Education in Anaesthesia Critical Care & Pain* 6 (2): 63–66.

Perry, A.G., Potter, P.A., and Ostendorf, W.R. (2014). *Clinical Nursing Skills and Techniques*, 8e. Missouri: Elsevier.

Pratt, R.J., Hoffman, P.N., and Robb, F.F. (2005). The need for skin preparation prior to injection: point –counterpoint. *Journal of Infection Prevention* 6 (4): 18–20.

Public Health England (2013). Immunisations procedures: the green book, chapter 4 https://www.gov.uk/government/publications/immunisation-procedures-the-green-book-chapter-4 (accessed 16 September 2022).

Raban, M.Z. and Westbrook, J. (2014). Are interventions to reduce interruptions and errors during medication administration effective? a systematic review. *BMJ Quality and Safety* 23 (5): 414–421.

Rang, H.P., Dale, M.M., Ritter, J.M., and Moore, P.K. (2003). *Pharmacology*, 5e. Edinburgh: Churchill Livingstone.

RCN (2020). Medicines Management. https://www.rcn.org.uk/Professional-Development/publications/pub-009018 (accessed 01 November 2022).

Reising, D.L. and Neal, R.S. (2005). Enteral tube flushing: what you think are the best practices may not be. *American Journal of Nursing* 105 (3): 58–63.

Resuscitation Council (UK) (2011). *European Paediatric Life Support Course. Provider Manual for Use in the UK*, 3e. London: Resuscitation Council (UK).

Royal College of Nursing (RCN) (2022). Non-medical prescribers. https://www.rcn.org.uk/Get-Help/RCN-advice/non-medical-prescribers (accessed 16 September 2022).

Royal College of Paediatrics and Child Health (2002). *Position statement on injection technique*. London: RCPCH.

Royal Pharmaceutical Society (RPS) (2021). A Competency Framework for all Prescribers. https://www.rpharms.com/resources/frameworks/prescribing-competency-framework/competency-framework (accessed 01 November 2022).

RPS and RCN (2019). Professional Guidance on the Administration of Medicines in Healthcare Settings. https://www.rpharms.com/portals/0/RPS%20document%20library/open%20access/professional%20standards/SSHM%20and%20Admin/Admin%20of%20meds%20prof%20guidance.pdf?ver=2019-01-23%20145026-567

Santos, J.M.S., Poland, F., Kelly, J., and Wright, D.J. (2012). Drug administration guides in dysphagia. *Nursing Times* 108 (21): 15–17.

Saul, R., Peters, J., and Bruce, E. (2016). Assessing acute and chronic pain in children and young people. *Nursing Standard* 31 (10): 51–61.

Selwood, K. (2008). Side effects of chemotherapy. In: *Cancer in Children and Young People* (eds. F. Gibson and L. Soanes), 35–72. Chichester: Wiley.

Shin, H. and Kim, M.J. (2006). Subcutaneous tissue thickness in children with type 1 diabetes. *Journal of Advanced Nursing* 54 (1): 29–34.

Taddio, A., Ilersich, A.L., Ipp, M. et al. (2009). Physical interventions and injection techniques for reducing injection pain during routine childhood immunisations: systematic review of randomised controlled trials and quasi-randomised controlled trials. *Clinical Therapeutics* 31 (Supplement B): 48–76.

Westbrook, J.L., Woods, A., Rob, M.I. et al. (2010). Association of interruptions with an increased risk and severity of medication administration errors. *JAMA Internal Medicine* 170 (8): 683–690.

White, R. and Bradnam, V. (2015). *Handbook of Drug Administration Via Enteral Tubes*, 3e. London: Pharmaceutical Press.

Williams, N.T. (2008). Medication administration through enteral feeding tubes. *American Journal of Health-System Pharmacy* 65: 2347–2357.

World Health Organization (2010) WHO best practices for injections and related procedures toolkit. https://www.ncbi.nlm.nih.gov/books/NBK138495 (accessed 16 September 2022).

Chapter 18

Mental health

Sharon Philips[1] and Caroline Grindrod[2]

[1]Formerly Ward Sister, Adolescent Mental Health Unit, Great Ormond Street Hospital, London, UK
[2]Formerly CNS, Eating Disorders Team, Adolescent Mental Health Unit, GOSH

Chapter contents

What is mental health?	406
How common are mental health difficulties?	406
Somatoform disorders and medically unexplained symptoms	407
Anxiety disorders	407
Psychosis	408
Eating disorders	408
References	413

Procedure guideline

18.1 Managing meal times	412

The Great Ormond Street Hospital Manual of Children and Young People's Nursing Practices, Second Edition. Edited by Elizabeth Anne Bruce, Janet Williss, and Faith Gibson.
© 2023 John Wiley & Sons Ltd. Published 2023 by John Wiley & Sons Ltd.

This chapter provides a brief overview of mental health disorders and how they present and are treated in children and young people (CYPs). The second part of the chapter focuses on eating disorders and how these manifest and are best managed in young people. The management of CYPs with learning difficulties is covered in Chapter 16: Learning (Intellectual) Disabilities.

What is mental health?

The World Health Organization (WHO) defines mental health as 'a state of well-being in which every individual realises his or her own potential, can cope with the normal stresses of life, can work productively and fruitfully, and is able to make a contribution to her or his community' (WHO 2022).

Mental health affects all aspects of a CYP's development including their cognitive abilities, social skills, and emotional well-being. Good mental health allows CYPs to develop the resilience to cope with whatever life throws at them and grow into well-rounded, healthy adults.

CYPs can experience many pressures from today's society; for example, from family, friends, school, and the media. In some CYPs, certain life events and challenges can 'trigger' difficulties or increase the likelihood of mental health difficulties occurring. Some of these factors include:

- Having a long-term physical illness.
- Having a parent who has had mental health problems, problems with alcohol, or has been in trouble with the law.
- Experiencing the death of someone close to them.
- Having parents who separate or divorce.
- Having been severely bullied or physically or sexually abused.
- Living in poverty or being homeless.

Things that can help a young person maintain good mental health include:

- Feeling loved, trusted, understood, valued, and safe.
- Being in good physical health.
- Being able to learn and play and have opportunities to succeed.
- Recognising what they are good at and having this acknowledged by others.
- Having a sense of belonging to their family, school, and community.
- Feeling that they have some control over their life.
- Having the ability to cope when something is wrong (resilience) and being able to problem solve.

(*Source:* Mental Health Foundation 2015)

How common are mental health difficulties?

Approximately 850 000 young people in the United Kingdom are estimated to have mental health problems (Young Minds 2022a). The British Child and Adolescent Mental Health Survey in 2004 found that 1 in 10 young people under the age of 16 had a diagnosable mental disorder (Office for National Statistics 2005). Additionally:

- One in five young adults show signs of an eating disorder.
- One in 12 young people deliberately harm themselves, with 25 000 hospitalised each year as a result.
- Nearly 80 000 young people suffer from severe depression.
- 3.3% (approximately 290 000) of young people have an anxiety disorder.

(*Source:* Young Minds 2022a)

Mental health is an important part of a young person's well-being, is closely connected with physical health, and significantly affects a young person's ability to engage with education, make and keep friends, have positive relationships with their family, and find their way in the world (Association for Young People's Health 2015). Mental health problems contribute to the global burden of disease (Whiteford et al. 2013), with untreated problems likely to become very expensive for health services as young people grow into adults. A study by Woodgate and Garralda (2006) suggests that the most common problems referred to psychiatry by paediatric ward staff include adjustment to illness, somatoform disorders, disturbed behaviour, anxiety disorders, and depression. Other difficulties that may be encountered by nursing staff on a paediatric ward include self-harm, enuresis, encopresis, psychosis, eating disorders, medically unexplained symptoms, and perplexing presentations.

What help is available?

Child and Adolescent Mental Health Services (CAMHS), both community and in-patient based, include psychiatrists, clinical psychologists, nurses (usually mental health nurses), psychotherapists (both individual and family), and social workers. CAMHS teams offer assessment and treatment when CYPs have emotional, behavioural, or mental health difficulties.

CAMHS work within a four-tiered framework:

Tier 1 (universal services):	Services whose primary remit is not that of providing a mental health service. They assess and support CYPs who have mental health problems as part of the duties they are routinely involved with. Universal services include GPs, health visitors, schools, early years' provision, and others.
Tier 2 (targeted services):	Services for CYPs with milder problems. These services may be delivered by professionals who are based in schools or children's centres. Targeted services also include those provided to specific groups of CYPs at increased risk of developing mental health problems (e.g. paediatric clinical psychologists based in acute-care settings).
Tier 3 (specialist services):	Multidisciplinary community teams of child and adolescent mental health professionals providing a range of interventions. Access to these teams is usually via referral from a GP.
Tier 4 (specialised services):	Highly specialist day and inpatient services, and some highly specialist outpatient services.

(CAMHS Tier 4 Report Steering Group 2014)

Liaison psychiatry provides consultation, assessment, and treatment to patients attending general hospitals (via Accident and Emergency department [A and E]) or those who are admitted to inpatient wards. This service is also known as paediatric liaison. The service provided and means of referral will vary depending on the Trust involved.

Adjustment to illness

Receiving a diagnosis of an acute or chronic illness can be the beginning of a challenging journey for both the CYP and their family (Christie and Khatun 2012). They may experience changes in their emotional life, education, peer relationships, lifestyle, and body image. The CYP may feel angry at being diagnosed with an illness and may look to blame others such as a parent. Sadness, denial, and grief (in both the CYP and their family) are common and a young person may struggle to adjust to illness to the extent that they refuse necessary treatment or assessment, for example, refusing to allow blood samples to be obtained or to take medication. Nursing staff can support the CYP by allowing them time to express their feelings around the illness and acknowledging these feelings as real and valid. Encourage problem solving to help the CYP to maintain a sense of control/mastery over their situation. Maintaining a structure that includes education and play can provide them with some stability at a time when many things may feel uncertain.

Somatoform disorders and medically unexplained symptoms

Somatoform disorders occur when stress is thought to be a major cause of symptoms, especially when symptoms continue for a long time or are particularly severe. Symptoms can be wide-ranging, varied, and differ in severity. They can include pain, paralysis, and loss of sensation or increased sensitivity.

Medically unexplained symptoms are symptoms that cannot be explained by an obvious physical cause. This does not mean that the symptoms are fake or 'all in the mind': They are real and can cause great suffering and distress. Such presentations are difficult to diagnose and manage and necessitate referral to mental health services. Nursing staff can support the CYP and their family by acknowledging that the symptoms are real and by providing opportunities for them to express their feelings and worries.

Occasionally there are inconsistencies in the presentation (e.g. the nurse may observe the CYP using a 'paralysed' limb). It is unhelpful to point these out. Encourage the CYP to complete tasks as independently as they can, in order to maintain as much function as possible. Physiotherapy colleagues can be consulted for advice on desensitisation and exercise programmes, and should be involved with CYPs with somatoform disorders and medically unexplained symptoms, particularly where mobility is affected.

Disturbed behaviour
CYPs (and adults) with learning disabilities, autism, or mental health difficulties may display 'problem' or 'unusual' behaviours. These can include:

- Aggression (e.g. hitting)
- Self-injury (e.g. head banging)
- Destruction (e.g. throwing)
- Other (e.g. rocking).

Challenging behaviour can be a result of disorders such as attention deficit and hyperactivity disorder (ADHD) or oppositional defiant disorder, or can be related to fear, confusion, a cognitive deficit, or a psychotic episode. CYPs who have a diagnosis of learning disability or autism spectrum disorder can exhibit behaviours or ways of interacting that are challenging. Where behaviour is disturbed, possible organic causes must be ruled out.

Why does it happen?
There is always a reason for challenging behaviour. In many cases, it's a way for a person to control what is going on around them and to get their needs met. They might also be ill, in pain, or want something. It is important to understand the reasons behind challenging behaviour to enable change to happen.

What can be done?
Although there is no quick fix, much can be done to prevent or reduce challenging behaviour:

- Work out if the person is in pain or bored.
- Is there a way of teaching the person to show you what they want in another way?
- Develop their communication skills.
- Keep a record of the behaviour.
- When safe to do so, ignore it and distract the person.
- Signpost the family to their GP/social worker to be referred for a 'functional assessment' to better understand the reasons behind their behaviour.

(Adapted from Challenging Behaviour Foundation, https://www.challengingbehaviour.org.uk/)

It is essential to determine whether there is a health reason behind a behaviour change as this is a common reason for such behaviour. Please see Chapter 16: Intellectual (Learning) Disability for further guidance on how to work with people with a learning disability. Paediatric liaison colleagues can offer advice on the management of a behaviourally disturbed CYP but there are several strategies that can be used by paediatric nursing staff. These include:

- Consistency in approach: This is essential, especially in how staff and family members respond to challenging behaviour.
- An individualised programme: This can be invaluable, providing the CYP with structure and appropriate stimulation.
- Structure: This provides the CYP with stability and consistency and can help to alleviate anxiety and boredom. An effective structured programme should include opportunities for play, learning, meal times, socialising, and relaxation. Incorporating medication times/assessments/interventions into the timetable can be helpful to help the CYP to prepare themselves.
- The use of a positive behaviour programme (a reward chart) can be helpful, in rewarding desired behaviour and boosting self-esteem.
- Using short sentences with simple language in a calm voice can be helpful; ensure only one adult speaks at a time to avoid overwhelming the CYP.
- Consider the physical environment; changes may need to be made to ensure the safety of a disturbed patient. Reduce stimulation for an overaroused CYP by limiting background noise, dimming the lights, and ensuring no disruption for a period of time.

Anxiety disorders

Anxiety is a normal response to a worrying or threatening situation and can be helpful to protect us from danger. If the anxiety is constant or very strong, it can be problematic. Most CYPs have times of feeling worried or frightened about things; it is a normal part of growing up. For example, a young child might feel anxious about being separated from their parents or carers, a child might be afraid of the dark, or a young person might be anxious about their appearance or meeting new people. If these worries or anxieties begin to impact on the CYP's life, help should be sought.

There are many types of anxiety disorders, including generalised anxiety disorder, social anxiety disorder, post-traumatic stress disorder, panic disorder, obsessive–compulsive disorder, and phobias (e.g. needle phobia, vomiting phobia, agoraphobia). Nearly 300 000 young people in Britain have an anxiety disorder (Royal College of Psychiatrists 2022c).

People often experience physical, psychological, and behavioural symptoms when they feel anxious or stressed. Individual or group cognitive behavioural therapy (CBT) is the intervention of choice when treating anxiety in CYPs and must be delivered by a competent practitioner (National Institute for Health and Clinical Excellence [NICE] 2013b). CAMHS colleagues and paediatric clinical psychologists are able to offer advice and support to staff and the CYP on managing anxiety in hospital. Ward nursing staff can provide support by encouraging relaxation through a variety of techniques including deep breathing, muscle relaxation, and visualisation. Talking through the CYP's fears and anxieties can be helpful and there are a wide range of online resources and scripts that parents and staff can use to promote calm and relaxation (NHS 2022; Kids Relaxation 2016).

Depression

Feeling sad or fed up is a normal reaction to experiences that are difficult or stressful. Sometimes, feelings of sadness can continue for some time and start to interfere with everyday life. At these times, low moods become part of an illness; 'depression.' Depression is thought to occur in around 1–3% of CYPs and can be caused by a number of factors. It can run in families, as it has a genetic component, can be triggered by a specific event such as bullying or bereavement, and is more likely to occur when CYPs feel under stress and lack support (Royal Society of Psychiatrists 2022d).

If depression is suspected while a CYP is in hospital, assessment should be sought from paediatric liaison/CAMHS colleagues. An urgent referral must be made if the CYP is self-harming, or expressing suicidal ideation or suicidal thoughts, which occur when they become preoccupied with thinking about suicide. If the CYP is expressing suicidal ideation while at home they must be seen by the GP or in A and E as a matter of urgency.

Depression is treatable, and ward nursing staff can support treatment by recognising that it is an illness, and by giving clear information to the CYP that recovery is possible. Encourage the CYP to take part in activities even though they may not want to. Spend time with them, listening, watching TV, or just sitting together.

A CYP in hospital who is expressing wishes to end their life can be supported by one-on-one observations and the maintenance of a safe environment (such as removing sharps, toxic liquids, potential ligatures, etc.). Psychiatry colleagues can offer support and guidance around this. At home, the principles are the same, as the CYP should not have access to any sharp or potentially dangerous substances, including medicines, if they are thinking about suicide. Keeping a close eye on the CYP is also important at home. The parent or carer needs to know to take them to the GP, or to the local A and E out of hours, if they are very concerned about their ability to keep them safe.

Self-harm

Self-harm is an umbrella term for any behaviour, action, or habit that can cause damage to health. Examples of self-harm include cutting, burning, pulling hair, picking skin, pinching, hitting/punching, and deliberate bruising. Actions such as these can also be referred to as 'self-injury.' Self-harming behaviour can also include actions that cause short- and long-term damage, e.g. over- or undereating, substance misuse, smoking, and other actions that may impact on the quality of life later. Overdosing and poisoning are also forms of self-harming. The management of poisoning and overdose is covered in Chapter 28: Poisoning and Overdose. It is important to note that while CYPs who self-harm are at greater risk of suicide, they do not necessarily self-harm because they want to commit suicide. One in 12 young people are said to self-harm and it has been reported that over the previous 10 years, inpatient admissions for young people who self-harm increased by 68% (Young Minds 2022b).

The need to self-harm usually comes from emotions that are difficult for the individual to manage. CYPs may harm themselves as this helps them to manage angry and aggressive emotions toward other people. Low levels of self-worth can prompt some to self-harm, while others use it as a way of feeling in control of the world around them. Harming causes the body to produce endorphins, which can produce an adrenaline type rush. Some people do not find harming addictive in a physical sense, but may become dependent on it emotionally.

If a CYP is self-harming while in hospital, an urgent assessment should be sought from paediatric liaison colleagues or a referral made to CAMHS. If a CYP is being treated as an out-patient or in their own home, a referral must be made to the local CAMHS, who will be able to assess and work with the CYP (and their family) to keep them safe. It can be difficult to broach the topic of self-harm. If you are worried that a CYP is hurting themself, a way to approach the topic could be: 'I noticed earlier that you had some scratches on your arms and wondered if it was something we could talk about. I would like to be able to understand and help.' Ward nursing staff can support the CYP by being nonjudgemental and nonconfrontational. Avoid saying things like 'that's silly,' 'you shouldn't do that,' 'that doesn't make sense.' Being able to talk about self-harming is vitally important, as learning to cope with the emotions they experience can help the CYP begin to reduce or stop self-harming.

There are a number of alternative coping strategies that could be suggested to and used by CYPs, though these should not be suggested in place of referral to mental health services. NICE Guidelines (2013a) state that the CYP who self-harms should be treated with respect, understanding, and be offered choices.

Psychosis

Psychosis is having unusual experiences/perceptions that are not shared by others, the two main symptoms being hallucinations and delusions (Young Minds 2022c). Hallucinations can be auditory (hearing voices that others don't), visual (seeing people or things that others don't), or can involve tastes, smells, and sensations that have no apparent cause, such as feeling insects crawling on the skin. A delusion is a fixed belief that is clearly untrue; for example, the sufferer may believe he is related to the Queen (when he is not); controls the weather, or that people are plotting to kill him/her (paranoia). Males are more likely to experience their first psychotic episode in their late teens/early twenties. With females, this is more usually experienced in the early twenties. Psychosis is a symptom of an underlying condition, so assessment is vital. Psychotic episodes in CYPs are relatively rare, so thorough and prompt assessment is essential.

Eating disorders

Eating disorders are understood to result from a complex integrated model of bio-psycho-social factors, with evidence for the impact of social and cultural factors related to body image and media influence (Nicholls and Grindrod 2012). There is a difference between eating disorders and disordered eating secondary to another illness or stressor. CYPs struggling with emotionally difficult situations may demonstrate changes in eating patterns due to separation, illness, and changes in routine contributing to eating difficulties of some kind. Stress can lead to under- or overeating. These temporary changes in eating should not cause long-term concern and they usually resolve alongside physical recovery and a return to usual routine. There are significant differences between brief periods of emotional eating disturbance and psychiatric disorders such as anorexia or bulimia nervosa.

Common conceptions of eating disorders include:

- Eating disorders are about 'feelings not food,' with CYPs struggling to regulate and express emotions in the usual way. This theory supports eating difficulties as an unintentional emotional communication with possible difficulties with identity development, emotional regulation, separation, and growing up (Lewer 2006).
- Eating disorders are about a CYP struggling with control (Button and Warren 2001).
- Clinicians are researching the area of brain functioning in eating disorders (Rose et al. 2014).

The characteristics of the two most common feeding disorders are outlined in Table 18.1.

Table 18.1 Characteristics of anorexia and bulimia

Condition	Physical symptoms	Behavioural symptoms	Psychological symptoms	Long-term effects
Anorexia nervosa	• Laxative misuse may cause loose stools and can result in electrolyte disturbance. • Abdominal cramps.	• Determined efforts to avoid or restrict eating. • Efforts to lose weight or avoid gaining weight by avoidance of eating and/or drinking, or avoidance of certain foods. • Purging methods: self-induced vomiting, compulsive exercising, laxative misuse. • Excessive standing, small repetitive movements of the body. • Trying to keep body temperature low. • Unusual behaviour around food and eating, e.g. ritualistic eating, cutting food up into small pieces, smearing, hiding food, eating foods separately, very slow eating, spoiling food, avoidance behaviours, refusal, and visible distress. • Asking to eat alone and disposing of food. • Hiding body in big baggy clothes. • Avoiding help, understanding, or a desire to engage in conversation, denial of behaviours or emotions observed by others. • Body checking, measuring, excessive use of mirrors. • Refusal to show body, e.g. avoidance of revealing clothes, swimsuits, or changing in front of others. • Compulsion to exercise, e.g. jiggling legs while sitting, star jumps in the bathroom, refusing to sit down. • Going to the bathroom directly after meals, smell/evidence of vomit in bathroom, vomit smell on breath are indicators that the child is purging.	• Conversations about meals/eating cause distress or concerns around food/eating and body image. • Anxiety, preoccupation and negative emotions prior to meals. • Intense fear of fatness. • Poor concentration, depression, rigid thinking, anxiety, obsessive thinking, mood swings. • Inability to see the seriousness of low weight and physical condition. • Rejection of help, with conflict between the CYP and family/staff team arising because of this.	• Mortality: 5–10% of patients across age groups die within 10 years of diagnosis. • Causes of death include starvation, suicide or electrochemical imbalance. • Low bone density • Osteopenia/ osteoporosis • Stunted growth • Delayed puberty/ amenorrhea
Bulimia nervosa	• Frequent weight change • Stomach pains • Dry or poor skin • Sore throat • Swollen salivary glands • Mouth infections/ulcers • Heart burn/ acid reflux • Electrochemical imbalance (low potassium) • Gastrointestinal effects • Hypokalemia and electrolyte disturbance	• Binges • Purging behaviours (vomiting, overexercising, laxative misuse) • Secretive eating • Periods of food avoidance • Dieting	• Weight and shape concerns • Preoccupation with food • Low self-esteem • Guilt and shame • High impulsivity • Anxiety and depression • Mood swings	• Mortality 0.3% Long-term physical effects include: • Dental erosion/ tooth decay (usually occurs after 6 months plus of vomiting) • Amenorrhea • Oesophagitis

(*Sources:* Nicholls and Grindrod 2012 and Lewer 2006)

Assessment

Where a CYP has a suspected eating disorder, referral to CAMHS is important, as research shows that early intervention results in better prognosis (Steinhausen 2009). NICE (2017) recommend that assessment includes an exploration of physical, psychological, and social need, and risk to self. Level of risk to the CYP's mental and physical health should be reassessed and monitored as treatment progresses. Risk may increase at times of weight change or transition between services. The assessment process should be seen as an opportunity for engagement, collaboration and information gathering, and an opportunity for a family and CYP to assess professionals' levels of skill and understanding (Nicholls and Grindrod 2012).

Specific questions can be used as a simple initial screen for the need for a formal assessment for eating disorders:

- Do you worry excessively about weight?
- Do you have concerns with your body?'
- Do you think you have an eating problem?
- How do you feel about your current weight?

(*Source:* Nicholls and Grindrod 2012)

Challenge and confrontation should be avoided; instead, use empathetic listening and provide information and guidance. Assessment should include time with the family, individual time with the young person, and time with parents.

Time with the family is important to:

- Discuss the history, development of eating difficulty, and how each person understands the problem.
- Describe current eating issues, including daily food intake, eating behaviours, how mealtimes are organised, and strategies used by the family to manage difficulties.
- Take a family history in order to understand relationships, emotional support in the family, and physical & mental health problems and eating disorders.

Time with CYP: It is important to discuss confidentiality prior to starting the interview. Alongside a full physical assessment, a mental state assessment should be undertaken, including an exploration of their view of the difficulty This could include talking about hopes for the future, motivation to change, and risk assessment of self-harm, suicidal ideation, and any harm to the CYP from others (current or past).

The Eating Disorder Examination (EDE) provides a framework for talking with a young person about their eating difficulty (Cooper and Fairburn 1987) and physical assessment is best carried out using Junior Marsipan guidelines (Royal College of Psychiatrists 2012). NB. Please also see the new Medical emergencies in eating disorders (MEED) guidelines, which were published this year and provide the latest evidence and recommendations, in an attempt to improve the diagnosis and treatment of eating disorders (Royal College of Psychiatrists 2022a, b).

Time with parents is used to take a developmental history, paying particular attention to early feeding and premorbid social development. It also provides time to discuss any concerns or feedback that the parents wish to discuss without the CYP present.

Eating disorders treatment

Treatment for eating disorders in CYPs involves physical factors, including nutrition, alongside psychological and psychiatric factors. Initial treatment in anorexia nervosa focuses on normalising eating in order to prioritise weight gain; early weight gain leads to a better prognosis (Lock et al. 2006). The initial treatment focus in bulimia is on normalising eating in order to interrupt the binge-purge cycle and stabilise weight (Ebeling et al. 2003; Gowers and Bryant-Waugh 2004), and to establish a more usual eating pattern with regular meals. Lethal medical complications are rare in bulimia nervosa but trauma to the gastrointestinal tract, fluid and electrolyte imbalance, and renal dysfunction can occur. NICE suggest that CYPs with anorexia and bulimia should ideally be managed and can be successfully treated in out-patient settings. With those affected by both anorexia and bulimia, attention to the adverse dental effects of vomiting and specific preventative guidance on oral hygiene is recommended (NICE 2017).

Throughout eating disorder treatment, close attention is paid to reducing both physical and psychiatric risk. Admission should only be considered if a CYP is at risk of severe self-harm or suicide (Schmidt and Treasure 1997) or of significant medical complications.

The decision to admit a CYP to hospital is usually made when there is:

- A rapid deterioration in medical state.
- Marked psychiatric risk, e.g. suicidal ideation/intent or marked depression.
- Acute food or fluid refusal unmanageable in out-patient setting.

(*Source:* Nicholls and Grindrod 2012)

Decisions to admit to a psychiatric inpatient unit are not taken lightly, as these admissions are usually intense and longer term, and often a distance away from home with limited social contact and disruption to the usual family, peer, and education contact. NICE (2017) recommend the involvement of an expert physician or paediatrician for all individuals who are medically at-risk. When treating young people with an eating disorder on general paediatric wards, it is important that locally agreed protocols between paediatric and mental health services are in place. The aims and goals of admission should be specific and agreed collaboratively prior to admission.

Family members should be involved in the treatment of CYPs with eating disorders; interventions may include sharing of information, advice on behavioural management, and facilitating communication (NICE 2017). Most CYPs with eating disorders (particularly anorexia) are ambivalent about change and may not be able to safely manage the risks if they are in charge of their eating and recovery. The Family Based Treatment (FBT) model holds control with parents supported by professionals. As the CYP recovers, and gains motivation to change, control is gently and gradually handed back.

Parents of CYPs with an eating disorder describe feelings of fear, helplessness, stress, shame, guilt, negative judgement from others, feeling excluded, depression, and anxiety (Weaver 2012). Weaver highlighted that parents want increased communication with caring, knowledgeable professionals who will intervene effectively with their child, and identified the 'persisting (and invalid) belief of family dysfunction as cause of eating disorders to be an underlying cause for tension between parents and health professionals' (Weaver 2012, p. 408).

Medication

Use of psychotropic medication has increased over the past 10 years, but these medications are not approved for use with CYPs with eating disorders. Psychiatrists should assess the CYP using a mental state examination, and assess for use of medication. Treatment guidelines suggest that medication should not be used as the primary treatment for CYPs with anorexia but for symptomatic control of comorbid symptoms (American Psychiatric Association 2013; NICE 2017). Management of anxiety, low mood, or agitation may have the added benefit to allow for psychological engagement, and ability to implement other therapeutic strategies. There is little evidence for the use of antidepressants in treating anorexia, while research on their use in bulimia demonstrates good effect, and they are recommended to have a 'legitimate but limited role' (Mitchell et al. 2007, p. 96).

Treatment recommendations for CYPs with bulimia are Cognitive Behavioural Therapy for Bulimia Nervosa (CBT BN), offered as first-line treatment, with fluoxetine added as adjunct (NICE 2017).

Specific risk management plans and close supervision are required when CYPs are taking medications, to ensure that they are swallowed. If they refuse or it is found that they are not taking their medication (e.g. hiding, spitting out, and hiding in cheeks), a discussion around consent and the CYP's concern around medication should be carried out with the psychiatrist, patient, and parents.

Nutritional management
Protocols on nutrition and risk management strategies should be used. CYPs at higher risk need to have prescribed meal plans monitored by a dietician using the Junior Marsipan guidelines for refeeding (Royal College of Psychiatrists 2012; 2022a, b).

In most underweight CYPs with anorexia, NICE guidelines recommend that meal plans allow for an average weekly weight gain of 0.5–1 kg in inpatient settings, compared with 0.5 kg per week in outpatient settings (NICE 2017).

Weight measurement
Weight should be measured at frequent regular intervals, on the same scales, with the CYP wearing similar clothes each time, and at the same time of day. The CYP should empty their bladder before being weighed. Inpatients are more likely to be weighed twice weekly. Privacy and dignity is paramount when acquiring an accurate weight. It is necessary to have vigilance over the weighing process as weight falsification is not uncommon. CYPs may water load before weighing, wear extra clothes, or hide heavy items in their pockets or on their bodies. It is best practice to pat pockets and visually scan for anything unusual before weighing. CYPs should not have access to unlimited fluids before weighing days.

Therapeutic relationship
Building a trusting therapeutic relationship with the CYPs and parents is a vital component of the nursing role and involves openness, honesty, and effective empathic communication. Listening to the CYP and developing an understanding of their symptoms, and a belief in family strengths and resources is essential to combat these illnesses. Nurses need a good understanding of the aetiology of eating disorders, the ability to build up a collaborative relationship with parents, and be aware of falling into the trap of believing that anyone is the 'problem'. It is the nurse's role to promote a neutral stance with family members and understand the concerns of each family member, as they may struggle with the situation in different ways. Goals of treatment should be agreed on collaboratively between team and family, with consideration to risk assessment and management at all times (Ramjam 2004; Snell et al. 2010; Wright 2010).

CYPs with eating disorders often show difficulties in knowing their own feelings and in being able to put them into words, particularly around feelings such as anger, frustration, sadness, and loss. Nurses have a role in modelling effective emotional communication skills and supporting a CYP to practice this. Providing time for the CYP to start to express themselves is vital, promoting healthy expression of feelings through words and other creative (drawing, clay, music, loom bands) or physical ways (hitting pillows, tearing up newspaper, kicking bean bags). Helping CYPs to develop coping and problem-solving skills, and an understanding of themselves helps development of future effective relationship skills.

Nurses and parents are likely to need to help the CYP to structure their spare time, as eating disorder thoughts can take over a CYP's mind in quiet times, and can become overwhelming and unpleasant. Spending 'illness free time' with a CYPs allows nurses to get to know them aside from the eating disorder, and in less confrontational interactions. Activities may include board games, crafts, jigsaws, puzzles, computer games, etc.

Boundaries are very important for CYPs with eating disorders, both boundaries to relationships and mealtimes, and to unhelpful eating disorder behaviours. Managing personal boundaries is an area nurses need to be able to negotiate, often finding themselves in a role that balances advocacy and authority. Nurses need to give of themselves enough to build relationships while maintaining a clear professional boundary between themselves and the CYP as patient. Nurses need to protect themselves from allegations about inappropriate conduct by ensuring that their practice is always safe. If CYPs need emotional comfort, refer to hospital policies, and always provide any personal care for the CYP alongside another member of staff. Snell et al. (2010) give clear guidance into the use of boundaries within the therapeutic nursing of patients with eating disorders.

Influence of peers
It is vital to support CYPs to maintain their peer relationships throughout treatment and hospitalisation. Young people with anorexia, when talking about the helpfulness of interaction with peers with eating disorders, expressed a dichotomy between helpfulness and competitiveness. Treatment providers must capitalise on the positive aspects and find ways of managing the negative effects (Bezance and Holliday 2013).

Observing for risk
Nurses working with CYPs need to understand the psychological and behavioural risks associated with eating disorders, e.g. low mood, self-harm, suicidal ideation, violence, food refusal, and the potential to make allegations. A psychiatrist will be responsible for regular risk assessment, clearly documented in the CYP's health care record, and nursing care plans should identify any specific risks and the required actions to manage them. A zero-tolerance approach should be taken to any violence displayed by the CYP, e.g. kicking or hitting out at parents or staff. Meetings should be held with senior staff and the family if this occurs to reset boundaries.

Staying close to a CYP's distress can be emotionally challenging for parents and nurses. Professional supervision is important to support nurses to manage high levels of psychiatric distress. If nurses are not self-aware of the feelings they can experience when with patients with eating disorders, these can be acted out in the relationship with the CYP through impatience, dislike, misunderstanding, and rejection. Nurses working with CYPs with eating disorders need to develop strategies to avoid personalising difficult behaviours that CYPs may show. Nurse peer support can be helpful. It is likely that once a CYP recovers they will acknowledge great respect for nurses who 'stick' with them through illness, and do not take things that have been said as indicative of the 'whole truth' about their relationship with the CYP (Lewer 2006; Snell et al. 2010).

Meal management
The primary aim of meal management is to support the CYP to eat adequate amounts of healthy food appropriate for necessary weight gain. Secondary aims include normalising eating behaviours: interaction styles that encourage and facilitate eating and help the CYP to feel understood. If staff can remain clear on their expectations, remain consistent, be firm but supportive, and have clear, nonnegotiable rules, this will give the best potential environment for a CYP to be able to eat. Be aware of the mechanisms that CYPs may use to induce vomiting, such as fingers, toothbrush, or a spoon. As the CYP becomes proficient at vomiting, it is likely that they will be able to vomit reflexively without mechanical stimulation. Gentle toothbrushing and use of fluoride mouthwash immediately after a vomiting episode helps to prevent dental caries (Mehler 2011).

Role of parents and nurses
At home, parents are the main support for the CYP. On a hospital ward, it is optimal if parents can be supported to continue in their usual role, supported by staff to increase their skills, confidence, and competence. Research shows that maternal and paternal self-efficacy scores around their confidence at mealtimes is predictive of eating disorder recovery and outcome (Robinson et al. 2013).

If nurses are to support the CYP, they can consider themselves 'in loco parentis' at mealtimes, but will always need to consider their limitations in this role, and should act in a way that does not undermine the CYP's parents.

Procedure guideline 18.1 Managing meal times

Statement	Rationale
1 CYPs with eating disorders should be supervised when eating and drinking.	1 To observe how much they eat and break the binge–purge cycle.
2 They will require the emotional support of an adult.	2 To distract, support, and encourage them to eat, and help them to manage anxiety at meals.
3 Mealtimes should be agreed on. A time limit should be set for the meal: 20–30 minutes for a main meal; and 10–15 minutes for dessert.	3 To allow a CYP to restore emotional energy used at mealtimes and provide a sense of control through knowing when the mealtimes begin and end.
4 CYPs should eat at a table, away from their bed if possible.	4 To provide a more normal eating environment, set boundaries, and minimise the chance for eating disorder behaviours to occur.
5 Adults should serve the food to the CYP according to a prescribed meal plan, with intake accurately recorded.	5 To minimse anxiety and introduce a regular, normal eating pattern.
6 Adults should be informed, firm, and clear regarding the amount a CYP is expected to eat and drink, and remain consistent in this expectation.	6, 7 To help the CYP feel emotionally contained, with little chance for negotiation or manipulation by the eating disorder.
7 Avoid discussions/negotiations around portion sizes.	
8 Do not be tempted to offer the CYP more food if they have eaten a whole meal or snack within the time limit.	8 Offering more food may cause undue anxiety to the CYP. It may affect how much they can eat at the next meal. CYPs with eating disorders should not be presented with surprises at mealtimes.
Interaction styles	
1 Show that you believe and trust the CYP but are also aware of the 'tricks' that the illness may play.	1 CYPs feel contained by staff that know about eating disorders tricks, and who recognise that there is a separation between the CYP and the eating disorder.
2 Be sensitive around conversation topics at mealtimes. Avoid food or body image talk. It is best to stick to neutral topics. Try to talk about normal age-appropriate topics, such as films, TV, news items, music, and weekend plans.	2 To reduce anxiety at the table, distract the CYP from eating disorder thoughts, and normalise the eating environment.
3 Be sensitive when giving feedback to the CYP on how they managed the meal. Check what they find helpful.	3 Many CYPs find praise around eating difficult, as this can produce guilt and a sense of failing the eating disorder, which can in turn have the negative effect of increased determination not to eat.
Emotional support	
CYPs differ in the types of emotional support they find helpful. Ask the what works best for them.	
1 However upset a CYP is, avoid discussing feelings about eating at the table. Advise them on more appropriate times to talk about eating and food.	1 This models that feelings and food are separate and promotes mealtimes as a time to focus on eating.
2 Beware of conversations that result in a CYP talking in place of eating.	2 To prevent distraction aimed at delaying/avoiding eating.
3 Emotional support may be required before and after meals. These support sessions should be kept brief, approximately 15 minutes.	3 To enable the CYP to express feelings and feel understood. The session should be kept short to prevent it becoming a preoccupation.
4 Premeal sessions can be used to plan how the nurse or parent can be most useful during a meal.	4 To find out what strategies are more and less helpful, and what roles to take if there is more than one adult with the CYP.
5 A CYP may need close supervision after meals. Distraction may help, as may peer or family contact. What is helpful will need to be discussed and understood and will be different for each CYP.	5 This helps if there is concern that they may be at risk of purging, exercising, or low mood following meals. Distraction may help, as may peer or family contact.

Consent

When a CYP with anorexia nervosa refuses treatment that is deemed essential, consideration should be given to their mental capacity (Department of Health 1983) and the right of those with parental responsibility to override the CYP's refusal (NICE 2017).

It is not advisable to rely on parental consent to over-ride refusal for treatment indefinitely. Clinicians should take legal advice at the point that a CYP is not consenting to treatment, with nonconsent clearly documented alongside team decisions about subsequent actions. When consent issues are highlighted, NICE (2017) recommend that a second opinion be sought by the treatment team.

Food refusal

If a CYP refuses to eat/ drink all of their meal, be clear that they are expected to make up the refused amount by the end of the day. Discuss how they would like to do this. Discuss with medical team and make a risk assessment. Agree on the level of physical observations needed.

If the CYP is not able to make up missed amounts of food/drink, discuss with dieticians whether supplements could be used as 'top-ups'. In this case the CYP is presented with their usual meal, and anything to make up is provided in a supplement drink, and presented to them immediately following the meal, with a 10-minute time limit.

If the CYP is not able to manage a meal plan with either food or supplements, a planning meeting needs to be held with professionals and parents, and the CYP should be involved as much as possible. Assessing risk and capacity is essential.

Nasogastric (NG) feeding may be considered if all options for oral intake have been explored. This decision may have long-term consequences in CYPs with anorexia, as they can become easily reliant on NG feeding, which can prolong the length of illness and hospitalisation. NG use needs to be discussed with the CYP. Feeding with consent and for short periods is safer and better for prognosis, so consent should be negotiated whenever possible and by a professional skilled in this area. Some CYPs accept NG feeding as it gives them a brief break from eating, and helps them regain physical health.

If a CYP does not consent to being fed, a second opinion should be sought in order to guide decisions around treatment, and inpatient treatment may be required (Tan et al. 2003).

References

American Psychiatric Association (2013). Diagnostic and statistical manual of mental disorders (5th edition). Washington, DC: American Psychiatric Association.

Association for Young People's Health (2015). Improving young people's health and well-being A framework for public health. https://assets.publishing.service.gov.uk/government/uploads/system/uploads/attachment_data/file/773365/20150128_YP_HW_Framework_FINAL_WP_3_.pdf (accessed 13 August 2022).

Bezance, J. and Holliday, J. (2013). Adolescents with anorexia nervosa have their say: a review of qualitative studies on treatment and recovery from anorexia nervosa. *European Eating Disorders Review* 21 (5): 352–360.

Button, E.J. and Warren, R.L. (2001). Living with anorexia nervosa: the experience of a cohort of sufferers from anorexia nervosa 7.5 years after initial presentation to a specialised eating disorders service. *European Eating Disorders Review* 9: 74–96.

CAMHS Tier 4 Report Steering Group (2014). Child and adolescent mental health services tier 4 report. NHS England. https://www.england.nhs.uk/wp-content/uploads/2014/07/camhs-tier-4-rep.pdf (accessed 13 August 2022).

Christie D and Khatun H. (2012). Adjusting life to chronic illness. The British Psychological Society. The Psychologist. 25(3):194–197.

Cooper, Z. and Fairburn, C.G. (1987). The eating disorder examination: a semistructured interview for the assessment of the specific psychopathology of eating disorders. *International Journal of Eating Disorders* 6: 1–8. https://doi.org/10.1002/1098-108x(198701)6:1<1::aid-eat2260060102>3.0.co;2-9.

Department of Health (DH) (1983). Mental Health Act 1983, London, HMSO. Available online at: www.legislation.gov.uk/ukpga/1983/20/contents (accessed 7 June 2018).

Ebeling, H., Tapanainen, P., Joutsenoja, A. et al.; Finnish Medical Society Duodecim. (2003). A practice guideline for treatment of eating disorders in children and adolescents. *Annals of Medicine* 35 (7): 488–501.

Gowers, S. and Bryant-Waugh, R. (2004). Management of child and adolescent eating disorders: the current evidence base and future directions. *Journal of Child Psychology and Psychiatry* 45 (1): 63–83.

Kids Relaxation (2016) Kids Relaxation; helping parents & educators activate children's highest potential. http://kidsrelaxation.com (accessed 7 June 2018).

Lewer, L. (2006). Nursing children and young people with eating disorders. In: *Child and Adolescent Mental Health Nursing* (ed. T. McDougall), 88–115. Oxford: Blackwell Publishing.

Lock, J., Couturier, J., Bryson, S., and Agras, S. (2006). Predictors of dropout and remission in family therapy for adolescent anorexia nervosa in a randomized clinical trial. *International Journal of Eating Disorders* 39: 639–647.

Mehler, P. (2011). Medical complications of bulimia nervosa and their treatments. *International Journal of Eating Disorders* 44 (2): 95–104.

Mental Health Foundation (2016). Fundamental facts about mental health 2016. https://www.mentalhealth.org.uk/publications/fundamental-facts-about-mental-health-2015 (accessed 13 August 2022).

Mitchell, J., Agras, S., and Wonderlich, S. (2007). Treatment of bulimia nervosa: where are we and where are we going? *International Journal of Eating Disorders* 40 (2): 95–101.

National Institute for Health and Clinical Excellence (NICE) (2013a). Self-harm. Quality standard (QS34). www.nice.org.uk/guidance/qs34 (accessed 13 August 2022).

National Institute for Health and Clinical Excellence (NICE) (2013b). Social anxiety disorder: recognition, assessment and treatment. CG159. www.nice.org.uk/guidance/cg159 (accessed 13 August 2022).

National Institute for Health and Clinical Excellence (NICE) (2017). Eating disorders: recognition and treatment. CG69. London: NICE. https://www.nice.org.uk/guidance/ng69 (accessed 13 August 2022).

NHS (2022). Mental health for children, teenagers and young adults. https://www.nhs.uk/mental-health/children-and-young-adults/ (accessed 13 August 2022).

Nicholls, D. and Grindrod, C. (2012). Behavioural eating disorders. *Paediatrics and Child Health* 23: 11–17.

Office for National Statistics (2005). Mental health of children and young people in Great Britain, 2004. https://digital.nhs.uk/data-and-information/publications/statistical/mental-health-of-children-and-young-people-in-england/mental-health-of-children-and-young-people-in-great-britain-2004 –(accessed 13 August 2022).

Ramjam, T. (2004). Nurses and the therapeutic relationship caring for adolescents with anorexia nervosa. *Journal of Advanced Nursing* 45: 495–503.

Robinson, A., Stratten, E., Girz, L. et al. (2013). I know I can help you'. Parental self –efficacy predicts adolescent outcomes in FBT for eating disorders. *European Eating Disorders Review* 21: 108–114.

Rose, M., Frampton, I., and Lask, B. (2014). Central coherence, organizational strategy, and visuospatial memory in children and adolescents with anorexia nervosa. *Applied Neuropsychology: Child* 3 (4): 284–296.

Royal College of Psychiatrists (2012). Junior MARSIPAN: Management of Really Sick Patients under 18 with Anorexia Nervosa. https://www.rcpsych.ac.uk/docs/default-source/members/faculties/eating-disorders/marsipan/junior-marsipan-cr168.pdf?sfvrsn=65e82800_2 (accessed 13 August 2022).

Royal College of Psychiatrists (2022a). From Marsipan to MEED. https://ellernmede.org/2022/03/24/from-marsipan-to-meed/ (accessed 13 August 2022).

Royal College of Psychiatrists (2022b). Medical emergencies in eating disorders (MEED). Guidance on recognition and management. https://www.rcpsych.ac.uk/improving-care/campaigning-for-better-mental-health-policy/college-reports/2022-college-reports/cr233 (accessed 13 August 2022).

Royal College of Psychiatrists (2022c). Anxiety, panic and phobias. https://www.rcpsych.ac.uk/mental-health/problems-disorders/anxiety-panic-and-phobias (accessed 13 August 2022).

Royal College of Psychiatrists (2022d). Depression in young people - helping children to cope: information for parents and carers. https://www.rcpsych.ac.uk/mental-health/parents-and-young-people/information-for-parents-and-carers/depression-in-young-people---helping-children-to-cope-for-parents-and-carers (accessed 13 August 2022).

Schmidt, U. and Treasure, J. (1997). *Clinician's Guide to Getter Better Bit(e) by Bit(e): A Survival Guide for Sufferers of Bulimia Nervosa and Binge Eating Disorders*. Brighton: Psychology Press.

Snell, L., Crowe, M., and Jordan, J. (2010). Maintaining a therapeutic connection: nursing in an inpatient eating disorder unit. *Journal of Clinical Nursing* 19 (3–4): 351–358.

Steinhausen, H. (2009). Outcomes of eating disorders. *Child & Adolescent Psychiatric Clinics of North America* 18: 225–242.

Tan, J.O., Hope, T., Stewart, A., and Fitzpatrick, R. (2003). Control and compulsory treatment in anorexia nervosa: the views of patients and parents. *International Journal of Law and Psychiatry* 26: 627–645.

Weaver, K. (2012). Loving her into well-being one day at a time. Narratives of caring for daughters with eating disorders. *Open Journal of Nursing* 2 (2): 406–419.

Whiteford, H., Hegenhardt, L., Rehgm, J. et al. (2013). Global burden of disease attributable to mental and substance use disorders: findings from the Global Burden of Disease Study 2010. *Lancet* 382: 1575–1586.

Woodgate, M. and Garralda, M.E. (2006). Paediatric liaison work by child and adolescent mental health services. *Child and Adolescent Mental Health* 11 (1): 19–24.

World Health Organization (WHO) (2022). Mental health: Overview. https://www.who.int/health-topics/mental-health#tab=tab_1 (accessed 13 August 2022).

Wright, P. (2010). Therapeutic relationships: developing a new understanding for nurses and care-workers within an eating disorder unit. *International Journal of Mental Health Nursing* 19 (3): 154–161.

Young Minds (2022a). Young Minds: Fighting for young people's mental health. www.youngminds.org.uk –(accessed 13 August 2022).

Young Minds (2022b). A guide for young people: Self-harm. https://www.youngminds.org.uk/young-person/my-feelings/self-harm/ (accessed 13 August 2022).

Young Minds (2022c). A guide for young people: Psychosis. https://www.youngminds.org.uk/young-person/mental-health-conditions/psychosis/ (accessed 13 August 2022).

Chapter 19

Moving and handling

Kathleen Owen[1] and Janet Brooks[2]

[1] Formerly Back Care Advisor and Moving and Handling Trainer, Great Ormond Street Hospital, London, UK

[2] Back Care Advisor, GOSH

Chapter contents

Introduction	416
Why is the legislation important?	416
Moving and handling risk assessment	416
Musculoskeletal health and wellbeing	417
Education and training	418
Documentation	421
Equipment	421
References	425

Principles tables

19.1 General guidelines	422
19.2 Patient assessment	423
19.3 Equipment	424
19.4 Positioning	424
19.5 Risk assessment	424
19.6 Hoisting	425

The Great Ormond Street Hospital Manual of Children and Young People's Nursing Practices, Second Edition. Edited by Elizabeth Anne Bruce, Janet Williss, and Faith Gibson.
© 2023 John Wiley & Sons Ltd. Published 2023 by John Wiley & Sons Ltd.

Introduction

Every day, healthcare practitioners (HCPs) move and handle a variety of items, including equipment and people. This can vary from carrying small pieces of medical equipment, to pushing beds and trolleys and moving and handling children and young people (CYPs). Each of these activities presents a unique challenge and, if not undertaken safely, has the potential to cause harm to the HCP, CYP, or others. Moving and handling practice is determined by legislation, this being The Manual Handling Operations Regulations 1992 (as amended) (MHOR 1992). The legislation dictates the duties of employers and employees in terms of moving and handling practice. The goal of safe moving and handling is to ensure that any risks are proportionate to the care and support needs of the individual CYP. All moving and handling activities need to be properly managed; CYPs with life-limiting conditions are supported with medical advancement and at times, the CYP's moving and handling needs may present significant challenges to the HCP.

The Health and Safety Executive (HSE) states that "Health and safety legislation does not prohibit all moving and handling; rather it requires employers to adopt a risk management approach. Employers need to focus on enabling, rather than prohibiting" (HSE 2022). There could be times when the clinical need of the CYP may impact the handling procedure prescribed. In cases such as this it is important that all members of the multi-disciplinary team are involved in undertaking a risk assessment that reduces the risks to the lowest level reasonably practicable. It is important that organisations own and acknowledge the moving and handling risks and have systems and processes in place to support the reduction of these risks. These need to be disseminated so that staff are aware of the safe systems of work within the sphere of their practice.

Staff may struggle to implement safe moving and handling if parents and carers undertake moving and handling techniques that put themselves at risk of injury. It can be difficult to intervene and promote techniques that are deemed current and best practice when parents are undertaking controversial techniques. However, staff have a personal and professional responsibility to adopt best practice and to support parents to do the same, through dialogue and discussion with family members and the CYP. With this in mind, staff need to have a basic understanding of the requirements of MHOR 1992 (as amended), as well as the impact of controversial techniques on their musculoskeletal health. For advice on restrictive physical interventions and clinical holding (formerly restraint) please see section 8 in the Introduction to this book.

Why is the legislation important?

Over time, moving and handling legislation has been interpreted heavily towards the HCP undertaking the handling, as opposed to having a balanced approach to risk assessment. It is important when supporting CYPs with moving and handling to have a balanced approach. The National Back Exchange publication *Manual Handling of Children* states that "focusing on one person, group or aspect when considering safer moving and handling carries the possibility that other areas may be under-emphasised or not given the importance deserved" (Alexander and Johnson 2011). The legislation surrounding health and safety can be confusing; however there are six key regulations that interlink and are known as the six-pack of health and safety legislation, being:

1 Management of Health and Safety at Work Regulations 1999: Requires employers to carry out risk assessments, make arrangements to implement necessary measures, appoint competent people, and arrange for appropriate information and training.
2 Workplace (Health, Safety and Welfare) Regulations 1992: Covers a wide range of basic health, safety, and welfare issues such as ventilation, heating, lighting, workstations, seating, and welfare facilities.
3 Health and Safety (Display Screen Equipment) Regulations 1992: Sets out requirements for work with Visual Display Units (VDUs).
4 Personal Protective Equipment at Work Regulations 1992: Requires employers to provide appropriate protective clothing and equipment for their employees.
5 Provision and Use of Work Equipment Regulations 1998: Requires that equipment provided for use at work, including machinery, is safe.
6 Manual Handling Operations Regulations 1992 (MHOR 1992): Covers the moving of objects by hand or bodily force.

The MOHR (1992) determines how organisations are to manage moving and handling practice in their establishments. The legislations imposes duties on the employer and employee. The main aim of the MHOR is to reduce the incidence and prevalence of musculoskeletal disorders (MSDs) arising from the manual handling of loads at work.

This chapter focuses primarily on the moving and handling of CYPs; however, in terms of the legislation "a load" is an inanimate object, a person, or an animal, so it is equally important to consider the regulations when using and moving equipment. The MHOR sets out a hierarchy of three duties on employers:

1 "The employer shall so far as is reasonably practicable, avoid the need for his employees to undertake any manual handling operations at work which involve a risk of injury (reg.4(1)(a));
2 Where (1) above is not possible, the employer shall make a suitable and sufficient assessment of all such operations which cannot be avoided, taking account of Schedule 1 (reg.4(1)(b)(i)); and
3 The employer shall take appropriate steps to reduce the risk of injury during those operations to the lowest level reasonably practicable (reg.4(1)(b)(ii))." (MHOR 2002)

When assessing the risk of moving and handling, the legislation guides staff to undertake an ergonomic risk assessment. This could be a formal documented risk assessment, or a dynamic risk assessment undertaken at the time of handling a load. Dynamic risk assessments are particularly pertinent to moving and handling CYPs, as their needs can change during an activity or task.

Over time, much work has been undertaken to develop and design people moving and handling techniques that are safe for all concerned; this includes hoists to move people from one surface to another instead of lifting them, and slide sheets to move people in the bed. These techniques are safer for all concerned and reduce the risks to the lowest level that is reasonably practicable. These techniques are usually known as "safe systems of work" or "moving and handling procedures". All health and social care services will include these as part of their moving and handling policy. Employers and employees need to have a clear understanding of their duties under the MHOR and it is important that this information is easy to access and understand. Training is seen as a key hierarchy of control and is important; however, it is not the main focus for moving and handling risk reduction methods. An embedded risk assessment and risk reduction culture within an organisation is important; staff need to feel empowered to undertake moving and handling in a correct and safe manner. It is important that managers and senior staff receive advice, guidance, and support in relation to legislation, policies, and best practices that have been endorsed by the organisation.

Moving and handling risk assessment

If a moving and handling task cannot be avoided, a risk assessment will be required. The risk assessment should follow an ergonomic approach and be suitable and sufficient to the CYP's needs. Following the risk assessment, an individualised plan should be documented to inform staff how best to support the CYP with the moving and handling task. Many organisations have a generic risk assessment tool and a set way to record the handling plan and the needs of the CYP. For many CYPs, their handling needs will fall within safe handling techniques. These are evidence-based and reduce the risks for all concerned. There may be a small number of CYPs, however, whose handling needs fall outside of these safe techniques; for example, with conjoined twins, a multidisciplinary approach to managing handing will be required. The handling techniques in cases like this may pose a higher risk to the handlers, and it is important that any risks to the HCP are clearly identified and acknowledged. Staff with existing health conditions may need to modify the handling they participate in. When supporting CYPs with moving and handling it is important to enable them to be as independent as possible. A simple tool to support this is described later in the chapter.

We often undertake an ergonomic risk assessment without formalising the process. The process is simply breaking the risk assessment into factors that may affect the handling being undertaken. We undertake risk assessment all the time, often subconsciously; a good example is when crossing the road. We are assessing the speed of the traffic, the road surface, the step down from the kerb, whether it is raining, or whether there is debris in the gutter.

The MHOR categorises the factors for a moving and handling risk assessment into five areas, which give us the acronym TILEO: the **T**ask being undertaken; the **I**ndividual undertaking the task; the **L**oad (inanimate load, person, or animal being moved, i.e. the CYP), the **E**nvironment in which the handling is being undertaken, the **E**quipment being used and any **O**ther aspect that may impact on the handling.

The following table identifies some of the risk factors that could be considered with determining the moving and handling risk factors.

Task	What are you trying to achieve? Does the task involve twisting, stooping, bending, and reaching upwards? Is there insufficient rest or recovery between tasks? Will the child move suddenly? Are there issues in taking hold of the load? Does the task involve static postures? Is the handler supporting a number of CYPs with handling tasks during the day? Is there a repetition of tasks?
Individual	(This part refers to the people undertaking the handling task.) Do they know how to undertake the task safely? Does the task pose a risk to someone with health issues? Does it call for special information or training? Do you have the correct clothing and footwear? Is the handler wearing full PPE? Is the handler hindered in their movement because of the PPE? Is the handler pregnant?
Load	Does the CYP have delicate skin? Is the CYP at risk of fractures? Does the CYP have capacity to consent to the handling activity? Does the CYP want to be supported in this manner? Does the CYP have additional needs that may impact on the handling task? Is the CYP's weight recorded accurately?
Environment	Is there enough space? Are there slip, trip, and fall risks? Is the area cluttered? Are there poor floor surfaces? Is the area too hot or too cold? What are the lighting conditions, especially when undertaking handling at night?
Equipment	Is the right equipment available in the place it is needed? Is the equipment functioning and ready to use? Is the equipment clean?
Other	Do the handlers feel they are supported? Do they feel there is a lack of consideration of the planning and scheduling of the tasks? When handling smaller children who may be considered for long-term hoisting, do the handlers feel it is easier just to lift the child? Has there been a sudden change in workload?

When undertaking the risk assessment, be it a dynamic or a formal, documented risk assessment, it is important to acknowledge that the handler will lift, move, and carry babies and small children in line with what is expected in society. The handler needs to be mindful of the risks associated with their role in these tasks; if they are supporting a number of babies and small children in the day this will increase the risks significantly. It is imperative that HCPs who identify handling hazards or risks report them to managers, and that managers ensure that these risks are then dealt with appropriately before the risk is reassessed, to ensure that the manual handling task is now safe. To comply with the MHOR (1992, amended 2002) this process should be documented in the CYP's records.

As mentioned earlier, it is important to encourage the CYP to do as much for themselves as possible, to maintain their mobility and independence. Another way to undertake a person-centred risk assessment for moving and handling is to be guided by the Manual Handling Questions (MHQs) (Steed and Kennedy 1999). MHQs are a hierarchy of questions that the handler can ask to determine the degree of moving and handling care and support a CYP needs. The questions are:

1. What is normal movement for the task?
2. Can I teach the person to do this unaided?
   a. If no go to Q3
3. If no, is there any small handling equipment that can help the person do this unaided?
   a. If no go to Q4
4. What is the assistance of one or two handlers?
5. Are there any unsafe methods I need to avoid?

MHQs encourage the HCP to work through the needs of the individual and encourage the CYP to do as much for themselves as possible. It is important to give the CYP verbal encouragement initially to help them achieve their goal and remain as independent as possible while also minimising the degree of moving and handling required by the HCP. Although the task may take longer, the benefits include maintaining the CYP's functioning and confidence. At other times, especially in an acute phase, the CYP may need more support from the HCP; it is helpful to identify parts of the task where the CYP can assist, or do things for themself, as this increases the CYP's confidence in their ability to be as independent as possible.

When assessing moving and handling CYPs, it is not uncommon for people to dismiss the risks associated with the task because the assumed weight of the CYP is much less than that of an adult. This is a dangerous assumption to make, as the load associated with CYPs can vary immensely, depending on the risk assessment factors identified. Utilising the MHQs as part of the risk assessment process will enable a safe outcome for all concerned.

Musculoskeletal health and wellbeing

The main focus of the MHOR (1992) is the reduction of work-related back injuries. The legislation imposes duties to support the reduction of work-related moving and handling risks. As well as implementing a risk assessment process and safe systems of work for moving and handling, organisations can put proactive systems in place to support staff. There is a growing emphasis on the workplace agendas of health and wellbeing. Promoting effective health and wellbeing programmes and supporting staff to engage in these promotes a healthy work place and workforce. Smith (2011) highlights the importance of developing an understanding of the biomechanics principles which promote best practice. This will enable staff to develop effective strategies for managing their own musculoskeletal health and wellbeing.

Moving and handling techniques are designed using a dynamic and normal movement approach to reduce the stress and strain on muscle groups, in particular the back. The human spine consists of 24 vertebrae that sit on top of each other and are separated by a thin cartilage disc that has a fibrous outer layer and a viscous centre (Figure 19.1). These discs act as shock absorbers and prevent the vertebrae from rubbing against each other when moving. There are 7 cervical vertebrae, 12 thoracic vertebrae, and 5 lumbar vertebrae. The vertebrae are held in place by ligaments and muscles that run the length of the spinal column and provide stability and movement throughout. Running inside the vertebral bodies is the spinal cord. This originates at the brain stem and concludes at the cauda equina at the sacral level. Exiting from each vertebral level from the space between the vertebrae are nerve roots that provide the nerve supply to each part of the body.

The lumbar spine is the most likely area to be injured in manual handling (HSE 2011). The lumbar spine is very stable in its closed packed position of neutral or slightly extended, i.e. standing upright. It has specific muscular support that assists in providing the important stability required in the area and allows the many movements that this area of the back offers. The lumbar spine has a good range of movement of forwards, backwards, and sideways. When flexing forward, the bony stability of the lumbar spine is lost, and the ligaments and muscles become responsible for its stability. In the first 45° of flexion there is a 'shear' force that acts on the joints of the lumbar spine. This force is magnified if there is increased weight in position forward of the person's centre of gravity. If there is a pre-existing weakness in the joints or if the muscular strength is insufficient to stabilise the movement this force can result in injury to the tissue. In moving and handling, this position of slight to moderate lumbar flexion is common, and especially so when working with CYPs. This posture is often adopted when supporting CYPs, repositioning in the bed or cot, playing on the floor, or undertaking personal care. HCPs may find they are undertaking tasks in these positions for extended periods of time under stressful loads and in difficult environments. This is why the lumbar spine is prone to injury when moving and handling. Injury to the lumbar spine can include damage to the muscles, joints, discs, nerves, or, commonly, a combination of these. The continuum of lumbar spine injury ranges from a slight strain, which can cause discomfort for a few days, to a ruptured disc and/or nerve compression, which can require surgery or months of rehabilitation (Roland et al. 2002).

The neck, thoracic spine, and upper limbs make up the majority of the remaining manual handling injuries (HSE 2010). Once again, posture in relation to the task, individual capabilities, load, and environment are the most common risk factors and cause of injury. HCPs are not only undertaking moving and handling care and support of CYPs; there has been a significant increase in the use of electronic patient records. The HCP may be using palm-held devices to record care at the bedside. When doing so they will flex the neck and look at the device for periods of time; when hunching over, the head leans forward; this is also known as "text-neck" (HSE 2010).

Looking after your musculoskeletal health is important; many organisations provide HCPs with moving and handling training which identifies the risks and the actions staff need to take to minimise these risks. This training is only part of the process; an effective health and wellbeing service provided by dedicated occupational health professionals is also essential. These services may include reduced-price gym membership, on-site Pilates, yoga sessions, and high-intensity training (HIT) classes, and should focus on all levels of health and fitness. Following any musculoskeletal injury, timely rehabilitation is vitally important in returning the HCP to full health. Research has shown that early intervention from a physiotherapist or similar HCP, and early return to work, results in reduced pain levels, improved function, and a more effective return to full duties than would otherwise occur (Boorman 2010). HCPs with an injury should seek advice as early as possible and attempt to maintain their mobility throughout the early stages of their injury. Lambeek et al. (2010) found that an integrated approach to rehabilitation, supported by occupational health, was the most effective and efficient way of returning employees to work and their full duties. The main goal of treatment should be to restore function in the HCP's working and personal life, and pain should be managed, rather than be the primary focus. Lambeek et al. (2010) utilised the skills of occupational nurses, doctors, and physiotherapists to offer a range of support structures to enable the worker to return to work earlier, with less cost to the organisation. The Boorman Review (Boorman 2010) advocated an integrated bio-psychosocial approach to rehabilitation following a work injury, which addressed biological, psychological, occupational, and compensation factors. Throughout the injury-healing process, an employee should be in constant contact with their manager and occupational health department. Early return to work is an important part of the rehabilitation process and can be facilitated through phased return to work programmes, utilising modified duties, and/or restricted hours. Organisations need to have comprehensive systems and processes in place for supporting all staff in managing the risks of moving and handling. These need to be interlinked and support the application of the MHOR.

When supporting CYPs with moving and handling it is important to consider any harm that may inadvertently occur as a result of the moving and handling. CYPs for the most part are significantly smaller than adults and require an altered level of force when being supported with moving and handling. Correct or incorrect moving and handling can result in soft tissue damage to the CYP. This can be due to difficult handholds, the application of too much pressure, residual joint and soft tissue tenderness, aggravation of pressure areas, or discomfort from poor positioning. The CYP may move suddenly or unpredictably; they may be fearful or not fully comprehend what you are trying to achieve; equipment used may cause injuries, such as bruising or marks. If any injuries occur it is imperative that these are recorded as part of the organisation's incident-reporting process.

Education and training

Induction training introduces employees to the working practices related to moving and handling and should ensure that they understand clearly how manual handling operations have been designed to ensure their safety. Regular updates enable an organisation to communicate changes in practices, policies, and procedures. It ensures that staff are aware of new equipment in their working environment and any changes to systems of work, and that they are able to assess a CYP with new or unexpected handling issues. Moving and handling advisors are seeking ways to develop blended approaches to moving and handling training. Many have developed risk assessment workshops, ward specific sessions, and competency assessment frameworks, as well as the traditional face-to-face training. It is important to remember that each individual HCP learns in a different way. The Health and Safety Executive (HSE 2004) states that courses should be suitable for the individual, tasks, and environment involved, use relevant examples, and last long enough to cover all the relevant information. Such information is likely to include advice on:

- Manual handling risk factors and how injuries can occur.
- How to implement safe moving and handling with good technique.

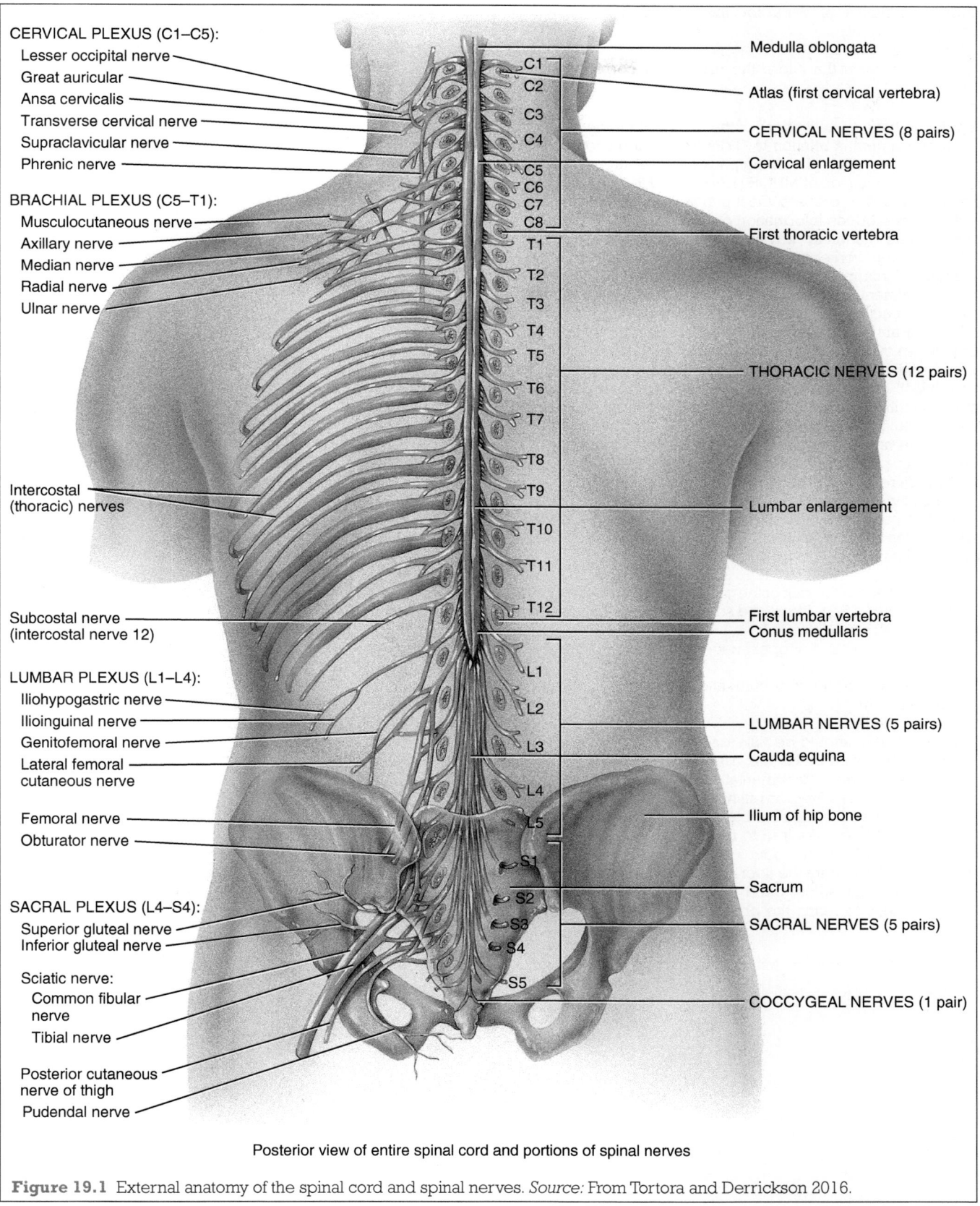

Figure 19.1 External anatomy of the spinal cord and spinal nerves. *Source:* From Tortora and Derrickson 2016.

- Appropriate policies of work for the individual's task and environment.
- Use of mechanical aids.
- A practical component that allows the instructor to correct unsafe habits.

HCPs need to have an awareness of the basics of biomechanics and normal movement in relation to CYPs. This information could be presented as part of an eLearning package. Resources on legislation, and the application of MHOR (1992) could form part of the organisation's induction process. Occupational health physiotherapy services can produce information on MSK and injury prevention; moving and handling advisors can undertake targeted practical application workshops, so staff can top up their skills on bed techniques. A competency assessment framework focusing on basic risk assessment processes can be developed to support the HCP in clinical practice. It is important to make moving and handling education and training relevant to the HCP role, as well as engaging and enjoyable. Education and training should enable the HCP to raise additional role specific concerns with the moving and handling advisor, and they should feel empowered to contact the moving and handling advisor if they have any queries or concerns regarding the moving and handling needs of a CYP in their care.

Because of the varied nature of the many job roles within a health care setting (e.g. phlebotomy, ICU nursing, physiotherapists, porters), all of which require manual handling of different items (CYPs, adults, machinery, equipment, etc.), it is not within the scope of this chapter to give advice on all of these. However, there are some general principles that should be followed to ensure safe and effective moving and handling. This includes:

- Stop and think: Assess the risk of the procedure prior to attempting the task (Figure 19.2). Abort and seek assistance if unable to complete the task safely.
- Assess the CYP care and support needs in relation to moving and handling.
- Ensure that the point above is documented in the correct manner in the clinical notes.
- Wear appropriate clothing.
- Load-handling tasks should be risk-assessed and documented. HCP's should be aware of the risk assessment and have ready access to the assessment documentation.
- When lifting, moving, pulling, or pushing, ensure that the load is kept as close to the body as possible. There is a direct relationship between the force required to move a weight and the distance that weight is from the body.
- When lifting an object from the floor, maintain a neutral (straight/in alignment) lumbar spine, bend forward from the hips, and bend at the knees to reach the object. Once in control with a sound grip, reinforce the straight/aligned back, push through the legs, and extend hips and knees (Figure 19.3).
- Always move the load within your base of support.
- The lumbar spine should not flex forward when lifting objects; it should remain straight. Avoid twisting or jerking movements (Figure 19.4).
- Avoid neck holds, bear hugs, and pivot transfers to mobilise a patient. HCPs should avoid holding CYPs on their hips.
- When tending to a CYP in bed where it is required to lean over, have the CYP move as close to the edge as possible. If they are unable to move, consider using slide sheets to reposition them.

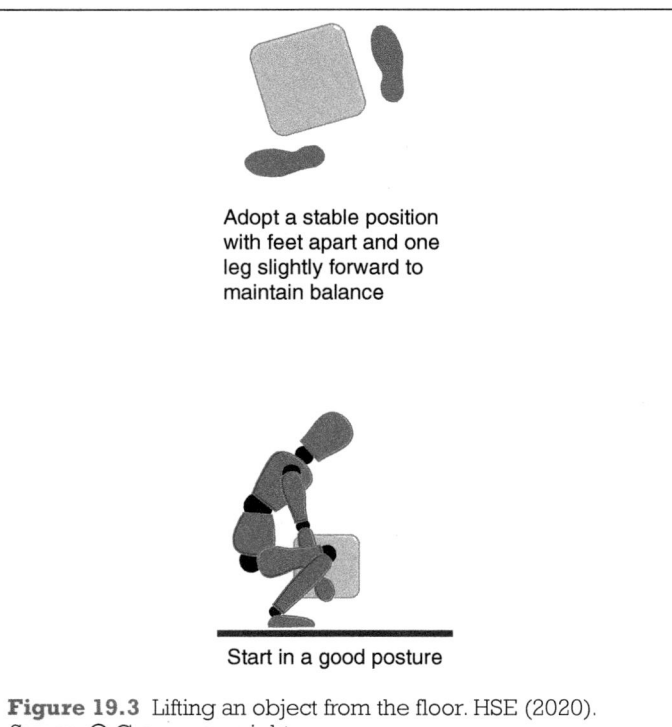

Figure 19.3 Lifting an object from the floor. HSE (2020). Source: © Crown copyright.

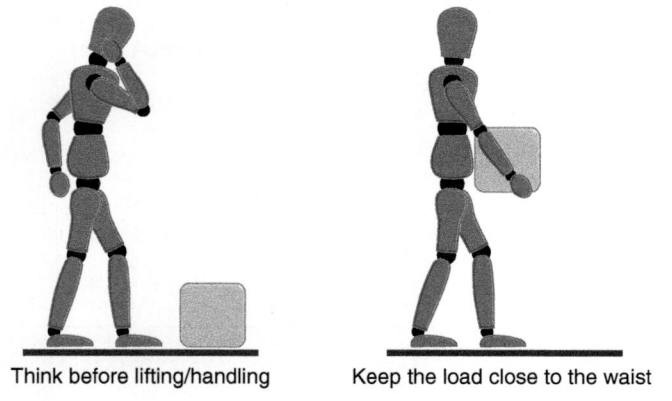

Figure 19.2 Rules for manual handling. HSE (2020). Source: © Crown copyright.

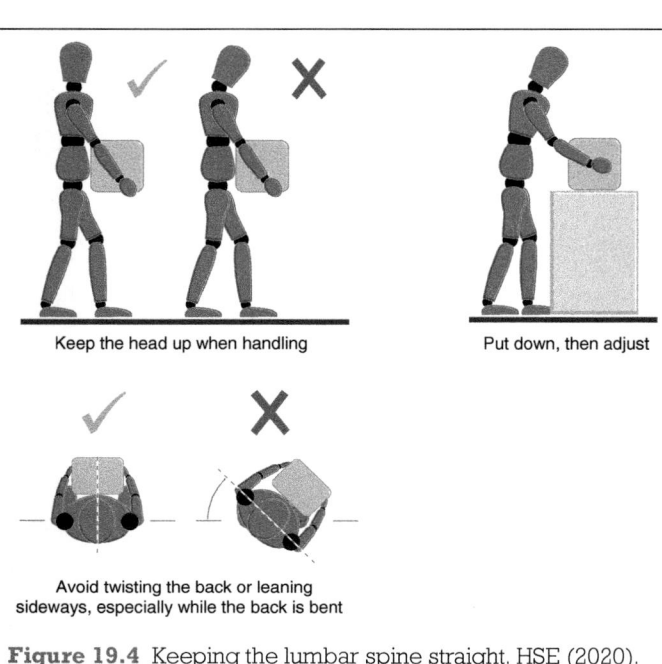

Figure 19.4 Keeping the lumbar spine straight. HSE (2020). Source: © Crown copyright.

- Ensure that the bed height is adjusted so that the area requiring access is within easy reach without leaning.
- The HCP should be close to the side of the bed to perform the procedure.
- Babies are often seen as easy to manually handle; however, they may be attached to medical equipment, which can make them heavy or difficult to handle. Planning should take this into account.
- When required to perform a task over a prolonged period, attempt to assume a position that is comfortable, but which also allows repositioning at regular intervals.

Whatever system of handling the HCP chooses based on the risk assessment, they must ensure that the CYP's airway can be maintained at all times and where necessary, one HCP is allocated to take control of the CYP's airway at all times.

Documentation

For each CYP, staff must complete an initial moving and handling risk assessment (as provided by their organisation), which identifies and reflects the CYP's handling needs, the people required to assist, and the equipment and procedures that will be used. This enables the HCP to maintain consistency in handling, reduce unnecessary handling, and ensure that nursing records reflect the moving and handling care and support needs of the CYP while maintaining accurate documentation (NMC 2015, updated 2018). The assessment should be read by all staff before supporting the CYP with moving and handling, be reviewed on a regular basis, and updated each time the CYP's handling needs change.

Documentation should reflect the observed effects, both positive and adverse, of each handling episode. Adverse incidents should be reported immediately to the relevant reporting system of the organisation senior staff member and the relevant incident/accident forms completed in line with local policy and the Reporting of Incidents, Diseases and Dangerous Occurrences Regulations (RIDDOR) (HSE 2013a). This will facilitate early detection of faulty equipment or user error and ensure the HCP or CYP is supported appropriately.

Equipment

Manual handling equipment is often used by the HCP in the adult population and should also be used for CYPs. Table 19.1 details the type of equipment that can be utilised for manual handling. It is important to remember that equipment or aids should reduce the load on the HCP, be easy to operate, be able to safely mobilise the CYP within the environment in which it is being used, and should be kept in good condition through regular maintenance. As stated previously, the risk of injury from a manual handling task is increased when workers do not have the information or training necessary to enable them to work safely. It is therefore essential that where equipment for manual handling or mechanical handling aids is available, appropriate support and guidance is provided. Legislation states that staff must be offered and take up support and guidance as required in their local policy (Health and Safety at Work etc. Act [HSWA] 1974; MHOR 1992, Provision and Use of Work Equipment Regulations [PUWER] 1998, and Lifting Operations and Lifting Equipment Regulations [LOLER] 1998). The guidance and support should enable staff to identify the advantages and risks of each piece of equipment, how and when to use it, equipment storage, where to find emergency/replacement equipment, how to buy new equipment, and how to identify and report faulty equipment.

There are various types of hoist that may be used when moving CYPs. Ceiling track, mobile, standing, bath, and walking hoists can all assist the HCP with various moving and handling tasks. Hoists utilise slings, which should be regularly checked, cleaned, and maintained, as they hold the load of the patient while being hoisted. Staff must have received guidance and support in the use of the hoists available in their area of work and ensure they use the appropriate sling and have 'sized' the CYP before applying the sling (LOLER 1998; PUWER 1998).

When using a hoist, staff must ensure that it has been serviced in the last year and inspected/load tested in the past six months. A label with the date and signature of the tester are usually visible on the hoist. The CYP and their family should receive an explanation as to why a hoist is being used. Patient hoists should be used only after completion of a risk assessment with CYPs who cannot weight bear. Faulty equipment must be identified, taken out of use, and reported as per local procedure.

HCPs often move small pieces of equipment such as infusion pumps, infusion poles, specialised seating, beds, and cots, all of which have handling risks associated with their weight and the HCPs ability to handle them. All HCPs should be able to apply the principles taught in a blended manner so that they can move equipment safely. Risk assessments should be updated when new equipment is introduced or if user instructions change. In hospital wards, height-adjustable beds should be left at the lowest height unless clinical assessment requires otherwise, in which case the bed should be adjusted for the individual HCP. On some electric beds and cots, it is possible to lockout the use of the backrest or bed height from the handset, ensuring that only HCPs can adjust them. This may help reduce the risk of injury due to misuse of equipment, especially with younger children. For babies and CYPs who do not understand the level of risk in falling from a height, the safety side on the cot or bed must be raised before carers leave the immediate environment. For CYPs outside this category, a full risk assessment may need to be written and agreed, to ensure that the use of cot sides or bed rails is not perceived as restraint.

In the operating theatre there is a predominance of top heavy patterns of movement, such as holding a limb for skin prepping, leaning over an abdomen holding a retractor, or leaning over a trolley during a patient transfer (Wicker 2000). These actions present considerable risk when performed for prolonged periods or repetitively. To reduce some of the risk, theatre staff should use equipment, such as lateral transfer boards with slide sheets, limb-holding slings, and theatre table attachments.

To maintain a safe environment, all moving and handling equipment should be stored clean and dry, away from the CYPs, in an easily accessible place for staff. All handling equipment must be latex free and stored away from latex containing products to reduce the potential for accidental exposure to latex-containing products, which can induce a reaction in sensitive individuals. To reduce the risk of cross-contamination, HCPs must wash their hands and cleanse the equipment according to local policy, before and after

Table 19.1 Types of equipment that can be utilised for manual handling

Type of manual handling	Types of equipment
Equipment to be used to assist in sitting to standing	Raised chair, raised toilet seat, tip-up chairs/cushions, grab rails
Equipment to be used to encourage independent transfers	Transfer boards, sliding boards, turntables, transfer belts, transfer netting
Equipment to be used for bed mobility	Hand block, trapeze, bed ladder, transfer sheets, sliding sheets, hoist
Equipment to be used in transfers when manual handling cannot be avoided	Handling slings, transfer sheets, sliding sheets, hoist
Equipment for a bathing	Bath seats, bath hoists

use, and when loaning equipment to other areas or sending equipment for repair or servicing (MHRA 2014).

Fabric equipment, slide sheets, and hoist slings should be labelled with the ward/area name to ensure they are returned after laundering. All fabric equipment should be laundered prior to use, when soiled, or when the CYP no longer needs it, to reduce the risk of cross infection. Hard-surfaced items, such as lateral transfer boards, wheelchairs, and handling aids, should be cleaned according to the manufacturer's instructions and local policy and procedures, and this must be documented. Single use and patient-specific use items must be disposed of according to the local infection control and environmental policies and must not be used on other patients (MHRA 2014). All staff must know where replacement items are kept, how to order further equipment, and where to seek advice to ensure that there is an adequate supply of appropriate equipment for future patients.

Principles table 19.1 General guidelines

Principle	Rationale
1 Read and understand the local Manual Handling Policy (may be called Moving and Handling, Safer Handling, Minimal Handling Policy).	1 To enable employer and employees to comply with current legislation and local policy. To provide staff with safe systems of work (HSWA 1974; MHOR 1992, amended 2002; MHSWR 1999).
2 Staff should know their limitations and refer to specialists (Back care Adviser, Handling Adviser/Trainer, Ergonomist, Occupational Physiotherapist, Physiotherapist Manager, etc.) where necessary.	2 To minimise the risk of injury to staff, CYPs and carers.
3 Staff should identify new and existing injuries (both work and non-work-related) to their manager at the earliest opportunity and seek advice from the Occupational Health Department.	3 Identified problems can be assessed to minimise the risk of further injury. Staff must be physically able to carry out given tasks (MHOR 1992 amended 2002).
4 Staff should attend training relevant to their employment and daily work activities.	4 To update skills and knowledge to undertake activities safely.
5 Wash your hands before and after handling episodes.	5 To reduce cross-infection (Trigg and Mohammed 2010).
6 Encourage independent movement where possible.	6 Mobility influences all systems of the body to function to their full potential, in particular skin, digestion, skeleton, cardiovascular and central nervous system.
7 Where possible, the environment should be prepared with appropriate equipment before the CYP arrives. NB: This may not always be possible in areas such as outpatients and X-ray.	7 To avoid unnecessary delays.
8 Know where the manual handling equipment is kept and how to use it.	8 To maintain a safe and responsive environment. To minimise the risk of injury to staff, CYPs and carers.
9 Gather equipment and check it is clean, intact, and working before taking it to the CYP.	9 To ensure the equipment is available and in good working order before starting the handling activity.
10 Complete, read, and update the risk assessment and ensure documentation is completed in conjunction with all relevant parties including the CYP, carer, and other HCPs.	10 To maximise adherence and encourage independence and family-centred care. To ensure documentation reflects current practice and the CYP's mobility and abilities.
11 Plan moving and handling into the CYP's activities of daily living and seek assistance of other staff where necessary. Use age-appropriate language and include an explanation of what the CYP may feel, see, and/or hear. A play therapist may be useful to help prepare the CYP if necessary.	11 To ensure a positive experience, consistency in handling, and to maintain effective communication. Use as many forms of communication as possible to maximise communication and minimise misunderstandings.
12 Agree and use instructions, such as "ready, steady, stand".	12 Standardisation of instructions minimises the risk of confusion for all involved and reduces the risk of injury.
13 Handling may take place throughout 24 hours. Therefore, the CYP will need to be assessed for moving and handling care and support during a variety of daily living functions.	13 To ensure the handling is integrated into the total care package. Handling decisions may be different if the CYP is receiving rehabilitation, palliative, or long-term care, or has fluctuating psychological or verbal responses.
14 Approach the CYP, parent/carer, and other staff with a positive attitude and listen to their concerns. Be honest, understanding, and confident. Discuss any concerns openly.	14 To maintain honesty, understanding, and cooperation.
15 Take time, especially when using equipment that the CYP/carer has not encountered before.	15 To reduce feelings of anxiety and being rushed.
16 Ensure dignity and privacy during handling.	
17 When a CYP is discharged, ensure that other relevant HCPs are aware of the handling needs and any risks associated with their care.	17 To maintain effective communication and a safe environment for the CYP, carers and staff.

Principles table 19.2 Patient assessment

Principle	Rationale
1 The assessment should be undertaken by a registered HCP who has undergone training and is deemed competent (MHOR 1992, amended 2002). In some cases, this may be a Health Care Assistant/student who has undergone training and is appropriately supervised and supported.	1 To ensure the safety of the CYP and other staff during the handling activity and that the assessment is performed thoroughly and systematically.
2 The initial Patient Handling Risk Assessment should be explained to the CYP and family, including why the assessment is necessary and identify when further assessment(s) might take place.	2 To identify the CYP's needs and risks and plan and implement a safe system of work, with or without the use of equipment.
3 Assess the degree of the CYP's understanding, mobility, and ability to move independently.	3 To maximise adherence and encourage, where possible, independence and family-centred care.
4 Weigh and record the CYP's weight at the earliest opportunity and before placing on weight-sensitive equipment such as high/low electric beds/cots. Remember unlike adults, children growth and weight can be underestimated.	4 To determine whether the use of moving and handling equipment is necessary. To establish if weight sensitive equipment is appropriate. The weight may influence the choice of equipment used. To comply with the MHOR (1992, amended 2002), LOLER (1998) and PUWER (1998).
5 Establish what, if any, moving and handling practices and equipment are used at home or school.	5 To ensure continuity of care, where possible, within a framework that the CYP is familiar with. Those with long-term handling issues may have an existing regimen, which may require little or no adaptation for their new environment.
6 Ensure there are no contraindications to continuing an existing handling regimen or proposed new regimen.	6 To reduce the likelihood of confusion and risk of injury to all parties involved in the handling activity. To obtain cooperation and consent.
7 Decisions should be made after full discussion and with the full agreement and involvement of the CYP, parent/carer, and other healthcare professionals where possible.	7 To answer any questions they may have and to ease concerns. To assist with continuity, safety and partnership in care.
8 CYPs presenting with a number of risks must have their handling needs discussed with the named nurse, medical team, and all relevant HCPs, e.g. physiotherapists, occupational therapists, tissue viability and infection control Nurse Specialists and Moving and Handling advisers/Trainer as appropriate.	8 To enable the multi-professional team approach. To prevent the CYP/parent/carer from receiving conflicting information. To negotiate and implement appropriate care.
9 Ascertain from medical record and/or family how the CYP's medical history has influenced their mobility and current handling practices.	9 To assist in the formulation of a safe system of work.
10 Ascertain whether an interpreter (sign or language) is required.	10 To enable the CYP and their family to communicate their needs effectively.
11 Speech and language or play therapists may be able to assist with communication issues when staff are having difficulty eliciting the CYP's wishes because of communication difficulties.	11 To enable the CYP to communicate their needs/wishes to staff through the most appropriate medium.
12 Play specialists may assist in communicating information in a child friendly way. They can also provide distraction therapy or complex information through the medium of play. For more information see Chapter 27, Play as a Therapeutic Tool.	12 To reduce anxiety
13 Where necessary, ensure the CYP has received appropriate and adequate pain relief prior to handling activity.	13 To minimise pain during the procedure.
14 Review handling needs whenever the CYP's condition changes.	14 To promote high standards of care and to monitor and record changes.

The Great Ormond Street Hospital Manual of Children and Young People's Nursing Practices

Principles table 19.3 Equipment

Principle	Rationale
1 Moving and handling activities must only be performed by staff who: a) Are conversant in the organisation's policy and procedures. b) Are competent in assessment and familiar with the risks and contra-indications of the equipment to be used. c) Received induction/update training. d) Received extra supervision (if applicable). e) Wearing appropriate footwear and clothing which allows freedom of movement and is compatible with the activity to be undertaken. f) Have sufficient time and resources to undertake the activity safely. g) Are aware of the actions to be taken in the event of an incident. h) Allow time for debriefing with CYP/carer other staff, as required.	1 a) In line with MHOR (1992, amended 2002) Guidelines. b) To ensure techniques are appropriately and safely applied to given situation to reduce the likelihood of injury to staff, the carer, or the CYP. c)-d) To establish and maintain the required level of skill and knowledge and comply with current legislation, MHOR (1992, amended 2002) and HSWA (1974). f) Ensures time is allowed for all involved to express their views, concerns and feed into an effective action plan. g) To facilitate early detection and action of any adverse effects of the handling activity.
2 Use equipment that is: a) Clean and usable b) Latex free c) Serviced and tested (where applicable)	2 To maintain a safe environment. a) To minimise the risk of infection. b) To reduce the risk of sensitisation to latex. c) To adhere to health and safety legislation (LOLER 1998).
3 Only use equipment on CYPs who have: a) Been weighed. b) A signed, updated and completed Risk Assessment. c) An understanding (age appropriate) of what is about to take place. d) Where appropriate, been given a choice of handling procedure to be used.	3 To comply with MHOR (1992); know the weight of the load being handled and undertake a risk assessment. b) To minimise risk. c) d) To decrease anxiety and facilitate a successful outcome while working in partnership with the CYP to promote a trusting relationship and promote independence.
4 Use equipment that is: • Regularly serviced and checked • Bought by the trust and asset marked • Of the appropriate weight and/or has been risk assessed prior to moving it.	4 To prevent harm to CYP, family, and staff.

Principles table 19.4 Positioning

Principle	Rationale
1 Risk assess any specific positions the CYP favours, or which meet the specific needs of their mobility problem.	1 Some positions may be detrimental to the CYP's long-term health and positioning.
2 Ensure that the CYP is left in final equipment (bed/chair) in a comfortable position.	2 Correct positioning reduces muscle contractures, pressure sores, physical or psychological stress.
3 Ensure limbs and joints are supported where necessary. Seek advice from other HCPs as appropriate.	3 For comfort and to maintain spinal alignment.
4 Ensure correct placement of the CYP on pressure relieving equipment.	4 To prevent pressure sores.

Principles table 19.5 Risk assessment

Principle	Rationale
1 All equipment has risk attached to it. Staff need to establish the risk for each CYP and situation and ensure everyone is aware of this.	1 Handling aids should be used wherever they can reduce the risk of injury in line with MHOR (1992 amended 2002) guidelines.
2 Regular skin assessments should be carried out to detect skin break down, bruising, or marking.	2 To minimise trauma and identify cause of skin marking and ensure that it is not confused with intentional marking.
3 Examples of equipment:	3 Examples of risks:

Principles table 19.5 Risk assessment (continued)

Principle	Rationale
a) Beds/cots – static height/variable height	a) Leaning, reaching, non-adjustable sides, moving around equipment attached to child/bed, prolonged positions leaning over a child in poor position.
b) Slide sheets	b) Heavy CYP, unable to assist, poorly positioned slide sheet, no additional assistance.
c) Hoists – various	c) No assistance, poor positioning of hoist, lack of room to accommodate hoist, awkward positions required to access CYP/hoist, poor pre-planning of hoist.
d) Wheelchairs/commodes.	d) Inadequate space, poorly planned transfer, sedated/heavy CYP, poor positioning for HCP to access the CYP.
4 Individual staff groups may have a greater risk of injury, e.g. pregnant, physiotherapist and other rehabilitation therapist, staff with existing musculoskeletal disorders or illness/injuries work or non-work related.	

Principles table 19.6 Hoisting

Principle	Rationale
1 A hoist should be used if a completed risk assessment indicates the need for hoisting and all individuals agree.	1 To maintain the safety of the CYP and staff during lifting.
2 Assistance must be sought from other healthcare professionals if completed assessment indicates use of hoist.	2 To maintain a safe working environment and safe systems of work for all. To gain a consensus, to allow forum for discussion, debate, and resolution.
3 Discuss the procedure and the choice of hoist and sling with the CYP and their family (if present).	3 To obtain consent and cooperation.
4 Check size and apply the appropriate sling, ensuring it is compatible with the hoisting system.	4 To prevent injury and discomfort to the CYP.
5 Ensure the hoist can be positioned under the equipment on which the CYP is placed.	5 Hoisting position may be unsafe if access to the hoist and CYP is restricted.
6 Wash hands and gather equipment.	6 To reduce the risk of cross-infection.
7 Undertake the hoisting as per local policy and training. All staff using the hoist must be trained in its use and be aware of the risks involved when using the specific hoist.	7 To minimise risk.
8 Record untoward incidents as per local policy.	8 As per HSE (2013b) and PUWER (1998).
9 Faulty equipment must be reported to the appropriate department, all staff informed, and alternative equipment sought.	9 To minimise risk of harm to staff and CYP.

References

Alexander P, Johnson C (2011). Manual Handling of Children. National Back Exchange.

Boorman, S. (2010). "Health and well-being of the NHS workforce", Journal of Public Mental Health, Vol. 9 No. 1, pp. 4–7. https://doi.org/10.5042/jpmh.2010.0158.

Health and Safety at Work etc. Act (HSWA) (1974). https://www.legislation.gov.uk/ukpga/1974/37/contents (accessed 05 July 2022).

Health and Safety Executive (HSE) (2004). Manual Handling Operations Regulations 1992. Guidance on Regulations. London, HMSO

Health and Safety Executive (HSE) (2010). Musculoskeletal disorders. https://www.hse.gov.uk/msd/ (accessed 05 July 2022).

Health and Safety Executive (HSE) (2011). https://www.hse.gov.uk/msd/backpain/ (accessed 05 July 2022).

Health and Safety Executive (HSE) (2020). Manual handling at work. A brief guide. https://www.hse.gov.uk/pubns/indg143.htm (accessed 05 July 2022).

Health and Safety Executive (HSE) (2013a). RIDDOR – Reporting of Injuries, Diseases and Dangerous Occurrences Regulations 2013. https://www.hse.gov.uk/pubns/indg453.htm (accessed 05 July 2022).

Health and Safety Executive (HSE) (2013b). Ergonomics and human factors at Work. A brief guide. https://www.hse.gov.uk/pubns/indg90.htm (accessed 05 July 2022).

Health and Safety Executive (HSE) (2022). Management of moving and handling in Health and Social Care. https://www.hse.gov.uk/healthservices/moving-handling.htm (accessed 05 July 2022).

Lambeek, L.C., Van Mechelen, W., Knol, D.L. et al. (2010). Randomised controlled trial of integrated care to reduce disability from chronic low back pain in working and private life. British Medical Journal 16: 340.

Lifting Operations and Lifting Equipment Regulations (LOLER) (1998). https://www.hse.gov.uk/work-equipment-machinery/loler.htm (accessed 05 July 2022).

Management of Health and Safety at Work Regulations 1999 (MHSWR). https://www.legislation.gov.uk/uksi/1999/3242/contents/made (accessed 05 July 2022).

Manual Handling Operations Regulations 1992 (MHOR) (as amended). https://www.hse.gov.uk/msd/backpain/employers/mhor.htm (accessed 05 July 2022).

MHRA (2014). Managing medical devices – guidance for healthcare and social services organisations on managing medical devices in practice.

https://www.gov.uk/government/publications/managing-medical-devices (accessed 05 July 2022).

Nursing and Midwifery Council (2015, updated 2018). The Code Professional standards of practice and behaviour for nurses, midwives and nursing associates. https://www.nmc.org.uk/standards/code/ (accessed 05 July 2022).

Provision and Use of Work Equipment Regulations (PUWER) (1998). https://www.hse.gov.uk/work-equipment-machinery/puwer.htm (accessed 05 July 2022).

Roland, M., Waddell, G., Moffett, J.K. et al. (2002). *The Back Book: the Best Way to Deal with Back Pain; Get Back Active*, 2e. Stationery Office Books.

Smith J (ed). (2011). The Guide to the Handling of People – 6th Edition (HOP6). National Back Pain Association.

Steed R, Kennedy C. (1999). Safer Handling of People in the Community. Teddington, National Back Pain Association, produced by BackCare.

Tortora, G. and Derrickson, B. (2016). *Principles of Anatomy and Physiology*, 13e. Hoboken: Wiley.

Trigg, E. and Mohammed, T.A. (2010). *Practices in Children's Nursing. Guidelines for Hospital and Community*, 3e. Edinburgh: Churchill Livingstone.

Wicker, P. (2000). Manual handling in preoperative environment. British Journal Preoperative Nursing 10 (5): 255–259.

Chapter 20

Neonatal care

Heather Parsons[1], Marie-Anne Kelly[2], Monika Sedlbauer[3], and Jane Burgering[4]

[1]RN (child), BSc (hons) Neonatal Nursing; Ward Sister NICU, Great Ormond Street Hospital, London, UK
[2]RN (child), ENB 405; Formerly Neonatal Clinical Nurse Specialist, GOSH
[3]MSc AdvPaedN, Formerly Practice Educator, NICU, GOSH
[4]Formerly Practice Educator, NICU, GOSH

Chapter contents

Introduction	428
Neonatal thermoregulation	428
Developmental care	433
Vitamin K administration	435
Umbilical cord care	436
Newborn blood spot screening	438
Phototherapy – neonatal jaundice	443
Neonatal fluid management	444
References	449

Procedure guidelines

20.1 Preparation for umbilical care	437	
20.2 Care of the umbilicus if soiled or sticky	437	
20.3 Newborn blood spot screening	439	
20.4 When to undertake newborn blood spot screening	439	
20.5 Collecting the blood spot sample	440	

Principles tables

20.1	Monitoring temperature	428	20.10 Noise management		435
20.2	Environment: incubator	429	20.11 Involve the family		435
20.3	Environment: Babytherm®	429	20.12 Vitamin K administration		435
20.4	Environment: open bassinette/cot	430	20.13 Management of Vitamin K		436
20.5	Prevention of heat loss	430	20.14 Repeating the newborn blood spot test		443
20.6	Interventions: cold stress	431	20.15 Phototherapy – neonatal jaundice		445
20.7	Interventions: heat stress	433	20.16 Care of neonates receiving phototherapy		448
20.8	Positioning	433	20.17 Fluid regime		448
20.9	Light management	434	20.18 Electrolyte and glucose requirements		449

The Great Ormond Street Hospital Manual of Children and Young People's Nursing Practices, Second Edition. Edited by Elizabeth Anne Bruce, Janet Williss, and Faith Gibson.
© 2023 John Wiley & Sons Ltd. Published 2023 by John Wiley & Sons Ltd.

Introduction

The neonatal period is the first 28 days after birth and is not determined by gestational age. Babies who are born prematurely have many additional requirements, so will need careful management and handling. This chapter provides some guiding principles on the care of neonates and support for their families.

The 'Toolkit for High Quality Neonatal Services' has the following as the first statement in the executive summary:

> "Well-organised, effective neonatal sensitive care, can make a lifelong difference to premature and sick newborn babies and their families. Getting this early care right is the responsibility of the NHS at all levels" (Department of Health [DH] 2009, p. 9).

The guidelines that follow have been included in this chapter as they are considered the most pertinent areas of neonatal care:

1 Neonatal thermoregulation
2 Developmental care
3 Vitamin K administration
4 Umbilical cord care
5 Newborn blood spot screening (formerly known as Guthrie testing)
6 Phototherapy – neonatal jaundice
7 Fluid management (for information regarding breastfeeding, please see Chapter 22: Nutrition and Feeding).

Neonatal thermoregulation

Temperature control (thermoregulation) is a critical physiological function and is one of the most fundamental principles in neonatal care. Thermoregulation is strongly influenced by physical immaturity, extent of illness, and environmental factors (Thomas 1994). The neonate's susceptibility to temperature instability needs to be recognised and understood in order to limit the effects of cold or heat stress.

It is essential that neonates are nursed within their 'neutral thermal environment' (NTE), a temperature range within which heat production is at the minimum needed to maintain normal body temperature (Lissauer and Fanaroff 2006), to ensure a minimal metabolic rate with minimal oxygen consumption, and thereby promote growth and well-being.

The preterm neonate is at a significant disadvantage compared to term babies and older children. They not only have reduced stores of brown fat, but also have decreased glycogen stores, an immature hypothalamus, immature skin, poor vascular control, and a lower maximum metabolism (Waldron and MacKinnon 2007). They thus have little to no ability to regulate their own temperature (Smith et al. 2013).

Cold and heat stress can have significant implications for this vulnerable patient group. (See Principles Tables 20.6 and 20.7 and Figure 20.5). The maintenance of the NTE should prevent thermal stress, which is the ultimate aim of neonatal temperature control and management.

Principles table 20.1 Monitoring temperature

Statement	Rationale
1 The acceptable set-point temperature is an axilla temperature of range 36.7–37.3°C (Merenstein and Gardner 2006).	1 To allow normal physiological function and body metabolism (Thomas 1994).
2 A single-use thermometer, such as a tempadot™ is recommended for use.	2 These are safe, quick and non-invasive to use (Leick-Rude and Bloom 1998) and reduce the risk of cross infection.
3 A central temperature is obtained by insertion of the thermometer at the axilla site for 3 min, placing the dots against the trunk. It must be read within 10 seconds following removal.	3 To ensure accurate temperature recording.
4 The axilla temperature should be checked and recorded 1–3 hourly in the sick neonate, or 4 hourly in the healthy term neonate (Merenstein and Gardner 2011).	4 The axilla is the safest and most common place for temperature measurement (Merenstein and Gardner 2011; Smith et al. 2013).
5 If the temperature falls outside the normal range, readings must be taken more frequently (every 30–60 minutes). This should be continued until the temperature has normalised.	5 To determine whether the temperature is deteriorating or improving.
6 If a neonate undergoes any change of environment or increased exposure, they may require 30-minute temperature checks for the first few hours until the temperature is stable (Merenstein and Gardner 2011).	6 It can take up to 2 hours for a central and peripheral temperature to stabilise following a change to the thermal environment or prolonged exposure in relation to nursing or medical procedures (Mok et al. 1991).
7 a) For neonates receiving intensive care, peripheral skin temperature is monitored continuously by use of a probe placed on the sole of the foot (Turnbull and Petty 2013). b) Peripheral temperature is recorded hourly and the probe site should be changed every 4–6 hours.	7 a) Peripheral temperature gives an early indication of cold stress (Lyon 2008). b) To maintain and monitor skin integrity under the probe site.

Principles table 20.2 Environment: incubator

Statement	Rationale
1 Any neonate <1.6 kg should be nursed within an enclosed incubator (Turnbull and Petty 2013).	1 To minimise heat loss by radiation, convection, conduction, and evaporation (Figures 20.1–20.4), while allowing clear visibility and access to the patient (Waldron and MacKinnon 2007).
2 Any neonate <30 weeks gestation and/or <1 kg in weight and in the first 14 days of life should be nursed in a closed incubator with added humidity as per local policy.	2 The preterm neonate has high 'trans-epidermal' water loss due to thin, poorly keratinised skin. Trans-epidermal water loss is a major cause of heat loss in the premature neonate (Marshall 1997). Humidification has been shown to decrease fluid requirements and decrease the incidence of electrolyte imbalance (Merenstein and Gardner 2011).
3 Set and maintain incubator temperature and check/record this hourly.	3 To minimise the neonate's oxygen and energy consumption and maintain homeostasis (Sheeran 1996).
4 Alter set incubator temperature according to the neonate's temperature and adjust by 0.5–1°C each time, depending on the extent of temperature instability.	4 To avoid rapid over- or underheating or sudden swings in temperature.
5 Care and interventions, e.g. suction, nappy care, should be carried out via portholes, avoiding opening the side of the incubator completely.	5 To avoid sudden loss of heat from inside the incubator.
6 Where appropriate, the incubator should be changed every 14 days (guided by local policy), particularly if humidity is being used, and documented accordingly.	6 To minimise the risk of infection.

Principles table 20.3 Environment: Babytherm®

Statement	Rationale
1 Babytherms® provide heat by a combination of conduction and radiation.	1 They limit heat loss during exposure and interventions because of easy access and radiant heater responsiveness (Seguin and Vieth 1996).
2 Most neonates >1.6 kg can be nursed in an open Babytherm.	2 To allow for easy access to the neonate.
3 a) When preparing a Babytherm for use, the mattress is switched to 'on' at a set temperature of 37°C. b) Ensure that the Babytherm is turned on at least an hour before it is needed.	3 a) To meet manufacturer's recommendations. b) It will take an hour to heat the Babytherm to the set temperature.
4 If the neonate is hypothermic, the initial settings should be higher (i.e. range 37–38.5 C, with overhead heater bars 6–10). This also applies to a neonate already established in a Babytherm who needs extra heat.	4 To avoid the complications associated with cold stress.
5 If the neonate requires cooling, turn the radiant heater off and choose extended lower range for the mattress, indicated by <37, i.e. 30–35°C).	5 To avoid the complications of heat stress.
6 Once established in the Babytherm, there are two heater options, which determine what the neonate is laid on and covered with: **Option One:** Both mattress and radiant heater on: a) The neonate should lie directly on one sheet covering the gel mattress. b) Nesting should be provided around, not under, the neonate. c) The neonate receiving ventilator support can then be covered with bubble wrap, bubbles downwards or left exposed. d) In self-ventilating neonates, bubble wrap should be used with great care or avoided completely. **Option Two:** Mattress with no radiant heater. As option one, but the neonate should be covered with a blanket.	 a) To achieve optimum heat transfer from the heat pad, via the gel mattress, to the neonate (conduction). b) Extra sheets may block heat transfer from the mattress to the neonate. c) Bubble wrap provides an insulation layer to prevent heat loss from convective air currents. The bubbles placed downwards maximise the air trapped between the sheet and neonate. d) To minimise the risk of suffocation. When there is no radiant heat from above, a blanket can be used.
7 When transferring a neonate in a Babytherm, the transfer should take a maximum of 15 minutes before re-connecting to mains supply.	7 Once switched off, the mattress retains heat for 15 minutes.

Principles table 20.4 Environment: open bassinette/cot

Statement	Rationale
1 A well neonate, >1.6 kg, who no longer requires close monitoring or intensive care and can maintain a stable central temperature in 26–28°C room temperature, can be transferred to an open bassinette or small cot (New et al. 2011).	1 If well insulated by clothes, hat, blankets, and/or swaddling, in the ideal room temperature, a well neonate will be able to maintain an adequate central temperature (Medoff-Cooper 1994).
2 Weaning a well neonate from an incubator or Babytherm should be done gradually, turning the incubator or mattress temperature down by 0.5–1°C every 4–8 hours, to maintain a normal central temperature (Merenstein and Gardner 2011).	2 The environmental temperature must be altered slowly due to the immature heat conserving mechanisms at this age and limited ability to adapt to sudden or extreme changes (Medoff-Cooper 1994; Merenstein and Gardner 2011).
3 Larger neonates, i.e. >4 kg, who require warming can be nursed in an open cot with a bear-hugger blanket.	3 Some larger babies are not an appropriate weight for an incubator or Babytherm but still require additional heating.

Principles table 20.5 Prevention of heat loss

Statement	Rationale
1 Before transferring a neonate to theatre or preparing them for procedures or general transportation, ensure they have dry blankets, dry gamgee, an appropriate-sized bonnet, and a clean nappy.	1 To provide optimal insulation and prevent heat loss during transfer/change to the NTE (Altimier et al. 1999).
2 During transfers, neonates should remain in their incubator or Babytherm. While unoccupied, the incubator/Babytherm should be left switched on, at the same setting, ready for the neonate to return.	2 To maintain an NTE at all times.
3 Temperature must continue to be monitored during transfers and procedures.	3 To assess for cold stress due to frequent handling and exposure.

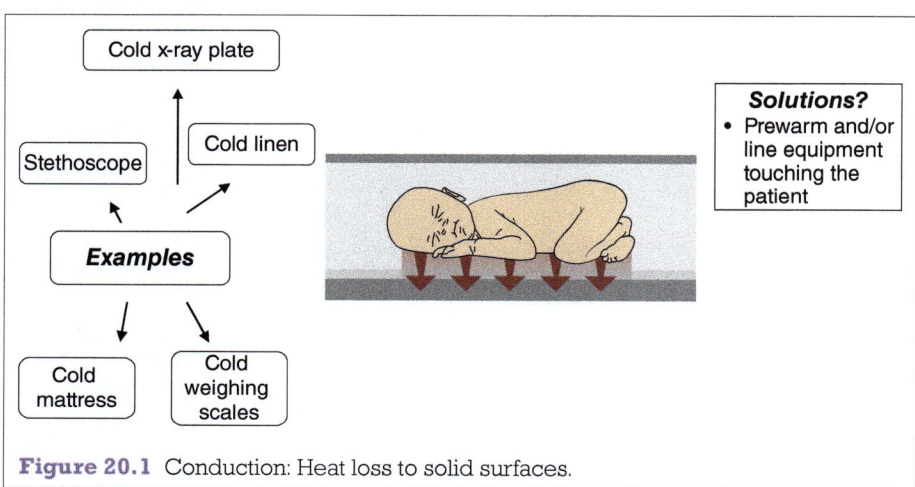

Figure 20.1 Conduction: Heat loss to solid surfaces.

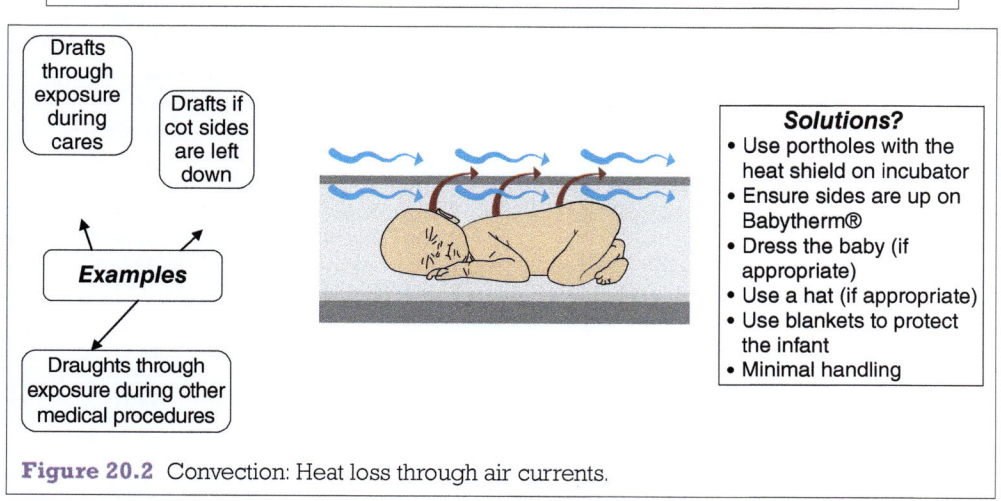

Figure 20.2 Convection: Heat loss through air currents.

Chapter 20 Neonatal care

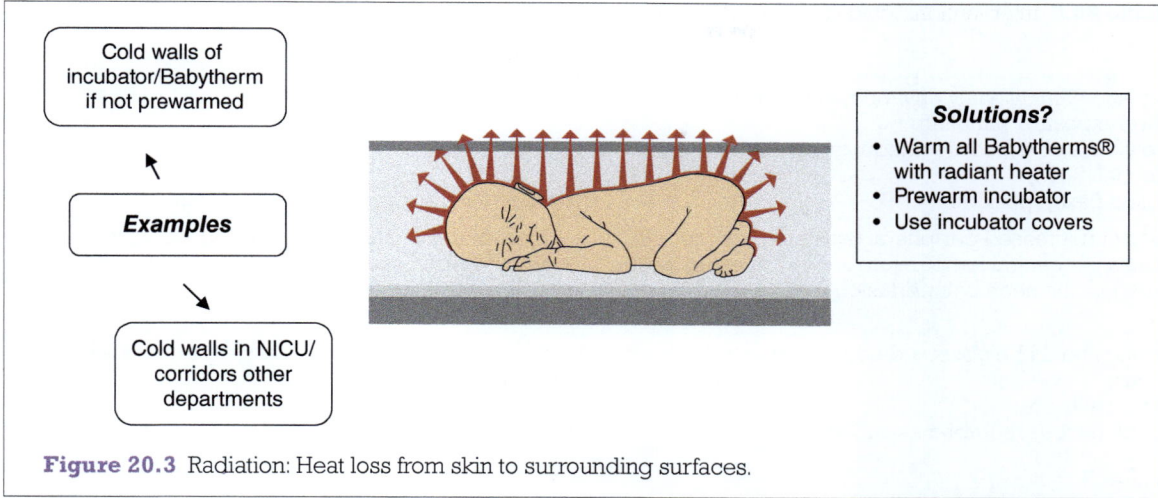

Figure 20.3 Radiation: Heat loss from skin to surrounding surfaces.

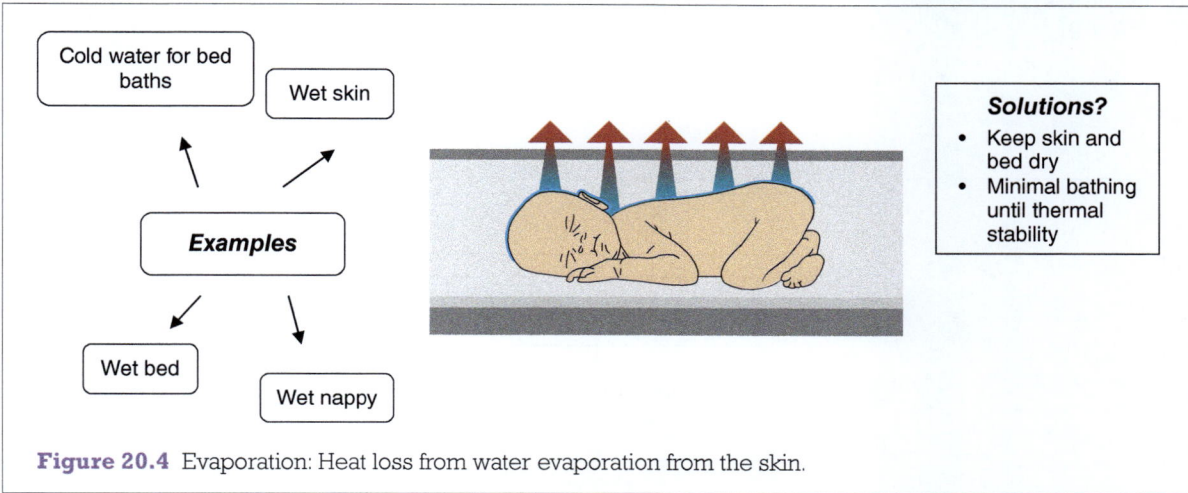

Figure 20.4 Evaporation: Heat loss from water evaporation from the skin.

Principles table 20.6 Interventions: cold stress

Cold stress is the process of extreme heat loss in neonates, leading to compensatory mechanisms to regulate their core body temperature. A decrease in body temperature to lower than the normal core temperature (36.7–37.3°C) will result in cold stress, if left untreated, can have serious adverse complications for the neonate (see Figure 20.5).

Statement	Rationale
1 Neonates should be observed for signs and associated problems of cold stress. These are: • Central temperature <36.5°C • An increase in toe-core (peripheral to central temperature) gap >2°C • Mottled and pale skin • Increased capillary refill time, i.e. >2 seconds • Increased oxygen requirements • Metabolic acidosis • Tachycardia • Hypoglycaemia • Apnoeas • Bradycardia	1 To enable quick recognition and prevention of adverse consequences (Waldron and MacKinnon 2007; Turnbull and Petty 2013).
2 To intervene in this situation: a) Place a neonate of <1.6 kg in an incubator at the upper range, i.e. >37°C. b) If using a Babytherm, for babies >1.6 kgs, set the temperature at the upper range, using both radiant heater and gel mattress, and follow guidelines for Babytherm use (Principles Table 20.3). c) Monitor temperature every 30–60 minutes until the neonate is warmed to an acceptable temperature.	a–e) To rewarm the neonate and avoid the complications of cold stress.

(continued)

Principles table 20.6 Interventions: cold stress *(continued)*

Statement	Rationale
d) Identify and eliminate any environmental causes, e.g. wet bed, overexposure, handling. e) Ensure ventilator gases are adequately warmed (Rennie and Kendall 2013). f) Promote a flexed position.	f) To decrease surface area for heat loss.
3 If the cause of decreased peripheral temperature is not due to cold stress, i.e. central temperature stable but an increase in toe-core gap, the neonate's perfusion status should be assessed.	3 Other possible causes include vasoconstriction from shock, hypovolaemia, postoperative stress, or handling.
4 The following should be observed and documented at least every 4 hours: a) Capillary refill time b) Colour of mucous membranes and extremities c) Skin d) Heart rate e) Peripheral pulses f) Blood pressure	4 To ensure early detection and treatment of any deterioration in the neonate.

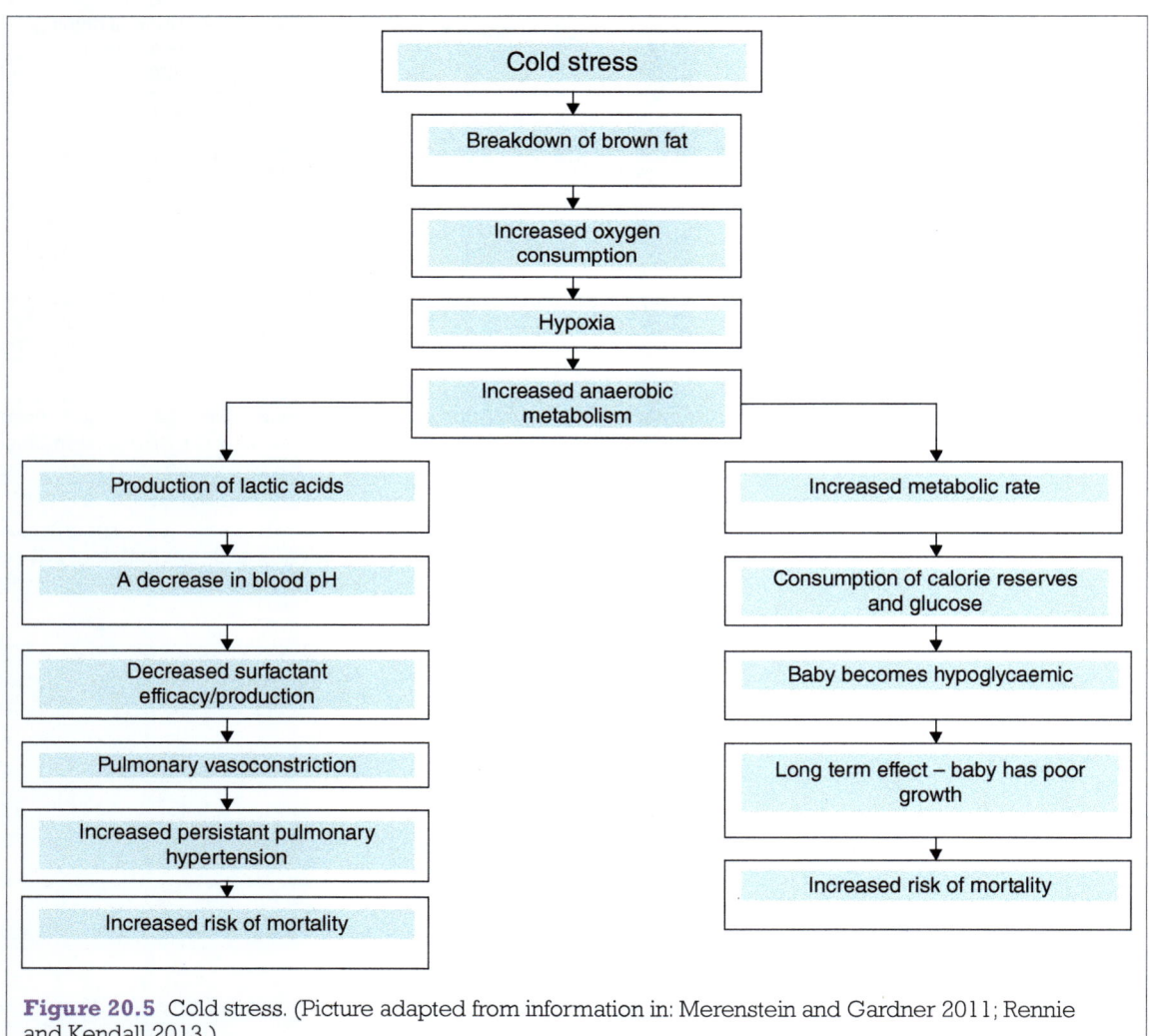

Figure 20.5 Cold stress. (Picture adapted from information in: Merenstein and Gardner 2011; Rennie and Kendall 2013.)

Principles table 20.7 Interventions: heat stress

Neonates are also prone to overheating as a result of limited sweating ability, sepsis, hypermetabolism, neonatal abstinence syndrome, maternal hyperthermia at delivery, and physical immaturity (Thomas 1994; Waldron and MacKinnon 2007).

Statement	Rationale
1 Observe the neonate for signs and associated problems of heat stress. These are: • Central temperature above 37.5°C and rising (Rennie and Kendall 2013). • Increased peripheral temperature and decrease in toe-core gap, i.e. <1°C. • Tachycardia. • Tachypnoea. • Restlessness. • Dehydration. • Stress.	1 To enable quick recognition and prevention of adverse consequences (Smith et al. 2013).
2 To intervene in this situation: • Check environmental temperature and reduce by 0.5°C at 15–30 minute intervals. • Remove excess layers and clothing. • In a Babytherm, turn radiant heater off and choose the extended lower range (<35°C). • Turn the temperature down by 0.5°C at 15–30 minute intervals. • Monitor temperature every 30–60 minutes until the neonate is warmed to an acceptable temperature.	2, 3 To gradually reduce the neonate's temperature to within normal limits and avoid the complications of heat stress.
3 If the cause is not environmental, infection is the most likely cause and should be investigated (Waldron and MacKinnon 2007).	

Developmental care

Developmental care for the neonate relates to a broad category of interventions designed to minimise the stress of the neonatal unit environment. It is an approach to caring for neonates in which an environment is created to maximise neurological development and reduce long-term behavioural problems (Hamilton and Redshaw 2009). This is achieved by ensuring adequate sleep for growth and development of the neonate, minimising stress and pain by appropriate positioning, management of noise and light, and inclusion of the family with an agreed plan of care (DH 2009). Assessment of the neonate, considering age and illness, is important to determine their individual developmental needs (Auckland District Health Board 2004).

Principles table 20.8 Positioning

Statement	Rationale
1 Position neonate for comfort and support. This includes: Nesting to create boundaries (Figure 20.6–20.8).	1 To promote sleep for growth and development. To conserve heat and energy. To minimise stress.
2 Alternate positions and use of pressure relieving equipment in line with individual unit policy.	2 To relieve pressure areas. To avoid head moulding/flattening. To avoid shoulder retraction and leg abduction.
3 Lie neonate with head slightly elevated. They may be placed in the following positions: a) Supine (Figure 20.6). b) Prone (Figure 20.7) (only if monitored). c) Side lying (Figure 20.8).	3 To aid digestion and prevent reflux. a) Helps avoid narrow head shape. Safe sleeping position for healthy babies (Kennedy Shriver 2007). b) Supports sternum and rib cage; optimal for oxygenation, and assists with breathing. c) Comfortable for neonate. Helps to develop hand-to-mouth co-ordination.

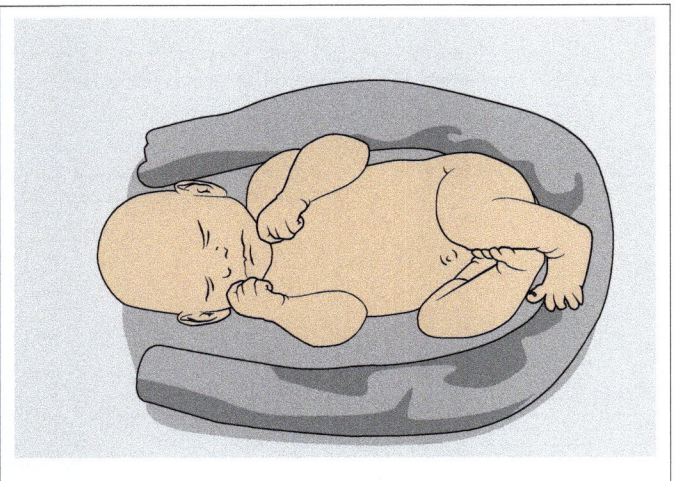
Figure 20.6 Nesting to create boundaries: Supine.

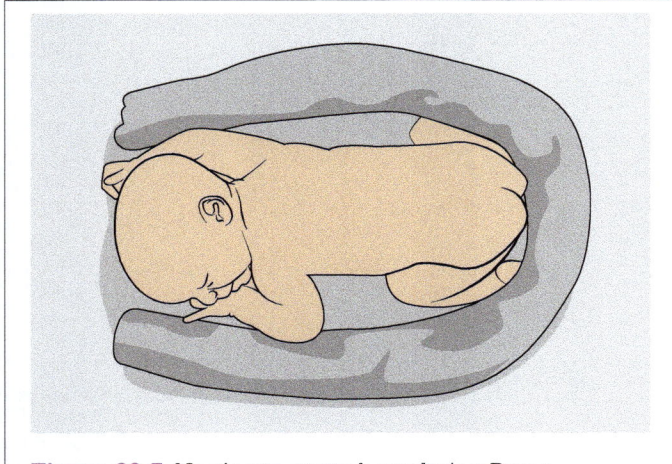
Figure 20.7 Nesting to create boundaries: Prone.

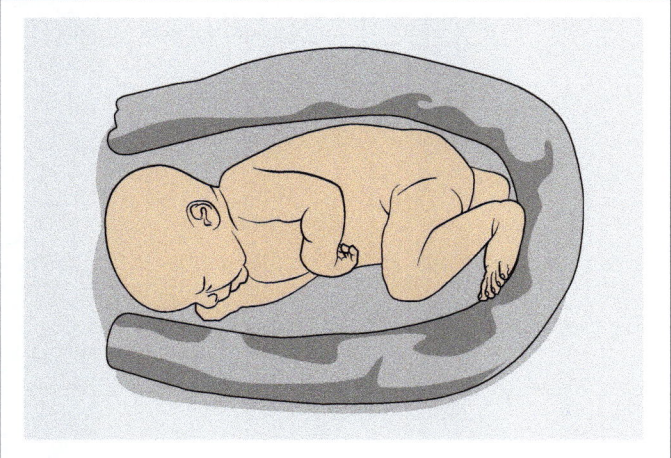
Figure 20.8 Nesting to create boundaries: Side lying.

Principles table 20.9 Light management

Statement	Rationale
1 Protect from bright light by dimming lights.	1 To promote sleep, growth and development.
2 Establish light and dark cycles.	2 To help build a sleeping pattern.
3 Shade neonate's face when undergoing procedures.	3 To avoid retinal damage.

Principles table 20.10 Noise management

Statement	Rationale
1 Reduce background noise.	1 To promote sleep, growth, and development.
2 Avoid intermittent loud noise.	2 To prevent startling the neonate.
3 Encourage parents to talk to their neonates softly and read stories.	3 Important for language development and recognition of family voices.
4 Establish quiet times on ward.	4 To help develop a routine.

Principles table 20.11 Involve the family

Statement	Rationale
1 Plan care with parents and encourage participation.	1 To empower the family to meet the needs of their neonate and encourage bonding.
2 Encourage and support parents involvement with decisions regarding all aspects of care (National Institute for Health and Care Excellence [NICE] 2020).	2 To support families' understanding of their babies' healthcare needs and support them in taking an active role in any decision making.
3 Encourage kangaroo care; the neonate is nestled in an upright position between the mother's breasts or on the father's chest and facing the mother.	3 This has been shown to help regulate vital signs in the neonate, help with breast milk production and encourage bonding (Baker-Rush 2016). Kangaroo care can also be carried out by the father.
4 Encourage non-nutritive sucking (NNS) from either breast or dummy.	4 To provide comfort (Liu et al. 2010) Also benefits feeding development by reducing transition time from nasogastric to oral feeds (Foster 2016). NNS encourages development of the sucking reflex and promotes readiness for oral feeding.

Vitamin K administration

The DH (1998) and NICE (2021) recommend that all parents should be offered vitamin K prophylaxis for their babies to prevent vitamin K deficiency bleeding (VKDB), a rare but serious and sometimes fatal disorder. Vitamin K is essential for the formation of prothrombin, factor VII, IX, and X, and the coagulation inhibitors protein C and protein S (Lippi and Franchini 2011; Blackburn 2012). VKDB occurs in approximately 1 in 10 000 babies. It occurs unpredictably in some babies, but others are recognised as being at high risk (Lippi and Franchini 2011).

VKDB can present in three ways:

- Early VKDB (<24 hours); this is thought to be due to abnormal maternal vitamin K metabolism.
- Classical VKDB (two to seven days); occurs in premature and/or breastfed babies. Exclusively breastfed babies are at higher risk of VKDB due to insufficient vitamin K in the breast milk. Formula-fed babies have a higher level of protection as formula milks are fortified with Vitamin K.
- Late VKDB (after seven days); occurs in babies who have some risk factors as with classical presentation and in addition may have missed a later oral dose of Vitamin K, and in those babies with hepatic disease.

Studies have shown that in half of those affected, bleeding occurs late. Of babies with late VKDB, about half suffer bleeding into the brain, leading to death in about one fifth of these babies or causing brain damage in many of those who survive (DH 1998).

There were concerns following studies in the early 90s that suggested a link between Intramuscular (IM) administration of vitamin K given to newborn babies and childhood cancers. Further research published in 2003 by the UK children's cancer study group concluded that there is no convincing evidence that neonatal vitamin K administration, irrespective of the route by which it is given, influences the risk of children developing leukaemia or any other cancer (Fear et al. 2003).

Principles table 20.12 Vitamin K administration

Statement	Rationale
1 Local protocols may vary, and an appropriate regime should have been discussed with parents antenatally.	1 To ensure informed consent.
2 All parents should be offered vitamin K prophylaxis for their babies.	2 To prevent VKDB; a rare but serious and sometimes fatal disorder.
3 Vitamin K is usually given at delivery or shortly after following stabilisation of a sick neonate.	3 A single dose of vitamin K 1 mg at birth effectively prevents VKDB in virtually all babies (NICE 2021).
4 The preferred method of vitamin K administration is a single dose of 1 milligram (mg) intramuscularly at birth.	4 This is the most clinically and cost-effective method of administration. A single dose of vitamin K 1 mg at birth effectively prevents VKDB in virtually all babies (NICE 2021).

(continued)

Principles table 20.12 Vitamin K administration (continued)

Statement	Rationale
5 Preterm neonates may be given 400 micrograms per kilogramme of body weight, up to a maximum of 1 mg. (British National Formulary for Children [BNFC] 2022).	
6 If parents decline intramuscular vitamin K for their neonate, oral vitamin K should be offered as a second-line option.	6 Parents should be advised that oral vitamin K must be given according to the manufacturer's instructions for clinical efficacy and will require multiple doses.
7 The intravenous (IV) route may be used in preterm neonates of very low birth-weight, if intramuscular injection is not possible (BNFC, 2022). However, it may not provide the prolonged protection of the intramuscular injection; any babies receiving IV vitamin K should be given subsequent oral doses.	7 To ensure effective absorption of the drug.
Subsequent doses	
8 The initial IV or oral dose is usually given at birth. If given orally, one or two subsequent oral doses should be given. The first subsequent dose should be given at 4–7 days.	8 Further information on administration can be found in the BNFC (2022).
9 A further oral dose should be given at 1 month of age for exclusively breastfed babies.	9 Vitamin K is added into formula feeds, so an additional dose is not required in bottle-fed babies (Lippi and Franchini 2011).
10 During any admission to hospital during the neonatal period it is important to ascertain: • Has vitamin K been given? • What dosage was given? • Which route was used? • How many doses have been given?	10 To ensure babies receive the correct dose and doses are not missed.
11 This information should be recorded on the birth history form or in the healthcare record.	11 To maintain an accurate record and ensure healthcare workers are checking and recording this information on admission.
12 When looking for information, check in the personal child health record (PCHR), drug administration record, or on the neonatal discharge letter.	12 To ensure all sources of information are checked to avoid the risk of a neonate missing Vitamin K prophylaxis.
13 If IV or oral doses were given, discuss with medical staff, as further doses may be needed.	13 To ensure an effective dose is given.

Principles table 20.13 Management of vitamin K

Statement	Rationale
1 If intramuscular vitamin K has been given there is no need for further action.	1 The effective dose to prevent VKDB has been already given.
2 If there is uncertainty about the previous administration of vitamin K: • Contact the referral hospital. • Refer to medical staff.	2 To clarify the situation.
3 If vitamin K has not been given: a) Notify the child's doctor. b) Discuss with the child's parents/carers the need for vitamin K. c) Obtain a prescription for the appropriate medication. d) Administer the medication as prescribed according to the medicines administration policy. e) Document the administration in the child's healthcare records.	a) To initiate appropriate treatment. b) To obtain consent. c) To enable Vitamin K to be administered. d) To prevent VKDB. e) To maintain an accurate record.

Umbilical cord care

The umbilical cord plays an essential part in foetal development, connecting the growing foetus with the maternal placenta. It supplies nutrients and oxygen needed for growth and carries away metabolic waste and carbon dioxide (Coyne et al. 2010). The umbilical cord is normally translucent due to Wharton's jelly, but can be stained green due to meconium or yellow if the neonate has hyperbilirubinaemia (Levene et al. 2008).

At birth, the cord is clamped to prevent bleeding and then cut using a sterile technique. The cord and placenta are then examined by a midwife. The cord is examined to ensure it contains two arteries and one vein (Levene et al. 2008); the number of vessels present is then recorded in the maternity notes. Approximately 1% of babies have a single umbilical artery and this is reported to be associated with growth retardation and congenital malformations, especially of the renal tract (Rennie and Roberton 2005).

Chapter 20 Neonatal care

Procedure guideline 20.1 Preparation for umbilical care

Statement	Rationale
1 Inform the family of the following: a) That the cord needs to be assessed. b) The reason for the assessment. c) What it will entail. d) The likely duration of the procedure. e) Advise the family to keep the cord clean and dry.	1. a) To ensure that parents/carers understand why this is being performed. b) To assess umbilical site for bleeding and infection. c) To provide information and support to relevant family members (Coyne et al. 2010). e) To provide evidence-based information related to umbilical cord care (McConnell et al. 2004).
2 Co-ordinate procedures to minimise handling the neonate.	2 To conserve energy, minimise oxygen consumption, and reduce stress and overstimulation of the neonate.
3 Collect equipment: a) Clean nappy. b) Umbilical swab and request form for microbiology if there are signs of infection. c) Appropriate personal protective equipment (ppe), including apron and gloves as a minimum. d) Sachet of sterile water. e) Gauze – two packs.	c) to minimise risk of cross infection (Mullany et al. 2006) d) there is no reliable evidence to suggest that anything other than water should be used on the umbilical area (Zupan et al. 2004; Imdad et al. 2013).
4 Wash hands immediately prior to and after handling neonate.	4 To minimise the risk of infection (World Health Organisation (WHO) 2007).
5 Observe the umbilicus and surrounding area for: • Inflammation or pus • A swollen cord • Offensive odour from the cord • Any abnormality, e.g. granuloma, hernia • A red flare around the cord stump	5 To identify any potential infection or abnormalities requiring prompt treatment. Infection in this area can lead to severe complications, including fever, meningitis and septic foci (Zupan et al. 2004). Abnormalities detected may need surgical intervention.
6 Document procedure and report any abnormalities.	6 To maintain an accurate record of care.

Procedure guideline 20.2 Care of the umbilicus if soiled or sticky

Statement	Rationale
If there are no signs of infection, leave the umbilical area clean and dry. Only carry out the procedure if the area is soiled or sticky.	
1 Perform a hand-wash before commencing the procedure.	1 To minimise the risk of cross infection (WHO 2007).
2 Standard precautions must be applied.	2 Standard precautions reduce the risk of transmission of bloodborne and other pathogens from unrecognised and recognised sources (WHO 2007).
3 Prepare the neonate: lay them supine, remove the nappy, but keep the neonate warm.	3 To access the whole area while maintaining the neonate's temperature, as babies lose heat quickly (Chamley et al. 2006).
4 To clean the umbilicus:	4
a) If there are signs of infection, take an umbilical swab for microbiology. b) Pour water onto an open gauze pack, ensuring that the water container does not touch the gauze. c) Open the other pack of gauze, ensuring materials stay dry. d) Work from clean to dirty area. e) Gently wipe around the stump with a wet piece of gauze. Use a new piece of gauze each time. f) Using a dry clean gauze, pat the cord area dry – do not rub or pull at the stump; any residue that remains should be left to fall off in time. g) The cord stump should be kept clean and dry. This can be facilitated by turning down the front of the nappy when fastening it, so that it does not cover the stump. h) Involve the parents/cares in reapplying the nappy and making the neonate comfortable.	a) To detect whether the area is infected and to ensure the correct medical regime is prescribed (Trotter 2004). b) To reduce the risk of contamination. d) To keep the procedure as clean as possible (Breathnach 2005). e) To prevent cross infection. f) To prevent trauma. g) To leave the cord clean, dry, and exposed to air (Trotter 2004). h) To encourage family-centred care and minimise discomfort to the neonate.

(continued)

The Great Ormond Street Hospital Manual of Children and Young People's Nursing Practices

Procedure guideline 20.2 Care of the umbilicus if soiled or sticky *(continued)*

Statement	Rationale
5 Dispose of used equipment according to local waste policy.	5 To prevent contamination of area and adhere to hospital policy.
6 Perform a hand-wash.	6 To minimise the risk of cross-infection (WHO 2007).
7 Record the completion of the procedure and any abnormalities identified in the child's healthcare records.	7 To provide an accurate record of the care given and promote continuity of care (Nursing and Midwifery Council 2015).
8 Send any bacterial swabs with a request form to microbiology.	8 To ensure that any infection is recognised quickly.
9 If the cord becomes detached it should be disposed of in a waste bag for incineration as per local policy.	9 To prevent contamination of the area and adhere to hospital policy.
10 If the parents/carers wish to keep the cord, it should be placed in a specimen container.	10 The parents/carers may wish to keep the cord as a memento.
11 Inform an experienced nurse or doctor of any abnormalities found.	11 To promote effective communication and ensure appropriate treatment of the problem.

The cord stump normally dries, epithelialises, and detaches from the neonate within 15 days of birth. Following delivery, the umbilical cord stump is colonised, usually with bacteria that are nonpathogenic (Broom and Smith 2013). Until the cord stump detaches and the umbilical area heals, it is recommended to keep the area dry and clean to prevent infection.

For the first few days after birth, the umbilical vessels are still patent and may be cannulated for arterial or venous access to allow administration of drugs and IV fluids, invasive blood pressure monitoring, blood sampling, or an exchange transfusion. The associated risks of cannulation include obstructed blood flow to major vessels, which can cause ischaemia to lower limbs, infection, thrombosis, and necrotising entero-colitis (Rennie and Roberton 2005).

Newborn blood spot screening

In the UK, all babies are offered screening for a number of rare but serious conditions including phenylketonuria (PKU), congenital hypothyroidism (CHT), sickle cell disease (SCD), cystic fibrosis (CF), and medium-chain acyl-CoA dehydrogenase deficiency (MCADD), as recommended by the UK National Screening Committee (UK NSC) and UK Newborn Screening Programme (Public Health England (PHE) 2014a, 2014b). In 2014 four new conditions were added to the screening programme; homocystinuria (HCU), maple syrup urine disease (MSUD), glutaric acidemia type 1 (GA1), and isovaleric acidemia (PHE 2014a, 2014b) see Table 20.1.

Screening aims to identify babies with these rare but serious conditions to ensure prompt referral and treatment. Early diagnosis and treatment can prevent or reduce the risk of the devastating consequences of untreated conditions mentioned above and may allow improved health outcomes for neonates with SCD and CF.

Table 20.1 Conditions for which newborn screening is offered

Condition and incidence	Description
Phenylketonuria (PKU) Incidence: Approximately 1 in 10 000	Babies born with PKU cannot process the amino acid phenylalanine. Effective processing of this amino acid is essential for normal brain development after birth. Untreated PKU can result in severe neurological disability (Williams et al. 2008). If diagnosed early, PKU can be managed with a special diet.
Congenital hypothyroidism (CHT) Incidence: 1 in 3000	Babies born with CHT have low levels of the hormone thyroxin. Without this hormone they do not grow properly and can develop serious intellectual/learning disability. Once diagnosed, patients can be treated with thyroxin (Olney et al. 2010).
Sickle cell disease (SCD) Incidence: 1 in 2000	SCD is an inherited condition that affects the haemoglobin in red blood cells. The condition causes the red blood cells to change shape, blocking small blood vessels. These blockages cause pain and can result in damage to the body and even death (Streetly et al. 2010).
Cystic fibrosis (CF) Incidence: 1 in 2500	CF is an inherited condition that affects the lungs and digestive system. Screening these babies means that treatment to improve digestion and reduce chest infections can be started early potentially slowing down the effects of the disease (Castellani et al. 2009).
Medium-chain acyl-CoA dehydrogenase deficiency (MCADD) Incidence): 1 in 10 000	Babies with this condition have problems breaking down fats to make energy for the body; this is particularly dangerous during periods of fasting or illness. Untreated, the condition can result in neurological disability and death. Once diagnosed, MCADD can be managed with diet and emergency regimes for times of illness (Leonard and Dezateux 2009).

Table 20.1 Conditions for which newborn screening is offered *(continued)*

Condition and incidence	Description
Homocystinuria (HCA) Incidence: 1 in 144 000	Babies with this condition have problems breaking down an amino acid called methionine from the food they eat. Without treatment, most children will have learning difficulties and problems with their eyes. They may also develop osteoporosis, blood clots, or strokes (Moorthie et al. 2013; PHE 2014a, 2014b).
Maple syrup urine disease (MSUD) Incidence: 1 in 116 000	MSUD is a disorder in the body's ability to use three of the essential amino acids in protein. This disease presents very dramatically in the newborn period with symptoms such as poor feeding, lethargy and convulsions occurring within the first few days of life. Without treatment MSUD can lead to coma and permanent brain damage (Moorthie et al. 2013; PHE 2014a, 2014b).
Glutaric acidemia (GA1) type 1 Incidence: 1 in 110 000	GA1 is an inherited disorder in which there is an absence or inefficiency in the enzyme needed to break down certain amino acids. This causes a build-up of amino acids and their intermediate breakdown products. Without treatment GA1 can result in brain damage (Moorthie et al. 2013; PHE 2014a, 2014b).
Isovaleric acidemia Incidence: 1 in 155 000	Isovaleric acidemia is a rare metabolic disorder which disrupts or prevents normal metabolism of the branch-chain amino acid leucine. Without treatment this can cause brain damage (Moorthie et al. 2013; PHE 2014a, 2014b).

This information was originally developed by the UK NSC Screening Programmes; www.screening.nhs.uk.

Procedure guideline 20.3 Newborn blood spot screening

Statement	Rationale
Preparation 1 Explain the procedure to parents. Parents should have access to the 'Screening Tests for Your Baby' booklet (PHE 2014a, 2014b). Ensure the booklet is in the appropriate language for the parents.	1 To ensure informed consent (NMC 2015).
2 Verbal consent is adequate in England – see national guidance if outside of England. The parents' consent decision should be documented in the medical notes. If the parents' consent, continue with the procedure.	2 Good record keeping is an integral part of nursing and midwifery practice (NMC 2015).
If parents decline screening: 3 For each condition declined record 'declined' and reason for decline (if known) in the PCHR. Complete the empty blood spot card and mark 'declined' in the comments box. Send the card to the screening laboratory.	3 To monitor rate of consent and declines and to ensure the GP and health visitor are informed that the neonate has not been screened.
4 The UK Newborn Blood Spot Screening Centre produces parent/carer information about the test and this should be used to supplement oral information (PHE 2014a, 2014b).	

Procedure guideline 20.4 When to undertake newborn blood spot screening

1 Routinely, newborn blood spot screening should be performed on day 5 of life. Day of birth is classed as day 0.	1 To screen for the conditions described in Table 20.1. (For local information and national booklets, see PHE 2014a, 2014b.)
2 In exceptional circumstances the full newborn screening sample can be collected between days 5–8. **All** babies must have a sample sent by day 8 regardless of feeding status, medical condition, or prematurity.	2 To enable timely detection of abnormal results and initiation of appropriate treatment.

(continued)

Procedure guideline 20.4 When to undertake newborn blood spot screening *(continued)*

3 For neonates requiring a blood transfusion: For the purposes of newborn screening a transfusion is classed as exchange transfusions, red cell transfusions, platelets, and fresh frozen plasma, i.e. any blood product that will affect the circulating concentration of the measured metabolite. Babies admitted to hospital at less than five days of age: a) All neonates admitted to hospital at less than five days of age should have a single blood spot sample taken on admission. b) Keep the sample taken to test for SCD with the neonate and send with routine day 5 blood spot. c) Mark the card 'pretransfusion' in the comments box.	a) This one spot sample will be used to test for SCD if the baby receives red cells prior to the day 5 sample being taken. Screening for SCD must be done before the neonate receives a blood transfusion. b) To ensure the blood spot sample remains with the neonate until all blood spots are ready to forward to the laboratory. c) To ensure that the laboratory staff know why a separate sample was taken.
4 Use a separate card for each sample (pre transfusion, day 5 etc.).	4 To enable accurate interpretation of screening results.
5 If a neonate is transfused at less than five days old, the routine blood spot sample should be taken on the fourth day post-transfusion.	5 Transfusions may affect the concentration of measured metabolites for several days.
6 If the neonate requires numerous transfusions, a sample must be taken by day 8, and a necessary repeat will be required.	6 To reduce the chance of the neonate missing screening.
7 The date of transfusion and what was transfused should be recorded on the screening card.	7 To enable accurate interpretation of screening results.
Preterm:	
8 Babies born at <32 weeks (less than or equal to 31 weeks +6 days) gestation will need a two-spot repeat sample taken when they reach 28 days (day of birth is day 0) or on discharge home, whichever is sooner.	8 Prematurity can mask congenital hypothyroidism.
9 Mark the card 'CHT preterm' in the comments box.	9 To ensure the lab know the reason for the sample.
Older babies:	
10 All neonates over five days and babies less than one year old should be checked on admission to hospital to ensure that blood spot screening has been done. If the test has not been done, consent should be obtained, and screening should be performed.	10 To ensure that no babies miss screening, and that affected babies are diagnosed promptly and treatment is commenced as soon as possible.
11 Newborn blood spot screening is offered to infants up to a year of age. However, blood spot screening for CF can only be performed up to 56 days of age.	11 To identify any affected infants and ensure that treatment is initiated as soon as possible. Blood spot screening for CF is not reliable after 56 days old.

Procedure guideline 20.5 Collecting the blood spot sample

1 The newborn blood spot test is usually done by a capillary blood sample. Blood obtained via venepuncture or venous/arterial blood sampling from an existing line is acceptable if it is not contaminated with EDTA and the line is free of infusate.	1 To co-ordinate screening with other blood tests where possible to reduce interventions and accessing of lines.
2 Take the sample according to local practice guidelines.	2 To ensure the sample is taken in line with best practice and to avoid contamination which can affect results.
3 Ensure comfort measures are used. Suggested comfort measures include: • Swaddling/cuddling/skin-to-skin care during the procedure • Breastfeeding • Non-nutritive sucking • Sucrose	3 To reduce the pain/discomfort of the procedure (Johnston et al. 1997; Shah et al. 2012; Stevens et al. 2016).

Procedure guideline 20.5 Collecting the blood spot sample *(continued)*

4 Gather equipment: • Gloves and an apron • Sachet of water • Clean pot for water • Gauze • Automated incision device designed for use on newborns • Newborn bloodspot screening card • Waxed envelope	4 To enable a timely uninterrupted procedure.
5 Wash hands and apply gloves and apron.	5 To minimise the risk of infection.
6 Clean the heel by washing thoroughly with plain tepid water. The heel should be allowed to dry completely before taking the sample.	6 Soap can irritate the neonate's skin (BNFC 2022).
7 Do not use alcohol or alcohol wipes to clean the heel.	7 Contamination of the sample may affect the results. The use of alcohol for skin preparation in neonates and premature babies can cause burns and blisters (Reynolds et al. 2005; Scales 2009; BNFC 2022).
8 Additional prewarming of the foot is not required.	8 There is no evidence that warming aids blood flow (Glenesk et al. 2006).
9 Perform the test using an automated incision device designed for use on newborns. Manual lancets must not be used. Skin puncture must be no deeper than 2.0 mm.	9 Newborn automated incision devices reduce pain and bruising, allow users to obtain the sample more quickly, and reduce the risk of accidental injury from manual lancets (Shepherd et al. 2006).
10 For full-term and preterm neonates, the external and internal limits of the calcaneus are the preferred puncture site (see Figure 20.9).	10 To minimise the risk of calcaneal puncture, which may lead to calcaneal osteomyelitis (Arena et al. 2005).
11 Avoid the posterior curvature of the heel.	11 The skin to calcaneus depth is greater in these areas. To minimise the risk of calcaneal puncture that may lead to calcaneal osteomyelitis (Arena et al. 2005).
12 Allow the heel to hang down.	12 To assist the blood flow.
13 Before activation place the automated incision device against the heel in accordance with manufacturers' instruction.	13 To ensure the device is used correctly and reduce the need for repeat incisions. This reduces the soft tissue damage and pain from repeated heel punctures in the same area. To ensure the correct depth of incision is achieved.
14 The aim is to fill each circle on the newborn bloodspot card, using a single drop of blood (see Figure 20.10).	14 To ensure the bloodspot card is completed effectively.
15 Wait for the blood to flow. Allow one spot of blood to drop onto each of the circles of the card. Do not allow the heel to make contact with the card.	15 To prevent contamination.
16 Do not squeeze the foot to try to increase blood flow.	16 This may cause pain and bruising.
17 Allow the blood to fill the circle by natural flow, and seep through from front to back.	17 This gives the optimum amount of blood for the laboratory to utilise.
18 Fill each of the four circles completely and do not layer the blood.	18 Layering of the blood is unacceptable for testing because too much blood can cause erroneous results (PHE 2014a, 2014b).
19 Do not compress the blood spot in order to ensure the blood has soaked through to the reverse of the card.	19 Applying pressure reduces the density of the sample and can lead to a 'suspected' result being missed.
20 If the blood flow ceases: a) The congealed blood should be wiped away firmly with cotton wool or gauze. b) Gently 'massage' the foot, avoid squeezing, and drop the blood onto the card. c) If the neonate is not bleeding, a second puncture will be necessary. d) The second puncture should be performed on a different part of the same foot or on the other foot, as marked by the shaded areas in Figure 20.9.	20 a) To disturb the clot and encourage blood flow. b) To reduce the amount of pain and bruising caused by the procedure. d) The original site is avoided to prevent the sample from containing excessive tissue fluid and to reduce pain.

(continued)

Procedure guideline 20.5 Collecting the blood spot sample *(continued)*

21 When the sample collection is complete, wipe excess blood from the heel and apply gentle pressure to the wound with cotton wool or gauze.	21 To prevent excessive bleeding and bruising and to protect the wound.
Completing the screening card:	
22 All parts of the screening card must be completed, including the neonate's NHS number.	22 Labs have a zero-tolerance policy in accepting cards that are incomplete and screening cannot be processed without this information.
23 Information that should be recorded on the Newborn Blood Spot Screening card in the 'comments' section includes: • Neonate's known medical conditions. • Relevant family history, e.g. PKU, CF, etc. • Mother's carrier status for SCD. • Reason for sample not taken on day 5–8 (e.g. pre transfusion, preterm CHT).	23 To ensure results are interpreted correctly. To assist newborn screening laboratory with linking antenatal and newborn screening results.
24 Ensure the sample is dry before being placed in the waxed paper envelope.	24 Wet samples can stick to the envelope and the test will be reported as compressed and a repeat will be requested.
25 Place the card in the special 'waxed paper' envelope for transportation to the laboratory.	
26 Send the card to the local Newborn Blood Spot Screening test centre.	26 To ensure it arrives promptly for processing.
27 The completion of the newborn blood spot screen and forwarding to the laboratory should be recorded: • In the child's healthcare record. • In the child's parent-held record when available. • On discharge and transfer documentation.	27 To provide accurate information. To ensure screening status is known and responsibility for screening is transferred.

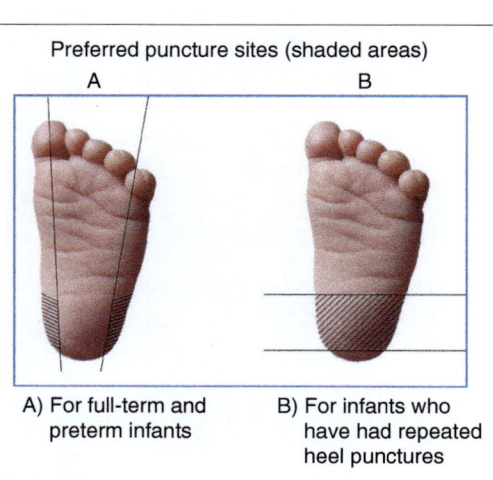

Figure 20.9 Preferred puncture sites for blood sampling (Public Health England 2014b, adapted from Jain and Rutter 1999).

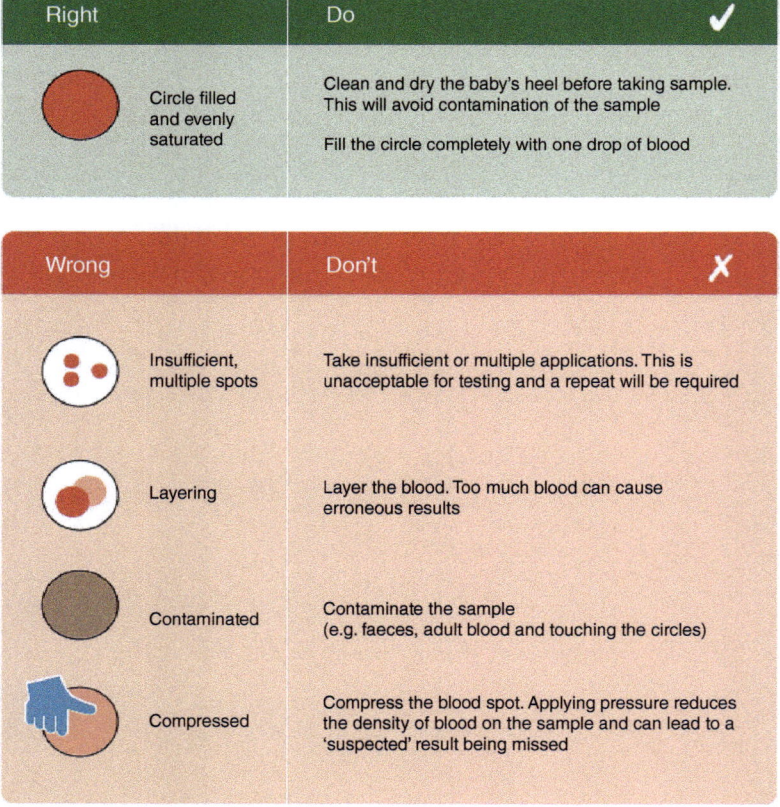

Figure 20.10 Taking a good quality sample. – Screening Programmes at www.screening.nhs.uk (PHE 2014b).

Principles table 20.14 Repeating the newborn blood spot test

Statement	Rationale
Repeat samples The newborn screening lab will inform the healthcare professional responsible for screening that a repeat is required.	
1 **Unavoidable repeats:** a) Borderline thyroid stimulating hormone (TSH) or inconclusive CF (follow advice on repeat request letter as to timing of repeat sample). b) Babies who require ongoing transfusions.	1 a) An interval of one week is required to detect any meaningful change in TSH levels. b) If a neonate does not have three clear days without transfusion between days 5–8 they will require a sample on day 8 and a repeat once they are three clear days post transfusion.
2 **Avoidable repeats:** These may be caused by: a) Incomplete data on card. b) No NHS number (or equivalent). c) Insufficient or layering of blood. d) Delay in sample getting to lab (send sample straight away). e) Sample taken too early (day of birth is day 0). f) Contamination of the card.	2 a) Labs have a zero-tolerance policy. b) Unique identifier required for each neonate. c) Not enough blood or risk of erroneous result. d) May lead to invalid result. e) May give false positive CHT. f) May give incorrect result.
3 When the test has been taken, it will be recorded in the regional centre. Currently regional centres cannot see if samples were taken outside of their region, so for screening results for babies transferred from out of region, their local screening lab will need to be contacted if there is no documentation in the PCHR or transfer documentation.	3 Regional nieonatal screening centres have been set up throughout the UK. To ensure no babies miss screening.
4 **Results:** a) Parents should be informed of results within six to eight weeks. If a neonate screens positive for a condition they will be contacted sooner. b) Results will be received via post or the health visitor. **If a positive result is detected:** c) Arrangements will be made for the neonate to be seen by a paediatric specialist, who is contacted by the regional screening centre, to instigate investigations. d) Treatment will be started as soon as possible after the diagnosis is confirmed. e) The child's GP will be contacted and informed of the child's investigations and results when available. f) The family should be advised of the support groups available for babies with CF, PKU, hypothyroidism, sickle cell disease, and MCADD, and they should be given a leaflet specific to the condition, from the UK Newborn Screening Programme Centre Website (PHE 2014a, 2014b).	a) To ensure that further tests and follow-up can be arranged as soon as possible following diagnosis. c-d) To enable urgent specialist referral, inform the family, confirm the diagnosis and commence appropriate treatment. e) To ensure that the primary healthcare team is aware of the potential diagnosis. f) To provide advice and support.

Phototherapy – neonatal jaundice

Jaundice refers to yellow colouration of the skin and the sclerae, which is caused by a raised level of bilirubin in the circulation; a condition known as hyperbilirubinaemia. It is one of the most common conditions needing medical attention in newborn babies. Approximately 60% of term and 80% of preterm babies develop jaundice in the first week of life. For the majority of babies, this is harmless and will require no treatment. However, a few babies develop very high levels of bilirubin, which can be dangerous if not treated (NICE 2010; Vandborg et al. 2012).

Bilirubin is produced when red blood cells are broken down. This initial bilirubin, known as unconjugated bilirubin, cannot be excreted. Unconjugated bilirubin is carried in the plasma bound to albumin, metabolised in the liver to form conjugated bilirubin, then carried in the bile and is excreted in the stool (Blackburn 2012).

Newborn babies have a higher level of red blood cells at birth than adults and these blood cells have a shorter life span. These factors, coupled with a relatively immature liver, result in a raised level of unconjugated bilirubin during the first few days of life, as the liver struggles to process and excrete the bilirubin. This is part of the normal adaption from intrauterine to extra uterine life and is often referred to as physiological jaundice (Stokowski 2011; Blackburn 2012).

It is thought that unconjugated bilirubin is generally safe while bound to albumin. However, once the rate of haemolysis outweighs albumin-binding sites and the processing capabilities of the liver, the level of unconjugated bilirubin not bound to albumin rises; this is described as free bilirubin. Free bilirubin can cross the blood–brain barrier, resulting in bilirubin encephalopathy and subsequently kernicterus, with permanent devastating neurological damage and hearing loss (NICE 2010; Stokowski 2011; Blackburn 2012).

All babies who are visibly jaundiced should have a total bilirubin level taken and plotted on the appropriate NICE treatment threshold graph (NICE 2010). However, it is noted by NICE (2010) that visual assessment is not a reliable method of assessing jaundice. It is important to determine whether there is a pathological cause for the jaundice in all babies who require phototherapy, who present with jaundice at less than 24 hours of age, those with jaundice that presents or remains after 14 days, and those with high levels of conjugated bilirubin.

Treatment

Phototherapy is the most common treatment for significant unconjugated hyperbilirubinaemia. This uses blue light to convert unconjugated bilirubin into harmless isomers that can be eliminated without conjugation in the liver (NICE 2010; Stokowski 2011; Blackburn 2012). (See Figure 20.11 for care of neonate undergoing phototherapy.) If phototherapy fails to reduce the bilirubin and it continues to rise an exchange transfusion may be required; this must be carried out within an ITU environment and is a consultant-led decision. Immunoglobulin is also used as a treatment method in babies with haemolytic disease with rapidly rising bilirubin levels.

In 2010 NICE published guidance on the management of neonatal jaundice within the first 14 days of life. This guidance aimed to ensure a more consistent approach to jaundice management in neonates. The guidance below is adapted from the NICE Neonatal Jaundice guideline CG98 (NICE 2010) and include the recommended changes from the 2016 updates.

NOTE: If positioning aids and boundaries are used, ensure they do not obstruct the phototherapy light. (See developmental care section of this chapter for advice regarding positioning.)

Neonatal fluid management

This section covers fluid intake for all neonates. It will briefly explain the significance of sodium (Na), potassium (K+), calcium (Ca), and glucose in the first few days of life (see Table 20.2).

For guidance related to growth and nutritional requirements, breastfeeding, and different neonatal formulas, please see Chapter 22: Nutrition and Feeding. Physical assessment of fluid balance will not be covered in this section. However, if a neonate gains weight in the first days after birth, when weight loss would be anticipated, further investigations will be required (Rennie 2005).

In the first week of life, a physiological contraction of extracellular fluid volume occurs with diuresis. This is reflected in a weight loss of 5–10% in term neonates, and up to 20% in preterm neonates. It is generally recommended to use birth weight, rather than current body weight, to calculate fluids on a per kilogramme basis until birth weight is reachieved (Halbardier 2010).

The goal of fluid therapy is to permit physiological, adaptive fluid and electrolyte changes to occur appropriately (Davis et al. 2002; Kerr et al. 2006). If fluid therapy is required, glucose 10% in water is used initially. Electrolytes are not usually added to maintenance IV fluids for the first 24–48 hours after birth. Serum electrolyte levels and urine output are used to determine when to add electrolytes to IV fluids (Halbardier 2010). In general, fluid management in the first few days of life is adjusted primarily on serum sodium values and changes in weight.

Fluid management requires the understanding of physiological water losses in the neonate, which results from either renal or extra renal causes - see text box below.

> **Sources of water loss**
> Renal losses may be due to:
> - Decreased glomerular filtration rate (GFR)
> - Reduced proximal and distal tubule sodium reabsorption
> - Decreased capacity to concentrate or dilute urine
> - Decreased bicarbonate, potassium, and hydrogen ion secretion
>
> Extra renal losses due to evaporation from the skin and respiratory tract are called insensible water losses (IWL). These may be due to:
> - Increased environmental and body temperature
> - Activity
> - Skin breakdown
> - Radiant warmers (e.g. phototherapy)
> - Prematurity
> - Crying
>
> *Source:* Adapted from Doherty (2012).

The emphasis in fluid therapy should be on the prevention of excessive insensible water loss rather than replacement of increased insensible water loss (Doherty 2012).

Prevention of over infusion of intravenous fluid in the neonate

To avoid over infusion in neonates who require IV fluids, National Patient Safety Agency (NPSA) advice should be followed (NPSA 2010).

This states: 'Due to a neonate's weight and size, and the often critical nature of their condition, fluid overload can prove fatal. There is evidence that the majority of cases of fluid overload are associated with user error of the infusion device' (NPSA 2010 p. 6). The NPSA (2010) recommends education, training, and assessment for staff who administer and monitor IV infusions, regular monitoring of the neonate, and effective handover of care to reduce the risk of over infusion and fluid overload in neonates. In addition, the NPSA (2010) reports that smart IV infusion pumps are effective in reducing medication errors associated with infusion pump user error. The main points are as follows and should be included in local standards for education, training, and assessment, and subject to audit, to ensure clinical practice is in accordance with the local policy (NPSA 2010):

- When using a syringe pump to administer IV fluids or medicines to neonates, a bag of fluid should not be left connected to the syringe. (This action does not apply to the administration of blood components.)
- All clamps on IV administration sets must be closed before removing the administration set from the infusion pump or switching the pump off. This is required regardless of whether the administration set has an anti-free-flow device.

- The frequency and responsibility for monitoring: (i) the IV infusion device, (ii) the infusion administration equipment, and (iii) the patient receiving IV infusion is clearly outlined.

In caring for a neonate receiving IV fluids,

- The infusion rate and the total volume should be checked against the prescription by two registered nurses.
- As a minimum, hourly check of the infusion rate and total volume infused, fluid balance calculation, pulse, and respiratory rate must be made and recorded in the healthcare record.
- If the infusion contains glucose, check and record the blood sugar within an hour of the start of the infusion, and then as determined by local management plan.

Chapter 20 Neonatal care

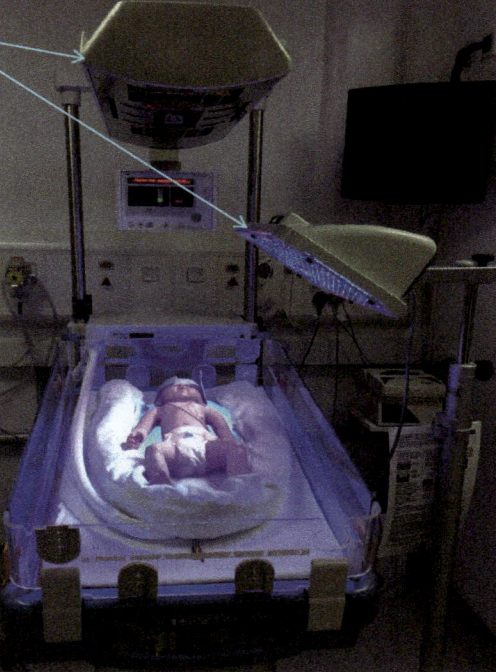

Figure 20.11 Neonate undergoing multiple phototherapies.

Principles table 20.15 Phototherapy – neonatal jaundice

Statement	Rationale
1 All newborns should be examined for jaundice at every opportunity, especially within the first 72 hours of life.	1 To ensure prompt recognition, diagnosis and treatment of neonatal jaundice and investigation of potential cause.
2 A colour assessment should be performed every time vital signs are recorded and documented or once per shift as a minimum.	2 To ensure a regular visual check is made of the neonate
3 During a visual inspection check the neonate, naked, in bright, preferably natural light. Examine the sclerae, gums, and blanched skin.	3 Artificial light can make it difficult to assess jaundice appropriately.
4 Clinical recognition of jaundice can be difficult, particularly in babies with dark skin tones.	
5 NICE (2010) recommend that babies who are at increased risk of significant hyperbilirubinaemia should receive an additional examination by a healthcare professional within 48 hours.	5 To detect significant hyperbilirubinaemia, i.e. that requiring treatment.
6 Babies at increased risk of significant hyperbilirubinaemia include those: • Born prior to 38 weeks gestation. • With a previous sibling with neonatal jaundice requiring phototherapy. • With visible jaundice within 24 hours of life. • Exclusively breastfed (NICE 2010).	
7 Other factors may also increase the risk of significant hyperbilirubinaemia.	

(continued)

Principles table 20.15 Phototherapy – neonatal jaundice *(continued)*

Statement	Rationale
8 If a neonate appears jaundiced, a total serum bilirubin measurement must be taken to determine the bilirubin level.	8 This is the most accurate method for guiding treatment.
9 Do not rely on visual assessment alone.	9 Visual assessment is not an accurate method of determining the level of bilirubin.
10 Take a sample of capillary, venous, or arterial blood and send for total bilirubin.	10 See local blood sampling policy for guidance.
11 The result of the total bilirubin must be plotted on an appropriate treatment threshold graph.	11 See NICE (2010) guidelines for jaundice for treatment threshold graphs.
12 Select appropriate graph for neonate's gestational week at birth to guide treatment for the first 14 days of life.	12 Treatment and exchange thresholds vary greatly.
13 Plot the total bilirubin results on the graph according to the neonate's postnatal age in hours (see Figure 20.12).	13 To ensure treatment is provided appropriately allowing for the normal pattern of bilirubin metabolism in the newborn and to ensure prompt diagnosis and investigation of neonates jaundiced at <24 hours of age.

Treatment threshold graph

14 Treatment of jaundice should be guided by treatment threshold graph.	14 To ensure consistent treatment of all jaundiced neonates and ensure no neonates miss treatment.
15 Other investigations may be needed; please refer to medical staff, local and NICE (2010) guidance.	15 To ensure correct investigations are undertaken allowing prompt and appropriate treatment to be delivered.

Treatment: Phototherapy

16 Phototherapy should be started when the total bilirubin plotted on the appropriate treatment threshold graph for gestation is on or above the treatment line.	16 Treatment should be guided by treatment threshold graph (NICE 2010)
17 If a neonate requires phototherapy further screening is required: • Clinical examination • Serum bilirubin • Blood packed cell volume • Blood group of mother and neonate • Direct antiglobulin test.	17 To eliminate pathological causes of jaundice
18 Consider: • Full blood count and examination of blood film. • Glucose-6-phosphate dehydrogenase deficiency. • Microbiological cultures of blood, urine, and cerebrospinal fluid.	

Monitoring total bilirubin

19 The bilirubin level should be repeated 4–6 hourly after commencing phototherapy and until the level is stable or falling.	19 To ensure escalation of treatment as appropriate.
20 Repeat the bilirubin level 6–12 hourly once the level is stable or falling.	20 To monitor levels and adjust treatment appropriately.
21 Repeat level 12–18 hours after stopping phototherapy.	21 To check for rebound.
22 Record all bilirubin levels on appropriate treatment threshold chart.	22 To ensure an accurate record is maintained.

Types of phototherapy at Great Ormond Street:

Single phototherapy

Single phototherapy can be provided via:
- Natus Neoblue lights
- Fibre optic blanket

23 Use your clinical judgement to allow breaks of up to 30 min for neonates undergoing single phototherapy to allow for feeds, cuddles, cares, etc.	23 To maximise surface area exposed to light. To enable establishment of breastfeeding and bonding and attachment.

Principles table 20.15 Phototherapy – neonatal jaundice (*continued*)

Statement	Rationale
Intensified phototherapy	
24 Commence continuous intensified phototherapy if: 　a) The bilirubin level is rising more than 8.5 micromol/l/h. 　b) The bilirubin level is within 50 micromol/l of the level for exchange transfusion. 　c) The bilirubin level continues to rise or does not fall within six hours of starting phototherapy.	24 To improve efficiency of treatment.
25 Continuous intensified phototherapy should be given using the 　a. Natus blue lights (with the double phototherapy switch on). 　b. It can also include the addition of a fibre optic blanket or additional Natus blue lights.	25 To ensure the most effective light source is used. To maximise surface area exposed.
26 Intensified phototherapy should be continuous; nutrition should be provided either intravenously or via nasogastric tube, cup, or bottle.	26 To ensure no gaps in the delivery of phototherapy reduce the efficacy of the treatment. See local policy for feeding guidance.
27 If the serum bilirubin falls to a level 50 micromol/l below exchange level during intensified phototherapy, the phototherapy can be stepped down to single.	27 Intensified phototherapy is no longer needed.
Stopping phototherapy	
28 Phototherapy should not be stopped until the bilirubin level is at least 50 micromol/l below the phototherapy treatment line.	28 To adhere to NICE (2010) recommendations.
29 The NICE website has quick reference guidance with clear pathways guiding recognition and treatment of jaundice. These can be printed to keep at the neonate's bed space.	29 To provide easy access to appropriate guidance NICE (2010).

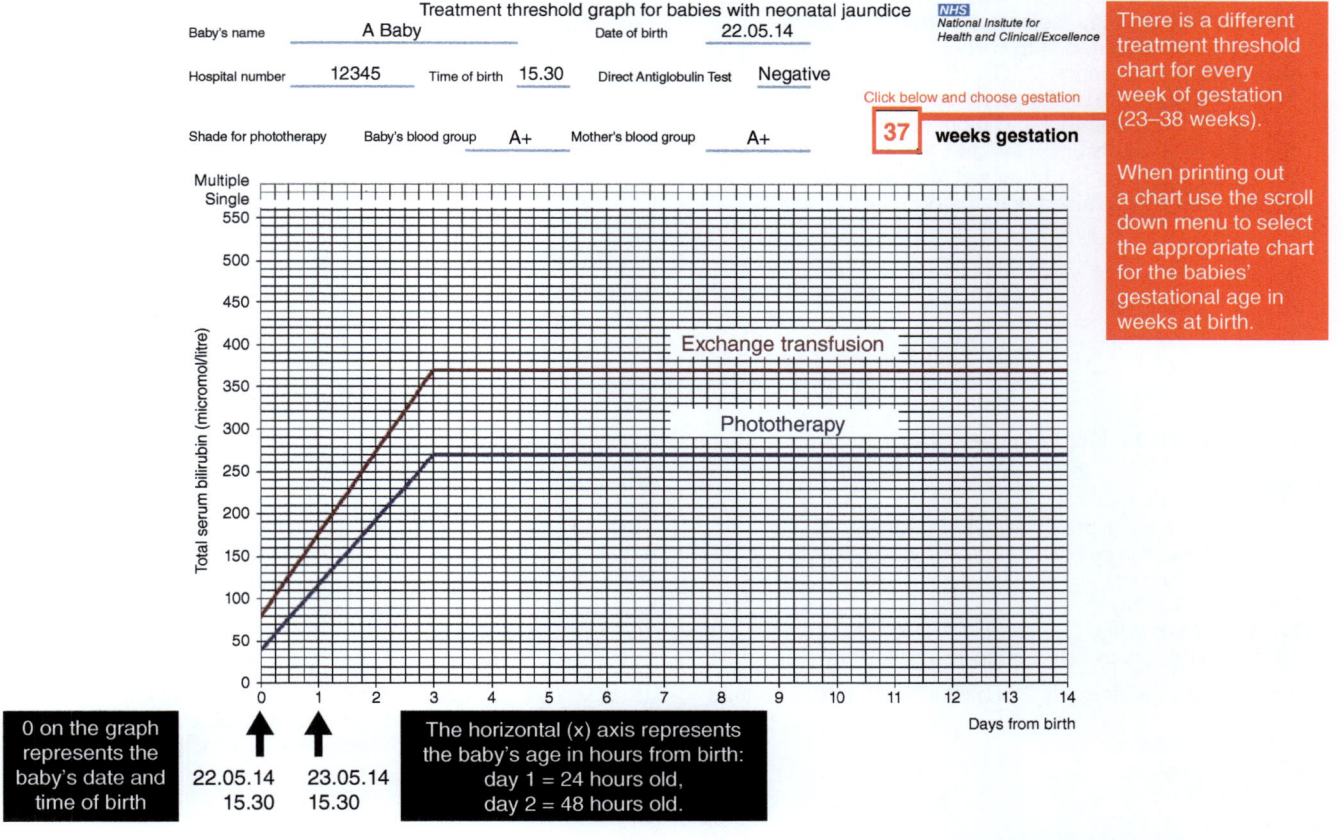

Figure 20.12 Example: NICE treatment threshold graph. *Source:* Reproduced from: National Institute for Health and Care Excellence/National Collaborating Centre for Women and Child Health. Neonatal Jaundice. Clinical Guideline No. 98. London: NICE; 2010, with the permission of the Royal College of Obstetricians and Gynaecologists.

Principles table 20.16 Care of neonates receiving phototherapy

Statement	Rationale
The effectiveness of phototherapy is dependent on three main factors:	
1 Surface area exposed to light a) Babies should be nursed in only a small nappy. b) Their eyes should be covered with appropriate protection (see Figure 20.11). Routine eye care should be performed. c) Position the neonate in the supine position unless clinical condition dictates otherwise. d) Do not routinely use white sheets or reflective materials around the incubator/Babytherm to increase surface area exposed to light.	1 a) To ensure maximum surface area covered by phototherapy. b) Appropriate eye protection should be worn due to risk of photochemical damage (NICE 2010; Stokowski 2011). c) To maximise surface area exposed to light. d) This could obstruct your view of the baby.
2 Colour of light Phototherapy units comprising of lights in the blue/green spectrum should be used.	2 Light in the blue/green spectrum is most effective in reducing total serum bilirubin level. (NICE 2010; Stokowski 2011; Vandborg et al. 2012).
3 Distance from light source Ensure that the light source is at the distance from the neonate recommended by the manufacturer.	3 To ensure maximum efficiency. To ensure the neonate does not overheat and the equipment is used in line with manufacturer's recommendations.
4 General care a) Monitor neonate's temperature closely and ensure a thermo neutral environment. b) Extra fluids should not be given routinely. c) Monitor hydration by weighing daily and assessing fluid balance d) Observe for pale stools and dark urine and report these immediately to the nurse in charge/medical team. e) Keep parents updated with verbal updates backed up with written information (NICE 2010). f) NICE guidance (2010) for jaundice covers the first 14 days of life. Treatment and monitoring beyond this time should be consultant led and allow appropriate timely investigation of prolonged jaundice and follow up of neonates with a raised conjugated bilirubin level.	a) To prevent hypo/hyperthermia. b) Extra fluids given routinely could impact on establishment of breastfeeding. Fluids should be adjusted according to individual needs. c) To ensure the baby is adequately hydrated. d) To ensure swift detection of potential complications. Pale stools and dark urine are suggestive of liver disorder, which requires prompt treatment (NICE 2010b). f) To enable prompt treatment of underlying cause.

Principles table 20.17 Fluid regime

Statement	Rationale
1 Fluid regime in a term, uncomplicated neonate: • Day 1: 60 millilitres per kilogramme of body weight per day (ml/kg/day) • Day 2: 90 ml/kg/day • Day 3: 120 ml/kg/day • Day 4: consider increasing up to 150 ml/kg/day	1 Any fluid therapy recommendation for a neonate must be adjusted to match the neonate's individual requirement. Variables such as insensible water loss, which occur through the skin, stool, and the respiratory system, must be taken into consideration (Chukwu et al. 2011).
2 Fluid regime in an extremely low birth weight and premature neonate: Day 1: 90 ml/kg/day Day 2: 120 ml/kg/day Day 3: 150 ml/kg/day Day 4: 180 ml/kg/day	2 Increased fluid intake is required for extremely low birth weight neonates and premature babies as a result of larger insensible water loss due to large surface area relative to body weight (Chukwu et al. 2011).

Chapter 20 Neonatal care

Table 20.2 Electrolyte values

Electrolyte	What does it do?	Normal values
Sodium (Na)	Major osmotic solute of extracellular fluids Action potential of muscle/ nerve cells	136–145 mmol/l
Potassium (K+)	Action potential of muscle/nerve cells	3.8–5.0 mmol/l
Calcium (Ca)	Formation of bones/teeth Blood clotting, muscle contraction Muscle/nerve action potentials Endo- and exocytosis Cell division	2.25–2.65 mmol/l
Glucose	Energy source for organs, especially for brain cells Essential for normal growth, activity, and development	2 mmol/l in first 2 hours of life, but it will rise to adult levels (4–7 mmol/l) within 2–3 days

Principles table 20.18 Electrolyte and glucose requirements

Statement	Rationale
1) **Day 1:**	1) No electrolytes administered routinely.
2) **Day 2 and onwards:**	2) Start administration after postnatal diuresis has been established.
3) **Sodium (Na) requirements:** Term neonate: 2–3 mmol/kg of body weight per day (mmol/kg/d) Preterm neonate (30–36 weeks): 4 mmol/kg/day Preterm neonate (<30 weeks): 4-8 mmol/kg/day	3) Low serum sodium levels may indicate that the neonate requires less fluid, or that the neonate has high sodium losses. Premature neonates have greater requirements for sodium because of the immaturity of renal tubular reabsorption (Shina et al. 2012).
4) **Potassium requirements:** Term neonate: 2 mmol/kg/d Preterm neonate (30–36 weeks): 2 mmol/kg/d Preterm neonate (<30 weeks): 2–4 mmol/kg/d	4) Potassium should not be given until adequate renal function has been established. Preterm babies require higher intake due to poor potassium regulation and leakage from immature cells after 48 hours of life.
5) **Calcium requirements:** Term neonate: 0.5 mmol/kg/d Preterm neonate (30–36 weeks): 0.5–1.5 mmol/kg/d Preterm neonate (<30 weeks): 1.5 mmol/kg/d	5) Regulatory mechanisms that maintain serum calcium levels may not be entirely adequate (American Academy of Pediatrics Committee on Nutrition 1999).
6) **Blood sugar requirements:** Term neonate: Keep levels above 2.6 millimols per litre (mmol/l) Or above 2.5 mmol/l in neonates who are at risk of hypoglycaemia, such as: • Premature babies • Extremely low birth weight neonates • Post-mature neonates (>42 weeks) • Neonates of diabetic mothers • Large for gestational age babies • Infection • Beckwith-Wiedeman syndrome • Birth asphyxia • Polycythaemia • Hypothermia	6) On the basis of different studies, the lower limit of normo-glycemia is 2.6 mmol/l, although levels below this do not necessarily mean that damage will occur (Shina et al. 2012).

References

Altimier, l., Warner, B., Amlung, S., and Kenner, C. (1999). *Neonatal thermoregulation; bed surface transfers. Neonatal Network* 18 (4): 35–37.

American Academy of Pediatrics Committee on Nutrition (1999). *Calcium requirements of infants, children, and adolescents. Pediatrics* 104 (5): 1152–1157.

Arena, J., Emparanza, J.I., Nogués, A., and Burls, A. (2005). *Skin to calcaneus distance in the neonate. Archives of Disease in Childhood. Fetal and Neonatal Edition* 90 (4): F328–f331.

Auckland District Health Board (2004). Developmental care - an overview. https://starship.org.nz/guidelines/developmental-care-an-overview (accessed 23 September 2022).

Baker-Rush, M. (2016). *Reducing stress in infants: kangaroo care. International Journal of Childbirth Education* 31 (3): 44–48.

Blackburn, S.T. (2012). Maternal, Fetal and Neonatal Physiology: A Clinical Perspective. London: Elsevier.

Breathnach, A. (2005). *Nosocominal infections. Medicine* 33 (3): 22–26.

British National Formulary for Children (BNFC) (2022). https://bnfc.nice.org.uk (accessed 23 September 2022).

Broom, M.A. and Smith, S.L. (2013). *Late presentation of neonatal omphalitis following dry cord care*. Clinical Pediatrics 52 (7): 675–677.

Castellani, C., Picci, L., Tamanini, A. et al. (2009). *Association between carrier screening and incidence of cystic fibrosis*. JAMA: The Journal of the American Medical Association 302 (23): 2573.

Chamley, C.A., Carson, P., Randall, B., and Sandwell, W.M. (2006). Developmental Anatomy and Physiology of Children: A Practical Approach. Edinburgh: Elsevier and Churchill Livingstone.

Chukwu, J., Gorman, W., and Molloy, E.J. (2011). Fluid and electrolyte balance in the newborn. In: Newborn Surgery (ed. P. Puri), 133–145. London: Hodder.

Coyne, I., Neill, F.B., and Timmins, F. (2010). Clinical Skills in Children's Nursing. Oxford: Oxford University Press.

Davis, I.D. and Avner, E.D. (2002). Fluid, electrolytes, and acid-base homeostasis. In: Neonatal-Perinatal Medicine- Disease of the Foetus and Infant, 7e (eds. A.A. Fanaroff and R.J. Martin), 619–627. St. Louis: Mosby.

Department of Health (DH) (2009). Toolkit for High-Quality Neonatal Services. https://www.londonneonatalnetwork.org.uk/wp-content/uploads/2015/09/Toolkit-2009.pdf (accessed 23 September 2022).

Department of Health Circular (1998) PL/ CMO/98/3. PL/CNO/98/4: Vitamin K for Newborn Babies. London, Department of Health.

Doherty, E.G. (2012). Fluid and electrolyte management. In: Manual of Neonatal Care, 7e (eds. J.P. Cloherty, E.C. Eichenwald, A.R. Hansen and A.R. Stark), 269–283. Lippincott, Williams & Wilkins. http://www.ypeda.com/attachments/article/150/manual%20of%20neonatal%20care%207th.pdf (accessed 23 September 2022).

Fear, N.T., Roman, E., Ansell, P. et al. (2003). *Vitamin K and childhood cancer: a report from the United Kingdom Childhood Cancer Study*. British Journal of Cancer 89 (7): 1228–1231.

Foster, J. (2016). *Non-nutritive sucking for increasing physiological stability in preterm infants*. Cochrane Neonatal Reviews 2016 (10): CD001071. https://doi.org/10.1002/14651858.CD001071.pub3.

Glenesk, A., Shepherd, A., Niven, C., and Mackenzie, J. (2006). *Blood spot testing: comparing techniques and automated devices*. British Journal of Midwifery 14 (2): 96–99.

Halbardier, B.H. (2010). Fluid and electrolyte management. In: In: Core Curriculum for Neonatal Intensive Care Nursing, 4e (eds. M.T. Verklan and M. Walden), 156–171. Saunders, Elsevier.

Hamilton, K.E.S.C. and Redshaw, M.E. (2009). *Developmental care in the UK: a developing initiative*. Acta Paediatr. 98 (11): 1738–1743.

Imdad, A., Bautista, R.M., Senen, K.A. and Uy, M.E. (2013). Umbilical cord antiseptics for preventing sepsis and death among newborns, online resource. http://onlinelibrary.wiley.com/doi/10.1002/14651858.CD008635.pub2/full (accessed 23 September 2022).

Jain, A. and Rutter, N. (1999) *Ultrasound study of heel to calcaneum depth in neonates*. Arch Dis Child Fetal Neonatal Ed, 80(3): p. F243–5.

Johnston, C.C., Collinge, J.M., Henderson, S.J., and Anand, K.J.S. (1997). *A cross-sectional survey of pain and pharmacological analgesia in Canadian neonatal intensive care units*. Clinical Journal of Pain 13 (4): 308–312.

Kennedy Shriver, E. (2007) Infant Sleep Position and SIDS. U.S Department of Health and Human Services. National Institutes of Health

Kerr, B.A., Starbuck, A.L., and Block, S.M. (2006). Fluid and electrolyte management. In: In: Handbook of Neonatal Intensive Care, 6e (eds. G.B. Mernstein and S.L. Gardner), 351–367. St. Louis: Mosby.

Leick-Rude, M.K. and Bloom, L.F. (1998). *A comparison of temperature-taking methods in neonates*. Neonatal Network 17 (5): 21–37.

Leonard, J.V. and Dezateux, C. (2009). *Newborn screening for medium chain acyl Coa dehydrogenase deficiency*. Archives of Disease in Childhood 94 (3): 235–238.

Levene, M.I., Tudehope, D.I., and Sinha, S. (2008). Essential Neonatal Medicine, 4e. Oxford: Blackwell Science.

Lippi, G. and Franchini, M. (2011). *Vitamin K in neonates: facts and myths*. Blood Transfusion 9: 4–9.

Lissauer, T. and Fanaroff, A.A. (2006). Neonatology at a Glance. Oxford: Blackwell Publishing.

Liu, M.F., Lin, K.C., Chou, Y.H., and Lee, T.Y. (2010). *Using non-nutritive sucking and oral glucose solution with neonates to relieve pain: a randomised controlled trial*. Journal of Clinical Nursing 19 (11–12): 1604–1611.

Lyon, A. (2008). *Temperature control in the neonate*. Paediatrics and Child Health 18 (4): 155–160.

Marshall, A. (1997). *Humidifying the environment for the premature neonate*. Journal of Neonatal Nursing 3 (1): 32–36.

McConnell, T., Lee, C.W., Couillard, M., and Sherrill, W.W. (2004). *Trends in umbilical cord care: scientific evidence for practice*. Newborn and Infant Nursing Reviews 4: 211–222.

Medoff-Cooper, B. (1994). *Transition of the preterm infant to an open crib*. Journal of Obstetric, Gynecologic, and Neonatal Nursing 23 (4): 329–335.

Merenstein, G.B. and Gardner, S.I. (2006). Handbook of Neonatal Intensive Care, 6e. St Louis: Mosby.

Merenstein, G.B. and Gardner, S.I. (2011). Handbook of Neonatal Intensive Care, 7e. St Louis: Mosby.

Mok, Q., Bass, C.A., Ducker, D.A., and McIntosh, N. (1991). *Temperature instability during nursing procedures in preterm neonates*. Archives of Disease in Childhood 66 (7): 783–786.

Moorthie, S., Cameron, L., Sagoo, G., and Burton, H. (2013). Birth Prevalence of Five Inherited Metabolic Disorders: A Systematic Review. London: PHG Foundation.

Mullany, L., Darmstadt, G.L., Katz, J. et al. (2006). *Development of clinical sign based algorithms for community based assessment of omphalitis*. Archives of Disease in Childhood. Fetal and Neonatal Edition 91: 99–104.

National Institute for Health and Care Excellence (NICE) (2020). Specialist neonatal respiratory care for babies born preterm Quality Standard [QS193]. London: National Institute for Health and Clinical Excellence. https://www.nice.org.uk/guidance/QS193 (accessed 23 September 2022).

National Institute for Health and Care Excellence (NICE) (2010). Jaundice in newborn babies under 28 days. Clinical guideline [CG98]. https://www.nice.org.uk/guidance/cg98 (accessed 23 September 2022).

National Institute for Health and Care Excellence (NICE) (2021). Postnatal care: NICE guideline [NG194]. https://www.nice.org.uk/guidance/ng194 (accessed 23 September 2022).

National Patient Safety Agency (2010). Prevention of over infusion of intravenous fluid and medicines in neonates. NPSA/2010/RRR015. National Patient Safety Agency. https://www.networks.nhs.uk/nhs-networks/staffordshire-shropshire-and-black-country-newborn/documents/1264_RRR_Prevention_of_over_infusion__FINAL.pdf (accessed 23 September 2022).

New, K., Flenady, V., and Davies, M.W. (2011). *Transfer of preterm infants from incubator to open cot at lower versus higher body weight*. Cochrane Database of Systematic Reviews 7 (9): CD004214. https://www.cochranelibrary.com/cdsr/doi/10.1002/14651858.CD004214.pub4/full (accessed 23 September 2022).

Nursing and Midwifery Council (2015). The code: Professional standards of practice and behaviour for nurses and midwives. The Nursing and Midwifery Council. London. https://www.nmc.org.uk/standards/code/ (accessed 23 September 2022).

Olney, R.S., Grosse, S.D., and Vogt, R.F. (2010). *Prevalence of congenital hypothyroidism – current trends and future directions: workshop summary*. Pediatrics 125 (Suppl 2): S31–S36.

Public Health England (PHE) (2014a). Newborn blood spot screening: programme handbook. https://www.gov.uk/government/publications/health-professional-handbook-newborn-blood-spot-screening (accessed 23 September 2022).

Public Health England (PHE) (2014b). Guidelines for Newborn Blood Spot Sampling. https://www.gov.uk/government/publications/newborn-blood-spot-screening-sampling-guidelines (accessed 23 September 2022).

Rennie, J.M. (2005). Fluid management. In: Roberton's Textbook of Neonatology, 4e (ed. J.M. Rennie). Elsevier.

Rennie, J.M. and Kendall, G.S. (2013). A Manual of Neonatal Intensive Care, 5e. London: CRC Press.

Rennie, J.M. and Roberton, N.R.C. (2005). Roberton's Textbook of Neonatology, 4e. Edinburgh: Churchill Livingstone.

Reynolds, P.R., Banerjee, S., and Meek, J.H. (2005). *Alcohol burns in extremely low birth weight infants: still occurring*. Archives of Disease in Childhood. Fetal and Neonatal Edition 90 (1): F10.

Scales, K. (2009). *Correct use of chlorhexidine in intravenous practice*. Nursing Standard 24 (8): 41–47.

Seguin, J.H. and Vieth, R. (1996). *Thermal stability of premature infants during routine care under radiant warmers*. Archives of Disease in Childhood. Fetal and Neonatal Edition 74 (2): F137–F138.

Shah, P.S., Herbozo, C., Aliwalas, L.L, and Shah, V.S. (2012). Breastfeeding or breast milk for procedural pain in neonates. The Cochrane Collaboration. The Cochrane Library, Issue 1. https://www.cochranelibrary.com/cdsr/doi/10.1002/14651858.CD004950.pub3/full (accessed 23 September 2022).

Sheeran, M.S. (1996). *Thermoregulation in neonates; obtaining an accurate axillary temperature measurement*. Journal of Neonatal Nursing 2 (4): 6–9.

Shepherd, A.J., Glenesk, A., Niven, C.A., and Mackenzie, J. (2006). *A Scottish study of heel-prick blood sampling in newborn babies*. Midwifery 22 (2): 158–168.

Shina, S., Miall, L., and Jardine, L. (2012). Essential Neonatal Medicine, 5e. Wiley Blackwell.

Smith, J., Alcock, G., and Usher, K. (2013). *Temperature measurement in the preterm and term neonate: a literature review*. Neonatal Network 32 (1): 16–25.

Stevens, B., Yamada J., Lee, Ohlsson, A., Haliburton, S., Shorkey, A. (2016). Sucrose for analgesia in newborn infants undergoing painful procedures. The Cochrane neonatal group. The Cochrane Library. https://www.cochranelibrary.com/cdsr/doi/10.1002/14651858.CD001069.pub5/full (accessed 23 September 2022).

Stokowski, L.A. (2011). *Fundamentals of phototherapy for neonatal jaundice*. Advances in Neonatal Care 11 (5s): s10–s21.

Streetly, A., Latinovic, R., and Henthorn, J. (2010). *Positive screening and carrier results for the England-wide universal newborn sickle cell screening Programme by ethnicity and area for 2005-2007*. Journal of Clinical Pathology 63 (7): 626–629.

Thomas, K. (1994). *Thermoregulation in neonate*. Neonatal Network 13 (2): 15–21.

Trotter, S. (2004). *Care of the newborn: proposed new guidelines*. British Journal of Midwifery 12 (3): 152–157.

Turnbull, V. and Petty, J. (2013). *Evidence-based thermal care of low birthweight neonates. Part one*. Nursing Children and Young People 25 (2): 18–22.

Vandborg, P.K., Hansen, B.M., Greisen, G., and Ebbesen, F. (2012). *Dose response relationship of phototherapy for Hyperbilirubinaemia*. Pediatrics 130 (2): e352–e357.

Waldron, S. and MacKinnon, R. (2007). *Neonatal thermoregulation*. Infantry 3 (3): 101–104.

Williams, R.A., Mamotte, C.D., and Burnett, J.R. (2008). *Phenylketonuria: an inborn error of phenylalanine metabolism*. Clinical Biochemistry Reviews 29 (1): 31–41.

World Health Organisation (2007). Standard precautions in healthcare. https://www.who.int/docs/default-source/documents/health-topics/standard-precautions-in-health-care.pdf (accessed 23 September 2022).

Zupan, J., Garner, P. & Omar, A.A. (2004). Topical umbilical cord care at birth. https://www.cochranelibrary.com/cdsr/doi/10.1002/14651858.CD001057.pub2/full (accessed 23 September 2022).

Chapter 21

Neurological care

Nicola Barnes[1], Sophie Boella[2], Lindy May[3], Ainsley Moven[4], and Jody O'Connor[5]

[1]RN (Child), MSc Paediatric Advanced Practice, Advanced Nurse Practitioner for Epilepsy Surgery, Great Ormond Street Hospital, London, UK

[2]RN (Child), Neurology Nurse, GOSH

[3]RN (Adult), RN (Child), MSc (Neuroscience), Diploma in Counselling, PhD, Formerly Nurse Consultant, Neurosurgery, GOSH

[4]RN (Child), PGDip, Nurse Practitioner, Neurosurgery, GOSH

[5]RN (Child), DIPHE, BSc (hons) Neuroscience, MSc ANP, Advanced Neurosurgical Nurse Practitioner, GOSH

Chapter contents

Introduction	454
Section 1: Neurological observations	454
Types of painful stimuli	462
Section 2: Seizures	463
Physiology of seizures	464
Care of the CYP with seizures	465
Classification of seizures	468
Section 3: External ventricular drainage	470
References	479

Procedure guidelines

21.1	Neurological observations	454	21.9 Drain management: patency of drain: repairing a catheter	476
21.2	Nursing management of the CYP during seizures	466	21.10 Drain management: patency of drain: unblocking of catheter	476
21.3	Introduction to external ventricular drainage	471	21.11 Drain management: fluid and electrolyte balance	477
21.4	Inform the CYP and family	472	21.12 Accessing the drain: CSF sampling	477
21.5	Neurological assessment	473	21.13 Accessing the drain: giving intrathecal drugs	478
21.6	Drain management: positioning of drain	473	21.14 Exit site care	478
21.7	Drain management: drainage	474	21.15 Removal of the drain	479
21.8	Drain management: connecting or changing the system	475		

Principles tables

21.1	Introduction to neurological observations	457	21.5 On admission: documentation	465
21.2	Inform the CYP and family	458	21.6 Management and goals	466
21.3	Signs of raised intracranial pressure	458	21.7 Status epilepticus	467
21.4	Education and training	458		

The Great Ormond Street Hospital Manual of Children and Young People's Nursing Practices, Second Edition. Edited by Elizabeth Anne Bruce, Janet Williss, and Faith Gibson.
© 2023 John Wiley & Sons Ltd. Published 2023 by John Wiley & Sons Ltd.

Introduction

This chapter is divided into three sections; neurological observations, including the Glasgow Coma Score (GCS), seizures and seizure management, and external ventricular drainage (EVD). Specific investigations utilised within neurology and neurosurgery include computerised tomography (CT) and magnetic resonance imaging (MRI), which are discussed in Chapter 15: Investigations. Neurovascular observations are covered in Chapter 23: Orthopaedic Care.

Section 1: Neurological observations

Introduction

Formal neurological observations should be undertaken as part of an overall physical assessment of the child or young person (CYP) in conjunction with systemic observations. The CYP's surroundings, activities, and the presence/absence of parents/carers must also form part of the assessment. The young child poses challenges when assessing level of consciousness due to factors including cognition, limited verbalisation, regression secondary to the illness itself, the effects of hospitalisation, separation from family and home environment, and fear (May and Carter 1995). The parent's unique knowledge and understanding of their child should be utilised whenever possible and where relevant, in helping to assess the CYP's behaviour and response. Appropriate documentation should include the use of a paediatric coma scoring system (Reilly et al. 1988) and an early warning system (Chapman et al. 2016). Early warning systems have now been adopted nationally and attempts continue to be made to standardise the tools used across the NHS (Royal College of Paediatrics and Child Health 2018).

Consciousness is described as a state of awareness, which combines two separate aspects; arousal or wakefulness, and cognitive functioning (Smith and Martin 2009). This 'higher brain function' can be assessed by the subjective observation of arousability and behaviour in response to stimuli (Ellis and Cavanagh 1992). Assessment of consciousness is closely linked to the assessment of pupil reaction; the reticular activating system (RAS) is situated just above the brainstem and is responsible for arousal; the anatomical proximity of the brainstem to the nuclei of cranial nerves III, IV, and VI is also significant as together these nerves control pupillary responses and eye movement (Disabato and Burkett 2007). The nurse should attempt to first rouse the CYP and then undertake assessment of pupil reaction to light. Once the CYP is roused, awareness is controlled in the cerebral cortex. The primary goal for the nurse is to identify changes that may indicate deterioration so that early intervention can be implemented.

A neurological assessment chart, known as the Glasgow Coma Scale (GCS), was first introduced by Jennet and Teasdale in 1974 (Teasdale 2014) and has been adapted worldwide as a standardised assessment for patients with central nervous system dysfunction. The scale is divided into three categories comprising eye opening, best verbal response, and best motor response. Each category is further divided, and the resulting graph and numerical score is used in conjunction with vital signs to identify the patient's clinical status. The lower the numerical score, the lower the level of consciousness.

Many of the responses required when utilising the GCS involve an adult neurodevelopment response, specifically the development of language and the ability to localise pain; the Adelaide scale (Reilly et al. 1988) was devised for use in children and further adaptations of the scale have since been produced by the Paediatric Neuroscience Benchmarking group to provide standardisation of the chart across the UK. Neurological assessment of the CYP in the Intensive Care Unit is outlined by Marcoux (2005), who describes the neurological assessment, pathophysiology, and management of increased intracranial pressure in the critically ill CYP who has sustained an acute neurological injury.

Procedure guideline 21.1 Neurological observations

Statement	Rationale
1 Observe the CYP from a distance. a) Assess for: • Eye opening • Appropriateness of vocalisation • Motor activity	a) To identify level of consciousness.
b) Determine if the family considers these actions normal for their child.	b) The family knows what normal behaviour is for their child.
c) If the CYP does not open his/her eyes or the family considers that actions are abnormal, then continue assessment as described in A–C below.	c) Spontaneous eye opening can only be achieved without any stimulation from the nursing staff (Armon et al. 2003).
d) The CYP must be fully woken to assess GCS.	d) To ensure an accurate assessment is made.
A) Eye opening	
Score 4: Spontaneous eye opening	Demonstrates that arousal mechanisms are intact (RAS) (Appleton and Gibbs 1998; Bateman 2001).
Score 3: Eye opening to speech Speak to the CYP using appropriate language and familiar names. Involve the family to encourage them to respond to verbal stimuli.	Demonstrates that the cerebral cortex is processing information (Armon et al. 2003). A CYP may not open their eyes for unfamiliar adults and this could be behavioural rather than neurological (Barrett-Goode 2000).
Score 2: Eye opening to painful stimuli If the CYP is not opening their eyes to speech, a central painful stimulus will need to be applied. (See Figure 21.3a–d: Response to painful stimuli.)	The necessity of painful stimuli to elicit eye opening suggests a decrease in level of consciousness.

Procedure guideline 21.1 Neurological observations *(continued)*

Score 1: No eye opening to either speech or painful stimuli
It is essential to note if a CYP is unable to open their eyes due to orbital swelling or a ptosis, rather than suggestion of a reduced level of consciousness, in which case a '**C**' should be inserted in the appropriate space on the assessment tool.

Indicates that there is a marked depression of the arousal system (Barrett-Goode 2000).
To prevent an unnecessary painful stimulus being applied.

B) Verbal response

This part of the assessment is scored from 1 to 5 and contains a description for the infant/preverbal child and the verbal CYP. Involve the family to use appropriate familiar words to encourage the CYP to verbalise.

Verbal response assesses consciousness and cognition (Appleton and Gibbs 1998).

An appropriate fear of strangers may lead some CYPs to not respond to unfamiliar adults.

Score 5
Infant/preverbal child: Smiling or contented infant who may coo or babble.
Verbal CYP: Orientated.

Orientation in a young child has been defined as an awareness of being in hospital or an ability to give his/her name (Birdsall and Greif 1990).

Score 4
Infant/preverbal child: Crying.
Verbal CYP: Disorientated.

Consider cognitive status when assessing verbal score.

Score 3
Infant/preverbal child: Inappropriate cry.
The pitch of the cry is important (Barrett-Goode 2000). A high-pitched cry should be recorded within the significant events.
Verbal CYP: Monosyllabic responses.

It is important to involve the family who will be able to identify if the cry is inappropriate for their child.
To ensure accurate recording of the CYP's condition.

Score 2
Infant/preverbal child: Occasional whimper.
Verbal CYP: Incomprehensible sounds.

At this stage, both verbal and painful stimuli may need to be used to obtain a response (Appleton and Gibbs 1998).

Score 1
All ages: No verbal response to both verbal and painful stimuli.
If a CYP is unable to speak as a result of damage to the speech centres of the brain (dysphasia), then a '**D**' should be placed in the appropriate space on the assessment tool (Appleton and Gibbs 1998).
If a CYP has a tracheostomy or an endotracheal tube in situ, a '**T**' should be marked in the appropriate space on the assessment tool (Aucken and Crawford 1999).

C) Best motor response

a) This part of the assessment is scored from 1 to 6. Upper limbs are used to assess motor response. The motor response of the best arm is recorded.
b) Limbs with an obvious injury such as a fracture are not assessed (Armon et al. 2003).

a) Lower limbs can be inconsistent and there may be a spinal reflex (Appleton and Gibbs 1998).
b) If a limb is broken it may not respond to a painful stimulus.

Score 6
a) An infant moves the arms spontaneously.
b) A CYP is able to obey commands.
c) Questions to be avoided when assessing a CYP's ability to obey commands are:
'Squeeze my fingers.'
'Open your eyes' (Armon et al. 2003).
Questions one might ask are age/cognition dependent but could include: 'Can you see Mummy?' or 'Where is Mummy?'
d) Involve the family to encourage the CYP to obey commands.

a, b) Demonstrates that the brain is able to receive and interpret sensory information and then coordinate a response (Armon et al. 2003).
c) The results could be either a reflex grasp or a coincidental action (Armon et al. 2003).
d) CYPs may refuse to obey commands for a stranger but may obey commands given by a family member or voice they recognise (Barrett-Goode, 2000).

Score 5
a) When an infant does not move limbs spontaneously or a CYP does not obey commands a central painful stimulus will need to be applied.
b) Level of neurological maturity determines the level of best response in a CYP (Bouffet et al. 1996). A CYP's responses to and understanding of pain is dependent on their age and cognition (Gaffney et al 2003).

a) To evoke and observe a localised response (Armon et al. 2003). If a CYP is localising spontaneously applying a painful stimulus will not be necessary.
b) Due to neurological immaturity, it is thought that an infant below six months is unable to localise to pain (Bouffet et al. 1996). However, there is now substantial evidence that neonates do exhibit certain pain behaviours such as crying and withdrawing of limbs (Fitzgerald 2005).

(continued)

Procedure guideline 21.1 Neurological observations *(continued)*

c) The best methods of central painful stimulus to evoke a localised response are: • Trapezius squeeze • Supraorbital pressure	c) To encourage the CYP to localise to pain (see Figure 21.3(a–d)).
d) The arm will move toward the source of the pain in an attempt to remove it. To qualify as localising, the CYP must bring their hand up beyond the level of the chin (Appleton and Gibbs 1998).	d) Localising to pain indicates that the brain is able to receive sensory information by feeling pain and can coordinate a motor response to attempt to remove the source of the pain (Appleton and Gibbs 1998).
e) Do not use a sternal rub.	e) This will not show a true localising response, as the CYP will not have to bring their arm up to chin height (Appleton and Gibbs 1998).
f) Use of an oxygen mask or nasogastric tube should be avoided as these may cause irritation and the CYP may localise spontaneously to these sources.	f) To prevent an unnecessary painful stimulus being applied.

Score 4

a) Normal flexion. b) CYP – not localising to a central painful stimulus but can bend their arm toward the source of the pain. c) The arm bends at the elbow and the wrist extends rapidly in response to pain but does not attempt to remove the source of the painful stimulus (Appleton and Gibbs 1998).	a–c) Indicates the brain is receiving sensory sensation and making an appropriate response.
d) Scores below 4 are considered abnormal responses.	d) Scores below 4 indicate varying degrees of cerebral damage.

Score 3

Abnormal flexion: Decorticate posturing describes abnormal flexion of the upper limbs and extension of the lower limbs; the arms are flexed over the chest (Talvik et al. 2012).	This is indicative of brainstem compression and potential life-threatening deterioration (Brown and Tallur 2005).

Score 2

Extension to central painful stimulus: Decerebrate posturing describes abnormal extension of all four limbs (Talvik et al. 2012).	Indication of continued compression of the mid brain, which may result in a loss of consciousness due to reduction in arousal of reticular activating system (Brown and Tallur 2005).

Score 1

a) No response to central painful stimulus.	a) Indication of extreme depression of brain stem function resulting in no possible sensory input and/or motor output (Armon et al. 2003).
b) If a CYP is paralysed, e.g. as a result of paralysing agents, then a '**P**' should be inserted in the appropriate space on the assessment tool.	b) To prevent any unnecessary painful central stimulus being applied.
c) When assessing best motor response, it is important to observe for any asymmetry or inability to move a particular limb.	c) To ensure accurate assessment and recording of the CYP's condition. An inability to move a particular limb may indicate a hemiplegia.

Overall score and recording:

a) Add up the total from the three categories to give the Glasgow Coma Score. Record this total on the assessment chart.	a) To ensure accurate assessment and recording of the CYP's condition.
b) Report any alteration to senior nursing staff/medical staff.	b) To enable prompt and appropriate action to be taken as required.
c) Assess the CYP's pain score (see pain assessment guideline) and record total on assessment chart.	c) To ensure accurate assessment and recording of the CYP's condition.
Although not part of the GCS, vital signs, papillary reaction and limb movement are an important part of the neurological assessment and should be recorded in addition to the CYP's conscious level.	
d) Record temperature, pulse rate, respiration rate, and blood pressure as condition dictates, together with neurological observations.	d) An irregular respiratory rate with associated bradycardia and hypertension (Cushing's triad) is a late sign of raised intracranial pressure in CYPs and requires urgent intervention (Paul et al. 2013). Control centres for blood pressure, heart rate, and respiration rate are located in the brain stem (Aucken and Crawford 1999).

D) Pupil reaction

a) The size of both pupils should be observed and noted before applying a light stimulus.	a) This is the pupil size that is recorded on the neurological assessment chart. Unequal pupil size usually indicates a compression of the oculomotor nerve and should be reported to the senior nurse or doctor immediately (Smith and Martin 2009).

Procedure guideline 21.1 Neurological observations *(continued)*

b) Document any medication that may affect pupil size on the significant events chart.	b) Drugs that cause constriction or dilation of pupils must be noted and accurately recorded (Smith and Martin 2009).
c) A pen torch with a bright narrow beam should be used to test both pupils individually. Both pupils should constrict when light is shone in either eye.	c) Both pupils should react briskly and constrict equally. If both pupils are not constricting, this may indicate damage to the optic nerve. Fixed, dilated pupils indicate a neurosurgical emergency and should be reported immediately.
d) Encourage the family to participate in the recording.	d) Young children may be more cooperative with family members.
e) Record pupil reaction in the appropriate space on the chart. Brisk reaction = **+** No reaction = **−** Sluggish reaction = **SL**	e) An absent or sluggish reaction may indicate damage to the occulomotor nerve as a result of raised intracranial pressure.
f) Report any change to senior nursing staff.	f) To enable prompt and appropriate action to be taken as required.
g) Document any known visual problems, e.g. blindness, on the significant events chart.	g) To ensure accurate assessment and recording of the CYP's condition.

E) Limb movement

1 The strength of both limbs is measured: a) In young babies: Observation of movement will provide an indication of muscle tone and strength. b) In younger children: Limb strength can be assessed through play, e.g., getting them to kick a ball. c) In older CYPs: Where possible, ask them to respond to commands, e.g. ask the CYP to push and pull against the assessor.	1 To assess for symmetry/asymmetry of limb function.
2 Document limb strength on the assessment chart. If there is a difference between the two sides, document the right (R) and left (L) sides separately.	2 A developing hemiparesis can be an indication of raised intracranial pressure as a result of damage to the motor cortex (Aucken and Crawford 1999).
3 Report any alteration to senior nursing staff.	3 To enable any prompt and appropriate action to be taken as required.
4 If a CYP is paralysed, for example, as a result of paralysing agents, then a **P** should be inserted in the appropriate space on the assessment tool. If they have a fracture, then a hash (**#**) sign should be entered in the appropriate space.	4 To ensure accurate assessment and recording of the CYP's condition.

Principles table 21.1 Introduction to neurological observations

Statement	Rationale
1 Neurological observations should be performed as a baseline observation, on those with or at risk of developing an impaired level of consciousness.	1 Early recognition of changes in conscious level is paramount in the prevention of secondary injury associated with raised intracranial pressure (Norman 2000).
2 Frequency of neurological observations is dictated by the CYP's condition and can be decided by either medical or nursing staff as appropriate. Each CYP should have an individualised monitoring plan documented and signed by a healthcare professional.	2 To enable appropriate, individualised assessment to be performed and to identify any acute deterioration.
3 All staff performing neurological observations should be trained in both the theoretical and practical aspects of these observations.	3–4) To ensure accurate assessment and recording of the CYP's condition.
4 An appropriate assessment tool is required that considers the physical and neurodevelopment age of the CYP. The neurological coma score assessment tool in use at GOSH incorporates an adaptation of the GCS (Jennet and Teasdale (1974) and the Adelaide Paediatric Coma Scale (Simpson and Reilly 1982), as well as the GOSH pain assessment chart (Figures 21.1 and 21.2).	

(continued)

The Great Ormond Street Hospital Manual of Children and Young People's Nursing Practices

Principles table 21.1 Introduction to neurological observations *(continued)*

Statement	Rationale
5 The GCS demonstrates level of consciousness by assessing a CYP's ability to perform three activities: a) Eye opening b) Verbal response c) Motor response Each activity is given a score and the three scores are added together to give a score between 3 and 15. A score of 15 indicates a fully alert, orientated CYP, whilst a score of 3 indicates a deep coma.	
6 The GCS is documented in the form of a graph and demonstrated by a series of joined-up dots.	6 To enable quick and easy evaluation of trends in a CYP's condition (Aucken and Crawford 1999).
7 When undertaking neurological assessment, it is essential that a baseline be established in relation to the individual CYP's cognitive development. For example, a nonverbal CYP cannot achieve a score of 15, only a deviation from the score that is normal for them would give rise for concern.	7 To ensure accurate assessment and recording of the CYP's condition.
8 Any alteration in the CYP's GCS should be reported to senior nursing/medical staff.	8 To enable prompt and appropriate action to be taken as required.
9 A CYP who is asleep should always be woken for neurological assessment.	9 To ensure accurate assessment and recording of their condition at prescribed times.

Principles table 21.2 Inform the CYP and Family

Statement	Rationale
1 Inform the CYP and family: a) That neurological observations are necessary. b) Why they are necessary. c) What they entail, and how often they are performed.	1 To prepare them for regular assessments, to inform and educate the family, and to encourage concordance.
2 Encourage the family to participate in the assessment.	2 Fear of strangers may affect the CYP's response and increase their stress.

Principles table 21.3 Signs of raised intracranial pressure

Statement	Rationale
1 Observe for the following: i) High pitched cry ii) Irritability iii) Lethargy iv) Vomiting v) Headaches. In infants and young children, the following may also be present: i) Tense or bulging anterior fontanel ii) Sunset eyes.	1 To identify signs of raised intracranial pressure.
2 Document these signs on the significant events chart and inform senior nursing staff.	2 To ensure accurate assessment and recording of the CYP's condition and enable prompt and appropriate action to be taken as required.

Principles table 21.4 Education and training

Statement	Rationale
1 Staff should receive a theoretical and practical training session from a children's nurse with neuroscience experience. Theoretical sessions should include the Trust training video: 'Paediatric Coma Charts – A Guide to Assessment' (Mooney and Comerford 2003).	1 To ensure correct assessment is performed reliably.
2 Staff should receive supervised practice and assessment.	2 To ensure correct assessment is performed reliably.

Name	
Hosp. No	
DOB	(Affix patient label)
Ward	

Coma Scale

Great Ormond Street **NHS**
Hospital for Children
NHS Foundation Trust

Consultant		Referring Hospital		Weight	Kg

The coma scale is scored on a total of 15 points. A score of less than 12 should give rise for concern. This is a universally accepted tool for measuring coma. A decrease in coma scale will be associated with a decreased level of consciousness. This needs to be considered along with the child's vital signs. Further information about the coma scale can be found in the related clinical procedure guideline.

A. Eyes Open
If the eyes are closed by swelling, please write 'C' in the relevant column, thus indicating the reason for a lower score.

B. Best Verbal Response
In the left hand margin are two separate scales: on the far left is the scale for babies and infants and on the right is the scale for older children.
The following section gives an explanation of the best verbal response of infants.

  a. Smiles
  This can be used to describe an alert, contented infant as not all will smile at a stranger. The interaction between parents/carers and the infant should therefore be taken into account.

  b. Appropriate Cries
  The infant may be unable to settle.

  c. Inappropriate Cries
  The infant may have periods of being drowsy, but at times is heard to cry out. This is not always associated with being disturbed. The cry may be high pitched.

  d. Occasional Whimper
  Less frequent than above and may be associated with deep painful stimuli, required to gain a motor response.

  e. None
  No verbal response.

C. Best Motor response to Stimuli
The age and cognitive abilities of the child must be taken into account.

D. Pupils
When recording pupil size it is important to remember the effects of drugs, e.g. morphine will cause pinpoint pupils and atropine drops will dilate pupils for up to 6 hours.

E. Limb Movements

  a. If a child has a permanent hemiparesis please indicate this in the relevant column, e.g. weakness, even though it is normal for the child.
  b. A child with a severe developmental delay may score lower on the coma scale, as his motor response may be poor.

Figure 21.1 Example of a GOSH coma chart including pain assessment and a record of significant events.

The Great Ormond Street Hospital Manual of Children and Young People's Nursing Practices

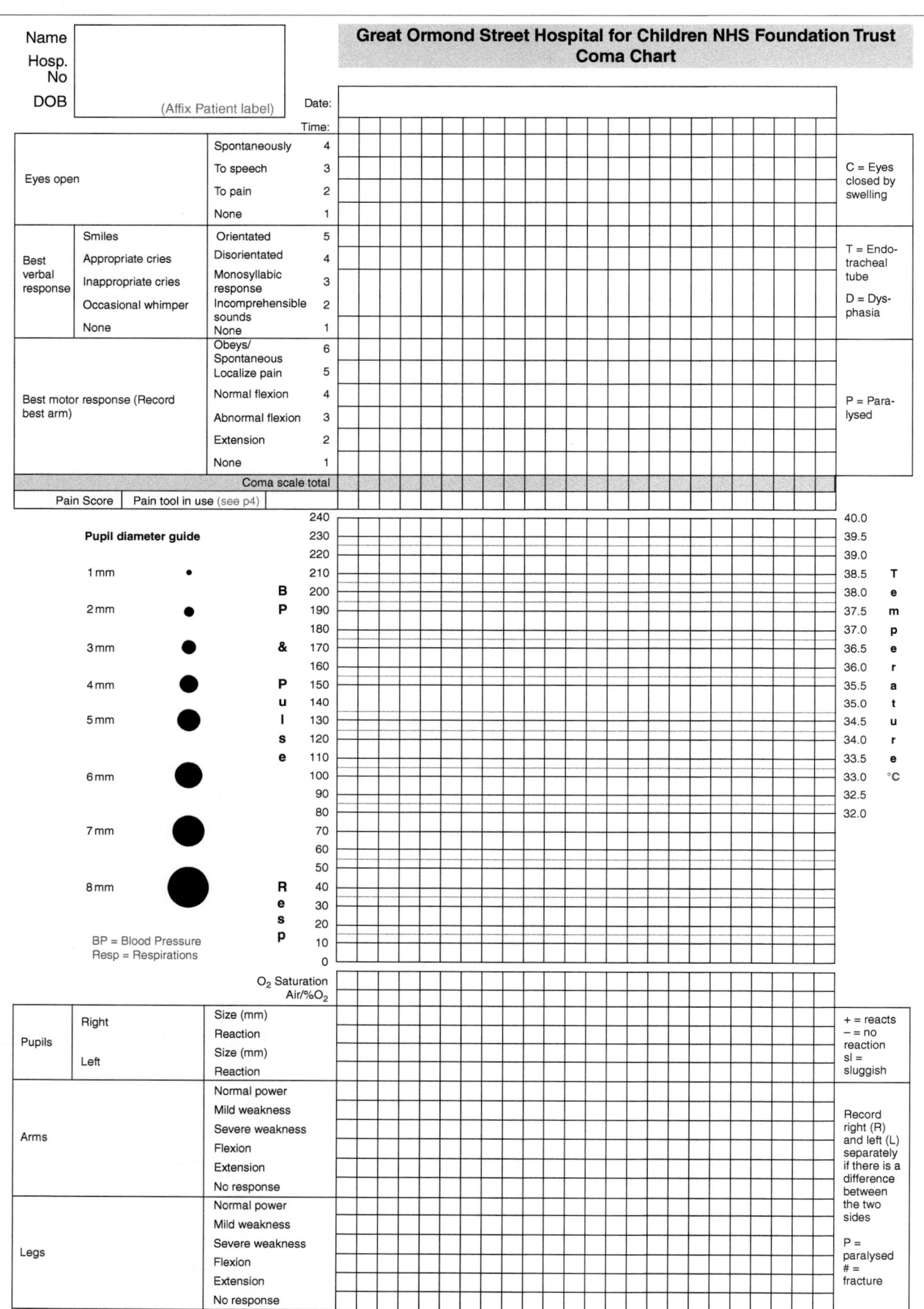

Figure 21.1 (continued)

Record of Significant Events

Developmental Age:

Coma Scale Prior to Illness:

Date	Time	Description of Significant Event (E.g. post seizure, pain, headache, vomiting etc.)	Signature

Figure 21.1 *(continued)*

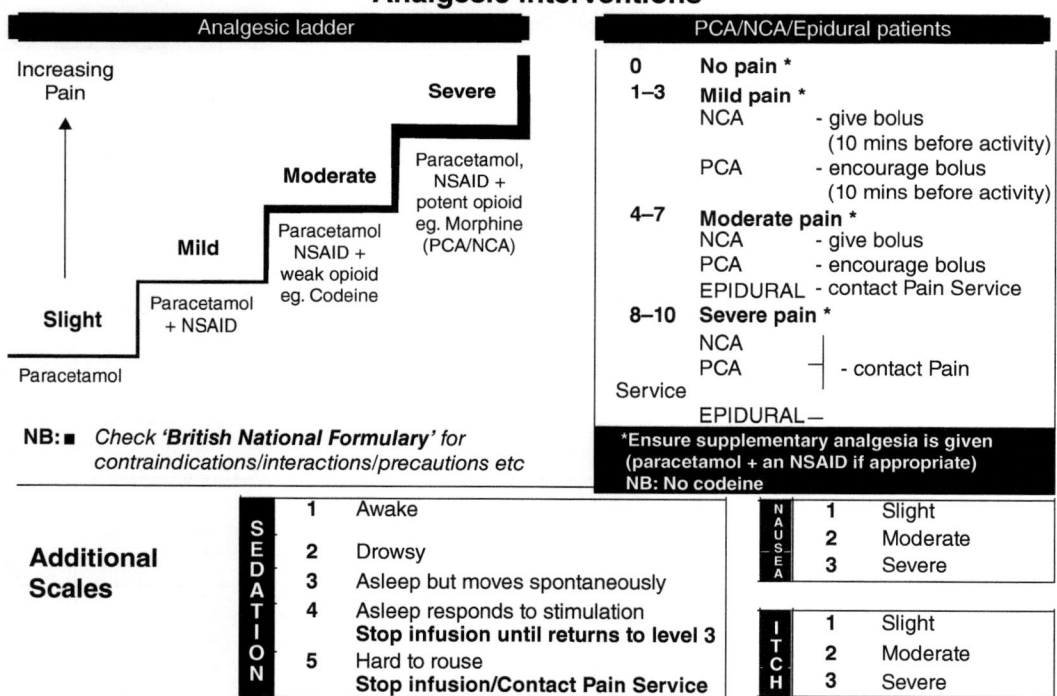

Figure 21.2 Pain assessment.

Types of painful stimuli

The type of painful stimulus used is a controversial issue, although it is generally agreed that a central painful stimulus is required to assess eye opening and verbal and motor response in CYPs who have a decreased level of consciousness (Appleton and Gibbs 1998). A central stimulus can be applied in one of three ways:

Trapezium Squeeze

Using a thumb and two fingers, hold and twist the trapezius muscle of the shoulder (Appleton and Gibbs 1998).

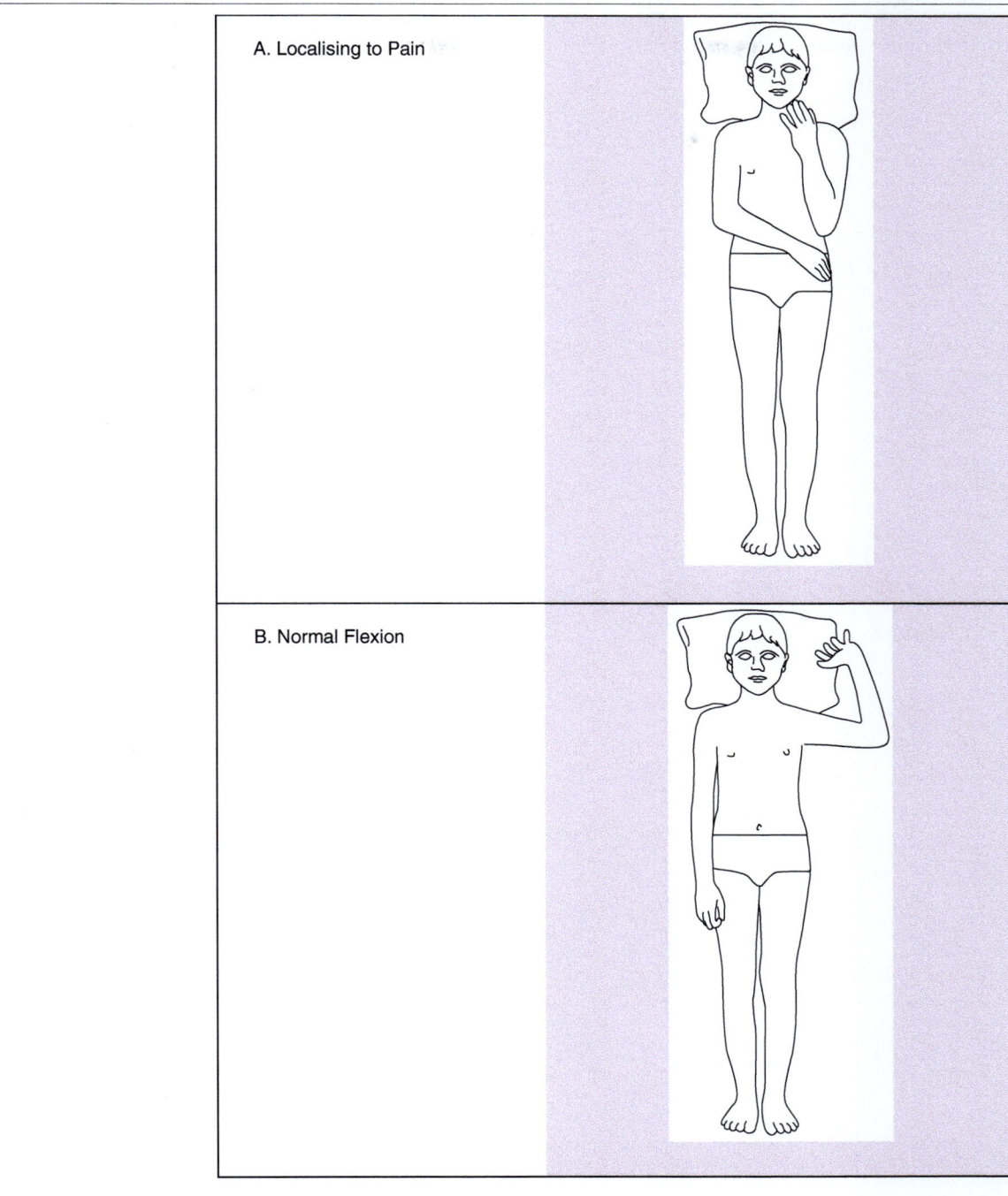

Figure 21.3 (a–d) Response to painful stimuli.

Supraorbital Pressure
Using a finger or thumbnail, apply pressure in the supraorbital groove. Applying supraorbital pressure can sometimes make a CYP grimace and close their eye rather than open it. If this is the case, another form of central stimulus may be required. Supraorbital pressure is also not recommended in CYPs who have facial fractures (Appleton and Gibbs 1998).

Sternal Rub
Using the knuckles of a clenched fist, vertically rub the centre of the sternum (not recommended) (Appleton and Gibbs 1998).

When applying a central painful stimulus, it is important to use caution as pressure on the supraorbital groove or sternum may cause unnecessary injury. Peripheral stimulus can also be used to elicit a response. The most common peripheral stimulus is to apply pressure to the nail beds and observe for a motor response. However, peripheral stimulus may only elicit a spinal reflex, which may not be an accurate assessment of the CYP's condition.

Section 2: Seizures

Introduction

These clinical guidelines incorporate the nursing care of CYPs with known reoccurring seizures (epilepsy) and those presenting with seizures for the first time. Seizures vary in classification. There are various management approaches for different types of seizures; e.g. in epilepsy, myoclonic seizures are dealt with differently from tonic–clonic seizures (see section on Classification

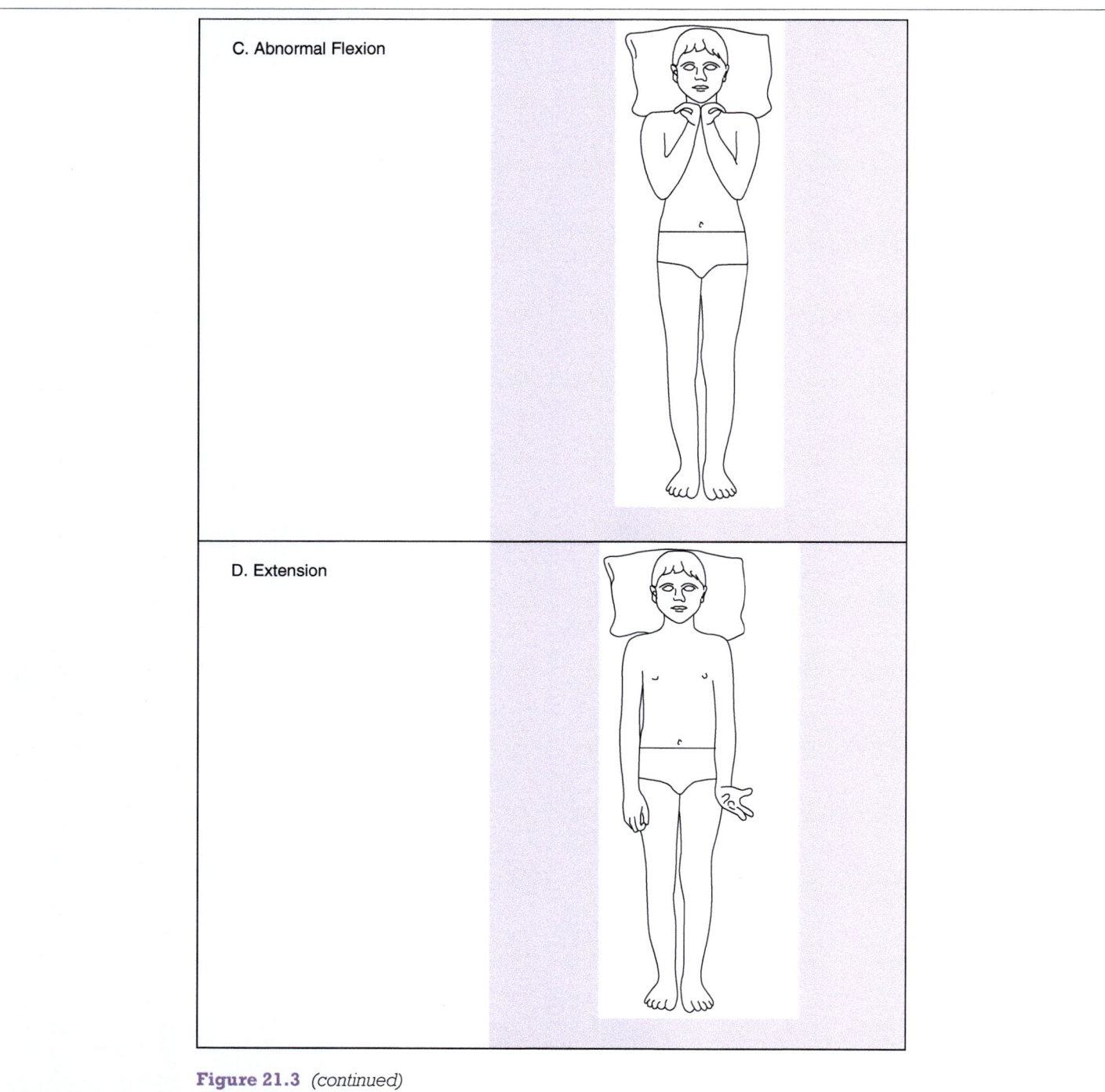

Figure 21.3 *(continued)*

of Seizures). Seizures occur due to abnormal excessive or synchronous neuronal activity within the brain. This will present as signs and symptoms of altered consciousness, which may be perceived by the CYP or witnessed by others, and may involve body motor movements, sensory feelings, autonomic changes, loss of memory, or behavioural changes (Panayiotopoulos 2011). When a CYP has a seizure, it is important to distinguish whether the episode was an epileptic or nonepileptic seizure. There can be several reasons for a seizure to occur (see Table 21.1). Some seizures result from an acute medical or neurological illness and cease once the illness is treated, e.g. febrile convulsions; electrolyte imbalances such as hypocalcaemia, hypernatraemia; hypoglycaemia – (typically seen in neonates); infection; and drugs (Matta et al 2011). Other seizures may already have been diagnosed as epilepsy.

Physiology of seizures

The brain has both inhibitory gamma-aminobutyric acid (GABA) and excitatory, glutamate neurotransmitters. When balanced, both may prevent the prolonged excitatory neuronal activity that is seen in seizures. Failure of this mechanism will result in increased excitatory activity of the neurons and decreased inhibitory neurotransmitter effect and thus cause the potential for a seizure to occur (Matta et al 2011).

Systemic physiological changes occur early in a seizure to prevent the effects of damage to the brain. These changes include:
- Increased cerebral blood flow with increase in oxygen and glucose delivery to the brain and increased removal of toxic metabolites, with the aim of protecting neurons against damage.
- Increased heart rate and/or blood pressure.
- Increased blood plasma glucose levels (Woodford and Mestecky 2011).

Chapter 21 Neurological care

Table 21.1 Types/causes of seizures

Seizure disorders – epilepsy	A common neurological disorder characterised by recurring seizures (NICE 2022).
Infection	Intracranial infections can lead to cerebral oedema, which can be the focus for seizures. Systemic (sepsis), CNS, encephalitis, meningitis, febrile convulsion. Focal infection – abscess.
Head injury	Seizure may be indication of raised intracranial pressure, a depressed fracture of the skull, or when anoxia has occurred.
Structural lesions – space occupying lesion or tumour	Focal seizures may present from structural abnormalities such as cortical dysplasia to tumour; e.g. a tumour may act as a focus for seizures.
Cerebral infarction, haematoma, intraventricular haemorrhage (IVH). Hypoxia – hypoxic ischaemic encephalopathy (HIE)	Any incident that interferes with normal blood flow can be a focus for seizures.
Acidosis, metabolic disturbance, electrolyte imbalances: hypocalcaemia, hypoglycaemia, hyponatraemia, hypernatraemia, dehydration, toxic ingestion	Depolarisation is associated with ionic imbalances that alter the chemical environment of the neurons with an intracellular accumulation of sodium, as well as a depletion of intracellular potassium. Depolarisation is followed by hyperpolarisation; the cell begins to fire repeatedly, producing sustained membrane depolarization and seizure activity (Hickey and Strayer 2020).
Genetic	Certain types of epilepsy are known to have a genetic cause and may be inherited, or occur as a spontaneous genetic pathogenic variant, for example SCN1A; Dravet syndrome.

At the same time, constant muscle contraction and relaxation increases tissue oxygen requirements in the rest of the body, leading to an increase in cellular respiration and glycolysis. This can also occur as a result of the metabolic changes from hypoxia leading to acidosis. As seizure continues, hyperthermia may be seen as core body temperature increases. After about 30 minutes these physiological mechanisms fail and potentially contribute to any neurological damage that may occur. Eventually this will lead to hypoxia, pulmonary oedema, hypertension, cardiac failure, electrolyte imbalance, and acute hepatic or renal failure (Walker and Shorvon 2013). Respiratory depression may also occur as a secondary effect from administration of antiepileptic medication to terminate seizures. Transfer of the CYP to intensive care for prompt ventilation and anaesthesia to manage and reduce complications is therefore needed.

A prolonged seizure must be treated; status epilepticus can be defined as a seizure of duration of 30 minutes or recurrent seizures within a 30 minute duration in which the person does not regain consciousness. Most seizures are self-limiting, although as status epilepticus progresses this becomes more sustained and difficult to treat. The International League Against Epilepsy (ILAE) acknowledges that treatment of status epilepticus should commence from five minutes of seizure activity, or if there is increased deterioration in the person's normal seizure pattern (Walker and Shorvon 2013).

Care of the CYP with seizures

Principles table 21.5 On admission: documentation

Statement	Rationale
1 Accurately observe any/all seizures and describe their features.	1 This is an important nursing clinical skill. The more detailed these descriptions, the more valuable they are for assessment and to therefore treat appropriately.
2 For a CYP presenting for the first time with seizures the following should be documented: a) A description of the manifestation of the seizures should be obtained from the eyewitnesses, i.e. nurse, doctor, parent, carer, etc. b) Any impairment or loss of consciousness. c) Motor effects, muscular contractions. d) Eye movements. e) Which parts of the body are affected; whether laterality is present. f) Typical duration of seizures and/or occurrence of 'clusters' of seizures. g) The CYP's past medical history and any relevant clinical findings should be evaluated.	a) This will assist medical staff to classify whether the seizure is focal or generalised. b) To aid characterisation of the seizure. c)–e) To help identify which side of the brain is affected. f) Individual seizures may be treated after a specific duration of time or amount/ number. g) To ascertain and clarify if there is any underlying cause for the seizures.
3 Information should be clearly documented in the CYP's healthcare records to describe seizure patterns.	3 To ensure good communication between all members of the multidisciplinary team.

(continued)

Principles table 21.5 On Admission: documentation *(continued)*

Statement	Rationale
Predisposing factors	
Any significant results of tests and investigations should be considered.	
4 For a CYP with a previous history of seizures or epilepsy document a full assessment of the types of seizures, which includes: a) The number of different types of seizure presentations with description of each type. b) Any altered behaviour during the event. c) Typical duration of seizures and/or occurrence of 'clusters' of seizures. d) Any aura experienced. e) Any impairment or loss of consciousness. f) Which parts of the body are affected; are changes in motor movement affecting only one side of the body? This may include muscular contractions, facial expression or change in eye movements. g) Sensory involvement, visual symptoms, pins and needles epigastric rising. h) Whether cyanosis is present. i) Triggers or precipitating factors to seizures e.g. lack of sleep and fatigue, activity, pre-meals, noise, bright flashing lights, loud noises, etc (Couffignal et al. 2001). j) Time when seizure normally occurs, e.g.-early morning, nocturnally, during sleep. When parents would administer as required medication i.e. after what time lapse. k) Post-ictal state.	4 For classification of seizure and to enable appropriate treatment of seizures when they occur. c) Seizures may be treated after a specific duration or number. f) Abnormal motor movements on one side of the body may indicate where in the brain abnormal electrical activity is occurring. g) This may indicate which part of the brain the abnormal electrical activity commences from. h) To determine whether oxygen is required. i) To prevent unnecessary factors that may trigger the seizures. j) To ensure continuity of care. k) To recognise end of seizure.
4 Ensure that a recent weight is documented on the CYP's prescription chart.	4 To ensure correct doses of medications are prescribed and to reduce the risk of medication errors.

Principles table 21.6 Management and goals

Statement	Rationale
1 Treatment of a CYP with seizures requires: a) Maintenance of vital functions. b) Termination of seizures. c) Elimination of any precipitating factors. d) Reversing correctable causes.	a) Due to the physiological changes that occur in the body as a result of seizure activity. b, c) It may not always be possible to abolish seizures completely but controlling seizures may be a more realistic goal for some. d) Management and treatment of correctable reversible underlying causes may terminate seizure activity.
2 The initial treatment is directed toward: a) Airway: Maintaining an airway. b) Breathing: Supporting breathing and administration of oxygen. c) Circulation: Support and maintenance of vital functions. d) Drugs: Administration of drugs (see below) e) Environment: Ensure safety of the CYP and others.	2 For more information, see Chapter 9: Early Recognition and Management of the Seriously Ill Child and Chapter 30: Resuscitation.

Procedure guideline 21.2 Nursing management of the CYP during seizures

Statement	Rationale
1 Nurse the CYP near: • Working oxygen • Working suction • Appropriate size bag-valve-mask, e.g. Ambu-bag • Appropriate size airway	1 They may need assistance to maintain a clear airway and breathing, due to the potential for respiratory depression caused by either seizure activity or administration of anticonvulsant medication.

Chapter 21 Neurological care

Procedure guideline 21.2 Nursing management of the CYP during seizures *(continued)*

Statement	Rationale
2 Administer oxygen if required. Carry out a risk assessment (see local policies and Chapter 19: Moving and Handling).	2 To determine whether portable oxygen and suction will need to be taken to the CYP if it is not safe to move them.
3 Nurse the CYP on his/her side.	3 To assist the maintenance of a clear airway in cases of vomiting, choking, and/or aspiration.
4 Ensure that the environment is safe, i.e. cot sides are in place, that they cannot bang limbs or head on objects. Positioning a blanket or soft object or padding may help prevent injury occurring.	4 To prevent the CYP from causing injury to him/herself.
5 Call for assistance, but never leave any CYP having a seizure.	5 To minimise the risk of airway obstruction, vomiting, or cyanosis.
6 Ensure the seizure is timed.	6 Treatment of the seizure after four to five minutes is important to prevent changes in the body's physiological mechanisms and minimise the risk of status epilepticus - see section on Physiology of Seizures.
7 Administer rectal/buccal/intravenous medication if required, according to clinical service guidelines, ensuring the correct dosages are administered.	7 To treat the seizure appropriately and minimise the risk of drug errors.
8 Closely monitor the CYP's physiological observations and vital functions. If necessary: • Use a saturation monitor to observe oxygen saturations, heart rate, and respiration rate. • Monitor consciousness level using the GCS.	8-9 To ensure early detection and intervention if condition deteriorates.
9 If required, administer further doses of rectal/buccal/intravenous medication according to hospital policy, continuing to carefully monitor CYP's vital signs (as stipulated above).	9 To treat the seizure while minimising the risk of respiratory depression.
10 Document seizures on the seizure events chart. If the seizure has not terminated or is not abating, the CYP may require further repeat doses of medication.	10 To ensure an accurate account is documented in the CYP's health record.

Principles table 21.7 Status epilepticus

Statement	Rationale
Definition of status epilepticus	
Status epilepticus can be defined as a seizure of a duration of 30 minutes or recurrent seizures within a 30-minute duration in which the person does not regain consciousness. Most seizures are self-limiting, although as status epilepticus progresses this becomes more sustained and difficult to treat.	Seizures that last at least 5–10 minutes are unlikely to stop spontaneously, and will continue for at least 30 minutes unless there is an appropriate intervention (Walker and Shorvoan 2013).
1 **STATUS EPILEPTICUS is a *MEDICAL EMERGENCY*.**	1 Status epilepticus requires immediate intervention to prevent possible brain injury or death, as sustained convulsions can increase cerebral blood flow and metabolic requirements and result in physiological sequelae - see section on physiology of seizures.)
2 The initial treatment for status epilepticus includes: • Monitoring of vital signs • Maintaining an airway • Administration of oxygen	2 To maintain the CYP's safety by preventing/detecting and treating any deterioration in condition promptly.
3 Check glucose before administering anticonvulsants. Administer prescribed buccal midazolam/rectal diazepam/paraldehyde/intravenous medication according to APLS clinical guidelines or local hospital trust guidance, if required, ensuring the correct dosages are administered (Bacon et al. 2022; NICE 2022).	3 To cease seizure activity. Buccal midazolam is now considered a first-line effective medication for use in both the hospital and community setting (NICE 2022). For a parent information leaflet regarding buccal midazolam go to: www.gosh.nhs.uk/conditions-and-treatments/medicines-information/buccal-oromucosal-midazolam/ (GOSH 2017).
4 Ensure secured intravenous access.	
5 Support and maintain vital functions.	

(continued)

Principles table 21.7 Status epilepticus (*continued*)

Statement	Rationale
6 Administer intravenous anticonvulsants if seizure activity continues.	
7 Ensure adequate hydration, e.g. intravenous fluids if required.	
8 The CYP must be closely monitored during administration of intravenous anticonvulsants.	8 To observe for respiratory depression.
9 Monitor level of consciousness, vital signs of respirations, heart rate, blood pressure, and temperature.	9 To determine whether the seizure is abating and ensure early detection of the deteriorating CYP.
10 If first-line drugs are ineffective, progress to second-line drugs.	10 To manage the seizure as quickly as possible.
11 Refer to local and national guidelines (Advanced Life Support Group 2016; Bacon et al. 2022; NICE 2022).	
12 The CYP may need respiratory support of intubation and ventilation on a paediatric intensive care unit.	
13 Outcome is related to aetiology and duration of the status epilepticus.	
14 Provide support to family and ensure that carers are aware of the CYP's seizure management care plan prior to discharge. A community care plan should be completed.	14 To ensure familie's full understanding and ability to manage seizures in the community.

Classification of seizures

There are several systems of classification of seizures. The International League against Epilepsy (ILAE) reviewed and proposed some new concepts and terminology to aid classification of the epilepsies (Scheffer et al. 2017).

The previous classification of the ILAE in 1989 was based on two major features (Panayiotopoulos 2007); first, whether the seizure type was focal or generalised, and second, whether the aetiology is idiopathic (with genetic predisposition), symptomatic (structural), or cryptogenic (probably symptomatic). These divisions shaped the first two major groups of epileptic syndromes.

A third group covered syndromes with seizures of uncertain type (often the case with nocturnal seizures) and a fourth group covered seizures associated with a specific situation (fever, drugs, metabolic imbalance).

The advancement of neuro imaging, molecular cell biology, genetics, and advancements in neurophysiology of electroencephalography (EEG), both on the scalp and intracranially, has aided our knowledge of the brain's working, seizure generation, and propagation, thus replacing the previous classification with a more flexible approach and the terms idiopathic, symptomatic, and cryptogenic are no longer used.

The ILAE have included a useful diagnostic online tool to aid classification of seizures and recommended treatments (www.epilepsydiagnosis.org). Recommended new terminology and concepts include the following.

Focal seizures are thought to commence at one point within a network in only one cerebral hemisphere of the brain. Focal seizures may be described by their semiology, the features of seizures observed, such as motor movements, and sensory involvement (Figure 21.4). Symptoms may identify seizure origin and propagation within the brain (Figure 21.5). They may involve the following signs and symptoms:

- Sensory aura, a subjective sensation; this may include the visual– occipital lobe.
- Auditory – temporal lobe or epigastric aura – parietal operculum and insula.
- Autonomic features of focal seizures may include cardiovascular – palpations, vasomotor – flushing or pallor.
- Thermoregulatory – feelings of hot or cold.

The term complex partial seizures has now been replaced with focal seizures with impaired awareness.

Focal seizures may continue to spread to both hemispheres and become bilateral tonic clonic.

Epilepsia partialis continua (EPC)

EPC is described as 'spontaneous regular or irregular clonic muscle twitching of cerebral cortical origin, sometimes aggravated by action or sensory stimuli confined to one part of the body and which could continue for a period of hours, days, or weeks'.

Generalised onset seizures are thought to commence at one point and rapidly engage bilateral networks within the brain's hemispheres. Seizure onset may not be consistent from one seizure to another and may involve motor or nonmotor components.

Seizure types
Tonic–Clonic

In the *tonic* phase, characterised by stiffening, there is rolling of the eyes upwards and immediate loss of consciousness. The CYP stiffens in a generalised and symmetric tonic contraction of the entire body. The arms usually flex, whereas the legs, head, and neck extend. This tonic phase lasts about 10–20 seconds, during which the CYP is apnoeic and may be cyanotic. In the *clonic* phase, characterised by rhythmic jerking, the tonic rigidity is replaced by intense jerking movements as the body undergoes rhythmic contraction and relaxation. As the seizure ends, the movements become less intense; this clonic phase lasts about 30 seconds. In the postictal stage, the CYP may be confused, poorly coordinated, and may sleep.

Chapter 21 Neurological care

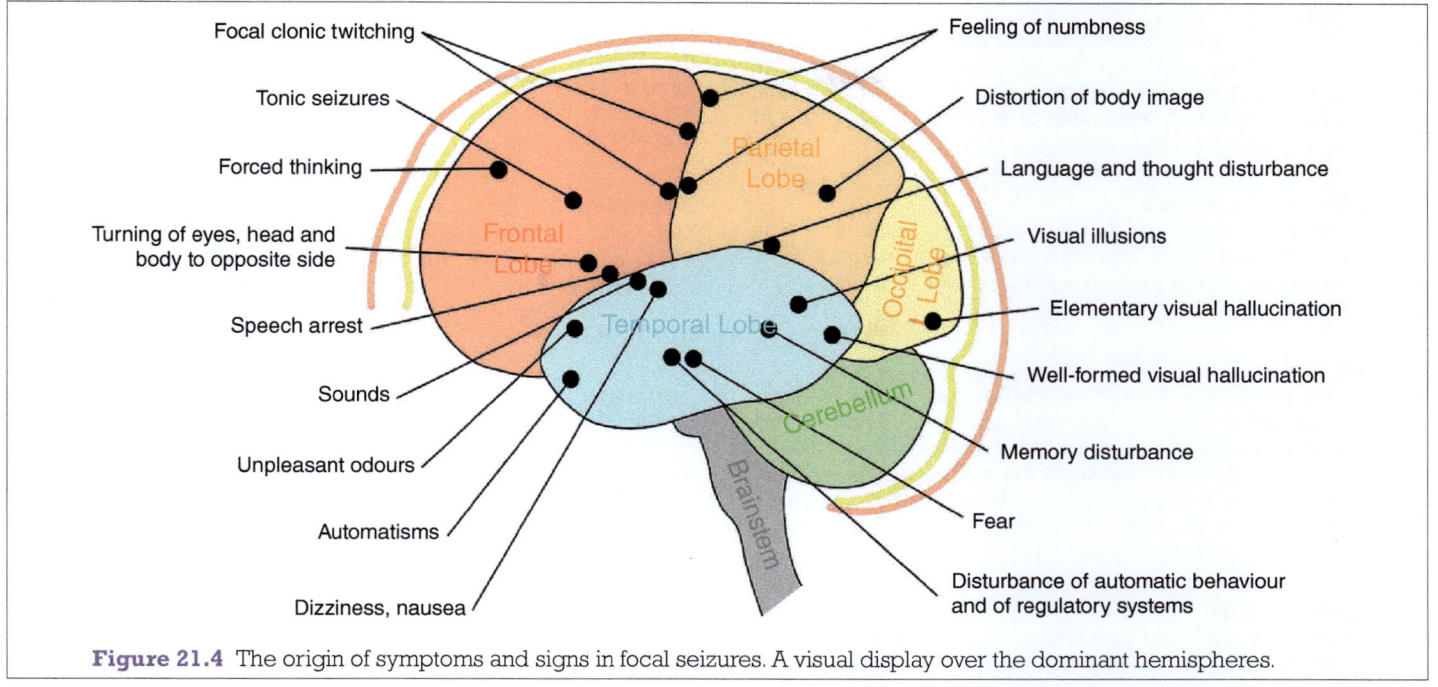

Figure 21.4 The origin of symptoms and signs in focal seizures. A visual display over the dominant hemispheres.

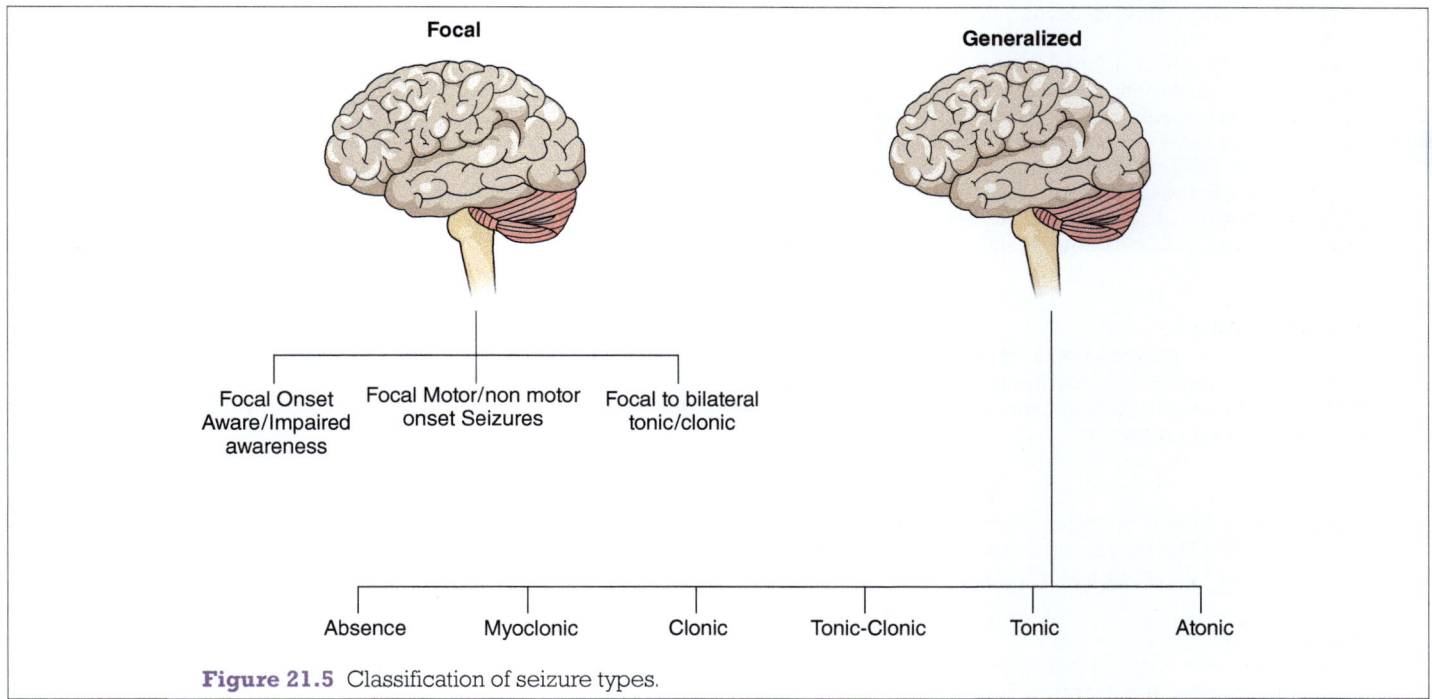

Figure 21.5 Classification of seizure types.

Clonic
Rhythmic jerking muscle activity

Absence
Typical absence: Brief generalised epileptic seizures usually lasting for 5–10 seconds with abrupt onset and abrupt termination. There is an impairment of awareness. The absence consists of sudden cessation of motor activity, followed by a blank stare and loss of awareness. The CYP then returns to the original activity.

Atypical absence: Possible atypical features of these absences include longer duration, incomplete loss of awareness, and atypical EEG changes.

Myoclonic absence: This manifests with impairment of consciousness, which varies from mild to severe and rhythmic myoclonic jerks, mainly of the shoulders, arms, and legs, with a concomitant tonic contraction. The jerks and tonic contraction may be unilateral or symmetrical.

Eyelid myoclonia
Consists of marked jerking of the eyelids, often associated with jerky upward deviation of the eyeballs. This may be associated with or followed by mild impairment of consciousness. The seizures are brief three to six seconds and consistently occur many times per day. Eyelid myoclonia can occur with or without absences.

Tonic
Stiffening of the body.

Myoclonic
Myoclonic means a quick movement of a muscle. These seizures are characterised by sudden, brief jerks of muscle groups and occur either in clusters or several times during the day. Flexor muscles are often involved on both sides of the body, resulting in sudden falls in older CYPs, and infantile spasms in infants.

Negative myoclonus
Seizure with brief loss of muscle tone lasting only a 500th of a millisecond. These may cause loss of posture and subsequent voluntary movement to restore posture and can occur as a single event or in a cluster.

Atonic
These involve a sudden loss of muscle tone and consciousness. Onset is between two and five years of age. During a mild seizure the CYP may experience several sudden brief head drops. During a severe episode they will suddenly fall to the ground, will lose consciousness briefly, and then get up. Frequent falls can result in injury, particularly to the face. Atonic seizures are also known as 'drop attacks' (Panayiotopoulos 2011).

Epileptic spasm
Epileptic spasms cause sudden flexion or extension of proximal and truncal muscles lasting one to two seconds; they normally present in a cluster of events and are usually seen on waking. They may involve bilateral symmetric, asymmetric, or unilateral movements (Scheffer et al. 2017).

Epilepsy Syndromes ILAE (Scheffer et al. 2017) informs diagnosing epilepsy by underlying aetiology (cause), which remains important, but the epilepsies can be organised into epilepsy syndromes. Syndromes have a typical age of onset, specific seizure types, and specific EEG characteristics. Diagnosing syndromes accurately can enable the correct choice of antiepileptic medication (AED). Appropriate choice of AED can reduce risk of seizure aggravation, e.g. the use of carbamazepine can increase generalised seizures.

Epilepsy Aetiology
As noted previously, advancements in our technology have increased understanding of causes of the epilepsies. ILAE (Scheffer et al. 2017) have reviewed potential causes; examples of each are included in the following sections.

Genetic
Aetiology may be the result of known or presumed gene or chromosomal abnormality. This may be inherited or a de nova mutation, e.g. Trisomy 21, Ring 20 Syndrome, or SCN1A.

Structural
Enhancements in neuroimaging have allowed more accurate diagnosis. Structural causes of epilepsy may include acquired or developmental disorders and may originate from trauma, infection, or stroke. Structural origin causes include tuberous sclerosis and malformations of cortical development, focal cortical dysplasia, benign tumours, ganglioglioma, or dysembroplastic neuroepithelial tumour (DNET). CYPs presenting with drug-resistant seizures would benefit from early referral to a specialist service for evaluation of epilepsy surgery (NICE 2022).

Metabolic
Metabolic disorders have a genetic origin, ILAE (Scheffer et al. 2017) early treatment optimises outcome and may inform treatment choice, cerebral folate deficiency, pyridoxine dependence, or glucose transporter disorders (GLUT1), which may respond to use of ketogenic diet.

Immune
Immune mediated causes with evidence of central nervous system inflammation; treatment choice can be targeted immunotherapies, Rasmussen's syndrome.

Infection
This is a common cause of epilepsy particularly in low and middle income countries; infections of the central nervous system can cause both acute symptoms of seizures particularly at initial infection – viral encephalitis, bacterial meningitis, HIV, and cerebral malaria.

Unknown epilepsies
The ILAE (Scheffer et al. 2017) state that the underlying cause of epilepsy syndrome may still be unknown; it may not fit into any one syndrome and may not fit typical EEG characteristics, but with time may evolve and allow diagnosis.

Section 3: External ventricular drainage

Introduction

An external ventricular drain (EVD) is the temporary diversion of cerebrospinal fluid (CSF) from the fluid-filled cavities of the brain (lateral ventricles) to a closed collection system outside the body (Cartwright and Wallace 2007). The indications for an EVD are; to relieve raised intracranial pressure, to divert infected CSF, or blood-stained CSF following surgery or haemorrhage or to divert the flow of CSF (Nielsen and Breedt (2007).

CSF will sometimes be drained through an external lumbar drain, for example following a dural tear during craniofacial surgery/CSF leak following transphenoidal surgery/spinal surgery. The position of the drain will be in accordance with Trust policy and set to drain a specific volume/be set at a specific level/specific pressure. The care of the drain is similar to care of an EVD (Ling et al 2017), but occasionally nerve irritation can occur and necessitate removal of the drain.

Procedure guideline 21.3 Introduction to external ventricular drainage

Statement	Rationale
EVDs should only be cared for by nursing and medical staff who are trained and competent to do so.	To ensure safety for the CYP.
1 The EVD is inserted in theatre under a general anaesthetic. NB. GOSH now uses NR-FIT EVDs as per government recommendations.	
2 There are two types of EVD system: a) The distal end of an existing shunt system may be externalised at the distal end and connected to an external drainage system. This shunt system contains a pressure valve. b) The most frequently used system is a new catheter placed into the ventricle through a small hole (burr hole) made in the skull. Once inserted, the scalp incision is sutured and covered with a sterile dressing. c) The new catheter is tunnelled under the skin, exiting on the abdominal wall and connects to an external drainage system. This system does not have a pressure valve, so drainage depends upon gravity.	2 a) To control the amount of drainage from the ventricles (Smith and Martin 2009). b) To prevent an unsightly scar, reduce the risk of infection and reduce risk of accidental removal (Smith and Martin 2009; Cartwright and Wallace 2007). c) The exit site must be planned carefully to prevent an unsightly scar, reduce the risk of infection, and reduce the risk of accidental removal (Smith and Martin 2009; Cartwright and Wallace 2007).
3 The ventricular catheter is connected to an external drainage system. The system has several components. See Figure 21.6. These include: a) A sampling/access port. b) An antireflux collection chamber. c) A drainage bag. d) A pressure scale.	3 a) To provide access to the catheter. b) To observe CSF drainage. c) To enable on-going collection of CSF. d) To facilitate accurate positioning.
4 a) Nonmetal clamps, gauze, and chlorhexidine impregnated wipes, e.g. Clinell® **must** be positioned by the CYP's bed to enable the system to be clamped if the drainage system accidentally becomes disconnected. b) The line must be clearly labelled, preferably near the injection and sampling port. Ideally a stopcock protection box will be placed over the access point to reduce the risk of accidental administration of intravenous medication.	4 a) To prevent loss of CSF. b) To minimise risk of inappropriate use.
5 The prescribed instructions of the neurosurgeon should be followed for either of the following: a) Position/pressure level of the drain. b) Expected hourly amount of CSF drainage.	5 To ensure desired CSF drainage.
6 The EVD system should be changed according to specific medical treatment under conditions of strict asepsis, according to microbiological advice/local policy. a) The drainage bag should be changed when three quarters full.	6 To minimise the risk of infection/further infection (Cartwright and Wallace 2007). a) Overfilling of the drainage bags impairs drainage (Cartwright and Wallace 2007).
7 For cases of infected CSF, intrathecal antibiotics are prescribed according to microbiological advice and administered through the injection and sampling port of the external ventricular drain. This should only be undertaken by a trained and competent healthcare professional.	7 To provide effective treatment by administering the antibiotics directly into the cerebral spinal fluid.

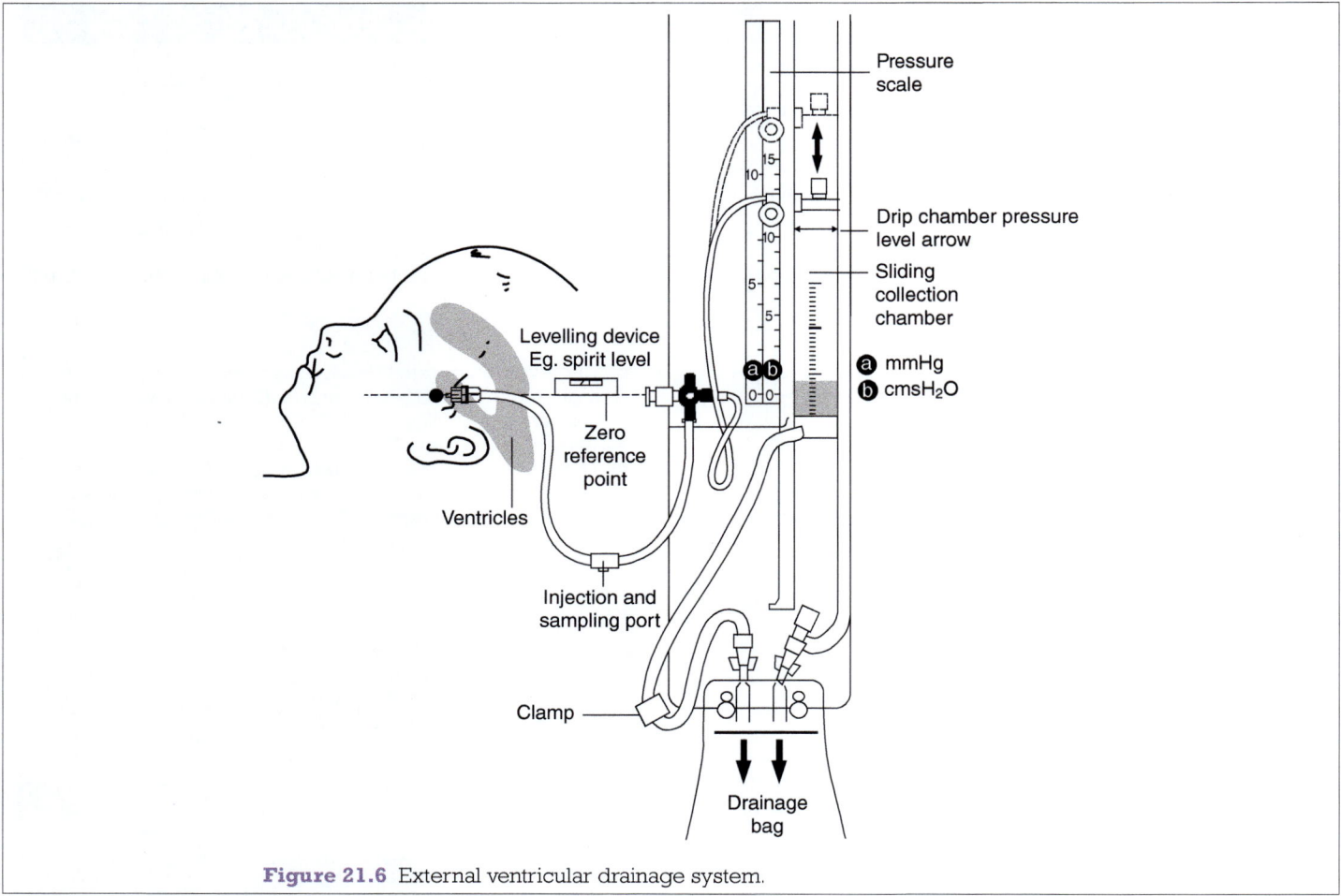

Figure 21.6 External ventricular drainage system.

Procedure guideline 21.4 Inform the CYP and family

Statement	Rationale
1 Explain the entire procedure and management to the CYP and family, avoiding medical and nursing jargon and language. Information must be given according to the CYP's age, condition, and cognition. Explain the following: a) Why the EVD is necessary. b) The reason for the EVD. c) What it entails. d) The likely length of placement of an EVD. e) The associated problems of an EVD (Smith and Martin 2009).	1 To ensure that the CYP and family understand the procedure and are psychologically prepared, and to ensure that informed consent is obtained.
2 Parents/carers should be given the EVD Parents Information Leaflet to reinforce the verbal information given.	2 This is available online at www.gosh.nhs.uk/conditions-and-treatments/procedures-and-treatments/external-ventricular-drainage/
3 If appropriate provide play preparation, involving the play specialist (Smith and Martin 2009). Consider involvement of a clinical psychologist if appropriate, particularly if previous procedures have been stressful for the CYP or if he/she is known to have or exhibits signs of anticipatory anxiety or distress (Salmon 2006).	3 To give the CYP the opportunity to express fears in a familiar environment.

Procedure guideline 21.5 Neurological assessment

Statement	Rationale
1 The following observations should be carried out on return from theatre. They must be performed according to the CYP's condition and hospital policy, but at least every four hours and in conjunction with paediatric early warning scores (PEWS).	1 To establish the baseline for future observations. To monitor change and identify any necessary changes in treatment, which may include changing the drain height to reduce/increase the volume of CSF draining.
2 Observe for a change in the CYP's neurological condition by assessing the following: a) Level of consciousness. b) Pupil reaction. c) Limb movement and strength. d) Heart rate. e) Blood pressure. f) Respiratory rate. g) The fontanelle should be checked in infants.	2 To identify changes on act on these findings appropriately. Changes can indicate a change in intracranial pressure and treatment may need to be implemented. For more information see Section 1 in this chapter. d) Bradycardia can be a sign of raised intracranial pressure; tachycardia can be a sign of low intracranial pressure. e) Hypertension can be a sign of raised intracranial pressure; hypotension can be a sign of low intracranial pressure. g) A bulging fontanelle indicates raised intracranial pressure; a dipped fontanelle indicates low intracranial pressure. For further information, refer to the previous section, Neurological Observations.
3 A change in body temperature.	3 Pyrexia could indicate an infection, the source of which should be identified and treated.
4 The frequency of nausea and vomiting should be monitored and documented in the significant events section of the coma chart.	4–5) To provide accurate information on which the CYP's clinical picture can be based.
5 The frequency, duration, and severity of any headaches should be monitored and documented in the significant events section of the coma chart.	
6 The family should be included in general observation of their child.	6 To use their knowledge of what is 'normal' for the CYP.

Procedure guideline 21.6 Drain management: positioning of drain

Statement	Rationale
1 The system must be positioned accurately according to medical instructions documented in the operation notes or medical notes. a) Ensure drain is clamped prior to any repositioning to avoid overdraining.	1 It is the responsibility of the neurosurgeon to give instructions on the level at which the drain is to be set or the amount of drainage required each hour. To ensure desired amount of CSF drainage.
2 Unless otherwise prescribed the drain is measured from the foramen of Monro, which is midway between the outer aspect of the CYP's eye and the external auditory meatus (Woodward et al. 2002). a) The midpoint of this line is the zero point for the EVD system. (See Figure 21.6 and 21.7.) b) Use a levelling device, e.g. spirit level, to estimate the zero point position against the pressure scale, which is either mounted on an intravenous (IV) pole or on a pressure scale mounting panel. (See Figure 21.6.) c) Position and secure the pressure scale, on either the IV pole or the system mounting panel with 0 cms being the estimated zero point.	2 To calibrate/determine the zero reference point for the drain, i.e. the level of the ventricles for positioning the EVD system (Cartwright and Wallace 2007). b) To ensure accuracy. c) For ease of accurate positioning.
3 Position the pressure level arrow at the top of the drip chamber at the prescribed height. a) The position of drain should be documented on the CYP's fluid chart and/or their neurological observation coma chart. If the height of the drain is changed for any reason, then this must be documented on the neurological observation coma chart and the medical notes.	3 To ensure correct CSF drainage. The difference in height between the ventricles and the drip chamber creates both a pressure gradient and a safety valve. The height of the drip chamber equates to the pressure inside of the head or intracranial pressure (ICP). This pressure must be reached before any CSF will drain into the collection chamber (Cartwright and Wallace 2007). a) To ensure an accurate record.

(continued)

Procedure guideline 21.6 Drain management: positioning of drain *(continued)*

Statement	Rationale

4 When moving or repositioning the CYP:
  a) Clamp both the three-way tap nearest the CYP and the EVD itself.
  b) Re-zero drain.
  c) Unclamp drain immediately after repositioning.
	4 The position of the drain always corresponds with the CYP's ventricles.

5 Parents should be advised of the importance of the following aspects of care when a drain is in situ.
  a) The importance of repositioning the drain.
  b) To clamp the drain if their child is being moved, crying excessively, or vomiting.
  c) To ask for the assistance of a healthcare professional who has been trained and has achieved competence in EVD management, to rezero/reposition the drain once their child has been moved (Cartwright and Wallace 2007).
  d) That the drain should not be clamped for longer than one hour unless otherwise specified and prescribed.
	5 To encourage parental involvement and promote safe management.
	  a) To ensure CSF drains as required.
	  b) To prevent over drainage of CSF.
	  c) To ensure correct CSF drainage.
	
	  d) To minimise risk of blocked catheter and to prevent raised intracranial pressure.

6 This instruction must be documented in the CYP's healthcare record.	6 To provide an accurate record.

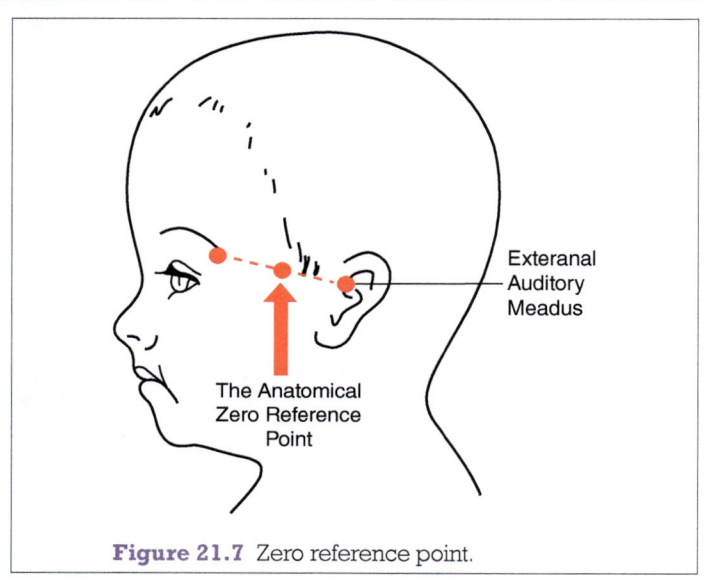

Figure 21.7 Zero reference point.

Procedure guideline 21.7 Drain management: drainage

Statement	Rationale
1 EVD systems should be connected in theatres when first inserted (Smith and Martin 2013).	1 To minimise the risk of infection. To prevent blockage of catheter.
2 Once the drain is connected and positioned, an initial assessment of CSF drainage should be made.	2 To ensure CSF is draining at the correct rate.

3 Subsequently, hourly checks should be made of:
  a) Amount of drainage
 	
  b) Colour of CSF – should be colourless.
 	
  c) Exit site.
	3 To promote safe management of the CYP.
	  a) To ensure CSF drainage rate is as prescribed. A sudden increase in drainage may result from inaccurate zeroing of the drain or could signify a rise in ICP. A decrease in drainage could also indicate inaccurate zeroing of the drain or that the tubing may be kinked, blocked, disconnected, or the ports are closed
	  b) Bloodstained CSF could indicate blood in the ventricles. Cloudy CSF may indicate the presence of an infection.
	  c) To ensure CSF is not leaking.

4 Record the CYP's intake and output on the fluid balance chart hourly and the neurological observations on the coma chart: Also document:
  a) The amount of CSF drainage.
  b) The position of the EVD and patency of the drain by observing dripping of CSF into the chamber or momentarily lowering the drain.
	
	  a) To ensure CSF drainage rate is as prescribed.
	  b) To ensure position of drain is correct, to provide an accurate record, and to ensure drain is patent.

Procedure guideline 21.7 Drain management: drainage *(continued)*

Statement	Rationale
5 The neurosurgeon will specify a drain height postoperatively and whether this is to be maintained or adjusted to drain a certain amount of CSF an hour.	5 The CYP's age and condition and prescription dictate the amount of drainage.
	An approximate guide to CSF drainage is:
	Infants: 2–5 ml/hr
	Children: 5–10 ml/hr
	Adolescents: 10–15 ml/hr.
6 If the CYP is crying excessively: a) the drain should be clamped off. b) It **must not** be clamped off for more than one hour.	6 a) To prevent over drainage. b) To prevent blockage and increase in intracranial pressure.
7 If there is no CSF drainage: a) Observe for pulsation movement of CSF in the tubing of the EVD. This should be a clear rise and fall, not just a flicker. b) Ensure system is not clamped or kinked. c) Lower chamber momentarily below head level. d) Advise neurosurgeon immediately if there is no drainage.	a) To determine whether drainage is slow. b) This will reduce or stop flow. c) To encourage flow and/or release an air lock. d) The system may need flushing.
8 If a catheter becomes disconnected: a) Clamp catheter close to CYP. b) Place end in sterile wrapping/container. c) Lie CYP down. d) Thoroughly clean exposed tip using a sterile chlorhexidine impregnated swab and connect a new system aseptically. e) Record event in CYP's healthcare records and inform their doctor.	8 a) To prevent excess CSF loss. b) To reduce infection risk. c) To prevent excess CSF loss. d) To reduce infection risk. e) To provide an accurate record.
9 Contact the neurosurgical team immediately if there are concerns about: a) The amount of drainage. b) The condition of the CYP.	9 The position of the drain may need to be re-evaluated.

Procedure guideline 21.8 Drain management: connecting or changing the system

Statement	Rationale
1 Newly inserted EVD's will be connected to the drainage system in theatres (Smith and Martin 2009).	1 To minimise the risk of infection.
2 Inform the CYP and family that the procedure is to be performed.	2 To gain understanding and co-operation.
3 The system should be connected by, or under the supervision of a healthcare professional who has been trained and has achieved competence. • Prepare equipment: • Dressing trolley • Clamps and gauze • A pair of sterile gloves and an apron • EVD system • Two chlorhexidine impregnated wipes, e.g. Clinell®	
4 To change the drainage system: a) Clamp catheter close to CYP using nonsterile gauze and clamps. b) Put on apron and perform a ward aseptic procedures handwash. c) Open new drainage system and put on sterile gloves. d) Assemble drainage set closing clamps. e) Disconnect the old system. Clean the newly exposed catheter connection with a chlorhexidine impregnated wipe and allow it to dry f) Connect new system. g) Check connections. h) Position system as prescribed by the neurosurgeon. i) Release clamps on new system and those close to the CYP. j) Clear away equipment according to Waste Policy. k) Wash hands. l) Record the procedure in the CYP's healthcare records.	a) To prevent loss of CSF on disconnection. To protect tubing. b) To prevent contamination. c) To prepare for procedure. d) To prevent CSF drainage until repositioned. e) To minimise the risk of infection. f) To establish new system. g) To prevent CSF loss. h) To establish instructed drainage. i) To commence CSF drainage. j) To maintain a safe environment. k) To minimise the risk of cross infection. l) To provide an accurate record.

Procedure guideline 21.9 Drain management: patency of drain: repairing a catheter

Statement	Rationale
1. If a catheter splits: a) Clamp catheter close to CYP using gauze and clamps. b) Place end in sterile wrapping/container, e.g. Clinell®. c) Lie CYP down.	a) To prevent excess CSF loss. b) To reduce risk of infection. c) To prevent excess CSF loss.
2. The catheter should be repaired by, or under, the supervision of a competent healthcare professional.	
3. Gather and prepare the following equipment: a) Dressing trolley b) A pair of sterile gloves and an apron c) EVD system d) EVD connector e) Sterile scissors f) Alcohol impregnated wipes, e.g. Clinell®	a) To provide a clean work surface. b) To minimise the risk of infection. c) To allow CSF drainage. d) To connect system safely. e) To minimise the risk of infection.
4. To repair a split catheter: a) Put on apron and perform a ward aseptic procedures hand-wash. b) Open new drainage system and put on sterile gloves. c) Assemble new drainage set closing clamps. d) The practitioner cleans the exposed catheter end with a sterile chlorhexidine impregnated wipe and allows it to dry. e) Using sterile scissors cut just above the split/broken catheter. f) Insert EVD connector into the catheter lumen. g) Connect new system. h) Check connections. i) Position system as prescribed by the neurosurgeon. j) Release clamps on new system and those close to the CYP. k) Clear away equipment according to Waste Policy. l) Wash hands according to local policy. m) Record the procedure in the CYP's healthcare records.	a) To minimise the risk of infection. b) To prepare for procedure. c) To prevent loss of CSF until repositioned. d)–e) To minimise the risk of infection. e) To create a clean end for connection. f) To establish new system. g)–h) To prevent CSF loss. i) To establish instructed drainage. j) To commence CSF drainage. k)–l) To minimise the risk of cross infection. m) To maintain an accurate record.

Procedure guideline 21.10 Drain management: patency of drain: unblocking of catheter

Statement	Rationale
1. If a catheter appears to be blocked: a) Exclude damage to the EVD system. b) Lower drain and observe for CSF movement.	a) Connections may be faulty. b) Air lock may be present.
2. If no CSF movement is observed, seek **urgent** advice from a neurosurgeon.	2. The catheter may be blocked resulting in raised intracranial pressure.
3. Catheters **must only** be aspirated by a healthcare professional who has undergone training and has achieved competence. To aspirate a drain please refer to guidelines for accessing the drain (see procedure guideline 21.12).	3. To minimise the potential risks of the procedure.
4. If the aspiration has been unsuccessful the EVD should be flushed. This **MUST ONLY** be done by a healthcare professional who has undergone training and has achieved competence.	4. To minimise the potential risks of the procedure. **This is a high-risk procedure.**
5. To flush the EVD: a) A competent clinician should draw up 4–5 ml of 0.9% sodium chloride into a syringe. b) Insert syringe into the injection port. c) Gently attempt to inject the sodium chloride.	c) To flush system.
6. After aspirating and/or flushing: a) Discard syringe. b) Connect new system. c) Check connections. d) Release clamps on new system and those close to the CYP. e) Gradually lower system. f) Position system as instructed by the neurosurgeon. g) Clear away equipment according to Waste Policy. h) Wash hands. i) Record the procedure in the CYP's healthcare records.	e) To check for drainage. f) To commence CSF drainage. g) To maintain a safe environment. h) To minimise the risk of cross infection. i) To maintain an accurate record.
7. If the flushing has not been successful, the neurosurgeon must be contacted.	7. A CT scan will need to be performed to determine the cause of the blockage.

Procedure guideline 21.11 Drain management: fluid and electrolyte balance

Statement	Rationale
1 For younger and sick children, CSF losses should be replaced ml/ml with intravenous 0.9% sodium chloride as prescribed, unless otherwise indicated (Nielsen and Breedt 2007).	1 To maintain fluid and electrolyte balance. CSF contains sodium.
2 Oral sodium chloride can be used if required.	2 If the CYP's oral intake is adequate.
3 CSF losses and intravenous fluid replacement should be recorded hourly on a fluid balance chart and reviewed every shift by the nurse in charge.	3 To ensure fluid balance is being maintained.
4 Serum electrolytes should be checked according to age, condition and CSF losses, but approximately twice weekly.	4 To monitor the CYP's electrolyte balance and treat as appropriate.

Procedure guideline 21.12 Accessing the drain: CSF sampling

Statement	Rationale

1 Routine CSF sampling is not advised due to the risk of introducing infection to an otherwise sterile circuit. However, when CSF samples are required, they must be taken by either nursing or medical staff who have undertaken training and achieved competence using an aseptic technique:
• Infected CSF samples should be taken in line with hospital policy and according to microbiological advice, until the CSF is sterile/infection free.
	1 CSF may be sampled to monitor:
	• CSF values including antibiotic levels in the CSF.
	• Progress in treatment of a known infection. The following can be utilised as a marker of infection,
	  i A raised cell and protein count.
	  ii A lowered glucose count.

2 CSF samples should be obtained by, or under the supervision of a healthcare professional who has been trained and has achieved competence.	2 To promote asepsis and to minimise the risk of infection.
3 The levels are checked daily to determine subsequent doses of antibiotics. This must be done in consultation with the microbiologist to avoid overdose of antibiotics.	3 Antibiotic levels should be as follows: • Vancomycin: less or equivalent to 15 mg/l • Gentamicin: less than 3 mg/l.

4 Gather the following equipment:
  a) Sterile paper
  b) Chlorhexidine impregnated wipe
  c) Two 10–30 ml syringes
  d) Two universal specimen containers:
    • 1 × Container = Protein count
    • 1 × Container = Cell count and antibiotic level (if required)
  e) Sterile gloves and an apron
  f) Request form.
	a) To provide a sterile field.
	b) To clean the entry port.
	c) Large syringe sizes reduce pressure exerted on catheter tubing of the EVD set
	d) To collect CSF specimen to determine the cell and protein count and the antibiotic level.
	e) To minimise the risk of infection.

5 To obtain a CSF specimen:
  a) Close clamps on drainage system close to injection port.
  b) Wash hands and put on apron.
  c) Prepare sterile field.
  d) Perform a ward aseptic procedures hand-wash and put on gloves.
  e) An assistant should hold the injection port/open and close the three-way tap.
  f) Clean injection port on EVD system with an alcohol impregnated wipe and allow to dry.
  g) Insert syringe into port.
  h) Slowly withdraw 5 ml of CSF, remove syringe and discard.
  i) Insert second syringe into port.
  j) Slowly withdraw 2 ml of CSF.
  k) Place 1 ml of CSF into each universal specimen container.
  l) Open clamps on drainage system close to injection port.
  m) Label samples and send them with completed request forms to the correct laboratory in accordance with local policy.
  n) Dispose of all used equipment according to Waste Policy.
  o) Wash hands according to hospital policy.
  p) Record the procedure in the CYP's healthcare records.
 	
NB: Should a CSF specimen be required from an EVD where the shunt valve remains in situ, the following protocol can be followed, with care being taken to withdraw the CSF gently and slowly.
	a) To prevent CSF aspiration from drainage system.
	b) To prevent contamination.
	c) To prevent contamination.
	d) To minimise the risk of infection.
	e) To minimise the risk of infection.
	f) To minimise infection.
	g) To access the system.
	h) To remove contaminated CSF sample.
	i) To access system.
	j) To obtain CSF sample for analysis.
	k) To facilitate analysis.
	l) To continue drainage of CSF.
	m) To facilitate analysis.
	
	n) To meet hospital policy.
	o) To minimise the risk of cross infection.
	p) To maintain an accurate record.

Procedure guideline 21.13 Accessing the drain: giving intrathecal drugs

Statement	Rationale

1 Intrathecal drugs, e.g. antibiotics, are administered to enable local treatment of the CSF (Barrett-Goode 2000).
  a) Antibiotic levels should be checked prior to administering each dose.
  b) Intrathecal antibiotics must only be administered by healthcare professionals who have undergone training and achieved competence.
	a) To ensure the correct dosage is administered.

2 Gather the following equipment:
  a) Sterile gloves and an apron
  b) Sterile paper sheet
  c) Chlorhexidine-impregnated wipe
  d) 1 or 2ml syringe
  e) 2 × 10–30ml syringes
  f) Blue needle
  g) Prescribed antibiotics
  h) Sodium chloride 0.9% for injection
  i) CYP's prescription chart
	a) To minimise risk of infection.
	b) To provide a sterile field.
	c) To clean the entry port.
	d) To administer small volumes of drugs.
	e) Large syringe sizes reduce pressure exerted on catheter.
	f) Use to draw up antibiotics.
	
	h) To flush catheter after antibiotics.
	i) To check drugs prescribed.

3 To administer intrathecal antibiotics:
  a) Close clamps on drainage system close to injection port.
  b) Put on apron and wash hands.
  c) Prepare sterile field.
  d) Perform a ward aseptic procedures handwash and put on gloves.
  e) Check drugs according to hospital drug policy.
  f) Prepare drugs using aseptic nontouch technique.
  g) Check CYP's identity according to the Drug Policy.
  h) Clean injection port on EVD system with an alcohol impregnated wipe and allow to dry.
  i) Slowly withdraw 5ml of CSF, according to Trust policy; remove syringe and discard.
  j) Insert syringe containing the antibiotic into injection port.
  k) Inject antibiotic according to manufacturer's guidelines.
  l) Remove syringe.
  m) Insert syringe containing 0.9% sodium chloride into port and gently flush catheter with 5ml 0.9% sodium chloride.
  n) Remove syringe
  o) Keep drainage system clamped for one hour only.
  p) Dispose of all used equipment according to Waste Policy.
  q) Wash hands according to hospital policy.
  r) Record the procedure in the CYP's healthcare records
	a) To prevent drug entering drainage system.
	b)–d) To prevent cross contamination and minimise the risk of infection.
	
	e) To ensure the drug is given safely.
	f) To minimise the risk of infection.
	g) To ensure that the drug is given to the correct CYP.
	h) To minimise the risk of infection.
	
	i) To meet prescription guidelines.
	
	j)–k) To facilitate drug administration.
	
	m) To facilitate flushing of system. To ensure drug given.
	
	o) To ensure absorption of antibiotic.
	p) To maintain safe environment.
	q) To minimise the risk of cross infection.
	r) To provide an accurate record.

Procedure guideline 21.14 Exit site care

Statement	Rationale
1 The CYP will return from theatre with a dressing over the exit site.	1 To keep wound clean and dry.
2 If exit site is dry it should be dressed with a clear, semipermiable, sterile dressing, e.g. IV3000™ or Opsite, to allow observation of the site.	2–4) To reduce the risk of infection.
3 Change the dressing weekly unless contaminated.	

4 The dressing should be changed if it becomes contaminated with CSF or blood (Woodward et al. 2002).
  a) If the exit site is oozing:
    a) It should be dressed with a nonadherent dressing, e.g. Solvaline N and steri strips.
    b) A microbiological swab may need to be taken for culture and sensitivity.
    c) The CYP's doctor should be kept informed.
	4 To exert a small amount of pressure to reduce drainage:
	  a) To soak up any oozing.
	  b) To identify any infective organisms.
	  c) To keep the CYP/family updated with the clinical situation.

5 Check exit site dressing hourly for:
  a) Redness
  b) Inflammation
  c) Oozing of blood
  d) Leakage of CSF
	5
	a) An indicator of infection.
	
	d) The drain may need repositioning.

6 Loop catheter once at exit site under dressing.	6 To reduce the risk of the catheter being accidentally removed.

Procedure guideline 21.15 Removal of the drain

Statement	Rationale
1 The length of time an EVD should remain in situs should be in accordance with local policy. The entire system should then be removed or changed in theatre.	1 To reduce the risk of further infection.
2 Preoperatively, it may be necessary to clamp the drain for a specified time prior to surgery.	2 To enlarge the ventricles for surgery. To facilitate insertion of catheter.
3 If the CYP's condition deteriorates due to clamping preoperatively, unclamp the drain and contact the neurosurgical team.	3 The CYP is likely to have raised ICP.
4 Post operatively, assess the CYP and dress the exit site.	4 To ensure recovery from the procedure and anaesthetic and to ensure there is no wound site infection, or CSF leakage.

References

Advanced Life Support Group (ALSG) (2016). *Advanced Paediatric Life Support: A Practical Approach to Emergencies (APLS)*, 6e. Wiley-Blackwell.

Appleton, R. and Gibbs, J. (1998). *Epilepsy in Childhood and Adolescence 2*. London: Martin Dunitz Ltd.

Armon, K., Stephenson, T., Gabri, V., and MacFaud, R. (2003). An evidence and consensus based guideline for the management of a child after seizure. Emergency Medical Journal 20 (1): 13–20.

Aucken, S. and Crawford, B. (1999). Neurological assessment. In: *Neuro Oncology for Nurses* (ed. D. Guerrero). London: Whurr;Barrett-Goode, P. (2000). Reliability of the Adelaide coma scale. Paediatric Nursing 12 (8): 23–27.

Bacon, M., Appleton, R., Bangalore, H., Brand, C., Browning, J. et al. (2022). Review of the new APLS guideline (2021): Management of the Convulsing Child. Arch Dis Child Educ Pract Ed Jun 22; edpract-2021-323351. doi: 10.1136/archdischild-2021-323351.

Bateman, D. (2001). Neurological assessment of coma. Journal of Neurology, Neurosurgery and Psychiatry 71 (1): i13.

Barrett-Goode, P. (2000) Reliability of the Adelaide Coma Scale. Paediatric Nursing 12 (8): 23–27.

Birdsall, C. and Greif, L. (1990). How do you manage external ventricular drainage? American Journal of Nursing 90: 47–49.

Bouffet, E., Douard, M.C., Annequin, D. et al. (1996). Pain in lumbar puncture. Results of a two year discussion at the French Society of Pediatric Oncology. Archives of Pediatrics 3 (1): 22–27.

Brown, K. and Tallur, T. (2005). Acute encephalopathies of childhood. In: *Paediatric Neurology* (eds. C.P. Panteliadis and R. Korinthenberg), 437–471. New York, Stuttgart: Georg Thieme Verlag.

Cartwright, C.C. and Wallace, D.C. (2007). *Nursing Care of the Pediatric Neurosurgery Patient*. Berlin: Springer.

Chapman, S.M., Wray, J., Oulton, K., and Peters, M.J. (2016). Systematic review of paediatric track and trigger systems. Resuscitation 109: 87–109.

Couffignal, B., D'Agate, B., and Bocquet, S. (2001). Are epilepsy seizures in patients with medial temporal lobe epilepsy influenced by participating factors. Epilepsies 13 (1): 49–52.

Disabato, J.A. and Burkett, K.W. (2007). Neurological assessment of the neonate, infant, child, and adolescent. In: *Nursing Care of the Pediatric Neurosurgery Patient* (eds. C. Cartwright and D. Wallace), 1–27. New York: Springer, Berlin, Heldelberg. https://doi.org/10.1007/978-3-540-29704-8_1.

Ellis, A. and Cavanagh, S. (1992). Aspects of neurosurgical assessment using the Glasgow Coma Scale. Intensive and Critical Nursing Care 8 (2): 94–99.

Fitzgerald, M. (2005). The development of nociceptive circuits. Nature Reviews Neuroscience 6 (7): 507–520.

Gaffney, A., McGrath, P.J., and Dick, B. (2003). Measuring pain in children: developmental and instrumental issues. In: *Pain in Infants, Children and Adolescents*, 2e (eds. N.L. Schechter, C.B. Berde and M. Yaster). Philadelphia: Lippincott Williams & Wilkins.

Hickey, J. and Strayer, A. (2020). *The Clinical Practice of Neurological and Neurosurgical Nursing*, 8e. Philadelphia, New York: Lippincott.

Jennet, B. and Teasdale, G. (1974). Assessment of coma and impaired consciousness. Lancet 2 (2872): 81–84.

Ling, L., Guo, L., Wang, J. et al. (2017). Nursing management of lumbar drainage in cryptococcal meningitis: a case report. The Journal of Neuroscience Nursing 49 (4): 198–202.

Marcoux, K. (2005). Management of increased intracranial pressure in the critically ill child with an acute neurological injury. AACN Clinical Issues 16: 212–231.

Matta, B., Menon, D., and Smith, M. (2011). *Core Topics in Neuroanaesthesia and Neurointensive Care*. Cambridge: Cambridge University Press.

May, L. and Carter, B. (1995). Nursing support and care: meeting the needs of the child and family with altered cerebral function. In: *Child Health Care Nursing* (eds. B. Carter and A. Dearman), 363–391. Oxford: Blackwell Science.

Mooney, G. and Comerford, D.M. (2003). Neurological observations. Nursing Times 99 (17): 24–25.

National Institute for Health and Care Excellence (NICE) (2022). Epilepsies in children, young people and adults. NICE guideline [NG217]. https://www.nice.org.uk/guidance/ng217 (accessed 26 September 2022).

Nielsen, N. and Breedt, A. (2007). Hydrocephalus. In: *Nursing Care of the Paediatric Neurosurgery Patient* (eds. C. Cartwright and D. Wallace), 39–89. Berlin: Springer. https://authorzilla.com/2e3No/hydrocephalus-springer.html (accessed 12 July 2022).

Norman, R. (2000). Controversies in pediatric emergency medicine. Pediatric Emergency Care 16 (4): 229–301.

Panayiotopoulos, C. (2007). *A Clinical Guide to Epileptic Syndromes and their Treatment*, 2e. Oxfordshire: Bladon Medical Publishing.

Panayiotopoulos, C.P. (2011). Epilepsies Vade Mecum Epileptic Seizures Medicinae. Oxford.

Paul, S., Smith, J., Green, J. et al. (2013). Managing children with raised intracranial pressure: part 1 (introduction and menegitis). Nursing Children and Young People 25 (10): 31–38.

Reilly, P.L., Simpson, D.A., Sprod, R., and Thomas, L. (1988). Assessing the conscious level in infants and young children: a paediatric version of the Glasgow coma scale. Child's Nervous System 4 (1): 30–33.

Royal College of Paediatrics and Child Health (2018). *Safe system framework for children at risk of deterioration*. https://www.rcpch.ac.uk/resources/safe-system-framework-children-risk-deterioration (accessed 26 September 2022).

Salmon, K. (2006). Preparing young children for medical procedures: taking account of memory. Journal of Pediatric Psychology 1 (8): 859–861.

Scheffer, I.E., Berkovic, S., Capovilla, G. et al. (2017). ILAE classification of the epilepsies: Position paper of the ILAE Commission for Classification and Terminology. Epilepsia 58 (4): 512–521. https://online.wiley.com/doi/full/10.1111/epi.13709 (accessed 12 July 2022).

Simpson, D. and Reilly, P. (1982). Paediatric coma scale. Lancet 2 (8295): 450. Neuroscience Nursing. December (6):347-55.

Smith, J. and Martin, C. (2009). *Paediatric Neurosurgery for Nurses. Evidence-Based Care for Children and Their Families*. London: Routledge.

Talvik, T., Kirkham, F., Metsvaht, T., and Talvik, I. (2012). Acute non-febrile encephalopathy. In: *Principles and Practice of Child Neurology in Infancy* (ed. C. Kennedy), 179–204. Mac Keith Press.

Teasdale G (2014). Forty years on: updating the Glasgow Coma Scale. Nursing Times; 110: 42, 12–16. https://www.nursingtimes.net/clinical-archive/accident-and-emergency/forty-years-on-updating-the-glasgow-coma-scale-10-10-2014/ (accessed 26 September 2022).

Walker, M.C. and Shorvon, S.D. (2013). Treatment of tonic-clonic status epilepticus. In: *Epilepsy 2013 from Membranes to Mankind – a Practical Guide to Epilepsy*, 14e (eds. F.J. Rugg-Gunn and J.E. Smalls), 331–342. Epilepsy Society UK.

Woodford, S. and Mestecky, A. (2011). *Neuroscience Nursing Evidence – Based Practice*. Chichester: Blackwell Publishing Ltd.

Woodward, S., Addison, C., Shah, S. et al. (2002). Benchmarking best practice for external ventricular drainage. British Journal of Nursing 11 (1): 47–53.

Chapter 22

Nutrition and feeding

Vanessa Shaw[1] and Sarah Kipps[2]

[1]MBE, MA, PG Dip Dietetics, RD, FBDA, Honorary Associate Professor of Paediatric Dietetics, Plymouth University, Honorary Senior Lecturer, UCL Great Ormond Street Institute, London, UK

[2]Formerly Practice Educator, Nursing Quality, Great Ormond Street Hospital, London, UK

The editors and authors would like to thank the following for their review of this chapter: Lauren Arpe, Marianne Forbes, Lucy Jackman, Kelly Larmour, Sarah Macdonald, Rory Philbin, Pamela Stepney and Natalie Yerlett.

Chapter contents

Introduction	482	Enteral feeding	489
Nutritional requirements	482	Parenteral nutrition	490
Nutrition from preterm to adolescence	483	References	515
Breastfeeding	488		

Procedure guidelines

22.1 Adding fortifier to EBM on the ward	496	22.5 Administration of enteral feeds	507
22.2 Inserting and managing the nasogastric tube	498	22.6 Monitoring CYPs on enteral feeds	509
22.3 Inserting and managing the nasojejunal tube	501	22.7 Delivery of PN in the hospital setting	510
22.4 Management where both a gastric and a jejunal tube are inserted	503	22.8 Sham feeding	513

Principles tables

22.1 Use of breast pumps	492	22.7 Handling of enteral feeds	497
22.2 Freshly expressed breast milk	493	22.8 Preparing the CYP and family (feeding tube insertion)	497
22.3 Frozen expressed breast milk	494	22.9 Nasogastric tube feeding	498
22.4 Dividing and decanting expressed breast milk	494	22.10 Nasojejunal tube feeding	501
22.5 Qualities of breast milk	495	22.11 Gastrostomy tube feeding	503
22.6 Increasing nutritional intake of preterm infants	495		

The Great Ormond Street Hospital Manual of Children and Young People's Nursing Practices, Second Edition. Edited by Elizabeth Anne Bruce, Janet Williss, and Faith Gibson.
© 2023 John Wiley & Sons Ltd. Published 2023 by John Wiley & Sons Ltd.

Introduction

Good nutrition is vital for the growth and development of all children and young people (CYPs) in both health and disease. It is important to have knowledge of the changing nutritional requirements throughout childhood and adolescence in order to assess whether intake is adequate. This chapter describes the nutritional requirements of CYPs from preterm to adolescence and outlines how these can be achieved through normal eating and drinking. Enteral and parenteral feeding, which are used when CYPs are unable to take adequate nutrition by mouth, are also discussed.

Box 22.1 Some conditions likely to cause impairment in nutritional status

- Preterm and low birth weight delivery.
- Inappropriately restrictive diets.
- Feeding problems; prolonged difficulties with ingesting or swallowing food.
- Vomiting, diarrhoea, or malabsorption.
- Severe or chronic catabolic illness, e.g. recurrent infections or multiple surgery.
- Child neglect/abuse.
- Eating disorders, e.g. anorexia nervosa.
- Diseases and therapies altering the normal pattern of eating, e.g. cancer and chemotherapy.

Nutritional requirements

A nutritionally adequate diet is essential for the normal growth and development of CYPs. During illness and recovery, requirements for nutrients increase. This may be due to factors such as increased losses, e.g. vomiting and diarrhoea, or increased metabolism, which expends energy stores, e.g. pyrexia, inflammation. Sick CYPs are particularly vulnerable to nutritional deficit and nutritional support is essential in the management of CYPs admitted to hospital (Joosten and Hulst 2008). Nutritional care must be a priority for all infants, and mothers, CYPs (National Institute for Health and Care Excellence [NICE] 2008).

Evidence that CYPs in UK hospitals have a poor nutritional status was first recognised in the 1990s. A study at Birmingham Children's Hospital found that 16% of the total population studied were severely stunted (chronic protein-energy malnutrition); 14% severely wasted (acute protein-energy malnutrition), and a further 20% were at risk of severe malnutrition. Chronically ill CYPs were significantly more stunted and wasted than those admitted with an acute/elective condition. Stunting was significantly more common in the cardiac, gastroenterology, and respiratory population, but not in oncology or renal patients. This study revealed an alarmingly high prevalence of both acute and chronic malnutrition in a cross-sectional survey of children in hospital (Moy et al. 1990).

Further study at the Royal Hospital for Sick Children in Glasgow revealed that 16% were underweight for age (<5th centile); 15% stunted (<5th centile height-for-age); 8% wasted (<80% weight-for-height); and 16% were moderately undernourished or at risk of becoming so. Only one-third of these malnourished children had previously been identified as such. Children with diseases of the digestive system (inflammatory bowel disease, cystic fibrosis, and coeliac disease) were most at risk of undernutrition (Hendrikse et al. 1997). A report by the British Association for Parenteral and Enteral Nutrition (BAPEN) looking at hospital food as a medical treatment found that 15% of children in the UK were malnourished on admission to hospital. Even more worrying, a majority who depended on hospital food for all their nutrition continued to lose weight while in hospital (Allison 1999). Nutrition screening over a three-day period in 2007 in 46 Dutch hospitals with a paediatric ward showed that 19% of children were undernourished on admission (Joosten et al. 2010). The overall prevalence of malnutrition was significantly higher in children with an underlying disease. A further study has shown that the largest proportion of malnourished CYPs were those with multiple diagnoses, learning disability, infectious diseases, and cystic fibrosis (Pawallek et al. 2008). The reported prevalence of acute malnutrition in infants, CYPs on admission to hospital over the last 30 years varies from 6.1% to 40.9% (Merritt et al. 1983; Hendricks et al. 1995; Hankard et al. 2001; Ozturk et al. 2003; Dogan et al. 2005; Marteletti et al. 2005; Rocha et al. 2006; Moy 2006; Pawallek et al. 2008; Hulst et al. 2010). The prevalence of chronic malnutrition in hospitalised CYPs has an incidence varying from 8% to 47%, depending on the definition used (Merritt et al. 1983; Hendricks et al. 1995; Ozturk et al. 2003; Rocha et al. 2006; Moy 2006; Pawallek et al. 2008; Hulst et al. 2010).

It is imperative to monitor the nutritional status of all CYPs in hospital closely to identify any signs of undernutrition. The Care Quality Commission has published essential standards of quality and safety that include a requirement for nutritional screening when an individual first starts to use a hospital service, in order to identify where there may be risk of poor nutrition or dehydration (Care Quality Commission 2010). The Council of Europe Resolution Food and Nutritional Care in Hospitals highlights 10 key characteristics of good nutritional care for all those in hospital, available from www.bapen.org.uk/pdfs/coe_leaflet.pdf. All guidance recommends the use of a screening tool. The benchmarking tool Patient-led Assessments of the Care Environment (PLACE), introduced on 4 January 2013, requires mandatory monitoring of nutrition (NHS England 2013).

Two nutrition screening tools have been developed and evaluated in the UK for use with children; the Screening Tool for the Assessment of Malnutrition in Paediatrics (STAMP) (McCarthy et al. 2012) and the Paediatric Yorkhill Malnutrition Score (PYMS) (Gerasimidis et al. 2010). Nutrition screening tools rely on height and weight measurements being taken on admission and interpreting these in the context of the CYP's intake of food or feed, underlying disease, and losses through vomiting and diarrhoea. This determines their risk for malnutrition.

Nutritional impairment in children is serious and may:

- Affect long-term health, growth and development in very young infants (Lucas et al. 1998, 2001).
- Impair health and growth, increase the rate of complications of disease or treatment and, in life-threatening illness, reduce the chances of survival (Hendrikse et al. 1997).
- Increase length of hospital stay (Joosten et al. 2010).

There are a number of conditions which are likely to cause impairment in nutritional status (see box 22.1). Energy, protein, and micronutrients (vitamins, minerals, and trace elements) are required for maintenance as well as growth. It is crucial that requirements are met during infancy, childhood, and adolescence. Deficiencies of energy and protein can cause poor growth and development and micronutrient deficiencies can lead to improper functioning of many of the body's systems. During and following illness and disease, requirements are raised due to hypermetabolism and anabolism. Total nutritional intake therefore needs to incorporate normal requirements and, in addition, requirements for catch-up growth. In these situations, requirements should be calculated individually for each CYP to ensure that sufficient nutrition is provided.

Table 22.1a Estimated average requirements for energy for healthy infants[a] (Scientific Advisory Committee on Nutrition 2011)

Age (months) Boys	Breastfed kcal/kg/day	Breastfed kcal/day	Breast milk substitute fed kcal/kg/day	Breast milk substitute fed kcal/day	Mixed feeding or unknown kcal/kg/day	Mixed feeding or unknown kcal/day
1–2	96	526	120	598	120	574
3–4	96	574	96	622	96	598
5–6	72	598	96	646	72	622
7–12	72	694	72	742	72	718
Age (months) Girls						
1–2	96	478	120	550	120	502
3–4	96	526	96	598	96	550
5–6	72	550	96	622	72	574
7–12	72	646	72	670	72	646

[a] The estimated average requirement (EAR) for energy is for a group of people. About half the group will usually need more than the EAR, and half less. It is important to remember that these figures are for populations, not individuals, and therefore serve as a guide only.

Table 22.1b Estimated average requirements for energy for healthy CYPs[a] (Scientific Advisory Committee on Nutrition 2011)

Age (years)	Boys	Girls
1	765	717
2	1004	932
3	1171	1076
4	1386	1291
5	1482	1362
6	1577	1482
7	1649	1530
8	1745	1625
9	1840	1721
10	2032	1936
11	2127	2023
12	2247	2103
13	2414	2223
14	2629	2342
15	2820	2390
16	2964	2414
17	3083	2462
18	3155	2462

[a] The estimated average requirement (EAR) for energy is for a group of people. About half the group will usually need more than the EAR, and half less. It is important to remember that these figures are for populations, not individuals, and therefore serve as a guide only.

The energy requirements for populations of healthy infants. (Table 22.1a), children. (Table 22.1b), and common dietary requirements for populations of healthy children (Table 22.2) are outlined below

Nutrition from preterm to adolescence

Breastfeeding is the optimum form of nutrition for infants and mothers should be supported in their decision to breast feed. Breastfeeding has significant short- and long-term benefits on the health of the mother and baby beyond the period of breastfeeding itself (Department of Health [DH] 2007; Royal College of Nursing [RCN] 2020). Supporting women to breastfeed will improve the quality of life for women and for children through reducing acute and chronic diseases (UNICEF 2012). The Scientific Advisory Committee on Nutrition (SCAN) recommends exclusive breastfeeding for the first 6 months or 26 weeks of life (SCAN 2018). The suck-swallow-breathe sequence that allows the newborn infant to feed is thought to be well developed by 37 weeks' gestation. Infants who are not able to coordinate this sequence, whether due to prematurity or clinical disorder, may need to be tube fed. The infants of mothers who are not able to breastfeed, or where breastfeeding is contraindicated, e.g. mothers who are HIV positive (practice in the UK), must receive a nutritionally complete infant formula that is appropriate for the age of the infant. Practices are variable; for further information about breastfeeding and mothers who are HIV positive, see https://www.laleche.org.uk/breastfeeding-hiv/. Solids should be offered from six months of age (SCAN 2018). Nutrient and energy requirements for healthy populations have been set by the government (DH 1991; SCAN 2011) (Tables 22.1a, and 22.2) and can be used as a guideline to assess the nutritional adequacy of energy, protein, vitamins, minerals and trace elements in an individual's diet. There are also recommendations concerning the amount of sugars, starch, nonstarch polysaccharides (NSP or fibre), and fats that constitute a healthy diet. There is recognition that young children may need a higher fat intake than the rest of the population in order to attain an adequate intake of energy. Recommendations for the population to lower its intake of fat do not apply before two years of age, but should be implemented after five years of age.

Feeding the premature infant

If the preterm baby is too young or too sick to breastfeed, the milk of choice is the mother's own breast milk, fed as soon after expression as possible. Preterm infants cannot tolerate the volume of expressed breast milk (EBM) that would be required to meet their nutritional requirements for growth and development.

Table 22.2 Summary table of selected dietary requirements (DH 1991). (© Crown copyright)

Age	Protein+		Sodium+		Potassium+		Vitamin C+	Calcium+	Iron+
	g/day	g/kg/day	mmol/day	mmol/kg/day	mmol/day	mmol/kg/day	mg/day	mmol/day	µmol/day
Males									
0–3 months	12.5	2.1	9	1.5	20	3.4	25	13.1	30
4–6	12.7	1.6	12	1.6	22	2.8	25	13.1	80
7–9	13.7	1.5	14	1.6	18	2.0	25	13.1	140
10–12	14.9	1.5	15	1.5	18	1.8	25	13.1	140
1–3 years	14.5	1.1	22	1.7	20	1.6	30	8.8	120
4–6	19.7	1.1	30	1.7	28	1.6	30	11.3	110
7–10	28.3	—	50	—	50	—	30	13.8	160
11–14	42.1	—	70	—	80	—	35	25.0	200
15–18	55.2	—	70	—	90	—	40	25.0	200
Females									
0–3 months	12.5	2.1	9	1.5	20	3.4	25	13.1	30
4–6	12.7	1.6	12	1.6	22	2.8	25	13.1	80
7–9	13.7	1.5	14	1.6	18	2.0	25	13.1	140
10–12	14.9	1.5	15	1.5	18	1.8	25	13.1	140
1–3 years	14.5	1.1	22	1.7	20	1.6	30	8.8	120
4–6	19.7	1.1	30	1.7	28	1.6	30	11.3	110
7–10	28.3	—	50	—	50	—	30	13.8	160
11–14	41.2	—	70	—	80	—	35	20.0	260
15–18	45.4	—	70	—	90	—	40	20.0	260

+ = RNI, Reference Nutrient Intake for protein or a vitamin or mineral. An amount of the nutrient that is enough, or more than enough, for virtually all people in a group. If the average intake of the group is at RNI, then the risk of deficiency in the group is very small.
It is important to remember that these figures are for populations, not individuals and therefore serve as a guide only.

Table 22.3a Fortifiers used for preterm infants

		per recommended dose	
		Energy (kcal)	Protein (g)
Breast milk fortifiers	Nutriprem breast milk fortifier (4.4 g/100 ml)	15	1.1
	SMA breast milk fortifier (4 g/100 ml)	17	1.4

Table 22.3b Feeds used for preterm infants

		Average composition per 100 ml	
		Energy (kcal)	Protein (g)
Preterm formulas	Nutriprem 1, Hydrolysed Nutriprem and SMA Gold Prem 1	80	2.7
Postdischarge nutrient dense formulas	Nutriprem 2, SMA Gold Prem 2	74	2.0

Table 22.4 Feeds for term infants

		Average composition per 100 ml	
		Energy (kcal)	Protein (g)
Whey-based formulas	Aptamil First, Cow and Gate 1, SMA 1	66	1.3
Casein-based formulas	Aptamil 2 Hungry, Cow and Gate 2, SMA Extra Hungry	66	1.6

Human milk fortifiers have been developed to provide additional protein, vitamins and minerals. They should be started according to local policy. Unless clinically indicated, fortified feeds are not used in preterm and surgical neonates at GOSH. Suitable products are given in Table 22.3a. Breast milk fortifiers (BMFs) meet the specific needs of preterm infants and should not be used to fortify EBM for babies born at term. If there is insufficient maternal expressed breast milk, donor expressed breast milk from a milk bank compliant with NICE recommendations can be considered as per local policy. If donor milk is not indicated then a preterm formula should be given (NICE 2010). These are highly specialised milks designed to meet the specific requirements of preterm infants. Nutritional adequacy may be achieved at a feed volume of 150 ml/kg (Table 22.3b). EBM with or without BMF and preterm formulas can be fed by tube or by mouth. On discharge from the special care unit, mothers should be encouraged to breastfeed on demand (the baby will need a multivitamin and iron supplement). If unable to do so, a nutrient-enriched postdischarge formula can be used to aid catch-up growth and bone mineralisation (Table 22.3b) (King and Tavener 2014).

Feeding the term infant

Ideally feed on demand or 150–200 ml/kg until weaning solids are established.

If mothers are unable to breastfeed, then whey-based infant formulas are recommended and can be used from birth (Table 22.4). Some mothers are swayed by advertising and prefer to use casein-based formulas when they perceive their infants to be hungry. The energy and nutrient profile of these two types of formulas are actually very similar and there is no nutritional benefit in changing from one formula to another. Some babies who do not feed well at the breast may be given their mother's EBM by bottle as a top-up.

Infants who are not breastfed should continue to receive an infant formula as the main milk drink until 12 months of age. Further information for parents/carers about breast feeding and bottle feeding may be found on the NHS website (NHS 2019).

Feed preparation and administration

Ideally infants will receive Ready to Feed (RTF) formulas when in hospital; these are sterile preparations. They need to be stored at cool temperatures, but do not need to be refrigerated. Hands should be thoroughly washed prior to feeding the infant. Warming of formulas for term infants prior to feeding is not necessary, but it is important to continue to provide feeds at the temperature that the baby is used to at home. The bottle may be put under warm running water or placed in an electric warming unit. If warm water baths are used, the bath should be cleaned and fresh water used on a regular basis according to local policy in order to avoid bacterial contamination (American Dietetic Association 2004). The water should not reach the level of the bottle's collar and the lid should not be submersed in the water. If the formula is warmed, the process should take less than 15 minutes (American Dietetic Association 2004). Microwave ovens must never be used for warming infant formulas because of the danger of formation of hot spots in the liquid (DH 1994) and overheating can reduce the activity of heat labile vitamins. The bottle cap should only be removed and the teat screwed on immediately prior to feeding the infant. The feed should be shaken to distribute the heat and to ensure that all the components are suspended. The temperature of the feed should be checked by testing a few drops on the inside of the wrist before giving to the baby. The infant formula manufacturers recommend that once opened, RTF formulas must be used within four hours. In the clinical situation, once a bottle has been warmed for feeding and the teat attached it is best practice to discard the feed once it has been at the bedside for one hour.

If the infant requires a formula that does not come in an RTF presentation, the formula will need to be reconstituted from powder. In large paediatric hospitals there will be a dedicated special feeds unit or milk room where formulas can be made up safely. In smaller paediatric units, feeds may be prepared at ward level. It is necessary to have a clean room with restricted access to personnel who are trained in the preparation of formulas. Strict protocols for reconstituting feeds must be adhered to, disinfected feed-making equipment and bottles must be made available, and adequate refrigeration of the prepared feed is necessary to ensure the microbial safety of feeds made at ward level. Guidelines for the requirements of feed-making areas are described elsewhere (Paediatric Group British Dietetic Association 2007; Watling 2014). Reconstituted feeds are not sterile and great care must be taken in their storage and handling prior to feeding. The administration of the feed to the baby is the same as described above. On discharge, mothers should be instructed how to make up a bottle of infant formula according to the manufacturer's instructions (1 level scoop of powder to 1 fluid ounce or 30 ml cooled boiled water). All feed-making equipment and bottles must be sterilised. The NHS website gives clear instructions on feed preparation at home (NHS 2022a).

Introduction of complimentary foods

In order to comply with the World Health Organization's (WHO) global recommendation on the duration of exclusive breastfeeding (WHO 2001) the current Department of Health guidelines suggest that solids (complimentary foods) should be offered from around six months of age; breast milk (or infant formula) provides all the nutrients that a baby needs until this time. Ensuring appropriate timing of complementary feeding ensures adequate development of the infant's gastrointestinal, immunological, and oromotor function. The European Society for Paediatric Gastroenterology, Hepatology and Nutrition recommends that weaning onto solid foods should begin by six months, but not before four months (Agostoni et al. 2008). Table 22.5 provides a guide for the introduction of complementary foods. Further information for parents/carers on how to feed their babies, toddlers, and older CYPs can be found on the NHS website www.nhs.uk/start4life/weaning/ (NHS 2019, 2022a). Each baby should be assessed on its need for solids individually. Some babies will not need solids until six months of age, whereas others may benefit from their introduction from four months (17 weeks) of age. It is recommended that preterm infants should be given solids sometime between five and eight months from their acutal birth date, (King and Tavener 2014), provided they have appropriate signs of readiness – for more information see www.bliss.org.uk. A suitable time frame of introduction would be that infants between 6–8 months of age should receive complementary foods 2–3 times a day, increasing to 3–4 times daily between 9–11 months. Additional, low-sugar, nutritious snacks should also be offered 1–2 times per day from 12–24 months of age https://www.who.int/health-topics/complementary-feeding#tab=tab_1. Baby-led weaning, traditional puree led weaning, or a combination of both, are all appropriate strategies for complementary feeding and should be decided by informed parental/ carer choice. Infants must be supervised when eating with all feeding strategies and only appropriate nutritious finger foods of correct size and texture should be offered. Foods should not added to bottle feeds. Salt must not be added to weaning foods at any time. A high salt intake may be associated with hypertension, heart disease, and stroke later in life. The government has made recommendations on the maximum daily salt consumption in CYPs: less than 1 g for infants aged up to 12 months; 2 g for one to three year olds; 3 g for four to six year olds; 5 g for 7–11 year olds; 6 g for CYPs over 11 years (NHS 2021).

To prevent dental caries, sugar should not be routinely added to complementary foods. Babies should be offered a variety of savoury and bitter flavours from the onset of feeding complementary foods and throughout childhood so they accept a wide range of flavours. Bitter flavours may need to be introduced more frequently before acceptance is achieved but this should be encouraged. White/brown sugar, or naturally derived sweet syrups such as maple syrup and date syrup, should not be added to foods given to infants and avoided /minimised wherever possible throughout childhood. All sugar and natural sugary syrups are cariogenic and, in addition, honey is contraindicated for infants under one year old as it may contain *Clostridium botulinum* spores. Infants should not be offered bottles or beakers of sugary drinks or any pure fruit juice offered. After 1 year of age drinks should have no added sugar and be well diluted to approx. 1:10 dilution. Water should be offered wherever possible in place of juices, especially in between meals.

The British Society of Allergy and Clinical Immunology (BSACI) currently recommend that infants with a known risk factor for food allergy (such as early onset atopic dermatitis or an existing food allergy) should be introduced to cooked egg and peanut (no added sugar smooth butter or ground) from 4 months of age followed by all allergens (https://www.bsaci.org/professional-resources/resources/early-feeding-guidelines/). Infants with a family member with food allergy or no risk of food allergy should include cooked egg and peanut (and then all allergens) at 6 months of age (not before 4 months). Whole nuts should be avoided until 5 years of age due to choking risk. More information on choking hazards during complimentary feeding can be found at https://www.nhs.uk/start4life/weaning/safe-weaning/choking/.

When infants are admitted to hospital for prolonged periods it is essential to start complementary feeding (if safe and medically appropriate). Infants should have access to highchairs at mealtimes, and age-appropriate spoons, bowls, and feeding cups should be used. If deemed necessary for high risk infants it may be safer from a microbiological view to give infants in hospital commercial weaning foods because they are sterile. However, there may be paediatric units that can safely provide infants with freshly cooked pureed and finger foods which should be prioritised if available. If the baby is already established on solids it is important to maintain their normal feeding routine as far as possible when in hospital.

Table 22.5 Complementary feeding for infants not at risk of allergies

	Foods	Milk
First stage Begin around 6 months, not before 4 months (17 weeks) of age	Smooth pureed or mashed fruit, vegetables, potatoes, baby cereals and soft and appropriate finger foods when the infant is able to grasp	Breast feeds or minimum 600 ml infant formula
Second stage 6–9 months	In addition to the above, mashed textures with soft lumps: meat, fish, cheese, well-cooked egg, pulses; cereals: rice, pasta, bread, suitable breakfast cereals	Breast feeds or 500–600 ml infant formula[a]
Third stage 9–12 months	Minced and chopped 'family foods' incorporating all of the above	Breast feeds or 500–600 ml infant formula[a]

[a] Follow-on formulas are not a necessary progression for infant formula fed babies. They can be used as an additional source of iron in babies after 6 months of age whose diet is deplete in iron-rich foods. Follow- on formula should not be used as a sole source of nutrition.

A schedule for the introduction of solids is given in Table 22.5.

1	Whole cow's milk	Pasteurised whole cow's milk is low in iron and should not be used as the main milk drink before 1 year of age. It can be used to cook and in cereal etc.
2	Semi-skimmed milk	Is lower in fat and energy than whole cow's milk; it may be used after two years of age if the child has an adequate intake of energy from food.
3	Water	Formula-fed infants may need additional water in some conditions; exclusively breastfed babies rarely need fluids other than breast milk; water given as a drink from a bottle for infants under six months must be either sterile or boiled and cooled; drinking water from a cup or beaker does not have to be boiled for infants over six months of age. It should be offered at each meal time during complementary feeding.
4	'Baby' juices	Should be avoided where possible due to their sugar content.
5	Squashes, juices, cordials, fizzy drinks	Should not be given to infants; their use in older children should be confined to meal times because of their high sugar content. Dilute in a ratio of 1:10 where appropriate.

From six months of age infants should be introduced to drinking from an open cup or beaker with each meal or snack. Bottle feeding should be reduced and discouraged from one year of age. Teeth should be cleaned after milk feeding in the evening before bedtime.

Diet throughout childhood and adolescence

By the time infants have reached their first birthday they should be able to take the family diet, albeit in a mashed-up form. Children need to be offered new tastes and textures to enable them to take a wide and varied diet that will provide them with the energy and nutrients needed for continued growth and development. Table 22.6 shows the food groups that meals for CYPs should be selected from. A healthy balanced diet for most CYPs is one rich in starchy carbohydrates, fruits, and vegetables with moderate amounts of meat and alternative protein foods, milk, and dairy foods. Most CYPs will not be able to meet their energy requirements for the day from the three main meals alone; they will need between-meal snacks. Care needs to be taken that these snacks do not rely on foods that are high in fat, sugar, and salt, e.g. crisps, biscuits, and chocolate, although these foods need not be banned and indeed can be useful sources of energy in sick CYPs who have small appetites. There are no mandatory standards for hospital meals for CYPs, but the government has given guidance on the menu choices that should be available for CYPs in hospital and acknowledges that they need between-meal snacks (NHS Estates 2003). Age-appropriate portion sizes are described elsewhere (Watling 2014). It is important that the environment in which meals are served is conducive to eating. Mealtimes should not be a solitary experience; CYPs will be more likely to try new foods and take a wider variety if they are eating with other people who are enjoying their food. Parents/carers friends and family should be encouraged to join the CYP at mealtimes. Furniture, cutlery, and crockery should be age appropriate.

Opportunities to provide dietary advice

Hospitalisation is an opportunity for healthcare workers to offer general advice to parents and indeed to CYPs. Health promotion

Table 22.6 Foods for CYPs

Food group	Examples	Comment
Cereals and starches	Bread, chapatti, pitta bread, rice, pasta, couscous, breakfast cereals, potatoes, sweet potatoes, yams, plantain	Meals should be based on these high-energy nutritious foods. Whole-grain varieties should be included to improve fibre intake.
Fruits and vegetables	Apples, bananas, pears, peaches, plums, satsumas, kiwi fruit, mango; broccoli, carrots, cabbage, green beans, sweet corn, peas, tomatoes	Aim for five portions a day to provide vitamins, minerals and antioxidants – portion size will depend on the age of the child. Fruit juice can be counted as one of the daily portions of fruit. The vitamin C content will help absorption of iron from breakfast cereals, green leafy vegetables and pulses.
Milk and dairy foods	Milk, cheese, fromage frais, yoghurt	Three portions a day will provide adequate calcium. From five years of age lower fat varieties should be used.
Meat, fish and alternatives	Meat, poultry, fish, eggs, nuts, pulses, e.g. lentils, dhal, chick peas, beans	Two to three portions a day will provide adequate protein and iron. At least two portions of fish per week is recommended, one of which should be oily. Oily fish (mackerel, salmon, sardines) contain beneficial omega 3 fatty acids. Boys may have up to four portions of oily fish per week; girls should have no more than two portions per week.
Drinks	Milk, water, fruit juice	Children need six to eight drinks a day, which should include 350 ml milk. To reduce its cariogenicity fruit juice should be given at mealtimes and diluted for young children to reduce its acidity and sugar content.
Fats and sugars	Biscuits, cakes, pastries, chocolate, ice cream, crisps, butter, margarine, oil	Can be offered as extra treats but should not replace the more nutritious foods described above. CYPs who are overweight should cut down on these high-fat, high-sugar foods.

opportunities must be grasped should they arise. Educational opportunities, which include information giving and counselling, will help to involve parents and empower CYPs in health decisions, in this case related to their nutritional needs. Childhood obesity is on a grand scale; nearly a third of CYPs aged 2–15 are overweight or obese (Health and Social Care Information Centre 2015). An admission to hospital might present an opportunity to discuss healthy eating: The UK government has an action plan for tackling childhood obesity in England (https://www.gov.uk/government/publications/childhood-obesity-a-plan-for-action).

Table 22.7 Sip feeds (oral nutritional supplements) for children

		Per 100 ml	
		Energy (kcal)	Protein (g)
Standard	PaediaSure	101	2.8
Increased energy/nutrient density	Frebini Energy	150	3.8
	Fortini	150	3.4
	PaediaSure Plus	151	4.2
	PaediSure Plus Juice[a]	150	4.2
	Resource Junior	150	3.0

[a] Does not contain any fat and therefore must not be used as a sole source of nutrition.

Continuing care

Some CYPs with complex needs may need a continuing care package delivered outside a hospital setting. A continuing care package will be required when a CYP has needs arising from disability, accident, or illness that cannot be met by existing universal or specialist services (Department for Health and Social Care 2016). For this population, nutritional care is essential, they may need assistance to ensure continuation of eating and drinking to meet their requirements. The range of care includes offering advice about diet, supervision and help with eating, and the use of other means of providing nutrition, such as parental or nasogastric feeding. The level of need is assessed, and care is planned to meet that need.

Supplementary feeding
Sip feeds

If CYPs have a poor appetite they will get insufficient energy and nutrients from the food that they eat and will experience a faltering in their growth. They may benefit from a sip feed (oral nutritional supplement) and a number are available for one to six year olds to enhance nutritional intake. The liquid ready-to-drink sip feeds are listed (Table 22.7) and these come in a variety of flavours.

There are no sip feeds specifically designed for those over six years of age. The above paediatric sip feeds can be given, or adult sip feeds may be used with caution. It is important to take into account the intake of food and drink to make sure that the total diet is nutritionally adequate and that intakes of protein, electrolytes, vitamins, and minerals are not excessive. It may be useful to supplement the diet with commercial drinks, such as milk shakes, to provide a source of energy, protein, and calcium, but these are not nutritionally complete.

Enteral feeds

All CYPs who are unable to feed adequately by mouth will require supplementary enteral feeding: enteral feeding may provide total nutritional requirements; or be used to supplement a poor oral intake. Enteral nutrition may be delivered via orogastric, nasogastric, gastrostomy, nasojejunal, or jejunostomy routes and guidelines for administration are given below:

- Infants: Feed volume 150–200 ml/kg/day. Infants should be fed either EBM or normal infant formula during the first year of life. If the infant has increased requirements that cannot be satisfied by increasing the feed volume, EBM and infant formula may be fortified to improve the energy and nutrient profile. Alternatively, commercial feeds may be used (Table 22.8).

Table 22.8 Enteral feeds for infants

		Per 100 ml	
		Energy (kcal)	Protein (g)
Standard	Expressed breast milk	69	1.3
	Infant formula	66	1.3
Increased energy and nutrient density	EBM + 3% infant formula	84	1.6
	15% infant formula	74	1.4
	SMA High Energy	100	2.6
	Infatrini	100	2.6
	Similac High Energy	100	2.6

Table 22.9 Enteral feeds for children

		per 100 ml	
		Energy (kcal)	Protein (g)
Standard	Frebini (8–30 kg)	100	2.5
	Nutrini (8–20 kg)	100	2.8
	PaediaSure (8–30 kg)	101	2.8
	Tentrini (21–45 kg)	100	3.3
Increased energy/nutrient density	Frebini Energy (8–30 kg)	150	3.8
	Nutrini Energy (8–20 kg)	150	4.0
	PaediaSure Plus (8–30 kg)	150	4.2
	Tentrini Energy (21–45 kg)	150	4.9

All feeds are available with added fibre.

- CYPs weighing 8–45 kg: Feed volume 85–110 ml/kg/day. There are a number of commercial feeds designed for children in this weight range. The feed manufacturers state the age range for which their feed is suitable, but there is some flexibility in which feed to use in a particular clinical situation. Some examples are given (Table 22.9). Some of these feeds are also available with added fibre.
- CYPs weighing > 45 kg: Feed volume 50–70 ml/kg/day. There are no commercial feeds designed for this age group. Adult enteral formulas may be used but care is needed to regularly check protein, electrolyte, vitamin, and mineral status to ensure that intakes are not excessive. Alternatively, paediatric enteral feeds can be used and fortified where necessary to improve the energy and protein profile.

Breastfeeding

Breastfeeding is the most suitable source of nutrition for the new born baby and the advantages for the baby and the mother are very well recognised. These include bonding of the mother and baby, the unique 'tailor-made' nutrient composition of breast milk, the reduction of infection owing to a range of immune factors in the milk, and the convenience of having the feed available at all times (Henschel and Inch 1996; Shaw and Lawson 2007). The mother too will find that she may lose weight more easily and regain her pre-pregnancy shape more quickly (UNICEF/WHO 1994). Research suggests that there is less risk of premenopausal breast and ovarian cancer and hip fractures in women who breastfeed (UNICEF/WHO 1994). WHO now recommends exclusive breastfeeding for the first six months of life for most healthy term babies (WHO 2001), and offers 10 factors to consider regarding breastfeeding (WHO 2015).

The global UNICEF/WHO Baby Friendly Initiative was launched in June 1991 and in the UK in November 1994. The 'Ten Steps to Successful Breast Feeding' formed the basis of this initiative, and hospitals have to demonstrate that they fully implement the steps and comply with the International Code on the Marketing of Breast Milk Substitutes (WHO 1981). There is no initiative for dedicated paediatric units at present, but the RCN document 'Promoting Optimal Breast Feeding in Children's Wards and Departments, Guidance for Good Practice' (RCN 2020) gives excellent guidelines and a checklist to enable the formulation of a policy that will provide a framework for supporting breast feeding. Ongoing, regular teaching for staff and the assistance for mothers at the bedside are essential (Lang 2002). It is important for staff to know that there are some contraindications to breastfeeding and mothers who are unable to breastfeed their baby must also be given support.

The lactation process commences shortly after the placenta separates during the third stage of labour. Where possible, the baby should be encouraged to suckle the breast as soon as possible after delivery. However, in some instances, this may not be possible because of the poor condition of the baby or because of a congenital anomaly.

Colostrum is produced from 12–16 weeks gestation; this is the 1st stage of lactogenesis. Some mums express colostrum pre birth. This clear liquid is high in protective immunoglobulins (especially IgA and IgE) and the sugar content helps to prevent hypoglycaemia. It is also a mild laxative so assists the baby to pass meconium.

Milk starts to be produced around the third to fourth day postpartum, but maternal stress and anxiety can delay the process. There are two main hormones involved: prolactin produces the milk in the milk ducts, and oxytocin expels it down the lactiferous sinuses to the nipple. The latter, known as the 'let down' reflex, occurs in response to the stimulation of the areola and the mother seeing and cuddling her baby. UNICEF (2012, 2013), Bliss (www.bliss.org.uk), and the RCN (2020) all recommend that the mother is able to express close to her baby as this helps with milk production. When the mother is not able to be present with her baby, this reflex can be replicated by her looking at her baby's photograph, or by her holding a special toy or piece of clothing while she expresses her milk.

The first milk produced by the breast at a feed is the fore milk and this is rather like a sugary drink, providing fluid to maintain hydration. Once the baby has settled on the breast and started rhythmic sucking and swallowing (at approximately one suck per second), the milk becomes richer and contains fat and protein – the hind milk. It is essential that the baby suckles long enough at each breast in turn to gain the benefits of both fore and hind milk.

Breast milk contains all the vitamins, minerals, and trace elements needed for growth and development in a bioavailable form. Together with its anti-infective properties, growth factors, lipase to aid fat digestion, and a host of other unique components it has many advantages over infant formula. In addition, it is also warm and always ready for the hungry baby.

Supporting the breastfeeding mother

The more the baby is able to suckle at the breast, the greater the volume of milk produced, so regular feeding is essential to establish the lactation process. If the baby cannot suckle, then breast milk must be regularly expressed to replicate the stimulation offered by demand breastfeeding. The mother will need much support and encouragement during this establishment phase of breastfeeding, particularly if she is separated from the baby and/or if her baby is unwell.

Practical assistance includes:

- Arranging for the mother to see a midwife regularly.
- Providing privacy when she is breastfeeding.
- Providing a suitable chair so that her back is supported and that her feet touch the floor.
- Providing a pillow for her lap so that the baby can lay more comfortably while feeding.
- Ensuring that she has a varied and well-balanced diet and drinks plenty of fluids.
- Encouraging her to rest as much as possible.

Demand feeding should be promoted whenever possible.

Leaflets should be available to give advice about breastfeeding. Links with the community team are essential, particularly when lactation and breastfeeding is not yet fully established. National support agencies, e.g. National Childbirth Trust, La Leche League, and the Association of Breast Feeding Mothers are also a great help, and mothers may wish to contact them.

Expressing breast milk

There are many special circumstances in the paediatric environment which make the establishment of breastfeeding more difficult. In some instances the mother cannot be with her baby for 24 hours a day because of her postpartum condition, social, or geographical reasons. Some babies have anatomical anomalies that may prevent the baby sucking at the breast. These include anomalies requiring surgery, e.g. oesophageal atresia, bowel obstruction or bowel motility problems; craniofacial anomalies like cleft palate or micrognathia; prematurity and the need for ongoing respiratory support; cardiac and renal conditions where fluids are restricted and breast milk alone cannot provide adequate nutrition; some rare metabolic disorders may preclude breastfeeding.

Some neonates need multidisciplinary input and a long period of hospitalisation, making it difficult for the mother and baby to establish a pattern of feeding. If the baby is unable to feed at the breast, it is important that lactation is established by the mother expressing her milk. Milk can be expressed either by hand or by using a breast pump. Hand expression is usually gentler than a breast pump and can be done anywhere. Hand expression appears to produce a better oxytocin response and milk ejection reflex (Renfrew et al. 2009). There are several types of pump available, both manual and electric. The mother will need much support with this, and she will need easy access to a pump in a congenial environment. Careful handwashing before expression is essential, and equipment should be sterilised before use.

Enteral feeding

Enteral feeding is the means of supplying nutrients directly to the gastrointestinal tract. The term is used to describe orogastric, nasogastric, nasojejunal, gastrostomy, and jejunostomy tube feeding. It is the preferred method of providing nutritional support to CYPs with a functioning gastrointestinal tract who fulfil the following criteria (Johnson 2014):

1. Inability to consume an adequate oral intake due to impaired sucking and swallowing, e.g. neurological and degenerative disorders, ventilated children.
2. Anorexia associated with chronic illness, e.g. malignancy, congenital heart disease, renal disease.
3. Increased nutritional requirements, e.g. cystic fibrosis, liver disease, short bowel syndrome, congenital heart disease, and increased work of breathing.
4. Congenital anomalies, e.g. oesophageal fistula, orofacial malformations.
5. Primary disease management, e.g. glycogen storage disease, very long chain fatty acid disorders.

A careful selection of the appropriate feeding route and equipment is essential to ensure optimal nutritional support and patient adherence. Nasogastric tube feeding is most commonly employed as a convenient and safe method of feed administration. However, it might not be suitable if long-term feeding is required or for patients with facial/oesophageal structural abnormalities, where gastrostomy tube feeding may be the route of choice. Nasojejunal tube feeding may be necessary if there is a significant risk of aspiration and delayed gastric emptying or jejunal tube feeding, if required for the long term.

Feeds may be given by bolus or pump-controlled continuous or intermittent feeding. Bolus feeding has considerable advantages as it mimics a physiologically normal feeding pattern and can be adapted to fit in with mealtimes. However, continuous feeds may be better tolerated in some circumstances and overnight feeding may release the daytime for other activities. Caution should be used when bolus feeding into the jejunum as bolus feeding is contraindicated due to the limited capacity of the jejunum.

Many of the problems associated with enteral feeding are preventable with a committed multidisciplinary team. It should consist of the CYP's dietician, paediatrician, and primary nurse. Nutrition and stoma nurse specialists may help with practical aspects of the CYP's care.

All health professionals and parents/carers should be aware of the negative aspects of enteral feeding and try to alleviate them. Hygienic storage and handling of both feed and feeding systems are essential in order to prevent microbial contamination and subsequent complications, such as diarrhoea, vomiting, malabsorption, or pneumonia. Safety guidelines have been developed by the National Institute for Health and Care Excellence [NICE] (2012) and should be referred to. All hospitals should have appropriate training packages in place for patients being discharged with non-oral enteral feed devices.

In collaboration with speech and language therapists and occupational therapists an oral stimulation programme should be developed to maintain and improve oromotor skills. The preservation of pleasant associations in connection with food and feeding is essential in order to avoid hypersensitivity to touch and taste and will facilitate the reintroduction of oral feeding if/when appropriate.

If enteral feeding is still necessary on discharge, it is essential that the parents/carers are fully trained so that they are competent in all aspects of feeding and equipment involved so that feeds can be administered safely. Feeds and feeding equipment are prescribed by the GP and are delivered directly to the CYP''s home by home enteral feeding companies. These companies will also provide an enteral feeding pump as needed. The community dietician and community paediatric nursing team, where available, can provide extra support to the families and so should be referred to before discharge.

Parenteral nutrition

Parenteral nutrition (PN) is the administration of nutrition directly into the bloodstream, therefore bypassing the gut. It is the method of providing nutrition for CYPs who, for a variety of reasons, cannot absorb enough energy and nutrients to support normal growth and development and maintain health and life (Hill and Long 2001). The need for PN may be on a short- or long-term basis, depending on the underlying medical condition. PN should be used only when feeding via the oral or enteral route cannot meet nutritional needs, as PN is an invasive treatment and can lead to physiological complications (Pennington 2000). Some CYPs require PN to supplement their nutritional requirements, while others may rely on PN as their sole source of energy and nutrients.

The following are all indications for PN:

- Prematurity.
- Autoimmune enteropathy.
- Inflammatory bowel disease.
- Intestinal failure due to: short gut, hollow visceral myopathy, radiation and/or cytotoxic therapy, postoperative paralytic ileus, protracted diarrhoea.
- Liver disease.
- Extensive burns.
- Severe trauma.

The nutrition support team

A Nutrition Support Team (NST) usually comprises a medical consultant with an interest in nutrition, a clinical nurse specialist, a specialist dietician, a specialist pharmacist, and a biochemist. The quality of care for CYPs requiring nutritional support is improved through the involvement of a NST (Hudson 2000). The NST should monitor the usage and effectiveness of PN in the hospital. There should be assessment by the team members as to the appropriateness of the referral, including nutritional assessment, height and weight measurement with subsequent plotting on a centile chart, other anthropometry as necessary, type of intravenous (IV) access available, gastrointestinal function, accurate fluid balance, diagnosis, and history of weight loss.

Regular ward rounds and discussion of the CYP's overall condition should be carried out in participation with the medical team managing the treatment for their underlying illness. As and when the CYP's condition, oral, or enteral intake improves, the NST will recommend how to reduce the PN until it can be discontinued.

Nutrient solutions

For a CYP requiring PN, it is important to establish a regimen that will provide adequate energy and nutrients to allow for tissue repair, as well as normal growth and development. The solutions are made up of amino acids, glucose, lipids, electrolytes, trace elements, and vitamins. Parenteral nutrition may be provided as bespoke solutions or as standard solutions with set composition.

Provision of PN

PN must be prescribed by a doctor. The NST will advise on the CYP's suitability for standard or bespoke PN. If bespoke, the prescription for preparing the PN is produced by the pharmacist and is compounded under sterile conditions in a laminar flow unit under supervision of the pharmacist (Hart 2008; Lamb and Dougherty 2008). The conditions in which PN is produced are strictly regulated due to the risks associated with contamination of the solutions by pathogens (Lee and Allwood 2001).

PN can be administered as a cyclical or continuous infusion. Cyclical PN is an ongoing treatment but it is routinely stopped for a set period of time, the length of which depends on the condition of the CYP. It is used for children from three months of age who are on a stable PN regimen and who perhaps can tolerate some enteral intake. It is particularly useful when the need for PN is long term, as is the case for CYPs who are receiving PN at home. The time spent off PN (usually during the day) allows the CYP and their family to live as normally as possible, given that activity is not as restricted as it is when the PN infusion is in progress. The infusion rate of cyclical PN must be steadily reduced over the last hour of the infusion to avoid rebound hypoglycaemia once the infusion stops. Depending on the functions of the IV infusion pump, this reduction can be in two stages, i.e. at two successive manually reduced rates at half-hour intervals or perhaps by an automatic gradual reduction in rate throughout the hour.

Continuous PN is a 24-hour continuous treatment. It is used when commencing PN treatment and when warranted by the condition of the CYP.

Methods of administration

PN can be administered either peripherally or centrally. It is important to determine how long the CYP is likely to require PN and consider the most appropriate route of administration. Peripheral lines should only be used for a very short time due to the potential for extravasation injury caused by the components of the PN. The maximum glucose concentration for peripheral use in children is recommended to be 10–12.5% (Sari and Rollins 1999). The use of peripheral lines for PN therefore reduces the amount of energy, in the form of glucose, which can be given. There is still some debate over the maximum glucose concentration permitted via the peripheral route (some centres will allow 20% glucose); therefore, local policies may differ.

CYPs may receive peripheral PN in certain circumstances, e.g. when awaiting insertion of a central venous access device (CVAD) or when receiving antibiotic therapy for a CVAD infection.

There are a variety of CVADs available and one must select a device suiting short- or long-term use. If it is anticipated that the CYP is unlikely to require PN for more than one month, then a peripherally inserted central catheter (PICC) may be useful.

If it is evident that the CYP is likely to require long-term PN, then a skin tunnelled central venous catheter, such as a Broviac or Hickman line, can be used. If possible a dedicated nutrition line should be established in order to minimise the risk of sepsis. Concurrent administration of IV fluids and medications may necessitate a double- or triple-lumen central venous catheter (DH 2001). Energy intake can be improved with the placement of a central catheter as a higher concentration glucose solution can be safely used. For further information, see Chapter 14: Intravenous and Intra-arterial Access and Infusions.

Home parenteral nutrition

When it is established that PN is likely to be required for at least two months, the option of going home on PN treatment is considered (Hill and Long 2001). Value rationality underpins discussion surrounding discharging the CYP on home parenteral nutrition (HPN), with the aim of achieving an improved quality of life at its core (Hill and Long 2001; Wang and Bernhard 2004). A psychosocial assessment is therefore included in the initial steps in this process. The importance of ensuring the CYP and family receive the support they require from local services at home should not be underestimated. The lifestyle of families with a child who is dependent on PN is altered significantly. Daily life must be organised such that the routine of cyclical PN is sustained and parents/carers need to readily respond to any possible problems consequential to PN treatment, including those associated with the CYP having an indwelling CVAD.

Prior to discharge, the clinical nurse specialist should carry out a home assessment, which is essential to ascertain that PN treatment can be carried out safely in the home setting. Plans can then be put in place for any necessary adaptations to the home. A constant supply of mains electricity to the home is necessary to supply power for a dedicated fridge for storage of PN, and for the IV infusion pumps. There must be sufficient space and suitable washing facilities available such that the Aseptic Non-Touch Technique (ANTT) or similar locally approved aseptic technique can be strictly adhered to.

A home care company can be used to supply the nutrients and equipment required for HPN once the pharmacist and the medical consultant have finalised an 'all-in-one' bag PN prescription. Parents/carers need to undergo an intensive training programme with the clinical nurse specialist. The HPN training programme must be carefully timed such that on completion of the training programme, all factors in the discharge planning process are in place, ready for the CYP to be discharged straight home. A discharge planning meeting should be held whereby the specific healthcare and social needs of the child and family are made explicit and the commencement of a shared care arrangement is formally marked. Funding needs to be identified and put in place.

The responsibility placed on the parent/carer is onerous and there are a number of very practical issues that need to be addressed. While the PN infusion is running overnight, parents'/carers' sleep can be interrupted by the CYP needing frequent micturition due to large volume of fluid intake. Parents/carers must also attend to the IV infusion pump when it alarms, to investigate and correct the cause for the alarm. The long-term impact of the responsibility of carrying out highly technical nursing care at home, the emotional stress of the fear of septicaemia, and the physical stress placed on the parents/carers necessitates the need for ongoing support from local services (Hill and Long 2001).

Sham feeding

This term is used to describe feeding a baby or young child with a cervical oesophagostomy by mouth while giving nutrition via a gastrostomy at the same time (DeBear 1996). The main indication for forming an oesophagostomy is in the baby with oesophageal atresia where a complete primary repair of the oesophagus is not possible. This is a rare situation today, as every effort is made to correct the defect by connecting the two blind ends of the oesophagus together in the primary repair.

An oesophagostomy is an artificial opening of the oesophagus onto the surface of the neck. It is formed by bringing the upper blind end of the oesophagus out onto the surface of the neck, thus forming a stoma. This allows drainage of the nasopharyngeal secretions and sham feeds. The oesophagostomy is closed when the oesophageal atresia repair is done, usually when the baby is aged six to nine months old.

The advantage of giving sham feeds is that it allows the baby to develop normal oral feeding behaviour. Sham feeds enable the infant to establish feeding by developing and maintaining sucking reflexes. Infants who need to remain nil by mouth until their corrective surgery is carried out do not experience normal oral feeding and this can lead to difficulties with sucking and swallowing after surgery and the development of oral hypersensitivity and food aversion.

Breastfeeding may be established once the oesophagostomy has been fashioned, or formula milk may be given by bottle. The milk will drain out of the oesophagostomy. Whenever possible the sham feed should be given at the same time as the gastrostomy feed so that the baby learns to associate a full stomach with the oral feeds.

The child may be discharged home, depending on their condition and tolerance of feeds, where sham feeding may continue if the parents/carers can cope with this care. The child's Health Visitor, GP, and Community Paediatric Nurse must be informed if sham feeds are to be given at home. The parents/carers will need much support and should be able to contact the ward at any time for advice.

Useful organisations and websites

Some useful website addresses for support of breastfeeding and infant feeding follow:

Breastfeeding

Association of Breastfeeding Mothers (ABM): https://abm.me.uk (accessed 18 July 2022)

La Leche League (Great Britain): www.laleche.org.uk (accessed 18 July 2022)

National Childbirth Trust (NCT): https://www.nct.org.uk/ (accessed 18 July 2022)

World Health Organization (WHO): https://www.who.int/western-pacific/health-topics/breastfeeding (accessed 18 July 2022)

Artificial feeding

PINNT: A support group for people receiving artificial nutrition: http://pinnt.com/ (accessed 18 July 2022).

BAPEN: A charity raising awareness about nutrition in hospital and the wider community: www.bapen.org.uk (accessed 18 July 2022).

The Great Ormond Street Hospital Manual of Children and Young People's Nursing Practices

Principles table 22.1 Use of breast pumps

Principle	Rationale
1 The benefits of human milk for preterm infants have been clearly described (Lucas et al. 1992). Advantages include not only long-term benefits in developmental indices, blood pressure, and lipoprotein profile, but a decreased risk of infection and neonatal necrotising enterocolitis (Lucas and Cole 1990; Lucas et al. 1992; Singhal et al. 2001; Singhal et al. 2004). a) Give the mother much encouragement to breastfeed, supplying her with information about its advantages. b) Encourage the mother to drink regularly (at least 8–10 glasses of fluid daily), and eat a good balanced and nutritious diet. c) Encourage the mother to rest and take some regular exercise. d) Privacy is usually appreciated while expressing, so provide a single room and/or curtains. e) Mothers must be taught correct use of the breast pump and shown how to safely handle their expressed breast milk. f) Information is available from the Bliss website and should be given to all mothers who are expressing. It provides information about hand and pump expressing and also about common problems encountered when expressing for a sick baby.	c) Sufficient rest, fluid, and a balanced diet create the optimum conditions for the initiation and maintenance of lactation. e) To initiate and maintain lactation if the baby is unable to suckle. Incorrect use of the breast pump may result in breast and nipple trauma. f) To provide information. Go to www.bliss.org.uk.
2 Single patient, reusable expressing kits are used at GOSH. These must be sterilised prior to use, then washed and sterilised after each use. They can be used for the duration of the baby's stay and after discharge. An aseptic nontouch technique should be adopted when handling expressed breast milk (EBM) (Rowley et al. 2010).	2 To avoid contaminating the EBM. For further information, see Chapter 13: Infection Prevention and Control.
3 Mothers should be given written and verbal advice on personal hygiene, and the collection and decanting of EBM (Rathwell and Shaw 2010).	3 Information can be confusing to mothers at times of stress. Written information can also help understanding or encourage questions to be asked.
4 A sterile collecting kit and sterile bottle in which to place EBM should be used each time milk is expressed.	4 Use of sterile equipment is essential when handling EBM (Balmer et al. 1997).
5 a) Milk should be expressed into sterile single use bottles. b) Mothers should be reminded not to overfill the bottles.	5 a) Sterile bottles should be used once only. b) Breast milk expands as it freezes.
6 a) Ideally milk should be expressed directly into the bottles which are to be used for feeding the baby. If this is not practical because of the small quantity and/or frequency of feeds required, sterile syringes and occlusion caps should be used. b) Feeds of 20 ml or less should be drawn up into a sterile syringe and capped with a sterile occlusion cap. c) Once the milk has been expressed, the mother should fill in the provided label. Details should include the ward, baby's name and hospital number and the mother should sign the label and provide details of any medications she is taking. Once complete, she should add her signature. A tamper evident sticker needs to be placed over the lid and down the side of the bottle.	6 To prevent contamination of the EBM. To facilitate the safe handling of small volumes of EBM. c) To ensure that the EBM is given to the correct infant. Breast milk is classified as a body fluid similar to blood or plasma, and contact with any type of body fluid carries a risk for transmission of infection (Drenckpohl et al. 2007; Zeilhofer et al. 2009).
7 Breast pumps should be maintained, cleaned with Clinell wipes after each use and sent for deep clean every 2 weeks.	7 To ensure safe and disinfected pumps are in use at all times.

Chapter 22 Nutrition and feeding

Principles table 22.2 Freshly expressed breast milk

Principle	Rationale
1 EBM is stored on the respective ward. If the amount stored is more than 20 bottles mothers are encouraged to take the milk home to store in their own freezers. Under exceptional circumstances EBM can be stored for a short time in the special feeds unit freezers, by arrangement with the unit manager. If a mother is expressing large volumes of milk or their baby is not feeding the option for donation should be discussed with them.	1 To enable fresh EBM to be used as much as possible (Lucas et al. 1992; Balmer et al. 1997).
2 The temperature of a refrigerator storing breast milk should be maintained at 2–4°C (Balmer et al. 1997).	2 To ensure safe refrigeration of the EBM.
3 The temperature should be monitored and recorded daily.	3 To provide an audit trail and ensure safe temperature control.
4 Once the milk has been expressed the lid should be replaced and the bottle placed in the refrigerator/freezer immediately.	4 To prevent contamination of the EBM.
5 All EBM must be handled using an aseptic nontouch technique (Rowley et al. 2010).	5 To prevent contamination of the EBM.
6 The bottle containing EBM should be opened once only and all the milk decanted at that time.	6 To reduce the risk of contamination with multiple openings of the bottle.
7 Feeds of 20 ml or less should be placed in a sterile syringe and capped with a sterile occlusion cap.	7 Smaller volumes of feed are more easily and accurately decanted if placed in syringes. An occlusion cap will prevent contamination.
8 Babies who are having continuous feeds of EBM should have the feed administered by: a) A 60 ml syringe with a maximum of 4 hours of feed. b) The bottle containing the feed should be agitated 1–2 hourly. c) In both instances, the EBM syringe or bottle should be changed 4 hourly.	8 a) To prevent colonisation of the EBM with bacteria. b) To disperse the fat throughout the feed. c) To prevent colonisation of the EBM with bacteria.
9 Each feed must be labelled using the baby's identification labels, and the date and time (Balmer et al. 1997).	9 To ensure that the EBM is given to the correct infant.
10 EBM feeds in syringes can be placed in cardboard trays after labelling and placed in the ward milk feed refrigerator.	10 To prevent the EBM falling off the shelves of the refrigerator.
11 The EBM in the refrigerator should be used as soon as possible after it has been divided.	11 To prevent colonisation of the EBM with bacteria.
12 It must be kept in the main section of the refrigerator until it is required. It should not be placed in the door.	12 Temperatures inside the door are higher than in the body of the refrigerator.
13 EBM should be stored at 2–4°C until used.	13 To prevent bacterial growth. This temperature is recommended for handling breast milk (Balmer et al. 1997).
14 Written guidelines should be available to assist the mothers. They should be used in conjunction with teaching by nursing staff.	14 Written guidelines help to reinforce oral advice and teaching.
15 Hand washing is essential before mothers express and handle their milk.	15 To prevent contamination of EBM from the hands.
16 Milk that is not used within 24 hours should be frozen in a designated freezer maintained at −18°C until required.	16 Frozen milk can be stored safely for three months (Balmer et al. 1997).
17 Occasionally there are instances when breastfeeding is contraindicated. These include mothers who are: a) Taking some medications. The current *British National Formulary* gives advice about prescribing in breastfeeding. b) Drug or alcohol abusers. c) HIV positive.	17 a) Some drugs transfer to the baby via EBM. b) Transmission of substances may occur. c) There is a risk of disease transmission.
18 Breast feeding is also contraindicated in babies with: a) Rare metabolic disorder of long chain fatty acid oxidation. b) Galactosaemia. c) Glucose-galactose malabsorption. d) A chylothorax. Any of the above situations should be discussed with medical staff before any decision is made.	18a a) This can cause developmental damage to the baby. b–d) Certain nutrients in EBM are contraindicated.
18 Routine bacteriology screening does not need to be carried out (Law et al. 1989).	19 This is not deemed necessary on a regular basis.

Principles table 22.3 Frozen expressed breast milk

Principle	Rationale
1 a) Fresh EBM, which is surplus to requirements for the following 24 hours, should be frozen as soon as possible after expression and stored frozen at −18°C. It can be stored at −18°C for up to three months for sick infants. b) Each syringe/bottle must be labelled with the patient name sticker, adding the date and time the milk was expressed.	1 a) To comply with recommended guidelines (Balmer et al. 1997; United Kingdom Association for Milk Banking 2022). b) To ensure correct EBM is given to the right baby once defrosted.
2 When frozen milk is required: • The oldest milk should be used first. • The milk should be left to defrost in the refrigerator or using a designated milk warmer. • The EBM bottle or syringe should be labelled with the time and date it was defrosted.	2 To ensure the EBM is defrosted safely. Rapid defrosting alters the heat labile vitamins.
3 Once defrosted, the EBM should be used within 24 hours.	
4 An aseptic nontouch technique must be used at all times by staff handling this milk (Rowley et al. 2010).	4 To prevent contamination of the EBM.
5 Milk, which is expressed outside the hospital that arrives frozen, should be placed in a designated freezer.	5 To comply with national guidelines (Balmer et al. 1997).

Principles table 22.4 Dividing and decanting expressed breast milk

Principle	Rationale
1 The division of EBM should take place on a clean surface in the breast pump room, in the ward milk feed room or at the bedside.	1 To prevent contamination of the EBM.
2 Where possible the mother should be encouraged to handle her own milk. There should be written guidelines for this procedure.	2 To minimise the handling of the EBM. Written guidelines complement oral instruction.
3 An aseptic nontouch technique must be employed whenever staff handle EBM (Rowley et al. 2010).	3 To prevent contamination of EBM.
4 To handle milk on behalf of the mother: a) An apron should be worn and hands washed thoroughly. b) Equipment should be assembled as required, e.g. sterile syringes, sterile occlusion caps, sterile quills, sterile EBM bottle, freshly expressed milk, patient name labels. c) Surface area should be cleaned, e.g. tray as used for giving IV medications, with an alcohol impregnated wipe. d) Hands should be washed thoroughly and nonsterile gloves worn. e) EBM should be drawn up, using a sterile milk straw or quill, as required into the syringes or sterile EBM bottles. f) Each syringe/bottle should be labelled with the patient name sticker, adding the date and time the milk was expressed. g) Feed(s) should be placed in the designated milk feed refrigerator. h) Feeds in syringes may be more easily accessed in a cardboard tray. i) All the feed should be decanted on one occasion. Half-decanted bottles of EBM should not be left on the wards.	4 a) To minimise the risk of infection (Rowley et al. 2010). b) To ensure all equipment is available. To minimise the risk of contamination. c)–d) To minimise the risk of contamination. e) To facilitate the use of EBM. f) To ensure correct EBM is given to the right baby within 24 hours of being expressed. g) To ensure EBM is safely stored. h) To facilitate easy use of EBM. i) To prevent contamination of open bottles of EBM.

Chapter 22 Nutrition and feeding

Principles table 22.5 Qualities of breast milk

Principle	Rationale
1 Human breast milk is the preferred source of nutrition for all infants (Sapsford 2000; Shaw and Lawson 2007).	1 It is species specific. • Provides the most appropriate balance and concentration of nutrients in a digestible form (Department of Health 1994). • Provides immunity against disease, and possibly protects against necrotising enterocolitis (NEC) and late onset sepsis (Sapsford 2000; Shaw and Lawson 2007). • There is greater enteral feed tolerance (Boyd et al. 2007) and more rapid weaning from parenteral nutrition (Lucas 1993). • Promotes the maternal–infant relationship (Lang 2002). It is always available, is at the right temperature and at no extra cost. • There is reduced risk of allergy when breast milk is exclusively used (Lucas 1993). • There are possible, but not proven, favourable effects on neuro-cognitive development (Lucas 1993; Sapsford 2000; Shaw and Lawson 2007).
2 However, breast milk may not fully meet the increased nutritional needs of the preterm infant, particularly energy, protein, sodium, calcium, phosphorus, and some vitamins (Lucas 1993; Edmond and Bahl 2007; Shaw and Lawson 2007).	
3 Fortification of expressed breast milk (EBM) can minimise these deficiencies in preterm infants (Lucas 1993; Sapsford 2000; Shaw and Lawson 2007). An extensively hydrolysed whey-based formula is sometimes used at GOSH instead of fortified EBM.	3 Breastfeeding is not usually possible in infants <34 weeks gestation; therefore, breast milk must be expressed (Lucas 1993).
4 Other babies may benefit from having their EBM fortified but their requirements will be different to those of the preterm infant. These include: • Babies who are fluid restricted, e.g. those with cardiac anomalies. • Babies who are failing to thrive due to increased requirements or losses, e.g. in malabsorptive states.	4 Preterm and term infants have different nutritional requirements.
5 When fortification is required, an aseptic nontouch technique must be used when handling the EBM (Rathwell and Shaw 2010; Rowley et al. 2010).	5 To prevent contamination of the EBM.

Principles table 22.6 Increasing nutritional intake of preterm infants

Principle	Rationale
1 The first step to improve nutritional intake should be to slowly increase the volume of EBM given.	1 Nutritional adequacy can be achieved if sufficient feed volumes are given (Shaw and Lawson 2007).
2 Well preterm babies >1.5 kg can tolerate up to 220 ml/kg (Shaw and Lawson 2007).	2 If the maximum volume of EBM tolerated provides inadequate nutrition then fortification should be considered.
3 A commercial breast milk fortifier (BMF) has the advantage over supplementing with a liquid preterm formula.	3 It will allow more of the mother's milk to be used (Lucas 1993; Shaw and Lawson 2007).
4 Supplementation with a source of energy alone is not advised (Shaw and Lawson 2007). A multinutrient BMF is recommended.	4 It will reduce the protein-energy ratio to an unacceptable level (Shaw and Lawson 2007).

Procedure guideline 22.1 Adding fortifier to EBM on the ward

Statement	Rationale
1 This procedure should be carried out as an aseptic, nontouch technique in a clean area of the ward (Rathwell and Shaw 2010; Rowley et al. 2010).	1 To prevent contamination of the feed.
2 The ward milk kitchen or a specific area should be used when available. a) It should be done as close to the feed time as possible.	2 a) To avoid loss of immunological factors. To prevent rise in osmolality of the feed, which can begin within 10 minutes of fortification (De Curtis et al. 1999).
3 The decision to fortify EBM for a preterm baby must be made by the medical consultant.	3 To ensure that addition of BMF is clinically indicated and safe.
4 The BMF must be prescribed by the medical staff on the infant's prescription chart.	4 To ensure the correct dose is given.
5 Urea and electrolyte levels must be carefully monitored.	5 Infants receiving BMF have shown raised urea, calcium, and phosphate levels.
6 Other vitamin and mineral levels may need to be routinely checked depending on which BMF is used.	6 To obtain baseline levels of these nutrients.
7 Serum levels should be repeated after two weeks and then monthly thereafter.	7 To monitor any decline in vitamin and mineral status.
8 Fortification of breast milk should be performed by a registered nurse/professional. In certain circumstances, this may also be done by the mother under supervision of a registered nurse.	8 To ensure that the prescription is accurately checked and administered.
9 Ensure that: a) The EBM is for the correct infant. b) The milk is in date. c) It is used in correct rotation. d) Milk, if frozen, is defrosted correctly (Rathwell and Shaw 2010; Balmer et al. 1997).	9 a) To ensure that this is a safe procedure. c) To prevent wastage of EBM. d) To prevent the risk of contamination of EBM.
10 The prescribed fortification is added to the correct amount of feed according to the manufacturer's instructions.	10 To ensure that the nutrient value of the feed is increased as prescribed.
11 The bottle is agitated gently.	11 To ensure an even distribution of fortifier in the breast milk.
12 The bottle is labelled and dated.	12 To ensure that the additives are recorded on the bottle and the time during which the feed can be used safely can be established.
13 The fortified EBM is fed immediately. Ideally the feed should be given within 10 minutes of fortification. a) If the fortified feed cannot be given immediately, it should be sealed and placed in the milk feed refrigerator on the ward. It must be used within 24 hours. b) Any excess defrosted EBM that has not been fortified must be discarded if not used within 24 hours. c) Any excess fresh EBM should be frozen for later use (see https://www.nhs.uk/conditions/baby/breastfeeding-and-bottle-feeding/breastfeeding/expressing-breast-milk/ (accessed 18 July 2022)).	13 To minimise bacterial growth and a rise in osmolality (De Curtis et al. 1999). a) To ensure that the feed is safely stored at the correct temperature. b) To minimise bacterial growth and prevent contamination. c) To ensure safe storage of the EBM.

Principles table 22.7 Handling of enteral feeds

Principle	Rationale
Storage	
A Sterile feeds (ready-to-use)	
1 Bottles, cans, or containers should be stored in closed, clean cupboards.	1 To keep feed container clean, dust free, and spoilage free.
2 Stock must be rotated regularly.	2 To prevent expiry dates of feed being exceeded.
3 Opened, unused sterile feeds must be discarded.	3 To prevent the contamination of opened feed containers.
B Modular feeds	
1 All modular feeds must be placed in a designated milk refrigerator (or designated area of the refrigerator if at home) immediately after arrival on the ward.	1 Ensure that the feed is stored at the recommended temperature as soon as possible.
2 The temperature of a refrigerator storing enteral feeds should be maintained at ≤4°C (Anderton 1995).	2 To ensure the safe refrigeration of enteral feeds.
3 The temperature should be monitored daily and recorded in a Temperature Log Book. This should be undertaken by housekeeping/nursing staff (or parent/carer at home) who will alert the nurse in charge to any problems.	3 To ensure that the temperature of all milk refrigerators is maintained accurately.
4 Partly decanted bottles of modular feeds must be discarded.	4 To prevent the contamination of opened bottles.
Infection control issues	
1 Good hygiene practices are essential to ensure that any feed given to a patient is safe.	1 To comply with the Food & Safety Act 1990 (Food Standards Agency 2009) and to minimise the risk of contamination. Bacterial contamination of enteral feeds may cause diarrhoea and vomiting. Contamination may also contribute to more serious infections including pneumonia and septicaemia (Anderton 1995).
2 Enteral feeds and feed administration systems must not be handled unnecessarily.	2 This minimises the risk of contamination.
3 An aseptic nontouch technique should be adhered to whenever feed administration systems are handled, including the wearing of nonsterile gloves (Rowley et al. 2010).	3 To minimise the risk of contamination. Poor hand hygiene is one of the most frequent causes of enteral feeds being significantly contaminated (Anderton 1995).
4 The feed reservoir used for continuous enteral feeding must not be topped up.	4 To prevent contamination of the feed reservoir while decanting.
5 Feeds for continuous enteral feeding should be given at room temperature. They must not be heated or given immediately from the refrigerator.	5 It is safer to give the feed at room temperature. If the feed is too hot this may damage the mucosal surface and if too cold this may cause the temperature of the baby/child to drop.
6 The feed administration set for continuous feeds must be changed every 24 hours (Anderton 1995).	6 To reduce the risk of infection

Principles table 22.8 Preparing the CYP and family (feeding tube insertion)

Principle	Rationale
1 CYPs need to be prepared for painful or uncomfortable procedures sensitively according to their needs.	1 Adequate psychological preparation is essential for both the CYP and the family in order to obtain informed consent, understanding, and co-operation.
2 Colouring booklets, training manuals and models, illustrated guides or videos can assist with these preparations (Paul et al. 1993; Holden et al. 1997).	2 Distraction techniques can help to reduce tension and anxiety during a procedure (RCN 2019).
3 Nurses or play specialist should explore the CYP's knowledge, interests, and past experience.	3 To identify the CYP's needs and plan the most appropriate method of distraction.

Principles table 22.9 Nasogastric tube feeding

Principle	Rationale
1 a) Nasogastric (NG) feeding is a method of feeding into the stomach and the common route for tube feeding. However, NG feeding can be associated with risks that must be assessed prior to initiation. The National Patient Safety Agency (NPSA, now the Patient Safety Learning Hub) recommends that the following questions should form part of a risk assessment for NG insertion (NPSA 2011): • Is nasogastric tube feeding the right decision for this patient? • Is this the right time to place the nasogastric tube and is the appropriate equipment available? • Is there sufficient knowledge/expertise available at this time to test for safe placement of the nasogastric tube? b) A nasal feeding tube (NGT) rather than an oral feeding tube (OGT) should always be inserted unless there is a documented contraindication to this procedure.	1 a) Nasogastric feeding is simple to initiate and manage and is associated with few complications if managed appropriately (Reilly 1998). However, a small but significant number of patients suffer complications and adverse effects from NG feeding (NPSA 2011). b) The risks of the tube migrating are reduced with nasal tubes.
2 Wide-bore polyvinyl chloride (PVC) tubes are suitable for short-term use only and must be changed at least every seven days. Fine-bore (polyurethane or 'Silk') tubes are designed for longer-term use. They need to be changed monthly.	2 Longer use may cause discomfort and nasal/oesophageal ulceration or irritations. There is a risk of the material of PVC tubes being eroded by gastric juices.
3 6–10 French gauge (Fr) sized nasogastric tubes are most commonly used in CYPs. The length of the tube depends on the size of the CYP. The smallest possible tube size should be chosen.	3 Larger size tube predisposes the CYP to gastroesophageal reflux (Noviski et al. 1999).
4 Enteral feeds via an NG tube can be administered as either bolus feeds or continuously.	
5 Medication (such as acid inhibitors) may alter the pH of the gastric aspirate. This may necessitate radiological confirmation of correct tube placement (Metheny and Titler 2001).	5 Bedside confirmation of correct placement relies on a clear pH reading (acid) using Universal Indicator Paper.

Procedure guideline 22.2 Inserting and managing the nasogastric tube

Statement	Rationale
1 Prepare the following equipment: a) Appropriate-sized wide-bore or fine-bore nasogastric tube. b) Sterile water to lubricate the tube. c) Foil bowl and tissue. d) pH strips. e) 20 ml oral syringe for CYPs and 2–5 ml oral syringe for neonates. f) Nonsterile gloves and apron. g) Tape suitable for the condition of the CYP's skin. h) Glass of water and straw or dummy if CYP is able to swallow.	1 c) In case of vomiting. d) To read the pH level of stomach content. e) Smaller syringes reduce the risk of vacuum trauma (Knox and Davie 2009) g) To secure the tube. h) Swallowing may support tube passage into the stomach.

Insertion

1 A risk assessment should have been performed before NG tube insertion is attempted using NPSA guidance (NPSA 2011).	1 To ensure that the risks are assessed and minimised.
2 The CYP and family should have been prepared by explaining the procedure.	2 To gain consent and co-operation.
3 Find the most appropriate position for the CYP depending on their age and ability. For example, older CYPs may wish to sit upright. Younger children and infants may sit on their parent's/carer's lap or lie down wrapped in a sheet.	3 To provide comfort and to prevent them from pulling their head back on insertion or pulling the tube out.
4 Choose the most suitable nostril. Ask the CYP if they have any preferences, where appropriate.	4 To involve them in the procedure and allow some control.
5 Wash hands thoroughly and dry. Put on an apron and nonsterile gloves.	5 To prevent cross-contamination (Anderton 1995).

Chapter 22 Nutrition and feeding

Procedure guideline 22.2 Inserting and managing the nasogastric tube *(continued)*

Statement	Rationale
6 Check the tube. If a guide wire is used, ensure the guide wire is not bent and is correctly inserted into the tube. The guide wire can be lubricated with 10 ml sterile water by flushing the tube prior to insertion.	6 To ensure the tube is patent. Guide wire NG/NJ tubes are not used on preterm babies and neonates unless under direct radiologic visualisation.
7 For neonates, measure from the nose to the ear and then halfway between the xiphisternum and umbilicus. For all other age groups, estimate the length of the tube by placing the exit port of the tube at the tip of the nose, then extend the tube to the earlobe and then to the xiphisternum (NPSA 2011).	7 To estimate the length to which tube should be inserted.
8 Lubricate the end of the tube in sterile water. Do not use K-Y jelly.	8 K-Y jelly may affect the pH measurement of the stomach content.
9 Gently pass the tip of the tube into the nostril and guide into the nasopharynx. a) If the CYP can safely swallow, offer a sip of water. Babies/toddlers should be offered a dummy. b) Slowly advance the tube until the required length has been passed.	9 a) This may support the passage of the tube into the stomach and ease discomfort.
10 Do not advance the tube against resistance, and should the CYP show any signs of distress, such as coughing or breathlessness, the tube should be removed immediately.	10 The tube might have passed into the trachea.
11 A distressed CYP should be allowed to have a break to rest at any time during the procedure.	
12 The tube is lightly secured with tape. Confirm the correct position of the tube by following the NPSA decision tree for infants and children (NPSA 2011). • Aspirate a small amount of stomach contents using a 20 ml or 50 ml syringe (except neonates, see above). • Test the aspirate on CE-marked pH indicator paper intended by the manufacturer to test human gastric aspirates. • For gastric tubes, the safe pH range is between 1 and 5.5. • Each test and test results must be documented on the nasogastric tube testing chart as appropriate and must be kept at the CYP's bedside.	12 The only safe methods of checking the tube position are: i) aspiration of gastric contents, which test at a pH of 1–5.5, or ii) visualisation of a radio-opaque tube on X-ray. The 'whoosh' test/air insufflation with abdominal auscultation (injecting air into the tube and listening for 'gurgling' noise over the stomach) must not be used to check tube placement as it is not reliable and must not be used (Lamont et al. 2011), and may result in serious harm, including death, for the patient.
13 The decision to confirm the correct tube placement by X-ray should be made by a senior clinician (NPSA, 2012). • The confirmation of feeding tube position by X-ray is a second-line intervention and should be used only when pH testing of feeding aspirates has failed. • The X-ray request form must clearly state that the purpose of the X-ray is to establish the position of a gastric or jejunal tube for the purposes of feeding or medication administration. • The X-ray must be interpreted by clinicians who have been deemed competent in assessing the position of feeding tubes by X-ray. • The assessment of feeding tube placement must be documented in the CYP's healthcare record.	13 To ensure the CYP is safe while not undergoing unnecessary X-rays.
14 Once the tube position is confirmed, remove the guide wire if present and safely secure the tube to the CYP's cheek. A hydrocolloid dressing should be used to protect the skin.	14 The adhesive tape to secure the tube should not extend beyond the size of the hydrocolloid dressing.
15 Record the indication for the tube, the size of tube, the length of the tube at the nostril, the appearance of the aspirate, and date of passing the tube in the CYP's healthcare record.	15 To provide accurate record of care and ongoing evaluation. To enable future checks of the tube position.
Tube management	
1 a) The nasal passages and surrounding skin should be checked at least daily to ensure they are not blocked. Clean with warm water and dry thoroughly. b) The skin around the nares should be checked daily and recorded in CYP's healthcare record to monitor for any signs of tissue damage.	1 a) To prevent build-up of dried mucus and promote comfort. b) Pressure damage can occur if the tube rubs on the nares.

(continued)

The Great Ormond Street Hospital Manual of Children and Young People's Nursing Practices

Procedure guideline 22.2 Inserting and managing the nasogastric tube *(continued)*

Statement	Rationale
2 The position of the tube must always be confirmed: • After insertion. • Before any liquid, feed, or medications are inserted via the tube. • When changing the feed during a continuous feed regime. • In the event of retching, vomiting, excessive coughing, respiratory distress, or the tube becoming partially dislodged. Signs of dislodgement of tube out of stomach include • Sudden decrease in residual volumes. • Bile stained feed. • Dislodged mark on the tube.	2 To ensure the tube is in the correct position and that the feed is going to the right place.
3 pH testing using pH indicator paper must be the first-line method of checking the tube position.	3 To safely check that the tube is in the right place. Caution: pH reading does not provide useful information during continuous feeding as the feed raises gastric pH. Consider the need for a radiological verification of tube placement (Metheny and Titler 2001).
4 For approved methods, see the following section. **If aspirate cannot be obtained OR if the aspirate is NOT between a pH of 1–5.5 for gastric tubes**: a) Change the CYP's position and try to aspirate again. b) Inject 1–5 ml air into the tube. c) Wait for 15–30 minutes and aspirate again. d) Advance or withdraw the tube by 1–2 cm. e) Give mouth care to patients who are nil by mouth f) NEVER use water to flush the tube before confirming the position.	4 This must be recorded in the CYP's healthcare record, indicating which alternate method worked. e) Mouth care stimulates gastric secretions of acid
5 If no aspirate is then obtained or the aspirate is still outside of the safe pH range (gastric tubes 1–5.5), the tube position must be checked by x-ray (second line testing)	5 This is the second line method and only used in the first line method has failed. It is better to base clinical decisions on one reliable test (pH indicator paper or radiography) than a combination of tests with varying reliability.

6 Neonates differ physiologically to children and the NPSA (2005) has recommended the following:
• None of the existing methods for checking feeding tube position is totally reliable
• Small bore feeding tubes are particularly difficult to gain aspirate from
• Tube markings should be used for all babies to enable accurate measurement of depth and length and the position of the tube documented.
• Although radiography is the most reliable indicator of feeding tube position, x-rays should not be 'routinely' used. However if the baby is going to have an x-ray as part of their clinical care, the feeding tube should be placed beforehand and checked for positioning.
• The NPSA flowsheet should be used to guide practitioners
• If the pH is outside the safe range AND an x-ray is not planned as part of routine care, a risk assessment should be performed and the following factors which may contribute to high pH considered:
  • the presence of amniotic fluid in a baby under 48 hours old
  • milk in the baby's stomach, particularly if they are on one to two hourly feeds
  • use of medication to reduce stomach acid	

7a) The tube should be flushed with 3–5 ml of sterile water: • Prior to and after each feed. • Prior to, in between multiple medications, and after the administration of medicines. • Four hourly if tube is not in use.	7a) To prevent blockage of the tube and bacterial contamination due to medicine and feed residues.

Procedure guideline 22.2 Inserting and managing the nasogastric tube *(continued)*

Statement	Rationale
b) An individual assessment of the flushing volumes must be undertaken for fluid restricted/small babies, taking into account the frequency and volume of feeds and medication. In preterm/neonates a flush may not be necessary following feeds as gravity feeding will be adequate and may only be needed after enteral medication. Only 0.5–2 mls of sterile water should be used when all medications are given.	b) To avoid fluid overload.
8 If aspirate cannot be obtained because the tube is blocked, fluid SHOULD NEVER be injected into the tube to unblock it. A blocked tube must not be manipulated using high pressure but should be removed and a new tube passed.	8 To avoid damaging the tube, which could lead to gut perforation or the instillation of feeds in the wrong place (Trigg and Mohammed 2006).

Principles table 22.10 Nasojejunal tube feeding

Principle	Rationale
1 Nasojejunal (or postpyloric feeding) is the method of feeding directly into the small bowel.	Jejunal access for feeding may be the preferred method in CYPs with: • Delayed gastric emptying. • Increased risk of aspiration. • Persistent vomiting. • During the postoperative period, before gastric emptying has resumed.
2 A long-length, fine-bore tube is passed via the nasogastric route, then through the pyloric sphincter and into the duodenum or jejunum.	
3 Hygienic handling of enteral feeds and feeding systems is paramount when using a jejunal route.	3 The stomach's barrier function is bypassed.
4 Jejunal feeds should be delivered continuously rather than as a bolus in order to avoid an overload of the small bowel.	4 The reservoir function of the stomach is bypassed.
5 Nasojejunal tubes are made of polyurethane and can remain in situ for 1 month. Weighted tubes encourage the tip of the tube to remain in the jejunum once passed.	5 Prolonged use affects the condition of the nasal passages.

Procedure guideline 22.3 Inserting and managing the nasojejunal tube

Statement	Rationale
Prepare the following equipment:	
1 a) An appropriately sized weighted tip tube with guide wire	1
b) Sterile water to lubricate the tube and flush the tube once correct placement has been confirmed	
c) Foil bowl and tissue	c) In case of vomiting.
d) pH strips	d) To read the changing pH of the aspirate as the tube passes through the stomach into the small bowel.
e) A 20 ml oral syringe	e) Smaller syringes reduce the risk of vacuum trauma (Knox and Davie 2009).
f) Nonsterile gloves and apron	
g) Tape suitable for the condition of the CYP's skin	g) To secure the tube.
h) Glass of water and straw or dummy if appropriate	h) If the CYP is able to swallow, this may support the tube passage into the stomach.
Insertion	
1 The CYP and family are informed of the following: • The indication for the nasojejunal (NJ) tube • The procedure to place the tube • The duration of the placement of the tube • The potential difficulties of this feeding route • The likely impact	1 To gain consent and co-operation.

(continued)

Procedure guideline 22.3 Inserting and managing the nasojejunal tube (continued)

Statement	Rationale
2 The NJ tube may be placed on the ward but positioning must be confirmed in fluoroscopy or an extended chest X-ray; however if the CYP has altered anatomy or has had previous failed attempts, then the procedure may need to be undertaken in fluoroscopy or interventional radiology.	
3 The NJ tube should be measured in two stages: a) The measurement of the tube from the nostril to the stomach: From the bridge of the nose to the ear and from the ear to the xiphisternum b) The measurement of the tube from the nostril to the jejunum • Neonates: From the bridge of the nose to the ankle of a fully extended leg. • Infants <1 year old: From the bridge of the nose to the ear, then to the midpoint between the xiphisternum and umbilicus, and then to the right iliac crest. • Children >1 year old: From the bridge of the nose to the mid xiphisternum and then to the right iliac crest.	3 To facilitate accurate placement of the tube.
4 **Follow steps 8–10 in passing an NG tube - see procedure guideline 22.2**.	
5 Aspirate the tube and check the pH using Universal Indicator Paper.	5 Aspirate: pH ≤ 5.5 and aspirate is grassy green, clear and colourless, or brown. Reposition the CYP if no aspirate can be obtained (Metheny and Titler 2001).
6 Once tube placement is confirmed to be in the stomach, flush the tube with 2 ml sterile water and advance the tube: • 1 cm every 15–30 minutes for neonates • 2–4 cm ever 5–10 minutes for infants and small children • 4–6 cm every 5–10 minutes for bigger children	6 To encourage peristalsis.
7 The tube should be flushed with 2 ml sterile water prior to advancing each time until the measurement from the nostril to the jejunum has been reached. Ideally the CYP should be positioned on their right side with the head of the bed raised 15–30° during this time. The tube should never be pushed against resistance. If resistance is felt, try flushing with water, and if resistance continues, then pull back a small amount and try again.	7 To assist passage through the pylorus.
8 A competent healthcare worker must confirm tube position with fluoroscopy or extended chest X-ray.	
9 The length of the tube at the nostril, date of insertion, confirmation that the X-ray has confirmed correct positioning, must all be recorded in the patient's healthcare records.	9 To provide accurate record of care and ongoing evaluation.

Tube management

1 The tube position must be confirmed by checking the measurement at the nostril is the same as documented at insertion. This must be recorded in the CYP's healthcare record. If dislodged, consider the need for radiological verification of the placement of the tube.	1 Aspirating the tube may cause the tube to collapse and recoil into the stomach.
2 It is preferable to avoid using jejunal tubes for the administration of drugs. If there is no alternative, only liquid medication should be used.	2 Drug absorption may be altered in the intestine and gastric acid may be required for activation (McIntyre and Monk 2014).
3 The compatibility of medicines with the small intestine should be discussed with pharmacy and medical staff.	

Procedure guideline 22.4 Management where both a gastric and a jejunal tube are inserted

Statement	Rationale
1 If both a gastric and jejunal tubes are in situ, each tube must be clearly identified using preprinted labels (Gastric/Jejunal) and documented.	1 To prevent inadvertent management (i.e. mixing up the jejunal with the gastric tube).
2 The length of each tube should be clearly documented; including the landmark which this is assessed against, this landmark should be marked on the tube with permanent marker at the time of confirmation of correct position (e.g. 15 cms to the right nostril).	
3 Testing of each tube should be documented on the appropriate testing/verification charts.	

Principles table 22.11 Gastrostomy tube feeding

Principle	Rationale
1 A gastrostomy is an opening formed through the abdomen directly into the stomach, bypassing the mouth and throat. A gastrostomy may be formed surgically under direct vision (open or laparoscopic), endoscopically (using a camera) or radiologically (using x-ray guidance).	1 A device inserted into the gastrostomy allows the delivery of supplemental nutrition and medications directly into the stomach. It also provides a mechanism to drain gastric contents, if required. In order for gastrostomy feeding to be successful the CYP must have a functioning gastrointestinal tract.
2 Use of a gastrostomy feeding device should be considered if the CYP: • Requires long-term enteral feeding support. • Has facial/oesophageal structural abnormalities that make NG tube feeding impossible. • is non-compliant with drug therapy. • Requires decompression of the stomach.	2 To maintain nutritional intake.
3 Gastrostomy tubes are made of either latex (malecots), polyurethane (PEGs), and balloon retained gastrostomy tubes are typically silicone. There are three main types: a) Temporary gastrostomy device tubes (e.g. latex Malecot® catheter). b) Percutaneous endoscopic gastrostomy devices (e.g Freka PEG or CORFLO™ PEG). These may also be placed as a radiologically inserted gastrostomy (RIG) or with a laparoscopic assist. c) Balloon retained gastrostomy devices. These may be low profile (e.g Mickey button and MiniONE button) or come in the form of balloon gastrostomy tubes. d) Other non balloon retained devices (e.g Capsule Monarch tube or non-balloon buttons)	3 a) Commonly used in patients having a concomitant fundoplication, obstructive oesophageal lesion, or expected difficult insertion. Usually replaced with a balloon retained gastrostomy device or non balloon device after six weeks. b) PEG devices are usually replaced every 18 months to two years, with Freka PEGs; a general anaesthetic (GA) is required to retrieve the internal fixator. CORFLO™ PEGs are designed to be traction removable but are commonly removed using a GA in paediatrics due to the level of traction required. c–d) Balloon and non balloon retained gastrostomy devices are commonly preferred by many as they obviate the need for an additional GA and can offer a low profile device. They may not, however, be suitable for CYPs who are more likely to pull the device out. Manufacturer's recommend that they are changed approximately every six months as long as both balloon and antireflux valve remain intact for this length of time.

Gastrostomy stoma care: newly formed stoma

1 Postoperative observations of temperature, pulse, respirations, and blood pressure must be performed in line with the Observations and PEWS policy.	1 To detect any postoperative complications and ensure effective escalation and management.
2 The child/young person should also have regular recording of their pain score and observation of the surgical wound for bleeding, leakage of gastric contents, or tube displacement. Administer pain relief as required. Any pain on feeding, prolonged or severe pain postprocedure, fresh bleeding, or external leakage of gastric contents must be escalated to the appropriate medical team. All feeding should stop immediately in these circumstances (NPSA 2010).	2 To keep the CYP pain free, allow a comfortable recovery period, and support easier handling and accessing of the device in the future.
3 On the CYP's return to the ward check that the external fixation plate is secure, and that it is not too tight or too loose.	3 If it is too tight the stoma will protrude through the fixation plate, causing pain and discomfort, and if it is too loose it will cause the tube to move back and forth. This would cause irritation to the tract, and could result in stretching of the tract diameter, and cause stomach contents to leak onto the skin.

(continued)

Principles table 22.11 Gastrostomy tube feeding (*continued*)

Principle	Rationale
4 The postoperative plan written in the operation notes/care pathway will give details of the type of device, size, make, and lot number, and these should be recorded in the medical and nursing records.	4 To ensure that the gastrostomy tube is used at the appropriate time postoperatively. There may have been other procedures carried out, e.g. biopsies, which influence when it is safe to use the tube.
5 The newly formed stoma should be left undisturbed for 24 hours and then be cleaned aseptically.	5 To minimise the risk of infection.
6 If the CYP is in discomfort the stomach should be decompressed by attaching a gravity bolus feed set to the PEG end. Ensure the feed set is held above the level of the stomach (usually shoulder height) and release the roller clamp. This will allow air to escape naturally from the stomach	6 To ensure the CYP is comfortable and pain free.
7 On return to the ward, there may be dry blood on the skin around the stoma, which is under the external fixation plate. This should be cleaned using sterile gauze and normal saline. This can be done without undoing the external fixation plate, by gently lifting the corners of the plate and cleaning in a circular motion around the stoma.	7 To keep the skin around the stoma site clean and dry.
8 For the first 14 days the stoma should be cleaned daily with a sterile saline solution and sterile gauze and inspected for signs of irritation or infection. At home this can be replaced with cooled boiled water and gauze swabs.	8 To help prevent infection while the wound is healing and to remove exudate.
9 The CYP can shower as normal or have a shallow bath. The stoma site should not be immersed fully in water until the site has healed.	
10 The stoma site needs to be checked regularly for tenderness, irritation, erythema, leakage of blood or gastric contents, or purulent exudate.	10 To detect signs of bleeding, infection, or tube migration.
11 No dressing is required as standard, but may be applied if needed. The dressing should be absorbent, non-adhesive, and antimicrobial. A clear plan should be in place for dressing changes and the site should continue to be properly monitored.	
12 It is important not to open the triangle for the first 14 days. This should be extended to 28 days in immune compromised CYPs or those with other conditions that affect clotting and healing. The first rotation of the tube should then take place and will require turning on a weekly basis.	12 To allow the stomach to adhere to the abdominal wall and form the tract. The stomach has been pulled up to the abdominal wall by the internal retention disc and is held in place by the external fixation triangle. Movement of the external fixator before the wound has healed can result in the stomach moving away from the abdominal wall, which can allow stomach content to leak into the peritoneum. The stoma should be healed and free of infection or discharge before rotating.
13 To rotate the tube: a) Wash hands with soap and water. Open the clamp of the fixation plate. Lift the tube free of the channel in the fixation plate, and move the plate away from the skin. Clean the stoma, surrounding skin, and fixation plate with gauze and water ensuring the area is dried thoroughly afterwards. b) Push the tube two to three centimetres into the stomach and rotate a full 360°. Pull the tube back gently until resistance is felt. Replace the fixation plate back into the original position above the stoma, reinsert the tube into the channel of the plate, and close the clamp. Check that the tube is not too tight or too loose. c) Care has to be taken when handling the tube as it takes two to three weeks for a fibrous tract to form (Peters and Westby 1994).	13 To avoid 'buried bumper' syndrome, where the internal fixator or balloon of the tube is taut against the abdominal wall and the internal fixation disc becomes buried, with the stomach lining growing around it.
Stoma care: established stoma	
1 When the stoma has healed it should be cleaned daily with mild soap and water and dried thoroughly.	1 To maintain skin integrity.
2 Bathing and showering is allowed as soon as the incision has healed.	
3 The stoma site should be monitored for signs of redness, bleeding, purulent exudates, pain, leakage, increase or change in consistency of stools.	3 To detect any complications and support early intervention.

Principles table 22.11 Gastrostomy tube feeding (*continued*)

Principle	Rationale
Tube management and troubleshooting **Checking tube placement** 1 Correct tube placement needs to be confirmed prior to the administration of the first feed after initial placement with all gastrostomies. Malecot tubes must have their position confirmed with a gastric acid aspirate prior to administration of all feeds or medications.	1 There is an increased risk of tube migration with Malecot tubes as it is only sutured at skin level and held in place by lugs.
Checking balloons 1 The balloon button device is held in place inside the stomach using an inflatable balloon; feeds are given by attaching an extension set. The buttons are made of silicone and the manufacturers recommend they are changed every three to six months.	
a) Ensure that the correct extension sets are used for feeding and giving medication.	a) There are many different manufacturers of balloon buttons and the extension sets are different for each.
b) The water used to inflate the balloon that holds the gastrostomy in place should be changed weekly as per manufacturer's instruction. A significant loss of water indicates a leakage and the device may need to be changed. NB. For a primary gastrostomy button it is advised to not change the water for the first six weeks to allow the gastrostomy to heal.	b) A small amount of water may be lost through the semipermeable membrane of the balloon.
c) Wash hands and wear nonsterile disposable gloves.	c) To avoid introduction of infection or cross infection. To comply with hospital policy on standard precautions when there is a possibility of contact with body fluids.
d) Remove the water from the balloon of the button to be changed, by attaching a syringe to the balloon port labelled BAL.	d) To ensure the CYP's comfort throughout the procedure. Failure to fully deflate the balloon before removal could cause pain or discomfort, which could cause noncompliance with future procedures.
e) Grip the external fixation hub, avoiding putting pressure on the CYP's abdomen.	
f) Withdraw the water; the balloon contains 3–5ml, depending on the size of the CYP.	
g) Recommended maximum filling volumes for balloons. • Under one year = 3 ml • Toddler = 4 ml • Older child/young person = =5 ml	
h) Check with the parent/carer if more or less water has been used.	
i) Avoid overfilling the balloon	i) To prevent damaging the balloon
j) Insert the new syringe with the clean water and inflate the balloon.	
k) The colour and volume of water removed from the balloon may be different to what was inserted	
l) Document the procedure in the CYP's health care record	
2 A spare device should always be supplied to the CYP.	2 To facilitate a quick change of the device.
3 Only syringes indicated for enteral use should be provided.	3 These are recommended to reduce the risk of inadvertent use of content through the intravenous route.
Preventing blockage 1 It is important that an appropriate device is in situ if planning to administer blenderised diet. This would usually be a 14fr balloon gastrostomy tube with an adequately healed tract that has already undergone it's first device change.	1 To avoid complications and hospitalisation.
2 Ensure that the device is working before administering a feed/medication.	2 To prevent interruptions to the feed once running, and to prevent the CYP being disturbed by the pump alarming due to blockage.
3 a) The tube should be flushed regularly prior to and after feeding/medicines with 10–20 ml of sterile or cooled, boiled water using a 20 ml enteral syringe. b) Liquid medicines should be used whenever possible. c) Drinking water can be used for flushing gastrostomy tubes. For children under one year or immune compromised CYPs the water should be boiled and cooled or sterile water may be used. Follow manufacturers' recommendations on flushing volumes and syringe sizes to be used.	3 a) To prevent the tube from becoming blocked by feed debris. b) To prevent damage of the tube by increased pressure due to build-up of deposits.

(*continued*)

Principles table 22.11 Gastrostomy tube feeding *(continued)*

Principle	Rationale

4 If the tube becomes blocked:
  a) Use a 50 ml enteral syringe with 10 ml warm water and pulsate water using a push/pull technique into the tube. High pressure should not be used while trying to unblock the device.
  b) Rotate and massage the tube between your fingers to try and dislodge the blockage.
  c) Carbonated water or preparations such as Corflo© Clog Zapper™ may be helpful in trying to clear the tube.
	4 a) To attempt to clear the blockage without causing any damage.

Dislodged gastrostomy devices

Principle	Rationale
1 If the tube is removed within the first two weeks after initial insertion the device may need to be replaced either surgically or endoscopically.	1 To maintain patency of the stoma.
2 A tubogram should be done following the procedure. Gastrostomy devices have to be replaced as quickly as possible in the early days as the tract will start to close within a short period of time. Once the tract is over six months old, it is stable for one to two hours.	2 To ensure that it is correctly positioned.
3 Routine changes of devices should be carried out as per manufacturer's instruction. Replacement tubes should not be used for the administration of feeds or medicines until correct placement has been confirmed by medical staff or X-ray.	
4 If necessary, a urinary catheter or NG tube can be used to maintain the stoma. If the same size replacement catheter is not available, the stoma might need to be dilated under general anaesthesia.	

Skin/stoma care
Infection

Principle	Rationale

1 The gastrostomy site should be cleaned every day and the site inspected for signs of infection and formation of granulation tissue.
  a) If the skin is clean and intact, dressings are not required. The stoma site should be observed for any signs of infection, such as irritation, erythema, purulent exudate, swelling, and oozing.
  b) If an infection is suspected, a swab should be sent for microscopy, culture and sensitivity (MC&S). Any infection should be treated before a device is changed.
  c) If leakage occurs from the site it is important to use a skin barrier product such as Cavilon®, detect the reason for leakage and resolve the problem. NB. A small amount of mucus discharge is completely normal, this usually appears yellow/green and 'crusty', and should be gently wiped away with daily cleans.
  d) The new gastrostomy should not be immersed in water until the tract is fully healed. Shallow baths can be taken, but swimming should be avoided.
  e) If granulation tissue has formed, early treatment is preferable. For small amounts of granulation, treat with Maxitrol® eye ointment topically twice daily. For larger amounts of granulation tissue, silver nitrate 75% caustic applicator sticks may be required. When using silver nitrate it is important to ensure contact is with the granulation tissue only. Protect the surrounding skin with a thick layer of yellow soft paraffin to prevent discolouration of peristomal skin.
  f) If excoriation of the skin occurs due to leakage of stomach contents a barrier product such as Cavilon (spray or individually wrapped sticks) or petroleum jelly can be applied.
	1 To protect the skin and allow healing to take place.
	
	a) To observe for any signs of infection.
	
	b) Bacterial or fungal infections are not uncommon. To identify any bacterial growth and establish sensitivities if antibiotics are required. Changing a device before the infection has been treated will lead to contamination of the new device. For further information regarding taking a swab, see Chapter 15: Investigations.
	c) To protect the peri-stomal skin: Any leakage from the stomach will contain acid which will burn the skin.
	
	d) To protect the site until the tract has healed.
	
	e) To prevent surrounding skin from damage.

Chapter 22 Nutrition and feeding

Principles table 22.11 Gastrostomy tube feeding *(continued)*

Principle	Rationale
Overgranulation	

1 If granulation tissue has formed, early treatment is preferable.
  a) For small amounts of granulation, treat with Maxitrol® eye ointment topically twice daily.
  b) For larger amounts of granulation tissue, silver nitrate 75% caustic applicator sticks may be required. When using silver nitrate it is important to ensure contact is with the granulation tissue only. Protect the surrounding skin with a thick layer of yellow soft paraffin to prevent discolouration of peristomal skin.
	1 To reduce the spread of granulation tissue. Over granulation around the stoma site may occur due to a predisposition of the CYP or friction on the tube. It can cause discomfort and bleeding.

Procedure guideline 22.5 Administration of enteral feeds

Statement	Rationale
Bolus feeds	
1 Intermittent bolus feeds are generally delivered by gravity over 15–30 minutes on a schedule of every two to four hours.	1 Administration of the feed should take the same length of time as it would take the CYP to have the same amount orally (Trigg and Mohammed 2006).
2 Bolus feeds are the preferred method of enteral feed administration (Holden et al. 2000).	2 Bolus feeds mimic a physiologically normal feeding pattern and can be adapted to fit in with meal times. CYPs on long-term feeding are given greater freedom and mobility (Johnson 2014).
3 Gravity feeding sets are single use only.	3 No attempt should be made to clean/disinfect and reuse any parts of a system that is marked for single use only (Anderton 1999). None of the tested cleaning methods are totally effective in removing bacteria from the lumina of feed administration sets (Anderton and Nwoguh 1991). The remaining bacteria and feed residues may provide an inoculum when the system is refilled with feeds (Anderton 1999).
4 The feed should be warmed to room temperature by placing the bottle in a jug of warm water. Do not heat continuous enteral feeds.	4 Feeds should not be heated in the microwave. Feed bottles may not be suitable and the feed may be too hot to use.
5 A clinical hand-wash should be performed according to guidelines and an apron and nonsterile gloves worn.	5 To prevent cross-contamination.
6 The feeding set should be assembled on a clean, dry surface and the reservoir/syringe filled with feed.	6 Air should be removed from the line by flushing the tube with water or feed.
7 The feeding tube is checked, and the CYP prepared and positioned.	7 To ensure the CYP gets the correct feed.
8 The feeding set is connected to the feeding tube. The clamp should be slowly released and the reservoir of the feed system raised to allow feed to flow into the tube.	
9 The young child should be encouraged to suck on a dummy or to play with food or feeding utensils.	9 To encourage normal socialisation associated with feeding and to maintain oromotor skills.
10 Gloves might be removed during feeding for nurturing interactions with the CYP or when oral stimulation is performed.	
Continuous feeds	
1 Continuous feeds are administered via an enteral feeding pump.	1 The continuous flow maintained by the pump prevents the blockage of tube/feeding set and avoids back-drainage of stomach/intestine content into the feeding system.
2 Continuous feeds are frequently chosen when enteral feeding is first started.	2 Small amounts of feed continuously infused are usually better tolerated (Holden et al. 2000).
3 Sterile feeds are the preferred feeds and should be used whenever possible.	3 To reduce the risk of giving feed to the patient that has already been contaminated during the process of preparation and decanting (Anderton 1999).

(continued)

Procedure guideline 22.5 Administration of enteral feeds *(continued)*

4 Sterile feeds in prefilled ready-to-use containers can be hung for up to 24 hours (check manufacture guidelines) provided that the system remains closed at all times.	4 To prevent the set being accessed frequently and therefore reduce the risk of bacterial contamination. Sterile feed containers remain free of bacterial contamination in closed systems for at least 24 hours (Beattie et al. 1996).
5 For diluted or decanted sterile feeds and reconstituted modular feeds the hanging time should not exceed 6 hours (Patchell et al. 1998). For CYPs on home enteral feeding in the community it is recommended that nonsterile reconstituted feeds should hang for a maximum four-hour period (NICE 2012).	5 To minimise the time during which the feed is exposed to room temperature.

Administering a continuous feed

1 The CYP is advised that an enteral feed is to be administered.	1 To psychologically prepare the CYP.
2 Put on a disposable apron. Perform a clinical hand wash and put on nonsterile gloves.	2 To minimise the risk of cross infection.
3 Ensure the feeding pump is wiped with an all-purpose detergent.	3 To decontaminate equipment.
4 Preparation area is cleaned and allowed to dry.	4 To minimise the risk of cross infection.
5, a) Gather equipment as required, e.g. feed containers/bottles, administration set. b) Type of feed, patient's name, and expiry date of feed checked.	5 To ensure the correct feed is administered safely and effectively.
6 Remove the feeding set from sterile pack and using the inside of the pack as the sterile field, use an aseptic nontouch technique.	
7 Decant the sterile (ready-to-use) feed into the feeding set reservoir or sterile bottle.	7 If a sterile bottle is used, the bottle must be attached onto the feeding set, taking care not to touch the top of the bottle or the spike set. This reduces the risk of contamination.
8 Prime the line, ensuring that all air is expelled.	
9 Insert the feeding set into the feeding pump.	
10 The feeding line should be labelled with a brightly coloured and clearly visible label, especially when simultaneous intravenous (IV) treatment is administered.	10 To prevent any confusion between IV and enteral feeding lines and ensure patient safety.
11 Check that the feeding tube is in the correct position; the CYP is prepared and correctly positioned.	11 To ensure safety and comfort.
12 Connect the feeding set onto the feeding tube using a nontouch aseptic technique (Anderton 1995; Beattie and Anderton 1998; Anderton 1999; Trigg and Mohammed 2006).	12 To minimise the risk of contamination.
13 The CYP's tube should be aspirated every four hours to reconfirm the correct tube location.	
14 The pump rate and alarm settings should be checked and adjusted as required.	14 To ensure that the correct amount of feeds is administered in the correct period of time.
15 When the feed is finished flush the tube with 5–10 ml water	
16 Any waste should be discarded according to local waste policy.	
17 Administration of the feed should be documented on the CYP's fluid balance chart and in their healthcare records.	17 To provide an accurate record.

Procedure guideline 22.6 Monitoring CYPs on enteral feeds

Statement	Rationale
1 Regular monitoring is a vital part of successful enteral feeding.	1 To prevent potential complications and to ensure that planned progress and improvement in nutritional status is achieved (Reilly 1998).

General observations

Statement	Rationale
1 The CYP should be observed daily for tube misplacement, nasal or stoma erosion and signs of aspiration. Tapes should be replaced when soiled, ensuring that the condition of the skin is checked.	1 To minimise complications and side effects of tube feeding.

Nutritional observation

Statement	Rationale
1 Height and weight should be measured before enteral feeding commences.	1 To provide a baseline with which to monitor the effectiveness of the feeding regimen.
2 At the initiation of enteral feeding the weight of infants should be recorded daily (older CYPs weekly) and thereafter plotted frequently on an approved growth chart.	2 Weight is the best short-term indicator of an improvement in nutritional status (Holden et al. 2000). The dietician or medical staff can change the nutritional composition of the feed to achieve appropriate weight gain and longer-term linear growth.
3 Length and height measurements should be monitored at agreed intervals and plotted on centile charts.	3 To indicate longer term improvements in nutrition and growth.

Monitoring gastrointestinal side-effects

Statement	Rationale
1 As enteral feeding may be an important part of disease management, symptoms such as diarrhoea, nausea, abdominal distension, and gastro-oesophageal reflux should be monitored.	1 To assess the improvement/change of symptoms during enteral feeding.
2 Diarrhoea may be caused by the enteral feed (Reilly 1998; Johnson 2014): • Too fast an administration rate • Bolus administration • Cold feed straight from the refrigerator • Bacterial contamination • High feed osmolality	2 Cause should be assessed and treated as quickly as possible.

Oral stimulation

Statement	Rationale
1 Prolonged absence of oral feeding can lead to the loss of oro-motor skills and the build-up of food aversion and anxiety.	1 The loss of normal socialisation associated with feeding and meal times as well as pleasant oral stimulation may cause a hypersensitivity to touch and taste (Trigg and Mohammed 2006).
2 Sucking, swallowing, and blowing should be encouraged through oral stimulation and in play, as well as the joyful exploration of food or feeding utensils at meal times.	2 This helps the CYP to associate food and meal times with pleasure.
3 There needs to be liaison with speech and language therapist, occupational therapist, or feeding nurse specialist regarding the implementation of feeding regimens.	3 This ensures the best outcome for the CYP and prevents complications later.

Procedure guideline 22.7 Delivery of PN in the hospital setting

Statement	Rationale
Inform the CYP and family	
1 Ensure the CYP and family are informed of the following: a) The reason for commencing PN. b) What it will involve. c) Likely duration of PN. d) Potential side effects of PN. e) Likely impact on CYP and family.	1 To obtain informed consent. a) To promote safe delivery of PN. c) To maximise effectiveness of PN.
2 The ward play specialist should be informed to enable them to prepare the CYP.	2 To help to psychologically prepare the CYP.
Refer to nutrition support team	
1 Once the medical team has decided that PN is indicated, the CYP should be referred to a member of the Nutrition Support Team (NST).	1 To determine the CYP's suitability for PN. To perform a nutritional assessment prior to PN being ordered. To allow the team to determine type of IV access present/required.
Baseline parameters	
1 The CYP's baseline parameters must be measured.	1 To determine effectiveness of PN.
2 Prior to starting PN the following observations should be recorded: • Temperature. • Heart rate. • Respiratory rate. • Blood pressure. For further information see Chapter 1: Assessment.	2 To establish the baseline for subsequent observations.
3 Weight and height should be recorded on the nursing record and centile chart.	3 To allow accuracy of PN formulation and to monitor growth.
4 The CYP should be weighed according to local policy, ideally unclothed and using the same scales for each weight obtained.	4 To obtain an accurate measurement.
5 'Nutritional' blood and urine samples should be taken according to the monitoring policy.	5 To monitor, assess, and correct any imbalance of electrolytes, vitamins, and trace elements (Puntis 2001). To prevent metabolic complications.
Venous access	
1 Long-term PN should be administered via a central venous access device (CVAD). Dextrose concentrations above 10% should be administered via CVAD. Local policy may differ.	1 To minimise risk of extravasation injury and phlebitis: a dextrose concentration above 10% is hypertonic and acidic.
2 The NST must be informed if a CVAD is not available for CYPs for whom PN is prescribed.	2 To determine appropriate course of treatment. To allow time to arrange for appropriate IV access.
3 A dedicated nutrition line should be used whenever possible, i.e. a single-lumen CVAD.	3 To reduce the risk of infection (DH 2003). Sometimes a double- or triple-lumen line will be necessary such as when giving cytotoxic therapy or blood products.
4 The intravenous device should be cared for according to the relevant local policy.	4 To reduce risks of infection and accidental removal or damage to the device.
Obtaining PN	
1 The requesting doctor should ideally liaise with the NST about the nutritional needs of the CYP. PN must be prescribed by the doctor.	1 To ensure that nutritional requirements are met and comply with legal requirements.
2 When the PN is delivered to the clinical area the following details must be checked: a) Name, date of birth, hospital number. b) That the bag is intact. c) PN has been stored in a fridge. d) The temperature of the fridge is recorded daily.	2 To avoid delay in treatment. a) To ensure correct PN has been delivered. b) To minimise risk of infection. c) To maintain stability of the PN. d) To provide a record for audit and accuracy and to detect equipment failure early.

Procedure guideline 22.7 Delivery of PN in the hospital setting *(continued)*

Statement	Rationale
3 The time to commence the PN should be negotiated with the CYP and family.	3 To promote a partnership in care and promote effective planning.
4 PN infusion should be prepared in a designated area.	4 To minimise the risk of infection. To provide access for resources.
5 Access to the room should be restricted while the PN infusion is being prepared.	5 To reduce the risk of error and contamination.
6 PN infusion should be prepared on an individual basis, i.e. immediately prior to connection. a) PN should be discarded after 24 hours. b) A new administration set and filter should always be used. c) PN should be administered via an appropriate administration set and a 1.2 μm filter.	6 To reduce the risk of infection and errors. a–b) To reduce the risk of infection. c) To ensure safe delivery of PN and avoid particulate contamination (Sari and Rollins 1999).
7 PN should be removed from the fridge 1–4 hours before use.	7 To ensure stability of PN. To avoid infusing a solution that is too cold (RCN 2016).
8 PN solution should be checked for leakage and precipitate.	8 To avoid infusion of contaminated PN and minimise the risk of infection for the CYP.
9 Check the following match when comparing the CYP's intravenous prescription chart against the PN solution and the pharmacy therapy sheet according to local Hospital Drug Policy: a) Full name, date of birth, hospital number. b) Route of administration. c) Dextrose concentration. d) Rate of infusion, duration of infusion, volume to be infused.	9 To ensure correct product is prepared for correct CYP. a) To ensure the correct prescription for the correct CYP.
10 If there is a discrepancy between the prescription sheet and the pharmacy therapy sheet: do not commence infusion, contact the relevant pharmacist and medical staff to resolve the problem.	10 To ensure appropriate nutrition is maintained. To detect errors and minimise risk to the CYP. An incident report should be completed.
11 An appropriate intravenous infusion pump must be used.	11 To ensure accuracy of infusion.
12 An aseptic nontouch technique (ANTT) (identified in local policy) must be followed when preparing the infusion.	12 To minimise the risk of infection (DH 2003). To comply with local policy.
13 Prime the IV administration set.	13 To prevent air embolism. To ensure IV administration set is patent.
14 When lipid is not prescribed water-soluble vitamins should be added in Pharmacy to the amino acid solution. In this case, the bag must be covered and protected from light.	14 Some water-soluble vitamins are light-sensitive.
15 If the CYP is having additional IV therapy, the administration set for that should be connected below the filter.	15 To minimise the risk of infection by reducing the number of times the CVAD is accessed.
16 Do not add any other drugs or solutions to the PN solution.	16 To minimise the risk of infection. To maintain stability of the PN.
Commencement of infusion	
1 If possible use the treatment room for connection to PN infusion.	1 To minimise number of procedures carried out at the CYP's bedside.
2 Check the CYP's identity against the PN prescription and solution according to hospital policy.	2 To reduce risk of drug error.
3 Use ANTT to access CVAD, to assess patency of CVAD and to connect to PN, according to local policy.	3 To minimise risk of infection.
4 The infusion pump should have the following set correctly: rate of infusion, volume to be infused, maximum pressure alarm limit.	4 To maintain patient safety. To ensure correct amount of PN is administered.
5 The infusion pump must be secured onto the appropriate infusion stand. The pump must be connected to the mains electricity whenever possible.	5 To ensure patient safety. To avoid the rechargeable battery from running down.

(continued)

Procedure guideline 22.7 Delivery of PN in the hospital setting *(continued)*

Statement	Rationale
6 The level of the pump should be positioned correctly and the pressure alarm set according to instructions attached to the infusion device.	6 To ensure alarm functions correctly.
7 Ensure all connections are secure in the administration system.	7 To prevent accidental disconnection.
8 Ensure all relevant clamps on the administration set and CVAD are open.	8 To facilitate flow of PN and avoid unnecessary alarms.
9 All equipment must be disposed of according to hospital waste policy.	9 To ensure safety of staff and patients.
10 Ensure prescription charts are signed on commencement of infusion and charted on the fluid balance chart.	10 To provide record of PN treatment.

Managing the infusion

Statement	Rationale
1 The NST should be contacted if there are any concerns about a CYP receiving PN.	1 To enable any issues to be resolved.
2 If there is accidental disconnection of the PN: a) Discard PN, flush and lock CVAD as per local policy. b) Inform medical staff.	2 a) To minimise risk of infection. b) To ensure safety of the CYP. Other fluids may need to be prescribed.
3 The PN infusion should not be interrupted if possible.	3 To ensure the CYP's nutritional needs are met.
4 If the filter blocks during the administration of the PN infusion: a) Stop the infusion; inform the CYP's doctor and pharmacist. b) Return the administration set and filter to pharmacy.	4 a) To obtain a standard PN solution from pharmacy as a replacement. b) To enable investigation of the problem.
5 While on PN treatment: a) Continue with normal oral hygiene and oral assessment. b) Encourage oral-motor stimulation in the CYP who is not eating. For further information see Chapter 11: Personal Hygiene and Pressure Ulcer Prevention.	5 a) To ensure a clean and healthy mouth and ensure appropriate oral hygiene regimen is used. b) To prevent problems with feeding and speech and language development.

Monitoring

Statement	Rationale
1 Frequency of monitoring and recording observations depends on the clinical condition of the CYP and any underlying disease process and includes: heart rate, respiratory rate, blood pressure, urinary electrolytes, glucose, and ketones, blood glucose, infusion pump pressure, infusion rate, and fluid volume infused.	1 To assess, monitor and document the response to therapy, observe for fluid overload and signs of infection, monitor tolerance of glucose and ensure accuracy of infusion pump.
2 If administering PN peripherally, check cannula site every 30 minutes for redness, pallor, swelling, inflammation, leakage, oozing, tenderness, temperature change. Record the visual infusion phlebitis score. Document this in the CYP's healthcare record. Stop infusion if any of the aforementioned appears.	2 To detect early signs of extravasation. For further information see Chapter 14: Intravenous and Intra-arterial Access and Infusions.
3 a) Obtain weight and height. b) Calibrate the equipment and use the same weighing scales each time. In the case of an infant, head circumference should also be monitored.	3 a) To monitor effectiveness of treatment and any fluid overload. To enable accuracy of PN formulation. b) To enable consistent measurement (Puntis 2001).

Completion of infusion: Continuous PN

Statement	Rationale
1 Record total volume infused on the CYP's fluid balance chart.	1 To maintain accurate fluid balance.
2 Change administration sets and new solutions without delay.	2 To maintain treatment regimen.
3 Clear the infusion pump settings – these must be reset when connecting new infusion.	3 To minimise risk of error on re-connection.
4 Follow guidelines for the specific infusion device when disconnecting and when connecting new infusion.	4 To ensure safe and effective use and maintenance of infusion device.
5 Record disconnection and new connection in the CYP's healthcare records.	5 To maintain accurate records.
6 Dispose of equipment according to Hospital Waste Policy.	6 Maintaining safe practice.

Procedure guideline 22.7 Delivery of PN in the hospital setting *(continued)*

Statement	Rationale
Completion of infusion: cyclical PN	
1 If cyclical regimen is new to the CYP, or if reducing duration of PN infusion, monitor blood glucose level.	1 To ensure cyclical regimen is tolerated.
2 Interventions by the multiprofessional team should be co-ordinated to suit PN infusion time and CYP's daily routine.	2 To promote family normality and improve quality of life. To maximise the quality and length of 'free' time available to CYP and family.
3 During the last hour of the infusion, reduce infusion rate in stages, according to the prescription.	3 To prevent rebound hypoglycaemia.
4 Record total volume infused on the CYP's fluid balance chart.	4 To maintain accurate fluid balance.
5 Clear the infusion pump settings – these must be reset when connecting new infusion.	5 To minimise risk of error on reconnection.
6 Follow guidelines for the specific infusion device when disconnecting and when connecting new infusion.	6 Safe and effective use and maintenance of infusion device.
7 Record disconnection and new connection in the CYP's healthcare records.	7 To maintain accurate records.
8 Dispose of equipment according to Waste Policy.	8 Maintaining safe practice.
Completion of PN treatment	
1 When PN is coming to an end the volume of PN to be infused should be decreased as the CYP's enteral intake increases.	1 To prevent fluid overload and establish enteral nutrition.
2 The CYP's doctor should inform the pharmacist when PN is no longer required.	2 To reduce wastage and unnecessary costs.
3 The intravenous access device should be removed when it is no longer required.	3 To minimise associated risks.
4 Height and weight should be recorded at the end of the PN treatment.	4 To audit effectiveness of treatment.
5 These and the CYP's enteral intake should continue to be monitored by the dietician.	5 To monitor progress and nutritional adequacy.

Procedure guideline 22.8 Sham feeding

Statement	Rationale
Inform the child and family	
1 Inform the child (if appropriate) and family of the following:	1 To increase understanding so facilitating shared care and family co-operation.
a) The reasons for feeding this way.	
b) The principles of an oesophagostomy and feeding using a gastrostomy.	
c) Why sham feeds are so important.	c) To encourage oral feeding.
d) The likely duration for the need for this procedure.	d) To help plan for a later surgical procedure.
2 The child's parents/carers must be taught all aspects of sham feeding and what to do if the gastrostomy becomes displaced.	2 To involve them in their child's care. To ensure the child's safety.
a) This instruction must be documented in the child's healthcare record.	a) To provide an accurate record.
Preparing to feed	
1 Prepare the following equipment:	1 To facilitate feeding.
a) Select appropriate feeding utensils, e.g. bottle and teat or teacher beaker.	
b) Prescribed milk feed (warmed).	
c) Tissues.	

(continued)

Procedure guideline 22.8 Sham feeding *(continued)*

Statement	Rationale
d) Towel. e) A new 'oesophagostomy sling'. f) Plastic sheeting. g) Barrier cream (if used).	e) A dressing used to soak up oesophageal secretions.
2 Prepare a clean 'oesophagostomy sling' for use after the procedure has been completed.	2 The 'sling' soaks up secretions thus protecting the surrounding skin. This can be made by cutting a length of tubular bandage long enough to cover the stoma and to be able to tie it in a knot underneath the arm. Two pieces of gauze need to be inserted inside the bandage.
3 The gauze is positioned over the stoma site and tied under the opposite arm.	

Feeding the child

Statement	Rationale
1 Before starting the sham feed: a) Remove the infant's upper clothing and 'oesophagostomy sling.' b) Observe the oesophagostomy site and check the stoma is pink and healthy. c) Check that saliva is draining from it. d) Inform the medical staff if there are signs of infection or thrush. e) If there is no saliva draining, **DO NOT** give the feed.	1 a) To prevent soiling of clothes. b) To ensure the blood supply is adequate and no prolapsed has occurred. c) To allow free drainage of the feed. d) Oral thrush may cause thrush at the oesophagostomy site. e) A lack of drainage may indicate a blockage or an oesophagostomy stricture.
2 An infant who is going to have the sham feed should be wrapped in a blanket allowing room to access the gastrostomy tube.	2 To prevent them from becoming cold.
3 Position the plastic sheeting around the baby's shoulders and cover with a towel.	3 To protect skin and prevent becoming wet and cold.
4 Prior to commencing the feed perform a social hand-wash and put on a disposable apron.	4 To minimise the risk of infection.
5 Where possible, two people should be available to assist with a sham feed.	5 To co-ordinate oral 'sham' feeding and gastrostomy feeding.
6 With the aid of the second person, simultaneously give the oral feed and gastrostomy feed.	6 To ensure the correct nutritional requirements are given for growth and development. The infant will associate a full stomach with oral feeding.
7 Observe the infant while feeding. If the infant becomes upset and distressed stop the oral feed but continue to give the gastrostomy feed slowly.	7 The infant, due to fatigue, may take less orally than via the gastrostomy, especially if this is a new procedure for the infant.
8 The oral volume of feed should be gradually built up as tolerated.	
9 Once the feed is completed the stoma site should be: a) Cleaned with warm water and gauze. b) Dried. c) Protected with an application of soft paraffin.	9 To prevent skin excoriation.
10 a) The new 'oesophagostomy sling' should be placed over the stoma and tied under the opposite arm. b) The knot should be checked to ensure it does not cause any pressure.	10 a) To soak up secretions thus protecting the surrounding skin. b) To maintain comfort and prevent sores.
11 The 'sling' should be changed whenever it becomes wet with saliva.	11 To prevent skin excoriation. To maintain comfort.

Procedure guideline 22.8 Sham feeding (continued)

Statement	Rationale
Completing the procedure	
1 On completion of the feed a hand wash should be performed.	1 To minimise the risk of cross-infection.
2 The infant should be made comfortable.	
3 Oral feeding equipment should be washed with warm, soapy water and decontaminated accordingly, e.g. in a dishwasher. Disposable equipment, e.g. gastrostomy feeding set, should not be reused.	3 To minimise the risk of cross-infection.
4 Disposable items and protective clothing should be disposed of according to the local policy.	
5 The quantity of feed taken orally and via the gastrostomy should be recorded on the child's fluid balance chart.	5 To assess how much feed the infant takes compared with its total requirements.
6 A child receiving sham feeds must: • be weighed at least twice weekly. • have their height/length measured monthly.	6 To determine the effectiveness of the child's feeding regimen.
7 Both recordings must be recorded in the child's healthcare records and plotted on their centile chart.	7 To maintain accurate records.

References

Agostoni, C., Decsi, T., Fewtrell, M. et al. (2008). Complementary feeding: a commentary by the ESPGHAN Committee on Nutrition. Journal of Pediatric Gastroenterology and Nutrition 46: 99–110.

Allison S. (1999). Hospital Food as Treatment. British Association for Parenteral and Enteral Nutrition (BAPEN) report. Redditch, BAPEN.

American Dietetic Association (2004). *Infant Feedings: Guidelines for Preparation of Formula and Breastmilk in Health Care Facilities*. Chicago: The American Dietetic Association.

Anderton, A. (1995). Reducing bacterial contamination in enteral feeds. British Journal of Nursing 4 (7): 368–375.

Anderton, A. (1999). *Microbial Contamination of Enteral Feeds. How Can we Reduce the Risk?* Birmingham: The Parenteral and Enteral Nutrition Group of the British Dietetic Association.

Anderton, A. and Nwoguh, C.E. (1991). Re-use of enteral feeding tubes – a potential hazard to the patient? A study of the efficiency of a representative range of cleaning and disinfection procedures. Journal of Hospital Infection 18 (2): 131–138.

Balmer, S.E., Nicoll, A., Weaver, G.A., and Williams, A.F. (1997). *Guidelines for the Collection Storage and Handling of mother's Breast Milk to Be Fed to Her Own Baby on a Neonatal Unit*. London: United Kingdom Association for Milk Banking.

Beattie, T.K. and Anderton, A. (1998). Bacterial contamination of enteral feeding systems due to faulty handling procedures: a comparison of a new system with two established systems. Journal of Human Nutrition and Dietetics 11 (4): 313–321.

Beattie, T.K., Anderton, A., and White, S. (1996). Aspiration of (gastric residuals)-a cause of bacterial contamination of enteral feeding systems? Journal of Human Nutrition and Dietetics 9 (2): 105–115.

Boyd, C.A., Quigley, M.A., and Brocklehurst, P. (2007). Formula versus donor breast milk for feeding preterm or low birthweight infants. Archives of Disease in Childhood 92: 169–175.

Care Quality Commission (2010) Essential standards of quality and safety. https://services.cqc.org.uk/sites/default/files/gac_-_dec_2011_update.pdf (accessed 19 July 2022).

De Curtis, M., Canduso, M., Pieltan, C., and Rigo, J. (1999). Effect of fortification on the osmolality of human milk. Archives of Diseases of Childhood Fetal and Neonatal Edition 81: F141–F143.

DeBear, K. (1996). Sham feeding: another kind of nourishment. American Journal of Nursing 86 (10): 1142–1143.

Department of Health (DH) (1991). *Report on Health and Social Subjects 41: Dietary Reference Values for Food Energy and Nutrition for the United Kingdom*. London: HMSO.

Department of Health (DH) (1994). *Report on Health and Social Subjects 45: Weaning and the Weaning Diet*. London: HMSO.

Department of Health (DH) (2001). Guidelines for preventing infections associated with the insertion and maintenance of central venous catheters. Journal of Hospital Infection 47 (supplement): S47–S67.

Department of Health (DH) (2003). *Winning Ways: Working Together to Reduce Healthcare Associated Infection*. London: DH.

Department of Health (DH) (2007). Implementation Plan for Reducing Health Inequalities in Infant Mortality: A Good Practice Guide. London, DH.

Department for Health and Social Care (2016). Children and young people's continuing care national framework. https://www.gov.uk/government/publications/children-and-young-peoples-continuing-care-national-framework (accessed 19 October 2022).

Dogan, Y., Erkan, T., Yalvaç, S. et al. (2005). Nutritional status of patients hospitalized in paediatric clinic. The Turkish Journal of Gastroenterology 16 (4): 212–216.

Drenckpohl, D., Bowers, L., and Cooper, H. (2007). Use of the Six Sigma methodology to reduce incidence of breast milk administration errors in the NICU. Neonatal Network 26 (3): 161–166.

Edmond, K. and Bahl, R. (2007). *Optimal Feeding of Low-Birth Weight Infants: Technical Review*. Geneva: WHO.

Food Standards Agency (2009). The Food safety Act 1990 A guide for food businesses. 2009 edition. https://www.food.gov.uk/sites/default/files/media/document/fsactguide.pdf (accessed 19 July 2022).

Gerasimidis, K., Keane, O., MacLeod, I. et al. (2010). A four-stage evaluation of the Paediatric Yorkhill malnutrition score in a tertiary paediatric hospital and a district general hospital. The British Journal of Nutrition 104: 751–756.

Hankard, R., Bloch, J.J., Martin, P. et al. (2001). Nutritional status and risk in hospitalized children. Archives de Pédiatrie 8 (11): 1203–1208.

Hart, S. (2008). Infection control in intravenous therapy. In: *Intravenous Therapy in Nursing Practice* (eds. L. Dougherty and J. Lamb). Edinburgh: Churchill Livingstone.

Health and Social Care Information Centre (2015). Health Survey for England 2014. http://content.digital.nhs.uk/catalogue/PUB19295/HSE2014-Sum-bklet.pdf (accessed 19 July 2022).

Hendricks, K.M., Duggan, C., Gallagher, L. et al. (1995). Malnutrition in hospitalized paediatric patients. Current prevalence. Archives of Pediatrics & Adolescent Medicine 149 (10): 1118–1122.

Hendrikse, W.H., Reilly, J.J., and Weaver, L.T. (1997). Malnutrition in a children's hospital. Clinical Nutrition 16: 13–18.

Henschel, D. and Inch, S. (1996). *Breast Feeding. A Guide for Midwives*, 1e, 58. Hale: Books for Midwives Press.

Hill, S. and Long, S. (2001). Home enteral and parenteral nutrition for children. In: *Intestinal Failure* (ed. J. Nightingale), 431–446. London: Greenwich Medical Media.

Holden, C., MacDonald, A., Ward, M. et al. (1997). Psychological preparation for nasogastric feeding in children. British Journal of Nursing 6 (7): 376–385.

Holden, C., Johnson, T., and Caney, D. (2000). Nutritional support for children in the community. In: *Nutrition and Child Health* (eds. C. Holden and A. MacDonald), 177–196. Edinburgh: Bailliere Tindall.

Hudson, J. (2000). The multidisciplinary team. In: *Total Parenteral Nutrition: A Practical Guide for Nurses* (ed. H. Hamilton). London: Churchill Livingstone.

Hulst, J.M., Zwart, H., Hop, W.C., and Joosten, K.F. (2010). Dutch national survey to test the STRONGkids nutritional risk screening tool in hospitalized children. Clinical Nutrition 29 (1): 106–111.

Johnson, T. (2014). Enteral nutrition. In: *Clinical Paediatric Dietetics*, 4e (ed. V. Shaw), 35–47. Oxford: Wiley Blackwell.

Joosten, K.F. and Hulst, J.M. (2008). Prevalence of malnutrition in paediatric hospital patients. Current Opinion in Pediatrics 20 (5): 590–596.

Joosten, K.F., Zwart, H., Hop, W.C., and Hulst, J.M. (2010). National malnutrition screening days in hospitalised children in the Netherlands. Archives of Diseases of Childhood 95: 141–145.

King, C. and Tavener, K. (2014). Preterm infants. In: *Clinical Paediatric Dietetics*, 4e (ed. V. Shaw), 83–102. Oxford: Wiley Blackwell.

Knox, T. and Davie, J. (2009). Nasogastric tube feeding-which syringe size produces lower pressure and is safest to use? Nursing Times 105 (27): 24–26.

Lamb, J. and Dougherty, L. (2008). Local and systemic complications of intravenous therapy. In: *Intravenous Therapy in Nursing Practice* (eds. L. Dougherty and J. Lamb), 167–196. Edinburgh: Churchill Livingstone.

Lamont, T., Beaumont, C., Fayaz, A. et al. (2011). Checking placement of nasogastric feeding tubes in adults (interpretation of x ray images): summary of a safety report from the National Patient Safety Agency. BMJ 342: d2586.

Lang, S. (2002). *Breast Feeding Special Care Babies, 2*, 4–5. London: Baillière Tindall.

Law, B.J., Urias, B.A., Lertzmaan, J. et al. (1989). Is ingestion of milk-associated bacteria by premature infants fed raw human milk controlled by routine bacteriologic screening? Journal of Clinical Microbiology 27: 1560–1566.

Lee, M.J. and Allwood, C. (2001). Formulation of parenteral feeds. In: *Intestinal Failure* (ed. J. Nightingale), 351–362. London: Greenwich Medical Media.

Lucas, A. (1993). Enteral nutrition. In: *Nutritional Needs of the Preterm Infant* (eds. R.C. Tsang, A. Lucas, R. Uauy and S. Zlotkin), 209–216. New York: Caduceus Medical Publishers.

Lucas, A. and Cole, T.J. (1990). Breast milk and neonatal necrotising enterocolitis. Lancet 336: 1519–1523.

Lucas, A., Morley, R., Cole, T.J. et al. (1992). Breast milk and subsequent intelligence quotient in children born pre-term. Lancet 339: 261–264.

Lucas, A., Morley, R., and Cole, T. (1998). Randomised trial of early diet in preterm babies and later intelligence quotients. British Medical Journal 317: 1481–1487.

Lucas, A., Morley, R., and Isaacs, E. (2001). Nutrition and mental development. Nutrition Reviews 59: S24–S32.

Marteletti, O., Caldari, D., Guimber, D. et al. (2005). Malnutrition screening in hospitalized children: influence of the hospital unit on its management. Archives de Pédiatrie 12 (8): 1226–1231.

McCarthy, H., Dixon, M., Crabtree, I. et al. (2012). The development and evaluation of the screening tool for the assessment of malnutrition in Paediatrics (STAMP©) for use by healthcare staff. Journal of Human Nutrition and Dietetics 25: 311–318.

McIntyre, C. and Monk, H. (2014). Medication absorption considerations in patients with post pyloric enteral feeding tubes. American Journal of Health-System Pharmacy 71: 549–556.

Merritt, R.J., Sinatra, F.R., and Smith, G.A. (1983). Nutritional support of the hospitalized child. Advances in Nutritional Research 5: 77–103.

Metheny, N.A. and Titler, M.G. (2001). Assessing placement of feeding tubes. American Journal of Nursing 101 (5): 36–45.

Moy, R.J. (2006). Prevalence, consequences and prevention of childhood nutritional iron deficiency: a child public health perspective. Clinical and Laboratory Haematology 28 (5): 291–298.

Moy, R., Smallman, S., and Booth, I. (1990). Malnutrition in a UK children's hospital. Journal of Human Nutrition and Dietetics 3: 93–100.

National Institute for Health and Care Excellence (NICE) (2008). (Updated 2014). Maternal and child nutrition. https://www.nice.org.uk/guidance/ph11 (accessed 05 October 2022).

National Institute for Health and Care Excellence (NICE) (2010). Donor milk banks: service operation. Clinical guieline [CG93]. https://www.nice.org.uk/guidance/cg93 (accessed 19 July 2022).

National Institute for Health and Care Excellence (NICE) (2012). (Updated 2017). Healthcare-associated infections: prevention and control in primary and community care. https://www.nice.org.uk/guidance/cg139 (accessed 19 July 2022).

National Patient Safety Agency (NPSA) (2005). Patient Safety Alert. Reducing the harm caused by misplaced naso and orogastric feeding tubes in babies under the care of neonatal units. https://webarchive.nationalarchives.gov.uk/ukgwa/20090706060315/http:/www.npsa.nhs.uk/nrls/alerts-and-directives/alerts/feedingtubes/ (accessed 20 July 2022).

National Patient Safety Agency (NPSA) (2010). Early detection of complications after gastrostomy. NPSA/2010/RRR01. Reference number 1214. https://media.gosh.nhs.uk/documents/NRLS-1214-Gastrostomy_RRR-2010.03.29-v1.pdf (accessed 20 July 2022).

National Patient Safety Agency (NPSA) (2011). Reducing the harm caused by misplaced nasogastric feeding tubes in adults, children and infants. London, NSPA (Available at Patient Safety Learning Team). https://www.pslhub.org/learn/improving-patient-safety/patient-safety-alert-npsa2011psa002-reducing-the-harm-caused-by-misplaced-nasogastric-feeding-tubes-in-adults-children-and-infants-r4525/ (accessed 19 July 2022).

National Patient Safety Agency (NPSA) (2012). Rapid Response report: Harm from flushing of nasogastric tubes before confirmation of placement. NPSA/2012/RRR001. https://www.cas.mhra.gov.uk/ViewandAcknowledgment/ViewAttachment.aspx?Attachment_id=101458 (accessed 05 October 2022).

NHS (2019). https://www.nhs.uk/conditions/baby/ (accessed 19 July 2022).

NHS (2019b). Expressing and storing breast milk. https://www.nhs.uk/conditions/baby/breastfeeding-and-bottle-feeding/breastfeeding/expressing-breast-milk/ (accessed 19 October 2022). [return]

NHS (2021). Salt: the facts. Eat well. https://www.nhs.uk/live-well/eat-well/food-types/salt-nutrition/ (accessed 19 July 2022).

NHS (2022a). Eat well. https://www.nhs.uk/live-well/eat-well/ (accessed 19 July 2022).

NHS (2022b). How to make up baby formula. https://www.nhs.uk/conditions/baby/breastfeeding-and-bottle-feeding/bottle-feeding/making-up-baby-formula/ (accessed 19 July 2022).

NHS (2019). Expressing and storing breast milk. https://www.nhs.uk/conditions/baby/breastfeeding-and-bottle-feeding/breastfeeding/ expressing-breast-milk/ (accessed 19 July 2022).

NHS England (2013). Patient-led assessments of the care environment (PLACE). www.england.nhs.uk/ourwork/qual-clin-lead/place (accessed 19 July 2022).

NHS Estates (2003). Better Hospital Food: Catering Services for Children and Young Adults. London, Department of Health NHS Estates. www.bapen.org.uk/pdfs/bhfi/bhfi_catering.pdf (accessed 19 July 2022).

Noviski, N., Yehuda, Y.B., Serour, F. et al. (1999). Does the size of nasogastric tubes affect gastroesophageal reflux in children? Journal of Pediatric Gastroenterology and Nutrition 29 (4): 448–451.

Ozturk, Y., Büyükgebiz, B. et al. (2003). Effects of hospital stay on nutritional anthropometric data in Turkish children. Journal of Tropical Pediatrics 49 (3): 189–190.

Paediatric Group British Dietetic Association (2007). *Guidelines for making up special feeds for infants and children in hospital*. London: Food Standards Agency.

Patchell, C.J., Anderton, A., Holden, C. et al. (1998). Reducing bacterial contamination of enteral feeds. Archives of Disease in Childhood 78: 166–168.

Paul, L., Holden, C., Smith, A. et al. (1993). *Tube Feeding and You*. Birmingham: Nutritional Care Department, Birmingham Children's Hospital NHS Foundation Trust.

Pawallek, I., Dokoupil, K., and Koletzko, B. (2008). Prevalence of malnutrition in paediatric hospital patients. Clinical Nutrition 27: 72–76.

Pennington, C. (2000). What is parenteral nutrition? In: *Total Parenteral Nutrition: A Practical Guide for Nurses* (ed. H. Hamilton). London: Churchill Livingstone.

Peters, R.A. and Westby, D. (1994). Percutaneous endoscopic gastrostomy. British Journal of Intensive Care 4 (3): 88–92.

Puntis, J.W.L. (2001). Paediatric parenteral nutrition. In: *Artificial Nutrition Support in Clinical Practice* (eds. J. Payne-James, G. Grimble and D. Silk). London: Churchill Livingstone, pp. 461–84.

Rathwell, A. and Shaw, V. (2010). *Clinical Practice Guideline. Expressing and handling breast milk*. London: Great Ormond Street Hospital for Children NHS Foundation Trust.

Reilly, H. (1998). Enteral feeding: an overview of indications and techniques. British Journal of Nursing 7 (9): 510–521.

Renfrew, M.J., Craig, D., Dyson, L. et al. (2009). Breastfeeding promotion for infants in neonatal units: a systemic review and economic analysis. Health Technology Assessment 13 (40) (e-pub).

Rocha, G.A., Rocha, E.J., and Martins, C.V. (2006). The effects of hospitalization on the nutritional status of children. Jornal de Pediatria 82 (1): 70–74. https://www.researchgate.net/publication/7246669_The_effects_of_hospitalization_on_the_nutritional_status_of_children (accessed 19 July 2022).

Rowley, S., Clare, S., Macqueen, S., and Molyneus, R. (2010). ANTT v2: an updated practice framework for aseptic technique. British Journal of Nursing (Intravenous Supplement) 19 (5): S5–S11.

Royal College of Nursing (2016). Standards for Infusion Therapy. 4th Ed. London, Royal College of Nursing. https://www.rcn.org.uk/-/media/Royal-College-Of-Nursing/Documents/Publications/Obselete/005704.pdf (accessed 19 July 2022).

Royal College of Nursing (RCN) (2019). Restrictive physical intervention and therapeutic holding for children and young people. https://www.rcn.org.uk/Professional-Development/publications/pub-007746 (accessed 19 July 2022).

Royal College of Nursing (RCN) (2020). Promoting Optimal Breastfeeding in Children's Wards and Departments. Guidance for good practice. RCN: London. https://www.rcn.org.uk/-/media/royal-college-of-nursing/documents/publications/2021/january/009-470.pdf?la=en (accessed 05 October 2022)..

Sapsford, A.L. (2000). Human milk and enteral nutrition products. In: *Nutritional Care for the High Risk Infant*, 3e (eds. S. Groh-Wargo, M. Thompson and J. Cox), 265–279. Chicago: Precept Press.

Sari, A. and Rollins, C. (1999). Principles and guidelines for parenteral nutrition in children. Parenteral Nutrition, Paediatric Annals 28 (2): 113–122.

Scientific Advisory Committee on Nutrition (2018). Feeding in the First Year of Life. https://www.gov.uk/government/publications/feeding-in-the-first-year-of-life-sacn-report (accessed 20 July 2022).

Scientific Advisory Committee on Nutrition (2011). *Dietary Reference Values for Energy*. London: SACN.

Shaw, V. and Lawson, M. (eds.) (2007). *Nutritional Assessment, Dietary Requirements, Feed Supplementation Chapter in Clinical Paeditric Dietetics*, 3e. Oxford: Blackwell Publishing.

Singhal, A., Cole, T.J., and Lucas, A. (2001). Early nutrition in preterm infants and later blood pressure: two cohorts after randomised trials. Lancet 357: 413–419.

Singhal, A., Cole, T.J., Fewtrell, M., and Lucas, A. (2004). Breastmilk feeding and lipoprotein profile in adolescents born preterm: follow-up of a prospective randomised study. Lancet 363: 1571–1578.

Trigg, E. and Mohammed, T.A. (eds.) (2006). *Practices in Children's Nursing. Guidelines for Hospital and Community*. Edinburgh: Churchill Livingstone.

UNICEF (2012). Preventing disease and saving resources: the potential contribution of increasing breastfeeding rates in the UK. https://www.unicef.org.uk/babyfriendly/about/preventing-disease-and-saving-resources/preventing_disease_saving_resources/ (accessed 19 July 2022).

UNICEF (2013). Assessment of breastmilk expression. Checklist. https://www.unicef.org.uk/babyfriendly/baby-friendly-resources/implementing-standards-resources/assessment-of-breastmilk-expression-checklist/ (accessed 19 July 2022).

UNICEF/WHO (1994). *Mothers Charter: Protecting Breast Feeding Rights*. London: UNICEF UK Baby-Friendly Initiative.

United Kingdom Association for Milk Banking (2022). Donating milk: 'Every drop counts.' https://ukamb.org/donate-milk/ (accessed 19 July 2022).

Wang, K.K. and Bernhard, A. (2004). Technology-dependent children and their families: a review. Journal of Advanced Nursing 45 (1): 36.

Watling, R. (2014). Provision of nutrition in a hospital setting. In: *Clinical Paediatric Dietetics*, 4e (ed. V. Shaw), 23–32. Oxford: Wiley Blackwell.

World Health Organization (1981). *International Code of Marketing of Breast Milk Substitutes*. Geneva: WHO.

World Health Organization (2001). *The Optimal Duration of Exclusive Breast Feeding – A Systematic Review*. Geneva: WHO.

World Health Organization (2015). *Ten Facts on Breastfeeding*. Geneva: WHO.

Zeilhofer, U.B., Frey, B., Zandee, J., and Bernet, V. (2009). The role of critical incident monitoring in detection and prevention of human breast milk confusions. European Journal of Pediatrics 168 (10): 1277–1279.

Chapter 23

Orthopaedic care

Nathan Askew[1], Edel Broomfield[2], Penny Howard[3], Carole Irwin[4], Deborah Jackson[5], and Nicola Wilson[6]

[1]MSc Adv P, BSc (hons), Dip HE Nursing (Child), formerly Lead Nurse and Advanced Practitioner, Surgery, Great Ormond Street Hospital, London, UK

[2]RN (Child), DipHE, BSc, MSc, Lead Spinal Advanced Nurse Practitioner, GOSH

[3]RN (Adult), RN (Child), Clinical Nurse Specialist, Orthopaedics, GOSH

[4]BSc (Hons), ENB 219, PGCE. Formerly Clinical Project Manager, GOSH

[5]BSc (Hons) in Physio, MSc in Advanced Physiotherapy, MCSP, SRP, Clinical Specialist Physiotherapist, GOSH

[6]MNurSci, PGCert Ed, DTN, Lead Practice Educator, GOSH

Chapter contents

Introduction	520
Traction	520
Skeletal pin site care	520
Neurovascular observations	520
Care of a plaster cast	520
Removal of plaster casts	520
Use of crutches	521
Orthopaedic traction	521
Care of a CYP in traction	521
Gallows traction	521
Modified gallows traction/abduction traction/hoop traction	527
Skin traction	527
Slings and springs suspension	528
Spinal traction	528
References	539
Further reading	540

Procedure guidelines

23.1	How to perform neurovascular observations	524	23.9	Performing basic care needs (CYP in a cast)	531
23.2	Management of acute compartment syndrome	526	23.10	Assessment (walking aid)	532
23.3	Handling a newly applied plaster cast	526	23.11	Checking safety of crutches	533
23.4	Preparation and equipment (cutting a plaster)	527	23.12	Education of CYP and carers (crutches)	533
23.5	Splitting a cast	529	23.13	Management of traction	536
23.6	How to window a cast	529	23.14	Applying skin traction	537
23.7	Reinforcing a cast	529	23.15	Nursing care of the CYP in traction	538
23.8	Removing a cast	530	23.16	Nursing care of the CYP receiving spinal traction	539

Principles tables

23.1	Inform CYP and family (Neurovascular observations)	521	23.6	Measure the CYP for crutches	534
23.2	Positioning of a CYP in a cast	530	23.7	Safe use of crutches on a flat surface	534
23.3	Mobilisation in a cast	531	23.8	Safe use of crutches on the stairs	535
23.4	Complications of a cast	531	23.9	Principles of assembling traction	535
23.5	Selecting an appropriate walking aid	532			

The Great Ormond Street Hospital Manual of Children and Young People's Nursing Practices, Second Edition. Edited by Elizabeth Anne Bruce, Janet Williss, and Faith Gibson.
© 2023 John Wiley & Sons Ltd. Published 2023 by John Wiley & Sons Ltd.

Introduction

Orthopaedic nursing requires the utilisation of core skills in caring for children and young people (CYPs). Any CYP in a cast or bandages, or following a fracture or orthopaedic surgery, is exposed to specific risks, including oedema, pressure ulcers, tissue damage, and neurovascular compromise. It is therefore essential that nurses are aware of the importance of recording and documenting neurovascular observations, and of taking prompt action when compromise is indicated. Early detection and action prevents the long-term damage that can occur in paediatric acute compartment syndrome (PACS).

Traction

The use of traction, especially skeletal traction, is in decline due to improvements in surgical fixation, which allows for quicker recovery times and earlier weight-bearing. A CYP in traction or a plaster cast will require care similar to that of any CYP on bed rest or with restricted mobility, will have additional hygiene and toileting needs, and be at increased risk of developing tissue damage and pressure ulcers. It is important that the nurse is able to identify these needs and any possible complications. Support and education must also be provided for families and carers.

Skeletal pin site care

Skeletal pins have been used for many years, but the increasing use of external fixators has meant that they are seen more frequently. It is important to be able to recognise the difference between the normal healing process and the development of an infection. Pin site infections can cause discomfort and pain, and if not promptly identified can lead to loosening of the pin site, deeper infection, and osteomyelitis. There is, however, a lack of strong evidence regarding the effective management of pin sites to prevent infection. Following a consensus meeting, the Royal College of Nursing (RCN) produced guidance on pin site care (RCN 2022), which should be reviewed alongside current literature to produce local pin site cleaning protocols.

Before any orthopaedic procedure, it is essential that the CYP and family are fully prepared through explanation and that analgesia is given if required. This will help to reduce anxiety, enable consent to be obtained, and increase the cooperation of the CYP and family.

This chapter covers the following practices:

1 Neurovascular observations
2 Care of a plaster cast
3 Removal of plaster casts
4 The use of crutches
5 Orthopaedic traction
6 Spinal traction

Neurovascular observations

Neurovascular observations are used to assess the sensory and motor function (neuro), and the peripheral circulation (vascular) of a limb (Schreiber 2016). As such they should be carried out when a CYP is at risk of neurovascular impairment as a result of either PACS or vascular limb interventions (Livingston et al. 2017). An insult to the arteriovenous gradient reduces perfusion, leads to tissue ischemia, and subsequently to nerve injury and muscle death (Livingston et al. 2017). Although this is not an exhaustive list, neurovascular observations should therefore be carried out in CYPs following:

- Angiography or cardiac catheterisation
- Deep vein thrombosis
- Bony or muscular trauma
- Burns, snake or insect bites, crush syndrome
- Infection
- Pre- or post orthopaedic/plastic surgery
- Traction/plaster cast or with circumferential dressings
- Application of an orthopaedic device
  (Krasemann 2015; Livingston et al. 2017; Wright 2009).

Delays in recognising neurovascular deterioration can lead to lasting nerve and muscle deficits, loss of a limb, and even death (Sedgwick and Richards 2015). In the case of PACS, ischaemia starts as quickly as four hours after a rise in intracompartmental pressure (ICP), and within eight hours necrosis of the tissues may be seen (Livingston et al. 2017). It has been suggested that the 'at risk' period of PACS is between two and 64 hours after trauma or surgery (Wall et al. 2010; Wright 2009).

Neurovascular observations must be analysed in conjunction with knowledge of the injury or intervention and other clinical observations, as decreased arterial blood flow may result in a cold, pale limb, whereas venous insufficiency may result in a warm limb (Schreiber 2016). It is important to note that although pulselessness and pallor may be early signs in vascular occlusion they are late signs in PACS. Current literature states that a more appropriate indicator of PACS are the three As: increased **A**nxiety, **A**gitation, and an increase in **A**nalgesia requirement (Bae et al. 2014; Noonan and McCarthy 2010). Other complications may include loss of limb, rhabdomyolsis (increasing the risk of renal impairment), and hyperkalemia (increasing the risk of cardiac dysrhythmias) (Fort 2003; Johnston-Walker and Hardcastle 2011).

Care of a plaster cast

Plaster casts are applied for a number of reasons; to immobilise and support bones and joints following fractures or surgery, to reduce pain, and to correct deformities by stretching muscles and ligaments. Casts may be made from plaster of Paris or a range of synthetic materials. Plaster of Paris is absorbent and easy to split, so it is often used for fresh fractures, following surgery, or where swelling or bleeding is likely to occur. Synthetic materials are lighter and more hardwearing than plaster of Paris but should be used with caution when swelling is expected, as they do not have the same level of flexibility as plaster of Paris (Miles 2012). A combination of the two materials is useful when the requirement is for a strong, light cast that is absorbent and easily moulded. The nurse caring for a CYP in a plaster cast must be aware of the reason for the cast and its function, the type of materials used, how to care for it, the duration of the plaster, and the mobility limitations it will cause.

Removal of plaster casts

In addition to removing casts at the end of treatment, staff may be required to split casts to relieve swelling, or to window casts to allow for inspection of the skin at wound sites or where pressure ulcers are suspected. This will involve the use of a plaster saw and/or shears, which must be checked prior to use to ensure they are in good working order. Staff must have had the relevant training to ensure safe and correct use (Miles 2012). Staff may also need to reinforce plaster of Paris casts for added strength.

Use of crutches

Crutches may be issued by a physiotherapist to improve the gait pattern of a CYP, to increase stability, and to reduce or eliminate weight bearing on the lower limb. If this is the case, a physiotherapist should assess the CYP for suitability for a walking aid then measure, supply, and teach the safe use of the appropriate walking aid. When the CYP is safe and independent with the crutches when getting on or off a chair, walking, and climbing stairs, they may be discharged from hospital. If a CYP is unable to go up and down stairs safely using crutches, they will either need to be supervised on stairs, taught to go up and down stairs on their bottom, or arrangements for single-level living will need to be considered.

Orthopaedic traction

Care of a CYP in traction

Traction is not a new concept; records from Aztec and Egyptian periods describe manual traction being used to reduce dislocations (RCN 2021) and equipment similar to that used today was developed during the eighteenth century. Orthopaedic traction is a 'pulling force exerted on a part of the body.' To be able to pull (or apply traction effectively), there must be something trying to 'pull' in the opposite direction. This is countertraction, without which traction is not effective. Countertraction may be provided by body weight (frictional force between the CYP and the bed) or by elevating the foot (where traction is on a lower extremity), or at the head of the bed (for example in cervical traction), in order to create a greater gravitational pull (Hockenberry and Wilson 2013; Wong et al. 2012).

There are two mechanisms of traction; **fixed**, which is a pull between two fixed points (e.g. Thomas Splint), and **balanced or sliding**, where the pull is balanced between weights and the body (e.g. Pugh's traction). Traction is applied directly to either the skin or skeletal system. **Manual traction** involves pulling a limb by hand and is a simple, temporary method of applying skin traction, which may be used to realign fractured bones (Lucas and Davis 2005). **Skin traction** exerts a force directly on the skin and indirectly on the underlying muscles and bones. Adhesive or nonadhesive strips, with an attached cord, are applied to the limb and secured with a bandage. The cord is either secured to a frame for fixed traction, or weights and pulleys are used for balanced traction. Skin traction can be applied to the long bones of the extremities, or using a sling or belt, to the spine or pelvis. **Skeletal traction** directly applies a pulling force to the skeletal structure by pins or wires that have been inserted surgically through the diameter of the bone (Hockenberry and Wilson 2013; Wong et al. 2012). The pins are attached to a loop or stirrup, to which cord is attached and weights are then secured to the cord. Skeletal traction can be used for long periods of time, or when a larger amount of weight is required.

Traction may be used:

- To reduce muscle spasm and pain.
- To maintain the correct alignment of the limb while ensuring rest and comfort.
- To restore and maintain the correct alignment of bone following fractures and/or dislocations, trauma, surgery, or as a result of the CYP's medical condition while allowing movement of the joints during the healing process.
- To prevent or gradually improve contracture deformities to the soft tissues caused by disease or injury.
- To allow the CYP to be moved with ease.
- To immobilise the CYP (Hockenberry and Wilson 2013; RCN 2021; Wong et al. 2012).

The type of traction applied is determined primarily by the age of the CYP, the condition of the soft tissue, and the type and degree of displacement of the fracture. Traction is used to immobilise the fracture in the correct position until there is sufficient healing to cast or splint the limb until fully healed. Splints and casts may be used in conjunction with skeletal traction.

Traction should be used with caution, as too much force may damage the nerves and soft tissues and too little force may produce painful muscle spasms and impair healing (RCN 2021). Traction is used less frequently today, as developments in orthopaedic fixation devices and other techniques allow CYPs to be partially or fully weight-bearing. These newer techniques reduce the period of immobility and the risks of the complications that are associated with this. The main forms of traction are described below.

Gallows traction

Gallows, or Bryant's traction is used to treat a fractured shaft of femur in the very young child (12 months or 10–16 kg) or to aid hip positioning prior to surgical reduction of developmental dysplasia of the hip (RCN 2021). Gallows traction can be fixed, with the cord secured to a frame above the cot, or balanced, with the use of pulleys and weights. The traction is always applied to both legs to maintain symmetry. The CYP lies supine with hips flexed to 90° so that the vertical pull to both legs maintains the correct alignment of the bones and hip joints. The knees are slightly flexed and the buttocks should be just clear of the mattress, with a gap to allow a flat hand to fit underneath. This allows the CYP's body weight to provide the counter traction (RCN 2021).

Principles table 23.1 Inform CYP and family (Neurovascular observations)

Principle	Rationale
1 The observations that will be carried out and the reason for them must be explained to the CYP and family.	1 To gain informed consent, improve cooperation, reduce fear, and provide reassurance.
2 The CYP should be encouraged to practice the movements shown on the chart regularly (see Figures 23.1 and 23.2). However, the CYP may be instructed by their physiotherapist to expand the range of movements.	2 To reduce fear of movement and the need for passive movement (i.e. physiotherapy). Movement reduces swelling, improves circulation, and promotes blood flow, which helps healing.
3 The CYP should have their pain assessed preprocedure and analgesia given if appropriate.	3 To determine whether the procedure is likely to cause pain or discomfort. To minimise pain.

The Great Ormond Street Hospital Manual of Children and Young People's Nursing Practices

Lower Limb Neurovascular Observation Chart

NHS Great Ormond Street Hospital for Children — NHS Foundation Trust

Patient Label

Left / Right (please circle)

Operation Date..................
Operation........................
....
Consultant.......................
Ward.............................

DATE:	
TIME:	
COLOUR:	PK = Pink P = Pale D = Dusky C = Cyanotic
WARMTH:	H = Hot W = Warm Cl = Cool Cd = Cold
SWELLING:	N = Nil S = Small M = Moderate MK = Marked
OOZE:	N = Nil S = Small M = Moderate L = Large
PULSES: 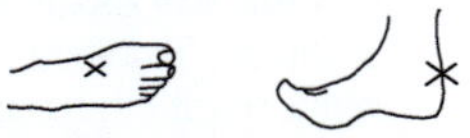	S = Strong W = Weak A = Absent
CAPILLARY REFILL:	1 = 1 sec 2 = 2 sec 3 = 3 sec 4+ = 4+ secs
PAIN SCORE:	0 - 10 (as per pain chart)
MOVEMENT:	A = Active movement without pain A* = Active movement with pain P = Passive movement without pain P* = Passive movement with pain — Peroneal Nerve (Dorsiflexion), Tibial Nerve (Plantarflexion)
SENSATION:	F = Full N = Nil PN = Pins and Needles P = Partial M = Moves to touch — Peroneal Nerve (dorsal surface), Tibial Nerve (plantar surface)
POSITION:	L = Left side R = Right side S = Supine P = Prone Sat = Sat up
COMMENTS:	
SIGNATURE:	

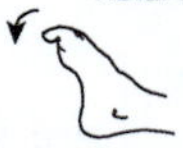

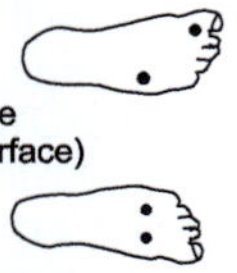

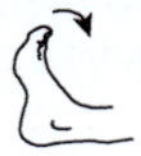

Adapted from RCH Melbourne

Figure 23.1 Neurovascular observations: lower limb.

Chapter 23 Orthopaedic care

NHS
Great Ormond Street Hospital for Children
NHS Foundation Trust

Upper Limb Neurovascular Observation Chart

Left / Right (please circle)

Patient Label

Operation Date.................
Operation.........................
....
Consultant......................
Ward...............................

DATE:	
TIME:	
COLOUR:	PK = Pink P = Pale D = Dusky C = Cyanotic
WARMTH:	H = Hot W = Warm Cl = Cool Cd = Cold
SWELLING:	N = Nil S = Small M = Moderate MK = Marked
OOZE:	N = Nil S = Small M = Moderate L = Large
PULSES:	S = Strong W = Weak A = Absent
CAPILLARY REFILL:	1 = 1 sec 2 = 2 sec 3 = 3 sec 4+ = 4+ secs
PAIN SCORE:	0 - 10 (as per pain chart)
MOVEMENT: A= Active movement without pain A= Active movement with pain P= Passive movement without pain P= Passive movement with pain	Radial Nerve (into extension) Median nerve Ulnar nerve
SENSATION: F = Full N = Nil PN = Pins and Needles P = Partial M = Moves to touch	Radial Median Ulnar
POSITION:	L = Left side R = Right side S = Supine P = Prone Sat = Sat up
VISUAL DISTURBANCE:	Y = Yes N = No (c spine patients only)
COMMENTS:	
SIGNATURE:	

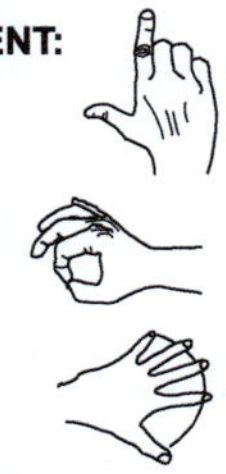

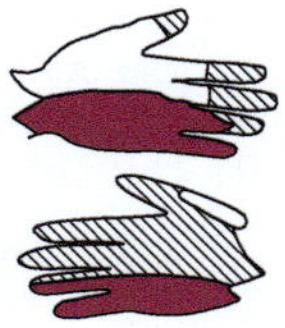

Adapted from RCH Melbourne

Figure 23.2 Neurovascular observations: upper limb.

The Great Ormond Street Hospital Manual of Children and Young People's Nursing Practices

Procedure guideline 23.1 How to perform neurovascular observations

Statement	Rationale
Colour, warmth, swelling, and ooze	
1 Visually assess the naked foot/hand, checking for colour, swelling, and ooze.	1 Colour and warmth are provided by a healthy blood supply. A cool pale limb is indicative of a reduced arterial supply, while a dusky, blue, or cyanotic limb is likely to be due to poor venous return. Swelling is an indicator for acute compartment syndrome and essential to observe. It is especially important if the limb is in any type of cast. Tense refers to a tight shiny limb/skin (Wright 2009; Leversedge et al. 2011).
2 Check for warmth with superficial touch.	2 Increased limb temperature can also be indicative of poor venous return (Altizer 2002).
3 If a chart refers to the colour 'pink,' limb perfusion should be checked in CYPs with darker skin.	3 'Pink' colour assessment is not accurate for all ethnic groups. In these circumstances, assess for a well-perfused limb.
4 Ooze requires monitoring for wound care and blood loss. It should be marked on a plaster cast for monitoring and documented.	4 To monitor for continuing or excessive bleeding.
Pulse and capillary refill	
1 Check foot/hand for presence and magnitude of pulses distal to the injury/affected area.	1 A pulseless limb is a late and unreliable sign of acute compartment syndrome as arterial flow may continue while the peripheral perfusion is compromised (Altizer 2002; Edwards 2004). An absent pulse is significant, however, as it may denote arterial stenosis, while an excessively strong pulse can suggest a distal occlusion.
2 Capillary refill should be measured by pressing on the digit for 5 seconds, then counting the seconds until the digit returns to its usual colour; this normally takes less than 2 seconds.	2 To assess peripheral perfusion and cardiac output.
Pain	
1 Pain score should be assessed in conjunction with movement.	1 To observe for compartment syndrome.
2 An increase in analgesia requirement should also be documented in the comments section.	2 Pain that is disproportionate to the injury and increases with passive extension is indicative of acute compartment syndrome (Altizer 2002; Edwards 2004). A more appropriate indicator of PACS is the three A's: increased anxiety, agitation, and analgesia requirement (Noonan and McCarthy 2010; Bae et al. 2014).
Movement of limbs	
1 It is essential that limbs are fully flexed and extended.	1 To detect early signs of acute compartment syndrome, which include pain or altered sensation on movement (Judge 2007; Johnston-Walker and Hardcastle 2011).
2 Where movement is restricted by a cast or orthotic device, the digits should still be flexed and extended, and the type of cast documented in the comments section.	2 This also stretches the muscles and demonstrates nerve function, although to a lesser extent.
3 If the CYP is asleep, full movement of the limbs should be carried out passively and documented as such. If the movement creates significant pain, assess efficacy of analgesia. If the pain is disproportionate to the injury further assessment is required.	3 To ensure that observations are carried out even when the CYP is asleep so that pain and complications are detected and treated promptly.
Foot movement	
1 The foot should be actively dorsiflexed as far as mechanically possible (see Figure 23.3a). If active movement is not possible due to language or developmental barriers then full dorsiflexion should be carried out passively (Altizer 2002).	1 To assess the function of the peroneal nerve. Active movement demonstrates nerve function (Duckworth and Blundell 2010). To assess the function of the peroneal nerve.
2 The CYP should then actively plantarflex the foot as far as mechanically possible (see Figure 23.3b). Where this is not possible due to language or developmental barriers this movement should be carried out passively.	2 To assess the tibial nerve function.

Chapter 23 Orthopaedic care

Procedure guideline 23.1 How to perform neurovascular observations *(continued)*

Statement	Rationale
Hand movement	
1 The thumb and first digit should be made into an L-shape and then extended upwards and backwards as far as mechanically possible (Figure 23.4a).	1 Active movement demonstrates nerve function. The extended L-shape tests the radial nerve function.
2 The thumb is then brought to meet the index finger in an OK sign (Figure 23.4b).	2 To test median nerve function.
3 The fingers are splayed and mild pressure applied to the external digits to ensure the position can be maintained (Figure 23.4c).	3 To test ulnar nerve function.
4 These tests should be done actively and can easily be made into a game. Where this is not possible, due to language or developmental barriers, these movements should be carried out passively (Altizer 2002).	4 To ensure that the limb is fully flexed and extended in order to assess for acute compartment syndrome.
Sensation	
1 All touchable/visible surfaces (including in-between digits) should be checked for presence and type of sensation.	1 To assess the peroneal (dorsal) and tibial (plantar) nerves in the foot (Figure 23.5a) and radial, median, and ulnar nerves in the hand (Figure 23.5b). Numbness or complaints of pins and needles/tingling can be indicative of nerve compromise (Judge 2007).
2 If possible, this should be done with the CYP's eyes closed/not watching.	2 It is more effective and accurate if the CYP is not watching.
Position	
1 The CYP's position should be altered regularly and documented as left, right, supine, prone, or sitting.	1 Regular changes in position are essential, as those requiring neurovascular observations commonly have reduced mobility and are therefore at a higher risk of pressure ulcers.
2 Regular assessment of the skin using a recognised assessment tool is required (see Chapter 11: Personal Hygiene and Pressure Ulcer Prevention).	2 To prevent or detect early signs of tissue/pressure damage.
Visual disturbances	
1 If there has been trauma or surgery to the neck (cervical spine) the CYP should be assessed for visual abnormalities such as blurred or double vision.	1 To check the effect of the cervical spine deformity or damage on the visual field and acuity.
2 Document the date and time of the observations in the CYP's healthcare records.	2 To maintain an accurate record (Nursing and Midwifery Council [NMC] 2018).

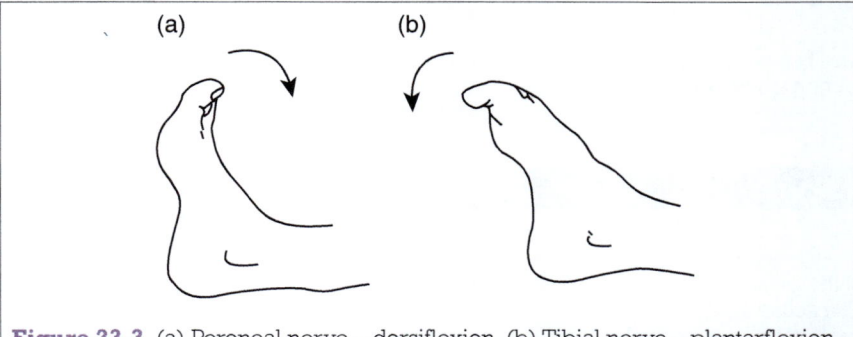

Figure 23.3 (a) Peroneal nerve – dorsiflexion. (b) Tibial nerve – plantarflexion.

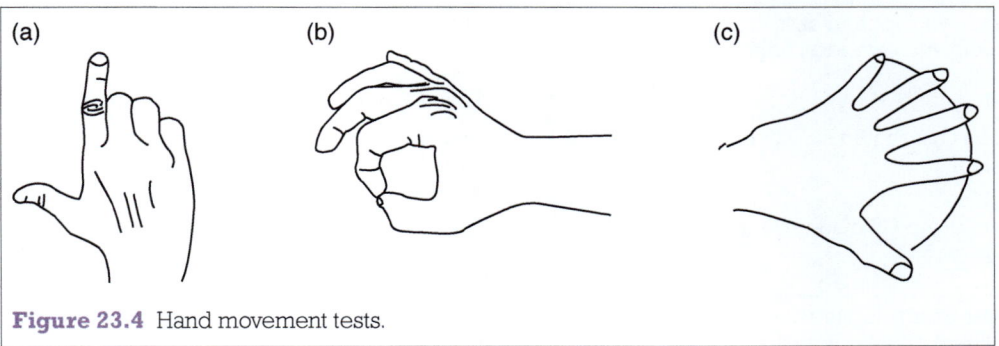

Figure 23.4 Hand movement tests.

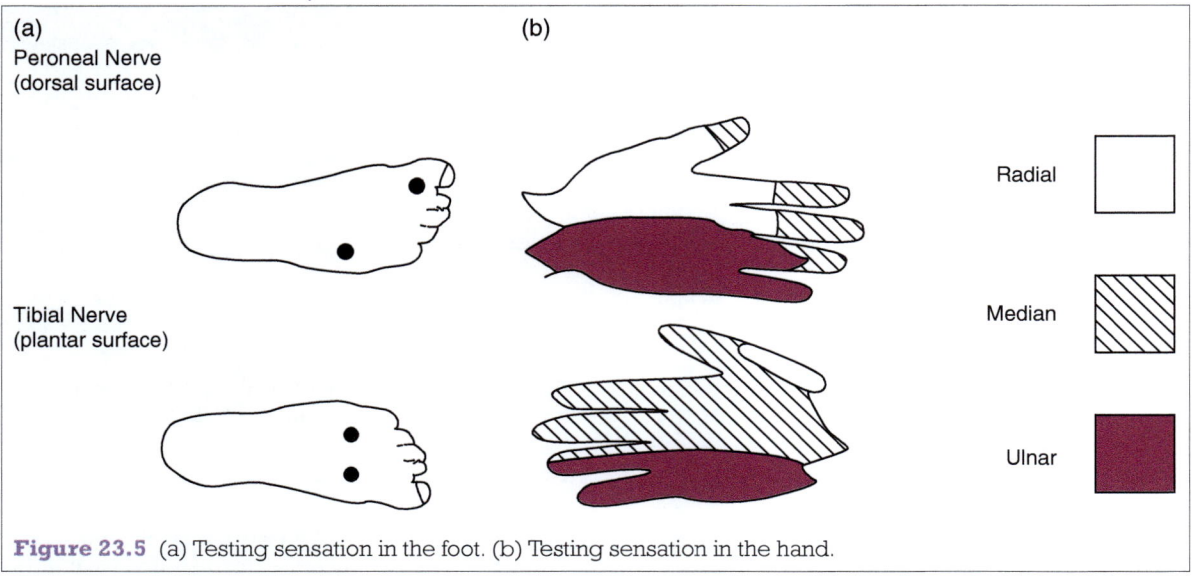

Figure 23.5 (a) Testing sensation in the foot. (b) Testing sensation in the hand.

Procedure guideline 23.2 Management of acute compartment syndrome

Statement	Rationale
If acute compartment syndrome is suspected:	
1 Call the CYP's medical team for an urgent review.	1 To instigate urgent investigation and treatment. The longer the delay, the greater the risk of muscle and nerve damage and tissue death.
2 If the limb has a bandage or plaster cast in situ completely split the cast and cut the dressing to skin level.	2 To relieve pressure.
3 Elevate the limb to the height of the heart.	3 If it is elevated higher, the vascular pressure will continue to increase and exacerbate the condition by increasing the ischemia (Judge 2007).
4 Carry out 15–30 minutes neurovascular observations.	4 To check on the condition of the affected limb.
If nerve compromise is suspected	
1 Contact the CYP's medical team if this is a new observation.	1 To instigate urgent investigation and treatment.
2 If acute compartment syndrome has been diagnosed the CYP will need to have an emergency fasciotomy in theatre.	2 The damage caused by acute compartment syndrome can occur extremely quickly and urgent surgery is required to reduce the amount of damage caused.

Procedure guideline 23.3 Handling a newly applied plaster cast

Statement	Rationale
1 Following application of a cast the plastered limb should be elevated if possible. This can be achieved by placing the cast on waterproof pillows covered with a towel or by elevating the foot of the bed (Trendelenburg position).	1 To aid venous return and minimise oedema to the affected limb.
2 When handling a newly applied cast, the carer should use the flat of their hand and extended fingertips.	2 To support the limb at all times and prevent accidental damage to the cast, which may cause pressure ulcers to develop under the plaster. Supporting the cast will also help reduce any pain or discomfort associated with the weight of the cast.
3 The newly applied cast should be left uncovered to aid effective drying.	3 A plaster of Paris cast can take up to three days to dry fully. Covering the cast with clothing or bed linen may inhibit this process.
4 Artificial means of drying should never be used.	4 Plasters dried artificially may become brittle and crack. Artificial methods of drying can also be harmful to the CYP, as plaster of Paris conducts heat and cold, which may cause burns or blisters.
5 Support and cover unaffected areas of the limb with clothing or bed linen.	5 Plaster of Paris casts can be cold and wet until they dry, which may cause discomfort.

Chapter 23 Orthopaedic care

Procedure guideline 23.4 Preparation and equipment (cutting a plaster)

Statement	Rationale
1 Prior to cutting into a cast, perform hand hygiene and put on gloves and an apron.	1 To prevent cross-infection and protect clothing.
2 It is advisable to wear appropriate personal protective equipment, i.e. eye or ear protection while splitting the cast.	2 To protect the person operating the saw and other staff/family members within the vicinity (Miles 2012).
3 Prepare a room/cubicle in which to perform the procedure, ensuring that it is safe and comfortable for the CYP and carer.	3 To allow privacy and to prevent disruption to other patients. Removing a plaster cast can create a lot of dust and noise.
Plaster saw	
1 When using the electric saw, hold the blade at 90° to the cast and cut through the plaster using an in and out motion.	1–3 The blade will cut the skin or become hot enough to create a burn if used incorrectly (Miles 2012).
2 Avoid sliding the saw up and down the cast and avoid bony prominences.	
3 If the saw becomes hot during the procedure stop and allow the saw to cool before continuing.	
4 The plaster saw must be used with extra caution if:	4
a) The plaster cast is not padded. b) The cast is stained with blood or has been applied following surgery. c) The limb is swollen.	a) To protect the CYP from harm. b) The padding may be too hard to cut (Bakody 2009). c) The plaster saw may easily cut taut skin (Miles 2012).
Plaster shears	
1 When using plaster shears, place the blades between the plaster and padding.	1 If the blade of the shear is tilted in either direction the point or the heel of the shears will dig in or nip the skin (Miles 2012).
2 Keeping the shears parallel to the skin, slowly depress the handles in a scissor like motion to cut through the cast (Figure 23.6).	
3 Avoid bony prominences.	
Plaster scissors	
1 Plaster scissors/blunt edged scissors should be used to split padding under plaster (Miles 2012).	1 To reduce the risk of injury to the CYP's skin.

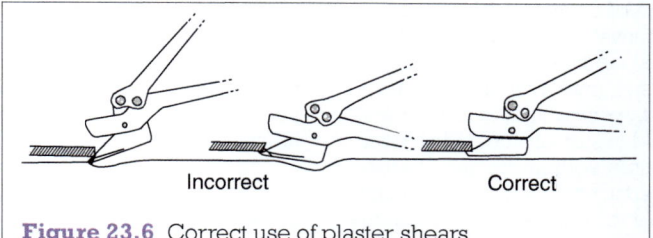

Figure 23.6 Correct use of plaster shears.

Modified gallows traction/abduction traction/hoop traction

Abduction traction can be used preoperatively in CYPs with developmental dysplasia of the hip prior to a closed reduction. Traction is applied in the same way as gallows traction, but after 24 hours with hips in a neutral position the child's legs are abducted daily, usually over a week or more to a maximum of 60° (Figure 23.7). There is some anecdotal evidence that abduction traction prior to closed reduction of the hip may reduce the risk of avascular necrosis of the femoral head. It is also believed to increase the probability of a successful closed reduction by stretching the soft tissues, but this is not proven (Weinstein 2014).

Skin traction

Skin traction (formerly known as Pugh's traction) is applied to either one or both legs using skin extensions. It is attached to a bar at the end of the bed, or to weights and a pulley (RCN 2021) (Figure 23.8). The foot of the bed is elevated to provide countertraction. A direct pull is applied in a plane that is in line with the body part to be treated. Skin traction may be applied preoperatively for a CYP with a slipped upper femoral epiphysis, following hip or lower limb surgery, or for developmental dysplasia of the hip, Perthes disease, or irritable hip. Medical staff should document in the CYP's health care record whether skin traction must be maintained continuously (e.g. following fractures and some types of surgery) or can be removed temporarily (e.g. for toileting, washing, and physiotherapy).

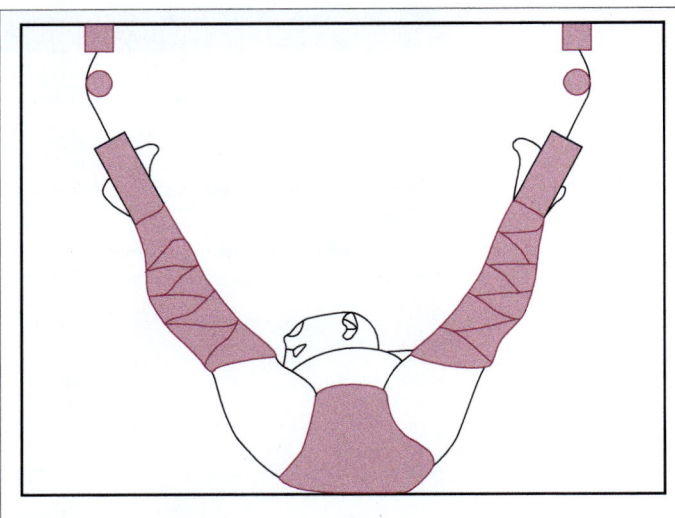

Figure 23.7 Abduction traction (modified Bryant's traction).

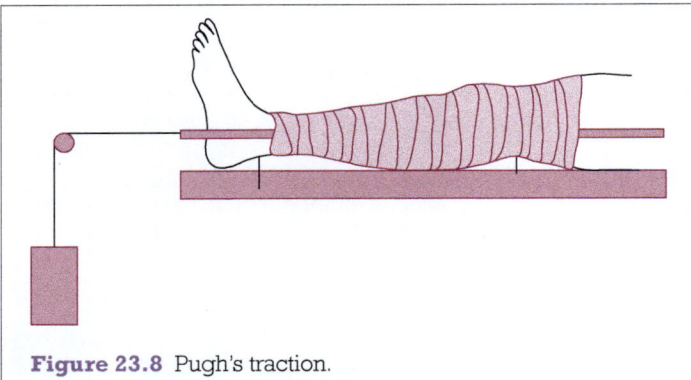

Figure 23.8 Pugh's traction.

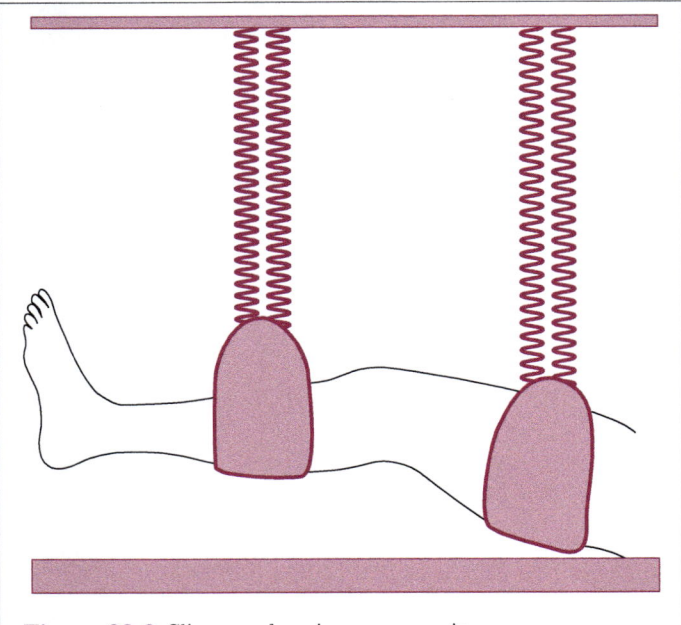

Figure 23.9 Slings and springs suspension.

Slings and springs suspension

Slings and springs are used in the care of CYPs with hip conditions such as Perthes disease, or post operatively following hip or lower limb surgery, and allow the CYP to rest the limb/joint while permitting gentle exercise and physiotherapy, and maintaining muscle strength and joint mobility. Slings and springs should not be confused with traction; here the limb is held in suspension and no countertraction is required. However, the same equipment may be used and slings and springs may also be used in conjunction with traction. The leg is supported by one sling under the thigh and one under the calf, both of which are attached to springs suspended from a traction frame (usually Balkan) (Figure 23.9). Padding must be placed under the slings to prevent the edges digging in and causing damage to skin, especially at pressure points. The principles of traction care should be applied to a CYP on slings and springs, as they are at risk of the same complications as a CYP in traction.

Spinal traction

CYPs with severe scoliosis may be unsuitable for a single stage spinal fusion and may first require a period of treatment with traction. The principle of spinal traction is to slowly increase the traction on the spine, increasing its flexibility and reducing the risk of spinal cord damage during definitive surgery.

Spinal traction uses a halo ring, which is attached to the skull with anterior and posterior pins and connected to a series of weights and pulleys (Figure 23.12). Spinal traction can involve a halo ring +/- tibia skeletal traction. This is applied under general anaesthetic and may be performed in conjunction with an anterior spinal release. The consultant spinal surgeon will determine the initial torque of the halo and traction weight prescribed. The traction force is usually increased by one kilogramme daily. This will be determined by the medical team and recorded in the CYP's healthcare record. The final traction force can be up to one third or one half of the CYP's body weight. Following application of traction and any increase in traction force upper and lower limb neurovascular observations must be performed and documented on the appropriate chart every 30 minutes for four hours. Any alteration in movement or sensation should be reported immediately to the medical team. For more information see the neurovascular observations section of this chapter and assessing the neurological system Chapter 1: Assessment.

If the CYP only has a halo ring they can be transferred to a traction chair. The CYP will be transferred from the traction bed to traction chair and back as determined and documented in their healthcare record by physiotherapy and OT teams. If the CYP has tibia-halo traction they must remain in bed.

The frequency and length of time that the CYP is allowed to sit in the traction chair is agreed by the multidisciplinary team. When not in the traction wheelchair, traction will continue on the CYP's bed.

Care should be provided in line with the manufacturers' recommendations and local guidelines. Extra care should be taken to ensure needs are met, including personal hygiene, pressure care, and administration of analgesia as required. It is essential to ensure that the CYP's psychological, play, and developmental needs are also met for the duration of treatment.

After approximately one to two weeks the skeletal traction is removed and the CYP will undergo a spinal fusion and instrumentation. Once traction therapy is complete the CYP will need to return to theatre for the definitive correction operation under a general anaesthetic and have the halo ring removed.

The psychology and play teams will utilise appropriate play therapies and visual education to prepare the CYP and family psychologically for halo application to minimise the CYP's distress, promote involvement, maximise compliance, and help the CYP and family develop coping strategies. All CYPs identified for halo traction will be assessed by the Occupational Therapist (OT) for appropriate postural needs/wheelchair size while attending the spinal investigation day.

Procedure guideline 23.5 Splitting a cast

Statement	Rationale
1 It may be necessary to split a plaster after application if circulation/neurovascular status is impaired.	1 A plaster cast forms a tight band around a limb and can inhibit circulation.
2 Always seek direction from medical staff prior to splitting the cast.	2 Splitting the case may compromise the post-surgical position of the limb.
3 Splitting of the cast should not be delayed if acute compartment syndrome is considered.	3 Acute compartment syndrome is a serious event which if left untreated can cause tissue necrosis and loss of a limb.
4 Splitting a synthetic cast may not relieve swelling, therefore bivalving (when a plaster is cut in two halves back and front) the cast may be necessary.	4 Synthetic material does not have the same level of flexibility as plaster of Paris (Miles 2012).
5 If a limb is expected to swell after surgery/trauma the plaster should be split immediately following application.	5 To protect neurovascular/circulatory status. It is easier to split plaster casts before swelling occurs (Miles 2012; RCN 2021).
6 Split the plaster by making one continuous cut from the top to the bottom of the cast.	6 Constriction will not be relieved unless the whole of the cast is split.
7 This is usually through the centre of the cast following a pencil line.	7 To ensure accuracy and to avoid bony prominences (Miles 2012; RCN 2021).
8 If splitting through the centre is contraindicated the surgeon should document in the CYP's health care record where to split the cast if this is required.	8 To prevent unnecessary injury to CYP and user. To avoid damage to wound sites.
9 The plaster must be split down to the skin. A finger should be run from the top to the bottom of split.	9 To ensure that no strands of padding or lining are left intact. Even one strand of fibre is sufficient to maintain constriction (Miles 2012).
10 Plaster spreaders may be required to prise apart the edges of the cast if the limb is very swollen. Extra padding should then be placed in the gap and cast position secured with crepe bandage.	10 To prevent tissue swelling into the split edge.
11 After oedema has subsided the plaster can be completed using synthetic cast bandage or a new cast can be applied.	11 To ensure that the plaster cast is secure and not too loose.

Procedure guideline 23.6 How to window a cast

Statement	Rationale
1 It may be necessary to cut a window into a plaster cast.	1 To observe a small area without affecting the integrity of the cast. This may be required to allow the nurse to inspect a wound, remove sutures, or check skin for suspected pressure ulcers (Miles 2012).
2 This should be done with direction from medical staff.	
3 A window may be cut using a hand or electric saw.	
4 The area to be windowed should be accurately marked to size prior to cutting.	4 To ensure that a whole section is removed, which can be easily replaced Miles (2012).
5 The removed section should be adequately padded with clean wadding.	5 To aid comfort and correct positioning once replaced.
6 Once the wound or skin has been inspected and treated, the window section should be replaced with synthetic plaster or plaster of Paris.	6 To prevent tissue swelling into the space made by the window (Miles 2012).

Procedure guideline 23.7 Reinforcing a cast

Statement	Rationale
1 When plaster of Paris is applied following trauma or surgery, the plaster may need to be reinforced using a synthetic material prior to weight bearing.	1 Plaster of Paris may not be durable enough to tolerate weight bearing.
2 The plaster should not be reinforced until neurovascular status is stable.	2 To allow easy splitting of a cast if required. Plaster of Paris can be split more easily than reinforced casts, which may require bivalving.

(continued)

Procedure guideline 23.7 Reinforcing a cast (continued)

Statement	Rationale
3 Use synthetic plaster materials in accordance with manufacturers' guidelines.	3 To ensure effective application.
4 The reinforcement bandages should be applied in a spiral pattern, overlapping by half a bandage width each turn.	4 To ensure even coverage and maintain original form of cast.
5 Take care not to stretch the bandages over the limb. Figure-of-eight bandaging should be used over heels and other areas of joint flexion.	
6 High impact areas, e.g. heels and base of foot should be doubly reinforced.	6 For added durability and protection.
7 Synthetic bandages should not come into direct contact with the skin.	7 The product will adhere to skin and cause irritation.
8 The reinforced cast should be smooth with no sharp edges (Miles 2012).	8 To prevent damage to skin of affected/adjacent limb.

Procedure guideline 23.8 Removing a cast

Statement	Rationale
1 When removing a plaster cast it should always be cut in to two halves (bivalving) (Miles 2012).	1 To avoid injury to the CYP, and to use as a splint if required.
2 A guide line should be marked medially and laterally prior to cutting the cast with plaster saw or shears (Miles 2012).	2 To avoid cutting over bony prominences and provide a useful splint.
3 Once the cast is cut on both sides, ease the cast open with plaster spreaders, then proceed to cut the padding.	
4 The limb should remain in the cast or the posterior aspect of the cast (back slab) until instructed by medical or physiotherapy notes (Miles 2012).	4 To avoid injury to the CYP.
5 After cast removal, inspect the skin for pressure areas, plaster ulcers, and injuries from foreign bodies. Give skin care as indicated.	5 To identify any complications from the cast.
6 Any pressure ulcers should be examined by the medical staff and recorded in the case notes. An incident report form must be completed and the development of the pressure sore investigated (Miles 2012).	6 To document the severity of the skin and tissue damage and enable staff to determine whether the pressure sore improves or deteriorates over time.
7 Any treatment prescribed and follow-up arrangements must also be documented.	7 To ensure an accurate record is maintained in the CYPs health care record.

Principles table 23.2 Positioning of a CYP in a cast

Principle	Rationale
1 Casted limbs should be elevated using pillows or Trendelenburg positioning for lower limbs to no more than 10cm above the heart (Miles 2012).	1 Elevation helps to prevent swelling of the affected limb and also provides support.
2 Slings, collar and cuff, or Bradford slings are used to elevate upper limbs.	
3 For children or babies in hip spica plasters, a bed of pillows or a beanbag is a useful way to help provide support.	
4 Areas that are vulnerable to pressure ulcers, including the heels and sacrum, should never receive direct pressure from the bed.	4 This may lead to pressure or plaster ulcers under the cast.
5 CYPs in large casts should be turned at least 2–4 hourly or repositioned using pillows or beanbags for support.	5 This helps the cast dry and minimises the risk of pressure areas developing.

Chapter 23 Orthopaedic care

Procedure guideline 23.9 Performing basic care needs (CYP in a cast)

Statement	Rationale
1 Cleanse the skin daily in the CYP's usual way using products of their choice. Pay particular attention to 'hard to reach' areas, such as the groin, underarm, and back.	1 These areas may be particularly difficult for the CYP to reach. Crumbs and debris can cause skin irritation, increasing the risk of plaster ulcers.
2 After washing, ensure that all exposed areas of skin are dried thoroughly and that any powders or creams used are not applied near or under the edges of the cast (McDermott and Nolan 2010).	2 Powders and creams may collect under the cast and encourage skin irritation and breakdown or may impede the strength of the cast.
3 Throughout the procedure it is imperative that the cast does not become wet or damaged in any way.	3 Wet or damaged casts do not provide adequate support and may cause further complications such as ulcers or skin irritation.
4 Ensure clothing is loose and comfortable. Some clothes may need to be altered to accommodate the cast; poppers and Velcro can be used at the seams to allow for easy dressing.	4 Tight clothing may cause restrictions and discomfort and will prevent moisture evaporating away from the surface of the skin.
5 CYPs in hip spicas, body casts, and bilateral long leg casts may need to use bedpans or urinal bottles for elimination and will probably need assistance with these.	5 To promote effective elimination while the CYP has reduced mobility. Toilets are rarely large enough to accommodate a CYP in a large cast comfortably.
6 a) Removable absorbent (not waterproof) tape should be applied to the edges of the cast and around the nappy area for protection. b) There should be sufficient padding around the edges of the casts.	6 a) Waterproof tape can create a channel, which allows moisture to track further into the cast and can damage the cast. Removable absorbent tape can be changed regularly if it becomes contaminated. b) To prevent denting or damage to the cast.
7 Nutrition is an essential component of care for CYPs in casts. Those in hip spicas or body casts should avoid large, heavy meals and be advised to eat smaller, more frequent meals to avoid a bloated or overfull feeling in a small space.	7 Hip spicas and body casts are usually quite snug-fitting in order to provide support; therefore, there is not a lot of room for expansion of the abdomen.

Principles table 23.3 Mobilisation in a cast

Principle	Rationale
1 Mobilising should only be undertaken when the cast is fully dry and reinforced.	1, 2 To prevent accidental damage or denting to the cast and injury to the CYP.
2 Adhere to weight bearing status as directed by medical staff.	
3 Protective plaster boots should be worn at all times (Miles 2012).	3 Plaster casts need protection even when reinforced, and can be very slippery to walk on.
4 The use of crutches or walking frames may be necessary to aid mobilisation (for more information see section on safe use of crutches).	4 To allow safe mobilisation when no or partial weight bearing is required.
5 If the CYP is not mobile, the affected limb should be put through a range of exercises above and below the affected area.	5 To prevent joint stiffness and muscle weakness and to help prevent swelling in the extremities.
6 All other limbs should be exercised and used as normally as possible (Jester et al. 2011).	6 To help promote independence and to prevent any unnecessary stiffness and weakness.
7 A physiotherapist should provide passive exercises, including giving verbal and written instructions.	7 To reinforce information and use for future reference.

Principles table 23.4 Complications of a cast

Principle	Rationale
1 Minor complications of a cast include: • Circulatory and nerve impairment • Excessive ooze or infection of surgical sites • Pressure or cast ulcers • Pain in casted limbs • Skin irritation from the cast	1 These complications can be caused by: • A cast that is too tight • Insufficient padding to allow for swelling, excessive swelling • Uneven tension on application • Local pressure on blood vessels or nerves • Insertion of foreign bodies into the cast • Excessive muscle stretching • Irritation from casting materials

(continued)

Principles table 23.4 Complications of a cast *(continued)*

Principle	Rationale
2 **Acute compartment syndrome**	2 For more information, see Procedure Guideline 23.2.
3 **Arterial compression**	
Extremities appear white initially, then blue and finally black. The beds of the toes and fingernails remain white when blanched and mobility to the digits is severely impaired (Miles 2012).	This is usually caused by constriction due to the cast being too tight, or pressure on an artery from some other source, such as poor positioning (Lucas and Davis 2005).
4 **Venous compression**	
Extremities appear very red, almost purple looking, pain is present, and sometimes swelling too (Miles 2012).	Usual cause of venous compression would be a constriction caused by the cast being too tight or pressure.
5 **Nerve compression**	
The CYP may complain of pins and needles, followed by numbness, reduced movement, and pain (Miles 2012).	Nerve compression or impairment is usually due to an injured nerve for example from surgery or constriction of a plaster cast.
6 Treatment of conditions 2–5 above is as follows: • Contact a member of the medical team immediately. • Split the cast through its entire length down to skin (see splitting a cast). • Once the cast is split the edges need to be opened with spreaders and the gap filled with padding to prevent tissue swelling into the gap. • The limb must then be elevated and movement encouraged in the extremities. • Monitor closely until normal colour and sensation resume and any pain settles (Miles 2012). • Document the incident and actions taken in the CYP's healthcare records.	

Procedure guideline 23.10 Assessment (walking aid)

Statement	Rationale
1 Read the medical notes prior to assessing the CYP.	1 To determine the surgeons' plan and the weight bearing status of the CYP. To determine lifestyle factors impacting on the choice of walking aid. To identify any medical history that would impact choice of walking aid, such as cognitive difficulties, upper limb deformity.
2 Determine the age of the CYP.	2 Children under the age of 6 are unlikely to cope with using crutches (see section on selecting an appropriate aid). Children who have used crutches to improve balance or gait may cope at a younger age.
3 Where possible, teaching in the use of crutches should be provided prior to surgery. If this is not possible, ensure that oral pain relief is given at least 45–60 minutes before the teaching (15–30 minutes if intravenous analgesia).	3 To ensure that the CYP is as free as pain as is possible when mobilising for the first time.

Principles table 23.5 Selecting an appropriate walking aid

Principle	Rationale
1 If the child is under six years old, or is lacking in coordination, crutches may not be appropriate. In this situation, a walking frame may be appropriate, or the child's parents/carers may prefer to carry the child or use a wheelchair or buggy.	1 To ensure that the safest and most appropriate method of mobilisation is provided in consultation with the child and family.
2 Elbow crutches are more commonly used in the UK and some hospitals no longer stock axillary crutches. Adapted handles may be required in the presence of upper limb abnormality.	2 Elbow crutches are more likely to be used correctly and have less potential complications if used incorrectly.

Principles table 23.5 Selecting an appropriate walking aid *(continued)*

Principle	Rationale
3 The decision to use axillary crutches should be based on the stability of the CYP and the ease with which they use the crutch.	3 Axillary crutches afford more stability to the user than elbow crutches.
4 A physiotherapist must assess a CYP who has been prescribed crutches.	4 To help them establish a suitable gait pattern. A physiotherapist is the most appropriate person to do this.
5 The person issuing the crutches needs to be aware that they all have weight limits. Although most CYPs weigh less than these limits, where there is doubt, consult the manufacturer. Most crutches have weight limits printed on them.	5 To ensure that the CYP has been issued with the appropriate crutches for their weight.

Procedure guideline 23.11 Checking safety of crutches

Statement	Rationale
1 Before issue check that: a) Ferrules (rubber tips) are not worn to the point where no tread is showing. b) Crutches are a matching pair. Do not issue a mismatched pair. c) Crutches are not cracked, warped, or damaged. d) Spring clip tips are located into both holes (for axillary crutches make sure the nuts and bolts are tight). e) The adjustment mechanism adjusts freely (elbow crutches). f) The holes on the adjustment legs are round and not worn into an oval shape (elbow crutches).	1 To ensure integrity of the walking aid and thereby ensure that the walking aid is in a fit state to be issued for use.
2 Before issuing the crutches, document the batch number of the crutches and record it in the CYP's healthcare records.	2 To enable recall of all crutches within a batch, in the unlikely event that one is found to be defective.

Procedure guideline 23.12 Education of CYP and carers (crutches)

Statement	Rationale
1 Explain to the CYP and their carers: • Why the crutches are needed, • How long they will be required for (if known). • The impact that using crutches will have on the CYP and family.	1 To gain informed consent for the intervention and correct use as instructed.
2 Be sure to explain the risks of improper use of the crutches and how to look for ferrule wear and integrity of the crutches.	2 To ensure that the CYP remains safe while using the crutches.
3 Make CYP and carers aware that they should not alter the crutches in any way, e.g. sticking foam onto the handles.	3 Alteration of crutch handles is classed as a customisation and if the crutches fail, the manufacturer will take no responsibility for the failure.
4 If the CYP is having problem with grip, cycling gloves may be recommended.	
5 If sore hands are a problem, the physiotherapist should be contacted to determine the availability of crutches with 'Fischer' handles (elbow crutches only).	

The Great Ormond Street Hospital Manual of Children and Young People's Nursing Practices

Principles table 23.6 Measure the CYP for crutches

Principle	Rationale
1 If able, measure the CYP when standing. They should stand with elbows flexed to 15°, with shoes on.	1 To ensure that the CYP is measured at the height that they will be when using the crutches.
2 The height of the crutch handgrips should be measured from the floor to the ulna styloid process using a tape measure.	2 The elbow is flexed to 15° when using the crutches to allow for propulsion.
3 If the CYP is unable to stand, the crutches should be measured when the CYP is supine.	3 To ensure that the CYP is safe and comfortable while being measured for crutches.
4 With the CYP lying flat, the height of the crutch handle should be measured, using a tape measure, from the ulna styloid process (with elbows as above) to the sole of the shoes the CYP is going to wear for walking.	4 To ensure that the crutches are the correct height for use with shoes on and that the elbow is flexed to approximately 15° when using the crutches.
5 If the CYP has a leg length discrepancy, the length of the crutches should normally be measured to the sole of the longest leg when wearing shoes.	5 This allows the long leg to stand with knee in neutral when stationary, and easy toe clearance of the longer leg when walking.
6 Once measured, alter the crutches to the correct height and check them alongside the CYP to ensure they have been adjusted correctly.	6 Measurement may not be fully accurate; this allows the physiotherapist to correct any error in the measurements.
7 Despite all the above, the crutches may still need to be altered once the CYP starts using them.	7 The correct height is the height at which the CYP feels confident and stable and may be slightly longer or shorter than the height measured.
8 If issuing axillary crutches, all the above applies for the handgrips but care must be taken that the axillary pad is two adult finger widths deep from the armpit (with the shoulders relaxed).	8 To avoid potential complications from misuse such as axillary artery aneurysms and radial nerve palsies (McFall et al. 2004; Lucas and Davis 2005).
9 If issuing elbow crutches with a height adjustable cuff, they should be adjusted so that they sit just below the elbows but allow the elbows to flex without any impingement.	9 To increase stability.

Principles table 23.7 Safe use of crutches on a flat surface

Principle	Rationale
1 The person issuing the crutches should explain, demonstrate and finally observe the CYP using the crutches.	1 To ensure that the CYP and carers understand how to use the crutches safely.
2 The CYP should stand up before putting on the crutches and take off the crutches before sitting down.	2 To avoid any injury to the arms from the crutches if the CYP slips while standing up or sitting down.
3 When standing, the crutches should be between 8 and 10 cm in front and to the side of the feet, making a triangle shape from the heels and around each crutch.	3 To enhance stability when stationary.

Non weight bearing

Principle	Rationale
1 Non-weight bearing means keeping the weight off the affected limb. Therefore, the CYP should be instructed to keep the affected limb off the ground and take weight through the unaffected limb and the crutches.	1 The crutches should not be in line with the feet because of the instability of this position.
2 Crutches should be placed one step ahead and level with each other.	
3 Putting weight through the crutches, the unaffected limb should be swung to land just in front of the crutches.	
4 Then the cycle should begin again.	

Partial weight bearing

Principle	Rationale
1 Partial weight bearing means taking some weight through the affected limb.	
2 The CYP is instructed to take the appropriate amount of weight through the affected limb, then place the crutches one step ahead and level with each other.	2 To ensure medical instructions for weight bearing status are adhered to.
3 The affected limb should be placed between the crutches, weight put through the limb and the crutches, then step through with the unaffected limb.	
4 Begin the cycle again.	

Principles table 23.8 Safe use of crutches on the stairs

Principle	Rationale

Non-weight bearing
 	
When going up stairs:
  i Put weight through the handrail and crutch.
  ii Hop up one step with the unaffected limb.
  iii Bring crutch up to the same step as the unaffected limb.
  iv Move hand forward on the handrail and start the cycle again.
  v The physiotherapist/parent should stand behind the CYP when ascending stairs.
 	
When going down stairs:
  i Put the crutch down one step.
  ii Put weight through the crutch and the handrail.
  iii Keeping the affected limb ahead of the body, hop down onto the same step with the unaffected limb.
  iv Move hand forward on the handrail and start the cycle again.
  v The physiotherapist/carer should stand in front of the CYP when descending stairs.
	This technique will minimise stress on joints and ensure the CYP's safety while avoiding any weight being placed through the affected limb.

Partial weight-bearing
 	
When going up stairs:
  i Put weight through the handrail and crutch.
  ii Step up one step with the unaffected limb followed by the affected limb.
  iii Finally bring the crutch up onto the same step.
  iv Move hand forward on the handrail and start the cycle again.
 	
To go down stairs, the partially weight-bearing CYP should:
  i Put the crutch down one step.
  ii Put weight through the crutch and handrail.
  iii Step down one step with the affected limb followed by the unaffected limb.
  iv Move hand forward on the handrail and start the cycle again.
 	
If there is no handrail then use both crutches instead of one and the handrail.
	This technique will minimise stress on joints, ensure the CYP's safety, and minimise the weight being placed through the affected limb.

Principles table 23.9 Principles of assembling traction

The type of traction required, including the number of weights and pulleys, must be prescribed and documented by medical staff. All equipment should be checked prior to use to ensure that it is clean and in full working order and the manufacturer's instructions must be followed at all times to ensure safe use. For further detailed information, see RCN (2021).

Principle	Rationale
1 The bed/cot must be compatible with the traction system and have a firm mattress.	1 To ensure traction is safe and efficient.
2 Set up traction with the bed in its lowest position.	2 To avoid strain injuries to staff. The weights will hang freely off the floor, once the bed is raised to the required height.
3 Traction cord must be used. The cord is threaded through the track in the pulleys which conveys the traction force.	3 To ensure the efficiency of the traction system. Traction cord will not stretch.
4 The correct diameter/strength of cord should be used to fit into the pulley.	
5 The cord must be a continuous single length, with the ends cut short (5 cm) and taped – knots should remain visible.	5 To prevent fraying and slipping.
6 The traction cord must not touch the traction frame or the bed.	6 To ensure the efficiency of the traction system and prevent cord from fraying.
7 Secure knots should be used to attach and suspend weights at the end of the cord. Knots should be a clove hitch, or two half hitches (see Figure 23.10).	7 These are nonslip knots.
8 Knots should be positioned away from the pulley.	8 To allow free movement of the cord.

(continued)

Principles table 23.9 Principles of assembling traction *(continued)*

Principle	Rationale
9 Ensure the prescribed weights are used and hang freely. They should not be in contact with the floor, the traction frame, or the bed.	9 To ensure the efficiency of the traction system and prevent discomfort to the CYP.
10 Where possible, weights should not hang directly over a CYP. If there is no option but to do this, then an extra safety cord must be used and checked regularly (RCN 2021).	10 To ensure the CYP's safety.
11 Apply guards (foam balls, squares, soft toys/puppets) over the ends of any protruding traction bars.	11 To prevent injury to the CYP, parents/carers, or staff.
12 Use bed cradles to keep heavy covers free from traction cords.	12 To maintain the efficiency of the traction system.

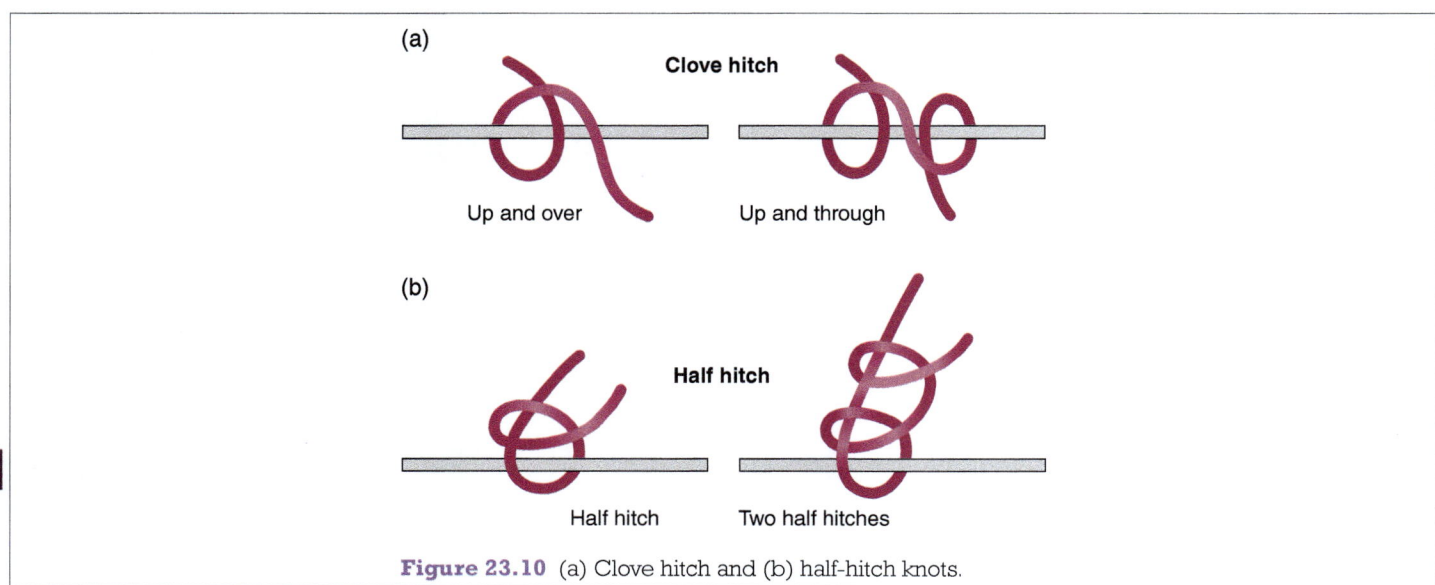

Figure 23.10 (a) Clove hitch and (b) half-hitch knots.

Procedure guideline 23.13 Management of traction

Statement	Rationale
1 Traction is maintained continuously, unless specified by the orthopaedic/spinal surgeon.	1 To ensure that the treatment programme is effective.
2 Check the traction equipment at the start of each shift, four hourly, and after each time the CYP is repositioned.	2–3 To ensure the integrity of the traction apparatus and the efficiency of traction.
3 Ensure that: • The frame, all clamps, and knots are secure. • The pulleys are running freely. • The weights are secure, hanging freely, and are off the floor.	
4 Ensure correct alignment of the body part in the traction system.	4 To maintain traction efficiency.
5 Ensure countertraction is maintained at all times.	5 Without countertraction, traction is ineffective (RCN 2021).
6 Assess the need to elevate the foot or head of the bed to increase countertraction.	6 To reduce friction on the sacrum and heels, which may lead to pressure ulcers. If countertraction is not present, the CYP will be pulled in the direction of the traction force and traction will not be effective.

Chapter 23 Orthopaedic care

Procedure guideline 23.14 Applying skin traction

Statement	Rationale
1 Administer analgesia if required.	1 To ensure the CYP is comfortable and aid adherence.
2 Place padding material over bony prominences.	2 To minimise the risk of a pressure ulcers
3 Unroll and stretch the skin extensions before removing the backing paper (if using adhesive extensions).	3 To remove any kinks and to ease handling.
4 The extensions should follow the contours of the limb. This can be facilitated by making nicks in the lengths of the adhesive strips.	
5 The extensions should be cut to length and the top edges rounded. Ensure the padding covers any bony prominences, and the adhesive strips are placed in position in accordance with traction prescribed.	5 To prevent pressure ulcers and neurovascular compression.
6 Bandages must be wrapped smoothly and evenly around the limb, maintaining even pressure, in a figure of eight, with the limb in internal rotation.	6 The 'figure of eight' wrap minimises the risk of slipping. The bandages keep the skin extensions in place, transfer the traction forces to the skin and underlying tissues, and encourage neutral rotation.
7 Avoid tight bandaging over pressure areas and vulnerable soft tissue areas (Figure 23.11).	7 To prevent neurovascular damage and allow limited movement of the joint.
8 Bandages are secured by a short length of tape.	8 The tape must not completely encircle the limb in order to avoid a tourniquet effect.
9 A gap should be left between the CYP's foot and the end of the skin extension, which allows the foot to touch the footplate when the toes are extended.	9 To allow plantar flexion of the foot (RCN 2021).
10 Allow for a gradual pull of traction by removing your hands slowly.	10 A sudden onset of traction can cause pain and muscle spasms.

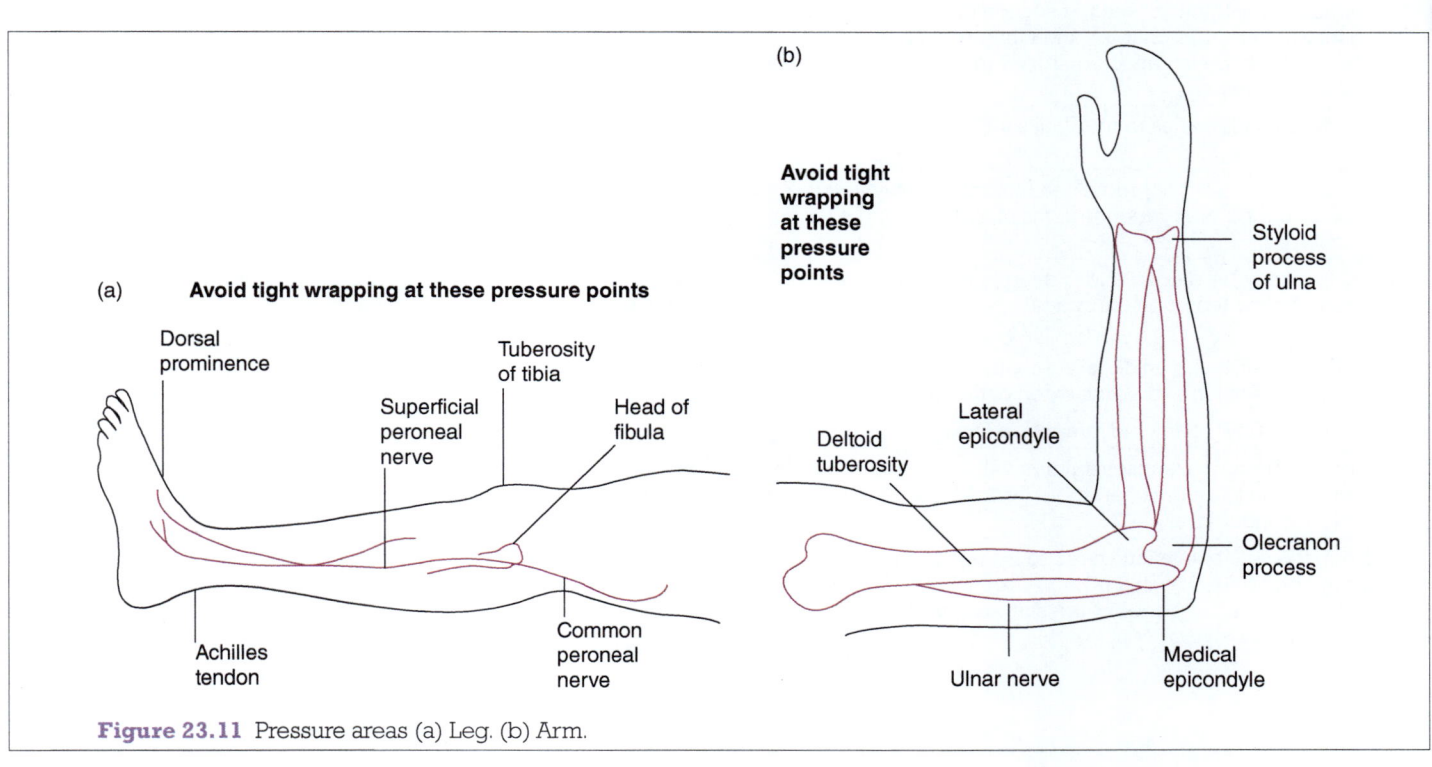

Figure 23.11 Pressure areas (a) Leg. (b) Arm.

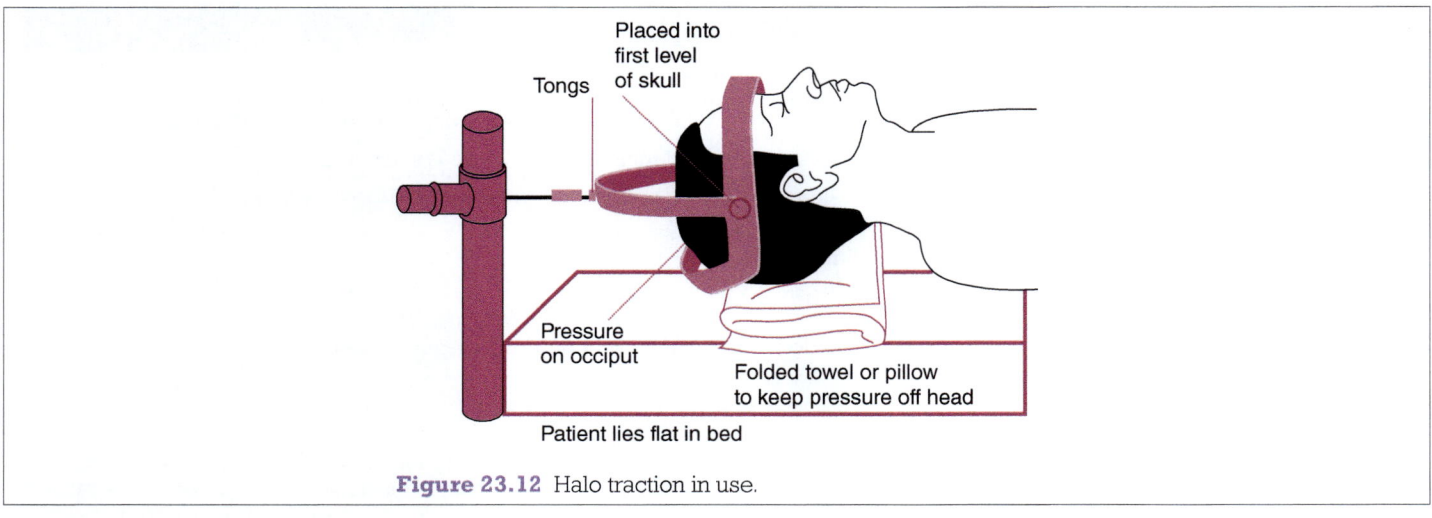

Figure 23.12 Halo traction in use.

Procedure guideline 23.15 Nursing care of the CYP in traction

For the most part, the nursing care of a CYP in traction is similar to that for any CYP on bed rest. The main aims are to meet the CYP's physical and psychological needs and prevent complications associated with bed rest and immobility, including pressure ulcers constipation, chest infection, etc. This section describes the specific nursing care related to traction.

Statement	Rationale
1 The CYP should be prepared for the application of traction using age appropriate language and pictures or photographs.	1 To obtain consent, aid adherence and facilitate successful treatment.
2 Neurovascular observations must be recorded prior to the application of traction (see the section on neurovascular observations in this chapter and Chapter 1 Assessment). Always compare the affected limb with the unaffected limb on each occasion.	2 To identify any complications promptly.
3 Report any anomalies to medical staff immediately.	3 Any compromise in neurovascular status is a medical emergency, requiring immediate intervention.
4 Bandages should be removed at least once daily and the skin should be observed for signs of irritation and allergic reaction.	4 To detect and treat complications.
5 A pillow may be placed under a leg in traction. It must extend below the popliteal space.	5 To relieve pressure on the heel and prevent bunching up of the pillow under the knee, which causes flexing of the joint and impairs venous flow.
6 Where possible the ankle joint should be left free to allow full plantar flexion and dorsiflexion of the foot.	6 To prevent stiffness and contracture deformity.
7 Inform the CYP of any movements to avoid.	
8 A physiotherapy exercise regimen will aim to maintain strength, muscle power, promote good circulation and prevent contractures (RCN 2021).	8 A prolonged period on traction may result in the loss of muscle power. Exercise also prevents muscle weakness in the unaffected limbs.
9 When the skin extensions need to be removed, these should be soaked off in the bath. Gently hold the skin taut and peel back the edges of the skin extensions slowly, using an adhesive solvent.	9 To reduce the risk of skin irritation and damage (RCN 2021).

Procedure guideline 23.16 Nursing care of the CYP receiving spinal traction

Statement	Rationale
1 The CYP should be prepared for the traction using age appropriate language and pictures or photographs.	1 To obtain consent, aid adherence and facilitate successful treatment.
2 Neurovascular observations must be recorded prior to the application of traction.	2 To identify any complications promptly.
3 Report any anomalies to medical staff immediately.	3 Any compromise in neurovascular status is a medical emergency, requiring intervention.
4 Inform the CYP of any movements they should avoid, such as sudden twisting of the body or head, or leaning forward.	4 To avoid any trauma.
5 A physiotherapy exercise regimen will aim to maintain strength, muscle power, promote good circulation, and prevent contractures (RCN 2021).	5 A prolonged period on traction may result in the loss of muscle power. Exercise also prevents muscle weakness in the unaffected limbs.
6 Medical staff must torque (tighten) the halo pins to the correct tension using the torque wrench.	6 The initial torque is determined by the spinal surgeon, based on the age and weight of the CYP.
7 Pin sites should be observed for signs of infection and any pain or discomfort, on each shift.	7 To identify problems at an early stage (RCN 2021, 2022).
8 The traction weight must be prescribed by the spinal surgeon and documented in the CYP'S health care record.	8 To ensure the correct traction weight is applied. To maintain accurate documentation.
9 The consultant determines the traction weight by X-rays, neurological function and the absence of pain.	9 To ensure neurovascular status is not compromised.
10 Ensure all aspects of the traction wheelchair is checked prior to the CYP using it.	10 To maintain safety.
11 The protocol for emergency management of any CYP on spinal traction must be approved locally and all staff must be appropriately trained in the appropriate action to be taken during emergency procedures such as resuscitation and ward evacuation.	11 To maintain safety.

References

Altizer, L. (2002). Neurovascular assessment. *Orthopaedic Nursing* 21 (4): 48–50.

Bae, D.S., Kadiyala, R.K., and Waters, P.M. (2014). Acute compartment syndrome in children: contemporary diagnosis, treatment and outcome. *Journal of Pediatric Orthopaedics* 34 (1): 50–54.

Bakody, E. (2009). Orthopaedic plaster casting: nurse and patient education. *Nursing Standard* 23 (51): 49–56.

Duckworth, T. and Blundell, C. (2010). *Orthopaedics and Fracture*, 4e. London: Wiley Blackwell.

Edwards, S. (2004). Acute compartment syndrome. *Emergency Nurse* 12 (3): 32–38.

Fort, C. (2003). How to combat 3 deadly trauma complications. *Nursing* 33 (5): 58–63.

Hockenberry, M.J. and Wilson, D. (2013). *Wong's Essentials of Pediatric Nursing*, 9e. Missouri: Elsevier Mosby.

Jester, R., Santy, J., and Rogers, J. (2011). *Oxford Handbook of Orthopaedic and Trauma Nursing*. Oxford: Oxford University Press.

Johnston-Walker, E. and Hardcastle, J. (2011). Neurovascular assessment in the critically ill patient. *Nursing in Critical Care* 16 (4): 170–177.

Judge, N.L. (2007). Neurovascular assessment. *Nursing Standard* 21 (45): 39–44.

Krasemann, T. (2015). Complications of cardiac catheterisation in children. *Heart* 101 (12): 915.

Leversedge, F.J., Moore, T.J., Peterson, B.C., and Seiler, J.G. III (2011). Compartment syndrome of the upper extremity. *The Journal of Hand Surgery* 36 (3): 544–559.

Livingston, K.S., Glotzbecker, M.P., and Shore, B.J. (2017). Pediatric acute compartment syndrome. *Journal of the American Academy of Orthopaedic Surgeons* 25 (5): 358–364.

Lucas, B. and Davis, P. (2005). Why restricting movement is important. In: *Orthopaedic and Trauma Nursing*, 2e (eds. J. Kneale and P. Davis), 105–139. Edinburgh: Churchill Livingstone.

McDermott, S. and Nolan, L. (2010). Musculo-skeletal system. In: *Clinical Skills in Children's Nursing* (eds. I. Coyne, F. Neill and F. Timss), 351–374. Oxford: Oxford University Press.

McFall, B., Arya, N., Soong, C. et al. (2004). Crutch induced axillary artery injury. *The Ulster Medical Journal* 73 (1): 50–52.

Miles, S. (2012). *A Practical Guide to Casting*, 3e. Hull: BSN Medical Ltd.

Noonan, K.J. and McCarthy, J.J. (2010). Compartment syndromes in the pediatric patient. *Journal of Pediatric Orthopaedics* 30 (2): 96–101.

Nursing and Midwifery Council (NMC) (2018). The code. Professional standards of practice and behaviour for nurses and midwives, NMC. www.nmc.org.uk/standards/code (accessed 25 July 2022).

Royal College of Nursing (RCN) (2021). *Traction Principles and Application*. London: RCN. https://www.rcn.org.uk/-/media/Royal-College-Of-Nursing/Documents/Publications/2021/July/009-816.pdf (accessed 25 July 2022).

Royal College of Nursing (RCN) (2022). Guidance on Pin Site Care. London: RCN. https://www.rcn.org.uk/-/media/Royal-College-Of-Nursing/Documents/Publications/2022/February/009-907.pdf (accessed 25 July 2022).

Schreiber, M.L. (2016). Neurovascular assessment: an essential nursing focus. *MedSurgNursing* 25 (1): 55–57.

Sedgwick, R and Richards, S. (2015). Neurovascular observations. Clinical guidelines (nursing). The Royal Children's Hospital Melbourne. https://www.rch.org.au/rchcpg/hospital_clinical_guideline_index/Neurovascular_observations/ (accessed 25 July 2022).

Wall, C.J., Lynch, J., Harris, I.A. et al. (2010). Clinical practice guidelines for the management of acute limb compartment syndrome following trauma. *ANZ Journal of Surgery* 80 (3): 151–156.

Weinstein, S.L. (2014). Developmental hip dysplasia and dislocation. In. In: *Lovell and Winter's Paediatric Orthopaedics*, 7e (eds. S.L. Weinstein and J.M. Flynn), 983–1111. Philadelphia: Lippincott Williams & Wilkins.

Wong, D.L., Whaley, L.F., and Wilson, D. (2012). *Whaley and Wong's Nursing Care of Infants and Children*, 9e. St Louis: CV Mosby.

Wright, E. (2009). Neurovascular impairment and compartment syndrome. *Paediatric Nursing* 21 (3): 26.

Further reading

DiFazio, R. (2003). Creating a halo traction wheelchair Resopurse Manuel: using the EBP approach. *Journal of Pediatric Nursing* 18 (2): 148–152.

Fleming, B.C., Krag, M.H., Huston, D.R., and Sughirara, S. (2000). Pin loosening in a halo – vest orthosis: a biomechanical study. *Spine* 25 (11): 1325–1331.

Middleton, C. (2003). Compartment syndrome: the importance of early diagnosis. *Nursing Times* 99 (21): 30–32.

Patterson, M. (2005). Multicentre pin care study. *Orthopaedic Nursing* 24 (5): 349–360.

Royal Children's Hospital (RCH) (2007). Orthopaedic fact sheet 19. Slings & Springs in Perthes Disease. https://www.rch.org.au/uploadedFiles/Main/Content/ortho/factsheets/SLINGS-AND-SPRINGS.pdf (accessed 25 July 2022).

Chapter 24

Pain management

Elizabeth Anne Bruce

RN (Child), RN (Adult), BSc (Hons), MSc, Clinical Nurse Specialist, Pain Control, Great Ormond Street Hospital, London, UK

Chapter contents

Introduction	542
General principles of pain management	542
Pain assessment	545
Administration of entonox	550
Epidural analgesia	555
Patient and nurse controlled analgesia (PCA/NCA)	565
Prevention and management of opioid-related complications	566
Sucrose	571
References	573
Further reading	575

Procedure guidelines

24.1	Pain assessment on admission	547
24.2	Pain assessment using a self-report tool	548
24.3	CYP assessment for use of entonox	551
24.4	Preparation for entonox use	552
24.5	Administration of entonox	553
24.6	Managing side-effects of entonox	554
24.7	After use	555
24.8	Storage	555
24.9	Transfer of the CYP following epidural insertion	557
24.10	Nursing care of an epidural (general)	557
24.11	Nursing care of an epidural (observations)	558
24.12	Epidural related complications	561
24.13	Technical problems	563
24.14	Discontinuing the epidural	564
24.15	Preparation for PCA/NCA use	566
24.16	Setting up a PCA/NCA infusion	567
24.17	Technical problems (PCA/NCA)	568
24.18	Care of the CYP receiving PCA/NCA	568
24.19	Prevention and management of opioid-related complications	569
24.20	Sucrose administration	572

Principles tables

24.1	General principles of pain management	543
24.2	Pain assessment	546
24.3	Pain assessment using a behavioural tool	549
24.4	Assessment and preparation for an epidural	556
24.5	Drug administration via an epidural	556

The author would like to acknowledge members of the pain team past and present who have contributed to the guidelines in this chapter, including but not limited to; Judith Middleton, Judith Peters, and Rebecca Saul.

The Great Ormond Street Hospital Manual of Children and Young People's Nursing Practices, Second Edition. Edited by Elizabeth Anne Bruce, Janet Williss, and Faith Gibson.
© 2023 John Wiley & Sons Ltd. Published 2023 by John Wiley & Sons Ltd.

Introduction

Pain is an unpleasant sensory and emotional experience, which is unique to individuals and usually associated with tissue damage. If left untreated it can have harmful physical and psychosocial effects and this can make future painful experiences much more difficult to manage (Weisman et al. 1998). Children and young people (CYPs) experience a wide range of painful situations and it is unlikely that any admission to hospital will be totally pain free. Nurses have an ethical and professional responsibility to ensure that pain is prevented and managed as effectively as possible (International Association for the Study of Pain [IASP] 2010). Since the mid-1990s there have been considerable developments in the management of pain in CYPs. An increase in research and education has improved knowledge, changed attitudes towards pain, dispelled myths, and prompted an increase in the use of opiates (Clinical Standards Advisory Group 2000; 2002; Howard 2003). Numerous guidelines and recommendations have been published that relate to the management of pain in CYPs (Box 24.1). Education of staff and audits of practice are essential components of safe, effective pain management (Department of Health [DH] 2004a b; Royal College of Anaesthetists [RCoA] 2022).

Effective pain management involves the use of a combination of pharmacological and nonpharmacological techniques to minimise both the emotional and sensory components of any potentially painful experiences. Pain in neonates and CYPs with special needs can be particularly difficult to assess and manage. A comprehensive pain management plan should be implemented for all CYPs on admission, reviewed/revised as needed, and continue until discharge. It should be child-focused, involving the CYP and family throughout, and various members of the interdisciplinary team as appropriate (DH 2004a,b).

This chapter contains the following nursing practice guidelines relating to the assessment and management of pain in CYPs:

- Pain management (general principles)
- Assessment of pain in CYPs
- Entonox administration®
- Epidural analgesia
- Patient-controlled and nurse-controlled analgesia
- Prevention and management of opioid-related complications
- Sucrose

It does not set out to describe all aspects of the management of pain in CYPs; for a general overview, see Twycross et al. (2014). For guidelines on the management of procedure-related pain, see Association of Paediatric Anaesthetists of Great Britain and Ireland (APAGBI) guidelines (2012). Further reading is recommended, particularly in relation to the management of chronic pain and pain in palliative care. For the prevention and management of opioid withdrawal, see Chapter 34: Drug Withdrawal: Prevention and Management. Preparation of CYPs for procedures and the use of distraction are discussed in Chapter 27: Play as a Therapeutic Tool.

General principles of pain management

This section provides an overview of the main principles of pain management.

Box 24.1 UK guidelines and recommendations for the management of pain in CYPs

- Association of Paediatric Anaesthetists of Great Britain and Ireland (2012). **Good practice in postoperative and procedural pain management. Paediatric Anaesthesia, 22(S1), 1–79.** https://onlinelibrary.wiley.com/doi/10.1111/j.1460-9592.2012.03838.x (accessed 25 November 2022).
- Faculty of Pain Management (FPM) (2021) **Core Standards for Pain Management Services in the UK**. Provides a framework for standards and recommendations in the provision of Pain Management Services for healthcare professionals (HCPs), commissioners, and other stakeholders to optimise care. https://www.fpm.ac.uk/standards-guidelines/core-standards (accessed 25 November 2022).
- Department of Health (2004b). **Ill Child Standard, National Service Framework for Children Young People and Maternity Services.** London, Department of Health. https://www.gov.uk/government/publications/national-service-framework-children-young-people-and-maternity-services (accessed 25 November 2022).
- National Institute for Health and Care Excellence (NICE) (2012). **Sickle cell disease: acute painful episodes in hospital. CG143.** www.nice.org.uk/guidance/cg143 (accessed 16 March 2022).
- National Institute for Health and Care Excellence (NICE) (2021) **Chronic pain (primary and secondary) in over 16s: assessment of all chronic pain and management of chronic primary pain NICE guideline [NG193].** https://www.nice.org.uk/guidance/NG193 (accessed 25 November 2022).
- Opioids Aware. A resource for patients and HCPs to support prescribing of opioid medicines for pain. This resource, which was developed by UK HCPs and policymakers, provides the information to support a safe and effective prescribing decision. http://www.fpm.ac.uk/opioids-aware (accessed 25 November 2022).
- Royal College of Anaesthetists (RCoA) (2020). **Best practice in the management of epidural analgesia in the hospital setting**. Includes a section on CYPs. https://fpm.ac.uk/fpm-release-updated-guidance-best-practice-management-epidural-analgesia-hospital-setting (accessed 25 November 2022).
- RCoA (2022) **Chapter 10: Guidelines for the Provision of Paediatric Anaesthesia Services 2022.** https://rcoa.ac.uk/gpas/chapter-10 (accessed 25 November 2022). Extensive paediatric guideline covering all aspects of paediatric anaesthesia. Recommends the establishment of a fully resourced children's inpatient pain service, delivered by an appropriately trained and experienced multidisciplinary team (MDT), with specific skills in children's pain management.
- Royal College of Nursing (RCN) and Palliative Care Forum (2015). **Pain Knowledge and Skills Framework for the Nursing Team**. Endorsed by the British Pain Society. https://www.rcn.org.uk/professional-development/publications/pub-004984 (accessed 25 November 2022).
- Royal College of Emergency Medicine (2017). **Management of Pain in Children**. https://rcem.ac.uk/search (accessed 25 November 2022).
- World Health Organisation (WHO) 2020) **Guidelines on the management of chronic pain in children.** https://www.who.int/publications/i/item/9789240017870 (accessed 25 November 2022).

Chapter 24 Pain management

Principles table 24.1 General principles of pain management

Principle	Rationale
1a) Pain management guidelines or protocols should be in place in all clinical areas, including ambulance services and accident and emergency departments. The involvement of pharmacists in protocol development is encouraged (DH 2004a; APAGBI 2012). b) Once guidelines or protocols have been introduced, regular audit should be carried out to determine whether they are being followed. c) They should be reviewed and updated every few years (DH 2004a; APAGBI 2012).	1a) To document the agreed standards for the provision of safe, effective pain management practices locally. To provide support and information for staff. b) To ensure that standards of care are met. c) To ensure that the evidence is up to date.
2 All staff caring for CYPs should receive education on the assessment and management of pain.	2 To ensure that staff are adequately trained to deliver safe, effective pain management for all CYPs (DH 2004a).
3 CYPs and their families should be actively involved in decisions regarding the assessment and management of pain (DH 2004a; RCN 2009; APAGBI 2012).	3 Pain is subjective. Involvement of CYPs and their families increases satisfaction with pain management (Franck and Bruce 2009).
4 Information regarding how any potentially painful experiences will be prevented and managed should be given to the CYP and family both prior to and on admission. A translator should be used if needed. Where procedures are planned and pain is likely, CYPs should be prepared through play and education. Picture-based leaflets can be used for CYPs with learning difficulties (https://patient.info/treatment-medication/nhs-and-other-care-options/accessible-leaflets).	4 To provide adequate information and psychological support (DH 2004a, RCN 2009). To facilitate CYP and family involvement in decision-making and informed consent (DH 2004a).
5 Pain assessment is an essential part of the pain management process and should be a routine activity (for more information, see Pain Assessment section).	5 To treat pain effectively (DH 2004a). Accurate information regarding the type, location and severity of pain is essential to determine the most appropriate intervention.
6 Pain assessments should be used as a guide to treatment. Intensity scores may be grouped into 'mild', 'moderate,' or 'severe' pain to assist decisions regarding the most appropriate intervention.	6 To encourage the use of stronger analgesia and a wider range of interventions when pain is more severe (see Figure 24.1).
7 The type of pain, its cause, and context must also be considered when deciding on the most appropriate intervention. For example, if a CYP indicates that they have abdominal pain, further investigation may be required to determine whether this is from a surgical wound, catheter, or drain, or another cause such as urinary retention or surgical complications.	7 To ensure that pain is managed effectively, using the most appropriate intervention(s) for the type and severity of pain experienced (APAGBI 2012).
8a) Pain should be prevented wherever possible. b) Treatment should combine drug and nondrug interventions, including psychological therapies such as distraction, coping skills, and cognitive-behavioural approaches (DH 2004a; RCPCH 1997; Stevens et al 2021).	8a) It is easier to prevent, rather than to treat pain once it occurs. b) The experience of pain is both sensory and emotional. For a review of nondrug techniques, see Schug et al. (2015) and Twycross et al. (2009).
9 If there is uncertainty regarding whether pain is present and there is a likelihood of pain, it may be appropriate to treat and reassess.	9 Behavioural and physiological responses are not always reliable. If the likelihood of pain is high, analgesia should be pre-emptive (RCPCH 1997; APAGBI 2012).
10 Pain management should be multi-modal where possible and specific to the type of pain experienced. The choice of drug will be determined by a number of factors including the duration of action and side effect profile of the drug, availability of route of administration, and acceptability.	10 Different groups of drugs work in different ways. For a more in-depth review, see Schechter et al. (2003), Twycross et al. (2014), and Schug et al. (2015). For more information regarding the routes and types of drugs used, see points 11–15 below.
11a) The route of administration of analgesia should be safe, effective and acceptable to the CYP and family. b) Verbal consent should be obtained. c) When using the rectal and epidural routes, ensure that the CYP/ family are aware of the risks and benefits. d) Cultural and developmental issues require careful consideration.	11a, b) To provide effective analgesia in partnership with the family. For more information, see Chapter 17: Administration of Medicines. c, d) Parents/carers may have limited knowledge of and be reluctant for drugs to be given via the rectal route (Seth et al. 2000).

(continued)

Principles table 24.1 General principles of pain management *(continued)*

Principle	Rationale
12 Simple analgesics, i.e. paracetamol and nonsteroidal anti-inflammatory drugs (NSAIDs) can be given alone for mild pain, in combination for moderate pain and combined with opiates for moderate to severe pain.	12 To provide effective pain relief with minimal complications. Simple analgesics have an opioid 'sparing' effect; if given regularly their use can reduce the amount of opioid analgesia required (Schug et al. 2015).
13 Local anaesthetics are used primarily to prevent procedure-related pain, but are also used to manage chronic pain. Routes of local anaesthetics include: • Topical/transdermal local anaesthetics applied to the skin, either as a cream or patch. • Local infiltration, which can be subcutaneous, or target a specific nerve or group of nerves. • Regional anaesthetic (e.g. caudal, epidural, spinal).	13 Local anaesthetics reversibly block conduction along the nerve fibres that they come into contact with (Neal 2002).
14 Opioids can be administered for moderate to severe pain. a) Morphine is generally considered the 'gold standard'. b) Fentanyl, oxycodone, and less commonly, diamorphine, and methadone are acceptable alternatives to morphine. c) Pethidine is generally avoided in CYPs, due to the risk of accumulation of the metabolite norpethidine. d) Codeine is a weak opioid with variable efficacy. Its use should be avoided in CYPs under 12 years and anyone with obstructive sleep apnoea (British National Formulary for Children (BNfC) 2022, Medicines and Healthcare Products Regulatory Agency [MHRA] 2013). e) Tramadol is the alternative opioid (for mild to moderate pain) used at GOSH. It is banned in some countries, including the USA.	14 For more information, see Twycross et al. (2009), APAGBI (2012), and Schug et al. (2015). a) The efficacy and side-effect profile are well documented. b) These opioids have different side-effect profiles and can be useful where morphine causes unmanageable side effects, or rotation is required to avoid tolerance (WHO 2012). c) Accumulation of norpethidine is associated with an increased incidence of convulsions. d) Individual CYPs may be poor or ultra-rapid metabolisers (Williams et al. 2002). Deaths have recently been reported in high risk groups, and CYPs with obstructed sleep apnoea are particularly at risk (Friedrichsdorf et al. 2013; MHRA 2013).
15 Adjuvants or 'coanalgesics' can also provide effective pain relief. These include: a) Ketamine. b) Clonidine. c) Antimuscarinics, e.g. Buscopan, oxybutynin. d) Anxiolytics, e.g. diazepam. e) Anti-neuropathic agents, e.g. carbamazepine, gabapentin, pregabalin, amitriptyline. f) Other drugs such as corticosteroids, chemotherapy, and bisphosphonates.	15 Coanalgesics either act on the cause of the pain, or exert their effect on a specific part of the pain pathway (APAGBI 2012; Schug et al. 2015). a, b) These can have an opioid sparing effect by providing multi-modal analgesia. c, d) For the management of painful spasms. e) For the management of neuropathic pain (Schug et al. 2015). f) These treat the cause of the pain; corticosteroids reduce inflammation in conditions such as Crohn's disease, chemotherapy drugs can reduce tumour size, and bisphosphonates increasing bone density.
16 Sedatives are used to reduce fear and increase adherence with procedures. The use of sedation alone is not sufficient when a procedure is likely to be painful. However, some sedatives also have analgesic properties.	16 For more information on sedation, see National Institute for Health and Care Excellence (NICE) sedation guidelines (NICE 2010).
17 Nondrug interventions should be widely employed and should range from information giving and building up a rapport, to the use of psychological techniques such as the use of distraction, breathing interventions, and cognitive behavioural therapy (CBT). The most appropriate intervention will vary depending on the age and cognitive ability of the CYP and the type of pain experienced.	17 To minimise pain (Sng et al. 2017; Birnie et al. 2018).

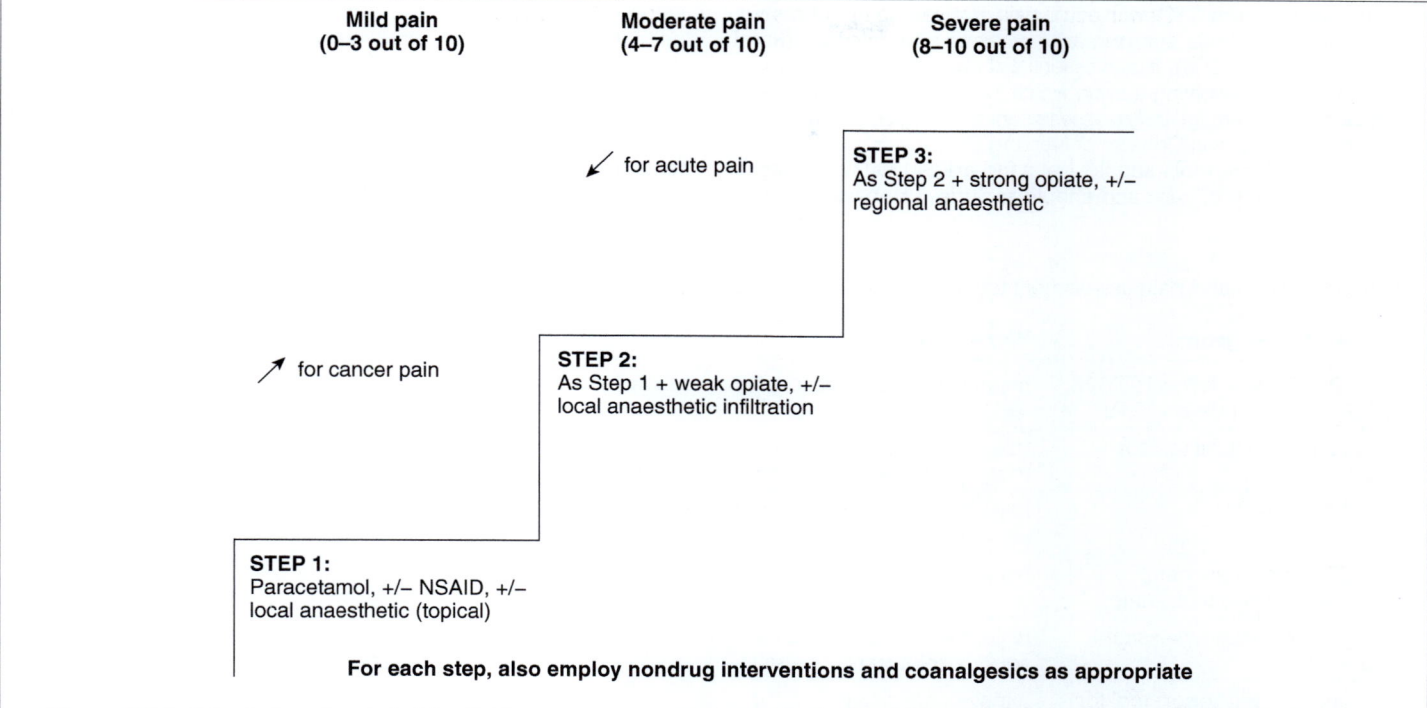

Figure 24.1 Adapted analgesic ladder linking assessment to treatment. The World Health Organization analgesic ladder (WHO 1986) was originally introduced to recommend a 'step-up' approach to managing cancer pain. For surgical or procedural pain, which can be predicted and prevented, the model can be adapted and used to provide a 'step-down' approach by anticipating the degree of pain likely. Although WHO have now moved away from this concept (WHO 2012) the ladder remains a useful tool for providing guidance on the range of interventions available to manage pain.

Pain assessment

Accurate assessment is an essential part of the pain management process. It enables HCPs to determine the nature and severity of a CYP's pain, to make decisions regarding the most appropriate action to relieve that pain, to determine whether a specific intervention has relieved pain and if not, to determine what further action is required. There are a wide range of tools available to facilitate accurate pain assessment. Within paediatrics, the range of pain assessment tools is particularly broad to encompass CYPs of all ages and stages of development with different types of pain. Research has demonstrated the validity and reliability of these tools and it is recommended that pain should be assessed and documented regularly, using a validated pain assessment tool (APAGBI 2012; DH 2002, 2004a, Royal College of Nursing [RCN] 2009).

The following pain assessment practices are based on published guidelines and standards and hence do not specify which tools should be used. When choosing a pain assessment tool for use with CYPs, HCPs should consider:

- The age and stage of development of the CYP.
- The type of pain to be assessed.
- The validity and reliability of the assessment tool.
- The clinical utility of the tool, i.e. ease of use, degree of burden on HCPs, etc.
- How frequently pain assessments will be carried out.
- Where these will be documented.
- How assessment will link to treatment decisions.
- The amount of education and ongoing support required to implement the tool.

Organisational support, adequate resources, and audit activities have been identified as essential for the successful implementation of improved pain assessment practices (Bruce and Franck 2004, 2005). The Department of Health have published standards for benchmarking pain (DH 2010).

Pain assessment in CYPs with acute pain involves the use of assessment tools or methods that primarily measure pain intensity (Royal College of Nursing 2009). It is an essential component of the pain management process involving a cycle which includes assessment, documentation, management and re-assessment of pain (see Figure 24.2).

Adapted from Royal College of Nursing (2009).

Pain assessment tools should be standardised within Trusts to provide continuity of care and should include a behavioural tool, self-report tools for younger and older CYPs, and a tool/tools for neonates (term, preterm, and ventilated neonates all require different tools). The assessment of CYPs with cognitive impairment is a particular challenge and tools have also been developed for use with this group (Breau et al. 2001; Hunt et al. 2003; Voepel-Lewis et al. 2008). Table 24.1 provides a list of validated pain assessment tools that can be downloaded from the internet (permission may be required before use).

Table 24.1 Validated pain assessment tools available on the internet (accessed 16 March 2022)

Tool and user group	Website address
Faces Pain Scale – Revised (FPS-R): Self-report tool for verbal CYPs	https://www.iasp-pain.org/resources/faces-pain-scale-revised/
FLACC: Behavioural tool for CYPs	(https://www1.health.gov.au/internet/publications/publishing.nsf/Content/triageqrg~triageqrg-pain~triageqrg-FLACC)
FLACC revised	https://www.gosh.nhs.uk/wards-and-departments/departments/clinical-specialties/pain-control-service-information-parents-and-visitors/download-documentation/
N-PASS: Neonates – pain, agitation, and sedation scale	http://www.anestesiarianimazione.com/2004/06c.asp
The Neonatal Pain Assessment Tool (PAT)	https://www.gosh.nhs.uk/wards-and-departments/departments/clinical-specialties/pain-control-service-information-parents-and-visitors/download-documentation/
The Oucher: Self-report tool for verbal CYPs	https://oucher.org/
Paediatric Pain Profile: CYPs with severe physical/learning impairment	www.ppprofile.org.uk/
Wong-Baker FACES Pain Rating Scale: Self-report tool	http://wongbakerfaces.org/

Principles table 24.2 Pain assessment
General Principles of Pain Assessment

Principle	Rationale
1 Involve the family in the assessment and documentation of pain.	1 Pain should be assessed in partnership with the family. Parents/carers are able to interpret behavioural cues (RCPCH 2001; DH 2002, 2004a,b; RCN 2009).
2 Pain should be assessed using validated pain assessment tools wherever possible. These should not be altered unless further reliability and validity testing is planned.	2 To increase the accuracy of assessments (RCPCH 2001; DH 2002, 2004a, b; RCN 2009). Any changes will invalidate the tool and make it less reliable.
3 Assessment should be multidimensional and should include: a) The CYP's self-report of pain wherever possible. b) Behavioural indicators. c) Physiological measures. d) Contextual factors.	3 To ensure accurate assessment of pain (RCPCH 2001; RCN 2009; Stevens et al. 2021). a) Pain is a subjective experience. Self-report is considered to be the 'gold standard.' b) Behaviour is a useful indicator of pain in CYPs as they may be unwilling or unable to self-report. c) Physiological measures are useful, but are not specific to pain and should not be used in isolation (RCN 2009). d) To consider potential causes of pain and and aid decision-making regarding the most appropriate intervention to manage the pain.
4 Accurate documentation of assessments is essential. Alongside intensity, space should be provided for documentation of the nature, location, and type of pain and any influencing contextual factors.	4 Accurate documentation is a legal and professional requirement (DH 2004a,b; NMC 2009). Most pain assessment tools measure pain intensity and should not be used in isolation (RCN 2009).
5 Pain assessments should be linked to and used as a guide to treatment (for more information, see section 24.1).	5 To ensure that assessment is used as an indicator for the need for treatment.
6 All HCPs caring for CYPs should be trained to recognise and assess pain.	6 To enable them to accurately assess and treat pain (RCPCH 2001; DH 2004a,b; RCN 2015)

Chapter 24 Pain management

Principle	Rationale
7 Pain assessment should be carried out: a) On admission. b) Whenever pain is suspected. c) Prior to and during any interventions that are likely to cause pain. d) Following an intervention. e) Alongside other care where possible. f) At regular intervals. Assessments should not be done rigidly (e.g. on the hour), but should reflect painful and/or pain-free episodes during a period.	7 a) To provide baseline information with which to compare future assessments. b) To confirm whether pain is present. c) To determine the most appropriate intervention. d) To determine whether an intervention has been effective. e) To provide minimal disruption; a sleeping CYP should not be woken to ask them about their pain (RCN 2009).
8 The minimum frequency of assessments should be agreed at local level but must be tailored to the individual CYP's needs / situation, including: a) The type and severity of pain experienced or anticipated. b) How long an intervention will take to have an effect.	8 To ensure that practice is standardised. a) Intense pain and pain related to surgical complications can be harmful and should be treated promptly. b) To determine the effectiveness of an intervention as soon as possible.

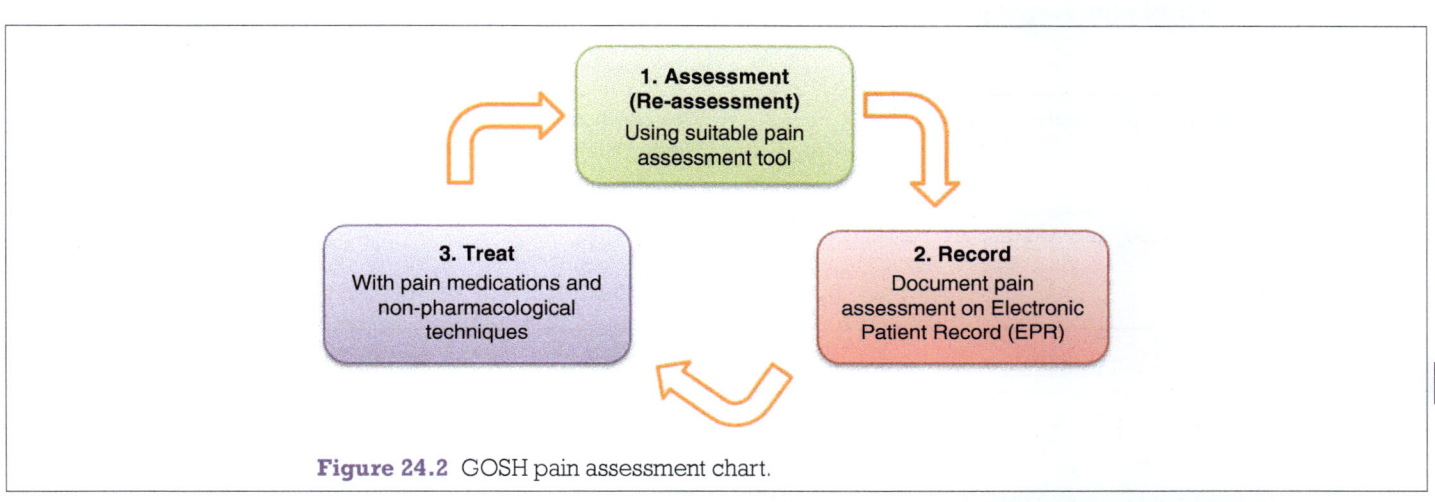

Figure 24.2 GOSH pain assessment chart.

Procedure guideline 24.1 Pain assessment on admission

Statement	Rationale
1 An accurate pain history should be taken on admission (see Figure 24.3 below). This should include: a) Previous experiences of pain and how these were managed. b) The words the CYP uses to describe pain. c) Usual behaviour when in pain. d) Information regarding comfort measures and analgesia used at home. e) A detailed history of any current pain.	1 To provide information that will assist in the assessment and management of pain during admission (RCPCH 2001; DH 2002, 2004a,b; RCN 2009).
2 Assessment of any current or illness-related pain should include: • Location, intensity, and duration of the pain. • The type/nature of the pain (e.g. spasms, burning, etc.). • Any factors that exacerbate or alleviate the pain.	2 To obtain a clear history of the pain and facilitate decision making regarding the most effective way to manage the pain.
3 If the CYP presents with pain on admission they may require: a) A physical examination. b) Prompt action to determine the cause of and treat the pain.	3 a) To determine the underlying condition/cause of pain. Severe pain can be difficult to manage and may be a sign of underlying pathophysiology (Schechter et al. 2003). b) To manage the pain quickly and effectively.
4 Pain assessment tools should be explained and the CYP/family should be taught how to use them wherever possible.	4 To familiarise the CYP/family with the tools and encourage their involvement in pain assessment.

My past experience of pain	More about pain management
What experiences of pain have you had in the past? What has helped to manage your pain in the past?	Please tell us about any pain in the past that you think we should know about. This information can help us to treat any pain that may occur after an operation or during a test or illness.
Do you have pain now? If yes, where is it and how often does the pain occur?	Yes ☐ No ☐
What score would you give your pain out of 10?	When scoring the pain, 0 = no pain, and 10 = the worse pain imaginable.
How would you describe the pain?	Describe how the pain feels to you, for example is it sharp, stabbing, or an ache?
Are you taking any medications for pain at the moment?	It also helps if you tell us what usually works to manage your pain, including medicines and distractions.

Figure 24.3 Initial assessment and history.

Procedure guideline 24.2 Pain assessment using a self-report tool

Statement	Rationale
1 CYPs should be encouraged to self-report pain wherever possible. The admitting nurse should consider factors such as age, language, cognitive ability, and willingness to report pain.	1 Self-report is considered the 'gold standard' of pain assessment. CYPs can self-report from an early age. Validated self-report tools can be used with children as young as four (Hicks et al. 2001; RCN 2009; Saul et al. 2016).
2 The CYP should be taught how to use any self-report tool on admission.	2 To familiarise the CYP with the tool and ensure that they are able to use it correctly.
a) The CYP's ability to use the tool should be checked by asking them to score previous painful experiences.	a) The CYP should be able to differentiate on the scale between something that hurts 'a little' and something that hurts 'a lot.'
b) Younger children should be taught how to use the tool to ensure that they can organise the faces/numbers, etc., into the correct order.	b) Younger children and those with learning difficulties may find more 'concrete' tools easier to use, but if explained correctly, faces scales can be used with children as young as four years old (Hicks et al. 2001), as well as adolescents.
c) If more than one tool is available, the CYP may help choose which tool to use. However, this should be linked to ease and accuracy of use, not just personal preference.	c) To facilitate choice and familiarity with the tool.
3 The original instructions and wording should be used to explain the tool if available.	3 To maintain validity and reliability.
4 The tool should be explained to the CYP in language that they understand and using the words they use to describe pain.	4 To facilitate accurate use. Younger children may not understand the word 'pain' (Jerrett and Evans 1986).

Procedure guideline 24.2 Pain assessment using a self-report tool *(continued)*

Statement	Rationale
5 There are a wide range of self-report tools available, which include: a) Concrete tools, e.g. Poker chip b) Faces scales c) Numeric or verbal rating scales d) Pain diaries	5 a) These may be easier for younger children to use. b) For example, Faces Pain Scale (Revised), the Oucher. c) Validated for older CYPs. d) For complex/chronic pain (Stinson et al. 2011; Saul et al. 2016).
6 It is important that a CYP is believed if they say that they DO have pain. If a CYP says that they DO NOT have pain, this should be verified by assessing behaviour and contextual factors.	6 CYPs rarely say that they have pain when they do not. However, they may be reluctant to admit it when they do have pain, due to fear of the consequences (e.g. foul-tasting medicine, worrying a parent/carer, or the possibility of prolonging their stay in hospital) (RCNI 1999).

Principles table 24.3 Pain assessment using a behavioural tool

Principle	Rationale
1 Behavioural assessment should be used in combination with verbal reports wherever possible. Physiological and contextual factors should also be considered.	1 To provide the most accurate assessment of pain (RCN 2009).
2 Behavioural indicators of pain are most accurate when assessing acute pain, particularly procedural pain.	2 Behaviour can be modified and pain behaviours are reduced within hours of surgery and shortly after a procedure (Beyer et al. 1990).
3 A validated tool should be used wherever possible. Examples of behavioural tools used at GOSH for different groups include: a) FLACC b) FLACC revised c) COMFORT d) PAT e) The Parents Postoperative Pain Measure (PPPM)	3 To ensure that assessments are valid and reliable (RCN 2009). For a list of tools available on the internet, see Table 24.1. a) Validated for use with children aged three months and over. (Voepel-Lewis et al. 2008). Some evidence of validity in critically ill patients (Voepel-Lewis et al. 2010). Translated into: French, Chinese, Portuguese, Swedish and Italian. b) For assessment of post op, procedural, and disease-related pain in CYPs with cognitive impairment (Malviya and Voepel-Lewis 2006). c) Ventilated and nonventilated CYPs, including neonates. (Van Dijk et al. 2000). d) Validated for use in neonates (Spence et al. 2005). e) Validated for use by parents/carers in the 1–12 year old age group (Chambers et al. 1996).
4 Where possible, observations should be recorded during handling or routine cares.	4 To provide a more accurate assessment. Pain is often greater on movement or handling.
5 a) All CYP should have a baseline measurement of their level of pain on admission to the trust (Royal College of Nursing 2017). Pain assessment should be measured whenever routine clinical observations are taken: • 4 hourly (or less frequently if clinically well) • 1-2 hourly if pain score indicates 'moderate' or 'severe' pain • before, during and after any painful procedures • Post-operatively pain assessment should be measured: • Every 15 minutes for the first hour • Hourly for the first 6 hours • 1-2 hourly if pain score indicates 'moderate' or 'severe' pain b) Pain should be re-assessed at an appropriate interval after any intervention.	5 a) To determine whether an intervention is required b) To determine whether the intervention as been effective.

Administration of entonox

The use of Entonox® has advanced the management of procedural pain in CYPs by providing effective short-term analgesia with minimal risk of adverse effects. Entonox is an inhaled mixture of 50% nitrous oxide and 50% oxygen. It can provide pain relief, some sedation, and reduce anxiety during painful procedures such as chest drain removal, pin site dressings, physiotherapy, and lumbar punctures (Bruce and Franck 2000; Bruce et al. 2006a; Association of Paediatric Anaesthetists of Great Britain and Ireland [APAGBI] 2012). Nitrous oxide is both rapidly absorbed and rapidly eliminated through the lungs, although small amounts are eliminated through the skin (Reynolds et al. 1996). Because of these properties, the onset of analgesia is extremely fast and, once inhalation ceases, analgesia and any adverse effects quickly subside. Although the mechanism of action is not clear, the analgesic, sedative, and anxiolytic effects of nitrous oxide are thought to be derived from its action at opioid receptors (Mason and Koka 1999). However, this issue remains the subject of debate, and involvement of other receptors has also been suggested (Zacny et al. 1999; British Oxygen Company [BOC] 2013).

Nitrous oxide is an anaesthetic gas and its continuous inhalation can result in moderate to deep sedation (National Institute for Health and Care Excellence [NICE] 2010). For this reason, when used in the UK outside of anaesthetics, dentistry or sedation services, Entonox is usually self-administered. To self-administer the gas a CYP must be able and willing to cooperate by holding the demand valve and inhaling the gas themselves. If they are unable to do this the use of Entonox should be abandoned and alternative analgesia given. The age at which a CYP is able to self-administer the gas will vary considerably. Concordance will depend on numerous factors, one of the main factors being the CYP's own coping style, degree of anticipatory fear, and their willingness to inhale the gas. Self-administered nitrous oxide offers several advantages over continuous flow administration, the main one being that it minimises the risk of over-sedation. It also requires the CYP to focus on regulating their breathing and offers them some control over the situation, both of which have been shown to have a positive effect on coping with pain (Hodgins and Lander 1997). Entonox should be administered alongside other drug and nondrug interventions to most effectively manage both the fear and sensation related to the procedure. A multimodal approach is particularly important for more painful procedures, such as chest drain removal, where Entonox alone may not be effective (Bruce et al. 2006a,b).

Healthcare professionals administering Entonox should have undertaken training, be competent in its use, and be familiar with the side effects and contra-indications (NICE 2010). Online training is available from BOC (2021). A list of staff trained and competent to administer Entonox should be kept on each ward. Entonox is a habit-forming drug and has been subject to abuse. Documented cases are rare, but provide evidence that long-term use can lead to myeloneuropathy and subacute combined degeneration (Reynolds et al. 1996). Nitrous oxide is not a controlled substance, but it is a substance of abuse and it is good practice to keep a log or audit of use (Figure 24.4) and a weekly check of cylinder levels.

DATE	CHILD NAME	GAUGE READING		TYPE OF PROCEDURE	DURATION OF USE	COMMENTS: State whether effective, if not why, details of any side effects, etc.
		AT START	AT END			

Figure 24.4 Audit sheet/log of use.

Training

Entonox must be administered only by staff who:

- Are competent in its administration and in basic life support.
- Are familiar with the side effects of Entonox and its contraindications.
- Are aware of the criteria for CYP selection (see Box 24.2).

These criteria will ensure that Entonox is administered safely and effectively and the likelihood of side effects and complications are reduced (NICE 2010).

To establish and maintain the required level of knowledge and skills (NICE 2010), staff should also have received:

- An Entonox training session.
- Supervised practice.
- Resuscitation training as per Trust policy.

A list of the staff on the ward who have been trained and are competent in the use of Entonox should be kept up to date, so that all ward staff know who can administer the gas.

Technical problems

It is vital that any faulty equipment is sent for repair and the safety of CYPs, staff, and environment is maintained. If any of the following technical problems occur, they should be reported to the hospital's engineering department immediately:

- Equipment not delivering gas.
- Leak at joint between regulator and cylinder valve.
- Demand valve leaks or does not shut cleanly.
- Demand valve does not stop giving flow after test button is released.

Box 24.2 Suggested competencies for training staff in the use of self-administered Entonox

All staff who use self-administered nitrous oxide during painful procedures should be trained and competent to do so. Staff should attend a training session and be familiar with hospital guidelines and protocols.
Aim of training: To enable staff to supervise the safe and effective self-administration of Entonox by CYPs undergoing painful procedures.
Competencies: Staff must be able to:
- Describe the characteristics of nitrous oxide and explain the rational for self-administered versus continuous flow delivery of Entonox.
- Give examples of the types of procedures where Entonox might be useful to provide pain relief.
- List the selection criteria for the use of Entonox.
- Describe the contraindications of nitrous oxide and its potential side effects.
- Explain why Entonox is not suitable for some CYPs or for prolonged or frequent use.
- Describe the nursing care of a CYP before, during, and after Entonox use.
- Demonstrate an understanding of the equipment and how it operates, including safety precautions and monitoring.
- Demonstrate the ability to instruct a CYP in the use of self-administered nitrous oxide, including indications, use, common side effects, and how these are prevented/managed.
- Describe the documentation used within the Trust.

The nurse should be responsible for arranging supervised practice sessions. Training is complete once both supervisor and trainee feel that the required level of competence has been achieved. A record of trained staff should be kept on the ward and regular update sessions made available for staff who need to refresh their skills (i.e. have not used nitrous oxide at least once in the past six months).

Procedure guideline 24.3 CYP assessment for use of entonox

Statement	Rationale
1 Assess the degree of pain and anxiety likely for the procedure to be carried out.	1 To determine whether Entonox is required.
2 Ensure that Entonox is not contraindicated for the CYP.	2 To reduce the likelihood of complications.
3 Entonox should not be used if the CYP has any condition where air is trapped in the body or an altered level of consciousness. These include: • Artificial, traumatic, or spontaneous pneumothorax. • Intestinal obstruction. • Head injuries with impaired consciousness. • Severe bullous emphysema. • Maxillofacial injuries. • Intoxication. • Following air encephalography. • Decompression sickness. • Air embolism. • Middle ear occlusion. • Following a recent underwater dive.	3 Nitrous oxide diffuses into air filled cavities, expanding the air to up to three times its original size. It is also thought to cause an increase in intra-cranial pressure (British Oxygen Company 2011; 2013).
4 To self-administer Entonox, a CYP must be able to: • Understand and follow simple instructions. • Hold the demand valve and inhale the gas through a mask or mouthpiece while breathing normally.	4 To ensure the CYP is able to use Entonox effectively.
5 Documentation of the assessment should be recorded in the CYP's healthcare record. See Figure 24.5 for GOS Entonox preassessment checklist.	5 To provide information (NICE 2010).

The Great Ormond Street Hospital Manual of Children and Young People's Nursing Practices

Pre Entonox Assessment	Date of Entonox Administration		
	Done Y/N	If NOT done – variance codes & comments	sign
Check ID band against prescription			
Check for any contraindications (bottom of prescription sheet)			
Check for any patient allergies?			
Oxygen and suction available at bedside?			
Well-ventilated room?			
Patient has been NBM (at least one hour)			
Pulse oximiter required? (if cardiac/respiratory condition)			
Analgesic administered prior to procedure?			
Anyone in the room in 1st trimester of pregnancy?			

Post Entonox Assessment	Done	If NOT done – variance codes & comments	sign
Any side effects?			
Good anaigesia?			
Safe environment maintained. (e.g. airway)			
Blood test required?			
(repeated Entonox administration, see CPG)			
Handover to patient's named nurse			
Documentation (prescription and audit book)			
Clean handset & tubing			

Figure 24.5 GOS Entonox preassessment checklist.

Procedure guideline 24.4 Preparation for entonox use

Statement	Rationale
1 Ensure the Entonox has been prescribed.	1 To adhere to hospital drug policy.
2 a) Liaise with the person carrying out the procedure.	2 a) To agree on a suitable time for the procedure.
b) The person administering the Entonox should not be involved with the procedure.	b) To ensure that the CYP is supervised throughout the procedure.
3 If Entonox is to be administered more frequently than every four days routine blood cell counts must be performed.	3 To observe for evidence of megaloblastic changes in red cells, reduced production of leucocytes and hypersegmentation of neutrophils (Amos et al. 1983; Nunn 1987).
4 Staff in the first trimester of pregnancy, or those trying to conceive may wish to avoid the area if Entonox is being administered for long periods in an area with no scavenging.	4 There is some evidence to suggest that exposure to very high levels of nitrous oxide can reduce fertility (Rowland et al. 1992) and may be harmful to the foetus during pregnancy (Aldridge and Tunstall 1986; Park et al. 1986).
5 The area should be well ventilated to prevent the accumulation of nitrous oxide.	5 To maintain a safe environment. The occupational exposure standard for long-term exposure is 1parts per million (ppm) (BOC 2014).
6 Gather and prepare the following equipment: a) Entonox cylinder and administration set: • Switch cylinder on and prime the administration set by pressing the test button on the back of the demand valve • Check the cylinder to ensure it is at least one-quarter full.	6 To ensure immediate availability of Entonox once inhalation commences.
b) A bacterial/viral filter (e.g. Hydroboy™) and mask or mouth piece: • Attach the filter to the mask or mouthpiece before attaching this to the demand valve.	b) To reduce the risk of infection. If no filter is used, the whole equipment needs to be cleaned thoroughly after use on each occasion.
7 Entonox cylinders must be checked carefully before use to ensure they contain the correct mix of 50% nitrous oxide and 50% oxygen.	7 To prevent drug errors. Stronger concentrations of nitrous oxide are available for anaesthetic use only.

Procedure guideline 24.4 Preparation for entonox use *(continued)*

Statement	Rationale
8 If the CYP has respiratory or cardiac problems, ensure that a saturation monitor is available.	8 To observe for post-inhalation hypoxia (BOC 2013).
9 To prepare the CYP: • Explain the procedure to be carried out and how Entonox will be used, including information about the side effects (see Procedure Guideline 24.6). • Reassure them that if side effects occur, these will wear off quickly once they stop inhaling the gas.	9 To provide information, relieve anxiety, and increase the level of cooperation/concordance.
10 The CYP should not eat immediately before the procedure. If they have been given sedatives, opioids, or already feel nauseous or sedated, a period of fasting is advisable.	10 To reduce the likelihood of vomiting and associated complications (e.g. aspiration). Vomiting is rare during Entonox use but the risk is increased if more than one sedative has been given (Gall et al. 2001).
11 Give supplementary analgesia as prescribed:	11 To provide additional pain relief.
a) Oral or rectal drugs should be given at least an hour before, and intravenous analgesia 20 minutes before starting the procedure.	a) To allow adequate time for absorption.
b) The CYP may continue to use their patient controlled analgesia (PCA) if this is in use.	
c) A bolus of intravenous opiate may be given if a high degree of pain is anticipated.	
d) It is important to ensure that the CYP's opiate intake is closely monitored.	d) If the CYP is too sleepy they will be unable to inhale the gas effectively.
12 The CYP should be allowed to practise using the Entonox before the procedure is started.	12 To ensure an effective technique is established.

If the CYP is unable to maintain an effective seal or inhale the gas effectively the use of Entonox should be abandoned and alternative analgesia should be prescribed.

Procedure guideline 24.5 Administration of entonox

Statement	Rationale
1 To administer the Entonox:	1
a) Calmly explain the procedure; tell the CYP that they should concentrate on breathing the gas normally.	a) To reassure the CYP and establish an effective inhalation technique.
b) Offer the demand valve to the CYP. If they have chosen to use a mask, they should hold it over their mouth and nose and, maintaining an airtight seal, breathe normally.	b) If they do not maintain a tight seal, the gas will not be delivered effectively.
c) If the CYP is not able to hold the face mask in place, they can try a mouthpiece, or the procedure must be abandoned.	c) To minimise the risk of oversedation: If the CYP becomes too sleepy they will be unable to maintain an effective seal around the mask.
No one should hold the mask in place for the CYP	
d) If the CYP has chosen the mouthpiece they should hold it between their teeth and breathe through their mouth. They may need considerable encouragement to start inhaling the gas. It is worth persevering, as any initial reluctance often disappears once they realise that the gas is working.	d) This technique can be harder for some CYPs. If so they may find the mask easier.
2 Inhalation should commence for at least six to eight breaths before the procedure starts.	2 To ensure Entonox has taken effect before introduction of painful stimuli.
a) Once administration has commenced the CYP should continue to use the Entonox as required throughout the procedure and should be encouraged to breathe slowly and deeply.	a–b) To provide effective analgesia with minimal side effects.

(continued)

Procedure guideline 24.5 Administration of entonox *(continued)*

Statement	Rationale
b) If the CYP hyperventilates, they should be encouraged to exhale slowly and then breathe normally.	
3 Observe the CYP throughout the procedure to determine: • Level of pain. • The presence of any side effects. • Whether the CYP is inhaling the gas effectively. • Oxygen saturation level should be monitored during the procedure if the CYP has an underlying cardiac or respiratory condition.	3 To provide adequate pain relief with minimal side effects.

NB: If use of Entonox is unsatisfactory at any stage, it may be necessary to stop the procedure until alternative analgesia has been prescribed and given.

Procedure guideline 24.6 Managing side-effects of entonox

Statement	Rationale
1 If the CYP experiences any Entonox-related side effects: a) Reassure them, and remind them that they may stop inhaling the gas until the side effects wear off. b) If necessary, negotiate with them to determine whether the procedure should be halted until they start to inhale the gas again.	1 To provide effective analgesia with minimal side effects.
2 **Earache:** If the CYP complains of earache, inhalation should be stopped and alternative analgesia prescribed.	2 Expansion of air trapped in the ear canal could cause perforation of the eardrum (BOC 2013).
3 **Dry mouth:** This is a common side effect which is not usually distressing and the CYP should be encouraged to continue inhaling the Entonox.	3 To provide effective analgesia.
4 **Dizziness and/or disorientation:** If the CYP starts to feel dizzy or disorientated, they may cease inhalation until the sensation starts to wear off. The CYP may choose to put up with these sensations and continue inhalation to maintain effective pain relief.	4 To provide effective analgesia with minimal side effects.
5 **Oversedation:** If the CYP becomes drowsy they will no longer inhale the gas. **The CYP should not be helped to keep the mask in situ**. If their level of sedation increases: • Monitor them closely. • The procedure may continue if their condition is stable. As the gas is self-administered it is unlikely that the CYP will become oversedated. However, if they are not responding to verbal commands, remove the Entonox and ensure that staff experienced in the management of sedation are contacted/nearby.	5 To prevent the onset of deeper stages of sedation and loss of protection of the laryngeal reflex. Self-administered Entonox should cause only minimal sedation (NICE 2010). For a definition of the levels of sedation, see Box 24.3.
6 **Nausea and vomiting:**	6
a) If the CYP complains of nausea they may choose to stop inhaling the gas for a while.	a) The side effects of Entonox wear off quickly once inhalation ceases.
b) Less commonly the CYP may vomit. If so remove the demand valve immediately.	b) To prevent inhalation of vomit.
c) Reassure the CYP and clear any obstruction to breathing.	c) To maintain a patent airway.
d) Clean or replace the face mask or mouthpiece.	d–e) To ensure the equipment is clean.
e) Clear vomit from the demand valve by vigorously shaking it using a 'flicking' downward action.	
f) Once the equipment has been wiped clean the CYP may then recommence administration if they wish.	f) The side effects of Entonox wear off quickly once inhalation ceases.
7 **Postadministration hypoxia:** If the CYP feels dizzy once they stop inhaling the gas they may benefit from oxygen therapy for 10–15 minutes.	7 To prevent post-administration hypoxia (BOC 2013).

Procedure guideline 24.7 After use

Statement	Rationale

1 Once the procedure has finished:
  a) Ensure that the CYP is comfortable.
  b) Order a new cylinder if required.
  c) Check and document the cylinder gauge level.
  d) Turn off the cylinder and depressurise the system fully by operating the test button.
	1
	
	b–c) To ensure there is an adequate supply for the next CYP.
	c–d) To prevent misuse and to maintain a safe ward environment.

2 Document that Entonox has been given:
  • On the audit form.
  • In the CYP's healthcare records.
	2 To document outcomes of care and promote evidence-based practice.

3 The CYP should not walk around unaided until any dizziness or disorientation has gone. Monitoring should continue for 30 minutes to ensure that the effects of the Entonox have completely worn off.	3 To prevent the CYP from injury.
4 If the Entonox is used infrequently the cylinder should be checked weekly and its contents recorded. A member of the ward staff should be responsible for ensuring that the equipment is checked regularly.	4 To maintain a safe environment and ensure that equipment is in good working order.

5 To clean the equipment:
  • Depressurise the system.
  • Clean the external surfaces of the demand valve with an alcohol based wipe.
  • If any contamination is suspected between the hose connection into the demand valve it must be sent to HSDU to be autoclaved.
  • Multiuse face masks and mouthpieces should be autoclaved at 121°C by HSDU.
  • Single-use face masks and mouthpieces should be discarded.
  • The external surfaces of the administration set should be cleaned with an alcohol based wipe.
  • Filters are for single use and should be discarded.
	5 To maintain a safe environment and prevent infection.

Procedure guideline 24.8 Storage

Statement	Rationale
1 Entonox cylinders should be stored in a secure environment, attached to a wall or trolley or in a locked cupboard, away from CYPs when not in use.	1 To maintain a safe environment.
2 If cylinders are stored outside in cold weather, they must be brought inside at least 24 hours before use and stored horizontally.	2 The gases will separate if cylinders are stored at temperatures below −6°C. Storing horizontally at 10°C for 24 hours will correct this (BOC 2011).
3 As with all pressurised gases, Entonox should not come into contact with a naked flame.	3 Nitrous oxide supports combustion and may produce toxic or corrosive fumes if exposed to fire.

Epidural analgesia

The epidural space is situated between the dura mater (the outer layer of the meninges) and the vertebral canal. It extends from the cranium to the sacrum and contains loose connective tissue, fat, lymph vessels, blood vessels, and nerves. Analgesics administered into the epidural space diffuse across the dura and the subarachnoid space and bind to receptors located in the substantia gelatinosa in the dorsal horn of the spinal cord. They also exert an effect on the nerve roots outside the dura mater, are absorbed systemically from epidural blood vessels, and may be distributed throughout the subarachnoid space in the cerebrospinal fluid (CSF). The epidural route is commonly used to manage intra-operative and postoperative pain associated with a variety of procedures. Less commonly, it is used to control nonsurgical or chronic pain. An epidural catheter is inserted into an anaesthetised CYP by a consultant anaesthetist with experience in inserting epidurals in CYPs, or an anaesthetic registrar under supervision. In infants under six months of age, or weighing less than 5 kg, the catheter is sometimes inserted via the sacral hiatus (caudal route) and threaded into the epidural space until the appropriate level has been reached.

Local anaesthetics and analgesics can be administered separately or in combination. Intraoperatively, these may be given either as a single bolus dose or as an infusion. Postoperative epidural analgesia is usually provided by a continuous infusion via a syringe driver or volumetric pump. The drugs most commonly used to provide analgesia include local anaesthetics and opioids. Each opioid has its advantages and disadvantages and different side effect profiles. Morphine has a slower onset, but longer duration of action than fentanyl or diamorphine (Rowney and Doyle 1998). In neonates, CYPs with sensitivity to opioids, and those at risk of opioid-related complications, local anaesthetic alone may be used. Less commonly, other drugs such as ketamine and clonidine are also administered via the epidural route.

All staff caring for CYPs with an epidural must be trained and competent to do so. Pumps should be standardised and training in their use should be provided (NPSA 2018). Infusion rates, syringe changes, and technical problems should be managed by staff who have had additional training and work within written local guidelines (DH 2004b; RCoA 2020).

Principles table 24.4 Assessment and preparation for an epidural

Principle	Rationale
1 Prior to insertion of an epidural the anaesthetist will consider: a) The benefits and risks of an epidural for the CYP. b) The effectiveness of epidural analgesia for the type of surgery/pain.	1 To ensure that potential risks are balanced against the benefits (Llewellyn and Moriarty 2007).
2a) Parents/carers should be given written and verbal information regarding available methods of pain relief. An anaesthetist will discuss the epidural with the CYP and family prior to theatre and obtain verbal consent for the procedure. b) If verbal consent is not obtained, alternative analgesia will be provided. NB: Other countries require written consent.	2a) To provide information and facilitate informed consent. An information leaflet is available online at https://www.gosh.nhs.uk/conditions-and-treatments/procedures-and-treatments/pain-relief-after-surgery-using-epidural/. b) To meet the family's needs and provide satisfactory analgesia.
3 The anaesthetist may choose not to insert an epidural if the CYP presents with: a) Local or generalised sepsis or a pyrexia of unknown origin. b) Coagulation disorders or anticoagulation therapy. c) Some diseases of the central nervous system. d) Spinal deformity.	3 To avoid the risk of epidural-related complications. a) To avoid the risk of an epidural-related infection. b) To avoid the risk of a subdural haematoma. c) To minimise the risk of exacerbation of the disease or other complications. d) This may make it impossible to insert the epidural catheter.
4 The CYP and family should be prepared for the epidural. They should be made aware that: • The epidural will be inserted once the CYP has been anaesthetised • If the procedure is unsuccessful alternative analgesia will be prescribed.	4 To meet information needs and minimise uncertainty and anxiety.
5 Nursing staff should also ensure that: • Any tools that will be used to assess pain are explained to the CYP/family on admission • Words the CYP uses for pain and the CYP's usual pain related behaviours are recorded on their care plan.	5 To provide knowledge and obtain information to facilitate accurate assessment of pain (see Pain Assessment section for further details).
6 The following baseline observations should also be recorded before the CYP goes to theatre: • Temperature • Heart rate • Respiratory rate • Blood pressure	6 To establish normal parameters with which to compare future observations. Deviation from baseline observations may indicate epidural related side effects or complications.
7 Any neurological abnormality (e.g. altered sensation, limb weakness) should be reported to the anaesthetist and recorded in the CYP's healthcare records.	7 To ensure that these are not attributed to, or exacerbated by the epidural at a later stage.

Principles table 24.5 Drug administration via an epidural

Principles	Rationale
1 A single bolus of local anaesthetic is usually given by the anaesthetist either through the epidural needle or once the catheter is in position.	1 To establish the initial block and provide effective analgesia.
2 Additional boluses may be given intraoperatively or an infusion commenced.	2 To provide effective analgesia.

Chapter 24 Pain management

Principles table 24.5 Drug administration via an epidural (*continued*)

Principles	Rationale
3 A continuous infusion may be administered either via a syringe driver or volumetric pump system according to local policy. In addition, the following principles should be applied:	3 To provide effective analgesia with minimal risk of complications.
a) Only appropriately trained staff working within written hospital guidelines should change epidural infusion rates and syringes or bags.	a–b) To minimise the risk of drug errors (NPSA 2018; RCoA 2020).
b) Pumps and infusion sets should be clearly identifiable as being for epidural use only.	
c) All syringes and equipment should be handled using an aseptic technique.	c) To minimise the risk of infection.
d) An epidural filter should always be used.	d) To minimise the risk of infection and nerve damage.
4 Since 2011, all epidural infusions and boluses should include connectors that cannot connect with intravenous Luer connectors or intravenous infusion spikes (NPSA 2011).	4 To reduce the risk of drugs being given via the wrong route.

Procedure guideline 24.9 Transfer of the CYP following epidural insertion

For other aspects of care of the CYP during the postoperative period, see Chapter 26: Perioperative Care.

Statement	Rationale
1 When collecting the CYP from theatre a verbal report should be obtained from the recovery nurse. This should include details of: • Any intraoperative analgesia and other drugs given. • The epidural solution and infusion rate. • Any pain or epidural related complications that have been experienced peri-operatively.	1 To provide adequate information.
2 The nurse collecting / taking over the care of the CYP should ensure that:	2
a) The drug being administered has been prescribed correctly and any medicine administration has been recorded.	a–b) To prevent drug errors. Any differences between the prescription and the pump settings/syringe label should, ideally, be rectified before the CYP leaves recovery.
b) The pump settings have been checked against the prescription.	
c) The CYP's pain is being managed effectively.	c–e) To provide effective analgesia with minimal side effects and determine whether the CYP is stable enough to be transferred to the ward.
d) The CYP is not excessively sedated.	
e) All other observations, including blood pressure, sensory and motor block are satisfactory.	
f) All documentation has been completed.	f) To provide adequate information.
g) For epidurals that contain an opioid, naloxone must have been prescribed BEFORE the CYP leaves recovery.	g) To facilitate immediate treatment of opiate-induced respiratory depression.

Procedure guideline 24.10 Nursing care of an epidural (general)

Statement	Rationale
1 A care plan/pathway should be available and should be adapted for each individual CYP.	1 To ensure that standards of care are maintained and tailored to need and that adequate information is recorded.
2 Supplementary analgesia, i.e. paracetamol and an NSAID if possible (e.g. diclofenac, ibuprofen, IV paracoxib) should be given regularly).	2 To provide optimal analgesia. Multimodal analgesia is more effective than single route analgesia (Schug et al. 2015).

(*continued*)

Procedure guideline 24.10 Nursing care of an epidural (general) *(continued)*

Statement	Rationale

3 The CYP should be encouraged to mobilise if their condition allows. Ensure that:
  a) The CYP is accompanied at all times while mobilising and is accompanied by a nurse if leaving the ward.
  b) Older CYPs are warned that they may experience some dizziness initially when mobilising.
	3 Early mobilisation improves circulation, respiratory effort and reduces the risk of complications.
	  a) To prevent falls, complications, and inadvertent catheter removal.
	  b) Local anaesthetics affect the sympathetic nervous system and can cause hypotension (Gunter 2002).

4 CYPs with numb or heavy legs, and those on bed rest or reluctant to mobilise should receive regular pressure area care.	4 To minimise the risk of pressure sores. For more information on pressure sore prevention, see Chapter 11: Personal Hygiene and Pressure Ulcer Prevention.

5 a) Intravenous access should be available throughout the duration of the epidural and for 6–12 hours after it has been discontinued.
  b) If the cannula has tissued, intramuscular naloxone may be given, but this is not the preferred route of administration.
	5 a) To enable the administration of naloxone by the quickest route if respiratory depression occurs. Morphine remains in the CSF for longer than fentanyl or diamorphine and the risk of respiratory depression is prolonged.
	  b) Onset of action is longer if the drug is given via the intramuscular route.

Procedure guideline 24.11 Nursing care of an epidural (observations)

Statement	Rationale

1 All observations should be documented in the CYP's healthcare record. This should include:
  • Pain scores.
  • Level of sedation.
  • Presence, incidence and severity of any epidural or opioid-related side effects.
  • Condition of the epidural entry site.
  • The height (dermatome level) and density (Bromage score) of the block (see points 2 and 3 below).
  • Respiratory rate, pulse and blood pressure.
  • Fluid balance.
	1 To provide accurate information and early detection of potential complications. See Figure 24.6 for an example of scoring tools. For the management of epidural and opioid-related side effects and complications, see the following sections.

2 The height of the block is most effectively checked using ice.
  a) Touch the ice on the arm or cheek and ask how it feels.
  b) Work down each side of the body, asking the CYP if they feel hot, warm, cold, or no sensation.
  c) If the block is above T3 (see Figure 24.7) STOP the epidural.
	2 To identify a patchy or unilateral block, or one that is too high or too low. The CYP needs to be able to communicate and willing to cooperate for this test to be effective.. For dermatome map, see Figure 24.6.
	  a) To identify that it feels cold.
	  b) There is no sensory block in areas where the CYP can feel cold.
	  c) To prevent complications. A high block can affect the muscles involved in respiration.

3 a) Assess the density of the block by asking the CYP to bend their knees or move their feet. The higher the Bromage score (Bromage 1978), the denser the block (Figure 24.6).
  b) If the score is 2 or 3, STOP the epidural infusion until the score is below 2.
  c) For thoracic epidurals, ask the CYP to squeeze your fingers, comparing the strength in both hands, then ask them to raise their arms.
  d) If they are unable to do this effectively, STOP the infusion.
  e) If motor function does not start to return within 2 hours the anaesthetist/pain team should be contacted.
	3a) To ensure early detection of complications. Loss of motor function could potentially be due to a haematoma/nerve damage.
	  b) A dense/heavy block (no movement) is unpleasant and greatly increases the risk of pressure sores.
	  c) To determine the height of the block.
	  d) A high block can affect respiratory function.
	  e) To rule out other causes such as an epidural abscess. For a summary of the management of a dense block see Figure 24.7.

Epidural Observations

Sedation Scores

- 0 Awake / alert
- 1 Sleepy / responds appropriately
- 2 Somnolent / rousable (light stimuli)
- 3 Deep sleep / rousable (deeper physical stimuli)
     Intervene
- 4 Unrousable to stimuli
     Stop infusion / Bleep 0577

BJA 88(2): 241-5 (2002)

Pressure Area Care

S = Sitting	M = Mobilising	
R = on Right side	F = on Front	
L = on Left side	B = on Back	

Nausea & Vomiting

- 1 None
- 2 Nausea
- 3 Vomited

Pruritus

- 1 Slight
- 2 Moderate
- 3 Severe

Pain Scores

- 0   No pain
- 1 – 3   Mild pain
- 4 – 7   Moderate pain
- 8 – 10 Severe pain *

Epidural Site

- R = Red
- S = Swelling / Lump
- L = Leaking
- P = Painful
- T = Related Pyrexia

© Pain Control Service, GOSH NHS Foundation Trust May 2014

Bromage Score

- 3 **Stop infusion & contact Pain Team:**
     Re-assess every 30 minutes

     Bromage 3 (complete) — Unable to move feet or knees

- 2 **Stop infusion & contact Pain Team:**
     Re-assess every 30 minutes
     (Extended role for senior nurses)

     Bromage 2 (almost complete) — Able to move feet only

- 1 **Observe hourly; consider reducing infusion rate if patient comfortable**

     Bromage 1 (partial) — Just able to move knees

- 0 **No intervention required**
     Patient may mobilise with supervision

     Bromage 0 (none) — Full flexion of knees and feet

Bromage PR (1978) "Epidural Analgesia" WB Saunders (ed), Philadelphia.

Dermatome Level

Should be documented:
- In recovery
- At the start of each shift
- If the patient is in pain
- 30 minutes after increasing or decreasing epidural infusion

N.B. Level should not be >T3

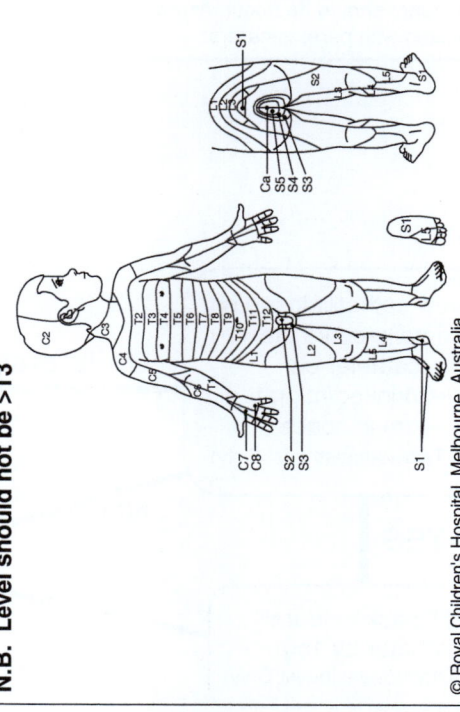

© Royal Children's Hospital, Melbourne, Australia

Figure 24.6 Epidural observations.

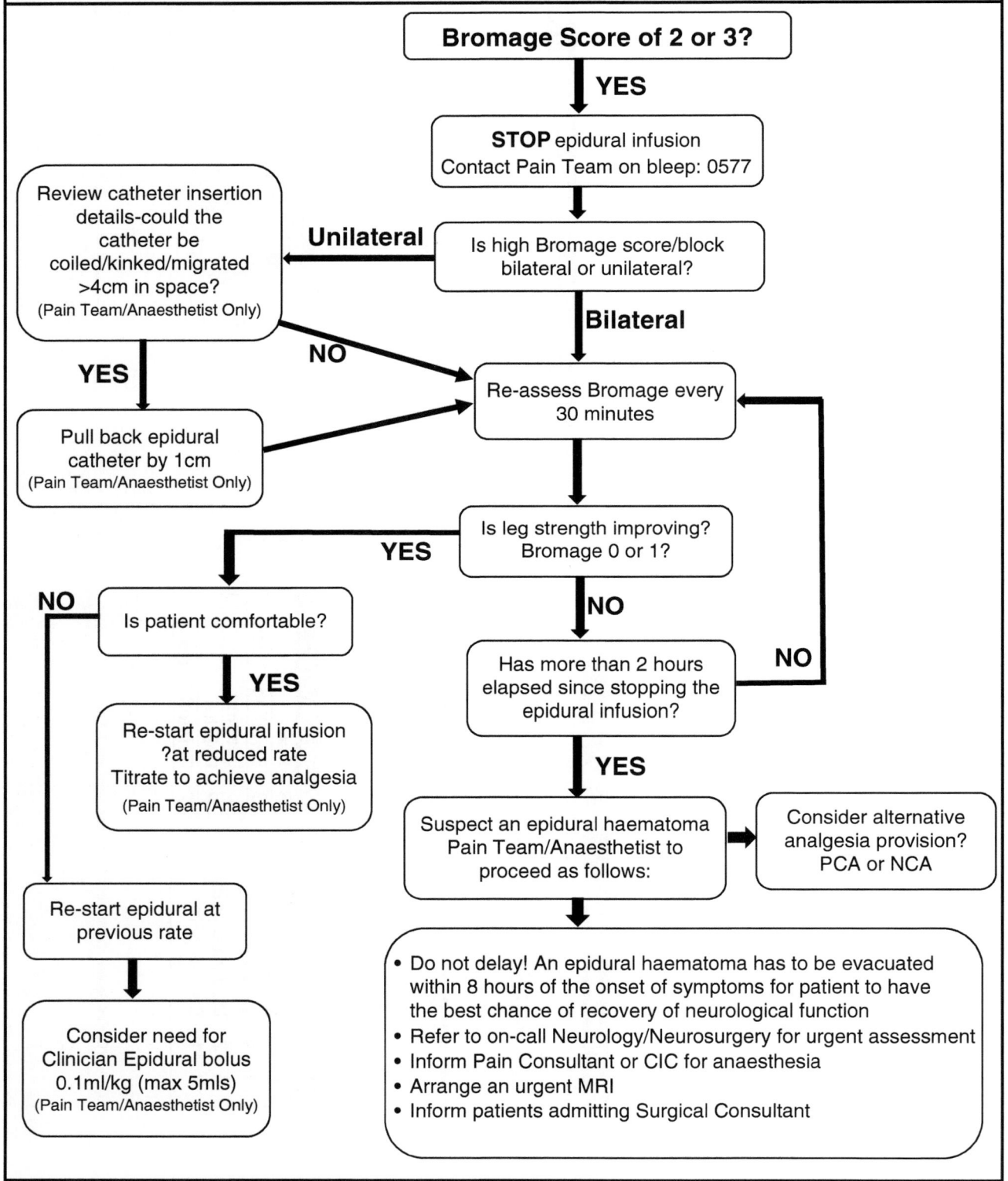

Figure 24.7 Management of High Bromage Score.

Procedure guideline 24.12 Epidural related complications

See also the section 'Prevention and management of opioid-related complications.'

Statement	Rationale
Pain	

1 Assess the level of the block.
  a) If it is too low and the CYP is not experiencing side effects the infusion rate could be increased.
  b) If it is unilateral or patchy an increase in the rate may also improve the level of pain relief. However, it may be necessary to carefully remove the dressing and pull back the catheter by 0.5–1 cm. This should only be done by an appropriately trained person, usually an anaesthetist.
	1 To establish whether the pain is due to a low, unilateral, or patchy block and rectify this if possible.

2 Administer simple analgesics, i.e. paracetamol and an NSAID if appropriate.	2 To provide optimal pain relief. Multimodal is more effective than a single mode of analgesia (Schug et al. 2015).
3 It may help to reposition the CYP.	3 To relieve pressure/discomfort.
4 Administer prescribed coanalgesics as appropriate (e.g. anti-spasmodic drugs).	4 To treat other causes of pain (e.g. bladder spasms).
5 Involve parents/carers, play specialist, and psychologist if the pain is anxiety related.	5 To manage the emotional component of the pain.
6 If the pain is unmanageable or indicative of surgical complications or other cause contact the surgeons, anaesthetist or pain team as appropriate.	6 To obtain advice regarding the cause of the pain and the most appropriate intervention.
7 Some CYP may benefit from having a plain epidural (local anaesthetic only) and either oral or intravenous opioids for breakthrough pain.	7 To provide effective analgesia with minimal side effects.
Urinary retention	
1 If the CYP has a urinary catheter this should remain in situ until the epidural infusion is discontinued.	1 To minimise the risk of retention. For care of the CYP with a urinary catheter, see Chapter 33: Urinary Catheter Care.
2 If the CYP has no urinary catheter, urine output should be monitored closely.	2 Opiates bind to receptors in the bladder, reducing the ability to detect changes in pressure as the bladder fills. Local anaesthetics will also have an effect on bladder sensitivity.

3 If the CYP has not passed urine recently the bladder should be palpated. Intervention is required if:
  • The CYP has a palpable bladder.
  • The CYP complains of discomfort/inability to pass urine.
	3 Urinary retention causes abdominal distension, pain, and can cause further complications. Increased discomfort or distress in a nonverbal CYPs may be mistaken for surgical pain when the cause is an overfull bladder.

4 Urinary retention should be treated as follows:	4 To maintain adequate urine output.
a) Administer naloxone (0.5 μg/kg) as prescribed.	a) To reverse opiate-induced retention. This is not the reversal dose, which is larger and only used for respiratory depression.
b) Four doses can be given at 10-minute intervals. This is half the reversal dose, so may reduce analgesic efficacy.	b) To partially block opioid receptors and stimulate enuresis.
c) If not effective, the doses may be repeated after an hour.	c) Naloxone is short acting.
d) A urinary catheter may need to be inserted. This should remain in situ until the epidural infusion is discontinued.	d) To prevent further complications.
Local anaesthetic toxicity	
1 Local anaesthetic toxicity is rare but is most likely in the following situations:	1
a) If the drug is accidentally administered intravenously.	a) Local anaesthetics are rarely given intravenously.
b) If the drug starts to accumulate (e.g. in a CYP with renal failure/a neonate).	b) Accumulation may occur in immature or reduced renal function.

(continued)

Procedure guideline 24.12 Epidural related complications *(continued)*

Statement	Rationale
2 Observe the CYP for a reaction to local anaesthetic. Signs include: • Tingling mouth and lips • Increased anxiety • Irritability • Sedation • Nausea • Hypotension • Respiratory distress • Cardiac arrhythmias • Convulsions.	2 To ensure prompt detection and intervention. Local anaesthetic toxicity is potentially fatal.
3 If any of the above are observed: a) Stop the infusion. b) Administer basic life support if necessary. c) Contact the anaesthetist, surgeon or pain team for advice regarding analgesia.	3 a) To prevent further accumulation. b) To stabilise the CYP. c) To identify an alternative method of analgesia.
4 After injection of a bolus of local anaesthetic, toxicity may develop at any time in the following hour. If local anaesthetic toxicity is suspected, the epidural infusion must be stopped immediately. If local anaesthetic-induced cardiovascular toxicity is suspected, follow guidelines from the BNFC (https://bnfc.nice.org.uk/treatment-summary/severe-local-anaesthetic-induced-cardiovascular-toxicity.html)	4

Epidural entry site

Statement	Rationale
1 The epidural catheter entry site should be observed when turning the CYP and at least four hourly.	1 To ensure prompt detection of leaking, swelling, or infection.
2 If leaking occurs: a) Observe the entry site more frequently, 1 to 2 hourly if possible. b) If the dressing starts to peel off, place a new one over the top. c) Removal of the dressing should be done only when absolutely necessary by a person with advanced training.	2 This is not uncommon and may not cause any problems, but has the potential to do so. a) To ensure the dressing remains intact and observe for signs of infection. b) To minimise the risk of leaking and infection. c) To prevent displacement of the catheter.
3 If the dressing falls off: a) Put a new sterile transparent occlusive hypoallergenic dressing on immediately. b) Contact a suitable trained individual to check the position of the catheter.	3 a) To prevent displacement of the catheter. b) The catheter may have become dislodged and will need to be removed if it is no longer effective.
4 If the epidural continues to leak the following actions may be carried out by an appropriately trained individual: a) Increase the epidural rate if the CYP is in pain. b) If the CYP has no surgical pain, reduce the rate. c) Redress the entry site. d) Remove the epidural and arrange alternative analgesia. e) Record actions in the CYP's healthcare record.	4 Excessive leakage may result in ineffective analgesia. a) To provide effective analgesia. b) To reduce the pressure, as this may prevent or reduce the leakage. c) If the catheter is kinked under the skin this may relieve the pressure and stop the leaking. d) Continual leaking increases the risk of epidural site infection. To provide effective analgesia with minimal complications. e) To ensure that an accurate record of care is maintained.

Procedure guideline 24.12 Epidural related complications (continued)

Statement	Rationale
Infection	
1 Prompt action should be taken if: • The entry site becomes red or swollen. • The catheter has become displaced. • The dressing has fallen off. • There is excessive leaking of fluid around the entry site. • The CYP has a pyrexia of unknown origin or other signs of unexplained infection, including neurological deterioration.	1 To ensure swift action to prevent/treat any potential infection.
2 If an epidural infection is suspected, inform the anaesthetist/pain team/surgeon. The following actions should be taken:	2 To ensure prompt, effective treatment and minimise the risk of complications.
a) Remove the epidural catheter.	a) To eliminate a potential source of infection.
b) Swab the entry site.	b) To identify the micro-organisms that need to be treated.
c) The catheter tip should only be sent to microbiology if a centralised infection is suspected.	c) Routine culture of catheter tips is not a good predictor of epidural infection (Seth et al. 2004).
d) Consider starting antibiotics if the CYP is clinically unwell.	d) To minimise the risks and potential complications of infection.
e) Follow up swab results.	e, f) To ensure that the correct antibiotic has been prescribed.
f) Commence antibiotics as appropriate for any micro-organisms isolated.	
g) Document and report the incident as per local policy.	g) To ensure effective communication.
3 Follow-up should continue until the infection has cleared. If an epidural abscess is suspected, an emergency scan should be arranged and a neurologist involved.	3 To minimise the risk of complications.
Neurological complications	
1 Neurological complications are rare, but can have serious consequences. Contact the anaesthetist, surgeon, or pain team if any of the following are observed:	1 Swift action is required to determine the cause (if possible), treat, and to prevent further deterioration. Symptoms may be indicative of:
a) Headache	a) Dural tap or centralised infection.
b) Loss of motor function, sensation or other signs of neurological deterioration	b) Nerve damage/abscess/haematoma.
2 Record symptoms and any action taken in the CYP's healthcare records.	2 To maintain an accurate record. Long-term follow-up may be required.
3 If neurological damage or an abscess is suspected: a) **Stop the infusion:** Do not remove the epidural catheter until certain that it is safe to do so.	3 a) To prevent worsening of the complications.
b) The CYP should be referred to a neurologist for further investigations.	b) To obtain specialist advice and ensure prompt diagnosis and treatment of the problem.

Procedure guideline 24.13 Technical problems

Statement	Rationale
Pump occlusion	
1 If the pump occludes:	1
a) Stop the infusion.	a) To determine the cause.
b) Check that the catheter is not kinked or trapped.	b) Kinked or trapped tubing can cause occlusion.
c) Ensure that the correct administration set is being used.	c–e) To prevent drug administration errors occurring due to the use of the wrong or faulty equipment.
d) Check the pump; pressures may need to be increased or the pump replaced.	
e) Any faulty pumps must be taken out of use and be reported in line with local procedures. Ensure that the pump serial number is documented in the CYP's health care record and any incident form.	

(continued)

The Great Ormond Street Hospital Manual of Children and Young People's Nursing Practices

Procedure guideline 24.13 Technical problems *(continued)*

Statement	Rationale
2 The following interventions should only be attempted by an anaesthetist or other suitably trained individual: a) Check the filter to ensure the connection is not too tight. b) Attempt to flush the catheter from the filter with 2 ml of 0.9% sodium chloride for injection in a 5 ml syringe. c) Observe and redress the entry site if necessary. If the catheter is kinked under the skin it may be possible to correct this by pulling the catheter back by 0.5–1 cm before redressing.	2 To safely determine the cause of the occlusion and attempt to correct it. a) A tight connection will increase pressure/resistance. b) To determine whether the source of the occlusion is below the filter. Flushing the line may also clear the occlusion. c) To relieve a kink under the dressing or skin.
3 If these interventions are unsuccessful the epidural may need to be removed and alternative analgesia prescribed.	3 To provide effective analgesia.

Catheter disconnection

Statement	Rationale
1 The filter should only be reconnected by appropriately trained staff working within written hospital/local guidelines.	1 To minimise the risk of errors and complications (RCoA 2020).
2 If the catheter becomes disconnected from the filter the following actions may be necessary: a) Wrap the filter and catheter in sterile paper. Do not lift the catheter up as this will allow air to be drawn in. b) Do not clamp the epidural catheter. c) Stop the infusion. d) The epidural catheter may be reconnected if: • The disconnection occurred less than two hours earlier and has been kept clean, • the fluid level within the catheter does not drop when held at CYP's level, • there is less than 2 inches of air in the catheter.	2 To minimise the risk of infection. These practices should be agreed at local level with microbiology. a) To minimise the risk of infection. If the catheter tip has/ may have been contaminated it MUST be removed. b) To prevent kinking of the catheter. c) To prevent further leakage. d) To provide effective analgesia while minimising the risk of infection (Langevin 1996; McNeely and Trentadue 1997; Kost-Byerly et al. 1998). N.B. Guidelines for reconnections must be approved locally in consultation with microbiology.
4 Reconnect the catheter using an aseptic nontouch technique (ANTT): • Clean the catheter with an alcohol impregnated swab and allow to dry completely. • With sterile scissors, cut off the section of catheter that contains air. • Reconnect catheter to the filter. • Dispose of used equipment according to local waste policy. • Record action in the CYP's notes.	4 To provide effective analgesia while minimising the risk of infection/air in the epidural space. For more information regarding ANTT see Chapter 11: IV & IA Infusions and Access
5 The epidural catheter must be removed if: • It has been disconnected for longer than two hours • The catheter is or could have been contaminated • This is a third disconnection.	5 To minimise the risk of infection. Local guidelines should be approved in discussion with microbiology.
6 If the epidural catheter has to be removed, alternative analgesia should be prescribed.	6 To provide effective analgesia via an alternative route.

Procedure guideline 24.14 Discontinuing the epidural

Statement	Rationale
1 An epidural catheter is usually left in situ for a maximum of 5 days. Local guidelines will vary. Policies should be agreed in liaison with microbiology.	1 The risk of infection increases the longer the catheter remains in situ. If an epidural catheter is required for a longer period for chronic/ palliative pain management it can be tunneled under the skin to reduce the risk of infection.
2 If rectal or oral analgesia is not appropriate or sufficient after this period, alternative analgesia (e.g. intravenous patient or nurse controlled analgesimust be provided.	2 To provide effective analgesia with minimal complications. Intravenous opiates may be required.

Procedure guideline 24.14 Discontinuing the epidural *(continued)*

Statement	Rationale
3 If the epidural catheter is pulled out inadvertently: a) Reassure the CYP. b) Put a spot plaster over the entry site. c) Check that the catheter is intact.	3 a) To reduce anxiety. b) To minimise the risk of infection. c) To ensure that none remains in the epidural space.
4 Prior to the removal of the epidural catheter: a) Prepare the CYP. b) Check that they do not have a clotting abnormality. c) If the CYP has abnormal clotting or is on anticoagulation therapy, discuss with a consultant / the pain team before removal.	4 a) To reduce anxiety and minimise the risk of complications. b–c) To minimise the risk of bleeding into the epidural space. A platelet infusion may be needed before the catheter is removed.
5 Only suitably trained and competent individuals, working with written local guidelines should remove an epidural catheter.	5 To minimise the risk of complications.
6 To remove the epidural catheter: a) Gather equipment: • Plastic apron and nonsterile gloves. • Spot plaster. • Plaster remover. • Microbiology swab. b) Put on a plastic apron and wash hands. c) Position the CYP comfortably, either on their side or sitting upright. d) Remove the dressing using plaster remover. e) Gently pull the catheter out. f) Check that the catheter tip is present. g) Swab the entry site if red or swollen. h) Place a small plaster over the site. i) Dispose of used equipment according to local hospital policy. j) The plaster should remain in situ for at least 24 hours, after which time the site should have healed.	6 a) To ensure procedure is carried out with minimal disruption and delay. b) To minimise the risk of infection. c) For ease of removal. d) To cause minimal distress to the CYP. e–f) To ensure that the catheter is removed intact. g) To ensure early detection and treatment of infection. h–j) To minimise the risk of infection.
7 Any pain, swelling, or redness that develops at the entry site after the catheter has been removed should be reported to the pain team or anaesthetist.	7 To ensure prompt detection and treatment of infection.
8 If the entry site has been swabbed: a) Microbiology results should be checked. b) The CYP's progress reviewed.	8 a) To ensure that the appropriate antibiotics are/have been prescribed. b) To detect and treat complications.

Patient and nurse controlled analgesia (PCA/NCA)

The use of patient-controlled (PCA) and nurse-controlled analgesia (NCA) has been shown to provide a safe and effective technique for the administration of intravenous or subcutaneous opioids for the relief of pain (Bray 1983; Doyle et al. 1993; Anderson et al. 1998; Howard et al. 2010). Patient-controlled analgesia refers to a method of pain control that allows the CYP to press a button to self-administer a preprogrammed amount of an intravenous or subcutaneous opioid (the bolus dose) after a set period of time (the lockout interval). The CYP may also receive a small background infusion of the opioid as the pump is programmed with a short lockout interval (5–10 minutes).

Nurse controlled analgesia refers to a technique by which the nurse may press a button to give the CYP a preprogrammed amount of an intravenous or subcutaneous opioid (the bolus dose) after a set period of time (the lockout period). The pump is programmed with a longer lockout interval (20–30 minutes), to allow time for the nurse to fully assess the effect of the opiod and its metabolites, and the CYP may receive a larger background infusion of the opioid. Neonates, CYPs with renal impairment, and those with sensitivity to morphine may require smaller boluses and no background infusion. Neonates in particular should be closely monitored, as they are at increased risk of sedation and respiratory depression (Howard et al. 2010).

PCA and NCA are most commonly used following surgery, but can also be effective for the management of nonsurgical pain such as sickle crisis, pancreatitis, and cancer-related pain and can also be used to manage pain prior to surgery. Staff should be aware that once pain is effectively managed its value as a diagnostic tool is weakened and other indicators of possible deterioration in the CYP's condition must be observed more closely. Morphine is considered to be the 'gold standard' for intravenous analgesia and is therefore usually the opioid of choice (Lloyd-Thomas 1999). The use of other opioids should be considered when morphine is contra-indicated.

A CYP's ability to use patient controlled analgesia depends on their cognitive and motor ability, and individual selection is essential, but the technique can be used by some CYPs as young a four to five years of age (Llewellyn 1993). The use of PCA and NCA requires a specially designed pump that allows for programming of a continuous infusion rate (if required), bolus dose and lockout interval. Pumps should be standardised and training in their use should be provided (DH 2004b). All personnel who care for CYPs receiving PCA or NCA must be trained and competent to do so. Additional training should be provided for staff who programme the pumps.

Prevention and management of opioid-related complications

The likelihood of opioid-related side effects and complications is affected by a number of factors, including the age, genetic makeup, the clinical condition of the CYP, the type of opioid administered, the dose and route of administration and the reason for its use. Prevention and early detection and treatment of unwanted side effects are paramount to ensuring the CYP's safety. Obtaining a history prior to use will minimise risk related to opioid sensitivity. The use of written guidelines, staff education and competencies for pump programming, plus frequent equipment checks will minimise the risk of an overdose related to pump failures and programming errors. It has been recommended that nurse:CYP ratios for CYPs with opioid infusions should be a minimum of a 1:4 ratio on a general ward, with a 1:2 or 1:1 ratio following major surgery (RCPCH 1997). This section relates to the prevention and management of complications related to intravenous and epidural opioids.

Procedure guideline 24.15 Preparation for PCA/NCA use

Statement	Rationale
1 Prior to surgery/setting up the infusion, the anaesthetist must consider the following: • The suitability of PCA/NCA for each individual CYP. • The effectiveness of PCA/NCA for the type of surgery/pain.	1 To ensure that potential risks are balanced against the benefits.
2 If the CYP is going to use PCA they must be: • Able to press the button on the handset. • Able to understand the technique. • Willing to use it.	2 To ensure that the technique will provide effective pain relief; if not the pump settings must be converted to NCA settings.
3 The anaesthetist will discuss the use of PCA/NCA with the CYP and family prior to surgery/setting up the infusion.	3 To provide information.
4 Written and verbal information should be given to prepare the CYP and family for the PCA/NCA: a) The nursing staff and/or play specialist should explain the technique to the CYP and family. b) The family should be made aware that if the CYP is unable to use PCA the pump can be changed to NCA programming. NCA may also be changed to PCA at a later date if the CYP is able and willing to press the button themselves. c) The CYP should be shown the pump and handset before going to theatre.	4 a) To meet information needs and reduce anxiety. A range of information leaflets are available on the hospital website (GOSH 2011). b) To provide the most suitable method of pain relief tailored to the individual CYP's needs.
5 Nursing staff should also ensure that: • Any tools that will be used to assess pain are explained to the CYP/family on admission • Words the CYP uses for pain and the CYP's usual pain related behaviour are recorded on their care plan.	5 To provide knowledge and obtain information, which will facilitate accurate assessment of pain (see 'Pain Assessment' section for further details).
6 The following baseline observations should be recorded before the CYP goes to theatre: • Heart rate • Respiratory rate • Blood pressure	6 To establish normal parameters with which to compare future observations.
7 Oxygen saturations should also be recorded for any CYPs: • Younger than 6 months. • With a respiratory or cardiac condition. • With a sensitivity to morphine. With an increased risk of, or signs of sedation/respiratory compromise.	7 To establish normal parameters with which to compare future observations. These CYPs will require oxygen saturation monitoring during opioid administration.

Procedure guideline 24.16 Setting up a PCA/NCA infusion

Statement	Rationale
1 The following principles are specific to setting up a PCA/NCA infusion. Detailed instructions for setting up infusions are included in Chapter 14.	1 For more information see Chapter 14: IV & IA Access and Infusions.
a) The PCA/NCA pump must only be programmed by a suitably trained person working within written hospital guidelines. Standardised hospital pump programming and drug concentrations should be used at all times.	a–b) To prevent drug errors and to provide effective analgesia with minimal risk of complications.
b) Local procedures for drawing up and administering a controlled drug will apply.	
c) If the intravenous route is not available the subcutaneous route may be used. However, this should be avoided if the CYP has poor peripheral circulation, infected or broken skin, or clotting problems.	c) To avoid the risk of intermittent or unreliable absorption, infection, or further damage to the skin.
2 Gather and prepare the following equipment:	2
a) 50 ml Luer lock syringe	
b) glucose solution OR 0.9% saline (saline must be used if the drug is being administered via the subcutaneous route)	
c) Morphine or other opioid, as prescribed	
d) An administration set with an anti-siphon valve for dedicated lines OR	d) To prevent free flow of fluid through gravity (Southern and Read 1994).
e) An anti-siphon and anti-reflux administration set, if running fluids via the same line.	e) To prevent the opioid backtracking and accumulating in other lines.
3 To make up the infusion:	3
a) Draw up the glucose or saline in the 50 ml syringe, add the opioid and mix well.	a) To ensure an even spread of the drug throughout the syringe.
b) Attach the anti-siphon or anti-siphon and anti-reflux administration set and prime the line.	b) To prevent siphonage and reflux.
c) Ensure that both the syringe and line are labelled.	c) To provide accurate information and prevent drug errors.
d) Place 50 ml syringe in pump and purge the solution through the line.	d) To prevent administration errors due to mechanical slack.
e) Flush the cannula or line and attach the infusion.	e) To ensure that the cannula and line are patent and prevent mixing of drugs.
f) Ensure that the pump programming is checked before starting the infusion.	f) To prevent drug errors.
4 When the infusion is commenced an initial 'loading' dose may be given by an appropriately trained person. This is particularly important for CYPs in severe pain, e.g. sickle cell crisis.	4 To establish initial pain relief (RCPCH 1997; Stevens et al 2021).
5 If the pump is set up on the ward the nurse should ensure that:	5
a) The drug being administered corresponds with the prescription chart.	a–b) To adhere to hospital drug policy and prevent drug errors.
b) The pump programming has been checked.	
c) Naloxone has also been prescribed.	c) To allow for immediate treatment of opioid induced respiratory depression.
d) These checks should be carried out at the handover of each shift to ensure that the correct drug is being infused at the correct rate, via the correct line.	d) To minimise the risk of drug errors.

(continued)

The Great Ormond Street Hospital Manual of Children and Young People's Nursing Practices

Procedure guideline 24.16 Setting up a PCA/NCA infusion *(continued)*

Statement	Rationale
6 If the pump has been set up in theatre/recovery, a verbal report should be obtained from the recovery nurse. This should include details of: • Intraoperative analgesia and other drugs given • Drug concentration and pump programming • Any pain-related complications that have been experienced peri-operatively	6 To provide adequate information.
7 Before leaving theatre the nurse should check: • The drug being administered corresponds with the prescription chart. • The pump programming is correct. • The CYP's pain is being managed effectively. • The CYP is not excessively sedated. • All documentation has been completed.	7 To prevent drug errors and minimise the risk of complications.
8 **Naloxone** should be prescribed **before** the CYP leaves theatre.	8 To facilitate the immediate treatment of opioid-induced respiratory depression.

Procedure guideline 24.17 Technical problems (PCA/NCA)

Statement	Rationale
1 If the pump alarms:	1

a) Stop the infusion.
  b) Check the display panel.
  c) If the line has occluded:
    • Check for kinks or closed clamps.
    • Flush the cannula.
    • Restart the infusion.
  d) If the syringe is empty a new syringe will need to be made up.
  e) If alarm is due to flat battery plug the pump into the mains.
	a–e) To determine and correct the cause of the problem.

f) If the pump is faulty it will need to be replaced and returned to biomedical engineering with a label describing the fault. g) If the cause of the alarm is unknown contact the engineer/pain team.	f, g) To prevent administration errors due to faulty equipment.
2 a) All faulty pumps must be removed from service and reported to the appropriate department (e.g. risk management, biomedical engineering).	2 a) To prevent administration errors due to faulty equipment.
b) If a pump fault has affected the analgesia that the CYP received this must be reported through the Trust's incident reporting system. Always include the pump serial number to enable further investigations to be carried out.	b) To report errors that affect / have the potential to affect treatment and to minimise the risk of future incidents.

Procedure guideline 24.18 Care of the CYP receiving PCA/NCA

Statement	Rationale
1 Record pain scores hourly.	1 To determine effectiveness of analgesia.

2 If the CYP is in pain:
  a) If using PCA, encourage the CYP to give a bolus and evaluate its effect after 10–15 minutes.
  b) If using NCA, administer a bolus and evaluate its effect after 10–15 minutes.
	2 To ensure optimal analgesia is provided.

Chapter 24 Pain management

Procedure guideline 24.18 Care of the CYP receiving PCA/NCA *(continued)*

Statement	Rationale
c) Administer prescribed simple analgesics, e.g. paracetamol and either diclofenac or ibuprofen, if appropriate.	c) Regular administration of simple analgesics has an opioid sparing effect (Schug et al. 2015).
d) Administer prescribed co-analgesics as appropriate, e.g. antispasmodic or anticonvulsant drugs.	d) To treat a specific cause of pain (e.g. spasms).
e) Involve parents/carers, play specialist to provide distraction and reassurance, particularly if the CYP is anxious.	e) To manage the emotional component of pain (i.e. fear).
f) If pain management is not satisfactory contact the pain service, anaesthetist or surgeon as per hospital policy.	f) To ensure that swift action is taken to minimise pain.
3 Hourly pump readings should be recorded. This should include:	3 To monitor hourly morphine consumption and prevent drug over/under administration errors.
a) Number of demands (tries).	a–b) To ensure that boluses are being used appropriately.
b) Number of good demands (good tries).	
c) Amount infused (hourly and running totals).	c–d) To ensure that the syringe pump is infusing correctly.
d) Four hourly syringe readings if using a syringe driver.	
4 Syringes and administration sets must be changed every 24–48 hours according to local policy.	4 To reduce the risk of infection. This should be agreed locally with pharmacy and microbiology.
5 The PCA/NCA may be discontinued when: • The background infusion has been reduced or stopped. • The CYP is requiring minimal bolus doses. • The CYP is able to take analgesia via an alternative route. • Alternative analgesia has been prescribed.	5 To ensure effective analgesia is maintained once the PCA/NCA has been discontinued.

Procedure guideline 24.19 Prevention and management of opioid-related complications

Statement	Rationale
Excessive sedation	
1 The CYP's sedation level must be observed and recorded hourly (see Box 24.4):	1 To ensure early detection and treatment of opioid-induced sedation.
a) While a PCA/NCA is in progress and for four to six hours after it has been discontinued.	a) The risk of excessive sedation continues until the drug has been eliminated (Kart et al. 1997).
b) While an epidural infusion is in progress and for 6–12 hours after it has been discontinued.	b) The clearance time of epidural opioids varies. Morphine has a prolonged duration of action, while fentanyl and diamorphine are cleared more quickly (Rowney and Doyle 1998).
2 Clear instructions should indicate the action(s) to be taken if the CYP is oversedated. If the CYP is difficult to rouse (moderate sedation):	2 To prevent further sedation and an increased risk of respiratory depression.
a) **Stop** the infusion.	a) To prevent further sedation.
b) Increase frequency of observations and introduce pulse oximetry if not already being recorded.	b) To ensure prompt detection of any further deterioration in condition.
c) Contact the pain team, anaesthetist or surgeon if appropriate.	c) The CYP may require a smaller or no background infusion.
d) The infusion may be recommenced once the CYP is rousable to normal stimulation (i.e. touch).	d) To continue to provide analgesia.
e) These actions must be recorded in the CYP's healthcare records.	e) To maintain an accurate record.
f) If the CYP is unrousable (deep sedation), administer naloxone. This may need to be repeated.	f) To reverse the sedative effects of the opioid. Naloxone is an opioid antagonist. Its half-life is shorter than that of most opioids (Reynolds et al. 1996).

(continued)

Procedure guideline 24.19 Prevention and management of opioid-related complications *(continued)*

Statement	Rationale
3 Routine oxygen saturation monitoring can be used. It should always be available for the following groups: • CYPs who continue to be excessively sedated (not rousable to touch). • CYPs with respiratory complications, an obstructed airway or a known sensitivity to opioids. • Infants under one year of age.	3 To ensure early detection and treatment of opioid-induced sedation in at-risk groups of CYPs (RCPCH 1997).

Respiratory depression

Statement	Rationale
1 The CYP's respiratory rate should be recorded hourly: a) While a PCA/NCA is in progress and for four to six hours after it has been discontinued. b) While an epidural infusion is in progress and for 6–12 hours after it has been discontinued. c) Increase frequency of observations if the CYP is excessively sedated or their condition deteriorates.	1 To ensure early detection and treatment of opioid induced sedation. a) The risk of respiratory depression continues until the drug has been eliminated (Kart et al. 1997). b) The clearance time of epidural opioids varies. Morphine has a prolonged duration of action, while fentanyl and diamorphine are cleared more quickly (Rowney and Doyle 1998).
2 The CYP's minimum satisfactory respiratory rate should be documented on the prescription chart or in the CYP's notes or care plan. a) This is for guidance only; it does not take into account: • Depth of respirations • Respiratory pattern and effort • Level of sedation • Oxygen saturation level	2 To indicate when it might be appropriate to administer naloxone. a) Deterioration in these may also indicate a potential respiratory depression/arrest.
3 If respiratory depression occurs: a) **STOP** the infusion. b) Administer intravenous naloxone as prescribed. This may need to be repeated. c) Observe the CYP closely. d) Contact the anaesthetist, pain team or surgeon. e) Document actions in the CYP's healthcare records. f) The event should be recorded as a critical incident/near miss, according to local hospital policy.	3 a) To eliminate the possible cause. b) Naloxone is an opioid antagonist. It has a shorter half-life than most opioids (Reynolds et al. 1996). c) To ensure prompt detection of further deterioration. d) To provide information and to review the CYP's analgesia. e) To maintain an accurate record. f) To learn from potential adverse events and minimise the risk of these reoccurring.
4 If respiratory arrest occurs: • Administer basic life support. • **STOP** the infusion. • Contact the clinical emergency team. • Follow steps (b–as for respiratory depression.	4 To ensure that respiratory arrest is treated promptly.

NB: Naloxone will only be effective if the respiratory depression/arrest is opiate induced.

Statement	Rationale
5 Once the CYP's condition has stabilised their analgesic regimen must be reviewed. If the respiratory depression/arrest was opiate induced: • A PCA/NCA can be recommenced with no continuous infusion (i.e. bolus only) and smaller boluses if necessary. • An epidural infusion can be recommenced with the opioid removed (i.e. local anaesthetic only).	5 To provide effective analgesia with minimal risk of complications.

Nausea and vomiting

Statement	Rationale
1 The CYP should be observed for nausea and/or vomiting at least four hourly (one to two hourly if they feel nauseous or have vomited). This should be recorded on the CYP's observation chart.	1 To ensure early detection of nausea and vomiting.
2 If the CYP complains of nausea, or has vomited, administer an antiemetic as prescribed and consider: a) Aspirating a nasogastric or gastrostomy tube or stopping oral intake. b) Use of an alternative anti-emetic if nausea/vomiting is not reduced. Dexamethasone may also be effective. c) Reducing the infusion rate, bolus size or speed of bolus delivery of a PCA/NCA.	2 To ensure effective treatment and prevention of nausea and vomiting. a) To empty the stomach. b) Numerous factors are involved in emesis. Each anti-emetic acts on a range of different receptors (Litman et al. 1994; Elhakim et al. 2003; Gan 2003). c,d) To minimise the amount of opioid given. This will only be effective if the nausea and vomiting is opioid induced.

Chapter 24 Pain management

Procedure guideline 24.19 Prevention and Management of opioid-related complications *(continued)*

Statement	Rationale
d) Reducing the continuous infusion rate of, or removing the opioid from an epidural.	
e) Use an appropriate assessment tool to monitor the degree of nausea and effectiveness of interventions.	

Pruritus (itching)

1 The CYP should be observed for itching at least 4 hourly (1–2 hourly if itching becomes a problem).	1 To ensure early detection and treatment of opioid-induced pruritus.
a) Nonverbal CYPs should be observed for an unexplained increase in distress or discomfort.	a) Nonverbal CYPs may display signs of distress/discomfort, which can be mistaken for surgical pain.
2 Pruritus should be treated as follows:	2

For epidurals:

a) Administer naloxone (0.5micrograms/kg) as prescribed.	a) To reverse opiate-induced pruritus without affecting the quality of analgesia provided (RCPCH 1997; BNFC 2022).
b) Four doses can be given at 10-minute intervals. However, if repeated doses of naloxone are required this may reduce the effectiveness of the analgesia.	b) This is equivalent to half the reversal dose and will start to affect analgesia as well as unwanted side effects.
c) The doses may be repeated after an hour if the pruritus returns. If this is effective, the epidural infusion rate should be reduced or the opioid removed from the epidural.	c) Naloxone is short-acting.
d) If naloxone is not effective an anti-histamine should be prescribed. Other causes of the itching should also be considered.	d) Both morphine and persistent itching increase histamine production.

For intravenous opioids:

e) Reduce background rate and/or bolus size.
f) Administer an antihistamine.
g) If the pruritus is severe and the above is not effective, consider switching to an alternative opioid.

Box 24.3 Levels of sedation

- **Minimal sedation**: A drug-induced state during which patients are awake and calm, and respond normally to verbal commands. Although cognitive function and coordination may be impaired, ventilatory and cardiovascular functions are unaffected.
- **Moderate sedation**: Drug-induced depression of consciousness during which patients are sleepy but respond purposefully to verbal commands (known as conscious sedation in dentistry, see further on) or light tactile stimulation (reflex withdrawal from a painful stimulus is not a purposeful response). No interventions are required to maintain a patent airway. Spontaneous ventilation is adequate. Cardiovascular function is usually maintained.
- **Conscious sedation**: Drug-induced depression of consciousness, similar to moderate sedation, except that verbal contact is always maintained with the patient. This term is used commonly in dentistry.
- **Deep sedation**: Drug-induced depression of consciousness during which patients are asleep and cannot be easily roused but do respond purposefully to repeated or painful stimulation. The ability to maintain ventilatory function independently may be impaired. Patients may require assistance to maintain a patent airway. Spontaneous ventilation may be inadequate. Cardiovascular function is usually maintained. (NICE 2010)

Box 24.4 GOSH Pain Control Service sedation score

0 – Awake/alert.
1 – Sleepy/responds appropriately.
2 – Somnulent/rousable (light stimuli).
3 – Deep sleep/rousable (deeper physical stimuli).
4 – Unrousable to stimuli (stop infusion).

Sucrose

Oral sucrose 24% sucrose solution (sucrose and water) (Sweet-Ease™) reduces distress behaviour and physiological response to painful procedures in babies less than three months of age (Morash and Fowler 2004; Lefrack et al. 2006; Stevens et al. 2016) and there is some evidence of its effectiveness in infants up to one year of age (Harrison et al. 2010; Kassab et al. 2012). It is safe and easily administered, but must be prescribed on the drug chart (as required) or administered under a patient group direction. Sucrose should be used in conjunction with other nonpharmacological comfort measures such as nonnutritive sucking, positioning, etc. and appropriate analgesia. It is not a substitute for analgesia or comfort measures. A recent study has suggested that sucrose does not affect nociceptive activity in the brain or spinal cord of a neonate and therefore might not provide effective analgesia (Slater et al. 2010). This article has generated considerable debate and further research, which will no doubt continue (Harrison et al. 2012). As there is currently no evidence to suggest that appropriate use of sucrose is harmful, its use alongside analgesia during painful procedures in neonates is still encouraged at GOSH. However, its use is avoided in neonates at risk of developing necrotising enterocolitis (NEC). For a list of contra-indications see box 24.6.

Procedure guideline 24.20 Sucrose administration

Statement	Rationale
Preparation:	
1 Assess pain prior to the procedure (see Procedure Guideline 24.1).	1 To provide a baseline for assessment of pain during and post procedure. To determine the most appropriate interventions to prevent/manage pain during the procedure.
2 Determine whether sucrose may be appropriate during the planned procedure (see Box 24.5) and identify any potential contra-indications for its use (see Box 24.6).	2 To minimise pain and ensure that sucrose is administered safely and effectively.
3 Determine whether analgesia should also be administered prior to the procedure. Analgesia should be given if: • The baby is already in pain. • The procedure is expected to be painful.	3 To provide effective analgesia. Sucrose is not a substitute for analgesia and comfort measures.
4 If analgesia is required, administer well before the procedure (e.g. 15–20 minutes for intravenous, 40–60 minutes for oral analgesia.	4 To allow for effective absorption prior to starting the procedure.
5 Ensure that staff and equipment are prepared and that the sucrose has been prescribed and is ready to use. If a parent or carer is present, ensure that they understand the procedure and that their role has been agreed.	5 To avoid delays.
Sucrose administration:	
1 To administer the drug: a) Swaddle or contain the baby as appropriate for their condition and the procedure. If appropriate, other comfort measures such as swaddling, rocking and nonnutritive sucking may also be used. b) Administer 1 drop or 0.1 ml of sucrose solution onto the anterior aspect of the tongue or inside the cheek, or the CYP's dummy. This may be done at the following intervals: • One to two minutes prior to procedure • When starting the procedure • At two-minute intervals during the procedure if required	1 a) To provide comfort b) To provide effective relief. The peak action of sucrose is 2 minutes and duration of action is 5–10 minutes.
2 The maximum dose that can be given during a procedure is dependent on gestational age: • 27–31 weeks: 0.5 ml • 32–36 weeks: 1 ml • 37+ weeks: 2 ml NB: no daily maximum has been identified.	
3 Offer a dummy if this is part of the baby's normal care.	3 This promotes nonnutritive sucking, which will enhance the effect of the sucrose.
4 During the procedure: a) Observe for gagging, choking, coughing and vomiting – if the solution is not tolerated, stop using it and reassess the CYP before continuing with the procedure. b) Assess for pain: If pain is poorly managed, halt the procedure, and consider the need for analgesia.	4 a) To minimise the risk of complications such as aspiration. b) To ensure that adequate analgesia is provided.
5 After the procedure: a) Reassess the CYP. b) Discard any remaining solution. c) All doses administered must be recorded on the CYP's prescription chart.	a) To determine efficacy of interventions and ensure that they are comfortable and safe. b) The containers are for single use only.

Box 24.5 Procedures for which sucrose may be effective

- Heel puncture, venipuncture, and cannulation
- Urinary catheterisation
- Eye examination
- Naso-gastric tube insertion
- Intramuscular and subcutaneous injections
- Lumbar puncture
- Colostomy bag change
- Removal of tape and dressing changes
- Scalp electrode placement
- Suturing
- Physiotherapy.

Box 24.6 Contra-indications

- Fructose or sucrose intolerance
- Unavailability of oral route (not effective via any other route)
- Paralysed and sedated patients

Caution with:

- Suspected or confirmed NEC
- Intubated patients

NB: Less evidence of efficacy in babies over three months in age.

References

Aldridge, L.M. and Tunstall, M.E. (1986). Nitrous oxide and the fetus: a review and the results of a retrospective study of 175 cases of anaesthesia for insertion of Shirokar suture. *British Journal of Anaesthesia* 58: 1348–1356.

Amos, R.J., Amess, J.A.L., Nancekievill, D.G., and Rees, G.M. (1983). Prevention of nitrous oxide induced megaloblastic changes in bone marrow using folinic acid. *British Journal of Anaesthesia* 56: 103–107.

Anderson, B.J., McKenzie, R., Persson, M.A., and Garden, A.L. (1998). Safety of postoperative paediatric analgesia. *Acute Pain* 1 (3): 14–20.

Association of Anaesthetists of Great Britain and Ireland (AAGBI) (2010) Guidelines for the Management of Severe Local Anaesthetic Toxicity. http://www.aagbi.org/sites/default/files/la_toxicity_2010_0.pdf (accessed 17 March 2022).

Association of Paediatric Anaesthetists of Great Britain and Ireland (APAGBI) (2012). Good practice in postoperative and procedural pain management. 2nd edition. *Pediatric Anesthesia* 22 (1): 1–79. https://onlinelibrary.wiley.com/doi/10.1111/j.1460-9592.2012.03838.x (accessed 25 November 2022)..

Beyer, J.E., McGrath, P.J., and Berde, C.B. (1990). Discordance between self-report and behavioral measures in 3–7 year old children following surgery. *Journal of Pain and Symptom Management* 5: 350–356.

Birnie, K.A., Noel, M., Chambers, C.T., Uman, L.S., Parker, J.A. (2018). Psychological interventions for needle-related procedural pain and distress in children and adolescents. https://www.cochranelibrary.com/cdsr/doi/10.1002/14651858.CD005179.pub4/full (accessed 21 December 2022).

Bray, R.J. (1983). Postoperative analgesia provided by morphine infusion in children. *Anaesthesia* 38: 1075–1078.

Breau, L.M., Camfield, C., McGrath, P.J. et al. (2001). Measuring pain accurately in children with cognitive impairments: refinement of a caregiver scale. *Journal of Pediatrics* 138 (5): 721–727.

British National Formulary for Children (BNfC) (2022). https://bnfc.nice.org.uk (accessed 17 March 2022).

British Oxygen Company (BOC) (2011). Medical Gases Datasheet: Entonox. https://www.bochealthcare.co.uk/en/quality-and-safety/safety-and-technical-data/safety-data-sheets/safety-data-sheets.html (accessed 17 March 2022).

British Oxygen Company (BOC) (2013). Entonox: the essential guide. https://www.boconline.co.uk/wcsstore/UK_BOC_Industrial_Ntl_Store/pdf/downloads/Entonox-essential-guide.pdf (accessed 17 March 2022).

British Oxygen Company (BOC) (2014). Medical nitrous oxide. Essential safety information. https://www.bochealthcare.co.uk/en/products-and-services/products-and-services-by-category/medical-gases/medical-nitrous/medical-nitrous-oxide.html (accessed 17 March 2022).

British Oxygen Company (BOC) (2021). https://www.bochealthcare.co.uk/en/products-and-services/products-and-services-by-category/services/education-and-training/education-and-training.html (accessed 17 March 2022).

Bromage, P.R. (1978). *Epidural Analgesia*. Philadelphia: WB Saunders.

Bruce, E. and Franck, L. (2000). Self-administered nitrous oxide (Entonox) for the management of procedural pain. *Paediatric Nursing* 12 (7): 15–19.

Bruce E, Franck L. (2004). Children's pain assessment: Implementing best nursing practices. In Shaw, T., Sanders, K. (eds), Foundation of Nursing Studies Dissemination Series, 2(8) London, FoNS. http://www.fons.org/resources/documents/DissSeriesVol2No8.pdf (accessed 17 March 2022).

Bruce, E. and Franck, L. (2005). Using the worldwide web to improve children's pain care. *International Nursing Review* 52: 204–209.

Bruce, E., Franck, L.S., and Howard, R.F. (2006a). The efficacy of morphine and Entonox analgesia during chest drain removal in children. *Pediatric Anesthesia* 16: 203–208.

Bruce, E.A., Howard, R.F., and Franck, L.S. (2006b). Chest drain removal pain and its management: a literature review. *Journal of Clinical Nursing* 15: 145–154.

Clinical Standards Advisory Group (2000, 2002). *Services for Children with Pain*. National Minimum Standards for Independent Health Care (ed. Department of Health (DH)). London: The Stationery Office, HMSO.

Chambers, C.T., Reid, G.J., McGrath, P.J., and Finley, G.A. (1996). Development and preliminary validation of a postoperative pain measure for parents. *Pain* 68: 307–313.

Department of Health (DH) (2004a). *Ill Child Standard, National Service Framework for Children, Young People and Maternity Services*. London: Department of Health.

Department of Health (DH) (2004b). *National Service Framework for Children, Young People and Maternity Services: Core Standards*. London: HMSO.

Department of Health (DH) (2010). *Essence of Care: Benchmarks for the Prevention and Management of Pain*. London: The Stationery Office.

Doyle, E., Harper, I., and Morton, N.S. (1993). Patient controlled analgesia with low dose background infusions after lower abdominal surgery in children. *British Journal of Anaesthesia* (6): 121–127.

Elhakim, M., Ali, N.M., Rashed, I. et al. (2003). Dexamethasone reduces postoperative vomiting and pain after pediatric tonsillectomy [La dexaméthasone réduit les vomissements et la douleur postopératoires après une amygdalectomie pédiatrique]. *Canadian Journal of Anesthesia* 50: 392–397.

Franck, L.S. and Bruce, E. (2009). Putting pain assessment into practice: why is it so painful? *Pain Research & Management* 14 (1): 13–20.

Friedrichsdorf, S.J., Nugent, A.P., and Strobl, A.Q. (2013). Codeine-associated pediatric deaths despite using recommended dosing guidelines: three case reports. *Journal of Opioid Management* 9 (2): 151–155.

Gall, O., Annequin, D., Benoit, G. et al. (2001). Adverse events of premixed nitrous oxide and oxygen for procedural sedation in children. *Lancet* 358: 1514–1515.

Gan, T.J. (2003). Evidence-based management of postoperative nausea and vomiting. *Canadian Journal of Anesthesia* 50: R5.

GOSH (2011). Clinical information. Information leaflets. Surgical pain. Pain relief after surgery using patient-controlled analgesia (PCA) or nurse-controlled analgesia (NCA). https://www.gosh.nhs.uk/wards-and-departments/departments/clinical-specialties/pain-control-service-information-parents-and-visitors/download-documentation/ (accessed 17 March 2022).

Gunter, J.B. (2002). Benefit and risks of local anesthetics in infants and children. *Paediatric Drugs* 4: 649–672.

Harrison, D., Stevens, B., Bueno, M. et al. (2010). Efficacy of sweet solutions for analgesia in infants between 1 and 12 months of age: a systematic review. *Archives of Disease in Childhood* 95 (6): 406–413.

Harrison, D., Beggs, S., and Stevens, B. (2012). Sucrose for procedural pain management in infants. *Pediatrics* 130 (5): 918–925.

Hicks, C., von Baeyer, C., Spafford, P. et al. (2001). The faces pain scale – revised: towards a common metric in pediatric pain measurement. *Pain* 93: 173–183.

Hodgins, M.J. and Lander, J. (1997). Children's coping with venepuncture. *Journal of Pain and Symptom Management* 13 (5): 274–285.

Howard, R.F. (2003). Current status of pain management in children. *Journal of the American Medical Association* 290 (18): 2464–2469.

Howard, R.F., Lloyd-Thomas, A., Thomas, M. et al. (2010). Nurse-controlled analgesia (NCA) following major surgery in 10 000 patients in a children's hospital. *Pediatric Anesthesia* 20 (2): 126–134.

Hunt, A., Mastroyannopoulou, K., Goldman, A., and Seers, K. (2003). Not knowing – the problem of pain in children with severe neurological impairment. *International Journal of Nursing Studies* 40 (2): 171–183.

International Association for the Study of Pain (IASP) 2010). Access to Pain Management: Declaration of Montreal. https://www.iasp-pain.org/advocacy/iasp-statements/access-to-pain-management-declaration-of-montreal/ (accessed 17 March 2022).

Jerrett, M. and Evans, K. (1986). Children's pain vocabulary. *Journal of Advanced Nursing* 11: 403–440.

Kart, T., Christupp, L.L., and Rasmussen, M. (1997). Recommended use of morphine in neonates, infants & children based on a literature review, part 2: clinical use. *Paediatric Anaesthesia* 7: 93–101.

Kassab M, Foster JP, Foureur M, Fowler C. Sweet-tasting solutions for needle-related procedural pain in infants one month to one year of age. *Cochrane Database of Systematic Reviews* 2012, Issue 12 (12 December). https://www.cochranelibrary.com/cdsr/doi/10.1002/14651858.CD008411.pub2/full (accessed 17 March 2022).

Kost-Byerly, S., Tobin, J.R., Greenberg, R.S. et al. (1998). Bacterial colonization & infection rate of continuous epidural catheters in children. *Anesthesia and Analgesia* 86 (4): 712–716.

Langevin, P.B. (1996). Epidural catheter reconnection – safe and unsafe practice. *Anesthesiology* 85 (4): 883–888.

Lefrack, L., Burch, K., Caravantes, R. et al. (2006). Sucrose analgesia: identifying potentially better practices. *Pediatrics* 118: 197–202.

Litman, R.S., Wu, C.L., and Catanzaro, F.A. (1994). Ondansetron decreases emesis after tonsillectomy in children. *Anesthesia and Analgesia* 78: 478–481.

Llewellyn, N. (1993). The use of PCA for post-operative pain management. *Paediatric Nursing* 5 (5): 12–15.

Llewellyn, N. and Moriarty, A. (2007). The national pediatric epidural audit. *Pediatric Anesthesia* 17 (6): 520–533.

Lloyd-Thomas, A.R. (1999). Modern concepts of paediatric analgesia. *Pharmacology and Therapeutics* 83 (1): 1–20.

Malviya, S. and Voepel-Lewis, T. (2006). The revised FLACC observational pain tool: improved reliability and validity for pain assessment in children with cognitive impairment. *Paediatric Anaesthesia* 16 (3): 258–265.

Mason, K. and Koka, B. (1999). Nitrous oxide. In: *Pediatric Procedural Sedation and Analgesia* (eds. B. Krauss and R.M. Brustowicz), 83–88. Baltimore: Lippincott, Williams & Wilkins.

McNeely, J. and Trentadue, N. (1997). Comparison of PCA with and without night-time morphine infusion following lower extremity surgery in children. *Journal of Pain and Symptom Management* 13 (5): 2268–2273.

Medicines and Healthcare Products Regulatory Agency (MHRA) (2013). Codeine for analgesia: restricted use in children because of reports of morphine toxicity. Drug Safety Update Volume 6, Issue 11. https://www.gov.uk/drug-safety-update/codeine-for-analgesia-restricted-use-in-children-because-of-reports-of-morphine-toxicity (accessed 17 March 2022).

Morash, D. and Fowler, K. (2004). An evidence-based approach to changing practice: using sucrose for infant analgesia. *Journal of Pediatric Nursing* 19 (5): 366–370.

National Institute for Health and Care Excellence (NICE) (2010). Sedation in under 19s: Sedation for diagnostic and therapeutic procedure. NICE Clinical Guideline 112. National Clinical Guideline Centre. UK. www.nice.org.uk/guidance/cg112 (accessed 17 March 2022).

National Patient Safety Agency (NPSA) (2018). Recommendations from National Patient Safety Agency alerts that remain relevant to the Never Events list 2018. https://www.england.nhs.uk/wp-content/uploads/2020/11/Recommendations-from-NPSA-alerts-that-remain-relevant-to-NEs-FINAL.pdf (accessed 17 March 2022).

National Patient Safety Agency (NPSA) (2011). Patient Safety Alerts NPSA/2011/PSA001 and NPSA/2009/PSA004B Safer spinal (intrathecal), epidural and regional devices – Part A and Part B. https://www.ukmi.nhs.uk/filestore/ukmiaps/NPSA-2011-PSA01(3).pdf (accessed 17 March 2022).

Neal, M.J. (2002). *Medical Pharmacology at a Glance*, 4e, 16–17. London: Blackwell Publishing.

Nunn, J.F. (1987). Clinical aspects of the interaction between nitrous oxide and vitamin B12. *British Journal of Anaesthesia* 59: 3–13.

Nursing and Midwifery Council (NMC) (2009). *Record Keeping: Guidelines for Nurses and Midwives*. London: Nursing and Midwifery Council.

Park, G.R., Fulton, I.C., and Shelly, M.P. (1986). Normal pregnancy following nitrous oxide exposure in the first trimester. *British Journal of Anaesthesia* 58 (5): 576–577.

Reynolds, J., Parfitt, K., Parsons, A., and Sweetman, S. (eds.) (1996). *The Extra Pharmacopoeia*, 31e. London: Royal Pharmaceutical Society of Great Britain.

Rowland, A.S., Baird, D.D., Weinberg, C.R. et al. (1992). Reduced fertility among women employed as dental assistants exposed to high levels of nitrous oxide. *New England Journal of Medicine* 327: 993–997.

Rowney, D.A. and Doyle, E. (1998). Review article: epidural and subarachnoid blockade in children. *Anaesthesia* 53: 980–1001.

Royal Children's Hospital (2000). Anaesthesia and Pain Management. Assessment of sensory block. Children's Pain Management Service. www.rch.org.au/anaes/pain_management/Assessment_of_sensory_block (accessed 17 March 2022).

Royal College of Anaesthetists (RCoA) (2020). Best practice in the management of epidural analgesia in the hospital setting. https://fpm.ac.uk/sites/fpm/files/documents/2020-09/Epidural-AUG-2020-FINAL.pdf (accessed 17 March 2022).

Royal College of Nursing (RCN) (2009). *The Recognition and Assessment of Acute Pain in Children: Update of Full Guideline*. London: RCN.

Royal College of Nursing Institute (1999). *The Recognition and Assessment of Acute Pain in Children: Recommendations*. London: RCNI.

Royal College of Paediatrics and Child Health (2001). *Guidelines for Good Practice: Recognition and Assessment of Acute Pain in Children*. London: RCPCH.

Royal College of Paediatrics and Child Health (RCPCH) (1997). *Prevention and Control of Pain in Children: A Manual for Health Care Professionals*. London: BMJ Publishing.

Saul, R., Peters, J., and Bruce, E. (2016). Assessing acute and chronic pain in children and young people. *Nursing Standard* 31 (10): 51–61.

Schechter, N.L., Berde, C., and Yaster, M. (2003). *Pain in Infants, Children and Adolescents*, 2e. New York: Lippincott Williams & Wilkins.

Schug, S.A., Palmer, G.M., Scott, D.A., Halliwell, R., Trinca, J. (2015). Australian and New Zealand College of Anaesthetists and Faculty of Pain Medicine Acute Pain Management: Scientific Evidence, 4th edition. ANZCA and FPM. https://www.anzca.edu.au/getattachment/4c3b03b7-52bf-4c10-9115-83d827c0fc38/Acute-Pain-Management-Scientific-Evidence.aspx (accessed 17 March 2022).

Seth, N., Llewellyn, N.E., and Howard, R.F. (2000). Parental opinions regarding the route of administration of analgesic medication in children. *Pediatric Anesthesia* 10 (5): 537–544.

Seth, N., Macqueen, S., and Howard, R.F. (2004). Continuous postoperative epidural analgesia in children: the value of catheter tip culture. *Paediatric Anaesthesia* 14 (12): 996–1000.

Slater, R., Cornelissen, L., Fabrizi, L. et al. (2010). Oral sucrose as an analgesic drug for procedural pain in newborn infants: a randomised controlled trial. *Lancet* 376 (9748): 1225–1232.

Sng, Q.W., He, H.G., Wng, W. et al. (2017). A meta-synthesis of Children's experiences of postoperative pain management. *Worldviews on Evidence-Based Nursing* 14 (1): 46–54.

Southern, D.A. and Read, M.S. (1994). Overdosage of opiate from patient controlled analgesia devices. *British Medical Journal* 309: 1002.

Spence, K., Gillies, D., Harrison, D. et al. (2005). A reliable pain assessment tool for clinical assessment in the neonatal intensive care unit. *Journal of Obstetric, Gynecologic & Neonatal Nursing* 34 (1): 80–86.

Stevens, B., Yamada, J., Ohlsson, A. et al. (2016). Sucrose for analgesia in newborn infants undergoing painful procedures. *Cochrane Database of Systematic Reviews* (7): CD001069. https://www.cochranelibrary.com/cdsr/doi/10.1002/14651858.CD001069.pub5/full (accessed 22 March 2022).

Stevens, B.J., Hathway, G., and Zempsky W.T., 2021) (eds) (2nd edition) Oxford Textbook of Pediatric Pain.

Stinson, J.N., Stevens, B.J., Feldman, B.M. et al. (2011). Using an electronic pain diary to better understand pain in children and adolescents with arthritis. *Pain Manag.* 1 (2): 127–137.

Twycross, A., Dowden, S.J., and Stinson, J. (eds.) (2014). *Managing Pain in Children: A Clinical Guide for Nurses and Healthcare Professionals*. Oxford: Wiley.

Van Dijk, M., de Boer, J.B., Koot, H.M. et al. (2000). The reliability and validity of the COMFORT scale as a postoperative pain instrument in 0 to 3-year-old infants. *Pain* 84 (2–3): 367–377.

Voepel-Lewis, T., Malviya, S., Tait, A.R. et al. (2008). A comparison of the clinical utility of pain assessment tools for children with cognitive impairment. *Anesthesia and Analgesia* 106 (1): 72–78.

Voepel-Lewis, T., Zanotti, J., Dammeyer, J.A., and Merkel, S. (2010). Reliability and validity of the face, legs, activity, cry, consolability behavioral tool in assessing acute pain in critically ill patients. *American Journal of Critical Care* 19 (1): 55–61. quiz 62.

Weisman, S.J., Bernstein, B.B., and Schechter, N.L. (1998). Consequences of inadequate analgesia during painful procedures in children. *Archives of Pediatrics & Adolescent Medicine* 152: 147–149.

Williams, D., Patel, A., and Howard, R. (2002). Pharmacogenetics of codeine metabolism in an urban population of children and its implications for analgesic reliability. *British Journal of Anaesthesia* 89: 839–845.

World Health Organization (2012). *WHO Guidelines on the Pharmacological Treatment of Persisting Pain in Children with Medical Illnesses*. Geneva: WHO.

World Health Organization (WHO) (1986). *Cancer Pain Relieef*. Geneva: WHO.

Zacny, J.P., Conran, A., Pardo, H. et al. (1999). Effects of naloxone on nitrous oxide actions in healthy volunteers. *Pain* 83: 411–418.

Further reading

Bach, D.M. (1995). Implementation of the Agency for Health Care Policy and Research postoperative pain management guideline. *Nursing Clinics of North America* 30 (3): 515–527.

Commission on the Provision of Surgical Services (1990). Report of the Working Party on Pain after Surgery. London, Royal College of Surgeons of England and the College of Anaesthetists.

College of Emergency Medicine (2013). *Management of Pain in Children*. London: The College of Emergency Medicine.

Franck, L.S., Greenberg, C.S., and Stevens, B. (2000). Pain assessment in infants and children. *Paediatric Clinics of North America* 47 (3): 487–512.

Gaffney A, McGrath PJ, Dick B. (2003) Measuring pain in children: developmental and instrument issues. In Schechter NL, Berde CB, Yaster M. *Pain in Infants, Children and Adolescents*, 2. Philadelphia, Lippincott, Williams & Wilkins, pp. 128–141

GOSH (2007). Protocol for the use of sucrose solution for procedural pain Management. Great Ormond Street Hospital Clinical Practice Guideline. https://www.gosh.nhs.uk/file/233/download (accessed 17 March 2022).

RCoA (2021) Chapter 11: Guidelines for the Provision of Anaesthesia Services for Inpatient Pain Management 2021. https://www.rcoa.ac.uk/gpas/chapter-11 (accessed 01/02/2022).

Royal College of Surgeons of England (RCSENG) (2007). *Surgery for Children: Delivering a First Class Service. Report of the Children's Surgical Forum*. London: RCSENG.

Simons et al (2020) Developing a framework to support the delivery of effective pain management for children: An exploratory qualitative study. https://pubmed.ncbi.nlm.nih.gov/33193925/ (accessed 21 December 2022).

World Health Organization (1997). *Looking Forward to Cancer Pain Relief for All. International Consensus on the Management of Cancer Pain*. Geneva: WHO.

Chapter 25

Palliative care

June Hemsley

RN (Child), BSc, MSc (Child); NMP, Advanced Nurse Practitioner, Louis Dundas Centre for Oncology Outreach and Palliative Care, Great Ormond Street Hospital, London, UK

Chapter contents

Introduction	578	Haemorrhage	582
Assessment of symptoms	579	Agitation	582
Pain in palliative care: PCA and proxy PCA	580	Seizures	582
Nausea and vomiting	580	Signs of impending death	583
Constipation and diarrhoea	581	Conclusion	584
Dyspnoea	581	References	591
Hydration and nutrition	582	Further reading	593

Procedure guidelines

25.1 Assessment of symptoms	584	25.6 Management of hydration and nutrition	588
25.2 Care of patient receiving PCA/PPCA for palliative care	585	25.7 Management of haemorrhage	589
25.3 Assessment and management of nausea and vomiting	586	25.8 Management of agitation	590
25.4 Assessment and management of constipation and diarrhoea	586	25.9 Management of seizures	591
25.5 Management of dyspnoea	587	25.10 Recognising signs of impending death	591

The Great Ormond Street Hospital Manual of Children and Young People's Nursing Practices, Second Edition. Edited by Elizabeth Anne Bruce, Janet Williss, and Faith Gibson.
© 2023 John Wiley & Sons Ltd. Published 2023 by John Wiley & Sons Ltd.

Introduction

Paediatric palliative care is widely accepted as 'an active and total approach to care, from the point of diagnosis or recognition, throughout the child's life, death, and beyond. It embraces physical, emotional, social, and spiritual elements and focuses on the enhancement of quality of life for the child or young person (CYP) and support for the family. It includes the management of distressing symptoms, provision of short breaks (formally known as respite), and care through death and bereavement' (Together for Short Lives 2013). This definition is concerned with maintaining quality of life, not just in the stages of dying, but throughout a CYP's life, from the point of diagnosis or recognition of a life-limiting condition (LLC), during the weeks, months, and years before a CYP's death, and beyond, as outlined in 'A Core Care Pathway for Children with Life-Limiting and Life-Threatening Conditions' (Together for Short Lives 2013).

Introducing palliative care to CYPs and families at the point of diagnosis or recognition of an LLC facilitates 'parallel planning', where plans are made both for life and death. Parallel planning is necessary when the prognosis is uncertain. Working alongside curative-directed treatments, parallel planning allows professionals to instigate discussions about palliative care, end-of-life care planning and symptom management (Mellor et al. 2012). Integrating palliative care with curative-directed treatments can reduce professional anxieties of when to refer to palliative care and empower families to make real and effective choices about preferred place of care and levels of medical/care intervention (Harrop and Edwards 2013). Parallel planning may also enable families to maintain hope for their child's future while accessing a wider network of support. Examples of parallel planning in practice include combining palliative care and rehabilitative approaches for CYPs with severe brain injuries (The Children's Trust 2011).

Technological advances in life-sustaining interventions and provision of palliative care can, on the surface, appear to be incongruous. However, considering principles of palliative care alongside life-sustaining treatments can offer better quality of care for CYPs receiving intensive care and offer greater choices and involvement in decision making. Approximately two thirds of CYPs who die in paediatric intensive care units (PICU) do so following withdrawal of life-sustaining treatment (Fraser et al. 2011), remaining in intensive care for end-of-life care. However, palliative care and PICU teams can work collaboratively to enable CYPs and families to return home or to a hospice for end-of-life care (Gupta et al. 2013; Laddie et al. 2014; Larcher et al. 2015; Needle 2010). The CYP can be transferred while remaining on a ventilator with support from PICU and paediatric palliative care professionals. Once the CYP has arrived at the preferred place of care, life-sustaining interventions are withdrawn, while palliation continues. A national care pathway exists that supports extubation within a CYP's palliative care framework, providing guidance around decision making to withdraw life-sustaining ventilation, the practicalities to be considered, and care at and around the time of death (Larcher et al. 2015; Together for Short Lives 2011).

The neonatal population (defined as a baby in the first 28 days of life) is under provided for in terms of palliative care. Over 80 000 babies are admitted to specialist neonatal units in the UK each year. Of these, just over 2100 die from causes likely to require palliative care and 98% of neonatal deaths occur in a hospital setting (Association for Children's Palliative Care [ACT] 2009). The high percentage of neonatal deaths within hospital is largely due to both the lack of neonatal palliative care service provision and the lack of staff awareness of palliative care services (Kelly et al. 2012). Palliative care for the neonate may be initiated when an antenatal appointment confirms that the unborn child has a LLC. For those families that wish to continue with the pregnancy, referral to a palliative care service can enable parents to explore advanced care planning, including preferred place of care of the child after birth and end-of-life care planning. In some cases, it may even help empower parents to articulate their hopes and wishes around the birthing process while involving effective multi-professional collaboration. Alternatively, referral to a palliative care service may occur shortly after birth. In either case, a multi-agency assessment of the family's needs, including consideration of postnatal care for the mother, is essential to formulate a multi-agency care plan (De Rooy et al. 2012; Mancini et al. 2014). The Neonatal Pathway for Babies with Palliative Care Needs (ACT 2009) describes a three-staged process outlining issues that should be considered, from breaking bad news of the baby's life limiting condition and planning for going home, through to assessment and planning of care needs, and finally, to end-of-life care and bereavement support.

Medical advances have enabled increasing numbers of CYPs with LLC requiring palliative care to survive into adulthood, resulting in a growing need to provide effective transitional care (Doug et al. 2011). Transition is a planned process that supports CYPs and their families to move from children's to adults' services. As such it involves fostering the CYP and family's trust in a new team and overcoming unique barriers such as lack of experience in the adult sector of conditions that were previously the sole remit of children's services; other barriers include service-based restrictions, such as a lack of equivalent services, and the desire to avoid transition to new services, which may be based on a previous experience of fragmented care that lacks coordination and collaboration (Mellor et al. 2012). Other more obvious barriers to transition include poor communication, poor planning, and lack of confidence in colleagues (Mellor et al. 2012). With these barriers in mind, it is not surprising that transitioning the CYP with an LLC such as a neuromuscular or metabolic condition can take between one and two years. The transition care pathway (ACT 2007) provides guidance on effective transition, identifying key stages including recognising the need to move on, moving on, and recognising the end of life, and builds on the core principles of involving the young person in decision making.

Palliative care aims to achieve optimal comfort and quality of life for the CYP and is not implemented only when curative treatment options have failed. As outlined above, it can be delivered in parallel with curative-focused treatments, or for some CYPs, palliation may be the only treatment option. Palliative care for CYPs can be provided at home or in a hospice or hospital, depending on the availability of services and community teams. Literature suggests that people rather than place are more important for families when deciding on a preferred place of care and death for their child (Bergstraesser 2013). To enable a family to make an informed choice about their preferred place of care they need to be provided with accurate information regarding available services and levels of support, as well as the expected progression of the disease. Experience of a familiar clinical environment and relationships with clinical staff may be considered a necessity to some families at the end of life and should be offered as an equally valid option as the perceived ideal of care at home (Bergstraesser 2013). Expert and effective palliative care requires a holistic approach by the multidisciplinary team (MDT) for the child and family (Liben et al. 2008; Mcculloch et al. 2008) attending not only to the physical symptoms of the child but also the hopes, anxieties, and expectations within the family. This would include talking with parents/carers, the CYP, and their siblings about what to expect, is dependent on their level of understanding, and should acknowledge and respect the family's cultural and religious beliefs.

Symptoms that may require management by a paediatric palliative care team may be the result of numerous different factors.

They may be specific to the disease process, such as anaemia and dyspnoea in haematological malignancies; part of the general deterioration of the body as death approaches, such as anorexia, cachexia, and fatigue; or they may be the side effects of medication and treatment, such as constipation associated with opioid analgesia (Goldman et al. 2012). To date, much of the paediatric palliative care research has been concerned with symptoms at the end of life and has focussed on the child with cancer. Pain and fatigue are identified as the most frequently reported symptoms (Rodgers et al. 2013). Other commonly reported symptoms include dyspnoea, nausea, vomiting, anorexia, drowsiness, constipation, anxiety, agitation, sadness, and fear (Rodgers et al. 2013). There is growing awareness that symptoms can occur in clusters of two or more occurring together, possibly causing a synergistic effect which leads to an increase in symptom intensity or an antecedent effect that leads to the development of additional symptoms (Rodgers et al. 2013). For instance, pain and fatigue have been associated with sleep disturbances, anxiety, depression, anorexia, and nausea and vomiting (Rodgers et al. 2013). It is therefore imperative that the nurse considers both the cause and effect of a symptom when planning effective management.

Caring for a CYP in hospital, hospice, or at home can pose specific and different problems for the professionals involved. Care of the CYP at home will be affected by local provision of care and the availability of drugs, equipment, children's community services, and parent/carer confidence. Palliative care, as with all aspects of care for CYPs, should be a partnership between family and professionals. Families who have provided care for a CYP with a life-threatening or LLC may have learned technical nursing skills and interventions such as nasopharyngeal suctioning, nasogastric/gastrostomy feeding, and even administration of intravenous (IV) medication. Some families will be happy to continue providing this level of care, and even to learn further skills. However, the high levels of stress and anxiety at this time in the CYP's life may influence parents' capacity and desire to learn new procedures. Furthermore, the family may feel that they want to relinquish and 'pass back' responsibility for the more technical aspects of their child's care. For many CYPs cared for at home, the children' community nurses or local palliative care teams will be able to support families in the practical aspects of care. When a CYP is cared for in hospital, staff may require support when the focus changes from curative to palliation. This particularly comes to light around issues such as monitoring and recording of vital signs. It may be helpful to remember that routine observations and investigations are only useful if they can influence the provision of care and comfort for the CYP.

It is outside the scope of this book to provide detailed guidelines on all aspects of palliative care for CYPs. Instead, the nurse can maintain their knowledge and competence in the following ways:

- Refer to a paediatric palliative care team for patient-specific guidance or advanced symptom management.
- Consider undertaking a relevant paediatric palliative care course to develop their knowledge and skills further or pursue a career in paediatric palliative care.
- Refer to texts such as The Rainbows Children's Hospice Guidelines for advice on basic symptom control (Together for Short Lives 2013).
- Keep up to date with online resources.
- Be aware of national guidance underpinning all aspects of care, such as that from National Institute for Health and Care Excellence (NICE 2016), and documents such as Ambitions for Palliative Care and End of Life Care, available online at: http://endoflifecareambitions.org.uk/wp-content/uploads/2015/09/Ambitions-for-Palliative-and-End-of-Life-Care.pdf. For information and guidance about supporting families after the death of a CYP see Chapter 35: When a Child Dies.

This chapter is intended to be a first point of information, with general guidance to help the nurse provide care for a CYP until expert advice is available. It includes the symptoms that are most commonly experienced, i.e. nausea, vomiting, constipation, diarrhoea, and dyspnoea. This chapter also describes the use of proxy PCA (PPCA) (for other aspects of pain management, see Chapter 24: Pain Management); provides information on situations that can often cause anxiety, namely bleeding, nutrition, and hydration; and describes the signs of impending death. There are other situations, such as spinal cord compression and acutely occurring airway obstruction, that will require rapid medical intervention to maintain life and optimise quality of life. It is again outside the scope of this chapter to discuss these in detail, but careful assessment of the CYP will ensure timely identification of concerns.

The vision for services of the future is that they will be commissioned and delivered in line with identified local need and national policy and driven by best practice (Department of Health (DH) 2008). This chapter presents some of the emerging evidence from practice, evidence that must, despite the challenges, begin to be mapped in terms of research-based practice.

Assessment of symptoms

Effective symptom management is dependent on undertaking a full and accurate assessment of the CYP, which starts with obtaining a comprehensive and concise history of the symptom or symptom cluster. There is a dearth of clinical assessment tools validated for use in the paediatric palliative care population and as a result, general tools are adopted and in some cases modified for the individual patient (Rajapakse and Comac 2012). One approach to symptom assessment is to use the biopsychosocial model (Figure 25.1). This model, first postulated by Engel (1977), considers symptoms in terms of biological (physical), psychological (emotional, thoughts, behaviours) and social (socioeconomic, sociocultural, and environmental) causes or influencing factors. For instance, nausea and vomiting may be caused by *biological factors*, such as gastric obstruction, medications, and raised intracranial pressure; *psychological factors*, such as anticipatory nausea and vomiting, anxiety, fear; and *social factors*, such as poor sanitation, or over-feeding. Using the biopsychosocial model enables the nurse to both assess and plan care holistically.

Other tools that may be useful to support an assessment of biological processes include:

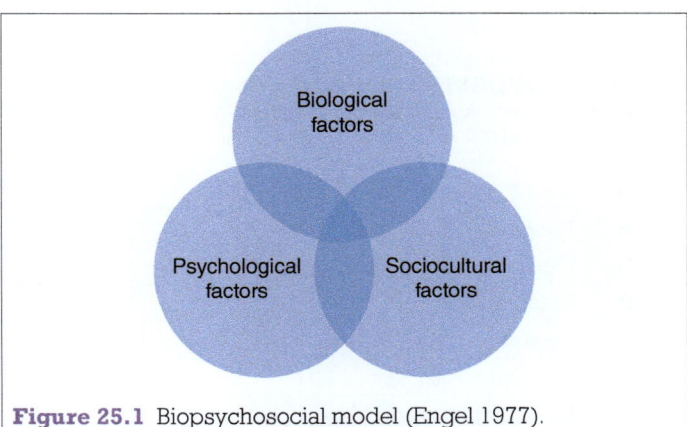

Figure 25.1 Biopsychosocial model (Engel 1977).

- ABCDE for consideration of the CYP's airway, breathing, circulation, disability, and exposure; for more information, see Chapter 9: Early Recognition and Management of the Seriously Ill Child.
- Symptom assessment in terms of body systems (respiratory, cardiovascular, neurological, gastrointestinal, etc.); each system can be considered in a generic nursing assessment or in terms of advanced assessment with appropriate training.
- Use of mnemonics such as SOCRATES (Table 25.1) or the OPQRSTU (Table 25.2) to aid history taking (Banicek 2010; Vera 2018).
- Existing validated pain assessment tools such as FLACC (World Health Organisation 2012, Royal College of Nursing, 2009).
- A Paediatric Coma Scale, such as the Adelaide Paediatric Coma Scale or the nationally accepted adaptation of the Glasgow Coma Scale (GCS) (Teasdale et al. 2014).
- Glamorgan Paediatric Pressure Ulcer risk assessment (Willock et al. 2007).
- The Bristol Stool chart (Lewis and Heaton 1997).

Patient self-report measures such as numerical rating scales (NRS), visual analogue scales (VAS), verbal rating scales (VRS), and categorical scales (CS) are essential when assessing subjective phenomena like pain and dyspnoea (Ekstrom et al. 2015). While they are easy to use, simple to understand, and inexpensive, they are heavily reliant on the CYP's concept of seriation and their ability to describe and rate a symptom, which varies with age, cognitive ability, and health status (Hunt 2012).

As with any assessment of the CYP, their needs should also be considered in the context of the family's previous experiences, as these may influence how the family view symptoms, compliance with planned interventions, and the effectiveness of their management. The nurse must balance the burden/intrusiveness of undertaking any assessment intervention against the perceived benefit/cost to the CYP, to ensure that quality of life is optimal and not compromised. Symptom assessment should be ongoing throughout the palliative phase, and used dynamically to plan and implement effective management (Klick and Hauer 2010).

Pain in palliative care: PCA and proxy PCA

Pain is a common symptom experienced by CYPs with an LLC. For general principles regarding pain management, see Chapter 24. As with any symptom, pain assessment should consider the CYP's diagnosis, previous pain experience, and explore the CYP's and family's perceptions of which interventions have been successful or not and why, to ensure effective pain management. Pain experienced by CYPs with LLCs is often complex, comprising both acute and chronic pain, and nociceptive, neuropathic, and existential pain, and should be assessed in terms of whether it is constant, episodic or recurrent pain, breakthrough or end-dose failure pain, and incident pain (World Health Organisation [WHO] 2012). As such, management may need to be equally complex, employing a variety of approaches including analgesic and adjuvant medications, consideration of routes of administration, and nonpharmacological approaches. Patient-controlled analgesia (PCA) and PPCA are one approach to managing pain.

PCA and nurse-controlled analgesia (NCA) have long been recognised as safe and effective methods of delivering opiates for postoperative, procedural and incidence pain relief, either intravenously or subcutaneously while the patient remains in hospital (Anghelescu et al. 2012). Use of PCA in palliative care practice in the home or community setting had, until recently, been limited to terminally ill adults with cancer. However, there is growing evidence that PCA and PPCA – defined as analgesia controlled by a parent or carer, is also effective and safe in managing the pain of terminally ill CYPs in both hospital and community settings (Zernikow et al. 2009). Assessment for PCA/PPCA for palliative care should be carried out by a paediatric palliative care team experienced in caring for CYP with escalating analgesia requirements and complex pain. The team needs to consider the suitability of PCA/PPCA for the CYP and family, the competency of staff administering the PCA/PPCA, the place of care (including transfers from one setting to another), the type of pain, disease profile, and expected/predicted pathway.

Table 25.1 SOCRATES mnemonic for obtaining pain history (Banicek 2010)

S	Severity: None, mild, moderate, severe
O	Onset: When and how did it start?
C	Characteristc: Is it shooting, burning, aching? Ask the patient to describe it.
R	Radiation: Does it radiate anywhere else?
A	Additional factors: What makes it better?
T	Time: Is it there all the time? Is there a time of day when it is worse?
E	Excacerbating factors: What makes it worse?
S	Site: Where is the pain?

Table 25.2 OPQRSTU mnemonic for obtaining history of symptoms (https://nurseslabs.com/nursing-health-assessment-mnemonics-tips)

O	Onset
P	Provocative/palliative factors
Q	Quality/quantity
R	Region/radiation
S	Severity
T	Time and treatment
U	Understanding and impact
V	Values

Nausea and vomiting

The causes of nausea and vomiting are numerous and varied (Figure 25.2), including the disease itself, its treatment, side effects of treatment, as well as unrelated comorbidities (Glare et al. 2011). In some cases, multiple aetiologies coexist (Glare et al. 2011). An assessment of the CYP's history, current symptoms, and previous management is essential for effective management (Klick and Hauer 2010). Nausea (a subjective sensation) may be experienced as a symptom in constipation, renal, or hepatic failure (Glare et al. 2011). Effortless early morning vomiting (or when moving from lying to sitting) associated with headache and positive neurological signs is typical of raised intracranial pressure (Miall et al. 2012). Nausea and vomiting related to toxins such as medications and biochemical abnormalities such as hypercalcaemia and uraemia should

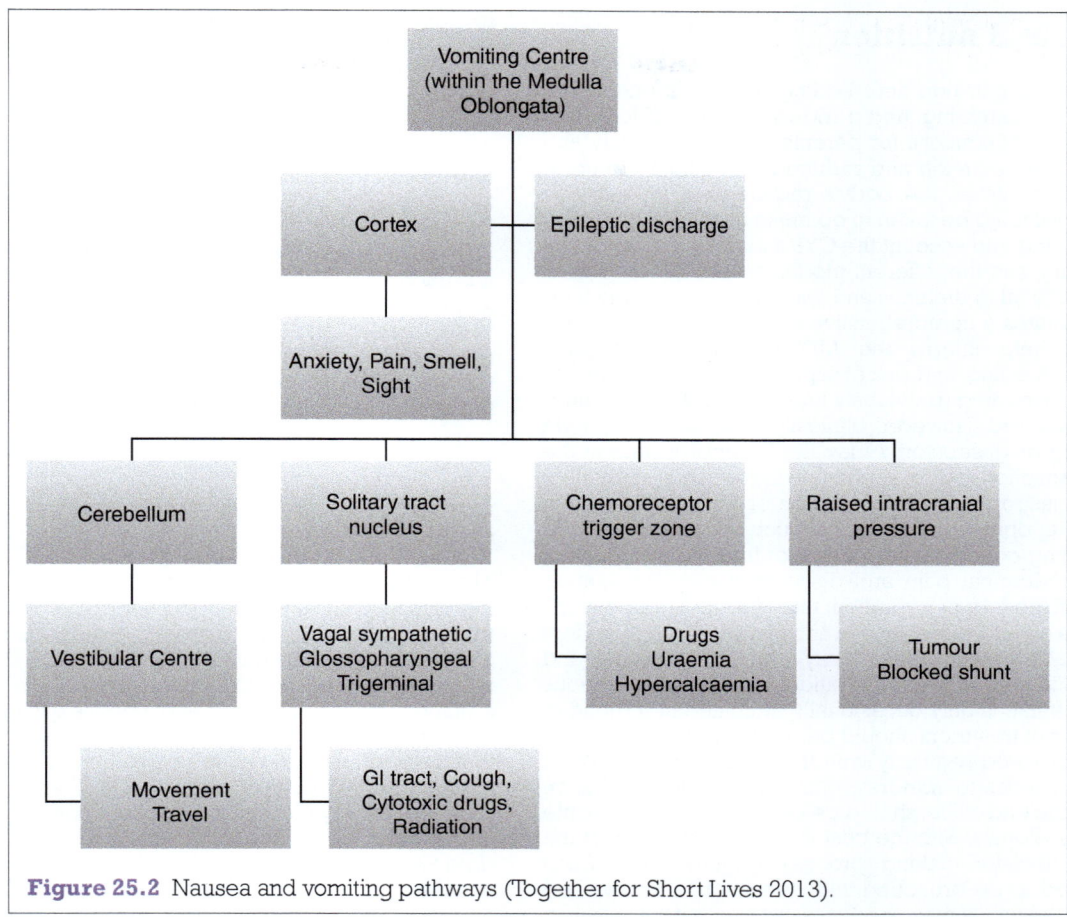

Figure 25.2 Nausea and vomiting pathways (Together for Short Lives 2013).

be considered, with subsequent correction of underlying cause where appropriate. Opioid-induced nausea and vomiting is reported to be less common in CYPs than previously thought (Mashayekhi et al. 2009). Vomiting without nausea may not be distressing for the CYP and may not require intervention. The choice of antiemetic prescribed is based on the perceived cause of emesis, anecdotal evidence, and professional preferences. The use of chemotherapy- and radiotherapy-induced or postoperative antiemetic regimes can have mixed results when used for palliative care (Davis and Hallerberg 2010). While further research is needed in this area, it is imperative that nurses assess and record the efficacy of any intervention used to optimise the management of this symptom.

Constipation and diarrhoea

Constipation is not just a measure of the frequency of bowel action but also refers to difficulty in defecation. It can be described as the inability to pass stools regularly or empty the bowels completely, resulting in infrequent, difficult, and often painful passage of hard stools (NICE 2014). In the palliative phase, constipation may be caused by poor food and fluid intake, reduced mobility, or as a direct result of the disease process (Klick and Hauer 2010). It is an almost universal and troublesome side effect of opioid medication, which reduces gastric propulsion, and relaxes the bowel, thus slowing stool passage (Miller and Karwacki 2012).

Diarrhoea is the passage of frequent loose stools, but the CYP may also describe a single loose stool along with frequent normal stools. Possible causes include problems with absorption of feeds, medications (such as antibiotics), infection, and overflow of liquid faecal matter as a result of impacted stool (Miller and Karwacki 2012).

Dyspnoea

Dyspnoea is defined as a subjective experience of 'breathing discomfort that consists of qualitatively distinct sensations that vary in intensity' (Parshall et al. 2012, p. 436). It is one of the most prevalent and distressing symptoms experienced by the CYP and observed by parents at the end of life (Schindera et al. 2014; Blume et al. 2014).

The latest neurophysiological model suggests dyspnoea is caused by an awareness of incongruity between the need to breathe and the ability to do so (Ekstrom et al. 2015). The cause of altered respiratory function and perception of work of breathing needs to be considered. For instance, breathlessness may be the result of deterioration of pre-existing conditions, such as spinal muscular atrophy (SMA), cystic fibrosis, or cardiac failure, or may be a symptom of progressive disease, such as anaemia in the CYP with cancer. It may also be exacerbated by anxiety or emotional distress (Brook et al. 2012). The causative factors, along with the overall condition of the CYP, will influence the MDT's decision to treat.

Hydration and nutrition

Providing adequate nutrition and feeding a child is one of the prime functions of parenting, and a reduced intake of food and fluid can cause great concern for parents or carers (Vesely and Beach 2013). While anorexia and reduced oral intake are common at the end of life as the body's requirement for nutrition decreases, steps should be taken to optimise the CYP's hydration and nutrition, taking into account the CYP's underlying condition, disease trajectory, and the different modes available (Thompson et al. 2012). A referral to dietetics and speech and language therapy (SALT) facilitates a comprehensive nutritional and oromotor assessment to help inform the MDT's management plan. Dysphagia, poor feeding, and risk of aspiration are indicators that clinically assisted feeding (previously known as artificial feeding) should be considered. However, clinically assisted feeding via nasogastric tube or gastrostomy may not be appropriate at the end of life, if absorption is diminished due to reduced gut motility, or if there is a gastrointestinal obstruction or intractable nausea and vomiting (Rapoport et al. 2013). In such cases, care should focus on providing comfort such as sips of fluid, or mouth care. Symptoms of abdominal pain and discomfort may be exacerbated by enteral feeding or hydration; therefore, detailed discussion about goals of care, expectations and symptom management should take place between the family and MDT (Vesely and Beach. 2013). Clinician-assisted hydration, such as subcutaneous fluids to satisfy thirst, is only occasionally indicated at the end of life and the goals of treatment should be established before commencing and reviewed regularly with the family and the CYP if appropriate. Decisions to withdraw clinically assisted hydration and nutrition at the end of life, should be made jointly between the family and professionals, with the best interests of the CYP at the centre of the decision-making process (Figure 25.3). Such discussions need to be broached with sensitivity and revisited as frequently as the family may need reassurance that the decision to withdraw clinically assisted hydration or nutrition was appropriate (Anderson et al. 2019; Larcher et al. 2015; Thompson et al. 2012).

Haemorrhage

Haemorrhage, although unusual in CYPs, can be a very frightening experience for everyone involved. There are certain conditions, including leukaemia, bone marrow transplant failure, pulmonary aspergillus infection, and solid tumours (nasopharyngeal rhabdomyosarcoma, liver tumours) that are associated with an increased risk of bleeding (Chan 2012). Fungating wounds in the CYP with a malignancy may result in bleeding due to abnormal tumour vasculature, erosion of blood vessels by cancerous cells, and thrombocytopenia (Chrisman 2010). Liaison with disease-specific medical and nursing teams for CYP with conditions such as epidermolysis bullosa (EB) is necessary to ensure that bleeding from fragile skin/tissues is minimised during dressing changes (Liang and Denyer 2012). CYP who are severely thrombocytopenic may be at risk of intracranial bleeding, which is more likely to cause sudden loss of consciousness or seizures rather than visible bleeding.

Treatment of mild external haemorrhage may include calcium alginate dressing, topical and systemic tranexamic acid, adrenaline sprays or adrenaline-soaked dressings (Liang and Denyer 2012). CYP with haematological conditions may benefit from regular transfusions of blood products to reduce the risk of haemorrhage. If bleeding is uncontrolled or frequent, a surgical referral to consider interventions such as cauterization, surgical diathermy or ligation may be appropriate. Alternatively, minimally invasive interventions such as radiotherapy or embolization may be useful in palliating bleeding. Providing dark towels and sheets is a simple but effective method of making the appearance of blood less frightening (Liang and Denyer 2012).

In the rare event that a catastrophic bleed occurs at the end of life it is unlikely it will be successfully controlled with any of the aforementioned interventions. Therefore, the focus of care shifts to providing comfort and sedation to the CYP and support for the family (Davies 2012). If there is a risk of catastrophic bleeding, it is important that the family are informed of this and how it will or will not be managed to ensure they are prepared.

Agitation

There appears to be no unifying definition of agitation, which is experienced by CYPs nearing the end of life. Signs of agitation may include crying, distress, restlessness, irritability, and aggressive behaviour, as well as confusion, altered speech, disrupted attention, and hallucinations (NICE 2016). The causes of agitation can vary widely and need exploration and targeted management of the underlying cause, although it is recognised that determining the cause of agitation can be difficult, particularly in the preverbal or nonverbal CYP and those with a neurological disability. Consideration should be given to psychological and emotional causes, such as unspoken fears, anxiety, and dreams possibly about death and dying, as well as physiological causes such as pain, adverse medication effects, constipation, dehydration, urinary retention, hypoxia, anaemia, raised intracranial pressure, or intracranial bleeds (NICE 2016). A management approach that aims to treat the underlying cause, as well as the symptom itself is likely to use both pharmacological and nonpharmacological interventions (NICE 2016). Professionals need to be cautious about sedating the agitated CYP without exploring cause, as sedation may mask symptoms such as pain, which is the primary cause of agitation. The distress and burden caused by agitation at the end of life not only affects the CYP but can have a detrimental impact on the family and professionals caring for them.

Seizures

Seizures at the end of life may affect CYPs with neurodegenerative diseases who may have suffered from seizures throughout their illness and CYP with brain tumours or metastatic disease of the central nervous system (Hauer and Faulkner 2012). Seizures may occur as a result of electrolyte imbalances (hyponatraemia), hypoglycaemia, intracranial haemorrhage, or high temperatures (febrile convulsion) (Hauer and Faulkner 2012). In some CYPs the seizure threshold may be lowered by intercurrent infection, fever, and medications such as amitriptyline, olanzapine, risperidone (Jassal and Aindow 2020). If reversible causes for seizures are suspected, these should be investigated and treated appropriately. Identifying those at risk of a seizure enables the nurse to prepare the CYP (where appropriate) and family to manage the seizures. The potential for

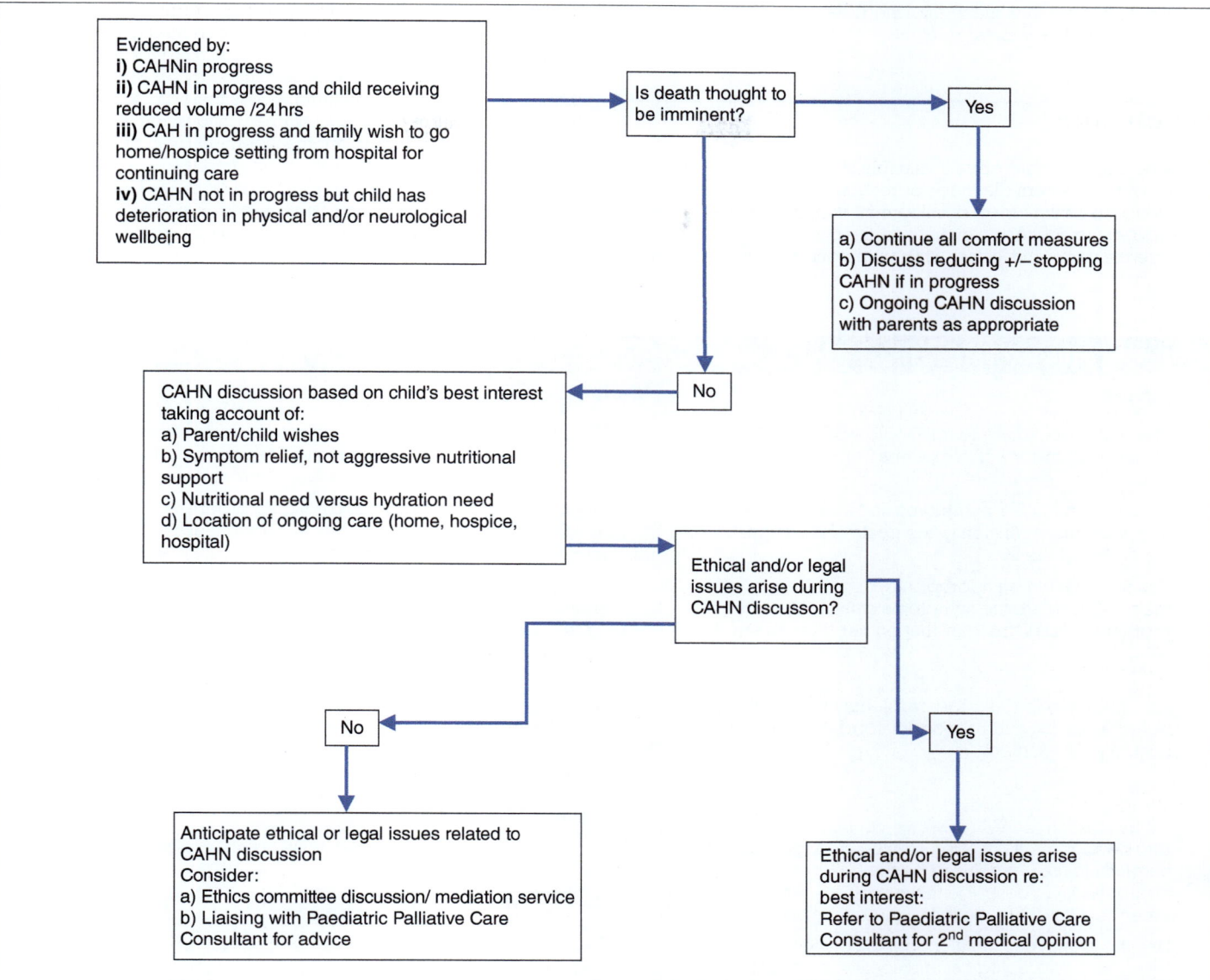

Figure 25.3 Decision-making algorithm for clinician-assisted hydration and nutrition (CAHN). Source: adapted from Paediatric Palliative Care Consultant Teams based at Evelina London Children's Hospital, Great Ormond Street Hospital for Children NHS Foundation Trust and The Royal Marsden NHS Foundation Trust, Surrey/Shooting Star Chase Children Hospice Care (2015).

the CYP to experience seizures may influence a family's decision making regarding their preferred place of care and death. Seizures can be a very frightening experience for families, especially if the seizure occurs at home and is unexpected.

Signs of impending death

Questions frequently posed by parents regarding impending death include 'How long do we have?', 'How will I know when it's time?', and 'What signs should I look out for?' In practice, it is very difficult to predict when death will occur. Signs and symptoms that predict imminent death in adults with cancer include periods of apnoea, Cheyne-Stokes breathing – defined as alternating periods of apnoea with gradually diminishing hyperpnoea (increased depth and rate of breathing), 'death rattle' caused by gurgling of secretions on inspiration or expiration, difficulty swallowing, decreased level of consciousness, peripheral cyanosis, weak or absent radial pulse on palpation, and reduced urine output (Hui et al. 2014). Empirical evidence suggests that the signs of impending death in CYP are not dissimilar to those in adults. Although it is difficult to broach these subjects with the family, addressing these questions openly and honestly and with sensitivity can empower families to care for their child and make informed decisions about place of care, and end-of-life wishes.

Conclusion

Paediatric palliative care plays a valuable integrated role in the care of CYPs with LLCs from diagnosis or recognition of the illness at any point along the continuum of development from the antenatal period through to young adulthood. In practice, the paediatric palliative care team interconnects and liaises with numerous professionals, often across a variety of settings, with the aim of promoting optimal quality of life wherever possible. Knowledge and experience has more often been built over time and learnt experientially. Paediatric palliative care practice is informed and underpinned by research, but more is needed to explore, measure, and assess the experience of patients holistically, as well as the impact of interventions from support around decision making and symptom management (both pharmacological and nonpharmacological). The goals must be to ensure that the voices of CYPs with LLCs are heard, acknowledged and acted upon, and that their needs and their families' needs are met.

Care practices most frequently associated with paediatric palliative care are outlined below.

Procedure guideline 25.1 Assessment of symptoms

Statement	Rationale
1 The multidisciplinary team should work together to obtain a full history of symptoms from the CYP and family.	1 Effective palliative care is best provided by a multidisciplinary approach as each profession brings its own expertise and individual approach to the problem (Klick and Hauer 2010).
2 Consider the CYP's symptoms and assess the value of interventions in relation to the goals of care agreed with the CYP and family.	2 Goals of care may change as the illness progresses, with the CYP and family perceiving previously acceptable assessment measures and interventions as burdensome or futile (Klick and Hauer 2010).
3 Ask the CYP (when appropriate) and the family what they consider are the symptoms causing them most problems and distress, or that bother them the most.	3 The CYP's self-report is considered to be the 'gold standard' and should be sought whenever appropriate (Klick and Hauer 2010). Symptom management in the palliative phase must focus on problems as seen by the CYP and family (Rajapakse and Comac 2012).
4 Ask the family to describe problems in as much detail as possible, giving prompts as appropriate to gain an accurate assessment.	4 Allowing CYP and families time to describe problems in detail provides a wealth of information and may highlight the occurrence of symptom clusters (Rodgers et al. 2013). It also ensures that professionals act on the concerns of the CYP and family rather than their own preconceived ideas of what the problems may be (Rajapakse and Comac 2012).
5 Use developmentally appropriate language and listen carefully to the words used by the CYP (when appropriate) to describe the symptoms. Ask the parent/carer how the CYP describes their symptoms.	5 To facilitate effective and meaningful communication (Klick and Hauer 2010).
6 Use the biopsychosocial model to consider the biological, psychological and social causes of the symptoms.	6 To ensure symptoms are considered holistically in the context of disease or treatment, as well as the social situation; to facilitate optimal management (Rajapakse and Comac 2012).
7 Obtain a clinical history of the symptoms, including their nature and quality, temporal factors, intensity, alleviating and exacerbating factors, as well as any associated symptoms.	7 To gain as full a picture as possible and ascertain the most appropriate management (Rajapakse and Comac 2012).
8 Where appropriate use a validated and age/developmentally appropriate symptom assessment tool to assess symptoms.	8 To gain as full a picture as possible of the symptom to inform effective symptom management (Rajapakse and Comac 2012).
9 Ask the CYP and family whether any medications or interventions have helped to relieve symptoms in the past.	9 To ensure that previously successful methods can be reinstigated.
10 Ascertain what has been tried but has not proved useful. Ensure that accurate information is taken regarding dosage, frequency and previously used medication.	10 To avoid the use of previously ineffective treatments and to ascertain if medication has been used optimally in the past.
11 Reassess daily (or as negotiated with the family) and adjust management as directed by further assessment.	11 Symptoms may not be fully controlled; a family may wish for less frequent contact with professionals at this palliative stage (Klick and Hauer 2010).

Procedure guideline 25.2 Care of patient receiving PCA/PPCA for palliative care

Statement	Rationale
1 Ensure the CYP and family have consented and received appropriate information and preparation prior to commencing PCA/PPCA.	1 To meet information needs and reduce anxiety.
2 If using PCA protocol, parents should be advised in a sensitive manner that they are not permitted to administer a bolus by pressing the button for PCA.	2 To ensure patient safety, only CYPs trained in the use of the PCA (and aware of potential side effects of opioids) may administer boluses. In PCA excessive opioid demands initiate sedation; the CYP falls asleep, thus allowing the opioid level to decrease.
3 Ensure the parents are aware that the PCA or PPCA programme can be changed to match the CYP's ability (or not) to use the PCA button.	3 PCA and PPCA programming differ.
4 Ensure the CYP and family can use an appropriate pain assessment tool.	4 To ensure the CYP understands and can use the tool effectively prior to the painful experience. Self-report is the gold standard for pain assessment and should be used whenever appropriate to do so considering the CYP's age and cognition (Ekstrom et al. 2015).
5 Administration sets used for PCA/PPCA should contain an anti-syphon/anti-reflux valve as recommended by the device manufacturer.	5 To prevent siphonage and reflux of medications.
6 Ensure appropriate safety checks including: • Check the CYP's PCA/PPCA protocol has been completed correctly. • Check the analgesic solution and additional drugs are prescribed.	6 To ensure patient safety. • To adhere to local medication policy. • To ensure effective analgesia with minimal side effects.
7 At an appropriate time and in a sensitive manner, discuss with the family end-of-life observable events due to disease (breathing changes, skin colour changes, depressed level of consciousness, and decreased responsiveness).	7 To ensure that the PCA/PPCA is not discontinued when changes (breathing, colour, level of consciousness, and responsiveness) associated with a natural death due to the underlying disease process occurs.
8 Regularly assess for symptoms of opiate toxicity such as increased sedation and respiratory depression that are unusual for the CYP or not thought to relate to the underlying disease process. If suspected: • **STOP** the infusion. • Contact the palliative care team (or relevant team managing the PPCA). • The infusion may be recommenced following assessment if appropriate.	8 To ensure early detection and treatment of opioid-induced sedation or opiate-induced respiratory depression.
9 Monitor the CYP for symptoms of nausea and/or vomiting, and pruritus, and contact the palliative care team (or relevant team managing the PPCA) if these symptoms are observed.	9 Nausea and vomiting, and pruritus may occur due to the disease process or PPCA medication. Discussion with the relevant team ensures appropriate investigation and treatment symptoms and underlying cause where appropriate.
10 Monitor the CYP's urine output. If the CYP has a reduced urine output or shows signs of discomfort when passing urine discuss with the palliative care team (or relevant team managing the CYP's care)	10 To ensure prompt investigation and treatment of urinary retention, including consideration of catheterization if needed. An audit of 10 000 CYPs receiving intravenous opioids urinary retention was rare (<2%) (Howard et al. 2010).
11 When a CYP is taking any opioid analgesia, liaise with medical staff about commencing a laxative with stimulant and softening action as prophylaxis.	11 Opioid analgesia effects gut motility and causes constipation (Miller and Karwacki 2012).
12 Discontinuing PCA/PPCA should only be done with guidance from the team managing the PCA/PPCA.	12 To minimise the risk to the CYP of periods without analgesia.
13 Return any pump that has technical problems, or has been dropped or damaged, to the Biomedical Engineering Department in your hospital, accurately describing the problem.	13 To prevent administration errors due to faulty equipment.

Procedure guideline 25.3 Assessment and management of nausea and vomiting

Statement	Rationale
1 Ask the CYP and family as appropriate to describe the nature, frequency and timing of the nausea and vomiting.	1 In order to determine the likely cause (Glare et al. 2011). Early morning vomiting is commonly seen in patients with CNS disease.
2 Obtain a history of recent bowel action.	2 Vomiting may be related to constipation (Klick and Hauer 2010).
3 Discuss with medical staff the possible need for further investigations, including biochemical abnormalities.	3 There may be an underlying cause of the nausea and/or vomiting, which could be treatable (Glare et al. 2011; Klick and Hauer 2010).
4 Discuss with medical staff the prescribing of appropriate anti-emetics drugs, depending on the cause of the nausea and vomiting.	4 Antiemetic choice depends on cause (Davis and Hallerberg 2010).
5 CYPs with CNS disease may find it helpful to sleep with their head raised.	5 To reduce the increase in pressure which occurs when the CYP is lying flat (Miall et al. 2012).
6 CYPs with signs of raised intracranial pressure may require a short-pulsed course of a steroid dose twice daily.	6 In MRI studies, dexamethasone has been shown to reduce water content of oedematous brain tissue (Sinha et al. 2004).
7 The CYP receiving enteral feeding may require a reduction of the volume or concentration of their feed.	7 Gut motility may be reduced in advanced illness (Miller and Karwacki 2012).
8 If the CYP is vomiting, provide a receptacle, which is changed frequently. Change clothes and sponge face as necessary. Offer mouthwash and sips of clear fluid.	8 To maintain comfort and dignity.
9 Reassure the family that attempts are being made to control the nausea and vomiting. Be honest with the family if it is likely to be impossible to completely control the symptoms.	9 To promote family confidence and recognition that in certain situations it may be impossible to completely control nausea and vomiting.
10 Consider nonpharmacological interventions in addition to pharmacological approaches, including complementary, psychosocial and behavioural therapies.	10 These may be helpful in optimising symptom management (Glare et al. 2011).
11 Avoid environmental stimuli such as certain sights, smells, or foods that cause the CYP to feel nauseous.	11 To reduce risk of nausea and vomiting (Glare et al. 2011).
12 If there is a discernible pattern to vomiting, try to time medication and food intake accordingly.	12 To facilitate the absorption of medication and maximise nutritional intake.

Procedure guideline 25.4 Assessment and management of constipation and diarrhoea

Statement	Rationale
1 Determine from CYP and family as appropriate, the CYP's usual bowel habit and whether current bowel action differs from normal.	1 To obtain baseline for assessment of current bowel actions and to facilitate decision making as to whether any treatment is necessary (Klick and Hauer 2010).
2 Ascertain whether CYP is taking any opioid analgesia, and liaise with medical staff about commencing a laxative with stimulant and softening action as prophylaxis.	2 Opioid analgesia effects gut motility and causes constipation (Miller and Karwacki 2012).

Management of constipation

Statement	Rationale
1 If current bowel action is abnormal, discuss with medical staff whether there is a need to investigate any underlying cause, e.g. radiological examination, etc.	1 Abnormal bowel actions may have some underlying treatable pathology which, if corrected, would improve the CYP's quality of life.

Chapter 25 Palliative care

Procedure guideline 25.4 Assessment and management of constipation and diarrhoea *(continued)*

Statement	Rationale
2 If the CYP has been constipated but has now started to pass small amounts of loose stool, discuss with medical staff whether clinical or radiological examination is necessary.	2 To exclude the possibility of impacted stools with overflow of liquid faecal matter (Miller and Karwacki 2012).
3 If history indicates that the CYP is constipated, offer dietary advice where appropriate and liaise with an independent prescriber for a prescription of laxatives with a suitable mode of action.	3 When a CYP is receiving palliative care it is often impossible to correct bowel action with dietary adjustments alone.
4 Ensure privacy, time and comfort for CYP when attempting to defecate.	4 To promote effective bowel action and minimise embarrassment.
5 If the CYP has not had a bowel action despite appropriate laxative, discuss with the family the appropriateness of rectal measures, e.g. suppositories, enema.	5 The CYP may require some rectal stimulant to open their bowels.
6 Do not discontinue oral laxatives.	6 It is important to continue to soften the stools and stimulate bowel peristalsis (Miller and Karwacki 2012).
7 When appropriate, encourage good fluid intake and high-fibre diet.	7 To maximise normal gastro-intestinal function.

Management of diarrhoea

Statement	Rationale
1 Obtain a stool specimen for culture and sensitivity and treat if appropriate (National Institute for Health and Care Excellence, 2014).	1 Acute onset may indicate infection, particularly if others are affected.
2 Review CYP's drug regimen with medical staff particularly if they are already taking antibiotics or laxatives.	2 To identify possible drug related causes of diarrhoea (Miller and Karwacki 2012).
3 Review CYP's feeding regimen including any errors in feeding and route, particularly if on clinically assisted feeding.	3 To rule out dietary causes of diarrhoea (Miller and Karwacki 2012).
4 Discuss with medical staff appropriate use of fluids and drugs.	4 To reduce peristalsis and number of bowel actions and maintain appropriate hydration.
5 Assist family and CYP in cleaning the anal area and application of barrier cream as necessary.	5 To minimise skin excoriation.
6 Ensure privacy for the CYP.	6 To minimise embarrassment.

Procedure guideline 25.5 Management of dyspnoea

Statement	Rationale
1 Obtain a detailed history from both CYP and family, observing and assessing the impact of dyspnoea on the CYP and their quality of life.	1 In order to identify potentially reversible underlying causes and decide the most appropriate treatment if any (Brook et al. 2012).
2 Discuss with medical staff the appropriateness of investigations and any active management, e.g. antibiotics, blood transfusion, or pleural tap.	2 To ensure that investigations and treatment are realistic given the CYP's condition and the disease progress and are beneficial rather than burdensome (Brook et al. 2012).
3 Allow the CYP to position him/herself as they prefer – this may not look comfortable to professionals or family. For instance, positioning the CYP upright as much as possible, leaning forward, resting arms on a pillow, the back of a chair, or table.	3 To improve ventilatory effort (Buckholz and Von Gunten 2009).

(continued)

The Great Ormond Street Hospital Manual of Children and Young People's Nursing Practices

Procedure guideline 25.5 Management of dyspnoea (continued)

Statement	Rationale
4 Discuss with medical staff whether oxygen may improve symptoms (see Chapter 29: Respiratory Care).	4 Evidence suggests that oxygen only improves dyspnoea caused by hypoxaemia (Abernethy et al. 2010; Brook et al. 2012).
5 Use a desktop or handheld fan.	5 Evidence suggests that 'fan therapy' reduces the sensation of breathlessness (Galbraith et al. 2010).
6 Consider use of low-dose opioids.	6 Low dose opioids (25–50% of usual analgesic dose) have been shown to significantly improve dyspnoea in adults receiving palliative care (Allcroft et al. 2013; Oxberry et al. 2011). In CYPs, evidence supporting low dose opioids for dyspnoea is limited (Harlos et al. 2013).
7 Discuss with medical staff the appropriateness of anxiolytics such as benzodiazepines.	7 To reduce the cycle of dyspnoea causing anxiety-agitation, which in turn increases dyspnoea (Together for Short Lives 2013).
8 Give appropriate explanation and reassurance.	8 To minimise anxiety of parents/carers and CYP.
9 Consider use of nonpharmacological strategies such as distraction, visualisation, gentle touch/massage, relaxation, and energy conservation through pacing of daily activities.	9 To optimise management of dyspnoea and empower CYP and family (Buckholz and Von Gunten 2009).

Procedure guideline 25.6 Management of hydration and nutrition

Statement	Rationale
1 Explore with the CYP (where appropriate) and the family their goals regarding hydration and nutrition at the end of life (Vesely and Beach 2013).	1 To elicit CYP and parental views and concerns, to inform hydration and nutrition management.
2 Discuss with the MDT how hydration and nutrition may be affected by CYP's declining health, considering benefits and burdens in the light of the CYP's declining physical health, illness trajectory (Thompson et al. 2012).	2 To inform individualised hydration and nutrition plan.
3 Consider appropriateness of different modes of providing hydration and nutrition, the acceptability of different modes to the CYP and family, and preferred place of care (Thompson et al. 2012).	3 To ensure hydration and nutrition management is tailored to the needs and wishes of the CYP and family and is delivered in their preferred place of care.
4 Observe for signs and symptoms of dehydration (thirst, dry mouth, sunken eyes, fatigue, vomiting) and hunger (rumbling stomach, feeling of an empty stomach, nausea, dizziness, faintness, headache, poor concentration, irritability).	4 To ensure prompt and early recognition of hunger and thirst.
5 Consider referral to dietetics and SALT for comprehensive nutritional and oromotor assessment.	5 To optimise nutrition where possible and to inform decision-making about the appropriateness of clinically-assisted hydration and nutrition.
6 If there is dysphagia, poor feeding, or risk of aspiration and the CYP is experiencing unsated hunger, consider clinician-assisted nutrition via alternative routes (e.g. nasogastric), exploring acceptability and appropriateness with the CYP and family.	6 To optimise nutrition where clinically appropriate to do so and alleviate unsated hunger.

Procedure guideline 25.6 Management of hydration and nutrition (continued)

Statement	Rationale
7 If the CYP is unable to tolerate enteral feeding (abdominal pain, reduced gut motility, reduced gastric absorption, intractable nausea and vomiting, or intestinal obstruction) consider cause, treat appropriately where possible, or shift focus of care to providing comfort through sips of fluids and mouthcare only.	7 To minimise distressing symptoms where possible and promote comfort (Rapoport et al. 2013).
8 Consider subcutaneous fluids if CYP is unable to sustain adequate hydration via enteral routes, and dehydration is contributing to CYP's symptom burden and/or causing distress.	8 To optimise hydration where clinically appropriate to do so.
9 Follow local policy regarding the administration of subcutaneous fluids and ensure that both the CYP (if appropriate) and family are aware of the benefits and risks.	9 To ensure that the CYP and family feel appropriately informed and supported.
10 Choose a suitable site for administration, e.g. abdomen or upper outer aspect of thigh, avoiding areas of tissue damage. Check site daily and rotate every 48–72h.	10 To minimise the risk of tissue damage. For more information on administration of subcutaneous medication see Chapter 17: Administration of Medicines.

Procedure guideline 25.7 Management of haemorrhage

Statement	Rationale
1 Obtain a detailed history if CYP's clinical condition permits, including previous episodes of haemorrhage, medical history, and diagnosis, considering factors which may contribute to increasing the risk of haemorrhage.	1,2 To determine the CYP's risk of haemorrhage, possible causes, and to inform optimal management.
2 Where possible, anticipate the risk of haemorrhage through discussion and liaison with CYP's lead team.	
3 Discuss with CYP (if appropriate) and family in a sensitive way if there is a risk of bleeding, informing them of anticipated severity, and likely location of bleeding (internal or external), expected signs and symptoms, and their management.	3 To ensure that they are informed of what to expect and how this will be managed.
4 Discuss sensitively with CYP and family the appropriateness of continuing regular blood sampling and transfusion of blood products in relation to their preferred place of care.	4 To ensure they are fully informed and have realistic expectations about what interventions are possible in their preferred place of care.
Management of minor to moderage haemorrhage	
5 Assess extent of bleeding and investigate cause, considering underlying diagnosis and medical history and treat reversible conditions.	5 To optimise management of haemorrhage.
6 Liaise with tissue viability team regarding treatment of bleeding from fungating wounds or pressure sores.	6 To optimise treatment.
Management of expected major haemorrhage at the end of life	
7 If there is a risk of a massive bleed, ensure the CYP (where appropriate) and family are informed that the priority will be to reduce anxiety, promote comfort, and manage distress.	7 To ensure CYP and family are informed of what to expect and how this will be managed.
8 Consider giving oral tranexamic acid prophylactically.	8 To reduce risk of severe bleeding.

(continued)

Procedure guideline 25.7 Management of haemorrhage *(continued)*

Statement	Rationale
9 Optimise gastric protection medications prophylactically.	9 To reduce risk of massive haematemesis.
10 Provide dark-coloured bedding and towels to reduce visual impact of bleeding. Advise use of dark bedclothes for CYP.	10 To reduce anxiety/agitation of CYP, family and professionals.
11 Ensure anxiolytics and opiate medications have been prescribed and are available to administer.	11 To ensure prompt palliation of anxiety and pain.
12 Remain with the CYP and family, providing support and symptom management.	12 To provide prompt palliation of symptom, reassurance, and comfort.

Procedure guideline 25.8 Management of agitation

Statement	Rationale
1 Ask CYP and/or family, as appropriate the nature, frequency, and events preceding episodes of agitation.	1,2 To identify possible causes of agitation and optimise treatment.
2 Investigate and explore underlying causes of agitation, considering psychological and emotional factors, as well as physiological and pharmaceutical causes.	
3 Assess CYP's physiological symptoms, particularly pain, hypoxia, urinary retention, nausea, and constipation, and treat accordingly (NICE 2016).	3 To ensure optimal treatment of possible underlying cause of agitation.
4 Provide opportunities for both CYP and parents to explore psychological factors that may be contributing to agitation, including unspoken fears, mutual pretence and family-oriented anxieties (NICE 2016).	4 To help address psychological and emotional factors that may be contributing to agitation.
5 Where services exist, consider referring CYP and siblings to a play specialist or youth worker and the whole family to psychosocial services.	5 To address holistically psychological and emotional factors that may be contributing to the CYP's agitation.
6 Obtain detailed list of medications being administered, reviewing for interactions and adverse effect. Consideration needs to be given to the benefit vs. burden profile of each medication, and the availability of suitable alternatives.	6 To determine whether any medications that might be causing agitation can be replaced with a more suitable medication.
7 Help the CYP and family identify and utilise nonpharmacological approaches for acute episodes of agitation, including guided imagery, comfort, reassurance, orientation to time, place, and person, storytelling, and distraction.	7 To optimise holistic management of agitation.
8 Consider appropriateness of pharmacological management with benzodiazepines and neuroleptic medications if CYP remains agitated and all possible causes have been appropriately addressed (NICE 2016).	8 To optimise palliation of agitation alongside treatment of underlying cause.

Procedure guideline 25.9 Management of seizures

Statement	Rationale
1 A detailed history should be obtained from the CYP and family including preceding factors, seizure type and duration, and post ictal sequelae.	1 To help inform diagnosis and management pathway.
2 CYP presenting with a seizure for the first time should be investigated and treated for reversible causes such as fever, infection, electrolyte imbalance, and drug interactions where appropriate.	2 To ensure treatment of reversible causes of seizure.
3 Where the CYP's diagnosis predisposes them to seizures, ensure family receive teaching about what seizures may look like and what actions to take, including ensuring CYP's safety and who to contact.	3 To ensure the family are prepared and know what to expect.
4 Liaise with the neurology team regarding a seizure management plan that considers the CYP and family's preferred place of care (NICE 2016).	4 To ensure the seizure management plan is achievable in their preferred place of care.
5 Give oxygen if CYP becomes grey or cyanosed and arrange home oxygen as necessary if the CYP is being transferred home.	5 To treat hypoxia secondary to seizures and ensure oxygen is available at home if needed.
6 Teach parents and family when and how to administer anti-epileptic medications, e.g. buccal and rectal medications.	6 To ensure family feel equipped to administer anti-epileptics safely.

Procedure guideline 25.10 Recognising signs of impending death

Statement	Rationale
1 Discuss altered respiratory rate or any changes in respiratory pattern. Identify that the respiratory rate may be reduced or there could be the onset of Cheyne–Stokes respirations; a form of periodic breathing associated with periods of apnoea (Hui et al. 2014).	1 To prepare the family and reduce anxiety.
2 a) Discuss noisy respirations (sometimes known as death rattle); an accumulation of secretions usually in the hypopharynx, which oscillate when the CYP breathes. Explain that this generally occurs in patients who are too weak to expectorate (Hui et al. 2014).	2 a) To prepare the family and reduce anxiety.
b) Noisy breathing may be improved by changing the position of the CYP (for instance, tilting their head to the side). Use of antisecretory medications such as hyoscine hydrobromide or glycopyrrolate may be effective in some patients (Campbell and Yarandi 2013).	b) To facilitate drainage of secretions and reduce production of secretions.
3 a) Discuss that the CYP may become agitated or restless as death approaches.	3 a) To prepare the family and reduce anxiety.
b) Consider any reversible causes of agitation such as pain, pruritus, urinary retention, drug side effects, or psychosocial issues and treat accordingly.	b) To facilitate appropriate symptom management.
c) Discuss with the family the use of sedating medication if symptoms prove refractory to optimal treatment (Korzeniewska-Eksterowicz et al. 2014). Consider sedative if all of the above have been excluded.	c) To reduce the CYP's distress.
4 Explain to the family that in the last few days prior to death many CYP sleep for longer periods and have a reduced level of consciousness (Hui et al. 2014).	4 To prepare the family and reduce anxiety.
5 Discuss with the family that the CYP may also have reduced peripheral circulation, leading to coldness and a discolouration of the extremities (Hui et al. 2014).	5 To prepare the family and reduce anxiety.

References

Abernethy, A.P., Mcdonald, C.F., Frith, P.A. et al. (2010). Effect of palliative oxygen versus room air in relief of breathlessness in patients with refractory dyspnoea: a double-blind, randomised controlled trial. *Lancet* 376: 784–793.

ACT (2007). The ACT Care Pathway: Transition. A Framework for the Development of Integrated Multi-Agency Care Pathways for Young People with Life-Threatening and Life-Limiting Conditions.

ACT (2009). A neonatal pathway for babies with palliative care needs [online]. https://www.neonatalnetwork.co.uk/nwnodn/wp-content/uploads/2017/06/ACTNeonatal_Pathway_for_Babies_5.pdf (accessed 3 August 2022).

Allcroft, P., Margitanovic, V., Greene, A. et al. (2013). The role of benzodiazepines in breathlessness: a single site, open label pilot of sustained release morphine together with clonazepam. *Journal of Palliative Medicine* 16: 741–744.

Anderson A., Burke, K., Bendle, L., Koh, M., McCulloch, R., and Breen, M. (2019) Artificial nutrition and hydration for children and young people towards end of life: consensus guidelines across four specialist paediatric palliative care centres. https://spcare.bmj.com/content/11/1/92 (accessed 3 August 2022).

Anghelescu, D.L., Faughnan, L.G., Oakes, L.L. et al. (2012). Parent-controlled PCA for pain management in pediatric oncology: is it safe? *Journal of Pediatric Hematology/Oncology* 34: 416–420.

Banicek, J. (2010). How to ensure acute pain in older people is appropriately assessed and managed. *Nursing Times* 106 (29): 14–17.

Bergstraesser, E. (2013). Pediatric palliative care – when quality of life becomes the main focus of treatment. *European Journal of Pediatrics* 172: 139–150.

Blume, E.D., Balkin, E.M., Aiyagari, R. et al. (2014). Parental perspectives on suffering and quality of life at end-of-life in children with advanced heart disease: an exploratory study*. *Pediatric Critical Care Medicine* 15: 336–342.

Brook, L., Twigg, E., Venables, A., and Shaw, C. (2012). Respiratory symptoms. In: *Oxford Textbook of Palliative Care for Children*, 2e (eds. A. Goldman, R. Hain and S. Liben), 319–327. Oxford: Oxford University Press.

Buckholz, G.T. and Von Gunten, C.F. (2009). Nonpharmacological management of dyspnea. *Current Opinion in Supportive and Palliative Care* 3: 98–102.

Campbell, M.L. and Yarandi, H.N. (2013). Death rattle is not associated with patient respiratory distress: is pharmacologic treatment indicated? *Journal of Palliative Medicine* 16: 1255–1259.

Chan, M.-Y. (2012). Haematological symptoms. In: *Oxford Textbook of Palliative Care for Children*, 2e (eds. A. Goldman, R. Hain and S. Liben), 344–351. Oxford: Oxford University Press.

Chrisman, C.A. (2010). Care of chronic wounds in palliative care and end-of-life patients. *International Wound Journal* 7: 214–235.

Davies, D. (2012). Care in the final hours and days. In: *Oxford Textbook of Palliative Care for Children*, 2e (eds. A. Goldman, R. Hain and S. Liben), 368–374. Oxford: Oxford University Press.

Davis, M.P. and Hallerberg, G. (2010). A systematic review of the treatment of nausea and/or vomiting in cancer unrelated to chemotherapy or radiation. *Journal of Pain and Symptom Management* 39: 756–767.

De Rooy, L., Aladangady, N., and Aidoo, E. (2012). Palliative care for the newborn in the United Kingdom. *Early Human Development* 88: 73–77.

Department of Health (DH) (2008). Better care, better lives. Improving outcomes for children, young people and their families living with life limiting and life threatening conditions. https://uwe-repository.worktribe.com/output/1015092 (accessed 31 October 2022).

Doug, M., Adi, Y., Williams, J. et al. (2011). Transition to adult services for children and young people with palliative care needs: a systematic review. *BMJ Supportive & Palliative Care* 1: 167–173.

Ekstrom, M.P., Abernethy, A.P., and Currow, D.C. (2015). The management of chronic breathlessness in patients with advanced and terminal illness. *BMJ* 349: g7617.

Engel, G.L. (1977). The need for a new medical model: a challenge for biomedicine. *Science* 196: 129–136.

Fraser, L.K., Miller, M., Draper, E.S. et al. (2011). Place of death and palliative care following discharge from paediatric intensive care units. *Archives of Disease in Childhood* 96: 1195–1198.

Galbraith, S., Fagan, P., Perkins, P. et al. (2010). Does the use of a handheld fan improve chronic dyspnea? A randomized, controlled, crossover trial. *Journal of Pain and Symptom Management* 39: 831–838.

Glare, P., Miller, J., Nikolova, T., and Tickoo, R. (2011). Treating nausea and vomiting in palliative care: a review. *Clinical Interventions in Aging* 6: 243–259.

Goldman, A., Hain, R., and Liben, S. (2012). *Oxford Textbook of Palliative Care for Children*. Oxford: Oxford University Press.

Gupta, N., Harrop, E., Lapwood, S., and Shefler, A. (2013). Journey from pediatric intensive care to palliative care. *Journal of Palliative Medicine* 16: 397–401.

Harlos, M.S., Stenekes, S., Lambert, D. et al. (2013). Intranasal fentanyl in the palliative Care of Newborns and Infants. *Journal of Pain and Symptom Management* 46: 265–274.

Harrop, E. and Edwards, C. (2013). How and when to refer a child for specialist paediatric palliative care. *Archives of Disease in Childhood – Education and Practice Edition* 98 (6): 202–208. edpract-2012-303325.

Hauer, J. and Faulkner, K. (2012). Neurological and neuromuscular conditions and symptoms. In: *Oxford Textbook of Palliative Care for Children*, 2e (eds. A. Goldman, R. Hain and S. Liben), 295–308. Oxford: Oxford University Press.

Howard, R.F., Lloyd-Thomas, A., Thomas, M. et al. (2010). Nurse-controlled analgesia (NCA) following major surgery in 10,000 patients in a children's hospital. *Paediatric Anaesthesia* 20: 126–134.

Hui, D., Dos Santos, R., Chisholm, G. et al. (2014). Clinical signs of impending death in cancer patients. *The Oncologist* 19: 681–687.

Hunt, A. (2012). Pain assessment. In: *Oxford Textbook of Palliative Care in Children*, 2e (eds. A. Goldman, R. Hain and S. Liben), 204–217. Oxford: Oxford University Press.

Jassal, S. and Aindow, A. (2020). The Association of Paediatric Palliative Medicine Master Formulary 2020 (5th edition) [online]. https://www.appm.org.uk/guidelines-resources/appm-master-formulary/ (accessed 3 August 2022).

Kelly, P., Twamley, K., Moss, R. et al. (2012). 'It's not just about death': changing attitudes and knowledge of palliative care in neonatal units. *BMJ Supportive & Palliative Care* 2: A20–A21.

Klick, J.C. and Hauer, J. (2010). Pediatric palliative care. *Current Problems in Pediatric and Adolescent Health Care* 40: 120–151.

Korzeniewska-Eksterowicz, A., Przysło, Ł., Fendler, W. et al. (2014). Palliative sedation at home for terminally ill children with Cancer. *Journal of Pain and Symptom Management* 48: 968–974.

Laddie, J., Craig, F., Brierley, J. et al. (2014). Withdrawal of ventilatory support outside the intensive care unit: guidance for practice. *Archives of Disease in Childhood* 99: 812–816.

Larcher, V., Craig, F., Bhogal, K. et al. (2015). Making decisions to limit treatment in life-limiting and life-threatening conditions in children: a framework for practice. *Archives of Disease in Childhood* 100 (Suppl 2): s3–s23.

Lewis, S.J. and Heaton, K.W. (1997). Stool form scale as a useful guide to intestinal transit time. *Scandinavian Jorunal of Gastroenterology* 32: 920–924.

Liang, Y. and Denyer, J. (2012). Skin symptoms. In: *Oxford Textbook of Palliative Care for Children*, 2e (eds. A. Goldman, R. Hain and S. Liben), 328–343. Oxford: Oxford University Press.

Liben, S., Papadatou, D., and Wolfe, J. (2008). Paediatric palliative care: challenges and emerging ideas. *Lancet* 371: 852–864.

Mancini, A., Uthaya, S., Beardsley, C., Wood, D., and Modi, N. (2014). Practical guidance for the management of palliative care on neonatal units [online]. https://www.sands.org.uk/sites/default/files/NICU-Palliative-Care-Feb-2014.pdf (accessed 3 August 2022).

Mashayekhi, S.O., Ghandforoush-Sattari, M., Routledge, P.A., and Hain, R.D. (2009). Pharmacokinetic and pharmacodynamic study of morphine and morphine 6-glucuronide after oral and intravenous administration of morphine in children with cancer. *Biopharmaceutics & Drug Disposition* 30: 99–106.

Mcculloch, R., Comac, M., and Craig, F. (2008). Paediatric palliative care: coming of age in oncology? *European Journal of Cancer* 44: 1139–1145.

Mellor, C., Heckford, E., and Frost, J. (2012). Developments in paediatric palliative care. *Paediatrics and Child Health* 22: 115–120.

Miall, L., Rudolf, M., and Smith, D. (2012). *Paediatrics at a Glance*. Chichester: Wiley-Blackwell.

Miller, M. and Karwacki, M. (2012). Management of the gastrointestinal tract in paediatric palliative medicine. In: *Oxford Textbook of Palliative Care for Children* (eds. A. Goldman, R. Hain and S. Liben), 271–283. Oxford: Oxford University Press.

National Institute for Health and Care Excellence (NICE) (2014). Constipation in children and young people. NICE Quality Standards [QS62]. https://www.nice.org.uk/Guidance/QS62 (accessed 4 August 2022).

National Institute for Health and Care Excellence (2016). End-of-life care for infants, children and young people with life-limiting conditions: planning and management. [NG61] [online]. www.nice.org.uk/guidance/NG61/chapter/Recommendations#managing-agitation (accessed 4 August 2022).

Needle, J.S. (2010). Home extubation by a pediatric critical care team: providing a compassionate death outside the pediatric intensive care unit. *Pediatric Critical Care Medicine* 11: 401–403.

Oxberry, S.G., Torgerson, D.J., Bland, J.M. et al. (2011). Short-term opioids for breathlessness in stable chronic heart failure: a randomized controlled trial. *European Journal of Heart Failure* 13: 1006–1012.

Paediatric Palliative Care Consultant Teams based at Evelina London Children's Hospital, Great Ormond Street Hospital for Children NHS Foundation Trust and The Royal Marsden NHS Foundation Trust, Surrey/Shooting Star Chase Children Hospice Care (2015) Artificial Nutrition and Hydration (ANH) guidelines for children and young people at end of life (unpublished).

Parshall, M.B., Schwartzstein, R.M., Adams, L. et al. (2012). 185 (4): 435-452. https://doi.org/10.1164/rccm.201111-2042ST.

Rajapakse, D. and Comac, M. (2012). Symptoms in life-threatening illness: overview and assessment. In: *Oxford Textbook of Palliative Care for Children* (eds. A. Goldman, R. Hain and S. Liben), 167–177. Oxford: Oxford University Press.

Rapoport, A., Shaheed, J., Newman, C. et al. (2013). Parental perceptions of forgoing artificial nutrition and hydration during end-of-life care. *Pediatrics* 131: 861–869.

Rodgers, C.C., Hooke, M.C., and Hockenberry, M.J. (2013). Symptom clusters in children. *Current Opinion in Supportive and Palliative Care* 7: 67–72.

Royal College of Nursing (RCN) (2009). The recognition and assessment of acute pain in children. Update of full guidance. RCN London. https://www.euroespa.com/wp-content/uploads/2014/10/003542.pdf (accessed 3 August 2022).

Schindera, C., Tomlinson, D., Bartels, U. et al. (2014). Predictors of symptoms and site of death in paediatric palliative patients with cancer at end of life. *American Journal of Hospice & Palliative Medicine* 31: 548–552.

Sinha, S., Bastin, M.E., Wardlaw, J.M. et al. (2004). Effects of dexamethasone on peritumoural oedematous brain: a DT-MRI study. *Journal of Neurology, Neurosurgery, and Psychiatry* 75: 1632–1635.

Teasdale, G., Allan, D., Brennan, P. et al. (2014). Forty years on: updating the Glasgow Coma Scale. *Nursing Times* 110 (42): 12–16.

The Children's Trust (2011). Care pathway for children and young people with life-threatening and life-limiting conditions related to severe acquired brain injury. The Children's Trust. London.

Thompson, A., Macdonald, A., and Holden, C. (2012). Feeding in palliative care. In: *Oxford Textbook of Palliative Care for Children*, 2e (eds. A. Goldman, R. Hain and S. Liben), 284–294. Oxford: Oxford University Press.

Together for Short Lives (2011). A care pathway to support extubation within a children's palliative care framework [online]. https://www.togetherforshortlives.org.uk/app/uploads/2018/01/ProRes-Extubation-Care-Pathway.pdf (accessed 4 August 2022).

Together for Short Lives (2013). A core care pathway for children with life-limiting and life-threatening conditions (3rd edition) [online]. https://www.togetherforshortlives.org.uk/app/uploads/2018/01/ProRes-Core-Care-Pathway.pdf (accessed 4 August 2022).

Together for Short Lives (2016). *Basic Symptom Control in Paediatric Palliative Care-The Rainbows Children's Hospice Guideline. 9th edition*, 5e. Together for Short Lives.

Vera, M. (2018). Making sense of health assessment and physical examination the easy way! Nursing Health Assessment Mnemonics & Tips. https://nurseslabs.com/nursing-health-assessment-mnemonics-tips/ (accessed 4 August 2022).

Vesely, C. and Beach, B. (2013). One Facility's experience in reframing non-feeding into a comprehensive palliative care model. *Journal of Obstetric, Gynecologic & Neonatal Nursing* 42: 383–389.

Willock, J., Baharestani, M., and Anthony, D. (2007). A risk assessment scale for pressure ulcers in children. *Nursing Times* 103 (14): 32–33. https://www.nursingtimes.net/clinical-archive/tissue-viability/a-risk-assessment-scale-for-pressure-ulcers-in-children-03-04-2007/ (accessed 4 August 2022).

World Health Organisation (WHO) (2012). *WHO guidelines on the pharmacological treatment of persisting pain in children with medical illnesses* [online]. https://www.apsoc.org.au/PDF/SIG-Pain_in_Childhood/WHO_Guidelines.pdf (accessed 4 August 2022).

Zernikow, B., Michel, E., Craig, F., and Anderson, B.J. (2009). Pediatric palliative care: use of opioids for the management of pain. *Paediatric Drugs* 11: 129–151.

Further reading

Department of Health (DH) (2007). Palliative and end of life care profiles: March 2022 data update. https://www.gov.uk/government/statistics/palliative-and-end-of-life-care-profiles-march-2022-data-update (accessed 31 October 2022).

National Palliative and End-of-life Care Partnership (2015). http://endoflifecareambitions.org.uk/wp-content/uploads/2015/09/Ambitions-for-Palliative-and-End-of-Life-Care.pdf (accessed 4 August 2022).

Rosen, D.S., Blum, R.W., Britto, M. et al. (2003). Transition to adult health care for adolescents and young adults with chronic conditions. *Journal of Adolescent Health* 33: 309–311.

Chapter 26

Perioperative care

Ciara McMullin[1], Anthony Baker[2], Claire Cook[3], Yvonne Hambley[4], and Melissa Silva[5]

[1] BSc Hons (Paediatrics), Dip Nursing (Adult): Head of Nursing and Patient Experience, GOSH
[2] Formerly Practice Educator, Theatres, Great Ormond Street Hospital, London, UK
[3] Team Leader for Spinal Surgery, GOSH
[4] RN (adult), DipHE (child health): Sister, Recovery, GOSH
[5] BSc (Nursing), MSc Nursing (Education): Formerly Assistant Practice Educator, Theatres, GOSH

Chapter contents

Introduction	596	Recovery	597
Preoperative preparation	596	References	617
Intra operative care	597	Further reading	619

Procedure guidelines

26.1	Pre-admission	598	26.4 Care in the anaesthetic room	601
26.2	Admission to hospital	598	26.5 Care in the operating theatre	602
26.3	Immediately prior to theatre	600	26.6 Care in recovery	609

Principles tables

26.1	Consent	599	26.3 Premedication	600
26.2	Fasting	599		

The Great Ormond Street Hospital Manual of Children and Young People's Nursing Practices, Second Edition. Edited by Elizabeth Anne Bruce, Janet Williss, and Faith Gibson.
© 2023 John Wiley & Sons Ltd. Published 2023 by John Wiley & Sons Ltd.

Introduction

Perioperative care is a term that incorporates the care given to children and young people (CYPs) before, during, and after surgical and invasive procedures (Steelman 2015). The operating theatre can be perceived as a very foreign environment (Shields 2010), where CYPs, their families, and carers can often feel quite vulnerable. It is also one of the only places in the hospital environment where parents are not able to be present during their child's stay, which can lead to heightened anxiety and a feeling of a loss of control. Because of this, CYPs, their families, and carers all require support, reassurance, and effective communication from the perioperative staff (Dreger and Trembeck 2006) and have the right to know that they will be cared for safely, with dignity and respect. This is especially true during intraoperative care, where the staff act as an advocate for the anaesthetised CYP. Intraoperative care is a team approach, which involves a variety of professionals all looking after different aspects of the CYP's specific needs in the operating department (Hughes and Mardell 2009). Effective communication and obtaining consent are important in all aspects of children's nursing care, particularly in the perioperative period. For more information regarding communication and consent see sections 7 and 8 of the Introduction. This chapter is divided into three sections; the first covers preoperative preparation, the second intraoperative care, and the final section, care in recovery.

Preoperative preparation

The preoperative period is a vital part of perioperative care, in which nurses play an important role in ensuring that the CYP and their family are fully prepared both physically and psychologically for the ensuing procedure. CYPs who are adequately prepared for their procedure and provided with the appropriate information often demonstrate increased coping and a reduction in anxiety (Brewer et al. 2006; Fortier et al. 2009). Preoperative preparation has increasingly been recognised as an important part of perioperative care and, as part of the National Health Service (NHS) Plan (Department of Health [DH] 2000), the NHS Modernisation Agency published recommendations for preoperative assessment to improve preparation and assessment of the patient (Royal College of Anaesthetists 2016). These guidelines incorporate both physical and psychological aspects of care and although they are adult focused, many of the principles apply to CYPs. For more information on the preparation of CYPs for procedures and investigations see Chapter 15: Investigations and Chapter 27: Play as a Therapeutic Tool.

The CYP should be as fit as possible before undergoing anaesthesia and an invasive procedure to minimise the risk of complications. A thorough assessment of their physical condition, medical history, and required and appropriate investigations should be undertaken. The anaesthetist is likely to use an established 'scoring' system developed by the American Society of Anesthesiologists (ASA) (2014) (Figure 26.1), which allows a subjective assessment of a patient's overall health.

Historically, investigations have been performed routinely as a precaution. However, the National Institute for Health and Care Excellence (NICE) issued guidelines aimed at streamlining preoperative investigations to avoid unnecessary tests, as these are time consuming and costly to the health service (Association of Anaesthetists of Great Britain and Ireland (AAGBI) 2010; NICE 2016). Whether investigations are required or not will be dependent on the type of surgery to be undertaken and the health of the CYP. Those with complex medical histories will require investigations and/or treatment to ensure they are in optimum condition prior to the invasive procedure. It is a recommendation of the Royal College of Surgeons (2007) that complex paediatric surgery should be centralised in units where this work is carried out routinely in order to provide the best outcomes for the CYP.

Although there is no consensus on the best way to prepare CYPs for surgery, most studies agree that some form of preoperative preparation is beneficial (Li 2007; Kain et al. 2007; Fortier et al. 2009; Royal College of Nursing [RCN] 2011) and may help reduce pain and other postoperative sequelae, including nightmares, bedwetting, and other regressive behaviour (Kain et al. 2006; Fortier et al. 2009). The psychological effects of surgery vary according to age and cognition and an understanding of a CYP's development is required to enable the best methods of preparation to be selected and undertaken. It is equally important that parents/carers are adequately prepared, as their anxiety can affect the way the CYP responds to stress. Information provided at this time should also cover what to expect on discharge from hospital.

Parents, carers, and CYPs are often well informed about procedures through access to the internet and services such as NHS direct. It is important to check any information obtained in this way and ensure the family has accurate information and has fully understood both the procedure and what to expect during the recovery period.

ASA I	A normal healthy patient
ASA II	A patient with mild systemic disease
ASA III	A patient with severe systemic disease
ASA IV	A patient with severe systemic disease that is a constant threat to life
ASA V	A moribund patient who is not expected to survive without the operation
ASA VI	A declared brain-dead patient whose organs are being removed for donor purposes

The addition of "E" denotes emergency surgery (An emergency is defined as existing when a delay in treatment of the patient would lead to a significant increase in the threat to life or body part)

Figure 26.1 ASA status (American Society of Anesthesiologists 2014).

Intra operative care

Prior to the arrival of the CYP in the theatre department, all members of the intraoperative team should have been informed of all relevant information and have appropriately prepared the environment. It is the responsibility of the intraoperative team; medical, nursing, and allied health professionals, to ensure that the environment is safe, so that the only trauma experienced by the CYP is the intended surgery. Appropriate risk assessments, using relevant risk assessment tools, are carried out where necessary (RCN 2011). The intraoperative team are dependent on the preoperative and anaesthetic assessments, the operator or surgeon's knowledge of the CYP, and their ward-based colleagues to ensure that all relevant information is communicated to them. This should be done before they are brought to the department, as omissions may compromise the quality of the intraoperative care. A preoperative checklist is often used to document that the required steps in the preparation have been undertaken. Examples include identification of loose milk teeth, the discussion and agreements for a Jehovah's Witness having major surgery, and precautions for individuals with latex allergy or a chronic condition. For the management of a CYP with latex allergy, both interoperatively and in recovery, see box 26.1. Some centres advocate the benefits of preoperative visits by theatre staff to enhance such information exchanges (Harris 2007) but this practice is not universal. All relevant information is disseminated to the intraoperative team in a safety briefing prior to the intended procedure. Procedural team briefing is an essential part of ensuring safe patient care in the intraoperative environment (World Health Organisation (WHO) 2009; NHS England Patient Safety Domain 2015). The WHO Safe Surgery Checklist is designed to minimise errors and incidents that occur during, or result from surgical procedures (WHO 2008). The introduction of the National Safety Standards for Invasive Procedures (NatSSIPs) in 2015 incorporated and added to this, and includes the safety briefing, the sign in, the time out and the sign out (NHS England Patient Safety Domain 2015). Intraoperative personnel should have been trained and have experience in routine and emergency care of CYPs (American Academy of Pediatrics 2015). The theatre environment and other areas where CYPs undergo general anaesthesia, should possess not only equipment required for routine procedures but also for emergency and unexpected events. A difficult intubation trolley, emergency trolley equipped with appropriate-sized resuscitation equipment, and appropriate paediatric concentrations of all relevant drugs must be available prior to induction of anaesthesia. Commonly, paediatric patients will be induced via inhalation agents. This may cause anxiety in some CYPs and various techniques are employed to help ease this, including scented masks, administering the inhalation agent directly from the circuit, anaesthetising the CYP on the parent/carer's lap where possible, and allowing preoperative play with the mask (Fortier et al. 2011). Background noise should be kept to a minimum during induction and intraoperative personnel should employ age appropriate methods of communication. The intraoperative setting also provides an opportunity to assess CYPs for any signs of abuse and neglect, as they will be exposed without parental supervision (Difusco 2015). Intraoperative staff should be able to recognise signs and symptoms and be aware of reporting arrangements, should they suspect any incidence of this. For more information regarding the signs and symptoms of abuse and neglect see Chapter 31: Safeguarding.

Recovery

The recovery room provides a way of smoothing the transition of care from the operating theatre to the ward area. The primary role of the recovery nurse is to safeguard the CYP until they have recovered from their anaesthesia and operative procedure. Recovery from anaesthesia is widely documented as one of the most dangerous periods during a surgical admission and therefore the CYP must be observed closely and never left unattended (RCN 2013). Many factors contribute to this danger; the CYP may be in the deeper stages of sedation and unable to maintain his/her protective reflexes and may also have received paralysing agents and/or opioid analgesia, which also increase the risk of sedation and airway compromise.

Recovery staff should be aware of the four stages of inhalational anaesthetic induction, as the CYP returns to consciousness through these stages in reverse. In particular, stage 2 poses a challenge during the recovery period due to the potential for laryngeal spasm and further airway compromise (Figure 26.2).

Box 26.1 Intraoperative care of CYPs at risk of latex allergy:

- All doors to the anaesthetic room and theatre must display 'Latex allergy' signs.
- All products must be checked for presence of latex. Latex containing products must be either removed or covered, e.g. latex tubing on equipment should have latex- safe tape wrapped around it in order to cover it completely. Theatre hats with elastic must not be worn.
- Following removal/ covering of latex products, in an operating room with standard air changes of at least 25 per hour, there should be an interval of at least 30 minutes to allow any latex particles to be sufficiently reduced to make the environment safe. N.B. There is limited evidence regarding whether this is necessary where all gloves are of non-powdered type.
- The CYP should be first on the list where possible, if this is not possible, follow the above instructions to create a safe environment.
- All staff must be aware of the CYP's status and this must be acknowledged during all phases of the WHO checklist.
- Non-latex surgical gloves must be used for all surgical procedures and preparation of instruments.

Postoperative care of CYPs at risk of latex allergy:
- CYPs can be recovered in the main recovery area, but where possible, recover those with confirmed latex anaphylaxis in theatre.
- Postoperative observations must include looking for signs or symptoms of potential allergic reaction, including swelling mucous membranes, rhinoconjunctivitis, increasing respiratory effort, wheezing, pruritis, and/ or rash.

Stage 1 : Analgesia or disorientation	CYP is sedated but conscious; breathing is slow and regular. This stages ends with loss of consciousness.
Stage 2 : Excitement or delirium	Airway reflexes remain intact and are often hypersensitive to stimulation. Risk of laryngospasm; spastic movements, vomiting, and rapid, irregular respirations can compromise the patient's airway.
Stage 3 : Surgical anaesthesia	Anaesthetic level for procedures requiring general anaesthesia. Airway manipulation is safe at this level. There are 4 "planes" in this stage; plane 3 is considered ideal for most surgeries as it involves relaxation of the intercostal and abdominal muscles and loss of the pupillary light reflex.
Stage 4 : Overdose	CYP receives too much anaesthetic in relation to the surgical stimulation. Without cardiovascular and respiratory support, this stage is lethal.

Figure 26.2 Stages of anaesthesia.
Source: Guedel (1937); Siddiqui and Kim (2021).

Procedure guideline 26.1 Pre-admission

Statement	Rationale
1 Where possible the family should be offered a preadmission visit.	1 To prepare them in a relaxed manner and allow them to familiarise themselves with the hospital environment.
2 Where a preadmission service is available the following should be undertaken: a) A physical assessment of the CYP. b) Relevant investigations (see NICE 2016). c) Psychological preparation of the CYP and family using age-appropriate methods. d) Information should be both written and verbal about the hospital and the procedure or surgery and its associated risks, including the risk of surgical site infection.	2 a) To ensure they are fit for surgery and identify any preexisting conditions that may increase the risk of anaesthesia/surgery. b) To ensure test results are available prior to surgery and action can be taken if abnormalities are found. c) To reduce anxiety and minimise adverse postoperative sequelae. d) To ensure that the family are fully informed of risks and benefits and can give informed consent for the procedure (NICE 2008a; DH 2009).
3 If a preadmission service is not available, information leaflets should be sent to the family prior to admission, including hospital details, what the procedure entails and what to expect afterwards, suggestions on how to prepare their child, fasting information, and a telephone number to ring if there are any queries.	3 To ensure they know what to expect both on admission and for discharge and can adequately prepare for the procedure. A range of information leaflets are available on the GOSH website at https://www.gosh.nhs.uk/conditions-and-treatments/conditions-we-treat/.

Procedure guideline 26.2 Admission to hospital

Statement	Rationale
1 The family should be greeted when they arrive on the ward and orientated as soon as possible.	1 To promote a welcoming environment and to put the family at ease.
2 If the CYP has been preadmitted, check that there has been no change in health status since the preadmission visit.	2–3 To ensure the CYP is fit for anaesthesia and surgery.
3 If the CYP has not been preadmitted they will need to be examined and a history taken, along with any relevant investigations.	
4 Check that the CYP's details are correct and apply an identity band, ensuring correct spelling of their name, date of birth and NHS/hospital number, and that these details correspond with information on the medical notes. If this is not possible (e.g. due to nonadherence/allergy, etc.) then an alternative method of identification must be used, as stated in local policy.	4 To ensure correct identification of CYP.
5 Check and record vital signs, including temperature, blood pressure, and where appropriate, oxygen saturation levels	5 To provide baseline observations as a reference point for observations during and after surgery. For more information on patient assessment see Chapter 1: Assessment.
6 If the CYP is pyrexial, the anaesthetist and surgical team must be informed.	6 It may be necessary to cancel the operation to prevent the risk of postoperative complications.

Procedure guideline 26.2 Admission to hospital (continued)

Statement	Rationale
7 Check that the CYP has not had a recent cough or cold.	7 To identify and prevent potential respiratory complications (Manley and Bellman 2000).
8 Check that there has been no contact with infectious diseases in past two weeks.	8 Incubation period of most childhood infectious diseases is between 12 hours and 21 days (e.g. norovirus and varicella respectively).
9 If the CYP has been in contact with a childhood infectious disease surgery should be postponed.	9 To avoid potential contamination of other patients and staff and the risk of anaesthetic complications.
10 Nose and throat swabs, skin lesion swabs and stool and urine samples may be taken on admission, depending on hospital policy.	10 To screen for antimicrobial resistance such as MRSA infection (DH 2007a) and for any abnormalities in the urine.
11 For females of menstruating age (this age is defined by local policy, usually from 12 years) undergoing surgery that poses a high risk to a foetus, pregnancy status must be checked in accordance with local procedures.	11 To protect any foetus from the adverse effects of surgery (Royal College of Paediatrics and Child Health 2012; NICE 2016). For more information, see Chapter 15: Investigations.
12 Weigh the CYP.	12 Accurate measurement of weight is required to prescribe appropriate drug dosages.
13 Complete relevant documentation, including weight, allergies, and relevant medical and social history.	13 To provide information and comply with legal and professional requirements.
14 Discuss with the family and the CYP, if appropriate, what they understand about why they have come to hospital.	14 To ascertain their level of comprehension and to correct any misunderstandings.
15 Where appropriate, use play therapy to prepare the CYP for their procedure.	15 To help them understand what is going to happen and allow them to work through any anxieties For more information see Chapter 27: Play as a Therapeutic Tool.

Principles table 26.1 Consent

Principle	Rationale
1 Consent should be obtained by a clinician who is capable of performing the procedure or has had specialist training in giving advice about the procedure (DH 2009).	1 To comply with legal requirements and to ensure that any queries can be fully answered. Ultimately it is the responsibility of the clinician performing the procedure to ensure that the family are fully informed and that informed consent has been obtained.
2 The consent form must be signed by a person with parental responsibility (if CYP is not able to give consent).	2 Only individuals with parental responsibility can legally give consent for surgery. For more information on consent and parental responsibility, see the Introduction.

Principles table 26.2 Fasting

Principle	Rationale
1 a) The following minimum fasting periods prior to surgery and anaesthesia are recommended by the Association of Anaesthetists of Great Britain and Ireland (2010): • Six hours for food, infant formula, and milk • Four hours for breast milk • Two hours for a clear drink b) At GOSH, the fasting policy for clear fluids is one hour before general anaesthesia, unless there is clear contraindication. c) The one hour fasting is contraindicated in CYPs with the following conditions: • GORD – either on treatment, (ranitidine, domperidone or omeprazole), or under investigation • Renal failure • Enteropathies – problems with digestion and absorption • Oesophageal strictures or those booked for oesophageal dilatation • Achalasia • Diabetes mellitus	1 a) To ensure minimal residual gastric volume and minimise the risk of vomiting and aspirating stomach contents into the lungs during induction of anaesthesia. Clear fluids are defined as water, lemon or orange squash, orange or apple ready-diluted drinks, and nonfizzy sports drinks. Clear fluids do not include fruit juice, milk including baby formula, fizzy drinks, red or purple drinks, caffeine drinks or hot drinks. Milk, sweets and chewing gum are considered as a **food**. b) With a 1-hour clear fluid policy, there is no increased risk of pulmonary aspiration and studies demonstrate the stomach is empty (Thomas et al 2018). c) To minimise the risk of aspiration in CYPs with slower gastric emptying.

(continued)

The Great Ormond Street Hospital Manual of Children and Young People's Nursing Practices

Principles table 26.2 Fasting (continued)

Principle	Rationale
2 a) It is essential that the period of fasting is not extended unnecessarily. Good communication with theatre staff regarding list changes and delays will help to avoid this. b) Premature infants and neonates may need an intravenous infusion prior to theatre.	2 a) Prolonged fasting can increase anxiety, irritability, dehydration, and postoperative healing times (Manley and Bellman 2000). b) This group are at greater risk of dehydration and hypoglycaemia, particularly with prolonged fasting times.
3 CYPs with certain metabolic conditions need careful consideration with regard to fasting times and placement on the list.	3 This group are at greater risk of metabolic imbalance if starved for too long.

Principles table 26.3 Premedication

Principle	Rationale
1 Premedication, when prescribed, should preferably be administered orally. The intramuscular (IM) route should be avoided wherever possible. However, it is used occasionally (eg. for atropine in high risk patients), as the effect is more reliable than by the oral route (British National Formulary for Children (BNFC) 2022).	1 Oral medications are more acceptable to CYP and family. IM injections are painful for the CYP and traumatic for all involved.
2 Sedative premedication, most commonly a benzodiazepine such as midazolam, may be prescribed if the CYP is anxious. This should be administered 30 minutes prior to going to theatre.	2 To reduce anxiety. The peak effect of midazolam is between 30 and 45 minutes.
3 Anticholinergic drugs such as atropine are rarely used, as modern inhalational anaesthetics are less irritant to the airways than previous agents. However, they may be required for certain conditions and procedures such as ear, nose, and throat (ENT) surgery.	3 To prevent reflex bradycardia and to reduce secretions.
4 Gastric motility drugs may be prescribed for those CYPs who are predisposed to gastro-oesophageal reflux.	4 To reduce the likelihood of vomiting and aspiration on induction of anaesthesia.
5 Local anaesthetic cream (e.g. EMLA or Ametop), where prescribed, should be applied to appropriate sites (e.g. back of the hands and antecubital fossa) 1 hour prior to theatre.	5 To allow time for cream to take effect to reduce the pain of cannula insertion.
6 CYPs with underlying conditions such as asthma or epilepsy may need medication prior to theatre.	6 To maintain therapeutic drug levels and minimise the risk of symptoms.

Procedure guideline 26.3 Immediately prior to theatre

Statement	Rationale
1 The CYP should have had a recent bath/shower/wash and hair wash prior to the procedure and will usually wear a theatre gown or dignity suit, although for some procedures it may be possible for them to wear their own clothes.	1 To minimise the risk of infection. To provide easy access to the operation site and easy attachment of monitoring equipment.
2 a) Any nail varnish should be removed. b) All jewellery, including body piercings should be removed or taped over. If piercings are left in situ, this must be documented in the CYP's notes and skin condition checked immediately before and after the surgical procedure.	2 a) Nail varnish prevents a clear view of the colour of the nail bed and may obscure observation of cyanosis. It also interferes with pulse oximetry. b) Jewellery increases the risk of accidental burns when diathermy is used.
3 The surgical site, if appropriate, must be marked before the CYP leaves the ward. This should be done by the operating surgeon or a nominated deputy.	3 To ensure correct site surgery. Wrong site surgery is a 'never event' (NHS England Patient Safety Domain 2015; NHS Improvement 2018).

Procedure guideline 26.3 Immediately prior to theatre *(continued)*

Statement	Rationale
4 Final checks and a preoperative checklist must be completed before leaving the ward to ensure that: a) The CYP is wearing an identity band and that the information matches that on the medical notes. b) The consent form is present with notes and has been signed. c) The CYP has been fasted for the relevant time period. **NB: If the CYP has not been fasted, the procedure will need to be delayed.**	4 a, b) To ensure that the CYP is identifiable and that all relevant documentation accompanies them to theatre. c) To minimise risk of aspiration.
5 A nurse or appropriately trained healthcare assistant should accompany the CYP to theatre.	5 To provide support for the family and handover the care of the CYP to the theatre staff.
6 If sedation has been given the CYP should be transferred to theatre on a trolley, with oxygen and suction available, and be accompanied by a registered nurse.	6 To minimise the risk of complications. Sedation may cause respiratory depression and loss of protective reflexes.
7 In the anaesthetic room the parents/carers can usually stay with their child until they are anaesthetised.	7 To provide reassurance.
8 The nurse or healthcare assistant should also remain until the CYP is anaesthetised and escort the parents/carers back to the ward.	8 To provide support for the family during and immediately after induction.

Procedure guideline 26.4 Care in the anaesthetic room

Statement	Rationale
1 The anaesthetic room should be fully prepared, with the necessary and appropriate sized equipment available, and the drugs already checked and ready for use.	1 To minimise delays.
2 Perioperative team members should have had training in minimising anxiety in CYPs and their families. Age appropriate methods of distraction should be available, e.g. washable pictures on walls and ceilings, washable toys, hand held tablets.	2 To focus the CYP's attention away from the stressful procedures and environment and ensure appropriate communication to alleviate any stress and anxiety (Dreger and Trembeck 2006).
3 The CYP should be allowed to bring a special toy or comforter with them. This item should either be stored safely during the surgical procedure on the trolley/bed or kept by the family so that it is available immediately afterwards. This may extend to objects of a religious nature.	3 To enhance comfort during induction and ensure that spiritual needs are being met without compromising safety.
4 It is important for the CYP and parents/carers to be put at ease in order to ensure that the induction goes as smoothly as possible.	4 To build up a rapport swiftly and to make the experience as stress-free as possible (Kristensson-Hallstrom 2000).
5 The anaesthetic team should carry out the WHO surgical safety Sign in check; a full check using the CYP's records and identity band prior to induction to ensure they have the: • Correct CYP • Correct procedure • Correct starvation time • Correct side/limb marked (if applicable) • Correct consent form signed and dated (WHO 2009).	5 To avoid an incorrect procedure being carried out (NHS England Patient Safety Domain 2015; National Patient Safety Agency [NPSA] 2009a).
6 Where possible, the removal of clothing/surgical gown should occur once the CYP is anaesthetised. This may need to be done beforehand if access for the anaesthetist is restricted.	6 To preserve dignity. To facilitate a safe and smooth induction and promote safe positioning on the operating table (Donnelly 2005).
7 Glasses and/or hearing aids should not be removed until the CYP is anaesthetised. These should be stored safely and returned to the CYP as soon as they are conscious.	7 To facilitate communication before and after the procedure and to minimise stress.
8 The CYP can, where appropriate, be offered a choice of route for the administration of induction agents, inhalation or intravenous, even if they have had a topical anaesthetic cream administered.	8 They are more likely to cooperate if they have been consulted and have some control over pending events (Tan and Meakin 2010).
9 The CYP should be in a comfortable position for the induction; if safe and feasible, this may be while sitting on the parent/carer's lap.	9 To minimise stress during induction and enhance the effect of the induction agent.

(continued)

Procedure guideline 26.4 Care in the anaesthetic room *(continued)*

Statement	Rationale
10 The parent/carer should be allowed the opportunity to briefly say farewell to their child before leaving the anaesthetic room.	10 To meet their emotional needs.
11 a) Intravenous access is mandatory during anaesthesia. b) This should be secured firmly, in an aseptic manner (DH 2007b; Walker and Lockie 2000).	11 a) To ensure there is a secure route for the administration of drugs and/or fluids during the surgical procedure. b) To minimise the risk of extravasation and cannula site infection in the postoperative period (Harris 2007).
12 If the identity band has had to be removed during cannulation, a new one with the correct patient details should be placed on an unaffected limb as soon as possible.	12 To facilitate safe checking throughout the CYP's stay in the operating department (Morse 2007; NPSA 2009a).
13 Equipment used for airway management will depend on the type of surgery to be carried out. It must be positioned correctly and securely maintained.	13 To ensure continued airway maintenance throughout the procedure.
14 Eyes should be taped shut or appropriately padded, depending on the position for and type of surgery, and unless ophthalmic surgery is to be carried out.	14 To avoid accidental damage to the cornea (Harris 2007).

Procedure guideline 26.5 Care in the operating theatre

Statement	Rationale
1 All equipment required for the operating list should be clean, tested, and set up in theatre before the CYP arrives. The requirements for the procedure should be discussed in the team safety briefing and confirmed as being available (WHO 2009; NHS England Patient Safety Domain 2015). This includes; sterile sets and supplementaries, implants, operating tables, diathermy machines, tourniquets, laparoscopic stacks, monitors, and microscopes.	1 To ensure that all equipment required for the procedure is available and in safe working order.
2 The theatre should be fully prepared to receive the CYP, with all the necessary and appropriate-sized equipment ready for use, including table attachments, positioning aids, and diathermy.	2 To provide a safe environment for the CYP and staff. Each CYP is different and will require different equipment according to procedure, size, weight, and duration of stay in theatre.

Throat Packs

Statement	Rationale
1 The decision whether to use a throat pack should be clarified during the Team Brief.	1 To ensure that the entire team is informed. The decision to use a throat pack should be clearly justified and jointly agreed by the anaesthetist and surgeon for each patient.
2 a) Throat packs must always be included as part of the surgical count and marked up on the surgical count board. b) A 'Throat Pack' sticker should be placed on the heat moisture exchange filter. Clearly document the time that the throat pack is inserted.	2 a) To ensure that the throat pack is identified as an item to be counted and removed at the end of the procedure. b) To ensure that there is a formal visual check and documented evidence to reduce the risk of leaving a throat pack *in situ* (NPSA 2009b).
3 The person who places the throat pack is also responsible for removing it. If they leave the theatre prior to this, a deputy must be nominated.	3 To ensure that there is a nominated person responsible for the throat pack and to ensure that the throat pack is removed at the end of the procedure.
4 If a swab must be placed as a secondary pack during surgery, this must be documented on the surgical count board separately.	4 To identify that there are now two throat packs in situ and prevent the retention of a secondary pack.
5 If the scrub practitioner needs to be replaced during surgery a full surgical count must be undertaken, including the counting of the throat pack, with the replacing scrub practitioner.	
6 The Sign Out cannot be completed until the throat pack has been removed by the person who placed it or the agreed deputy. The entire team must remain in the theatre until the Sign Out is complete.	6 To ensure that the throat pack has been removed prior to the patient leaving the theatre.

Procedure guideline 26.5 Care in the operating theatre (continued)

Statement	Rationale
Thermoregulation	See also Chapter 20: Neonatal Care.
1 The theatre environment should be maintained at 21°C and should not dip below 19°C, unless instructed by the surgical team.	1 To provide a suitable environment and minimise the risk of hypothermia.
2 Room temperatures may need to be increased for neonatal surgery and for CYPs with extensive tissue damage, such as burns/scalds.	2 Neonates have immature thermoregulation systems and require assistance to maintain optimum temperature. Hypothermia in neonates may destabilise blood sugar levels and lead to increased oxygen needs (Brown et al. 2000; Wilson and da Cunha 2010). Excess fluid loss with extensive tissue damage can result in hypoxia due to hypovolaemic shock (Methven et al. 2007).
3 The use of a forced air-warming device should be considered in both the anaesthetic room and theatre environment for all surgical procedures.	3 To maintain the CYP's temperature. NICE (2008b) states that the patient's temperature can drop to below 35.0°C within the first 20–30 minutes of induction.
4 Warm antiseptic skin preparations should be considered. The use of alcohol-based solutions should be avoided for preterm infants.	4 Alcohol-based solutions evaporate, which can increase the potential for hypothermia (Harris 2007).
5 Intravenous fluids (500 ml or more) should be warmed to 37°C using a fluid warming device prior to being administered to the CYP.	5 To maintain the CYP's temperature NICE (2008b).
6 All irrigation fluids used intraoperatively should be warmed in a thermostatically controlled cabinet to 38–40°C before being dispensed onto the surgical field, unless otherwise stated by the surgeon.	6 To maintain the CYP's temperature.
Manual handling	
1 Appropriately sized transfer aids should be used to move the CYP to and from the trolley and operating table.	1 To protect the CYP and staff from injury.
2 When transferring a CYP to and from the operating table there should be one person in charge (usually the anaesthetist) who takes the lead, ensuring that the CYP is moved in their natural alignment and that all extremities move together.	2 To minimise the risk of injury (Association for Perioperative Practice [AfPP] 2011a). *For more information see Chapter 19: Moving and Handling.*
3 Co-ordination and communication is key when transferring the CYP to the operating table to ensure that all intravenous lines, monitoring and catheters (where applicable) are not caught during transfer.	3 To minimise the risk of injury (AfPP 2011a).
4 Handling of preterm infants, especially extremely low birth weight babies, should be kept to a minimum.	4 To reduce the effects of prolonged environmental stress (Askin and Wilson 2014). Preterm infants are unable to differentiate different types of stimuli so elici a physiological response to all stimuli (Meeks et al. 2009).
5 When using any specific positioning aids or operating tables (e.g. Jackson table, seated position, etc.) it is essential that: • All staff know how to use the attachments, aids, and tables. • The attachments are all in theatre ready to use. • There are enough members of staff to turn the CYP.	5 To protect the CYP and staff from injury.
Positioning	
1 The CYP should be placed in an optimum position for the surgery to be performed, ensuring that limbs are moved and secured in a 'neutral' state.	1 To facilitate surgical access and avoid potential limb dislocation and nerve damage. To avoid injury from hyperextension of the joints. To avoid potential pressure damage and to avoid accidental disconnection of anaesthetic medical devices (Smith 2007).
2 Careful consideration should be taken with CYPs with physical abnormalities and/or fixed limbs to ensure that limbs are not forced into a position, but a compromise position is found.	2 To minimise the risk of injury (AfPP 2011a).
3 Skin should be protected from contact with all metal objects, including table attachments and jewellery. Theatre practitioners should ensure that correct placement of attachments and padding is used.	3 To avoid intraoperative contact burns as a result of using diathermy (AfPP 2011a).
4 The surgeon should confirm that they are happy with the CYP's position before prepping and draping can occur.	4 To ensure surgical access is correct and avoid the need for repositioning.

(continued)

Procedure guideline 26.5 Care in the operating theatre *(continued)*

Statement	Rationale
Pressure care	For more information, see Chapter 11: Personal Hygiene and Pressure Ulcer Prevention.
1 Care should be taken to ensure that all potential pressure points are protected using appropriate equipment and aids such as gel pads, etc.	1 To avoid the formation of intraoperative pressure injuries.
2 The scrub practitioner should ensure that the sterile drapes and surgical equipment do not pose a pressure risk for the CYP during the surgical procedure.	2 To minimise the risk of pressure ulcers (Radford et al. 2004; Schober-Flores 2012).
3 The theatre practitioner should check to make sure that no monitoring cables or intravenous lines are underneath the CYP or at risk of being caught in the drapes when removed at the end of the case. Ensure that padding is used to cover or pad when required.	3 To avoid the formation of intraoperative pressure injuries. To avoid accidental disconnection of medical devices and intravenous lines (AfPP 2011a).
4 Girls who have started menstruating and all CYPs over 12 years of age who are undergoing long procedures should wear compression stockings and the use of pneumatic compression pumps should be considered.	4 To avoid intraoperative pressure injuries and deep vein thrombosis (AfPP 2011a).
5 The CYP's skin integrity should be checked pre and postsurgery and any change documented in their care plan, handed over verbally, and reported as per local guidelines.	5 To identify any changes that may occur and monitor/treat appropriately (AfPP 2011a).
Privacy and dignity	
1 The CYP should remain covered until the start of the surgical procedure.	1 To maintain their dignity and to reduce the potential for hypothermia.
WHO Surgical Safety Checklist Time Out	
1 This should be led by a scrub practitioner and carried out before the start of the procedure.	1 To identify a clear leader and time to carry out the Time Out (NPSA 2009a; WHO 2009; NHS England Patient Safety Domain 2015).
2 The surgeon, anaesthetist and scrub practitioner should confirm: a) CYP's Identity b) Procedure c) Site d) Position	2 To minimise the risk of errors by ensuring that they have the: a) Correct CYP b) Correct procedure c) Correct site d) Correct position for the procedure (NPSA 2009a)
3 The surgeon should confirm: • Plan • Imaging (if any) • Concerns • Estimated blood loss	3 To ensure the whole team knows what is planned.
4 The anaesthetist should confirm: • American Society of Anaesthesiologists (ASA) physical status classification score (ASA 2014) • Allergies • Antibiotics • Concerns • Local anaesthetic dose	4 To ensure everyone knows the CYP's status and to minimise risk.
5 The scrub practitioner should again confirm that all equipment necessary for procedure is available or on standby.	5 To ensure that the whole team knows what equipment is available.
Blood loss	
1 Theatre practitioners should keep accurate blood loss records.	1 To avoid intra- and postoperative hypovolaemia and associated complications. CYPs have small circulating fluid volumes, so accurate calculations are essential.
2 Intraoperative cell salvage should be considered for CYPs where high levels of blood loss are expected as an alternative method of blood replacement.	2 To reduce the immunological and infection risks of allogeneic blood.

Chapter 26 Perioperative care

Procedure guideline 26.5 Care in the operating theatre *(continued)*

Statement	Rationale

3 Swabs may be washed during a procedure:
  a) A litre bag of 0.9% Normal Saline is decanted into a bowl.
  b) Bloody swabs must be weighed before they are put into the bowl of saline.
  c) Digital scales should be available within the sterile field; this can be achieved by using a transparent sterile drape to cover the scales.
  d) The scales should be zeroed prior to use.
  e) Swabs must be weighed in the multiples that they come in.
  f) The scrub practitioner should call out to the circulating practitioner the type and weight of the wet swabs, for them to be documented.
  g) The circulating practitioner must record the time, swab type, dry and wet weights, and calculate the blood loss on the Blood Loss Form, which is then communicated to the anaesthetist.
  h) The standard suction should also be checked every hour for blood loss.
  i) After the swabs have been weighed they can be placed in the bowl of saline and gently washed.
  j) It is important that this is done delicately.
  k) The scrub nurse will then gently compress the swabs dry and remove from the saline.
  l) When swabs are ready to be given off the sterile field they must follow the surgical count policy.
  m) Near the end of the case, the scrub practitioner will use the cell salvage suction to suck up all the swab wash solution and notify the anaesthetist. This can be done every hour if requested by the anaesthetist.
  n) If during the case the scrub practitioner requires fresh swab wash, they must notify the anaesthetist when sucking up the wash.
  o) The circulating practitioner must clearly document the new total of wash used on the blood loss form.
  p) At the end of the case the Blood Loss form should be included in the medical/nursing notes.
	3 Up to 50% of blood loss may be collected into swabs. By washing swabs, a large amount of this blood can be recycled by the cell salvage unit (UK Cell Salvage Group 2015).
	  b) To provide an accurate record of blood loss.
	  c) The blood absorbed by the swab is estimated by this formula: Weight of wet swab − weight of dry swab = blood weight. 1 g of weight in blood is approximate to 1 ml of blood (Ince and Skinner 2000).
	
	  i) To release any cells that can be returned to the patient
	  j) To avoid damaging the cells. Gentle handling can limit the number of blood cells damaged prior to recycling by the cell salvage unit (UK Cell Salvage Group 2015).

Electrosurgical diathermy

Statement	Rationale

1 a) The electrosurgical unit (ESU) must be inspected by a competent practitioner prior to use, including all safety features for the make of electrosurgical unit.
  b) All cables and electrosurgical application electrodes must be checked prior to use.
  c) The volume of the activation sound indicator should be maintained at an audible level.
  d) The ESU should not be used in the presence of flammable agents.
  e) It should be operated at the lowest effective power setting to achieve the desired effect for coagulation and cutting.
  f) The CYP's skin integrity should be evaluated and documented in the perioperative care plan before and after ESU use.
	1 a) To ensure that the unit is functioning and safe to use.
	
	  b) To ensure integrity of equipment and prevent short circuits and accidental application of electrosurgical current (Woodhead and Wicker 2005).
	  c) To immediately alert staff when the electrosurgical unit is activated.
	  d) Ignition of flammable agents by the active electrodes can resulted in injuries to patient and staff.
	  e) To minimise the electrical current and risk of injury.
	  f) To identify any injuries or burns.

2 a) If two ESUs are used simultaneously they must have the same technology, e.g. both must be grounded or isolated.
  b) Ensure that the return electrode mat or adhesive return electrode pad (whichever is used) is the appropriate size for the CYP's weight, as per manufacturer's instructions.
  c) Before the start of the procedure, the intraoperative team must ensure that no part of the CYP is touching any earthed objects, such as the trim of the operating table or drip stands.
	2 a) To prevent the electricity from taking alternative pathways, which would increase the potential for burns (AfPP 2011a).
	  b) A reduced surface area increases the impedance of the electrical current, increasing the risk of unintentional burns.
	  c) Contact with metal can cause the electrical current to travel through the metal rather than the return electrode and can cause an unintentional burn (Potty et al. 2010).

(continued)

Procedure guideline 26.5 Care in the operating theatre *(continued)*

Statement	Rationale
3 When using a return electrode mat there must be a minimum amount of material between the patient and the mat. This includes draw sheets, sliding sheets, blankets, gamgee, nappies, and any other clothing. The return electrode mat should be placed on the operating table before transferring the CYP onto the operating table. Ensure manufacturers' instructions are followed in regard to required contact (Association of Perioperative Registered Nurses [AORN] 2009).	3 To ensure that there is enough of the CYP in contact with the return electrode mat to allow the current to safely pass through them and be returned to the electro surgical unit to prevent unintentional burns.
4 Disposable return electrodes should be placed on a well-vascularised site as close to the operating site as possible. If using a disposable return electrode plate, it should not be placed over: a) A bony prominence b) Implanted metal prosthesis c) Areas distal to a tourniquet d) Scar tissue e) Hairy surfaces f) Pressure points/areas (Spruce and Braswell 2012)	4 To reduce impedance of the current to prevent unintentional burns. b) To reduce the risk of superheating above the site of an implanted metal prosthesis. c, d) Adequate tissue perfusion is not assured if the dispersive electrode is placed distal to tourniquets or over scar tissue. e) Hair at the contact site prevents skin contact with the CYP's skin and allows arcing of electricity between the skin and the dispersive electrode (AfPP 2011a). f) To eliminate risk of current concentration.
5 a) The return electrode should be connected to the ESU prior to draping to ensure adequate contact and then the lead disconnected from the ESU temporarily to allow for the draping of the patient and the positioning of the surgeon. b) The return electrode and its connection to the ESU should be checked if any tension is applied to the cable if the surgical team repositions the CYP. c) The cable should not be wrapped around metal objects, e.g. theatre table trims. d) Return electrodes plates should not be used on CYPs suffering from epidermolysis bullosa. A return electrode mat or bipolar electrosurgery should be used instead.	5 a) To ensure that there is an adequate connection to allow for safe return of current. b) To ensure that the return electrode is not inadvertently disconnected. c) The electrode cable wrapped around metal objects could induce a current and cause an electrical shock to staff. d) To avoid any skin trauma upon removal due to the nature of the condition.
6 The power settings of the electrosurgical unit are determined in conjunction with the manufacturers written recommendations, patient size and type of procedure (Medicines and Healthcare products Regulatory Agency [MHRA] 2011; 2015).	6 To reduce the potential for injury and operate the electrosurgical unit at the lowest possible setting.
7 The active electrode tip should be easy to clean, securely placed & be single use (AORN 2009).	7 Eschar build-up on the active electrode tip inhibits the electrosurgical unit from working safely and properly.
8 When not in use the active electrode should be placed in a clean well-insulated holster. This is the responsibility of the scrub practitioner (Woodhead and Wicker 2005).	8 To minimise the risk of accidental activation and burn injuries to the CYP or staff.
9 a) After use, the return electrode plate should be removed carefully. If the condition of the skin is acceptable, verbal confirmation should be given to all members of the operating team. The CYP's skin integrity should be evaluated and documented before and after ESU use. b) Following removal of the electrode, if the skin appears to be damaged, the following should be carried out: • Inform the surgeon. • Carry out any prescribed treatment. • Record in the health care records. • Complete an Incident Report Form. • Inform staff in Recovery Room or whoever takes over care. • It is the surgeon's responsibility to inform the family.	9 a) To avoid damaging the surface of the skin. b) To ensure accurate documentation and the prompt detection and treatment of any injuries.
10 Staff should take special precautions when using the ESU in the presence of pacemakers and automatic defibrillators.	10 To ensure that there is no interference to the pacemaker or automatic defibrillator device. The ESU may interfere with the pacemaker or defibrillator's circuitry.

Procedure guideline 26.5 Care in the operating theatre *(continued)*

Statement	Rationale
11 The following additional precautions should be observed for CYPs with pacemakers: • Ensure the distance between the active electrode and the dispersive electrode is as short as possible. • Keep all ESU cables away from the pacemaker and its leads. • Have a defibrillator immediately available for emergencies during surgery. • Use bipolar diathermy where possible. • Have a magnet or control unit available.	11 The pacemaker may interpret electrosurgical current as cardiac activity and prevent the pacemaker from initiating a heartbeat.
12 CYPs with automatic implantable cardioverter/defibrillator (ACID) should have the ACID device deactivated before the electrosurgical unit is activated and a defibrillator immediately available for use (Potty et al. 2010).	12 Using electrosurgery on a CYP with an activated ACID may trigger an electrical shock.
13 The following precautions should be observed for CYPs with cochlear implants: • Use bipolar diathermy where possible. • If monopolar diathermy is deemed necessary by the surgeon ensure that the distance between the active electrode and the return electrode is as short as possible (Potty et al. 2010). This can be achieved by using a return electrode mat.	13 To ensure that the current path between the surgical site and dispersive electrode does not pass through the vicinity of the stimulator or leads.

Tourniquet use in theatres

Statement	Rationale
1 The tourniquet should be checked prior to use, ensuring that the cuff is not leaking, connections are not loose, tubing is not worn, and the equipment is clean.	1 To avoid potential damage to the CYP.
2 A selection of appropriate cuffs, padding and occlusion dressings must be readily available.	2 To facilitate optimal operating conditions for the surgery.
3 Padding should be placed under the cuff, which should be positioned on the point of the limb which offers the largest amount of soft tissue.	3 To provide natural padding for the nerves and vessels, thus helping to prevent peripheral nerve and vessel damage (Rothrock 2015).
4 Occlusion dressings should be placed around the edge of the cuff to protect the CYP's skin from prepping solutions.	4 To prevent chemical burns (Rothrock 2015).
5 Exsanguination of the limb must be done using one of the following methods • An Esmarch bandage • A roll cylinder • Limb elevation prior to inflation	5 To facilitate the venous return of blood from the limb and aid in the prevention of blood pooling in the veins.
6 a) It is the surgeon's responsibility to approve the tourniquet pressure setting. b) The circulating practitioner should inflate the cuff to the required pressure, ensuring that the cuff has inflated and activate the tourniquet clock, recording the time inflation on the theatre count board. c) If the tourniquet is inflated for over one hour the scrub practitioner should inform the surgeon and continue to do so for every half hour afterwards until the tourniquet pressure is released.	6 a) To prevent injury to the CYP or inadequate use of tourniquet. b) Over inflation will cause injury to the CYP and under inflation will not provide a bloodless operating field. c) To minimise the risk of damage to the CYP's circulation (AfPP 2011a).
7 The ultimate responsibility for the application and release of the tourniquet is that of the operating surgeon.	7 To ensure clear designation and responsibility for the use of the tourniquet during surgery (AfPP 2011a).
8 Any compromise to the integrity of the skin underlying the tourniquet cuff must be reported to the surgeon, an incident form completed and a record of the incident record in the CYP's health care records.	8 To provide accurate documentation in accordance with trust policy.
9 An explanation of the incident should be given to the CYP and their family at the earliest opportunity.	9 In accordance with trust policy and to facilitate the risk management process.
10 At the end of every use the cuff, tubing and tourniquet unit should be checked for damage, soiling, and should be cleaned with detergent wipes.	10 To prevent cross infection (AfPP 2011a,b).

(continued)

Procedure guideline 26.5 Care in the operating theatre *(continued)*

Statement	Rationale
The surgical count	
1 Surgical items, such as instruments, swabs and sharps used by the surgical team to perform invasive procedures, are foreign bodies and must be accounted for at all times to prevent retention and injury to the patient (AORN 2006; AfPP 2011b; Rothrock 2015; NHS England Patient Safety Domain 2015).	1 Foreign bodies are potential sources of infection and can cause harm to the CYP. Retained foreign objects are viewed as 'Never events' (NHS Improvement 2018).
2 The surgical count must be undertaken by a scrub practitioner and a circulating practitioner, one of which must be a registered member of the intraoperative team, usually a registered nurse or operating department practitioner (AfPP 2011b). The count should not be completed between two circulators or two scrub practitioners.	2 To reduce the risk of an inaccurate count.
3 The theatre environment should have a dry-wipe white board, which is preprinted and displays all the significant items used. The board must be a permanent fixture within the theatre and be visible and accessible to every team member (AfPP 2011a,b).	3 To allow all staff to easily see the number of items in the surgical field.
4 A count should be performed: a) Prior to the surgery commencing (Radford et al. 2004; AfPP 2011b). b) Before the closure of a cavity or a cavity within a cavity, with subsequent counts for each cavity closed (AfPP 2011b). c) At the closure of skin or at the end of the procedure (Radford et al. 2004).	4 a) To establish a baseline reference for all subsequent counts. b) To identify any retained items prior to closing the cavity. c) To ensure that all items are accounted for before the patient leaves the operating theatre.
5 On completion of a cavity count and the final count, the scrub practitioner must communicate to the operating surgeon that the cavity/final surgical count is correct and that all items are accounted for. The operating surgeon should also verbally acknowledge the fact that he/she has heard the scrub practitioner (Woodhead 2009; AfPP 2011b).	5 To facilitate good communication and avoid any misunderstanding.
6 Swabs retained in the wound to act as packs intraoperatively must be documented on the wipe board designated for the surgical count (AfPP 2011b). If they are to remain *in situ* post operatively this must be documented in the CYP's notes and care plan.	6 To facilitate good communication and avoid any misunderstanding that may lead to an inaccurate swab count or a swab being retained in the cavity. To ensure that any purposely retained items are recorded to be removed at a later date.
WHO Surgical Safety Checklist Sign Out (WHO 2009)	
1 This must be completed at the end of the procedure, before operating surgeon leaves theatre, and before transferring the CYP to recovery.	1 To ensure that the surgeon is available to confirm details of sign out.
2 Sign out must confirm the following: a) What procedure(s) have been completed? b) Have all consented procedure(s) been completed and if not then why? c) Are all surgical counts correct? d) Are there any specimens, are they labelled correctly, and is the request form correct? e) Has all documentation been completed correctly? f) What information does the surgeon and anaesthetist want handed over to recovery?	2 To ensure that the correct procedure(s) have been done and that no procedure is mistakenly omitted. c) To ensure that all items used in the surgery are accounted for (see section on surgical counts). e-f) To ensure that all care is documented and that the next area caring for the CYP has all the necessary information to provide the best possible care.
3 At the end of the case any critical incidents, e.g. equipment failure, unexpected blood loss, unforeseen complications etc. should be discussed.	3 To encourage learning and highlight areas of best practice and ensure that staff are supported in their further development. To aid in prevention of these incidents in the future (WHO 2009).

Chapter 26 Perioperative care

Procedure guideline 26.5 Care in the operating theatre (continued)

Statement	Rationale
Transfer to recovery	
1 a) Trolley sides should be fitted with protective 'bumpers' to prevent the CYP from injuring themselves. b) Trolleys should be fitted with oxygen for transfer (AAGBI 2013).	1 a) The CYP may become restless as consciousness returns (Harris 2007). b) To prevent hypoxaemia.
2 All intraoperative care records should be completed and authorised by the appropriate staff prior to the CYP's transfer to recovery, including the surgical counts.	2 To ensure completeness of documentation and surgical equipment prior to the transfer.
3 All used equipment, soiled linens, and sharps should be disposed of in compliance with Trust waste regulations.	3 To ensure the safe decontamination and disposal of surgical equipment and devices.
4 Pulse oximetry, ECG, noninvasive, and invasive monitoring should be readily available in each theatre for transferring the CYP to the recovery room.	4 To ensure the safe transfer of the CYP to the recovery room and observation of vital signs while in transit.

Procedure guideline 26.6 Care in recovery

Statement	Rationale
Preparation of Recovery Area	
1 At the beginning of each shift, check that the: a) Reintubation trolley is checked against the contents list, all items are present, and emergency drugs are in date. b) Resuscitation trolley has been checked as per guidelines. c) Defibrillator is in full working order and has passed the daily user test. d) Suction equipment is clean, in full working order, and has passed safety tests. e) Oxygen supplies (high and low flow) are in full working order. f) Emergency alarm bells are working. g) Emergency breathing systems, e.g. Mapleson's F and Mapleson's C, are checked and in working order (Hatfield 2014). h) Sharps containers are available. i) A supply of clean gowns and warmed blankets are available. j) Quality control checks have been performed on near patient testing equipment such as glucometers, Haemacue® and blood gas analyser systems. k) Any CYP who poses an infection risk has been identified and allotted a recovery bed space and nurse. l) CYPs with learning difficulties have been identified the allotted bed space (i.e. quieter with lower lighting).	1 To ensure all equipment used in the postoperative period is available and in working order. h) To ensure safe disposal of sharps used in an emergency. For more information on the safe use of sharps see Chapter 14: Intravenous and Intra-arterial Access and Infusions. i) To maintain the CYP's comfort.
2 Before each CYP arrives check that: • A clean Yankauer sucker is switched on and working. • An oxygen mask is connected and ready for use. • Saturation monitoring is switched on and working. • Blood pressure monitoring equipment is working and ready to connect. • ECG and invasive monitoring are readily available, if required. • Emergency breathing systems are available with appropriate fitting facemask (Hatfield 2014).	2 To ensure all equipment used in the postoperative period is available and in working order.

(continued)

The Great Ormond Street Hospital Manual of Children and Young People's Nursing Practices

Procedure guideline 26.6 Care in recovery *(continued)*

Statement	Rationale
Reception of the CYP into Recovery	
1 The recovery practitioner must receive handover from the anaesthetist, nursing scrub staff and on occasion, the surgical team.	1 To gain a full understanding of the CYP's history and operative procedure. To enable them to plan effective, safe care in the immediate postoperative period.
2 Anaesthetic handover must include the following details: • Name • Age • Known allergies • Significant medical/behavioural problems • Indications for surgery • Operative procedure and name of surgeon • Details of vital signs: blood pressure, pulse, and respiratory rate • Untoward incidents during or before surgery • Analgesia given and anticipated analgesic needs • Blood loss/fluid replacement • Blood components used/available • Intravenous fluids given and future needs • Antibiotics given and when the next dose is due • Urine output during the procedure and expected output for the next few hours • Anxiety level and preoperative psychological problems • Further investigations required • How much oxygen is required and how to administer it • Monitoring required in the recovery room and on return to the ward • Possible language barrier • If a throat pack has been used and subsequently removed • Confirmation that all intravenous lines have been flushed and documented on the anaesthetic chart • Isolation precautions and the reason required	2 To plan safe, effective care in the immediate postoperative period and ensure that accurate documentation is maintained in preparation for the CYP's return to the ward (see Figure 26.3).
3 Intraoperative nursing staff handover should include: • Care and placement of drains • Precautions about dressings • Special nursing requirements, such as positioning of the CYP • Nursing problems such as pressure ulcers • Ensuring correct charts and investigation results accompany the patient • Personal belongings such as hearing aids and comforters, toys, etc. are present (Hatfield 2014) • Preoperative skin assessment	3 To plan effective care in the immediate postoperative period.

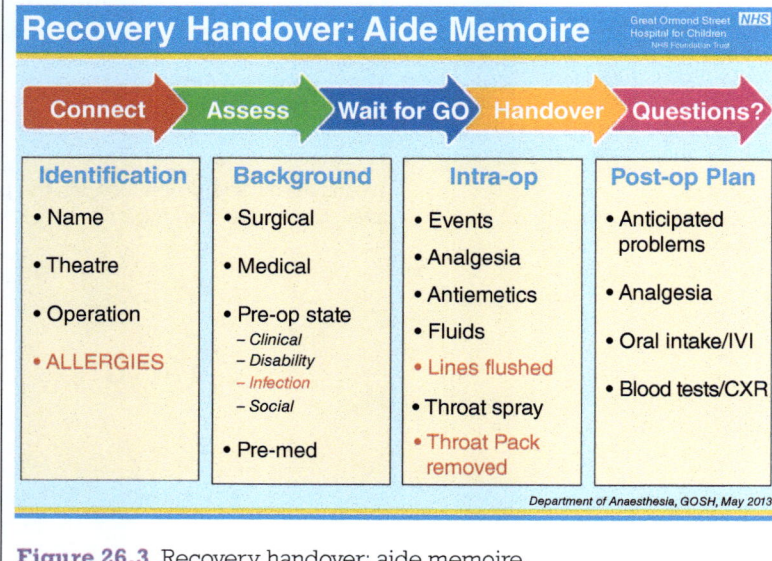

Figure 26.3 Recovery handover: aide memoire.

Procedure guideline 26.6 Care in recovery (continued)

Statement	Rationale
Reception of the CYP into Recovery	
4 Surgical handover should be included if there are specific surgical instructions.	4, 5 To minimise complications and plan effective care in the immediate postoperative period (Hatfield 2014).
5 Before the anaesthetist leaves the recovery room the CYP must be breathing spontaneously and have satisfactory oxygen saturation levels, and a stable blood pressure and pulse rate. The anaesthetist must provide a contact number and remain in close proximity while the CYP is in the recovery room or have handed care over to a colleague.	
Initial Assessment	
1 On arrival to the recovery unit, a thorough head to toe assessment of the CYP's physiological status must be conducted:	1 To assess their physiological status and detect and prevent deterioration in their condition.
Airway assessment	
1 Assess the airway; is the CYP self-ventilating/requiring assisted ventilation/maintaining own airway/requiring airway support?	1 To ensure the CYP has a clear airway, is breathing and air is moving freely and quietly in and out of the chest.
2 Observe for signs of partial or complete airway obstruction i.e. supracostal, intercostal, and subcostal retraction, inspiratory stridor, or crowing, nasal flaring, tracheal tug, or decreased/absent air entry (Hatfield 2014). • Common causes of airway obstruction include: • Tongue • Laryngospasm • Foreign bodies such as vomit, acidic gastric contents, mucous, blood/secretions, and dislodged teeth	2–4 To ensure the CYP has a patent airway.
3 Determine the need for techniques to open the airway and the continued use/insertion of airway adjuncts until the CYP begins to regain consciousness:	
4 Manual techniques: • Chin tilt: neutral position for neonates, 'sniffing the morning air' for small child • Jaw thrust for adolescents/adults	
5 Airway adjuncts: • Nasopharyngeal airway • Oral pharyngeal airway • Laryngeal mask airway • Endotracheal tube • Tracheostomy tube • Nasal stent	5 If manual actions do not open the airway, an artificial airway may need to be inserted (Rothrock 2015).
6 If there are secretions/vomit/blood present in the airway, gently suction the oral-pharynx/naso-pharynx/trachea.	6 To maintain a clear airway.
7 Administer oxygen 6 l/min (40%) via a clear facemask. If a laryngeal mask is used, administer oxygen at 10 l/min (40%) via Recovery T-kit.	7 To prevent hypoxaemia. The demand for oxygen is high and the protective responses to hypercarbia and hypoxaemia are limited (Litwack et al. 1991). Causes of hypoventilation include depression of the respiratory centres due to opiates and residual anaesthetic drugs (Hatfield 2014).
8 Attach pulse oximetry monitoring.	8 To assess oxygen saturation levels.
9 Observe the CYP closely for complications of anaesthesia such as laryngospasm. Indicative symptoms include noisy or shallow respirations, nasal flaring, retractions, stridor, dyspnoea, and cyanosis (Hatfield 2014).	9 To identify potential respiratory insufficiency at an early stage.
10 In the event of laryngospasm: a) Contact the anaesthetic team immediately. b) Apply positive pressure ventilation and reassure CYP. c) Prepare propofol 0.5–1 mg/kg ready for immediate use by the anaesthetist and be prepared for the possibility of an emergency intubation. d) If symptoms persist or severe hypoxaemia is observed, obtain a muscle relaxant such as suxamethonium (1 mg/kg).	10 a) To enable prompt and appropriate action to be taken if required. b) To provide 100% oxygen under positive pressure in an attempt to relieve the spasms. c, d) Emergency intubation may be required to reverse increasing hypoxaemia (James and Walker 2013).
11 Consider passing a nasogastric tube once the laryngospasm has resolved.	11 To decompress air from the stomach thereby aiding respiratory effort.

(continued)

Procedure guideline 26.6 Care in recovery *(continued)*

Statement	Rationale
Initial Assessment	
Breathing assessment	
1 Evaluate breathing by: • Listening to inspiratory breath sounds. • Observing the work of breathing by noting the adequacy of tidal volume and resultant chest expansion.	1 To ensure the CYP has a clear airway, is breathing, and air is moving freely and quietly in and out of the chest.
2 Determine the rate, depth, and rhythm of respirations in accordance with the CYP's age and clinical condition. The CYP's normal range should also be considered (Table 26.1).	2 To identify potential respiratory insufficiency at an early stage. Tachypnoea without other signs of respiratory distress is often an attempt to maintain a normal pH by increasing minute ventilation, thereby causing a compensating respiratory alkalosis.
3 Observe for signs of peripheral and central cyanosis: a) Peripheral cyanosis: indicated by blue hands, feet, and fingernail beds. b) Central cyanosis: indicated by blue lips, tongue, and mucous membranes.	3 a) Peripheral cyanosis without central cyanosis may indicate that the CYP is cold. b) Central cyanosis is a sign of severe hypoxaemia.
4 An anaemic CYP may not appear cyanotic despite the presence of profound hypoxaemia.	4 This is due to low haemoglobin levels.
5 Note oxygen saturation readings and maintain oxygen therapy (40–100%) to ensure oxygen saturations remain above 94%. The duration of oxygen therapy should be determined by the oxygen saturation values in the recovery unit.	5 To ensure adequate oxygenation. There is a greater risk of respiratory complications in CYPs, particularly those with a history of recent upper respiratory tract infection, who have required tracheal intubation; a history of prematurity; chronic obstructive sleep apnoea; passive exposure to tobacco smoke, or postintubation croup.
6 If required, provide ventilatory support as necessary: • Continuous positive airway pressure (CPAP) • Intermittent positive pressure ventilation (IPPV) • Bi-phasic intermittent positive airway pressure (BIPAP)	6 To provide 100% oxygen under positive pressure in the event of respiratory failure (hypoxia and hypoventilation).
Circulation assessment	
1 Observe the clinical presentation of the CYP and record: • Colour (central-peripheral) • Temperature (core/peripheral) • Capillary refill time • Peripheral pulses (volume/strength) • The carotid, axillary, radial, femoral, dorsalis pedis, and posterior tibial pulses	1 Restoration of circulating volume and fluid maintenance becomes a priority once airway patency and breathing have been established (Hazinski 2013). For more information see Chapter 1: Assessment and Chapter 9: Early Recognition and Management of the Child.
2 The CYP's normal range for heart rate should also be considered (Table 26.2).	
3 Monitor and record blood/fluid losses on arrival, and half hourly thereafter from wound sites and drainage systems.	3 To monitor fluid/blood losses and prevent hypovolaemic shock.
4 Routinely record the estimated blood volume (EBV) for all patients undergoing craniofacial surgery or those with significant losses. • Moderate blood loss = <10 mls/kg/hr • Significant blood loss = >10mls/kg/hr, as per local policy • For postoperative fluid replacement in CYPs after craniofacial surgery, see local policy.	4 If acute haemorrhage totals more than 15% of blood volume, signs of circulatory failure will be observed (American Heart Association/American Academy of Pediatrics 2011). See Table 26.3
5 If requested by the anaesthetist, administer immediate fluid replacement (blood products/colloids/crystalloids).	5 To maintain circulation
6 Routinely replace drainage losses for at risk groups (e.g. after craniofacial surgery) as per local protocol or anaesthetist's instruction.	6 To provide rapid resuscitation if compromise in systemic perfusion is detected. Craniofacial surgery in particular poses a high risk of bleeding postoperatively (American Heart Association/American Academy of Pediatrics 2011).
7 Bandage and protect any intravenous lines.	7 To ensure venous lines are secure as access in CYPs is often difficult to obtain and causes patient distress.
8 Apply an appropriate splint to arterial lines, leaving the cannula visible for regular inspection. Radial lines should be splinted with the wrist extended, as per local policy.	8 To facilitate easy observation of the cannula site and prevent movement, which may cause extravasation and phlebitis (Hatfield 2014).
9 Label arterial lines clearly.	9 To maintain patient safety.

Chapter 26 Perioperative care

Table 26.1 Normal respiratory rates in CYPs (Hazinski 2013)

Age	Rate (breaths per minute)
Infants	30–60
Toddlers	24–40
Preschoolers	22–34
School-aged CYPs	18–30
Adolescents	12–16

Table 26.2 Normal heart rates in CYPs (Hazinski 2013)

Age	Awake rate/min	Sleeping rate/min
Neonate	100–180	80–160
Infant (6 mo.)	100–160	75–160
Toddler	80–110	60–90
Preschooler	70–110	60–90
School-age	65–110	60–90
Adolescent	60–90	50–90

Table 26.3 Calculating circulating blood volumes in CYPs (Hazinski 2013)

Age of the child	Blood volume (ml/kg)
Neonates	85–90
Infants	75–80
CYPs	70–75
Adults	65–70

Table 26.4 Normal urine output in CYPs (Hazinski 2013)

Age	Ml/kg/hr
Neonate	2–3
Infant	2
Child	1–2
Adolescent	0.5–1

Procedure guideline 26.6 Care in recovery (continued)

Statement	Rationale
Vital signs monitoring	
1 Record vital signs, i.e. heart rate, respiratory rate/effort and blood pressure (invasive and noninvasive) and repeat assessments every 10 minutes to evaluate trends, taking into account the CYP's normal range and clinical condition.	1 Vital signs provide important information in the recognition of respiratory failure and shock. Sinus tachycardia is common response to stress (e.g. anxiety, pain, fever, hypoxia, hypercapnia, hypovolaemia, or cardiac impairment). For more information see Chapter 1: Assessment.
2 Monitor with an electrocardiogram (ECG), any CYP who has evidence of or is at risk of respiratory or cardiovascular instability (Hatfield 2014). This includes: • Known or suspected heart disease • Hypoxaemia and acidosis resulting from respiratory insufficiency or shock • Neonates • Heart-affecting drug therapy • Arrhythmias experienced during the anaesthetic • Electrolyte imbalances • History of lung disease/airway complications/poor oxygen saturations intraoperatively • Abnormal perfusion status • Cardiac surgery • Improperly reversed muscle relaxants • Hypothermia	2 To determine their cardiac rhythm and detect arrhythmias, which may compromise cardiac output (American Heart Association/American Academy of Pediatrics 2011).
3 Assess the CYP's diuresis, taking into account their intravenous input while in theatre and any fluid losses that may have occurred. Commence a new fluid balance record once they arrive in recovery.	3 To ensure early detection of complications. Measurement of fluid balance provides indirect evidence of the CYP's systemic perfusion. Hypovolaemia and shock are frequent prerenal causes of acute renal failure (Hazinski 2013).
4 The CYP's normal range for urine output should be considered, providing hydration is adequate (Table 26.4).	4 A small reduction in urine volume may indicate significant compromise in renal perfusion or function.
5 Administer volume therapy if indicated by the anaesthetist. Fluid resuscitation consists of a 20ml/kg bolus of 0.9% saline, Hartmann's solution, colloid, or blood as indicated per local policy.	5 To prevent hypovolaemic shock – for more information see Chapter 9: Early Recognition and Management of the Seriously Ill Child and Chapter 10: Fluid Balance.
6 Routinely monitor central venous pressure (CVP) in all CYPs having undergone renal transplantation, or if requested by the anaesthetist. Normal CVP should be between 2 and 5mm/Hg.	6 This measures right heart filling pressures and therefore provides an assessment of fluid balance (Hazinski 2013).

(continued)

Procedure guideline 26.6 Care in recovery *(continued)*

Statement	Rationale
Thermoregulation	
1 Measure and record body temperature on admission and document route of measurement.	1 To ensure early detection and treatment of hypo/hyperthermia.
2 Initiate measures to warm a hypothermic CYP (core temperature below 36°C) (Hockenberry and Wilson 2015) by applying warmed blankets to the body and head, and utilising active warming devises such as overhead radiant heaters, forced air warmers and BabyTherms®.	2 To actively warm the CYP to a normothermic temperature (36.1–37.8°C). For more information regarding thermoregulation in a neonate see Chapter 20: Neonatal Care.
3 Continue oxygen therapy until the CYP's temperature reaches normal levels.	3 Hypothermia increases oxygen requirements and can compromise systemic perfusion and cardiac output. The neonate is particularly at risk (James and Walker 2013).
4 Initiate measures to cool a hyperthermic CYP (temperature above 38°C) by: • Minimising clothing and blankets. • Exposing the skin to air. • Increasing air circulation.	4, 5 To reduce body temperature to normothermic values.
5 Consider the use of an antipyretic drug such as paracetamol.	
6 Consider the risk of malignant hyperthermia in CYPs with a rapid increase in temperature (2°C/hr), accompanied muscle rigidity, tachycardia, unstable rising blood pressure, brown or bloody urine, changes in skin colour from a flushed to mottled appearance, hypoxia, and/or tachypnoea (American Heart Association/American Association of Pediatrics 2011).	6, 7 Malignant hyperthermia is a genetic condition precipitated by the use of inhalation anaesthetic agents and depolarising muscle relaxants such as suxamethonium. If treated promptly, most patients recover, although a mortality rate of around 5% has been reported (James and Walker 2013).
7 If malignant hyperthermia is suspected, notify the anaesthetist immediately and assist in patient management as per local guidelines for the emergency management of malignant hyperthermia.	
Neurological assessment	
1 Evaluate the CYP's alertness and responsiveness to the environment.	1 To determine their conscious level. A CYP with a conscious level of less than 8 on the GOSH coma scale will have an unprotected airway. For more information see Chapter 21: Neurological Care.
2 Perform a rapid but thorough neurological assessment for all CYPs who have undergone neurological or neurosurgical procedures. This must incorporate an assessment of eye opening, verbal responsiveness, motor function and reflexes, and pupil size and response to light.	2 To detect potential complications of neurosurgery such as raised intracranial pressure and the presence of seizures (Hazinski 2013).
3 Continue neurological observations at 10 minute intervals alongside the recording of vital signs.	3 To identify any changes in condition.
4 Report any observations of rising intracranial pressure to the surgeon and anaesthetist immediately - see box 26.2.	4 To enable any prompt and appropriate action to be taken as required.
5 Routinely measure intracranial pressure on CYPs who have monitoring devices in situ.	5 To observe for normal intracranial pressure, i.e. approximately 4–15 mmHg (Hazinski 2013).
6 Immediately report any fluctuations in intracranial pressure outside normal parameters to the surgeon and anaesthetist.	6 To monitor/treat dangerous trends in the intracranial pressure.
7 Liaise closely with the surgical team in respect to postoperative instructions, i.e. positioning of the CYP, nil per oral times, position of surgical drains, and the commencement of ventricular drainage systems.	7 To enable any prompt and appropriate action to be taken as required.
8 If required, set up external ventricular drainage in accordance with local guidelines.	8 To adhere to specific instructions and prevent postoperative complications. For more information on external ventricular drains see Chapter 21: Neurological Care.

Box 26.2 Signs of increased intracranial pressure in CYPs

- Reduced level of consciousness.
- Irritability, then lethargy.
- Confusion, disorientation.
- Decreased responsiveness (decreased eye contact, decreased response to parents, and then to pain).
- Reduced ability to follow commands (e.g "hold up two fingers, wiggle toes, stick out tongue").
- Pupil dilation with decreased response to light.
- Reduced spontaneous movement or deterioration in reflexive posturing.
- Purposeful movement deteriorates.
- Decorticate posturing, then decerebrate posturing, then flaccid response to pain.
- Cushing's triad (hypertension, bradycardia, apnoea) – this may occur as a late sign.

(Hazinski 2013).

Procedure guideline 26.6 Care in recovery *(continued)*

Statement	Rationale
Nausea and vomiting	
1 Assess CYP's level of nausea and/or incidences of vomiting.	1 To ensure early detection and treatment of nausea and vomiting. Nausea, vomiting, and retching cause discomfort. Severe vomiting can cause tension and bleeding of suture lines, muscular fatigue, and tracheal aspiration of vomitus.
2 In the event of vomiting in the unconscious/semiconscious patient, roll them immediately onto their side, remove any pillows, gently suction out the oral-pharynx, and position the bed into the Trendelenberg (head down) position.	2 To prevent aspiration of gastric contents into the lungs and facilitate drainage of vomitus into the mouth (Hatfield 2014).
3 If nausea or vomiting occurs: a) Consider the cause of the vomiting and attempt to eliminate contributory factors, i.e. pain, hypotension, hypoxia, hypovolaemia, anxiety, early mobilisation, and swallowed blood (Hatfield 2014). b) Administer an antiemetic as prescribed and monitor efficacy.	3 a) To alleviate contributory factors. b) To treat nausea or vomiting.
4 If nausea or vomiting persists, consult the anaesthetic team and consider the use of an alternative or additional antiemetic.	4 To provide further treatment.
Pain	
1 Assess the CYP's pain and document pain scores using a validated pain assessment tool.	1 To determine effectiveness of intra-operative analgesia and assess need for further analgesia.
2 As well as severity, it is also important to document location and type of pain, where possible.	2 To identify the cause of the pain and guide decisions regarding the most appropriate intervention.
3 In the event of pain: • Determine details of intra-operative analgesia and other drugs given. • Administer analgesics as prescribed and monitor effectiveness. • Administer prescribed simple analgesics where appropriate alongside intravenous opioids/epidural analgesia. • Consider administering prescribed co-analgesics if appropriate, e.g. antispasmodics or muscle relaxants. • Involve parents and provide distraction techniques particularly if the pain is anxiety related. • Consider possible attributing factors, e.g. patient position, tightness of plaster cast, etc.	3 To minimise and/or treat the causes of the pain where possible. For more information see Chapter 24: Pain Management.

(continued)

Procedure guideline 26.6 Care in recovery *(continued)*

Statement	Rationale
Electrolyte, fluid balance and gastro-intestinal status	
1 Assess CYP's level of hydration by observing for moist mucous membranes, adequate urine output (1 ml/kg/hr), and evidence of good systemic perfusion.	1 To determine the need for maintenance fluid therapy.
2 Consider administering maintenance fluids in CYPs as per local policy, who: • Have undergone major surgical procedures. • Require a postoperative nil-per-oral status. • Have experienced prolonged fasting times. • Are experiencing postoperative nausea and vomiting. • Have compromised oral intake due to postoperative sedation. • Require electrolyte balancing. • Require kidney irrigation post urology procedures.	2 To meet normal physiological needs, to restore deficits and replace losses (Meyer-Pahoulis1994).
3 Administer all intravenous fluids through volume-controlled infusion pumps.	3 To ensure accurate fluid administration. For more information see Chapter 10: Fluid Balance.
4 Measure and record fluid balance hourly if: a) The CYP has undergone abdominal surgery; if indicated by the anaesthetist/surgeon, administer normal saline +10 mmols potassium chloride (500 mls) to replace nasogastric aspirates ml/ml. b) Fluid output exceeds intake; contact the anaesthetic team immediately.	4 To ensure hydration and fluid intake is adequate. a) To replace nasogastric losses, ensure adequate hydration and maintain satisfactory serum potassium levels. b) To prevent dehydration; an adjustment in fluid administration may be required.
5 Routinely measure blood glucose in all diabetic CYPs (normal blood glucose levels: 3.85–6.05 mmols) (Hazinski 2013).	5–8. To detect and treat hypo/hyperglycaemia and prevent further complications.
6 Administer fluid therapy and titrate insulin sliding scale in accordance with endocrine team instructions.	
7 Consider performing a blood glucose measurement on neonates or CYPs presenting with signs of hypoglycaemia, i.e. muscle twitching, an obtund conscious state, convulsions, or respiratory depression (Hatfield 2014).	
8 Document and report all results to the anaesthetic team.	
Psychological Care:	
1 Once the CYP arrives in recovery, contact the ward/ parents/ carers and ask them to wait in the designated parents' room.	1 To ensure that the parents can be with their child in recovery as soon as possible.
2 Ensure parents/carers are brought into recovery as soon as the CYP is emerging from anaesthetic.	2 To provide comfort and a familiar presence.
3 Provide information and reassurance about postanaesthetic behaviour, particularly if the CYP is experiencing emergence delirium (ED).	3 To relieve anxiety and provide reassurance. ED is a dissociated state of consciousness in which the CYP is irritable, uncompromising, uncooperative, incoherent, and inconsolably crying, moaning, kicking, or thrashing. ED can disrupt the surgical repair, be distressing for parents and staff and may cause parental dissatisfaction with their child's care (Reduque and Verghese 2012).
4 Ensure CYPs with learning disabilities receive a slow recovery with the parents in close proximity as soon as the airway is safe. They should be recovered in a designated area with lower levels of noise and lighting as per local policy.	4 To relieve anxiety and provide reassurance.
5 Encourage the use of comforters and favourite toys.	5 To provide comfort and distraction.
6 If permissible, offer thirsty CYPs a drink of water.	6 To provide comfort and relieve distress from thirst.

Procedure guideline 26.6 Care in recovery *(continued)*

Statement	Rationale
Discharge Criteria	
1 For non-ITU patients, consider discharging the CYP once the following targets have been met in agreement with the anaesthetist and ward nurse: • Spontaneous, regular respirations and a self-supporting airway. • The SpO2 is within normal limits for the CYP and oxygen has been prescribed if necessary. • Heart rate and blood pressure is stable and within preoperative limits. • The central temperature is within normal limits and they are warm peripherally. • The CYP is awake or easily rousable. • The Paediatric Early Warning System (PEWS) is 4 or below. • The CYP is comfortable and any pain is adequately controlled. • Nausea/vomiting is adequately controlled. • Wound is dry/exudates minimal. • Catheters/drains are patent and drainage is within anticipated limits. • Postoperative hydration therapy has been prescribed if required. • If appropriate, the CYP is free from neurovascular compromise. • The prescription has been checked and all medications prescribed. • Blood components have been given and/or prescribed as needed. • Documentation is complete, including the operation record and any notable postoperative instructions.	1 To ensure they have recovered from the effects of anaesthesia and are safe to return to the ward environment.
2 If the above criteria cannot be met the anaesthetist should review the CYP with the ward nurse. If they agree that the CYP is suitable for transfer this must be documented on the anaesthetic chart.	2 To minimise the risks of complications.
Handover	
1 The Recovery Nurse / Operating Department Practitioner must provide a comprehensive handover to the ward nurse utilising the SBARD communication tool to include any specific instructions to take place in the postoperative period. Handover should incorporate the details on the operation record, condition of the CYP while under anaesthesia, any problems that have occurred, any analgesia or other drugs administered, and the current PEWS. These instructions must also be documented in the CYP's health care record.	1–3. To ensure relevant information is passed on to ward staff to enable continuity of care. For more information regarding SBARD and PEWS, see section 8 in the Introduction, Chapter 1: Assessment, and Chapter 9: Early Recognition and Management of the Seriously Ill Child.
2 If medication or intravenous fluids have been administered in the recovery area these must be documented before the CYP leaves and reported verbally to the ward staff.	
3 The discharge checklist must be checked and signed by both the recovery practitioner and the receiving ward nurse.	

References

American Academy of Pediatrics (2015). Critical elements for the pediatric perioperative anesthesia environment. Pediatrics 136 (6):1200–1205. https://publications.aap.org/pediatrics/article/136/6/1200/33916/Critical-Elements-for-the-Pediatric-Perioperative (accessed 11 August 2022).

American Heart Association/ American Association of Pediatrics (2011). *Paediatric Advanced Life Support*. Dallas: America Heart Association.

American Society of Anesthesiologists (2014). ASA Physical Status Classification System (amended 2020). https://www.asahq.org/standards-and-guidelines/asa-physical-status-classification-system (accessed 9 August 2022).

Askin, D.F. and Wilson, D. (2014). Chapter 10. The high-risk newborn and family. In: *Wong's Nursing Care of Infants and Children*, 9the (eds. M.J. Hockenberry and D. Wilson). St Louis: Mosby Elsevier, 314–389.

Association of Anaesthetists of Great Britain and Ireland (2013). Immediate Postanaesthetic Recovery. https://associationofanaesthetists-publications.onlinelibrary.wiley.com/doi/full/10.1111/anae.12146 (accessed 9 August 2022).

Association of Anaesthetists of Great Britain and Ireland (AAGBI) (2010) Pre-operative Assessment and Patient Preparation – The Role of the Anaesthetist. https://anaesthetists.org/Portals/0/PDFs/Guidelines%20PDFs/Guideline_preoperative_assessment_patient_preparation_anaesthetist_2010_final.pdf?ver=2018-07-11-163756-537 (accessed 9 August 2022).

Association for Perioperative Practice (AfPP) (2011a). *Standards and Recommendations for Safe Perioperative Practice*, 3rde. Harrogate: Association for Perioperative Practice.

Association of Perioperative Practice (AfPP) (2011b). Swab, instrument and needle counts. Association of Perioperative Practice. In: *Standards and Recommendations for Safe Practice*. Harrogate: AfPP.

Association of Perioperative Registered Nurses (AORN) (2006). Recommended practices for sponge, sharp and instrument counts AORN. In: *AORN Standards, Recommended Practices and Guidelines*. Denver: AORN.

Association of Perioperative Registered Nurses (AORN) (2009). *Perioperative Standards and Recommended Practices*. Colorado: AORN.

British National Formulary for Children (BNFC) (2022). *British National Formulary for Children*. London: RCPCH Publishings. https://bnfc.nice.org.uk/ (accessed 9 August 2022).

Brewer, S., Gleditsch, S.L., Syblik, D. et al. (2006). Pediatric anxiety: child life intervention in day surgery. *Journal of Pediatric Nursing* 21 (1): 13–22.

Brown, K., De Lima, J., McEwan, A., and Sumner, E. (2000). Development and disease in childhood. In: *Paediatric Anaesthesia*, 2nde (eds. E. Sumner and D.J. Hatch). London: Arnold.

Department of Health (DH) (2000). *The NHS Plan, a Plan for Investment, a Plan for Reform*. London: DH.

Department of Health (DH) (2007a). *Saving Lives: Reducing Infection, Delivering Clean and Safe Care High Impact Intervention no 2: Peripheral Intravenous Cannula Care Bundle*. London: DH.

Department of Health (DH) (2007b). *Saving Lives: Reducing Infection, Delivering Clean and Safe Care High Impact Intervention no 4: Care Bundle to Prevent Surgical Site Infection*. London: DH.

Department of Health (DH) (2009). *Reference Guide to Consent for Examination or Treatment*, 2e. London: DH.

Difusco, L.A. (2015). *Pediatric surgery. In Alexander's Care of the Patient in Surgery*, 15the (ed. J.C. Rothrock), 1008–1080. MO: Elsevier Mosby.

Donnelly, J. (2005). Care of children and adolescents. In: *A Textbook of Perioperative Care* (eds. K. Woodhead and P. Wicker). Edinburgh: Elsevier Churchill Livingstone, 267–284.

Dreger, VA and Trembeck, TF (2006) Management of preoperative anxiety in children *AORM Journal* 84(5), 778–780, 782–786, 788-790 passim.

Fortier, M.A., MacLaren Chorney, J., YAffa Zisk Rony, R. et al. (2009). Children's desire for preoperative information. *Anesthesia and Analgesia* 109 (4): 1085–1090.

Fortier, M.A., Blount, R.L., Wang, S.-M. et al. (2011). Analysing a family centred pre-operative intervention programme: a dismantling approach. *British Journal of Anaesthesia* 106 (5): 713–718.

Guedel (1937) as cited in Hewer CL (1937)). The stages and signs of general Anaesthesia. *British Medical Journal* 2 (3996): 274–276.

Harris, S. (2007). Care of the child in the operating theatre. In: *Surgical Nursing of Children* (eds. M.A. Chambers and S. Jones). Edinburgh: Elsevier Churchill Livingstone.

Hatfield, A. (2014). *The Complete Recovery Room Book*, 5e. New York: Oxford University Press.

Hazinski MF (2013) *Nursing Care of the Critically Ill Child*. 3rd edition. St Louis, Mosby.

Hockenberry, M. and Wilson, D. (2015). *Wong's Nursing Care of Infants and Children*, 10e. St Louis: Missouri.

Hughes, S. and Mardell, A. (2009). *Oxford Handbook of Perioperative Practice*. Oxford: Oxford University Press.

Ince, C. and Skinner, A. (2000). Scientific principles in relation to monitoring equipment. In: *Fundamentals of Operating Department Practice* (eds. A. Davey and C. Ince). Cambridge: Cambridge University Press, 109–120.

James, I. and Walker, I. (2013). *Core Topics in Paediatric Anaesthesia*. New York: Cambridge University Press.

Kain, Z., Mayes, L., Caldwell-Andrews, A. et al. (2006). Preoperative anxiety, postoperative pain, and behavioural recovery in young children undergoing surgery. *Pediatrics* 118 (2): 651–658.

Kain, Z., Caldwell-Andrews, A., Mayes, L. et al. (2007). Family-centered preparation for surgery improves perioperative outcomes in children: a randomised controlled trial. *Anesthesiology* 106 (1): 65–74.

Kristensson-Hallstrom, I. (2000). Parental participation in pediatric surgical care. *AORN Journal* 71 (5): 1021–1029.

Li, H.C.W. (2007). Evaluating the effectiveness of preoperative interventions: the appropriateness of using the children's emotional manifestation scale. *Journal of Clinical Nursing* 16: 1919–1926.

Litwack, K., Saleh, D., and Schultz, P. (1991). Postoperative pulmonary complications. *Critical Care Nursing Clinics of North America* 3 (1): 77–82.

Manley, K. and Bellman, L. (2000). *Surgical Nursing Advancing Practice*. Eastbourne: Churchill Livingstone.

Medicines and Healthcare products Regulatory Agency (MHRA)(2011) Electrosurgery equipment safety poster. https://extranet.whh.nhs.uk/application/files/2714/7126/5029/Electrosurgery_Poster.pdf (accessed 9 August 2022).

MHRA (2015). Electrosurgery: top tips. https://www.gov.uk/government/publications/electrosurgery-top-tips (accessed 11 August 2022).

Meeks, M., Hallsworth, M., and Yeo, H. (2009). *Nursing the Neonate*, 3rde. Oxford: Blackwell Science.

Methven, A., Duncan, O., and Chambers, M. (2007). Burns and plastics. In: *Surgical Nursing Care of Children. Edinburgh* (eds. M.A. Chambers and S. Jones). Churchill Livingstone.: Elsevier.

Meyer-Pahoulis, E. (1994). Pediatric Postanesthesia care. *Plastic Surgery Nursing* 14 (2): 92–95. 107.

Morse, T. (2007). Day care surgery. In: *Surgical Nursing Care of Children* (eds. M.A. Chambers and S. Jones). Edinburgh: Elsevier Churchill Livingstone.

National Institute for Health and Care Excellence (NICE) (2008a). Surgical site infection. Prevention and treatment. www.nice.org.uk/guidance/cg74 -(accessed 9 August 2022).

National Institute for Health and Care Excellence (NICE) (2008b). Hypothermia: prevention and management in adults having surgery. http://guidance.nice.org.uk/CG65/NICEGuidance/pdf/English (accessed 9 August 2022).

National Institute for Health and Care Excellence (NICE) (2016). Routine preoperative tests for elective surgery. www.nice.org.uk/guidance/ng45/resources/routine-preoperative-tests-for-elective-surgery-pdf-1837454508997 (accessed 9 August 2022).

National Patient Safety Agency (NPSA) (2009a). WHO surgical safety checklist. https://www.who.int/teams/integrated-health-services/patient-safety/research/safe-surgery/tool-and-resources (accessed 11 August 2022).

National Patient Safety Agency (NPSA) (2009b). Reducing the risk of retained throat pack after surgery. Supporting information. https://www.medis-medical.com/content-files/NPSA-Report-Reducing-Risk-Retained-Throat-Packs-Surgery.pdf (accessed 9 August 2022).

NHS Improvement (2018). Never Events List 2018 (updated 2021). https://www.england.nhs.uk/wp-content/uploads/2020/11/2018-Never-Events-List-updated-February-2021.pdf (accessed 9 August 2022).

NHS England Patient Safety Domain (2015). National Safety Standards for invasive Procedures (NatSSIPs). https://www.england.nhs.uk/wp-content/uploads/2015/09/natssips-safety-standards.pdf (accessed 9 August 2022).

Potty, A., Khan, W., and Tailor, H. (2010). Diathermy in perioperative practice. *Journal of Perioperative Practice* 20 (11): 402–405.

Radford, M., County, B., and Oakley, M. (2004). *Advancing Perioperative Practice*. Cheltenham: Nelson Thomas.

Reduque LL, Verghese ST (2012). Paediatric emergence delirium. In Continuing Education in Anaesthesia, Critical Care and Pain. Oxford, Oxford University Press (on behalf of the British Journal of Anaesthesia).

Rothrock, J.C. (2015). *Alexander's Care of the Patient in Surgery*, 15the. Missouri: Elsevier Mosby.

Royal College of Anesthetists (2016). Guidelines for the provision of anaesthesia services. https://www.rcoa.ac.uk/safety-standards-quality/guidance-resources/guidelines-provision-anaesthetic-services (accessed 11 August 2022).

Royal College of Nursing (RCN) (2011). *Transferring Children to and from Theatre – RCN Position Statement and Guidance for Good Practice*. London: Royal College of Nursing.

Royal College of Nursing (RCN) (2013). Defining Staffing levels for Children and Young Peoples Services. Royal College of Nursing. https://www.academia.edu/33912568/Defining_staffing_levels_for_children_and_young_peoples_services_RCN_standards_for_clinical_professionals_and_service_managers (accessed 11 August 2022).

Royal College of Paediatrics and Child Health (2012). *Pre-Procedure Pregnancy Checking in under 16's: Guidance for Clinicians*. London: RCPCH. https://www.rcpch.ac.uk/sites/default/files/Guidance.pdf (accessed 9 August 2022).

Royal College of Surgeons (2007). *Surgery for Children – Delivering a First Class Service*. London: Royal College of Surgeons.

Schober-Flores, C. (2012). Pressure ulcers in the Paediatric population. *Journal of the Dermatology Nurse's Association* 4 (5): 295–306.

Shields, L. (2010). The psychosocial care of children in the perioperative area. In: *Perioperative Care of the Child: A Nursing Manual* (ed. L. Shields), 13–22. UK: Wiley Blackwell.

Siddiqui, BA. and Kim, P.Y. (2021). Anesthesia Stages in StatPearls [Internet]. https://www.ncbi.nlm.nih.gov/books/NBK557596/ (accessed 11 August 2022).

Smith, C. (2007). Care of the patient undergoing surgery. In: *A Textbook of Perioperative Care* (eds. K. Woodhead and P. Wicker). Edinburgh: Elsevier Churchill Livingstone, 161–180.

Spruce, L. and Braswell, M.L. (2012). Implementing AORN recommended practices for Electrosurgery. *AORN Journal* 95 (3): 373–387.

Steelman, V.M. (2015). Concepts basic to perioperative nursing. In: (ed. J. Rothrock). (ed.), Alexander's Care of the Patient in Surgery. St. Louis, MO: Elsevier, 1–15.

Tan, L. and Meakin, G.H. (2010). Anaestheisa for the uncooperative child. *Continuing Education in Anaesthesia, Critical Care and Pain* 10 (2): 48–52.

Thomas M, Morrison C, Newton R, Schindler E. Consensus statement on clear fluids fasting for elective pediatric general anaesthesia. Pediatr Anesth. 2018; 28:411-414.

United Kingdom (UK) Cell Salvage Action Group (2015). ICS Technical Factsheet: Swab Washing, Version 3. https://www.transfusionguidelines.org/document-library/documents/factsheet-1-swab-washing-version-3 (accessed 11 August 2022).

Walker, I. and Lockie, J. (2000). Basic techniques for anaesthesia. In: *Paediatric Anaesthesia*, 2nde (eds. E. Sumner and D.J. Hatch). London: Arnold.

Wilson, D. and da Cunha, M.F. (2010). Health problems of the newborn. In: *Wong's Nursing Care of Infants and Children*, 9the (eds. M.J. Hockenberry and D. Wilson). St Louis: Mosby Elsevier.

Woodhead, K. (2009). Safe surgery: reducing the risks of retained items. *Journal of Perioperative Practice* 19 (10): 358–361.

Woodhead, K. and Wicker, P. (eds.) (2005). *A Textbook of Perioperative Care*. Edinburgh: Elsevier Churchill Livingstone.

World Health Organisation (WHO) (2009). *Implementation Manual WHO Surgical Safety Checklist*. Geneva: World Health Organisation Publishing. https://www.who.int/publications/i/item/9789241598590 (accessed 11 August 2022).

Further reading

Aitkenhead, A., Moppet, I., and Thompson, J. (2013). *Smith and Aitkenhead's Textbook of Anaesthesia*, 6e. New York: Churchill Livingstone.

Alsop-Shields, L. (2000). Perioperative care of children in a transcultural context. *AORN Journal* 71 (5): 1004–1020.

Andersson, H., Zaren, B., and Frykholm, P. (2015). Low incidence of pulmonary aspiration in children allowed to intake fluids until called to the operating suite. *Pediatric Anesthesia* 25 (8): 770–777.

Ministry of Health (1959). The welfare of children in hospital, Platt Report. London, Her Majesty's Stationery Office.

Resuscitation Council (UK) (2006). *European Paediatric Life Support*, 2e. Resuscitation Council (UK).

Resuscitation Council (2013). *European Paediatric Life Support*. Resuscitation Council (UK).

Schmidt, A.R., Buehler, P., Seglias, L. et al. (2015). Gastric pH and residual volume after one and two hours fasting time for clear fluids in children. *British Journal of Anaesthesia* 114 (3): 477–482.

Simpson, P.J. and Popat, M. (2002). *Understanding Anaesthesia*, 4e. Oxford: Butterworth_Heinemann.

Steward, D.J., Lerman, J., and Cote, C.J. (2010). *Manual of Paediatric Anaesthesia with an Index of Pediatric Syndromes*, 6the. Edinburgh: Churchill Livingstone.

Watcha, M. (2013). The immediate recovery period. In: *Paediatric Anaesthesia*, 2nde (eds. E. Sumner and D.J. Hatch). London: Arnold.

Chapter 27

Play as a therapeutic tool

Jennifer Dyer[1], Janet Holmes[2], Denise Cochrane[1], and Nigel Mills[3]

[1] Play Specialist Team Leader, Great Ormond Street Hospital, London, UK
[2] BSC (Hons), NNEB, HPSET, Senior Health Play Specialist, GOSH
[3] Formerly Adolescent Nurse Specialist, GOSH

Chapter contents

Introduction	622
The development of play in hospital	622
Normal play for development	622
Types of play	623
Functions of play	623
Development of play	623
The importance of play for children in hospital	623
The functions of play in hospital	623
Siblings	624
The health play specialist (HPS)	624
HPS training	624
The play worker (PW)	625
Preparation for surgery and procedures	625
Aims of play preparation	625
Preadmission programmes	626
Preparation session	626
Postprocedural play	627
The reluctant CYP	627
Adolescents	627
Children and young people with additional needs or a learning disability (LD)	627
Distraction techniques	628
Distraction Tools and Resources	630
Relaxation	630
Guided imagery	631
Therapeutic play	631
Desensitisation	632
Arts in health	633
References	633
Further reading	634
Useful websites	634

Case studies

27.1 James; a Five-year-old with autistic spectrum disorder	628
27.2 Thomas: Distress and noncompliance with oral medication	631
27.3 Alex and the use of desensitisation	632

Procedure guideline

27.1 Using distraction during a painful/frightening procedure	629

The Great Ormond Street Hospital Manual of Children and Young People's Nursing Practices, Second Edition. Edited by Elizabeth Anne Bruce, Janet Williss, and Faith Gibson.
© 2023 John Wiley & Sons Ltd. Published 2023 by John Wiley & Sons Ltd.

Introduction

There have been many attempts to define play and why children and young people (CYPs) play. All who write on play agree it is virtually impossible to produce a concise definition (Burghardt 2005; Smith et al. 2003). To an adult, play suggests relaxation, but for a CYP, play is their work. A playing CYP is not simply idling away time until the next important event organised by an adult; they are practising and learning vital life skills. Role play, for instance, is a CYP's way of re-enacting observed adult behaviour. It helps them develop problem solving skills and an understanding of the world around them by building on first hand experiences.

Play enhances every aspect of a CYP's development, helping them to develop control of their body, to perfect physical skills and muscular coordination, and refine their sight, hearing, and other senses. Ginsburg (2007) suggests play contributes to the cognitive, physical, social, and emotional well-being of CYPs. Play begins at birth, providing the building blocks to independence and successful functioning. It is not a means to an end, and continues through to adult life; many adults continue to enjoy playing! Play is important at every stage of a CYP's life. It is important that all those with responsibility for CYPs ensure that adequate provision for play is made at home, in schools, and in the community. The *Charter for Play* states 'Play is an essential part of every child's life and is vital for the enjoyment of childhood as well as social, emotional, intellectual and physical development' (Play England 2020, p. 1). There are some trends in childhood that affect CYPs' opportunities to play, such as an emphasis on academic studies at the cost of play in school. In some areas there is inadequate environmental planning, which results in a lack of amenities provided for play. Whatever the reason, being deprived of time to play is thought to be detrimental to a child's development (Gleave and Cole-Hamilton 2012; Gray 2011; Richardson 2013).

Play is important for the sick CYP both at home and in the hospital environment. Play contributes to the holistic and multiprofessional approach to their care. The National Service Framework for Children (Department of Health [DH] 2003) commented that children are not the same as adults and that hospitals need to be child friendly. This means designing hospital services from the CYP's perspective. This understanding has had an impact on how we care for sick CYPs and their families, and underlines the importance of the continuing care and support CYPs need to enable them to achieve their full potential. The needs of hospitalised adolescents require particular consideration (DH 2003; Suris et al. 2004). Adolescence is a period of huge physical, social, and emotional change; of striving toward independence and preparing for adulthood. The impact of a hospital admission can compromise a young person's independence, challenge their self-esteem, and raise questions of self-determination. This, coupled with a greater understanding of the world and what the future may hold, can lead to heightened anxiety levels for young people, and to feelings of confusion and insecurity. Health Play Specialists (HPS) are trusted members of the multidisciplinary team, enabling the young person to voice and explore their anxieties and frustrations, and helping them to meet these challenges.

The development of play in hospital

Children's hospitals emerged in the mid-nineteenth century, their primary role being to deal with the large number of infections and deficiency diseases prevalent at the time. Until then, dispensaries gave advice and medicine to parents. In 1927, Sir James Spence opened a small mother and baby unit in Newcastle-upon-Tyne, and promoted an approach to care that encouraged mothers to stay with their babies (Spence 1946). The work of Bowlby (1953) and Robertson (1962, 1970) on maternal deprivation further highlighted the needs of children in hospital. A major breakthrough came with the publication of the Platt Report (Platt 1959). This resulted in attempts to make a stay in hospital for children more humane by offering open visiting, live-in facilities for parents and carers, and by encouraging parents to participate in the care of their child in hospital.

Since 1961 the National Association for the Welfare of Children in Hospital, now known as Action for Sick Children (http://www.actionforsickchildren.org.uk/), has monitored how the recommendations of the Platt Report have been implemented. Action for Sick Children has been a source of support to parents and carers, enabling them to stay with their child in hospital. In 1989 the Save the Children Fund (SCF) commissioned the report 'Hospital: A Deprived Environment for Children? – Case for Hospital Play Schemes' (SCF 1989). This report documented the progress of hospital play schemes since they were established by Susan Harvey in 1963, and looks at the state of play provision within hospitals. It found that despite positive changes, there was still much to be done to create an environment where CYPs' emotional and psychosocial needs were acknowledged and met. Christine Hogg (1990) produced a benchmarking tool 'Quality Management for Children: Play in Hospital' for the Hospital Liaison Committee. This allowed the HPS and others concerned to provide good quality play opportunities and facilities for children in hospital, and to monitor and evaluate services. Other drivers for change include the cases at Bristol Royal Infirmary (mid 1980s) and Victoria Climbie case (mid 1990) which highlighted the need for change, strengthened by the reports of Kennedy (2001) and Lord Laming (Laming 2003). The National Service Framework for Children, Young People and Maternity Services (DH 2003) set standards for CYPs throughout the health and social care services from prebirth to 19 years of age. The document acknowledged that CYPs benefit from play provision during a hospital admission and involvement of a HPS working as part of the multidisciplinary team (MDT). It also recognised that play provision in a hospital setting has a therapeutic value, hastens recovery, and recommended children in hospital have daily access to a HPS. 'Play for Health: Delivering and Auditing Quality in Hospital Play Services' (Walker 2006) succeeded Hogg's report, and acknowledged and promoted the ways that the Play Specialist role has evolved and developed since 1990, and provided a new set of standards for hospital play.

Normal play for development

All types of play are important for a CYP's physical, emotional, cognitive, and social development and are as vital as food and rest (Gleave and Cole-Hamilton 2012). Play is the way CYPs learn about themselves and their world, and enlarge their horizons, while reducing the world to manageable proportions. Play enables the CYP to make sense of the flood of impressions pouring in from the outside world, acting as an integrating mechanism for every aspect of their experience. Through play, CYPs create other worlds where they can test out reality and discover who they are. Piaget (1951) highlighted the significance of providing children with the opportunity to express their emotions by providing a CYP with a unique individual experience and language to express their feelings, thus laying down the foundations of normal emotional development.

Play is the medium through which the CYP can express positive emotions and channel negative ones. It provides a safe outlet for emotional stresses and may help them to cope with problems in a safe setting. Through play, CYPs are encouraged to explore, experience, discover, practise skills, develop ideas and interests, and to interact socially. Playing precedes serious 'doing', as they experiment and become confident with new skills and concepts.

Play:

- Is spontaneous, although it may be stimulated by an adult, and pleasurable.
- Comes from the child's own intrinsic motivation.
- Usually concentrates on a process not a product.
- Has no explicit rules, and no right or wrong way of performing.
- Is an activity where children have ownership of what takes place.
- The child is a willing and active participant.
- Builds on the child's first hand experiences.

(O'Hagan and Smith 1994, p. 43)

Types of play

Play can be categorised as:

- Spontaneous and active
- Exploratory and manipulative
- Imitative
- Constructive
- Imaginative
- Games with rules
- Hobbies

Functions of play

Play:

- Aids physical, emotional, cognitive, and social growth and development.
- Is an opportunity to learn about oneself and one's environment.
- Provides an opportunity to practice potential skills.
- Can be a useful tool in the assessment of children.

Development of play

CYPs develop through play, and play develops through stages:

- Solitary play: Independent play where the child plays alone with toys that are different from those chosen by other children in the area.
- Parallel play: Children play side by side with similar toys but there is a lack of interaction.
- Associative play: Involves a group of children who have similar goals, will play with the same toys but do not set rules and there is no formal organisation.
- Co-operative play: Play is organised by group goals.

(Tassani et al. 2005)

The importance of play for children in hospital

Play is a fundamental need of every CYP and the benefits and value of play to the hospitalised CYP should not be underestimated. The provision of normal play for development in hospital is as important as the provision of therapeutic interventions. Play and play facilities provided in hospital provide a significant part of the overall emotional and holistic care given to the CYP, and their family, during an admission.

When CYPs are admitted to hospital they may be separated from friends and familiar surroundings. Play in hospital aims to bridge the gap between the normality of home and the abnormality of the hospital environment. It provides a safe space for CYPs to face, work through, and learn to cope with traumatic or unpleasant aspects of their illness or hospital treatments. Play can increase co-operation, choice, and consent. It also alleviates boredom and makes time go more quickly (Ekra et al. 2012).

Participation in an organised play scheme may be a welcome normalising activity. Research shows that play reduces anxiety, facilitates communication, and helps speed recovery and rehabilitation. As Jun-Tai (2004, p. 4) states, 'A teenager with a head injury will require many forms of play and social opportunities in order to rebuild self-confidence and self-esteem, especially if their body image has been altered. The choice of activities and their participation in making decisions is key to the recovery process as they begin to regain some autonomy'. Play also enables CYPs to create an environment through blending fantasy and reality to give a sense of control, at a time when they have little or no control. Webster (2000, p. 27) stated, 'A fundamental philosophy of play in healthcare should be to seek to empower children with their families throughout their healthcare experience'.

Play in hospital does much more than keep CYPs happy and occupied; it provides a safety valve for their emotions, offers support where stress and trauma arise through illness and hospital experiences, and prepares them for some of the different and difficult experiences they may encounter during their stay. Play in hospital does not need to be limited to clean, quiet, and unexciting activities. For example, bedding can be covered with waterproof sheeting, making it possible to play with water, paint and other messy play materials. Play in hospital can provide an element of fun and enjoyment for the CYP and family, helping to make their hospital experience a more positive one, normalising the abnormal. Normal play in hospital is therapeutic in its own way.

Young people need to be given as much positive control as possible. They should be provided with age-appropriate information about what is about to happen, why it is going to happen, and techniques for coping. It is useful to explore normal coping mechanisms, and to work with and practice these. Techniques that work well include breathing exercises, listening to music of their choice, watching videos/DVDs, using guided imagery and/or relaxation techniques, or being coached, comforted, or massaged by their parents/carers or a chosen friend. Distraction techniques are discussed later in the chapter.

The functions of play in hospital

Aiding normality

The provision of play in hospital provides a sense of normality, giving opportunities for normal development in an abnormal setting. Menzies-Lyth (1982) recognised that when a child enters hospital there is a tendency toward developmental regression as a normal reaction to stress. The provision of appropriate play ensures that normal development is maintained, and that CYPs are not deprived of developmental life experiences. A number of authors acknowledge that play in hospital may actually help to make the experience of hospitalisation one of growth (D'Antonio 1984). Current thinking is that the emphasis should not be on the treatment of illness in isolation from the CYP's other needs. Medical needs should be taken into consideration alongside social and emotional concerns, an important aspect of fostering normality. Normalising and free play should be central to the care and support given. As Jun-Tai (2008, p. 2) states, 'Play should be provided in the hospital setting in order to maintain the emotional well-being of the child.'

Reducing anxiety

'Hospitalisation has long been recognised as a potentially stressful time for both children and their parents' (Darbyshire 1996, p. 1), and a major function of play in hospital is the reduction of stress and anxiety, not only for the CYP, but also for parents/carers and staff

(D'Antonio 1984; Jolly 1977, 1981; Poster 1983; Robertson 1958; Weller 1980).

If play were not provided, CYPs would inevitably become bored. Boredom is known to be a contributor to stress for both adults and CYPs alike. Play in hospital provides familiarity, choice, and control in situations where control is significantly reduced. Allowing CYPs to develop skills that lead to enhanced confidence and increased resilience enables them to cope with the challenges that a hospital admission may present.

Play can be used as a form of distraction for the CYP to engage in as a means of escape from what is happening to and around them. Through play, children can actively learn to deal with anxiety caused by a hospital admission or aspects of treatment (Barbour and Jun-tai 2014). It is an important part of the HPS role to recognise and anticipate the effects of hospitalisation on the CYP and respond effectively, using appropriate play activities to help reduce their anxiety and to maintain their emotional well-being. Involving parents and siblings in play can help reduce their anxiety as well. 'Play allows children to explore a world they can master, conquering their fears while practicing adult roles, sometimes in conjunction with other children or adult caregivers' (Ginsburg 2007, pp. 182–191).

Speeding recovery

Play accelerates recovery, and can reduce the need for interventions under general anaesthesia (Jolly 1975; Department of Health [DH] 2003), partly through an increase in the CYP's awareness of interest in the environment (Play Scotland 2012). A direct link between play and speed of recovery through a reduction in anxiety was noted by Garot (1986) and Jun-Tai (2008). Play is a normal part of any CYP's day, and the more settled they are and engaged in play activities, the more relaxed they become. This in turn helps promote recovery. See also http://www.playscotland.org/wp-content/uploads/Power-of-Play-Policy-Context.pdf.

Facilitating communication

For a CYP, verbal communication is easier when they are happily engaged in play in the company of a trusted adult. Projected play was introduced by Klein (1929) as a technique whereby a child could project anxieties through an object or toy. This process has been recognised as one that reduces the anxiety experienced by a CYP. It enhances a sense of mastery and self-confidence and, in turn, affects the extent to which they interact socially. Projective play can also offer insight into how the CYP is feeling, acting as a form of communication, regardless of whether their anxiety has been fully expressed. The HPS can gain valuable information through their observations of a CYP at play; these observations may contribute to clinical decisions. Using play as a communication tool, the HPS can assess the needs of the CYP and plan how best to meet those needs.

Play also serves to facilitate communication with the wider hospital environment. Play on the hospital ward has been shown to improve communication between staff, and between staff and parents/carers through the promotion of decreased anxiety levels.

Siblings

Working with siblings should be an established practice of any hospital play scheme. It is understood that when a CYP is admitted to hospital the whole family unit can be affected. Depending on their age, developmental level, emotional maturity, and previous hospital experience, siblings may adapt to their brother or sister being in hospital without difficulty. However, for some this may be traumatic. They may come to resent the sick CYP and the time their parent(s) spend caring for them; they may also demonstrate signs of jealousy or anxiety, particularly sensing parental anxiety, which may be evident in a change in their behaviour, regression, or an expression of feelings of guilt, or they may worry that they too may become ill. To help siblings make sense of the changes in their family circumstances they are encouraged to play in hospital, with their brother or sister where possible, and have time in the playroom where they can work through their feelings. Play may be directive or nondirective; 'Play Specialists acknowledge their feelings through play and conversation . . . recognising and meeting their needs' (Walker 2006, p. 34). The provision of play in hospital for siblings helps to reduce parental anxiety, allowing them to balance the needs of the sick CYP and their sibling(s). It also offers support to siblings if they need help to deal with their own feelings and experiences (Proctor 2007).

The health play specialist (HPS)

The Department of Health has recommended that all CYPs staying in hospital should have daily access to a play specialist (DH 2003).

HPSs work specifically on the potential effects of hospitalisation and illness on CYPs, and are trained to work therapeutically with sick or hospitalised CYPs. They are a distinct group of health professionals, and are seen as the main providers of play within the health service (Nuttall 2013). Using normalising play as a foundation, they carry out focused play support such as preparing the CYP for procedures. This helps reduce anxiety and stress in the CYP and family, empowering and supporting all concerned throughout the hospital experience. The support and interventions the HPS can bring to a wide range of situations are valuable, not only to the CYP and their family, but to the range of professionals whose work can be made easier by their patients' improved ability to cope. Jun-Tai (2008, p. 233) suggests that 'the collaboration between play specialists and MDT colleagues supports an integrated and co-ordinated service promoting the best interests of the CYP and family.' Providing normal play activities gives the HPS the opportunity to build a trusting relationship with the CYP. This may be an important factor in enabling the CYP to accept future medical treatments. The HPS can be a familiar, safe and trusted person, helping children come to terms with future illness and treatment. When the opportunity for normal play has not taken place and the CYP requires treatment, the HPS will be less able to provide support and gain their co-operation. 'HPS have the ability to provide a safe, therapeutic and healing environment for infants, children, young people and families' (National Association of Health Play Specialists (NAHPS) 2012, p. 2).

HPS training

The first course specifically designed for hospital play specialists was established in 1973. This developed from a certificate to a diploma and, since 2010, to a health play specialism foundation degree. To acknowledge the number of HPSs now working within the community and hospices, it was decided in 2012 to change the title from Hospital Play Specialist to HPS. As part of continuing professional development, all HPSs are required to reregister with the HPS Education Trust (HPSET) every two years.

The Role of the HPS in the hospital environment is:

- To work as part of the multidisciplinary team (MDT), sharing the unique expertise and training of the HPS in care planning and case reviews.
- To provide creative and social activities to assess patient's knowledge of their condition and treatments and measure anxiety levels.
- To prepare patients for procedures and treatments.
- To use distraction techniques to help and support CYPs through medical and surgical procedures and investigations, e.g. blood tests, cannulation, CT scans, dressing changes, and in the anaesthetic room.

- To support CYPs to recognise and form their own coping strategies to cope with hospital admission, treatments, and procedures.
- To undertake therapeutic play, e.g. bereavement play, developmental play, and adherence issues.
- To support and advise parents/carers on appropriate play for the sick or hospitalised CYP.
- To provide play sessions to help CYPs gain skills lost through regression or effects of illness and hospitalisation.
- To identify CYPs and family members who are distressed or having difficulty coping.
- To support siblings, providing strategies for them to deal with what may be happening with their brother or sister.
- To act as an advocate for the CYP and family.
- To put play on the agenda as an accepted and normal part of routine anywhere in a hospital.
- To provide teaching for other health care workers and students.

The play worker (PW)

The play worker (PW) role has been introduced into some hospital play departments to work alongside HPSs and is specifically trained to work with CYPs in a wide variety of settings. A play worker qualification can be either a level 3 NVQ in Children and Young People's Workforce/Child Care and Education or a degree in Early Childhood Studies. The training provides an insight and understanding of child development, how to encourage children to engage in spontaneous and naturally playful experiences, to understand the process of CYPs play, how to instigate free flow play of age-appropriate activities, and how a CYP's play can change. The play worker's role is one of play facilitator, involving the setting up and resourcing of an environment where play is freely chosen and intrinsically driven (Hughes 1984).

There are some similarities in the work undertaken by the Play Worker and HPS, such as the facilitation of normal and creative play activities. However, the HPS aims to guide CYPs to a higher and clearer level of understanding of their experiences by the means of a variety of play techniques. The PW role is generally noninterventionist (Hughes 1996). The HPS often uses play in a guided way to bring about a particular outcome, e.g. to distract a CYP through a stressful, invasive procedure, or by showing them what a blood test involves by 'playing it through', using a doll and a book of photographs (Hubbuck 2009).

The role of the play worker within the hospital environment is:

- To help to create and maintain a welcoming and age-appropriate play/recreation environment for CYPs and families.
- To provide creative, recreational, and social activities that bring entertainment and fun into a potentially stressful environment.
- To provide support for CYPs and family members in adjusting to the hospital environment, giving a reassuring experience to increase each individual CYP's confidence, self-esteem, and independence.
- To arrange play sessions to help CYPs gain skills lost through regression or effects of illness and hospitalisation.
- To work alongside the HPS and other members of the MDT.
- To support the HPS to implement play programmes.
- To act as an advocate for the CYP and family.
- To put play on the agenda so it is accepted as a normal part of routine.
- To provide teaching for other health care workers and students.

Preparation for surgery and procedures

The need for, and the benefits of, preparation for surgery and medical procedures is highlighted by many childcare and healthcare experts. Play preparation should be available to every CYP for any procedure they may undergo during their time in hospital; e.g. preparation for radiotherapy and scans (Grisson et al. 2016; Netzke-Doyle 2010). The role of the HPS is paramount in the preparation process, with the HPS being the key link between the CYP, family, and the wider MDT. Play preparation is more than just an information giving exercise; it is about assessing the needs of the CYP and family, and responding as appropriate. The guidance in the "United Nations Convention on the Rights of the Child" (UNICEF 1989) and the Children Act (1989) outlines clearly the necessity for the inclusion of children in important decisions affecting their lives. Preparation through play is a good example of the aims of this guidance as it provides opportunities for CYPs to be given information appropriate to their age, cognitive development, and abilities. This enables them to be included in decisions and give consent for their treatments. The opportunity for play before a procedure is another way of helping CYPs to achieve a relaxed state of mind. As stated by Lansdown, 'Patients who have been well prepared are reported less anxious, require less medication, exhibit less maladaptive behaviour, and cope more effectively with medical procedures' (Lansdown 1996, p. 64).

The effectiveness of introducing developmentally appropriate information about procedures through structured play has a strong research basis (Walker 2006) and is supported by the Department of Health, 'Play may . . . be used for therapeutic purposes, as part of the child's care plan, and as a way of helping the child assimilate new information; adjust to and gain control over a potentially frightening environment; and prepare to cope with procedures and interventions' and 'where procedures are planned and pain can be predicted, the opportunity should be taken to prepare children through play and education' (DH 2003, p.14). Carefully structured and directed play helps to inform the CYP of procedures, increases co-operation with treatment, and consent. Young people benefit from having procedures explained in an age, and developmentally, appropriate manner, before the procedure is carried out. They need to have privacy and permission to express their emotions and ask questions, preferably without a parent or carer present.

Preparation should ideally begin before the CYP is admitted to hospital. This can be done using books or websites that focus on admission to hospital. Some hospital web sites have information about how parents/carers can help their child to cope with hospital admissions and/or painful procedures. Play preparation requires good communication and close co-operation between the CYP, parent/carer, all members of the MDT, and the community or local hospital teams, providing a consistent team approach for the CYP/parent/carer and family.

Parents/carers should be actively encouraged to assist and participate in the preparation of their child. This allows them to be more involved in their child's care and to feel more confident and better informed to reassure them. Calmer, more confident parents/carers find it easier to give emotional support, and to be more considerate of the needs of siblings.

Young people should be given the choice as to whether and how they would like their parents/carers involved and in to what extent. Sibling needs should also be considered in the HPS assessment as they may need support or wish to be involved in the preparation process.

Aims of play preparation

- Ascertains what the CYP already knows.
- Helps the CYP understand their illness, the reason for admission, and medical/surgical procedures they will undergo, and other treatment.
- Gives the opportunity to express feelings, anxieties, and fears and in this way to alleviate fear of the known/unknown.
- Addresses misconceptions or fantasies.
- Encourages the CYP to trust hospital staff.

- Enables the CYP to develop coping mechanisms.
- Reduces the short/long term effects of hospitalisation.
- Aids recovery.
- Promotes confidence and self-esteem.
- Facilitates informed consent and choices in care.

Preadmission programmes

Some hospitals/units are able to provide preadmission programmes/clinics, providing an opportunity for the CYP to visit the hospital with their family's support, and allowing them to familiarise themselves with the environment, staff, and hospital routines. Preadmission programmes empower parents/carers through accurate information sharing and discussion, and provision of an opportunity to address questions or concerns they may have. Confusion, worries, misconceptions, and fears can be identified and addressed by the HPS and nursing staff. Common procedures and the roles of staff undertaking these can be explained. These programmes provide an opportunity for the CYP to ask questions through play using, e.g., hospital corners, and preparation equipment, such as story, picture, or colouring books.

How preadmission programmes or clinics run varies from hospital to hospital. Some hold a half-day event involving a number of families, allowing them to visit the ward where they will be staying, and to watch a video/DVD explaining what is going to happen during admission. They may meet relevant staff involved in their care, e.g. play specialist, nurse, doctor, physiotherapist, and have an opportunity to take part in hospital play facilitated by a HPS. This gives them hands-on experience of medical equipment and procedures particular to their admission and treatment, e.g. taking blood from a doll or teddy, tucking a hospital corner, dressing up in the different uniforms, using story or picture books, etc. This allows the CYP to play out and talk about their fears or worries in an age-appropriate manner and helps prepare them for their admission. Using discussion and appropriate preparation resources may also be beneficial for young people.

In other hospitals where CYPs have to travel a considerable distance for treatment, the HPS and other members of the MDT may attend an outpatient preadmission clinic where preparation for admission is carried out on an individual basis.

Where preadmission is not available or possible a leaflet/web link should be provided prior to admission. This should include:

- General information about the hospital, the ward, and its routines.
- Information regarding medical/surgical procedures that may be carried out.
- Names of key staff and their roles.
- A list of items that the CYP may bring, e.g. clothes, favourite toy, book, DVD/Video.
- Advice on preparation activities that the parent/carer can carry out at home.
- A ward contact name and telephone number.

Two essential components of preparation are the relationship between the HPS and the child, and the assessment of the needs of the CYP and their family/carers. The HPS should aim to build a trusting relationship with the CYP, establishing what their interests are and what play/recreational activities they enjoy. There are a number of considerations to be taken into account during the assessment. These include:

- Age of CYP.
- Cognitive development, level of understanding, and ability to retain information.
- Emotional maturity.
- Individual vulnerability.
- Cultural/religious background and language barriers that may be present.
- Medical history.
- Previous hospital/medical experiences – what they know and what would they like to know.
- Previous preparation/coping techniques used – including what was successful and whether techniques need to be modified.
- CYP/family anxieties.
- The ability of the CYP and family to cope in what may be stressful situations.
- CYP/parental wishes regarding treatments and procedures if choices are possible.

Preparation session

Resources

A quiet area with no interruptions should be made available for the play preparation. Most young children benefit from one-on-one preparation in a quiet area with no distractions and with a parent present. Young people might or might not wish for their parent to be present for a preparation session. The HPS should ensure that all preparation materials and resources are suitable for all age groups and needs. Preparation materials and resources, i.e. booklets, specially adapted preparation dolls, hospital play equipment, e.g. theatre scrubs, masks, bandages stethoscopes, syringes, DVDs, computer games, and touch screen devices should be regularly reviewed and updated. Consent for preparation should always be sought from the parents/carers and where appropriate, the CYP. The HPS should ensure all parties understand the philosophy of play preparation, giving clear explanation of their role prior to asking for consent. In some instances, parents may not give consent for preparation to take place: it may be that they do not know or understand what is going to happen; they may be afraid they will be unable to cope with their child's fears and responses as well as their own; or they may find a situation difficult to deal with. Where consent is not forthcoming, the HPS, nursing staff, or medical staff should explain the benefits of preparation: that the CYP will have time to prepare for the event and develop coping strategies. The HPS can explain that their child will trust them as parents, and trust hospital staff more if they are honest with them and they are well prepared. Play also encourages co-operation and creates a less stressful environment for all. Reassure the parent that staff will support them through this. Time should be given to build a trusting relationship with parents in the hope that they will feel able to confide in the HPS regarding their fears and anxieties. The issue of trust is particularly important for all concerned and the truth must be given. If parents still feel unable to consent to preparation, their wishes must be respected; and this should be documented in the CYP's notes.

Process/action
- Select an appropriate method of preparation to be used, using real equipment where possible, e.g. bandages, theatre masks, syringes, etc. (beware of latex allergies).
- Timing of the session is important: this will depend on the age of the CYP and time of the procedure.
- Ask questions to find out what the CYP knows and what they would like to know.
- Introduce preparation materials step by step. This is important particularly if a CYP is having surgery that requires them to have drips and drains post-theatre.
- Explanations should be honest and factual, using appropriate words and phrases.
- Go at the CYP's pace, using age-appropriate language.
- Allow time to process information and for the CYP to ask questions, and play with preparation materials (supervised). Young people may also wish to familiarise themselves with medical equipment by handling it.

- Feelings should be acknowledged and the CYP should be reassured that fears or worries are a normal reaction.
- Discuss coping strategies and distraction techniques.
- Offer the CYP choices where appropriate, e.g. walking to the anaesthetic room. Choices for younger children should be kept simple, i.e. either A or B.
- Reassure the CYP that a parent can stay with them at all times, if this is the case (apart from in the operating theatre and some high dependency areas).
- Document the session in clinical notes and communicate anxieties to appropriate staff.

CYPs due to undergo an operation or scan may benefit from the opportunity to visit the area beforehand, e.g. visiting the anaesthetic, recovery, or scanning room and practising going into the scanner, particularly if they are not having sedation or a general anaesthetic for the procedure. If a CYP requires surgery or a medical procedure of an intimate nature, it may be more appropriate for the preparation session to be carried out by a person of the same sex, with reassurance given that privacy will be maintained during the procedure. The younger child or a CYP having complex surgery may need more than one preparation session. Siblings should be involved in the preparation session, where appropriate. If not, then they should have a one-on-one session.

Following the procedure
- Provide praise and rewards as appropriate. Stickers and achievement certificates can be offered.
- Evaluate coping strategies used and effectiveness of preparation: discuss this with the child and parent/carer.
- Postprocedural role play should be offered to the young child; the older CYP should be given the opportunity to discuss the procedure.

Outcomes
- Through play preparation, fears or anxieties should be significantly reduced.
- The CYP should have a better understanding of the procedure and what will happen afterwards.
- The CYP and parent/carer will have coping strategies and a better understanding of the importance of co-operation during a procedure.
- The HPS should discuss outcomes and follow up required with the MDT.
- The work undertaken by the HPS and outcomes of the session and procedure should be documented and included in the CYP's health care record for future reference.
- As a result of effective preparation, length of stay in hospital may be reduced.
- A positive experience for the CYP and family.
- Effective communication is carried out between the CYP/parent and MDT.

No one method of preparation will best suit a particular age group; each CYP is an individual and must be treated as such.

Postprocedural play

The opportunity for CYPs to play out their hospital experiences is of great value to them, particularly for the younger child. It allows them to play out fears, express their anger, and relieve some of their anxieties. Rereading preparation books, dressing up or acting out what has happened to them, and encouraging them to talk about their feelings and come to terms with the experience, are helpful techniques. Misconceptions and anxieties that remain about procedures can be addressed during this type of play.

Advice and suggestions for ongoing support will be given. It can also be a measure of how successful the preparation has been.

The reluctant CYP

For some CYPs, preparation may greatly increase their anxieties; therefore offering support through each stage of the procedure and postprocedural play may be more beneficial to them. Others may choose not to engage in preparation, 'coping' with their worries by denying that anything is going to happen. They may find it easier to talk through a third party such as a parent, puppet, or doll, or to be a passive participant; this may be their way of managing the situation.

Adolescents

Although the aims of preparation for adolescents are the same, the process is different in that the initial approach is to talk one to one to the young person first, rather than to the parent. The following should be taken into account when preparing young people:

- Take time to build rapport.
- Assess coping strategies.
- Be aware of developmental age and emotional needs.
- Give appropriate information and time for the young person to process it.
- Give permission to express their emotions.
- Involve them in decision making.
- Do not judge, assume, patronise, tease, make fun of their fears, or use sarcasm.
- Do not make decisions on their behalf unless they want you to.
- Involve parents appropriately.

Children and young people with additional needs or a learning disability (LD)

CYPs with additional needs or a learning disability (LD) may have limited understanding and use different ways to express fears and anxieties. Parents and carers are integral to the process of preparing CYPs with complex needs, as they will have in-depth knowledge of how their child communicates and processes information. Although assessment and preparation principles remain the same, methods of preparation will depend on the CYP's level of understanding and ability to communicate. Preparation may require more than one session.

The following suggested methods can all be used:

- General preparation resources may be used and adapted to meet the CYP's needs.
- Explanation should be simple and symbolic, e.g. using a doll/teddy or pictures.
- Role play using doctor's tools, etc. is useful.
- Simple picture books/laminated picture cards/social stories showing what is going to happen and in what order, are helpful. This is beneficial for CYPs who have language/communication disorders.
- Makaton and British Sign Language can be used with the hearing impaired CYP.
- Use of tactile sensory/'feely' boards (objects can be attached with Velcro to board).
- Communication books – some CYPs may have their own.
- Taking the CYP to visit the area where the procedure is to take place, allowing them to meet the staff, touch and feel the different

uniforms and equipment, listen to particular sounds of equipment, e.g. X-ray machine.
- CYPs on the autistic spectrum range can be challenging to work with, as their levels of understanding and communication may vary, with no specific method being the right one. Many have set routines and may become distressed when these are altered, particularly at short notice. Preparation needs to be simple, visual, and repetitive with a clear plan of action that should be adhered to.
- A play tunnel can be useful in preparing for a MRI scan, as lying inside the tunnel can prepare them for lying in the scanner.
- Computer programmes can be used for older CYPs, and for younger children, simple pictures and dialogue.
- Both methods of distraction and pain relief need to be planned well in advance.

Case study 27.1 James; a Five-year-old with autistic spectrum disorder

James was five years old when referred to an HPS with anxieties about blood tests; a procedure he had to undergo regularly. James had been diagnosed with Autistic Spectrum Disorder (ASD) and Semantic Pragmatic Communication Disorder (SPCD), which meant he found it difficult to extract meaning from communication and difficulty understanding expectations.

The HPS made a 'Blood Teddy' which James named Jonathan. This allowed James to carry out blood tests on the teddy bear and 'play out' his anxieties. This helped the HPS to assess what his anxieties were, and facilitate an understanding of why he needed blood tests, and what the process involved.

With James and his mother, the HPS devised a procedure plan of what was going to happen before, during and after the procedure, and which distraction tools to use. James chose to blow bubbles. The use of the teddy bear and procedure plan were successful, and James managed to have blood tests done regularly without undue fear or anxiety.

James's medical condition deteriorated, requiring him to have frequent admissions to hospital for further tests, investigations, and surgery. This resulted in James developing a mistrust of hospitals and medical staff, as well as heightened anxieties around medical procedures.

Managing and supporting James and his family through admissions required different approaches and strategies over time. These included:

- Preparing him for each procedure/investigation/surgery using anatomically correct dolls and medical equipment. James engaged well with this approach as he was a visual learner.
- Increasing James' familiarity and comfort with hospital staff, environment, and routines. This included preadmission visits to the ward, theatre, and meeting staff involved in his care.
- Creating a photo book of places and staff within the hospital.
- Allowing James to have some control over treatment by using closed questions and concrete choices.
- Procedure plans in place.
- Time-out cards to use when he was feeling overwhelmed.
- Being admitted to the ward the day before any surgery or investigation requiring a general anaesthetic.
- Allowing him to have his own anaesthetic mask to decorate with stickers.
- Ensuring not too many people in the room when he is undergoing a procedure/treatment.
- Reward systems.

The approaches and strategies used provided consistency, routine, and predictability for James, enabling him to feel comfortable and safe, and allowing him to manage anxieties more effectively.

Distraction techniques

'During normal growth and development, children strive to be in control of their bodies and the world around them. Illness and the accompanying diagnostic and therapeutic procedures place an additional burden on CYPs' ability to cope. Providing children with cognitive strategies helps to lessen their discomfort and allows them some control in the medical procedure' (Kachoyeanos and Friedhoff 1993, pp. 14–19). Some procedures that CYPs experience in hospital are straightforward, causing little distress. Procedures that are anticipated to be painful or cause harm inevitably cause distress and anxiety to the CYP. How they cope with this distress or anxiety depends on the individual: some put on a brave face, others show signs of distress but remain co-operative, and for others it can be an agonising struggle from beginning to end. For more information regarding the management of painful procedures, see Bruce (2009).

Distraction is the facilitation of an effective coping strategy for CYPs undergoing treatment or procedures, according to the particular situation and the CYP's individual needs. It is a nonpharmacological method used to enable a CYP to reduce anxiety and pain, by focusing on something other than the procedure. Distraction enables the CYP to manage fears and anxieties during painful or traumatic procedures more effectively, giving them some control over the situation and helping medical and nursing staff to carry out procedures more effectively. Parents/carers and staff alike will be more comfortable if children cope without showing signs of distress. When children are relaxed, they can be treated more quickly, and are usually happier and less fearful of further treatment.

The perception of pain is an individual experience and should be acknowledged with reassurance in a positive way; it should not be the main focus of the procedure. CYPs who are allowed to cry can be significantly less stressed than those who are told to be brave. Distraction therapy and alternative focus activities help CYPs to cope with procedures by putting pain or distress at the 'periphery of awareness'. They are therefore less likely to be distressed and non-compliant, creating a safer clinical environment and can gain confidence in themselves and those who care for them. As a result of distraction therapy, the CYP may experience less pain: 'Play Specialists enable patients to cope with clinical procedures and investigations by providing alternative focus for their attention' (Walker 2006, p. 26).

The HPS uses distraction techniques in a number of ways to help and support CYPs through medical and surgical procedures and investigations, e.g. blood tests, cannulation, CT scans, dressing changes, and anaesthetic induction. Although many CYPs find needles one of the most frightening aspects of treatment, very few actually have 'needle phobia' and under the right conditions, children can learn that anticipatory fear is worse than associated pain. Distraction tools and techniques used depend on the age of CYP, their level of development, their interests, and the length and type of procedure. 'None of them are magical, although the effects can seem magical' (Lansdown 1987, p. 1).

Standards for distraction

Distraction techniques are very effective and should be incorporated into routine practice and offered to all CYPs undergoing medical treatments or procedures where appropriate and possible. Distraction should be carried out by a qualified play specialist or another appropriately trained adult.

Resources

The treatment room should be welcoming, well presented, and friendly. Each treatment room should contain a distraction box with a variety of equipment suitable for all ages such as:

- Bubbles

Chapter 27 Play as a therapeutic tool

- Musical toys, cause-and-effect toys, and musical books
- Search and find books for the different age ranges
- Music
- Sensory equipment
- DVDs (where suitable)

Outcomes
- The CYP is able to allow the procedure to be carried out with little or no distress.
- The anxious CYP is able to use coping strategies such as distraction to enable them to manage anxieties more effectively which they can use for future procedures.
- The use of distraction may help reinforce positive behaviours.

Procedure guideline 27.1 Using distraction during a painful/frightening procedure

Statement	Rationale
1 Liaise with medical and nursing staff in order to understand the procedure. Where possible build a 'platform of trust' with the CYP and family through play or conversation. If this is not possible, introduce yourself, and explain your role and the use of distraction techniques using age-appropriate language and examples.	
2 Assess the CYP's understanding of the procedure, offering appropriate information, such as preparation. Decide on appropriate distraction techniques to be used; consideration should be given to the CYP's coping strategies, cognitive development, attention span, previous experiences, and length of procedure.	
3 Only the people necessary for the procedure should be in the room, with the required equipment prepared before the CYP arrives. The environment should be calm and quiet.	
4 Prior to the procedure, the roles of all involved should be clearly defined. Ensure all medical equipment required for the procedure is prepared and ready and a selection of distraction tools has been chosen and is available.	4 To minimise confusion during the procedure for CYP and family, allowing all members involved to know what is expected of them.
5 For effective distraction to take place: • The position of the CYP and the distraction method must be carefully planned. • Body language and eye contact can help the engagement and distraction process (taking into account different cultures). • The CYP and parent/carer must be receptive toward the concept of distraction.	
6 A 'plan of action' should be made with the CYP/parent and medical team, regarding how the procedure is to be carried out. Choices should be made about what is going to happen before, during, and after the procedure, with agreed on and safe boundaries in place. Choices may include: • What topical pain relief to use. • What play activity to participate in prior to the procedure. • Whether the CYP would like to sit or lie down for the procedure (where possible). • Who they would like to accompany them during the procedure. • Choice of distraction tools. • Whether the CYP would like to watch the procedure or look away. • Whether they would like to know what is happening at each step of the procedure or not. • Where possible to help medical staff with the procedure, e.g. taking off plasters/dressings. The HPS will set up these 'plans of action' as part of a play preparation or therapeutic play session.	6 The key to success, particularly with very anxious children, is negotiation, so that the CYP feels they have choice and control wherever possible.
7 Before and during the procedure, ensure that all involved are aware you are providing distraction therapy.	7 To prevent others from trying to distract simultaneously, which will cause overstimulation and can increase distress for the CYP and parent/carer.
8 Timing of distraction is crucial: it should commence when the child is relaxed, before the procedure begins, or at an agreed on point in the process.	
9 CYPs who have been assessed as highly anxious before a procedure need experienced and familiar staff to carry out the procedure.	

(continued)

The Great Ormond Street Hospital Manual of Children and Young People's Nursing Practices

Procedure guideline 27.1 Using distraction during a painful/frightening procedure *(continued)*

Statement	Rationale
10 Parents' role should be to comfort, distract if the HPS is not present, and to hold (not restrain).	
11 Reassurance should be given to the CYP that it is acceptable to cry, sing, and shout etc. during the procedure, while emphasis is placed on keeping still.	
12 If the CYP becomes too distressed it may be necessary to withdraw distraction and offer comfort and support.	12 To provide comfort when distraction is not an option.
13 If after two attempts, it has not been possible to carry out the procedure, the professional should stop and either ask someone else to continue or allow for all involved to have a break.	13 To minimise distress and prevent increasing tension.

- Try to discuss with the CYP and parent/carer(s) the effectiveness of distraction used during the procedure. Give feedback to the child through praising and rewarding appropriate behaviour using specific achievements, e.g. 'well done, you kept really still.' Stickers and certificates of achievement can be offered to reinforce this.
- The use of distraction enables the multidisciplinary team to function more effectively in providing a team approach for the CYP/family.
- The distraction method used and its effectiveness should be documented and included in the CYP's health record for future reference.

In some cases, a parent/carer's fears and behaviours may influence the success of the procedure. If this is likely, it is advisable to suggest in a sensitive manner that they join the CYP after the procedure has finished. 'Many parents find it difficult to be present while "something nasty is being done" to their child, and yet they feel they must stay with them. They themselves may hate "needles" and cannot watch their child have a blood test, much less be expected to hold them during the procedure' (Cook 1999, p. 165).

Distraction Tools and Resources

Below is a list of recommended distraction tools and resources for children of different ages.

Infants:
- Dummy
- Cuddling
- Positive touch
- Rattles
- Noisy toys
- Bubbles
- Music
- Tactile soothing toys

Toddlers:
- Bubbles
- Sensory toys
- Pop-up/musical books
- Simple storybooks
- Noisy cause-and-effect toys
- Songs and rhymes

Preschool:
- Short storybooks/pop-up books/musical books/counting books
- Bubbles
- Puppets
- Songs/rhymes
- Noisy cause-and-effect toys
- Sensory toys
- iPad®/Tablet
- DVD

School-age children:
- Search and find books
- Kaleidoscope
- Songs/rhymes
- Guided imagery
- Talking, coaching
- Breathing techniques
- iPad®/tablet, DVD
- Handheld computer games
- Music
- Sensory toys
- Reading aloud
- Guided imagery

Young People:
- iPad®/tablet, DVD
- Handheld computer games
- Music
- Guided imagery
- Breathing and relaxation techniques
- Conversation, talking, coaching
- Word games
- Sensory toys

CYP with Special Needs:
- Fibre optic lights
- Musical/noisy toys
- Bubbles
- Sensory tactile toys and equipment
- iPad®/tablet, DVD
- Tac-pac®

It is important that the CYP's cognitive age, culture, and preference are taken into consideration when selecting distraction tools. The success of distraction is dependent on the person supporting and being able to engage the CYP, and adjusting the techniques used according to how they are interacting and responding. Some CYPs do not respond to distraction, and comforting and coaching allow for alternative successful outcomes.

Long waits can lead to anxiety; if the CYP has to wait in-between treatments and procedures, try to keep them occupied, or let them have a break to play in the play area.

Anxiety levels will increase if the CYP has to watch professionals drawing up medications. If they become too distressed and the procedure is not able to be carried out, stop, and give them time and space to calm down. Go back over the distraction plans before trying again. Most important, do not assume you know what is concerning or worrying them and decide how they should cope with a procedure. This often leads to more anxiety, frustration, anger, and an unsuccessful procedure.

Relaxation

Relaxation techniques can be used by the CYP, siblings, and parents during their hospital stay and in day-to-day life. Whether to help to sleep, to use during painful procedures, or for episodes of acute pain, or for just a 'switch off' from the hospital environment, these simple techniques can be hugely beneficial to the CYP and to those around them. Some CYPs find that listening to their favourite music or specific relaxation CDs is beneficial; others find that watching TV or playing computer games is enough to distract them and therefore allow them to relax. Specific techniques are easily taught, can be adapted for most situations, and can be extremely useful.

Relaxation techniques are, in most cases, a successful means of helping children to cope, with a procedure, taking into account the needs of the individual CYP. The aim is to enable them to feel confident and secure by being able to take control of the situation.

Box 27.1 Muscle relaxation

- Make yourself comfortable on your bed or chair. Ensure TV, music, etc. is switched off and, if possible, dim the lights or draw the curtains.
- Encourage the CYP to take slow, regular, deep breaths as before.
- Breathe slowly in and out five times before commencing exercise.
- Speak instructions slowly and calmly.
- Wiggle your toes, push them down, and arch your feet, then relax and let your feet and legs go floppy.
- Squeeze the big muscle in your thigh, hold it, then relax and let your leg go floppy.
- Squeeze your tummy muscles, breathe in really deeply, then relax
- Shrug and lift up your shoulders, pull your shoulder blades together, hold them, then relax.
- Straighten your arm, squeeze your fists tight, then relax and let your arms go floppy.
- Move your head slowly from side to side, then front to back, let your head 'hang' down toward your chest and hold it, feel the stretch in the back of your neck, then roll your head slowly around, one way, then the other, loosening all those muscles.
- Wrinkle your forehead, frown, and then relax.
- Wrinkle your nose, then relax.
- Finally, smile, clench your jaw really tight, hold it, then relax.
- Finish with five more slow, deep breaths, and then slowly open your eyes.

Muscle Relaxation

Flexing and relaxing the muscles of the body is another way to distract and relax. Try to ensure a warm and quiet environment and if comfortable, encourage the CYP to close their eyes. Ideally, the person talking should also close their eyes to show that they too are relaxed. Each move should be held for at least five seconds. Start with the right foot, then the left, before moving on to right then left thigh (see Box 27.1).

Passive or progressive relaxation videos are available online e.g. youtube.

Any of these techniques can be safely used for a sick CYP and/or their siblings and parents. It is important to know the CYP's medical history, as discussed earlier. For example, some steps may have to be omitted, for a CYP following abdominal surgery, as they may find it uncomfortable to tense their stomach muscles.

Guided imagery

Guided imagery is another technique that can be used to help with relaxation and coping. CYPs have very vivid imaginations and asking them to think of something they like doing and then gently asking them questions, so that they become immersed in the image or scenario, can distract many CYPs effectively and this can be easily carried out by parents or carers.

Using a CYP's imagination

- Ask the CYP to imagine their favourite place or imagine that they are playing with friends – give them ideas, e.g. playing on the beach, but the actual choice of 'imagery' must be their own.
- Encourage them to take nice, slow, deep breaths. Imagine breathing in as if smelling your favourite flower and breathing out as if you are gently blowing bubbles.
- Ask the CYP about their image, 'what are you doing/what can you see/what can you hear/is anyone with you?'
- Throughout, encourage the CYP to continue to breathe slowly and deeply.

Combining the techniques outlined can also be a therapeutic way of enabling CYPs to cope with their anxieties and/or pain when having medical procedures. The common thread in all approaches is the importance of developing a trusting relationship with the CYP and their families. Time spent with them following the procedure is just as important as the distraction. They need to be reassured that cooperative behaviour has been helpful and they have coped well. This will hopefully prepare them for the next time a procedure needs to be undertaken. Some CYPs, however, still find the procedure distressing and will need further help as discussed below. They need to be praised, however, for any little improvement that has been seen. The word 'brave' should be avoided as it reinforces the message that CYPs must not cry or show distress, which is not the case.

Therapeutic play

Some CYPs do not respond to preparation/distraction techniques, continuing to find procedures distressing (procedural anxiety and fear) to the extent that they are not able to comply with treatment. For these children, one-to-one therapeutic play sessions over a period of time may be necessary. Feelings linked to needle fear and anxiety can be explored through these types of play session (Jelbert et al. 2005).

Koller (2008, p. 7) states 'Research provides evidence for the effectiveness of therapeutic play in reducing psychological and physiological stress for children facing medical challenges'. Therapeutic play facilitates expression, coping, and mastery of healthcare experiences, and helps facilitate treatment and procedures. Anxiety may be around an aspect of the treatment/procedure or many aspects of the hospital experience. This type of play can be directive or nondirective, allowing a trusting relationship to be built between the CYP, family, and HPS, and subsequently the medical team. As with play preparation it enables the CYP to reflect and interpret feelings of what has happened in the past, as well as prepare for the future. Therapeutic play is concerned with both a CYP's feelings and behaviour. It allows them to express their feelings, anxieties and concerns, ask questions and to discuss and develop coping strategies.

In any kind of therapeutic play the first stage is the development of a relationship with the HPS or other staff member facilitating therapeutic play. This is usually developed through the provision of normal play; finding out what the CYP is interested in and providing stimulating activities that engage them, can enhance the development of a trusting relationship. Once this has been established, further work can continue.

Case study 27.2 Thomas: Distress and noncompliance with oral medication

Thomas, a four-year-old boy, was referred to the HPS by a metabolic clinical nurse specialist (CNS). He was refusing to take one of his medicines (40 ml medicine in total per day) and becoming very distressed each time his mother tried to give it to him, which was impacting on their relationship. He had previously been an inpatient at his local hospital, where there had been an attempt to pass a nasogastric tube. Thomas had no play preparation for this and subsequently pulled the tube out. His local consultant suggested a gastrostomy tube should be inserted, as he had not had his medication for seven weeks. However the CNS wanted to try therapeutic play first, as this had not been used before, and she did not want to put Thomas through a surgical procedure unnecessarily. Thomas was admitted to a ward for three consecutive days on three consecutive weeks. Play sessions included directive and nondirective approaches, negotiation of a contract with goals. Parents were not involved in the first two weeks of sessions. Interventions used were:

(continued)

Case study 27.2 *(continued)*

- Building a relationship using normal play
- Assessment
- Desensitisation through role play using puppets
- Mixing and tasting sessions with medicines
- Negotiation of a contract with goals
- Reward systems
- Collaboration with parents
- Increased medicines

Using normal play activities, the HPS built up a rapport with Thomas, he was a sociable and active little boy who engaged very well. Through this session the HPS was also able to assess Thomas's understanding of his medical condition and help him understand why he needed the medication. This was done using puppets, Thomas called one puppet 'the good doctor who took his medicines' and the other 'the bad doctor who did not take his medicine.' Through playing with puppets, and discussion and questions facilitated by the HPS, it was ascertained that Thomas did not like the taste of the medicine, and the amount he needed to take. Role play allowed Thomas to express some of his anger and frustration of the experiences of his admission at his local hospital and the stresses of the last few weeks. Using the puppets, the HPS was able to convey the importance of taking his medication to Thomas. At four years old Thomas did not have a complete understanding of his medical condition and the need to take his medicines. To enable him to be able to understand this, the HPS explained if he took them he would become bigger and stronger. This idea appealed to Thomas as he wanted to be big and strong like his Dad.

The next step was to carry out tasting sessions, starting with 0.5 ml at a time, allowing him, with supervision, to mix the medicine and measure the dose, finding out which of his favourite drinks tasted better with medicine. The medicine was not mixed into the drink; Thomas was encouraged to have a mouthful of drink first, then his medicine from a spoon rather than a syringe, then to have a drink afterwards. This strategy worked well, and a reward chart was instigated. Each time he was able to take his medicine, he received a sticker with lots of praise and positive re-enforcement. The negotiation of goals was set with Thomas, and the increase of medicines was set at his pace. As part of the reward system, Thomas was able to choose a specific play activity to do after taking the medicines. By the end of the second week Thomas was taking 9 ml three times a day, a big achievement for him, and he was proud to tell his mother about it.

The final step was to rebuild the relationship with his mother. This was done through play sessions, allowing Thomas and his mother to have fun; they engaged very well with this. As Thomas' mother was the main giver of his medicines, the HPS worked with her so that she would be able to take on board the techniques and strategies used to help Thomas take medicine. By the end of the three-week admission, Thomas was taking 11 ml three times a day without distress. After 10 days at home, he was able to take all of his 40 ml of medicine in one go.

The case study above is an example of the value of therapeutic play, showing how different techniques used were successful in helping Thomas, empowering him and giving him control, supporting him and his family to achieve the goals of his treatment plan; it also suggests that medical/surgical interventions are not always the right route to take.

Desensitisation

Desensitisation has long been used as an approach to tackle fears for adults, and is also very helpful with some CYPs. In one study, 92% of CYPs treated with desensitisation had a reduction in their fear of needles (Rainwater et al. 1988). The idea behind this therapy is that the more a CYP is exposed to the feared object, the more able they are to tackle the cause of anxiety and find out how to deal with their feelings and develop positive coping strategies.

The first step in desensitisation is to help the CYP to become relaxed. The next step is to approach the cause of the fear gradually, with the objective of allowing the feared object to become associated with feeling relaxed, rather than being associated with fear and dread. For example, if the fear you are tackling is one of needles, begin by subjecting the CYP to a controlled exposure of the object, i.e. a picture of the needle; allow them to look at it, and touch it; you could produce an outline drawing that the CYP can colour. The important aspect of this work is that they are free of fear or given time and space to overcome fear, with the CYP deciding the pace of the treatment. Once this is mastered, begin to show the CYP the real needle; maybe safely concealed within the packet to begin with, then move on to looking at the real needle, then to the CYP holding it, and then slowly allowing the needle to come nearer and nearer the skin, until they can tolerate the needle touching their skin. Once they are confident with holding needles, they can proceed on to carrying out a 'blood test' on a model hand or specially adapted doll, progressing to rehearsing the procedure. When undertaking this type of desensitisation work it is important to find out exactly what scares them the most about the needle, and work down to the least scary thing – your starting point.

Before embarking on this treatment a full discussion with the CYP and family needs to take place so that they fully understand what is being suggested. This kind of treatment can be very successful for some CYPs. The disadvantage is that it takes time before they are ready to accept the blood test or injection.

CYPs displaying needle anxiety/fear should be provided with therapeutic needle play session(s) in a controlled environment. A qualified HPS, who has competency in this area should undertake this type of play, and may involve the support of a clinical psychologist if necessary. Parental anxieties should be assessed, and discussed with the parents/carers in question. It can be useful to have this conversation away from the CYP, as parental anxiety will affect their child's mood.

Parents/carers may choose not to accompany their child during play sessions, but should be given the opportunity to, unless an older CYP has requested that they do not, or the HPS has assessed that their anxiety levels will prevent a positive outcome. This should always be carefully and sensitively explained to parents/carers, with support offered regarding managing their anxiety.

The HPS should have knowledge of and adhere to their Trust's policies relating to the use and disposal of sharps, and other relevant policies referring to needle stick injuries, when undertaking needle play. The HPS should discuss with the CYP the safety issues that need to be taken into account when handling needles. Desensitisation can be a lengthy process, it is not always successful or appropriate; it requires careful planning, with progress regularly reviewed.

Case study 27.3 Alex and the use of desensitisation

Alex, an 11-year-old boy, was referred to the HPS, as he had been refusing to have blood tests, which were required on a monthly basis. The HPS met Alex and his mother for an initial assessment to find out why he was refusing to have blood taken, what his anxieties and concerns were, and if any previous coping strategies had worked. He reported that his anxieties were related to the thought of a needle going into his hand, and he was not convinced that 'numbing cream' worked, and he often found the blood test painful. The strategies used to help Alex overcome these anxieties were:

- To build a rapport and find out his interests
- Graded desensitisation
- Use of a topical local anaesthetic cream

Case study 27.3 (continued)

- Having a procedure plan in place
- Distraction
- Liaising with nursing staff
- Support during the procedure
- Having a clear outcome

It was important that Alex dictated the pace of the preparation; he had five sessions before he was ready to have the procedure.

It was important to build a rapport with Alex to support his engagement in this process, and to give enough information so that he gained a full understanding of his medical condition and why he needed to have his bloods taken.

This was followed by graded exposure to the 'butterfly needles' used for blood tests. Alex was allowed to look at and handle the needle, and begin to explore what it was about the needle that made him anxious. He was facilitated to touch his skin with the needle and, when ready, to carry out a 'blood test' on a model hand; this enabled him to feel more relaxed and confident gaining control of his anxieties.

The use of the topical local anaesthetic cream and cold spray was explored: the differences between the two, how they work, and their benefits. This entailed allowing Alex to put the cream and then spray on the back of his hand, illustrating to him how it numbs the area. He decided to use the anaesthetic cream. It was important that Alex was allowed to have some choices regarding what he would like to happen, and when he was ready to have his blood test. This was done by creating a three-part procedure plan: what was going to happen before, during, and after the procedure. The HPS and Alex discussed different types of distraction, their benefits, and how to use these when having a procedure; Alex chose to use his iPad®.

The final step was for an appointment to be made for Alex to have his blood test. The HPS liaised with nursing staff regarding Alex's plan, ensuring that is was followed, and supported Alex throughout the procedure. Alex was able to have bloods taken, without undue fear or anxiety. He engaged in distraction of his choice. This worked well, and the cream was effective, as he reported the test was not painful. Following this positive experience Alex is now able to have his bloods taken with confidence and ease.

This case study demonstrates undertaking this type of desensitisation and needle play, shows the important role the HPS has, and the skills needed to carry out this form of therapeutic play.

Play is a powerful therapeutic tool, which used in the right way can help children to cope with hospitalisation, illness, and treatment:

Children need to play – it's a fundamental part of every child's nature. Children, who know how to play and have the opportunity, thrive, do well in life and develop into well-rounded individuals. Play is the parent of creativity, co-operativeness, and leadership. Children whose play is denied or restricted fail to thrive, their spirit dies, their potential is denied. There is a basic and healthy requirement for every child to be free to spend time doing what every child knows best – to play. Play requires opportunity, environment, resources and respect (Fair Play for Children 2000).

Arts in health

Arts in health have become more mainstream and are in evidence in many hospitals within the UK and elsewhere. Its contribution may seem obvious, where art is incorporated into the hospital environment, but the effect that active engagement in the arts can have on the health and well-being of individuals and communities is less obvious. Arts in health incorporate many different elements; e.g. participatory arts programmes, arts therapy, medical training, and medical humanities. GOSH Arts is just one example of an arts programme and is available online at https://www.gosh.nhs.uk/wards-and-departments/departments/gosh-arts/. It offers a wide range of activities designed to encourage creativity and improve the hospital experience for everyone. Staricoff and Clift (2011) undertook a review, and included children in their evaluation of the evidence relating to arts in health. Music, singing, drama, storytelling, and dance are just some of the interventions they identified that have been used to manage medical procedures, pain and anxiety in CYPs.

References

Barbour, F. and Jun-tai, N. (2014). Enhancing a resilience in children and young people. In: *Play in Healthcare: Using Play to Promote Child Development and Well-being* (ed. A. Tonkin), 93–109. Oxon: Routledge.

Bowlby, J. (1953). *Child Care and the Growth of Love*. Baltimore: Pelican Books.

Bruce, E. (2009). Management of Painful Procedures. In: *Managing Pain in Children* (eds. A. Twycross, J. Dowden and E. Bruce), 201–218. Wiley-Blackwell.

Burghardt, G.M. (2005). *The Genesis of Animal Play: Testing the Limits*. Cambridge, MA: MIT Press.

Children Act 1989. https://www.legislation.gov.uk/ukpga/1989/41 (accessed 6 September).

Cook, P. (1999). *Supporting Sick Children and their Families*. London, Bailliere Tindall.

D'Antonio, I.J. (1984). Therapeutic use of play in hospital. *Nursing Clinics of North America* 19 (2): 351–359.

Darbyshire, P. (1996). *Living with a Sick Child in Hospital*. London: Chapman & Hall.

Department of Health (DH) (2003). *Getting the Right Start: The National Service Framework for Children, Young People and Maternity Services*. Standard for Hospital Services. Crown Copyright.

Ekra, E., Blaaka, G., Korsvold, T., and Gjengedal, E. (2012). Children in an adult world: a phenomenological study of adults and their childhood experiences of being hospitalized with newly diagnosed type 1 diabetes. *Journal of Child Healthcare* 16 (4): 395–405.

Fair Play for Children (2000). Their Millennium Resolution. Journal of Fair Play for Children Association Trust Ltd (Reg. Charity 292134) by Premier Promotions.

Garot, P.A. (1986). Therapeutic play: work of both child and nurse. *Journal of Peadiatric Nursing* 1 (2): 111–116.

Ginsburg, K.R. (2007). The importance of play in promoting healthy child development and maintaining strong parent–child bonds. *The American Academy of Paediatrics* 119 (1): 182–191.

Gleave, J. and Cole-Hamilton, I. (2012). A world without play: A literature review. Play England. https://www.scribd.com/document/308544779/A-World-Without-Play-Literature-Review-2012 (accessed 6 September 2022).

GOSH Arts. https://www.gosh.nhs.uk/wards-and-departments/departments/gosh-arts/ (accessed 6 September 2022).

Gray, P. (2011). The decline of play and the rise of psychopathology in children and adolescents. *American Journal of Play* 3 (4): 443–463.

Grisson, S., Boles, J., Bailey, K. et al. (2016). Play based procedural and support intervention for cranial radiation. *Supportive Care in Cancer* 24 (6): 2421–2427.

Hogg, C. (1990). *Quality Management for Children. Play in Hospital*. London: Hospital Liaison Committee.

Hubbuck, C. (2009). *Play for Sick Children. Play Specialists in Hospital and beyond*. Jessica-Kingsley Publishers.

Hughes, B. (1984). Play: a definition by synthesis. In: *Play Provision and Play Needs*. Lancaster: Play Education.

Hughes, B. (1996). *Playworker's Taxonomy of Play Types*. London: Playlink.

Jelbert, R., Caddy, G., Mortimer, J., and Frampton, I. (2005). Procedure preparation works! An open trial of twenty four children with needle phobia or anticipatory anxiety. *The Journal of the National Association of Hospital Play Staff* 36 (Winter): 14–18.

Jolly H. (1975). How play in hospital helps a child's recovery. The Times (July 16): 13.

Jolly, J.D. (1977). How to be in hospital without being frightened. *Nursing Times* 73 (48): 1887–1888.

Jolly, J. (1981). *The Other Side of Paediatrics – A Quick Guide to the Everyday Care of the Sick Child*. Basingstoke: Macmillan Press.

Jun-Tai, N. (2004). Fact Sheet No.6 Play in Hospital, Children's Play Information Service, National Childrens Bureau.

Jun-Tai, N. (2008). Play in hospital. *Paediatrics and Child Health* 18 (5): 233–237.

Kachoyeanos, M.K. and Friedhoff, H.M. (1993). Cognitive and behavioural strategies to reduce children's pain. *The American Journal of Maternal Child Nursing* 18: 14–19.

Kennedy, I. (2001). Learning from Bristol. The report of the public enquiry into children's heart surgery at the Bristol Royal Infirmary. 1984–1995. Crown Copyright.

Klein, M. (1929). Personification in the play of children. *The International Journal of Psycho-Analysis* 10: 193–204.

Koller, D. (2008). Child Life Council evidence-based practice statement. Therapeutic Play in Pediatric Health Care: The Essence of Child Life Practice, 7.

Lansdown, R., Great Ormond Street Hospital, Department of Psychological Medicine (1987). Helping children cope with needles – a guide for parents and staff. London, Great Ormond Street Hospital.

Lansdown, R. (1996). *Children in Hospital*. Oxford: Oxford Medical Publications.

Laming, W. H. (2003). *The Victoria Climbie inquiry: Report of an inquiry by Lord Laming (Cm. 5730)*. London: The Stationery Office. https://www.gov.uk/government/publications/the-victoria-climbie-inquiry-report-of-an-inquiry-by-lord-laming (accessed 6 September 2022).

Menzies-Lyth I. (1982). The psychological welfare of children making long stays in hospital: an experience in the art of the possible. Occasional Paper No. 3. London, The Tavistock Institute of Human Relations

National Association of Health Play Specialists (NAHPS) (2012). National Association of Health Play Specialists Standards 2012. https://www.nahps.org.uk/wp-content/uploads/2018/08/NAHPS-Occupation-Standards.pdf (accessed 6 September 2022).

Netzke-Doyle, V. (2010). Distraction strategies used in obtaining an MRI in pediatrics: a review of the evidence. *Journal of Radiology Nursing* 29 (3): 87–90.

Nuttall, J. (2013). Inter-professional work with young children in hospital: the role of "relational agency". *Early Years* 33 (4): 413–425.

O'Hagan, M. and Smith, M. (1994). *Special Issues in Child Care. A Comprehensive NVQ – Linked Text Book*. London: Balliere Tindall.

Piaget, J. (1951). *Play, Dreams and Imitation in Childhood*. London: William Heinemann Ltd.

Platt, H. (1959). *The Welfare of Children in Hospital*. London, HMSO.

Play England, (2020). Charter for Play. https://www.playengland.org.uk/charter-for-play (accessed 6 September 2022).

Play Scotland (2012). Getting it right for play: The power of play: an evidence base. Edinburgh, Play Scotland. http://www.playscotland.org/wp-content/uploads/Power-of-Play-Policy-Context.pdf (accessed 6 September 2022).

Poster, E.C. (1983). Stress immunization techniques to help children cope with hospital. *Maternal-Child Nursing Journal* 12 (2): 119–134.

Proctor, I. (2007). Sibling days at the Royal Hospital for sick children, Edinburgh and western general hospital, Edinburgh. *The Journal of the National Association of Hospital Play Staff* 40: 14–15.

Rainwater, N., Davis, B., Sweet, A. et al. (1988). Systematic desensitization in the treatment of needle phobias for children with Diabetes. *Journal of Child & Family Behavior Therapy* 10 (1): 19–31.

Richardson H (2013). Play being 'pushed aside' in nurseries. BBC News. https://www.bbc.co.uk/news/education-23033496 (accesses 6 September 2022).

Robertson, J. (1958). *Going into Hospital with Mother*. London: Tavistock.

Robertson, J. (1962). *Hospitals and Children: A Review of Letters from Parents to 'the Observer' and the BBC*. London: Victor Gollancz.

Robertson, J. (1970). *Young Children in Hospital*. London: Tavistock.

Save the Children Fund (1989). *Hospital a Deprived Environment for Children?: The Case for Hospital Play Schemes*. London: Save the Children Fund.

Smith, P.K., Cowie, H., and Blades, M. (2003). *Understanding Children's Development*. Oxford: Wiley-Blackwell.

Spence, J.C. (1946). *The Purpose of the Family: A Guide to the Care of Children*. London: National Children's Homes.

Staricoff, R & Clift, S (2011). Arts and Music in Healthcare: An overview of the medical literature: 2004–2011. Chelsea and Westminster Health Charity. https://www.artshealthresources.org.uk/docs/arts-and-music-in-healthcare-an-overview-of-medical-literature-2004-2011/ (accessed 6 September 2022).

Suris, J.-C., Michand, P.-A., and Viner, R. (2004). The adolescent with a chronic condition part 1: development. *Archives of Disease in Childhood* 89: 938–942.

Tassani, P., Bein, K., Eldridge, H., and Gough, A. (2005). *Child Care and Education*. Heinemann.

UNICEF (1989). The United Nations Convention on the Rights of the Child. https://www.unicef.org/child-rights-convention (accessed 6 September 2022).

Walker, J. (2006). *Play for Health Delivery and Auditing Quality in Hospital Play Services*. NAHPS.

Webster A. (2000) The facilitating role of the play specialist. *Paediatric Nursing* 12(7): 24–27.

Weller, B.F. (1980). *Helping Sick Children Play*. London: Baillière Tindall.

Further reading

Action for Sick Children (2006). Consenting to Treatment for Children and Young People

Alsop-Shields, L. and Mohay, H. (1991). John Bowlby and James Robertson: theorists, scientists and crusaders for improvements in the care of children in hospital. *Journal of Advanced Nursing* 35 (1): 50–58.

Axline, V. (1991). *Play Therapy*. New York: Pelican.

Bolig, R. et al. (1991). Medical play and preparation: questions and answers. *CHC Fall* 20 (4): 225–229.

Bowlby, J. (1956). The effects of mother-child separation: a follow-up study. *British Journal of Medical Psychology* 29: 211.

Bowlby, J. (1990). *Child Care and the Growth of Love*. London: Penguin.

Cook, P. (1999). *Supporting Sick Children and Their Families*. London: Baillière Tindall.

Department of Health (DH) (1991). *Welfare of CYPs in Hospital*. London: HMSO.

Keenan, T. (2002). *Introduction to Child Development*. London: Sage.

Lerwick, J.L. (2013). Psychosocial implications of pediatric surgical hospitalization. *Seminars in Paediatric Surgery* 22: 129–133.

National Association of Health Play Specialists (NAHPS) (2012). *Play Focus Distraction*. National Association of Health Play Specialists.

National Association of Health Play Specialists (NAHPS) (2012). Play Focus: Preparation for Surgery and Medical Procedures. National Association of Health Play Specialists

Play in Hospital Liaison Committee (1990). *Quality Management for Children – Play in Hospital*. London: Save the Children Fund.

Power, T.G. (2000). *Play and Exploration in Children and Animals*. Mahwah, NJ/London: Lawrence Erlbaum.

Tonkin, A. (Ed) (various authors) (2014). Play in HealthCare: Using Play to Promote Child Development and Well-Being. London, Routledge.

Tonkin, A. (2014). The provision of play in health service delivery. Fulfilling children's rights under Article 31 of the United Nations Convention on the Rights of the Child: a literature review (NAHPS).

Useful websites

www.actionforsickchildren.org.uk
www.nahps.org.uk
www.childlife.org

Chapter 28

Poisoning and overdose

Robert Cole

RN (adult), RN (child), MA Ed, PGDip Ed, BSc (Hons) with ENB Higher Award, ENB 199, 998, and A53, APLS Instructor, Head of Nursing for Children and Young People, University Hospital Lewisham, Lewisham & Greenwich NHS Trust

Chapter contents

Nonaccidental ingestion and self-harm	636	Treatment of ingested poisons	640
Health promotion strategies	637	Gastric lavage	640
Common ingestions	637	References	644
Initial management following poisoning or overdose	639		
Care of the parent/carer	640		

Procedure guidelines

28.1 Patient consent and preparation	642	28.3 Procedure (gastric lavage)	642
28.2 Preparation of equipment (gastric lavage)	642	28.4 Postprocedure (gastric lavage)	643

Principles tables

28.1 Gastric lavage: initial assessment	641	28.2 Gastric lavage: training	641

The Great Ormond Street Hospital Manual of Children and Young People's Nursing Practices, Second Edition. Edited by Elizabeth Anne Bruce, Janet Williss, and Faith Gibson.
© 2023 John Wiley & Sons Ltd. Published 2023 by John Wiley & Sons Ltd.

Poisoning in children and young people (CYPs) falls into three categories; accidental, nonaccidental, and deliberate. Accidental poisoning is most commonly seen in children aged five or younger and older CYPs who have some form of developmental delay, specifically CYPs with learning and/or behavioural difficulties (Gordon et al. 2014). Older CYPs who self-harm or have suicidal thoughts may intentionally poison themselves. In older CYPs, it is estimated that around one in every four cases of poisoning is intentional (NHS Choices 2018).

The number of CYPs dying as a consequence of poisoning has fallen significantly over the past five years. This reduction is associated with better treatment, child-resistant container regulations, and the restriction in the sale of paracetamol to packs of 16 tablets or less. The reduction in accidental ingestions has also been linked to the introduction of childproof containers and tops for liquids such as paracetamol and ibuprofen. By law, manufacturers must package certain household items, including some medicines, cleaning products and gardening items, in child resistant packaging.(British Standards Institute (BSI 2016). The majority of ingestions are of relatively nontoxic substances and CYPs are usually discharged home from A&E or Children's Ambulatory Services (National Poisons Information Service [NPIS] 2015).

Around 75–99% of accidental poisonings in children less than five years of age occur in a domestic environment. This is usually the child's own home, but as many as 20% of domestic incidents occur in the home of a relative (often a grandparent) or friend (Royal Society for the Prevention of Accidents [RoSPA] 2017). The majority of children who have taken poisons do not have serious symptoms. Medicines may be of low toxicity, e.g. the oral contraceptive pill or antibiotics. Many of the household products children take may be relatively nontoxic, but a few, such as caustic soda and paint stripper, may cause serious harm.

During 2013–2014, national poisons centres saw a significant number of enquiries related to electronic cigarette (e-cigarette) poisonings. A total of 204 enquiries were received during the year. Children aged less than five years were involved in 22% of the enquiries (Gordon et al. 2014), the most common route was through ingestion and had no features of toxicity. However, two children had moderate to severe toxicity, while another had severe toxicity and required treatment in an intensive care setting. Clinical features of toxicity after ingestion of e-cigarettes include conjunctivitis, irritation of the oral cavity, anxiety, vomiting, hyperventilation, and changes in heart rate. The most alarming feature is the accidental nature of the ingestion and occurrence in young children. Additionally, the number of adolescents using e-cigarettes was reported to have doubled in the 5 years from 2012 to 2017 (Scientific Committee on Health, Environmental and Emerging Risks SCHEER 2021). The European Commission produced legislation in 2014 and a safety report in 2016, both of which relate to the use of e-cigarettes and they continue to monitor the implementation and efficacy of this legislation (European Commission 2021).

A campaign led by RoSPA has been initiated nationally to prevent poisoning in the home. The aim is to increase awareness of the dangers of household cleaning agents/products, and the importance of safe keeping of medicines and education (RoSPA 2017). Box 28.1 identifies the top 10 enquiries received by the London Poison Centre in 2019–2020 (NPIS 2020).

Box 28.1 Pharmaceutical agents: top 10 telephone enquiries to the national poisons information service in 2019/20 (NPIS 2020)

Paracetamol	Quetapine
Ibuprofen	Codeine
Sertaline	Pregabalin
Diazepam	Mirtazapine
Propranolol	Amitriptyline

This chapter will address the following topics:

- Nonaccidental ingestion and self-harm
- Health promotion strategies
- Common ingestions (paracetamol and ethanol)
- Initial management following poisoning or overdose
- Care of the parent/carer
- Treatment of ingested poisons
- Gastric lavage

Nonaccidental ingestion and self-harm

The two groups of CYPs who need specific consideration are those in whom poisoning may have been nonaccidental and those who self-harm by poisoning.

Nonaccidental poisoning

Careful consideration must be given to the possibility of nonaccidental poisoning; a serious though relatively rare form of child abuse (Pitettii et al. 2008). Numerous agents have been used to poison children intentionally, including opioids, anticonvulsants, salt, and tricyclic antidepressants (Davis 2013). Suspicion should be raised if the story of the incident is vague, lacking in detail, and/or inconsistent over time or from person to person and in addition, when unusual behaviour is observed in the carer or there is a delay or refusal to allow treatment, unprovoked aggression, or a history or evidence of repeated ingestions. Healthcare workers should follow local safeguarding policies and procedures if they have any concerns relating to a possible non accidental poisoning. CYPs who seem 'spaced out' or have had an unexplained fall and are behaving 'oddly' should have urine and blood samples taken for toxicology, and consideration given to the possibility of nonaccidental poisoning. Toxicology is the study of the nature, effects, and detection of poisons and the treatment of poisoning (Hodgson 2010). For more information about nonaccidental injury see Chapter 31: Safeguarding.

Self-harm

Hawton et al. (2003) suggest that the rate of self-harm is relatively low in early childhood, but increases rapidly with the onset of adolescence, with females being the most vulnerable. Unfortunately, most acts of self-harm in young people never come to the attention of care services (Hawton et al. 2002). The National Institute for Health and Care Excellence (NICE) set the gold standard in the care and management of CYPs aged eight years and over who self-harm and have updated their pathways for the management of self-harm (NICE 2004, 2022). CYPs who attend the emergency department having ingested a poison will undergo triage and be prioritised based on their clinical need. The triage system most commonly used in the UK is the Manchester Emergency Triage System (Mackway-Jones et al. 2013). This system requires assessment of the CYP against a simple flow chart for overdose and self-poisoning (see Figure 28.1). Following triage, CYPs who have self-harmed should receive the requisite treatment for their physical condition, and undergo a risk and full psychosocial needs assessment and mental state examination, with referral for further treatment and care as necessary (NICE 2022). It is recommended that a member from the Child and Adolescent Mental Health Services (CAMHS) team should undertake this assessment and provide consultation for the CYP, their family, the paediatric team and social services (NICE 2004). For more information on self-harm see Chapter 18: Mental Health.

Ongoing care and follow up of the CYP will depend on the reason behind the ingestion. Accidental ingestions are routinely referred to the health visitor if the CYP is under five years of age. This is normally facilitated via the paediatric liaison health visitor. CYPs who have self-harmed are usually admitted and referred to the CAMHS. In cases of suspected intentional poisoning the CYP will always be admitted, and the consultant on-call informed. Safeguarding procedures should be followed with referral to social care and the police.

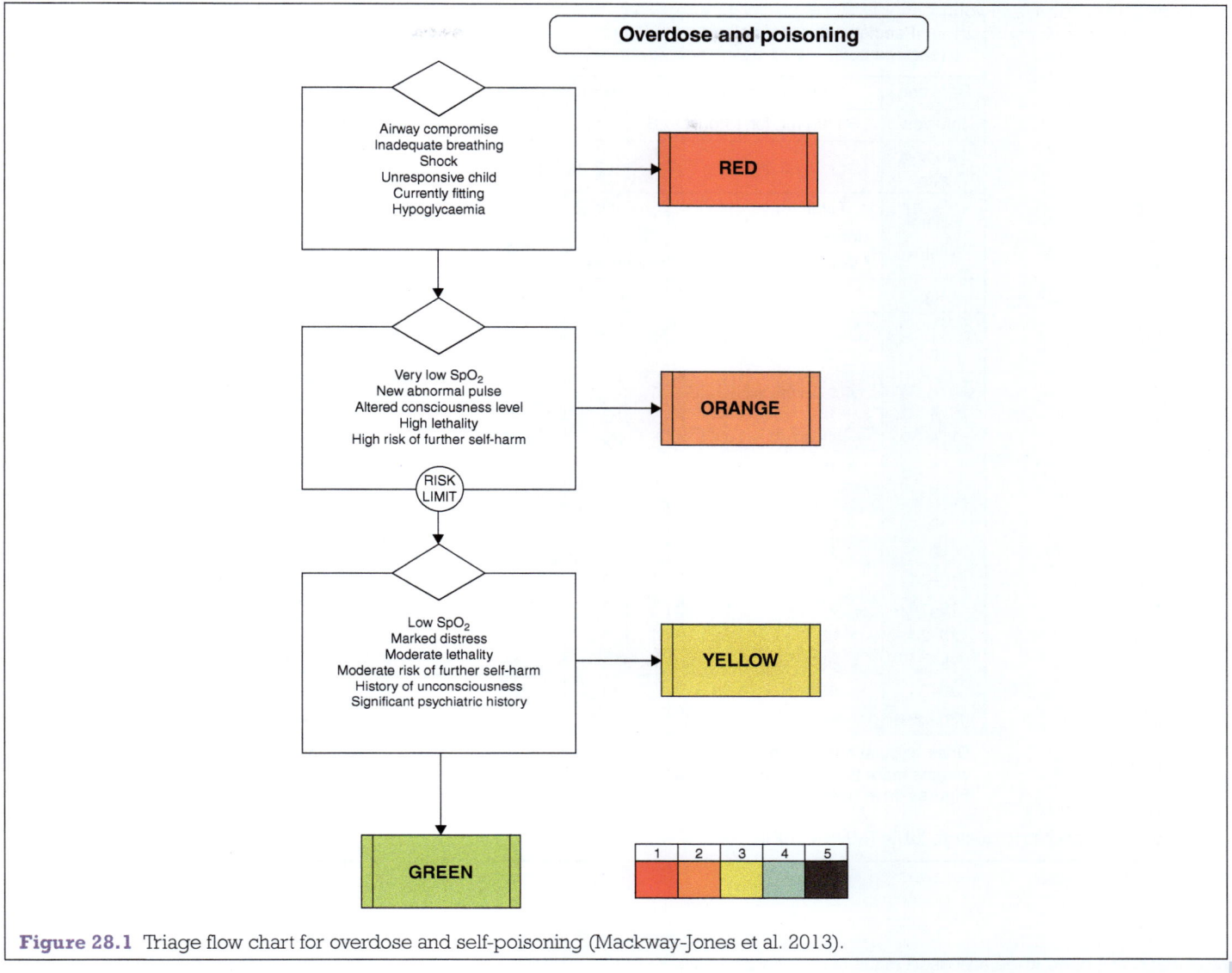

Figure 28.1 Triage flow chart for overdose and self-poisoning (Mackway-Jones et al. 2013).

Health promotion strategies

Current initiatives to reduce the number of accidental ingestions have focused on restricting access to containers by means of child-resistant lids and stoppers, or bungs for liquids. This has been found to be particularly effective in reducing the number of ingestions in children under the age of 5 years (Hawton et al. 2002). Based on the number of ingestions that occur in the home, the most obvious solution is to keep dangerous products out of the home. This unfortunately is not realistic and therefore parents/carers should be educated in safe practices and encouraged to keep dangerous products out of sight and reach. This change in behaviour can only be brought about by education and an appreciation of the risk, including with new products such as e-cigarettes.

Common ingestions

Paracetamol

Paracetamol is by far the most common poisonous substance ingested by CYPs. Unfortunately there are often no initial symptoms, although there may occasionally be nausea and vomiting. The effect on the liver indicated by raised liver function tests and prothrombin time can be detected after 24–48 hours, peaking after 72–96 hours. In 2012 the Commission on Human Medicines (CHM) reviewed the management of paracetamol ingestions and recommended that CYPs should be treated with the same dose of acetylcysteine and regimen as adults (Medicine and Healthcare Products Regulatory Agency [MHRA] 2014). The British National Formulary for Children (BNFC) (Paediatric Formulary Committee 2022) reflects these changes. However, the intravenous fluid volumes have been modified to take into account age and weight, as fluid overload is a potential risk in CYPs. Doses should be administered sequentially using an appropriate infusion pump, See Figure 28.2 for paediatric acetylcysteine doses and Figure 28.3 to view the nomogram providing guidance regarding how to assess the need for acetylcysteine (MHRA 2012, 2021). A summary of the key changes from the previous guidance can be accessed on the Royal College of Emergency Medicine (RCEM) website (https://www.rcem.ac.uk/) which includes copies of the paracetamol poisoning proforma to guide the management of all oral ingestions in patients aged >1 month and <16 years old.

If the CYP has ingested less than 75 mg/kg of paracetamol, it is unlikely that serious toxicity will occur (MHRA 2014). Children under six years of age seldom ingest sufficient amounts to be at risk of liver damage and may metabolise the drug differently from adults. However the most recent recommendations by the MHRA

Paediatric acetylcysteine prescription (each ampoule = 200 mg/mL acetylcysteine)							Please circle appropriate weight and volume.	
Regimen	First Infusion		Second Infusion		Third Infusion			
Infusion	50 mg/mL for 1 hour		6.25 mg/mL for 4 hours		6.25 mg/mL for 16 hours			
Infusion rate	3 mL/kg/h		2 mL/kg/h		1 mL/kg/h			
Patient Weight[1]	Total Infusion Volume	Infusion Rate	Total Infusion Volume	Infusion Rate	Total Infusion Volume	Infusion Rate		
kg	mL	mL/h	mL	mL/h	mL	mL/h		
1	3	3	8	2	16	1		
2	6	6	16	4	32	2		
3	9	9	24	6	48	3		
4	12	12	32	8	64	4		
5	15	15	40	10	80	5		
6	18	18	48	12	96	6		
7	21	21	56	14	112	7		
8	24	24	64	16	128	8		
9	27	27	72	18	144	9		
10–14	38	38	100	25	208	13		
15–19	53	53	140	35	288	18		
20–24	68	68	180	45	368	23		
25–29	83	83	220	55	448	28		
30–34	98	98	260	65	528	33		
35–39	113	113	300	75	608	38		

[1] Dose calculations are based on the weight in the middle of each band. If the patient weighs more than 40 kg use the adult dosage table. Figures have been rounded up to the nearest whole number

Figure 28.2 Paediatric dosage table (MHRA 2021).

insist that CYPs need to be assessed in the same way as adults following an ingestion of paracetamol (MHRA 2021).

The MHRA advises that all CYPs require medical assessment, including blood tests, if:

- They have taken a staggered paracetamol overdose (doses taken over more than one hour).
- They have taken more than the licenced dose, which is 75 mg/kg in any 24 hour period.
- The time of ingestion is uncertain and the dose is more than or equal to 75 mg/kg.

Historically, individual risk factors have been used in the assessment of paracetamol toxicity; However, CHM guidance states that individual risk factors should no longer be used in the assessment, and that treatment with acetylcysteine should be given in all staggered overdoses (MHRA 2021).

CYPs who have ingested more than 75 mg/kg of paracetamol need to have blood samples taken for paracetamol concentration four hours post ingestion. There is usually no indication to start acetylcysteine provided the results can be obtained and acted upon within eight hours of ingestion. If however, there is going to be an undue delay in obtaining these results or if more than 150 mg/kg paracetamol has been ingested, treatment with acetylcysteine should be started (MHRA 2021).

The treatment of choice is acetylcysteine if the CYP's blood paracetamol level is above the high-risk treatment line (Figure 28.3). Side effects of acetylcysteine include rashes and anaphylaxis. Activated charcoal may be considered if the CYP presents within one hour of ingestion and where the dose exceeds 150 mg/kg. The BNFC specifies the charcoal dose for CYPs as 1 g/kg (Paediatric Formulary Committee 2022).

Ethanol

Ethanol (alcohol) is a poison very commonly ingested in young people over the age of 14, but fortunately severe poisoning is uncommon. Symptoms include poor coordination, slurred speech, ataxia, drowsiness, hypoglycaemia, and acidosis (Dolan and Holt 2013). Care must be taken to exclude other conditions with similar symptoms, such as raised intracranial pressure, diabetic hypoglycaemia and drug overdose (Skinner and Driscoll 2013). Severe cases of alcohol ingestion; where the blood alcohol concentration is between 200 and 400 mg/l, can lead to coma, hypothermia, convulsions, respiratory depression and the risk of aspiration. Due to the risk of rapid central nervous system depression, induced emesis is not recommended. The NPIS recommends a period of observation of at least four hours following ingestion equivalent to 0.4 ml/kg (1 ml/kg body weight for 40% spirit, 4 ml/kg body weight for 10% wine, 8 ml/kg body weight for a 5% beer) (NPIS 2015). During this time blood sugar monitoring should be undertaken, and in the event of the

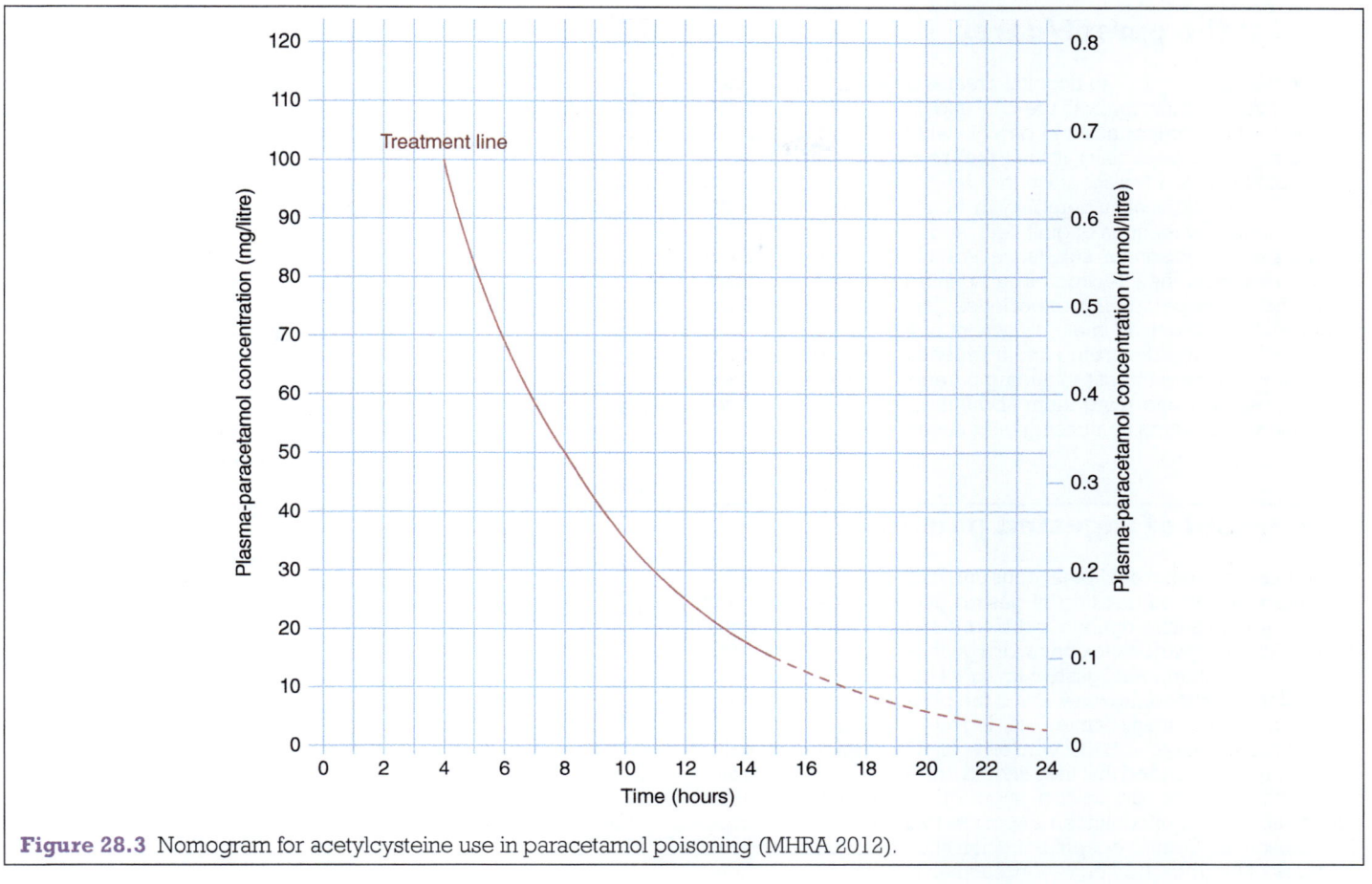

Figure 28.3 Nomogram for acetylcysteine use in paracetamol poisoning (MHRA 2012).

blood glucose dropping below 3 mmol, a bolus dose of 2 ml/kg of 10% glucose should be administered and the blood sugar repeated 30 minutes later (Advanced Paediatric Life Support [APLS] 2016).

Initial management following poisoning or overdose

The initial management of the CYP following any known or suspected poisoning is to assess and stabilise their airway, breathing and circulation, irrespective of what poison they have ingested. Only after this has been achieved should attention be given to the toxin involved. The airway may be compromised by swelling of the mouth and pharynx and depression of the central nervous system, and can cause reduced respiratory drive and an increased risk of aspiration. Adequacy of breathing should be continually assessed by clinical observation and oxygen saturation monitoring, supplemented by blood gas analysis if appropriate. Inadequate respiratory effort will require intubation and artificial ventilation (APLS 2016). The circulation can be compromised by excessive fluid loss from vomiting and diarrhoea and should be supported with appropriate fluid replacement. Some toxins cause vasodilatation and hypotension, so it is important to obtain intravenous access early in a potentially serious case of poisoning, as this can become more difficult in critically ill CYPs. Appropriate blood samples may be taken at this time. If intravenous access is difficult or unobtainable, using intraosseous access is a useful alternative in the younger child (APLS 2016).

'Shock' is often observed following serious poisoning and poor peripheral perfusion is an early sign, which may be followed by tachycardia and hypotension. It is essential, therefore, that continuous electrocardiography, blood pressure and temperature monitoring be carried out. Mild to moderate shock usually responds to intravenous fluids: initially a 20ml/kg bolus dose of 0.9% normal saline (isotonic) may be given and repeated as necessary. If fluid replacement is insufficient, the CYP may need inotropic support (McIntosh et al. 2008).

Arrhythmias are relatively uncommon in paediatric poisoning, and initial management involves adequate resuscitation and correction of any hypoxia, hypercarbia, and acid–base or electrolyte imbalances (McIntosh et al. 2008). Specific therapy need only be considered if supportive measures are inadequate. Metabolic acidosis is frequent, but only needs correction with fluids and bicarbonate boluses if severe. Correction of mild acidosis may reduce renal clearance of toxins. Central nervous system depression and convulsions are common features of poisoning. Convulsions induced by toxic agents are usually short-lived, but they may be more refractory to treatment than convulsions due to other causes.

At the earliest opportunity and once the type of poison is known, specific guidance on management should be sought from the NPIS, via TOXBASE (https://www.toxbase.org) or using the regional telephone number.

Care of the parent/carer

Any admission of a CYP to hospital creates a feeling of apprehension and vulnerability for both the CYP and the parent or carer. This can be further compounded in parents whose child has ingested something toxic, especially if they feel responsible and have, in their opinion, failed to recognise the dangers in their home environment or the signs of vulnerability in their child. Parents are often overwhelmed by feelings of guilt, fear, and anger when their child has ingested a poisonous substance. Providing an opportunity for them to express their feelings in a nonjudgemental atmosphere helps them to cope with this experience (James et al. 2012). Some aspects of treatment, such as placement of a gastric tube or support ventilation are disturbing and frightening experiences to parents. Explaining treatments, including parents in care-giving where appropriate, and informing them about their child's condition will go some way towards minimising their stress.

Treatment of ingested poisons

In the past, the removal of poisonous substances from the stomach fell under the broad heading of gastric decontamination through one of three possible options: induced emesis, activated charcoal (which absorbs various toxins or drugs, thus preventing gastrointestinal absorption), and gastric lavage. However there has been much debate and controversy about the place each of these methods has in the management of ingested poisons (Vale and Kulig 2004; Chyka et al. 2005; Benson et al. 2013; Hojer et al. 2013). It is now recommended that they should only be considered in situations where there are severe ongoing (or predicted) adverse effects as a result of continued exposure to the toxin, for example iron poisoning. Gastric decontamination should not be considered in cases of hydrocarbon ingestion, such as paraffin or white spirit, or with corrosive substances such as caustic soda, due to the risk of aspiration pneumonia (McIntosh et al. 2008).

Induced emesis had long been the favoured method of gastric emptying in CYPs (Hojer et al. 2013). A number of different emetics have been used in the past, but syrup of ipecacuanha (ipecac) has been the drug of choice for a number of years. Ipecac has a good safety record, which in part may account for its long use in the management of acute poisoning and it is quickly absorbed. However, there is a delay of up to 20–30 minutes before vomiting occurs, during which time absorption of the agent continues. If vomiting has not occurred after 20 minutes a second dose may be given. However, this method is not without its complications and contraindications (see Boxes 28.2 and 28.3). Over time this method has been the subject of many reviews and as a result, induced emesis using ipecacuanha paediatric mixture is no longer recommended (Hojer et al. 2013; British National Formulary 2022).

Gut decontamination with activated charcoal is being increasingly used in the management of childhood poisoning (Chyka et al. 2005). Activated charcoal absorbs toxic materials in the gut by offering binding sites and can been used for a variety of drugs including aspirin, carbamazepine and tricyclic antidepressant poisoning. However, it is ineffective in poisons relating to glycol, alcohol, metal and electrolytes. Its routine use is limited by its poor acceptance by children and it may not be effective more than one hour after ingestion (Chyka et al. 2005). The recommended dose is 1 g/kg for neonates and children aged 1 month to 11 years (max dose 50 g) and 50 g for 12– to 17-year-olds (Paediatric Formulary Committee 2022).

Conscious CYPs should be able to drink the charcoal, but if they find it impossible to do so, or are vomiting, it should be given via a nasogastric tube. Palatability of activated charcoal is often a problem and it may be mixed with soft drinks/fruit juices to disguise the taste. Combining activated charcoal with caffeine-free diet cola does not seem to affect the absorptive capacity of charcoal (Rangan et al. 2001). Its use is not without its complications and adverse effects, which are highlighted in Box 28.4. Contraindications include CYPs with a reduced Glasgow coma scale, reduced or absent bowel sounds, and use of antidotes that may be absorbed by the charcoal (Chyka et al. 2005).

Box 28.4 Adverse effects and complications of charcoal

- Aspiration
- Perforation
- Intestinal obstruction
- Rectal ulcer

Vale and Kulig (2004)

Box 28.2 Contra-indications and adverse effects of ipecac use

- Children <12 months
- Comatose or very drowsy children
- Ingestion of corrosive chemicals
- Sharp foreign bodies
- Agents causing rapid CNS depression
- Volatile chemicals
- Detergents

(Hojer et al. 2013)

Box 28.3 Adverse effects and complications of ipecac

- Mallory–Weiss tear of oesophagus
- Delay to administration of charcoal
- Retropneumoperitoneum gastric rupture

(Hojer et al. 2013)

Gastric lavage

Gastric lavage is the third method of gut decontamination and its use in CYPs has been poorly studied and more research is needed. If cold fluid is used, extra care should be taken when performing this procedure in children due to the increased risk of hypothermia. Electrolyte imbalance can occur if fluids other than water or isotonic saline are used. Large amounts of water used during the lavage may cause water intoxication, and therefore aliquots of up to 10–20 ml/kg should be used (Benson et al. 2013). Gastric lavage is absolutely contraindicated in the comatose CYP with a depressed gag reflex and unprotected airway. Elective intubation using an appropriate-sized endotracheal tube is recommended in these patients. Gastric lavage involves the passage of a large bore orogastric tube with sequential administration and removal of fluid for the purpose of removing toxins contained in gastric fluid (Benson et al. 2013). The orogastric tube should be as large as can be safely tolerated by the CYP (16–36 Fr) (3.5–8.5 mm). This technique of gastric decontamination has been used as a treatment for acute poison ingestion for over 200 years. Until the mid 1980s, the use of gastric lavage up to four hours post ingestion followed by the administration of activated charcoal was accepted as the standard of care. However, the types of drug ingestions today are dramatically different and the need and utility of gastric lavage remains controversial. In 2013 a systematic review of the literature concluded that at present there is no evidence showing that gastric lavage should be used routinely in the management of poisonings. Further, the evidence supporting its practice as a beneficial treatment in specific situations is weak, and it should only be performed by individuals with appropriate training and expertise (Benson et al. 2013).

The procedure for undertaking a gastric lavage is outlined below.

Chapter 28 Poisoning and overdose

Principles table 28.1 Gastric lavage: initial assessment

Principle	Rationale
1 While taking a history it is important to ascertain: a) What was ingested and the formulation. Ideally the parents/carers will have brought the container and remaining tablets with them. If berries or toadstools have been eaten they should bring a good sized, unchewed bit of plant where possible. b) How much has been ingested (calculate amounts per kg of body weight).	1 a) To determine exactly what type of drug/toxin has been ingested (RoSPA 2017). b) It is essential to calculate the maximum possible amount ingested assuming an initial full container and no toxin wasted (Mackway-Jones et al. 2013).
2 When telephoning a poisons information centre it is helpful to have the following information to hand: • Name, age, sex, weight (in kg) of the CYP. • The time since exposure. • The substance(s) to which the CYP has been exposed. • The amount taken or duration of exposure. • The constituents and the manufacturer's name of the product, if applicable. • Packing details and description of product. • The clinical condition of the CYP. • Any relevant pre-existing disease. • The normal daily dose if this is a drug ingestion of a medication the CYP is taking therapeutically.	2 To inform decision regarding whether and how to treat. The poisons information centre should be contacted if there is any doubt about toxicity of a substance a CYP has taken or the treatment that is needed (Dolan and Holt 2013; Mackway-Jones et al. 2013).
3 Gastric lavage should only be considered if the ingestion has occurred within 1 hour and following recommendations from a poison information centre.	3 Gastric lavage should NOT be carried out routinely as there is no evidence to support any improved clinical outcome or reduced mortality (Benson et al. 2013).

Principles table 28.2 Gastric lavage: training

Principle	Rationale
1 Gastric lavage must be performed only by experienced staff who:	1 To ensure safety and reduce the likelihood of side effects and complications (Bartlett 2003).
a) Are competent in performing the procedure and in basic life-support.	a) Strong vagal stimulation can induce cardiac dysrhythmias and cardiopulmonary arrest.
b) Are familiar with the indications and contraindications for the procedure – it should be considered only if the CYP has ingested a potentially life-threatening amount of poison and the procedure can be undertaken within 60 minutes of ingestion.	b) To identify CYPs who are at least at risk from the potential complications of this procedure and would benefit from it.
c) Have received: • Training on how to perform this procedure safely • Supervised practice • Resuscitation training as per trust policy	c) To establish and maintain the required level of competence.
d) Understand the potential complications of: • Aspiration pneumonia • Laryngospasm • Hypoxia and hypercapnia • Mechanical injury to the throat, oesophagus, and stomach • Fluid and electrolyte imbalance	
2 Gastric lavage should NOT be performed in CYPs who:	2 To ensure safety and reduce the likelihood of side effects and complications.
a) Have a reduced state of consciousness.	a) Loss of protective reflexes increases the risk of pulmonary aspiration. These patients should be intubated before the procedure.
b) Have ingested a corrosive substance such as a strong acid or alkali solution.	b) To prevent strong acids or alkalis causing further damage to the oesophagus and potential aspiration of a corrosive substance.
c) Have ingested a hydrocarbon (polish, paint stripper/thinner, insecticides, rubber, plastic, etc.).	c) Hydrocarbons have a high aspiration potential.
d) Are at risk of haemorrhage or gastrointestinal perforation due to recent surgery or other medical conditions.	d) To prevent further complications.

The Great Ormond Street Hospital Manual of Children and Young People's Nursing Practices

Procedure guideline 28.1 Patient consent and preparation

Statement	Rationale
1 Obtain consent for the procedure to be carried out. • Ensure the CYP is awake and cooperative. • Explain the procedure to the CYP (if able to understand) or young person and carer and allow time for any questions.	1 To gain consent from the carer who has parental responsibility and assent from the CYP (Lynch 2010).
2 To minimise complications. • Do not attempt to perform a gastric lavage in a completely uncooperative or aggressive CYP who refuses to swallow a gastric lavage tube.	• To prevent the risk of pulmonary aspiration and haemorrhage.

Procedure guideline 28.2 Preparation of equipment (gastric lavage)

Statement	Rationale
1 Assemble the appropriate equipment ensuring the following are available on the trolley prior to performing the gastric lavage: • Incontinence pads/plastic sheeting • Disposable plastic aprons and gloves, K-Y jelly • Sterile gastric tube with connector, funnel, and connecting tubing • Large jug and bucket for gastric washing • Towel and blankets • Universal container • 50 ml bladder syringe • pH paper <5.5 • Activated charcoal solution • Warm 0.9% saline (10 ml/kg)	1 To ensure the procedure is conducted as smoothly as possible without unnecessary delays.
2 Ensure that the following equipment is available and in good working order: a) Suction, oxygen, CYP/adult oxygen face mask, appropriate-size Yankauer, and a range of suction catheters. b) A bed with the facility to tilt the CYP head down.	2 To maintain a safe environment. a) To ensure that equipment available to maintain the CYP's airway if needed (Dolan and Holt 2013). b) To minimise the risk of aspiration.
3 Calculate the quantity of liquid required. For children, 10 ml/kg body weight of warm normal saline (0.9%) should be given. Water should be avoided in young children because of the risk of inducing hyponatraemia and water intoxication.	3 Small volumes are used to minimise the risk of gastric contents entering the duodenum during lavage. Warm fluids avoid the risk of hypothermia in the very young (Bartlett 2003).

Procedure guideline 28.3 Procedure (gastric lavage)

Statement	Rationale
1 In order to undertake the procedure safely and efficiently the following must be adhered to.	1 To ensure that the procedure is performed safely and effectively (Benson et al. 2013).
2 Ensure that there are a minimum of two staff available for the duration of the procedure.	2 One nurse with sole responsibility for managing the procedure and airway, the other comforting and supporting the CYP.
3 Explain the procedure to the whole family if appropriate and ensure they understand the procedure.	3 To gain the CYP's cooperation and reduce the risks of complications.
4 Ascertain whether a member of the family/carer wishes to be present.	4 To gain the cooperation of the CYP and offer reassurance.
5 Provide reassurance and support throughout the procedure.	5 To minimise any complications that may occur should the CYP become agitated.
6 Lay the CYP on their left side with the head end of the bed tilted 20° down.	6 Head-down tilt will aid the drainage of gastric contents and ensure that no secretions/vomit is inhaled.
7 Place disposable sheets and towels under the CYP's head and a plastic sheet over the floor.	7 To protect the nurse and the CYP should vomiting occur.
8 Turn on suction and place appropriate-sized Yankauer sucker near the CYP's head.	8 To ensure suction is immediately available to clear the airway should the CYP vomit.
9 Perform hand hygiene and put on plastic apron and non sterile gloves.	9 To adhere to standard precautions.

Procedure guideline 28.3 Procedure (gastric lavage) *(continued)*

Statement	Rationale
10 The length of the tube to be inserted is measured and marked before insertion. In CYPs, a size 16–36 Fr with a diameter of 3.5–8.5mm should be used. The tube should be for single use only.	10 To ensure the correct length of tube and minimise trauma while passing the tube.
11 Lubricate the tube and pass a few centimetres at a time while the CYP swallows.	11 To facilitate passage of the tube.
12 Check that the tube is in the stomach by aspirating some of the stomach contents and confirming acidity using pH paper is <5.5.	12 Ph testing is used as the first line test method to ensure the tube is in the stomach and to minimise the risk of aspiration. (National Patient Safety Agency 2011)
13 Place some of the stomach contents in a universal container and send off for toxicology analysis.	13 To identify the ingestion of any medications/substances that may be toxic to the body.
14 a) Attach the connecting tubing and funnel to the gastric tube. b) Slowly pour 0.9% saline solution at 37°C through the funnel to lavage the stomach. Administer in volumes of 10–20ml/kg.	14 a) To enable the fluid to be administered. b) To prevent sudden lowering of body temperature and possible shock (Benson et al. 2013).
15 Fluid is run through the tubing with the funnel held approximately 50cm above the CYP's shoulder, taking care not to introduce air into the tube.	15 To control the rate at which the fluid is installed.
16 Before the last of the fluid enters the tube, compress the tube and lower the funnel into the bucket to allow the lavage fluid to return.	16 A syphoning action is needed to recall the contents of the stomach.
17 Observe for tablet debris, which may be seen on the side of the tube or in the bucket. If possible these should be compared to the tablet ingested.	17 To confirm ingestion of suspected tablets.
18 As the last of the fluid drains out, care should be taken to compress the tubing to prevent air getting into the system.	18 To minimise the risk of the CYP vomiting and experiencing discomfort.
19 The lavage is repeated until the return is completely clear.	19 To maximise clearance of any tablets.
20 Activated charcoal may then be administered down the tube if recommended.	20 To absorb any tablets that may be left in the stomach.
21 Disconnect the funnel from the tube and gently but firmly remove the gastric tube. Level the head end of the bed.	21 Gagging and possible vomiting may occur when the tube is removed. As the tube reaches the pharynx, any fluid left may escape and infiltrate into the lungs.
22 Dispose of all equipment in line with local policy. Perform hand hygiene.	22 To minimise the risk of infection and adhere to local waste disposal policy.
23 Send sample of gastric contents to toxicology unit for analysis.	23 To try and identify the content of the ingested substance.

Procedure guideline 28.4 Postprocedure (gastric lavage)

Statement	Rationale
1 Sit the CYP up and make them comfortable, reassuring them and the carer all the time.	1 To minimise the distress to the CYP and carer.
2 Provide oral hygiene facilities as required.	2 To maintain a clean, moist mouth.
3 Document findings and outcome following gastric lavage.	3 To ensure effective communication and provide documentary evidence of care provided.
4 Reassure the parents following the procedure regarding any possible complications and encourage them to speak to the nurse caring for their CYP as soon as possible if they have any concerns.	4 To provide comfort, support, and reassurance. Parents/carers are likely to be very anxious regarding the possible consequences of the ingestion.

References

Advanced Paediatric Life-support Group (2016). *Advanced Paediatric Life Support: The Practical Approach*, 6th ed. London: BMJ Publishing.

Bartlett, D. (2003). The ABC of gastric decontamination. *Journal of Emergency Nursing* 29 (6): 576–577.

Benson BE, Hoppu K Troutman W G, Bedry R, Erdman A, Hojer J, Megarbane B, Thanacoody R, Carvati E. M. (2013) Position paper update: gastric lavage for gastrointestinal decontamination *Clinical Toxicology* 51, 140–146

British National Formulary (2022) Poisoning, emergency treatment. https://bnf.nice.org.uk/treatment-summaries/poisoning-emergency-treatment/ (accessed 14 September 2022).

British Standard Institute (BSI) (2016) Child resistant packaging – A consumer's guide to the standards for child resistant packaging. https://www.bsigroup.com/LocalFiles/en-GB/consumer-guides/resources/BSI-Consumer-Brochure-Child-Resistant-Packaging-UK-EN.pdf (accessed 7 September 2022).

Chyka, P.A., Seger, D., Krenzelok, E.P., and Vale, J. (2005). American Academy of clinical toxicology, European Association of Poisons Centres and Clinical Toxicologists. Position paper: single dose activated charcoal. *Journal of Toxicology. Clinical Toxicology* 43 (2): 61–87.

Davis, P. (2013). Deliberate poisoning in the context of induced illness in children. *Paediatrics and Child Health* 23 (9): 385–390.

Dolan, B. and Holt, L. (2013). *Accident & Emergency: Theory into Practice*, 3rd ed. London: Baillière Tindall.

European Commission (2021). Tobacco: Electronic cigarettes. https://health.ec.europa.eu/tobacco/product-regulation/electronic-cigarettes_en (accessed 14 September 2022).

Gordon, L., Jackson, G., and Eddleston, M. (eds) (2014). National Poisons Information Service Report 2013/14 (online). https://www.npis.org/Download/NPISAnnualReport2013-14.pdf (accessed 7 September 2022).

Hawton, K., Rodham, K., Evans, E., and Weatherall, R. (2002). Deliberate self-harm in adolescents: self-report survey in schools in England. *British Medical Journal* 325 (7374): 1207–1211.

Hawton, K., Hall, S., Simkin, S. et al. (2003). Deliberate self-harm in adolescents: a study of characteristics and trends in Oxford, 1990–2000. *Journal of Child Psychology and Psychiatry* 44 (8): 1191–1198.

Hodgson, E. (2010). *A Textbook of Modern Toxicology*, 4th ed, 10. Wiley.

Hojer, J., Troutman, W., Hoppu, K. et al. (2013). Position paper update: ipecac syrup for gastrointestinal decontamination. *Clinical Toxicology* 51 (3): 134–139.

James, S., Nelson, K. et al. (2012). *Nursing Care of Children: Principles and Practice*, 4th ed, 202–210. London: Elsevier.

Lynch, J. (2010). *Consent to Treatment*. Milton Keynes: Radcliffe Publishing.

Mackway-Jones, K., Marsden, J., and Windle, J. (2013). *Emergency Triage: Manchester Triage Group*, 3rd ed. Wiley Blackwell.

McIntosh, N., Helms, P., Smyth, R., and Logan, S. (2008). *Forfar & Arneil's Textbook of Pediatrics*, 7th ed. London: Churchill Livingstone.

Medicine and Healthcare Products Regulatory Agency (MHRA) (2012). Paracetamol overdose: Simplification of the use of intravenous acetylcysteine. Safety warnings and messages for medicines 3 September 2012. https://webarchive.nationalarchives.gov.uk/ukgwa/20150110162216/http://www.mhra.gov.uk/Safetyinformation/Safetywarningsalertsandrecalls/Safetywarningsandmessagesformedicines/CON178225 (accessed 7 September 2022).

Medicine and Healthcare Products Regulatory Agency (MHRA) (2014). Treating paracetamol overdose with intravenous acetylcysteine: new guidance Drug safety update. https://www.gov.uk/drug-safety-update/treating-paracetamol-overdose-with-intravenous-acetylcysteine-new-guidance (accessed 7 September 2022).

Medicine and Healthcare Products Regulatory Agency (MHRA) (2021). Acetylcysteine 200mg/ml Injection. Administration information for the healthcare professional. https://mhraproducts4853.blob.core.windows.net/docs/4ec94f1b9c69b5dc3f9f17d62fd0f6dac9b82ab9 (accessed 7 September 2022).

National Institute for Health and Care Excellence (NICE) (2004). *Self-Harm: The Short-Term Physical and Psychological Management and Secondary Prevention of Self-Harm in Primary and Secondary Care*. London: The British Psychological Society.

National Institute for Health and Care Excellence (NICE) (2022). Self-harm: assessment, management and preventing recurrence. NICE guideline [NG225]. https://www.nice.org.uk/guidance/ng225 (accessed 14 September 2022).

National Patient Safety Agency (NPSA) (2011). Patient Safety Alert NPSA/2011/PSA002: reducing the harm caused by misplaced nasogastric feeding tubes in adults, children and infants. NPSA (Online) NPSA. https://www.pslhub.org/learn/improving-patient-safety/patient-safety-alert-npsa2011psa002-reducing-the-harm-caused-by-misplaced-nasogastric-feeding-tubes-in-adults-children-and-infants-r4525/ (accessed 14 September 2022).

National Poisons Information Service (NPIS) (2015). TOXBASE (Online) NPIS. https://www.toxbase.org/ (accessed 14 September 2022).

National poisons Information Service (NPIS) (2020) National poisons Information Service Report 2019/20. https://www.npis.org/Download/NPIS%20Report%202019-20.pdf (accessed 14 September 2022).

NHS Choices (2018.) Poisoning. (Online) NHS Choices. https://www.nhs.uk/conditions/poisoning/ (accessed 14 September 2022).

Paediatric Formulary Committee (2022) BNF for Children (Online). London: BMJ Group, Pharmaceutical Press, and RCPCH Publications. https://bnfc.nice.org.uk/ (accessed 14 September 2022).

Pitettii, R.D., Whitman, E., and Zaylor, A. (2008). Accidental and non-accidental poisonings as a cause of apparent life-threatening events in infants. *Pediatrics* 122: e359–e362.

Rangan, C., Nordt, S., Hamilton, R. et al. (2001). Treatment of acetaminophen ingestion with a super-activated charcoal-cola mixture. *Annual Emergency Medicine* 37: 55–58.

Royal Society for the Prevention of Accidents (RoSPA) (2017). Preventing accidents in the home. https://www.rospa.com/home-safety/advice/general/preventing-accidents-in-the-home (accessed 14 September 2022).

Scientific Committee on Health, Environmental and Emerging Risks (SCHEER) (2021). Opinion on electronic cigarettes. https://health.ec.europa.eu/system/files/2022-08/scheer_o_017.pdf (accessed 14 September 2022).

Skinner, D. and Driscoll, P. (2013). *ABC of Major Trauma*, 4th ed. London: BMJ Publishing.

Vale, J. and Kulig, K. (2004). American Academy of clinical toxicology, European Association of Poisons Centres and Clinical Toxicologists. Position paper: gastric lavage. *Journal of Toxicology. Clinical Toxicology* 42 (7): 933–943.

Chapter 29

Respiratory care

Elizabeth Leonard[1], Charlotte Donovan[2], Emma Shkurka[3], Joanne Cooke[4], Heather Hatter[5], Maura O'Callaghan[6], Vicky Robinson[7], Catherine Spreckley[8], Ana Marote[9], Harriet Clark[10], and Jade Rand[11]

[1] RN (Adult), RN (Child), BA (Hons), MSc, Head of Education (Operational), Great Ormond Street Hospital, London, UK
[2] BSc (Hons) Physiotherapy, Paediatric Physiotherapist, PICU and NICU, GOSH
[3] BSc (Hons) Physiotherapy, MRes Clinical Practice, Paediatric Critical Care Physiotherapist and NIHR Clinical Doctoral Research Fellow, GOSH
[4] TD, MSc, BSc (Hons), RN (Adult), RN (Child), NT, Advanced Nurse Practitioner, ENT/Tracheostomies, GOSH
[5] RN (Adult), RN (Child), BSc (Hons), Dip Nursing, Practice Educator, Respiratory Medicine, GOSH
[6] RN (Adult), RN (Child), ANP, Lead Nurse, ECMO/VAD, Cardiorespiratory Unit, GOSH
[7] DipHe and BSc (Hons) Children's Nursing, RN (Child), CNS Non-invasive Ventilation, GOSH
[8] RN (Child), BSc (Hons), PGCE, PGDip, Former Practice Educator, Respiratory, GOSH
[9] Formerly Ward Sister, Respiratory, GOSH
[10] RN (Child) BSc (Hons) Children's Nursing, Respiratory, GOSH
[11] RN (Child) BSc (Hons) Children's Nursing, PG Cert Practice Education, Respiratory, GOSH

Chapter contents

Introduction	646
Airway suction	646
Nasopharyngeal airway	649
Oxygen therapy	657
Chest drain management	663
Noninvasive ventilation (NIV)	672
Long-term ventilation (LTV)	676
References	680

Procedure guidelines

29.1	Suction: training, assessment and preparation	647	29.14 Ongoing chest drain care and prevention of complications	669
29.2	Performing suction	648	29.15 Changing a chest drain chamber	670
29.3	Preparation for a NPA	651	29.16 Removal of a chest drain	670
29.4	Inserting the NPA	654	29.17 Preparation for NIV	673
29.5	Observations post NPA insertion	656	29.18 NIV mask placement and care	673
29.6	Ongoing care of an NPA and discharge planning	656	29.19 NIV humidification and oxygen	674
29.7	Education, assessment, and preparation for oxygen administration	660	29.20 NIV safety, tolerance, and compliance	675
29.8	Administration of oxygen therapy	660	29.21 Ongoing care of NIV	675
29.9	Continuous assessment of the CYP receiving oxygen therapy	661	29.22 Assessment for LTV and transitional care	676
29.10	Discharge planning for the CYP on long-term oxygen	662	29.23 Management of a CYP on LTV	676
29.11	Preparation for insertion of a chest drain	665	29.24 Leaving the clinical area with LTV	677
29.12	Postprocedure care of a chest drain	665	29.25 Discharge planning for a CYP with LTV	678
29.13	Specific chest drain observations	666	29.26 The management of acute illness in a CYP with a tracheostomy at home	680

The Great Ormond Street Hospital Manual of Children and Young People's Nursing Practices, Second Edition. Edited by Elizabeth Anne Bruce, Janet Williss, and Faith Gibson.
© 2023 John Wiley & Sons Ltd. Published 2023 by John Wiley & Sons Ltd.

Introduction

Respiratory care is one of the fundamental roles of the nurse, ranging from the regular observation of respiratory rate and assessment of effort to the management of longer-term airway support. Respiratory physiology consists of:

- **Ventilation**: The act of getting air into and out of the lungs.
- **Respiration**: The exchange of gases across the alveolar membrane, an essential function of the lungs, providing the body's cells with oxygen and the removal of carbon dioxide from the body.

Lung development starts at 26 days after fertilisation and proceeds through various stages of development (Schoenwolf et al. 2014). The lungs are usually mature at 36 weeks gestation and babies born prematurely can present with lung immaturity and reduction in the expected lung efficiency seen in full term babies. Respiratory issues can be linked to many other comorbidities and be part of group of clinical issues forming a syndrome or part of a genetic anomaly, e.g. Down Syndrome (Pandit and Fitzgerald 2012) or cystic fibrosis. The lungs are relatively immature at birth but continue to develop into childhood, with alveoli development complete around the age of seven years. Infants and small children have small resting volumes and low oxygen reserves. They also have a higher rate of oxygen consumption, which results in a rapid fall in blood oxygen levels when their respiratory state is compromised.

Clinical observation and assessment, effective and efficient airway management, and support of oxygen delivery are of primary importance to ensure that children and young people (CYPs) are able to maintain optimal respiratory function, either independently or supported. This is part of the assessment of basic and advanced life support, directing assessment and clinical support strategies. All clinical teams caring for the CYP need to be competent in clinical observation and assessment of children of all ages. Early recognition and effective management of respiratory failure or problems will prevent the majority of cardiorespiratory arrests in CYPs, and reduce associated morbidity and mortality (Royal College of Paediatrics and Child Health [RCPCH] 2014a). A standardised baseline assessment using a paediatric early warning score (PEWS) (Pearson and Duncan 2011; Royal College of Nursing [RCN] 2017) and the use of a communication tool such as SBARD (situation, background, assessment, recommendations, decision) enable concise and timely communication of problems such as deterioration in the child's respiratory function. This drives patient safety directives and aids assertive, effective communication, reducing the need for repetition in challenging communication situations between all staff levels. These tools also provide a standardised documentation of events (RCPCH 2018).

Skills and competence to manage all respiratory issues are essential for all nurses. CYPs who have a reduced ability to clear or maintain an airway or who require additional oxygen delivery as part of their ongoing care require ongoing assessment of their needs. This should be provided by a registered health professional or, for CYPs with a chronic stable condition, a parent, carer, or healthcare assistant who has received training and has the relevant skills, including the ability to recognise deterioration and provide life support to keep the CYP safe. This chapter has links with Chapter 1: Assessment, which covers respiratory assessment on admission, and Chapter 9: Early Recognition and Management of the Seriously Ill Child, which covers respiratory assessment in the deteriorating child.

Airway suction

Introduction

The aim of airway suction is to clear secretions to maintain a patent airway. Suction is used to clear retained or excessive respiratory tract secretions in those CYPs who are unable to do so effectively for themselves. This could be due to the presence of an artificial airway, such as an endotracheal or tracheostomy tube, or where the CYP, for a number of reasons, might have a poor cough, e.g. due to excessive sedation or a neurological condition. Having an artificial airway in situ impairs the cough reflex and may increase mucus production (Walsh et al. 2011). Therefore, in neonatal and paediatric intensive care units, suctioning of an artificial airway is likely to be a common procedure (Argent 2009).

Suction is a procedure that is regularly carried out by healthcare workers (HCWs) and in some cases by parents or carers. The aim is to clear the airway and in doing so to reduce work of breathing and the risk of atelectasis, thereby maintaining or improving gas exchange. In self-ventilating CYPs, the upper respiratory tract may need to be suctioned via the oro- or nasopharynx to enable them to breathe comfortably, particularly in the presence of increased secretions during a respiratory infection. It is performed so that the airway is not compromised; this is particularly important in young infants, who preferentially breathe through their nose, thus enabling natural humidification and reducing resistance (Walsh et al. 2011).

Those performing suction should be aware of the potentially harmful side effects and have the skills and competence to assess the need for suction and to perform it safely and effectively while minimising the potential side effects. The effects that need to be minimised during suction are:

- Tracheobronchial trauma
- Atelectasis
- Hypoxia
- Cardiovascular changes
- Alterations in intracranial pressure
- Pneumothorax
- Infection
- Formation of distal granulation tissue or ulceration.

(Argent 2009; American Association for Respiratory Care 2010; Davies et al. 2015; Edwards 2018).

Although care should be taken to minimise the occurrence of the above side effects it is of paramount importance that the objective, the maintenance of a patent airway, is achieved. When suctioning is indicated, the decision to withhold suction to avoid potential adverse events may result in, for example, a blocked endotracheal tube (ETT) and the risks associated with an emergency reintubation (American Association for Respiratory Care 2010; Davies et al. 2015).

The CYP and equipment should be prepared and the procedure should be carried out as quickly as possible to prevent loss of lung volume. This may be caused by taking too long to perform suction (Tingay et al. 2010).

Chapter 29 Respiratory care

Procedure guideline 29.1 Suction: training, assessment and preparation

Statement	Rationale
1 All individuals performing suction should receive training in: • Respiratory assessment. • Indications for suction. • Suction technique. • Potential side effects. • Signs of clinical deterioration.	1 To ensure the CYP receives suction that is appropriate, effective, and safe with minimal side effects.
2 All staff should have training in the required level of resuscitation skills.	2 To facilitate rapid clinical emergency interventions.

Assessing the need for suction

1 Assess the need for suction by observing and documenting the following: a) Increased work of breathing including: • Increased respiratory rate • Alteration in respiratory pattern • Recession • Nasal flaring • Tracheal tug • Head bobbing • Grunting • Altered level of consciousness b) Alteration in gas exchange including: • Decrease in the SaO_2 (oxygen saturation) • Pale and/or mottled appearance • Cyanosis • Decreased blood oxygen levels and/or increased carbon dioxide levels c) Evidence of secretions, either visible, audible, or on auscultation and/or palpation d) Examination of the chest X-ray e) Alteration of ventilator parameters f) Inability to effectively clear secretions independently (poor cough)	1 To ensure that suctioning is not carried out unnecessarily. Ongoing monitoring of the listed parameters should result in a timely intervention, thus minimising the risk of deterioration. This will also provide a baseline to use as a comparison when reassessing the CYP at the end of the intervention.
2 It is also important that other causes of respiratory distress that do not require suction are considered; e.g. a pneumothorax, fluid overload, or a misplaced artificial airway.	2 To ensure that suctioning is not carried out unnecessarily and that appropriate management is initiated in a timely manner.

Preparing the CYP and family

1 Ensure that the CYP, and the family if they are present, are prepared for the procedure: a) In a nonemergency situation, check that the CYP has not just been fed (approximately 30 mins) or, if on continuous feeds, ensure the feed is turned off prior to suction. b) In an intubated CYP, ensure they are receiving sedation. c) In an alert older CYP explain what is about to happen. d) Although not always required, in awake infants, there may be times when it may be advisable to wrap them securely in a sheet or blanket and place them in side lying position.	1 To facilitate understanding and co-operation. a) To minimise the risk of vomiting and subsequent aspiration. b) To minimise the stress and discomfort caused by the procedure. c) To facilitate understanding and co-operation. d) To facilitate quick suction with minimal interference, thereby reducing side effects. In the event of vomiting the side lying position will help to reduce the risk of aspiration.

(continued)

Procedure guideline 29.1 Suction: Training, assessment and preparation *(continued)*

Preparation of equipment: negative pressure

Statement	Rationale
1 The suction unit may be a piped vacuum system (as seen on the ward) or a portable system (as used in the nonclinical setting). Each must be checked and tested regularly. Suction should be checked daily for function and before use on a newly admitted patient.	1 To ensure system is in good working order and has been serviced for continued use. To minimise the risks of trauma, hypoxia and atelectasis.
2 Recommended pressure setting are: • 75–90 mmHg for <3 years of age, • 90–150 mmHg for aged 3–13 years and • 150 mmHg for >13 years.	2 To minimise the adverse effects of suction. There is little evidence to specify the optimal negative pressure. The lowest pressure that will effectively clear secretions should be used (American Association for Respiratory Care, 2010; Association of Paediatric Chartered Physiotherapists 2020).
3 The vacuum and suction setting must be checked prior to each procedure. Check the pressure by occluding the end of the suction tubing prior to use.	3 To avoid high pressure and the risk of hypoxia and airway trauma or too low pressure, which will result in ineffective suction.

Preparation of equipment: catheter selection

Statement	Rationale
1 Rigid suction catheters (e.g. a yankauer) may be used to clear the mouth of thick secretions.	1 The wide diameter and rigid design facilitates the removal of thick secretions. Due to the rigid nature, care must be taken not to advance the sucker into the pharynx.
2 In other circumstances, catheters must not exceed 50% of the internal diameter. Where there is an artificial airway, the size of tube should be half the catheter size used. For example, a 3.5 mm artificial airway will require a size 7 suction catheter.	2 To enable gas flow around the catheter and minimise the risk of hypoxia.

Procedure guideline 29.2 Performing suction

Statement	Rationale
1 Before performing suction, gather the equipment: • Catheters • Personal protective equipment (PPE) (nonsterile gloves, apron, mask and eye protection/visor) • Bowl of water (for flushing tubing).	1 To ensure that the procedure can be performed in a safe and timely manner.
2 Perform a clinical hand-wash. Gloves should be worn and should touch only the catheter and the airway.	2 Airway suctioning must be performed as a 'clean' procedure to minimise the risk of infections and contamination.
3 The distance the suction catheter is to be inserted is predetermined by measuring the length of the airway and connections (if artificial airway). For nasopharyngeal suction (without an artificial airway) the catheter is passed to a depth approximately the distance from the nostril to the mid part of the earlobe and down to the base of the neck. This should be sufficient to pass through the nasopharynx and stimulate a cough.	3 To prevent the catheter being inserted at an incorrect length to reduce the risk of tracheobronchial trauma, including bleeding, pneumothorax, and vagal stimulation leading to bradycardia (Morrow et al. 2006).
4 Be cautious in the younger population when/if passing through the larynx (Gillies and Spence 2011; Walsh et al. 2011; Association of Paediatric Chartered Physiotherapists 2020)	4 To reduce the risk of causing atelectasis, hypoxia, and trauma (American Association for Respiratory Care 2010).
5 Turn on the suction unit and insert catheter or yankauer into the airway to the predetermined length. Suction should be applied only on withdrawal, using the lowest pressure that will effectively clear secretions.	5 In infants and children, while there is little evidence to support the optimal negative pressure to be applied, the lowest pressure that will effectively clear secretions should always be used (Argent 2009; American Association for Respiratory Care 2010; Davies et al. 2015).
6 The duration of suction should be quick but effective enough to remove secretions and minimise complications. If the CYP is ventilated, they should be disconnected from the ventilator for the shortest possible time, or a closed suction system should be used.	6,7 To minimise the risk from the accompanying side effects and ensure that the CYP receives suction when needed, reducing the risk of secretions building up, and increasing discomfort and work of breathing.
7 Suctioning should not be performed on a routine basis and the need for suction should be assessed every time, thereby ensuring that suction is only performed when required.	
8 If the secretions are bloody, purulent, foul-smelling, or unusually thick, samples should be taken for analysis as required.	8 To detect any infection requiring treatment.

Procedure guideline 29.2 Performing suction *(continued)*

Statement	Rationale
9 Assess the CYP following the suction, with reference to the preintervention assessment. It may be necessary to repeat the procedure. If doing so immediately the catheters can be reused if the distal end is clear from secretions.	9 To ensure the airway is clear and the CYP is breathing/ventilated comfortably.
10 Following the procedure: a) The suction catheter should be wrapped around the hand and the glove removed ensuring the catheter is contained inside the glove. This is then disposed of in the appropriate waste bin. b) The suction tubing should be rinsed through with sterile water. c) The HCW should remove all PPE and undertake a hand-wash. d) Document the time of suction and the consistency of the secretions.	10 a) To prevent cross contamination. b) To ensure the tubing is clean and patent and to prevent cross contamination. c) To prevent cross contamination. d) To maintain an accurate record of care.

Special considerations

11a) Saline may be used in an effort to loosen and mobilise secretions. It may be instilled via an artificial airway, saline nebuliser, or nasal drops may be administered. This should be undertaken only by an experienced practitioner. b) Newly formed tracheostomies must be suctioned at least every 30 minutes in the first 12–24 hours and then regularly until the first tube change. c) CYPs with nasal stents and nasopharyngeal airways will need regular suction. d) If suction is not successful or secretions are tenacious consider increasing the suction pressure and/or increasing the size of catheter (Association of Paediatric Chartered Physiotherapists 2020). e) If repeated suction is needed or nasal trauma apparent, moisten the tip of the catheter with sterile water or apply a thin layer of aqua gel. f) Closed suction could be considered with the following intubated and ventilated patients: • Preterm infants • Known poor handling • High Frequency Oscillatory Ventilation (HFOV) • Peep >8 cmH$_2$O • Neuroprotected • Diagnosed of suspected respiratory infection.	11a) There is little evidence to support the use of saline intillation, although clinicians using saline say that they can clear secretions, particularly tenacious secretions, more effectively with saline rather than without it (Roberts 2009). b) To decrease the risk of airway obstruction following surgery. For more information, see Chapter 32: Tracheostomy Care and Management. c) To prevent occlusion; these narrow artificial airways often lead to excess secretions and an increased risk of obstruction. d) To increase the efficacy of the procedure e) To lubricate the tip of the suction catheter for easier insertion. f) The majority of literature regarding closed suction is on the pre-term population with evidence of improved stability and reduction in cerebral blood flow variance (Fisk 2018). There is some evidence to suggest that closed suction may be superior to open suction in offering: • Improved cardiovascular stability (Evans et al. 2014) • Quicker time to recover lung volume in HFOV patients (Hoellering et al. 2008) • Avoiding negative end expiratory pressure (Nakstad et al. 2016) • Safer method of suctioning for less experienced staff (Tume et al. 2017) • Avoiding an aerosol-generating procedure (Fisk 2018; Evans et al. 2014; Hoellering et al. 2008; Nakstad et al. 2016; Tume et al. 2017).

Nasopharyngeal airway

Introduction

A nasopharyngeal airway (NPA) is a flexible ETT designed to open a channel between the nostril and the nasopharynx to bypass any upper airway obstruction at the level of the nose, nasopharynx, or base of the tongue. It can be used in an emergency situation or for long-term care (Resuscitation Council 2016). A correctly placed NPA will sit just above the epiglottis, having separated the soft palate from the posterior wall of the oropharynx. This knowledge is vital if the NPA is to be sized correctly in patients: If the airway is too short it will fail to separate the soft palate from the pharynx; if too long it can pass into the larynx and aggravate cough and gag reflexes (Roberts et al. 2005).

The NPA primarily acts as a 'splint' to maintain the patency of the airway, preventing the tongue from falling back onto the posterior pharyngeal wall and occluding the airway, and therefore preventing airway obstruction, hypoxia, and asphyxia (Dinwiddie 1997). NPAs are generally well tolerated by conscious CYPs and are used in the management of CYPs with a variety of conditions (Tweedie et al. 2007). Indications for an NPA itself and the length required to relieve the obstruction must be determined on an individual basis for each CYP (see Box 29.1).

Sizing of the NPA

The size and length of the NPA is determined by:

- Measuring the child's crown to heel length, as there is a positive correlation between this and the length of the NPA (Figure 29.1)
- Referring to the lateral neck X-ray, if appropriate
- Clinical assessment
- Measuring the distance from the nostril to the angle of the mandible to determine length
- Using visual clinical judgement to assess suitable diameter of the NPA, based on CYP's nares.

Box 29.1 Indications for a NPA

Pierre Robin Sequence
Pierre Robin Sequence (PRS) is characterised by an unusually small mandible (micrognathia), posterior displacement or retraction of the tongue (glossoptosis), and upper airway obstruction. Incomplete closure of the roof of the mouth (cleft palate) is present in the majority of patients, and is commonly U-shaped.

In PRS, airway obstruction is mostly due to glossoptosis, whereby the tongue occludes the airway, resulting in difficulty breathing. Upper airway obstruction results in a failure of airflow into the lungs, despite adequate inspiratory effort. Increasing respiratory effort can worsen the obstruction, as increased intrathoracic pressure collapses the soft tissue structures inwards. PRS is seen in other syndromes including Stickler, Treacher Collins, and Velo-cardiofacial syndromes. The airway obstruction may be intermittent, and may also take time to develop, with some infants not presenting for days to weeks after birth, most commonly with failure to thrive due to ongoing increased work of breathing.

Craniofacial Syndromes
CYPs with craniofacial syndromes (e.g. Apert, Crouzon, Pfeiffer) may have an NPA for the treatment of obstructive sleep apnoea. The NPA may be used for months or years and often allows avoidance of a tracheostomy. These CYPs have anatomical midfacial hypoplasia, which includes narrowed nasal passages, underdeveloped and setback mid-facial skeletal structures, and malocclusion of the upper and lower jaws. Position of the tongue can occlude the airway. CYPs may present with symptoms of upper airway obstruction, feeding difficulties, and failure to thrive.

Postcraniofacial Mid-Facial Advancement Surgery
This surgery is carried out to advance the facial skeleton and involves multiple facial fractures and postoperative oedema (Hayward et al. 2004). The NPA is sutured in place and supports the airway.

Postadenotonsillectomy
CYPs are at risk of respiratory compromise following an adenotonsillectomy, due to postoperative oedema (Tweedie et al. 2007). The NPA in this group of CYPs is to maintain the airway during the early postoperative period.

Post Cleft Lip and Palate Repair
Occasionally a baby undergoing a unilateral or bilateral lip repair with anterior palate repair (vomerine flap) may require an NPA. Babies with isolated cleft palate, may have postoperative swelling requiring an NPA. This is usually left in situ for one to two nights postoperatively.

Emergency Airway
Airway obstruction is a common occurrence in paediatric resuscitation. An NPA can be used to maintain the airway.

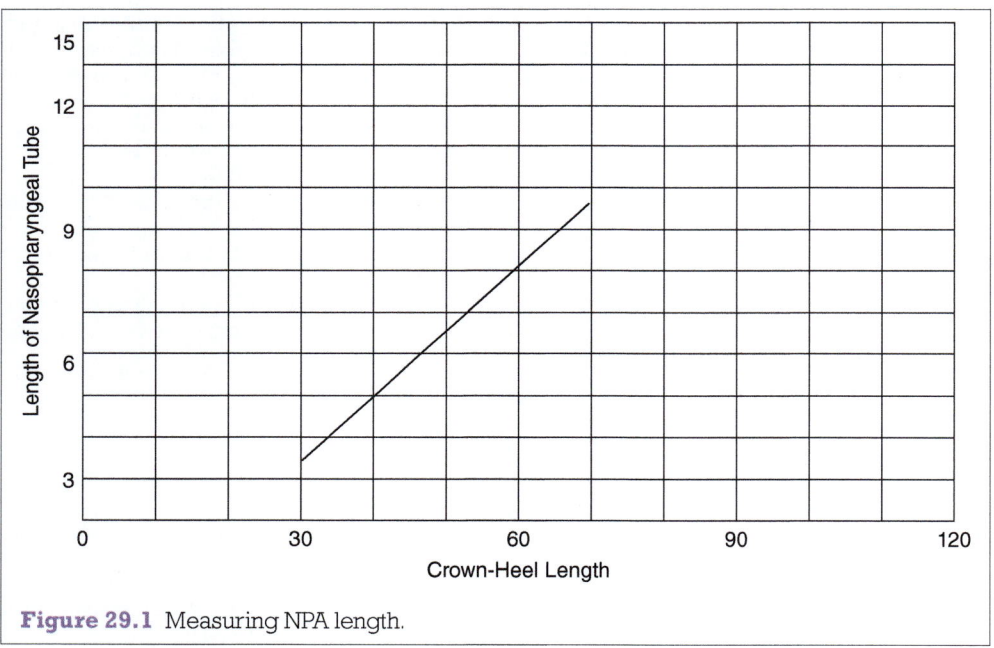

Figure 29.1 Measuring NPA length.

In an emergency situation the required length for the nasopharyngeal tube can be calculated by measuring the tube from tip of the child's nose to the angle of the mandible (Resuscitation Council 2016). The appropriate tube width/size can be estimated by matching its diameter against the opening of the child's nostril; when inserted, it should not cause blanching of the nostril on insertion as this indicates it is too large. The NPA should fit snuggly into the nostril with no gaping around the tube, as this would indicate the NPA is too small in width/size and be ineffective.

Chapter 29 Respiratory care

Procedure guideline 29.3 Preparation for a NPA

Statement	Rationale
1 Ensure that the CYP and family are informed of the following to obtain consent and to maximise the effectiveness of the procedure: • The reason for the NPA. • What it will involve. • The likely duration of the airway placement. • The potential difficulties of using an airway, the likely impact on the CYP and family. • The potential for trauma from insertion. If necessary, contact a play specialist or psychologist to help prepare the CYP.	1 To gain cooperation and understanding.

Preparation of equipment and environment

Statement	Rationale
1 The CYP's bed area must be made accessible to ensure safe and unrestricted access to emergency equipment. Correct emergency equipment must be readily available to facilitate an immediate response and possible resuscitation.	1 To maintain patient safety.
2 The CYP with an NPA should have an **emergency NPA equipment bag** by the bedside containing: a) A spare NPA of the same size internal diameter (ID) and length in case the NPA needs to be changed. b) An NPA (one size, 0.5mm ID, smaller), to the same length as the current NPA. c) A water-based lubricant. d) Round-ended scissors to cut tape and or suture.	a) In case of blockage, displacement, or accidental removal, a spare NPA of the same size can be repassed immediately. b) In case you are unable to repass usual size, due to oedema. c) To facilitate insertion.
e) Roll of the tape. (**Caution**: For CYPs with a latex allergy, an alternative medical adhesive tape must be sourced which is strong and durable enough to secure the NPA). f) Personal protective equipment (PPE).	e) To secure the flange to the CYP's face. The tape used must have good adhesive qualities if placed correctly over the hydrocolloid dressing. f) To minimise the risk of cross infection.
3 All equipment must be present and in working order.	3 To ensure patient safety.
4 A CYP with an NPA must be supervised at all times.	4 An NPA is an artificial airway and requires constant care to keep airway patent.
5 To ensure safety, the accompanying carer must be able to: • Recognise signs of airway obstruction. • Suction the NPA.	
6 Additional equipment required: a) Suction catheters – correct size (refer to suction section). b) Hydrocolloid dressing. c) Gauze. d) Saline solution for cleaning. e) Clean receiver with sterile bottled water to flush suction tubing. f) 2ml syringe and ampoule 0.9% sodium chloride for irrigation. g) Clinical waste bag. h) Working walled suction or portable suction machine.	b) To prevent excoriation by creating a barrier between the skin and adhesive tape.

Equipment to form a NPA

Statement	Rationale
1 Standard-sized NPA's are available that do not require customisation; these are used for short-term airway management (e.g. postoperation craniofacial patients, during/following resuscitation).	1 For some CYPs the standard NPAs will be too long and therefore unsuitable. CYPs requiring a specific length NPA will require a custom-made tube (see Figure 29.2).
2 To make an NPA the following equipment needs to be gathered: • Portex™ endotracheal (ET) tube of the appropriate size. • Portex tracheal tube holder (0.5mm smaller than ET tube size). • Nylon nonabsorbable suture to secure the ET tube to the tube holder • Round-ended scissors.	

(continued)

Procedure guideline 29.3 Preparation for a NPA (continued)

Statement	Rationale
Making a NPA (Figure 29.2)	
1 Cut endotracheal tube to measured length, to ensure it fits through the nostrils to sit just above the epiglottis.	1 Once the desired length is known, the ET tube is cut to size.
2 Shorten the length of the tracheal tube holder by half and insert over the ET tube. The tube should be facing downwards and aligned centrally, not veering off to one side.	2 To ensure that it doesn't increase the diameter of the ET tube, causing a pressure injury to the nares.
3 Suture the ET tube and tracheal tube holder together. Sutures should be circumferential.	3 To secure the tube holder to the ET tube.
4 Sutures must be neat and secured, around three to four stitches on each side as a guide. Avoid the sutures occluding the opening.	4 To ensure the sutures do not prevent the suction catheter from being inserted into the NPA.

(a)
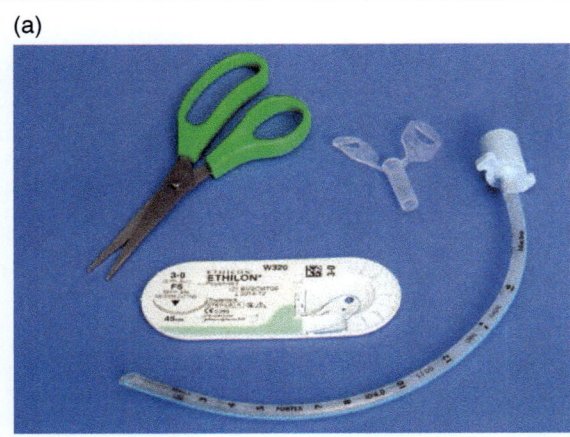
Equipment required to make a nasopharyngeal airway

(b)
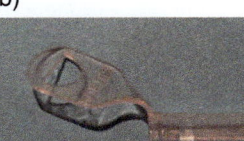
Cut here — preparation of equipment

(c)
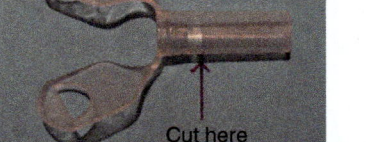
Cut tracheal tube holder

Making a nasopharyngeal airway

Figure 29.2 Making a NPA.

(d)

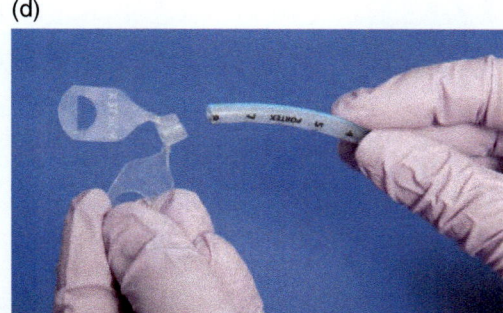

Fit tracheal tube holder onto cut end of endotracheal tube

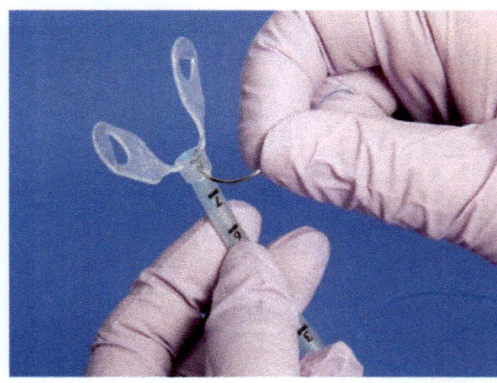

Sew tracheal tube holder into place on cut end of endotracheal tube

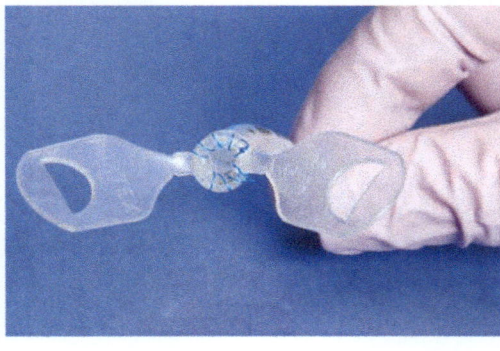

Sutures need to be placed circumferentially around the whole tracheal tube holder

Figure 29.2 Making a NPA. *(continued)*

Procedure guideline 29.4 Inserting the NPA

Statement	Rationale
Inserting the NPA	
The right-sided nostril is almost always used for NPAs because of the natural curve of the ET tube allowing the flange bevel to open into the pharynx. If a standard ET tube is used in the left nostril the bevel will sit against the pharyngeal wall and is more likely to become occluded. If long term, alternate nostrils may be used if tolerated clinically to prevent the overstretching of one nostril and preserving good tissue health. The insertion of the NPA should be parallel to the nasal floor, rather than upwards to the cribiform plate of the ethmoid bone (Roberts et al. 2005). Anatomically, the placement of the NPA should follow the natural downward curve of the nasal cavity.	

1 To insert the NPA:
  a) Gather all equipment required.
  b) Wash hands and put on personal protective equipment (PPE).
  c) Ensure the child is swaddled, if appropriate.
  d) Ensure the CYP's nostrils are clear from secretions.
  e) Ensure working oxygen and suction are available at the bedside.
  f) Lubricate the NPA and gently insert the tip of the tube into the right-hand nostril and gently thread the tube along the floor of the nasal passage, perpendicular to the face, until the flange is at the tip of the nose.
  g) Do not force the NPA at any stage.
	a) To facilitate a quick and safe procedure.
	b) To minimise the risk of infection.
	c) To contain the CYP and ensure the safe and timely placement of the tube.
	d) Pre-existing secretions are likely to become lodged in the NPA.
	e) To maintain safety and facilitate immediate suctioning of the NPA to ensure patency.
	f) Anatomically, the placement of the NPA should follow the natural downward curve of the nasal cavity.
	g) Forcing the NPA can cause trauma, pain, oedema, and incorrect placement.

2 If it is not possible to insert the NPA consider:
  a) Summoning more experienced help.
  b) Using a smaller NPA.
  c) Steroid-based nasal drops (as prescribed).
  d) Insertion in theatre under direct vision and general anaesthetic.
  e) Use a suction catheter (not attached to suction) to thread through or 'railroad' the NPA and insert into the nostril.
	a) There may be inflammation to the airway.
	
	e) To act as a soft guidewire and ease insertion.

3 a) While passing the NPA, observe for any undue respiratory distress.
  • General behaviour or colour
  • Oxygen saturations
  • Respiratory rate and effort
  • Heart rate
  • PEWS.
  b) If signs of distress are present, stop and treat accordingly with supportive measures, e.g. oxygen or suction, and summon assistance as appropriate.
	3 a) To ensure early detection and treatment of complications.
	
	b) Insertion may be distressing for the CYP and cause a change in the CYP's vital signs.

4 Once inserted, secure the NPA by passing the tape through the loops of the tracheal tube holder and then onto the hydrocolloid dressing on the cheeks. Note: This tape may also be placed prior to NPA insertion for ease and speed.	4 Use tape with good adhesive qualities to place correctly over the hydrocolloid dressing.
5 Clear away equipment and wash hands.	5 To minimise the risk of infection.
6 The insertion of a NPA and details of the length and diameter of the NPA and the size of the tube holder must be recorded in the CYP's healthcare record. This information should also be clearly visible at the patient's bedside. Practitioners should be familiar with and have access to the Emergency Algorithm (Figure 29.3).	6 To provide information to facilitate ongoing care. Documenting the length of the NPA allows practitioners to ensure suction doesn't occur distal to the tube tip, which may cause trauma. Bedside information ensures quick treatment in an emergency situation.

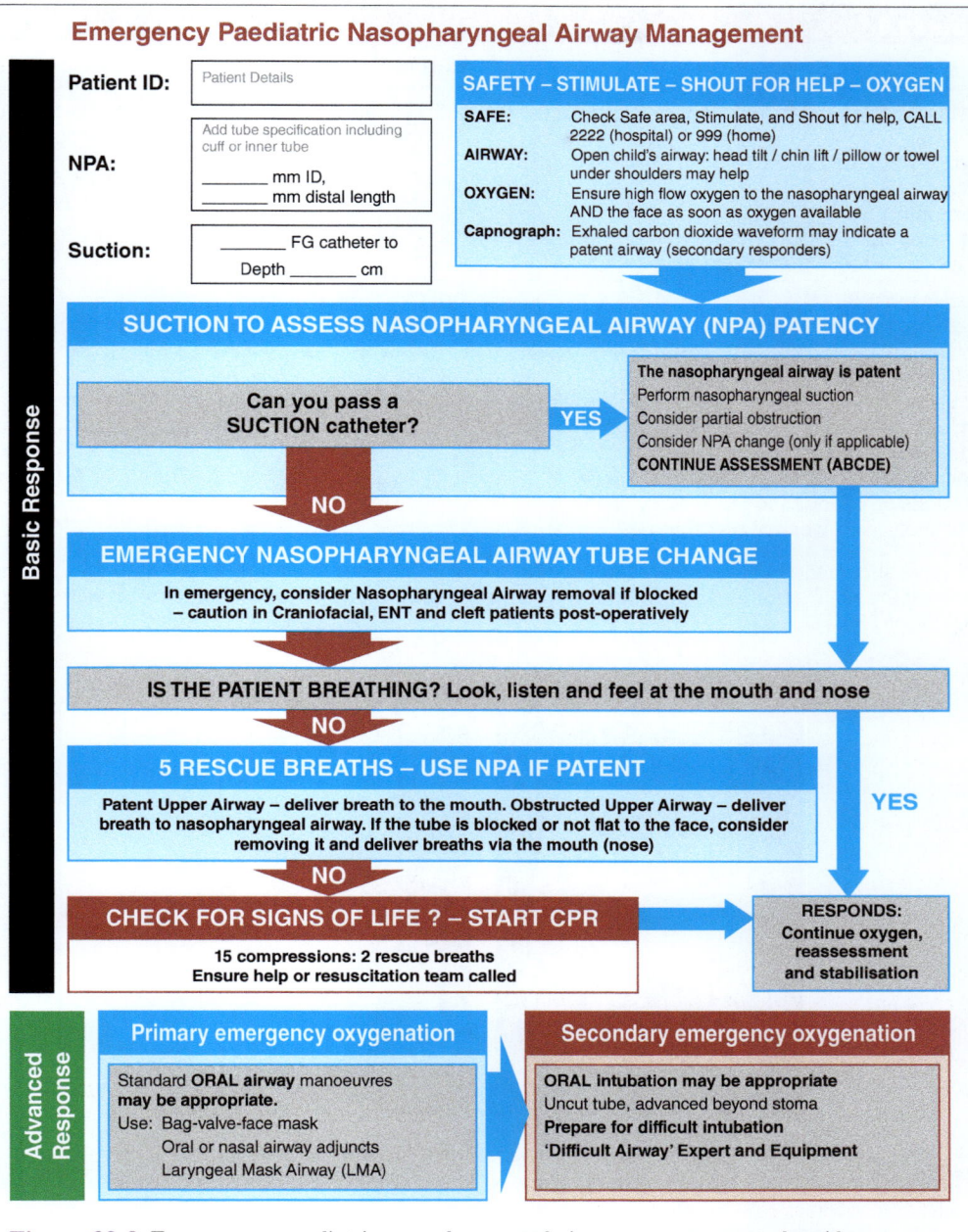

Figure 29.3 Emergency paediatric nasopharyngeal airway management algorithm.

Procedure guideline 29.5 Observations post NPA insertion

Statement	Rationale
1 Immediately after insertion observe and document any of the following: • Excessive bleeding from the nostril; contact medical team if bleeding persists. • Patency with suctioning. • Improvement of respiratory symptoms, monitored through regular observations and PEWS scoring.	1 To ensure swift detection and treatment of any potential complications and to maintain an accurate record.
2 Specific observations include: a) Blanching of nares, leading to pressure injury or skin breakdown around the nostril rim. This **must** be reported to the medical team immediately. b) Milk or food observed in the NPA before, during, or after feeds. If this occurs, keep the CYP nil by mouth until reviewed by the team who inserted NPA. c) The need for increased suctioning of the tube due to excessive secretions or changes in respiratory status. d) Any coughing or increased work of breathing.	a) Blanching is an early sign of vascular compromise and may occur as a result of the ET tube holder being too wide for the CYP's nostril. b) This may indicate that the NPA is too long, and interfering with the CYP's ability to swallow, causing food/milk to aspirate into the NPA. c, d) To assess the potential for the NPA to become blocked.
3 If the observations have shown the NPA to be too long, a 'donut spacer' may be used at the nostril rim until the NPA is removed/replaced (Figure 29.4).	3 To shorten the length of the NPA. This is a **temporary solution** to avoid having to remove the existing NPA. Caution should be used with donut spacers as they may be dislodged and be ingested by the CYP.

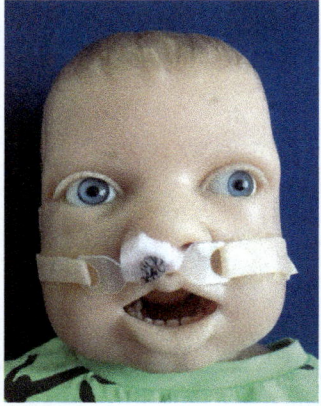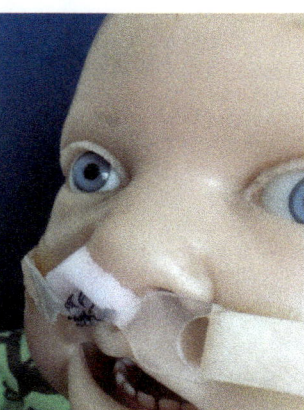

Figure 29.4 Position of a 'donut spacer' to shorten the NPA (in the short term).

Procedure guideline 29.6 Ongoing care of an NPA and discharge planning

Nursing actions during the few days following insertion of the NPA centre on:
- Maintaining the correct positioning and patency of the NPA.
- Maintaining skin integrity.
- Delivering parental teaching to support safe discharge.

Statement	Rationale
1 Care of the skin: a) Clean the nostrils as required to prevent excoriation. b) Change the tape daily or as required. The strong adhesive backing ensures a secure bond onto the tube holder and skin protector. NB: for CYPs with latex allergy, an alternative adhesive tape must be sourced which is strong and durable enough to secure the NPA.	a) To protect the skin from breakdown.

Procedure guideline 29.6 Ongoing care of an NPA and discharge planning *(continued)*

Statement	Rationale
c) Observe pressure areas for redness or breakdown, especially around the nostrils. d) Document and contact relevant team if concerned. e) Use hydrocolloid dressing to protect cheeks.	c,d) To identify any concerns early and allow for appropriate treatment. e) To protect the skin from breakdown.
2 Maintaining patency: a) Instillation of saline drops is a contentious area and there is little evidence to support this practice so this should not be used routinely (Ackerman and Gugerty 1990; Neil 2001). b) Secretions may become thick and tenacious, making their expulsion difficult. The CYP may require extra humidity. Humidification of the NPA must be provided artificially with saline nebulisers/water humidification and/or systemic hydration.	a) Instilling saline down the NPA may support the retrieval of secretions. This should be done on an individualised basis and only by experienced practitioners. b) The NPA bypasses the natural route for humidification – secretions will be thicker and more tenacious, which may lead to occlusion of the tube (American Thoracic Society 2000).
3 Ensuring good hydration: It is important that a CYP with a NPA remains systemically hydrated. The CYP's fluid intake may need to be increased during times of illness, particularly when vomiting, diarrhoea, and/or pyrexia occur. Alternative methods of hydration, such as intravenous fluids may be required, particularly in the postoperative period.	3 Dehydration may increase thickness of secretions.
4 Discharge: a) For CYPs who will be discharged with a long term NPA, early communication between the hospital and community health professionals must occur. Frequency of NPA changes should be discussed on an individual basis and included in the discharge plan. b) Liaison must take place with the CYP's local hospital and/or community team after insertion and a detailed equipment list provided. c) A CYP with an NPA may be discharged home whenever their condition is stable and the parents/carers have been trained and are competent to care for the NPA independently. The training record and documentation should be kept in the CYP's health care records. d) A follow-up appointment should be arranged according to the CYP and family's needs. e) A copy of the training booklet should be provided to the community team.	4 a) Early engagement with local hospital and community support is essential, so that discharge planning/obtaining the necessary equipment/training staff can be started as soon as possible. b) To ensure the local healthcare team has time to order the necessary supplies before the CYP is discharged. c,d) To ensure the CYP can be safely cared for after discharge. e) To facilitate effective communication.

Oxygen therapy

Introduction

Oxygen therapy is defined as 'the therapeutic use of oxygen and consists of administering oxygen at higher concentrations than those found in room air, with the aim of treating or preventing hypoxia' (Ortega et al. 2014).

The World Health Organisation (WHO) defines hypoxaemia as 'low levels of oxygen in the blood (low blood oxygen saturation or content)' and hypoxia as 'inadequate oxygen in tissues for normal cell and organ function. Hypoxia results from hypoxaemia' (WHO 2016, p. 4). Oxygen deprivation can have severe adverse effects, and can quickly lead to organ failure and death (WHO 2016).

Arterial oxygen saturation is referred to as SpO_2 when measured by pulse oximetry. The normal range of oxygen saturations (SpO_2) is 94–99%; however, this can be dependent on the CYP's underlying health condition and should be reviewed on an individual basis.

Oxygen is a very common drug used in medical emergencies and as part of ongoing clinical care utilised across a wide range of clinical conditions. The concentrations of oxygen required are dependent on the CYP's condition. The administration of inappropriate concentrations of oxygen can have potentially serious effects, leading to serious harm and death if not administered and managed appropriately (National Patient Safety Agency ([NPSA] 2009). Oxygen should be regarded as a medication and its use documented and prescribed within a range of agreed clinical parameters for each patient as part of their clinical care (British National Formulary for Children (BNFC) 2022). The safe and appropriate administration of oxygen is an important component of the nurse's role. Clinical observation is important and the escalation of clinical concerns, using a PEWS system and escalation policy, is required for the detection and effective management of clinical deterioration (RCN 2017).

The guidelines in this section of the chapter include:

- Education, assessment, and preparation for oxygen administration.
- Administration of oxygen therapy.
- Continuous assessment of the CYP receiving oxygen therapy.
- Discharge planning for the CYP on long-term oxygen.

Indications for oxygen therapy

Oxygen therapy should be administered to prevent cellular hypoxia caused by hypoxaemia and thus prevent potentially irreversible damage to vital organs.

It should be considered for any CYP with one or more of the following:

- Peri- and postcardiac or respiratory arrest.
- Hypoxia (oxygen saturation levels of <92%).
- Acute and chronic hypoxemia (SaO_2 < 92%), e.g. pneumonia, shock, asthma.
- Low cardiac output and metabolic acidosis.
- Acute blood loss.
- Chronic respiratory disease (hypoxia and hypercapnia). (Balfour-Lynn et al. 2009).

Despite a lack of supportive data, oxygen is also administered in the following conditions:

- Dyspnoea without hypoxemia.
- Postoperatively, if specifically instructed by surgical team (Kbar and Campbell 2006).
- Treatment of pneumothorax ((Robinson et al. 2009).

There remains a lack of consensus regarding fundamental issues in oxygen therapy for CYPs, but it differs considerably from adult oxygen therapy and the following issues must be taken into account:

- Assessment can be challenging; it is often difficult to obtain arterial/venous blood samples.
- Clinical conditions in infancy/childhood can be exclusive, although some overlaps exist in adolescents.
- Prognosis in infancy is usually positive – children often require oxygen therapy for limited periods.
- Many CYPs require long-term oxygen therapy overnight only – this differs from the requirement for 15 hours of oxygen therapy which forms the adult long-term therapy definition.
- Low-flow equipment is sometimes required.
- Supervision from a parent or carer is essential.
- Oxygen provision may be necessary within school (Balfour-Lynn et al. 2009).

Caution: There are conditions where the CYP's condition may be made worse by the administration of oxygen, e.g. complex congenital heart defects. In addition, oxygen administration for CYPs with chronic carbon dioxide retention may further increase respiratory acidosis and worsening Glasgow Coma Scale (GCS) score, e.g. cystic fibrosis, chronic neuromuscular disorders, and chronic lung disease of prematurity.

Oxygen measurement through pulse oximetry

Pulse oximetry allows reliable monitoring or detection of hypoxaemia with little distress to the CYP as long as the probe is correctly applied and it is moved frequently to prevent skin injury.

For CYPs requiring long-term oxygen therapy, most assessments are made using pulse oximetry measurement rather than arterial blood sampling. Oximeters from different manufacturers may give different ranges of oxygen saturation readings (Balfour-Lynn et al. 2009).

Types of oxygen therapy

High concentration oxygen therapy is usually given in an emergency situation through a bag mask valve (BMV) or high-flow oxygen mask. In ICU this can be given via a ventilator or on the ward through high-flow nasal prongs. In an emergency it is safe and used as a treatment in conditions such as pneumonia, pulmonary thromboembolism, pulmonary fibrosis, shock, severe trauma, sepsis, or anaphylaxis. In such conditions low arterial oxygen (PaO_2) is usually associated with low or normal arterial carbon dioxide ($PaCO_2$), and therefore there is little risk of hypoventilation and carbon dioxide retention. High concentration oxygen therapy can have detrimental effects on the respiratory system, particularly after prolonged usage and can lead to respiratory distress due to absorption atelectasis (collapse of alveoli due to blockage). However, it is lifesaving therapy. In the premature infant, retinopathy of prematurity can be a side effect due to vasoconstriction, and can lead to permanent blindness (Hellström et al. 2013).

Low concentration oxygen therapy (controlled oxygen therapy) is used to correct hypoxaemia by using an accurate amount of oxygen without depleting existing maintenance of carbon dioxide and respiratory acidosis. Blood gases are the most accurate measure to correct hypoxaemia.

Long-term oxygen therapy (LTOT): The aim of long-term oxygen therapy is to maintain oxygen saturation of at least 92%. CYPs (especially those with chronic neonatal lung disease) often require supplemental oxygen. For the provision of continuous oxygen therapy for CYPs with chronic hypoxaemia, requirements vary between 24-hour dependency, to dependency only during periods of sleep (BNFC (2022)). LTOT principally aims to improve symptoms and prevent harm from chronic hypoxaemia. Any CYP likely to require LTOT for longer than three weeks should be considered for domiciliary oxygen.

CYPs potentially affected by chronic hypoxaemia include those with:

- Chronic lung disease.
- Congenital heart disease with pulmonary hypertension.
- Pulmonary hypertension secondary to respiratory disease.
- Interstitial lung disease.
- Obliterative bronchiolitis.
- Cystic fibrosis and other causes of severe bronchiectasis.
- Obstructive sleep apnoea and other sleep-related disorders.
- Palliative care for symptom relief (Balfour-Lynn et al. 2009).

Prescribing oxygen

Oxygen should always be prescribed on the medicine administration system before it is administered, except in emergencies, when it should be documented after the event. The prescription should include a target oxygen saturation level.

Nasal cannula	Face mask	Non-rebreathe mask	Small ambu bag	Adult ambu bag	500ml Ayers t-Piece
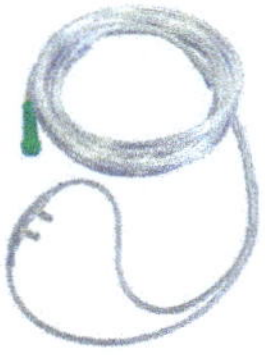	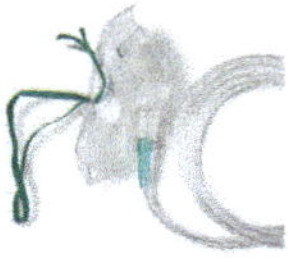	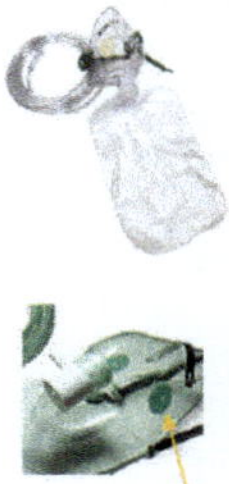 Ensure green valves are still in situ to ensure 'non-rebreathe function	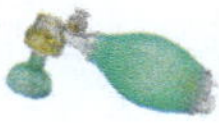	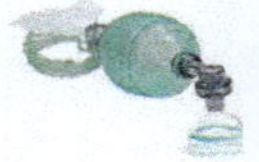	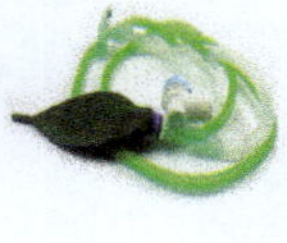
0-2 litres O₂	5-15 litres O₂	10-15 litres O₂	10-15 litres O₂	15 litres O₂	6-8 litres O₂

Figure 29.5 Minimum oxygen requirements for different types of delivery equipment

Methods and equipment for oxygen administration

The selection of the appropriate method of administration should take account of the CYP's clinical condition, preferences, and the aim of treatment. For the minimum oxygen requirements for different types of delivery equipment see Figure 29.5.

Oxygen delivery in an emergency situation:

High concentration oxygen masks with a large reservoir that allows oxygen only to be breathed in by the CYP. The approximate oxygen received is 90% (Resuscitation Council 2016)

- **Via an anaesthetic T-piece:** An open-ended bag, used by anaesthetists and other experienced practitioners. This administration set gives a reliable impression of the state of the lungs. It also allows manual application of positive end-expiratory pressure (PEEP). It is completely reliant on an effective oxygen source (Resuscitation Council 2016).
- **Bag valve mask:** These come in three sizes: generally 250, 500, and 1500 ml. The smallest one is ineffective even at birth. The two smallest bags have a pressure limiting valve set at 4.41 kPa (45 cm H_2O) to protect the lungs from barotrauma (i.e. damage caused to tissues by a change in pressure inside and outside the body). The reservoir bag enables the delivery of oxygen concentrations up to 90%. Without the reservoir bag it is not possible to supply more than 50% oxygen (Resuscitation Council 2016).

Oxygen delivery in non-emergency situations:

Oxygen can be delivered through either low-flow or high-flow delivery methods.

- **Low flow**

Face masks

These are supplied in children's sizes but they are not always tolerated by young children (WHO 2016).

The Simple oxygen mask has vents in the mask to allow for the dilution of oxygen (Wagstaff and Soni 2007). High concentrations of oxygen can be safely administered. When using the mask with high concentrations of oxygen over a long period of time, it should be humidified.

- **Simple nasal cannula:** This method can be used for long-term oxygen delivery, allowing the CYP to vocalise and eat. However, the concentration is often not controlled, resulting in low inspiratory oxygen concentrations. Only low-flow rates of up to 2l per minute can be given (Dougherty and Lister 2015). Nasal cannula oxygen does not need to be humidified. The use of nasal cannulae can produce dermatitis and mucosal drying (BNFC 2022).

- **Tracheostomy mask:** Oxygen can be delivered via the tracheostomy with a heat moisture exchanger (HME) connector in situ or via a ventilator tubing circuit if applicable.

- **Wafting:** When conventional delivery methods are not tolerated, wafting of oxygen via a face mask has been shown to deliver concentrations of 30–40%, with 10l of oxygen per minute to an area of 35 × 32 cms from the mask (Davies et al. 2002). A standard paediatric oxygen mask placed on the chest can give significant oxygen therapy with minimal distress to the CYP (Davies et al. 2002).

Wafting via green oxygen tubing has been assessed as appropriate for short-term use only, e.g. while feeding (Blake et al. 2014).

- **High flow**
NB: All high-flow systems require humidification

- **Via a ventilation circuit:** Oxygen can be delivered at various points throughout the ventilation circuit (Simonds 2007), before the humidification unit to allow the oxygen to be warmed and humidified. Ventilated patients receive oxygen via an artificial airway or noninvasive ventilation mask.
- **CPAP/BiPAP drivers**
- **High-flow nasal cannula:** Nasal cannula adapted to the size of nares deliver heated and humidified gas (usually with additional oxygen) at a high-flow rate. They are usually well tolerated and reduce the work of breathing (Lee et al. 2013).

Procedure guideline 29.7 Education, assessment, and preparation for oxygen administration

Statement	Rationale
1 Ensure that adequate education regarding the safe administration of oxygen by various methods is provided.	1 All staff using oxygen need training to ensure it is delivered safely.
2 Oxygen should not be delivered in the vicinity of any naked flames.	2 Oxygen is combustible.
3 A thorough clinical examination should be carried out to assess the reason for an oxygen requirement.	3 To ensure that oxygen is not administered unnecessarily. For example, repositioning a CYP may improve oxygenation.
4 Age-appropriate information must be given to the CYP and family about: • Why oxygen is required. • The method of delivery to be used. • The benefits of the treatment. • The side effects of the treatment. • Duration of the treatment. • Restrictions for the CYP while on oxygen, e.g. mobility, proximity to naked flames, etc.	4 To ensure they are prepared for oxygen and aware of the risks and benefits associated with the treatment. To provide reassurance.
5 Baseline observations and any signs of respiratory distress should be noted and documented before commencing therapy.	5 Acute oxygen therapy requires regular monitoring to ensure that any subsequent changes in the CYP's status will be noted and escalated accordingly.

To prepare the equipment:

Statement	Rationale
1 Ensure there is an adequate and working oxygen supply.	1 To facilitate reliable and effective treatment.
2 Where oxygen is to be provided via piped provision, check the correct valve in in place, connected to the oxygen supply and it is working in advance.	2 To facilitate effective treatment and prevent patient safety incidents where piped air is administered instead of oxygen, in error (NHS Improvement 2016).
3 The use of portable oxygen cylinders should be minimised (NPSA 2009). a) If portable oxygen cylinders are used, e.g. for patient transfer between departments, ensure the cylinder has adequate oxygen and ensure accessible provision of back-up cylinders. b) Check spare oxygen cylinders are full and working in advance. c) Check valves on portable oxygen cylinders are open.	3 Piped oxygen is preferred where possible to minimise the risks of oxygen not being immediately available (NPSA 2009). a) To ensure a continuous and safe delivery of oxygen to the CYP at all times. b) To ensure a continuous and safe delivery of oxygen to the CYP at all times. c) To ensure a continuous and safe delivery of oxygen to the CYP at all times.
4 a) Attach tubing from chosen method of delivery to the oxygen supply device. Note that increased length of tubing from oxygen source to patient can increase 'dead space'. b) Set up administration device to enable effective administration as per manufacturer's instructions.	
5 Ensure pulse oximetry is available to monitor the CYPs oxygen saturations (NPSA 2009).	5 To effectively monitor the CYP and reduce the risks associated with oxygen therapy.

Procedure guideline 29.8 Administration of oxygen therapy

Statement	Rationale
1 Prepare the CYP: Use age-appropriate language and information to explain: The need for oxygen therapy, • The rationale and explanation for method of delivery. • The positive/expected benefits of treatment. • The possible side effects of treatment. • The minimum duration of treatment.	1 To gain informed consent and provide reassurance and psychological support.
2 Undertake and record baseline observations for the CYP, including oxygen saturation, and document a full PEW score on the appropriate chart.	2 To record a baseline and allow for monitoring of the effectiveness of treatment.
3 a) Check the patient's individual prescription, including the target oxygen saturation for the CYP in line with local policy. b) Initiate and maintain oxygen flow rate and concentration as prescribed.	3 a) Oxygen is classed as a drug and should be prescribed by law. b) Administration of an inappropriate concentration of oxygen can have serious or even lethal consequences.

Procedure guideline 29.8 Administration of oxygen therapy *(continued)*

Statement	Rationale
4 Give the oxygen via the approved, or tolerated, method for the CYP. • For a face mask, ensure that there is a good fit to the face and that there are no large gaps which will prevent the full administration of the oxygen concentration. • For simple nasal cannula, the prongs should be the correct size for the age of the CYP. The tubing should be taken around the ears and then tightened at the front. For infants it is advisable to tape the tubing to the cheek to prevent movement. Using a barrier layer underneath the tubing protects the skin. • The tracheostomy mask must be the correct size for the tracheostomy to enable the desired concentration of oxygen to be inspired. Similarly, there must be the right size connected on the HME if oxygen is going to be added. • Wafting oxygen: placing with the tubing or a mask attached to the tubing near the patient. Although well tolerated, this is not recommended as it is impossible to measure how much oxygen is being given this way. This method relies on frequent patient assessment to judge clinical change. • A ventilator circuit can have oxygen added. Some ventilators are able to display the oxygen concentration as a percentage. • High-flow nasal prongs are attached as the simple nasal prongs. The cannula should never be cut to fit into the nares, however small the CYP. The prongs should be sized against the CYP before attaching.	4 To ensure that the established method for the delivery of oxygen is appropriate for the individual CYP's needs (RCN 2017). Delivery of oxygen therapy will depend of the developmental age; understanding and how individual CYPs react to this treatment.
5 Oxygen should be delivered at the lowest concentration possible and for the shortest possible time (Martin et al. 2015).	5 Oxygen toxicity can occur with oxygen concentrations of 50% or higher if administered for 24–48 hours or more.
6 Assess whether the delivery system requires humidification (Ricard and Boyer 2009)	6 This depends on the method of administration, only simple nasal cannula will not require humidification long term and in this instance if there is nasal congestion or tissue soreness at the nares, humidification may be considered.
7 Assess the CYP for adequate chest expansion. Consider if the CYP need repositioning or suction.	7 To ensure that oxygen therapy is effective.
8 Assess the CYP's level of anxiety and give explanations appropriate to their understanding and developmental stage. Be aware that the procedure may be frightening for the CYP.	8 To provide emotional support.
9 Follow the prescribed protocol for the individual CYP regarding acceptable oxygen saturations and prescribed oxygen therapy.	9 To ensure that individual prescriptions are adhered to and the CYP's needs are met. Each CYP has her or his own prescribed and clinical parameters.
10 a) Monitor oxygen saturation levels immediately after starting oxygen therapy for at least five minutes and then as dictated by the CYP's condition and early warning score. b) Record all observations on the appropriate observation chart. c) All oxygen therapy administered must be documented on appropriate chart. d) If the CYP is clinically stable the medical team may advise slow and safe weaning of oxygen while being monitored.	10 a) To identify if the prescribed oxygen therapy is maintaining the required saturation levels and allow for adjustment of the oxygen therapy as required or the need to escalate care needs. b) To provide information and effective communication. c) To provide information and effective communication. d) To ensure oxygen is used only when needed.

Procedure guideline 29.9 Continuous assessment of the CYP receiving oxygen therapy

Statement	Rationale
1 Pulse oximetry and frequent assessment and observation should continue during oxygen therapy, in line with the individual child's condition (Martin et al. 2015). Monitor oxygen saturation levels immediately after any change to oxygen therapy for at least five minutes and then as dictated by the CYP's condition and PEW score.	1 To provide an accurate picture of the CYP's condition and to assess the effectiveness of the oxygen therapy. Each CYP will need individual assessment as to his or her ongoing response to oxygen therapy. To identify if the prescribed oxygen therapy is maintaining the required saturation levels and allow for adjustment of the oxygen therapy as required (RCN 2017).

(continued)

Procedure guideline 29.9 Continuous assessment of the CYP receiving oxygen therapy *(continued)*

Statement	Rationale
2 Monitor effort of breathing and other signs of respiratory distress/failure including: a) Respiratory rate. b) Use of accessory muscles and head bobbing. c) Presence of wheeze. d) Presence of stridor. e) Grunting and/or nasal flaring. f) Signs of fatigue and tiring.	2 To be alert to early signs of a worsening condition and to enable early detection of the CYP's respiratory distress. a) To allow detection of increase work of breathing. b) Intercostal, subcostal, or sternal recession show increased effort, particularly in CYPs, resulting from their compliant chest walls. Head bobbing demonstrates use of the sternomastoid muscle with each breath. c) Indication of broncho-constriction, usually expiratory. d) Sound during respiration when there is a partial obstruction or collapse of the trachea or larynx. e) Sign of severe respiratory distress.
3 Assess heart rate and monitor any changes.	3 Hypoxia produces tachycardia. Bradycardia can be caused by severe or prolonged hypoxia and is a prearrest sign.
4 Assess skin tone, taking into account cardiac conditions and possible anaemia.	4 Hypoxia initially causes vasoconstriction and skin pallor. Visible cyanosis is a late sign of respiratory distress. Cyanosis could result from cyanotic cardiac disease. Profound cyanosis may not be visible in the severely anaemic CYP or in those with darker skin.
5 Consider mental status and conscious level, and use a recognised system of assessment such as APVU (alert, responds to voice, responds to pain, unresponsive to stimuli).	5 Hypoxia can cause the CYP to be drowsy and/or agitated.
6 If oxygen requirements increase or the CYP's condition deteriorates: • Check administration system to ensure the system is working and oxygen is being delivered. • Continue to monitor child. • Inform the nurse in charge and medical team as necessary, in line with local escalation guideline.	6 To assess the response to oxygen therapy and ensure effective detection, reporting, and management of any deterioration in the CYP's condition.
7 Record all observations on the appropriate chart/in the CYP's healthcare record.	7 To maintain an accurate record and facilitate good communication.
8 If oxygen saturation levels are at the target level for an extended period of time it may be possible to alter care by: • Reducing oxygen therapy in line with prescription. • Considering discontinuation of oxygen therapy. • If oxygen is discontinued, continue to monitor the CYP in line with escalation guideline.	8 To prevent oxygen toxicity and potential side effects.

Procedure guideline 29.10 Discharge planning for the CYP on long-term oxygen

Statement	Rationale
1 Discharge planning should begin on admission in line with national guidelines and should be consistent, systematic, and collaborative in manner (Balfour-Lynn et al. 2009).	1 To ensure a smooth transition to the home environment. Communication of information between professionals and families is vital in order to ensure the best follow-up care.
2 The CYP's community team should be contacted as soon as discharge planning is commenced.	2 Early planning ensures a smoother, co-ordinated discharge process, ensuring all team members are involved.
3 The clinical decision that a CYP will receive home oxygen is made by the consultant in charge of the CYP's care and should be documented in the CYP's healthcare record.	3 Oxygen therapy remains a prescribed treatment for the CYP wherever it is administered.
4 An indivdualised management plan should be written and should include the following: • Oxygen prescription. • Amount of oxygen required. • Sliding scale of parameters with details of when to seek advice and from whom. • Mode of delivery. • Delivery system required (Balfour-Lynn et al. 2009).	4 To provide information and ensure that each CYP has his or her own management plan, including guidelines for use and information relating to clinical signs and symptoms (Balfour-Lynn et al. 2009).

Procedure guideline 29.10 Discharge planning for the CYP on long-term oxygen (continued)

Statement	Rationale
5 A medical decision will be required regarding whether the use of a pulse oximeter and/or apnoea alarm is appropriate for the home environment.	5 There is limited evidence on whether routine use of saturation monitoring at home is of benefit or harm (Balfour-Lynn et al. 2009) and whether it improves patient care at home. Alarms are often activated by movement and can cause carers to change oxygen flow unnecessarily (Balfour-Lynn et al. 2009).
6 Parents/carers should understand the need for home oxygen therapy and be willing and competent to look after the CYP in the home environment.	6 Parents/carers should be confident in their abilities to care for their CYP in the home environment with the support of competency-based training by hospital staff.
7 The family must be aware of the risks involved in the CYP having home oxygen therapy. They should be advised to take safety precautions such as installing fire alarms and smoke detectors, notifying the local fire brigade that they have oxygen at home, and keeping the oxygen at least 3 metres away from any appliances that use an open flame and 1.5 metres away from electrical appliances (NHS 2020).	7 Oxygen is a potential source of combustion and increases the rate at which fire spreads.
8 Parents/carers must be able to assess their CYP's respiratory pattern, recognise respiratory distress, and be able to take relevant and appropriate action.	8 Parents/carers must be aware of early signs of hypoxia and respiratory distress in order to reduce the risk of further deterioration in the CYP's condition.
9 Ensure the CYP on home oxygen therapy receives all relevant equipment.	9 To maintain quality of life and to ensure that equipment is providing desired outcomes.
10 Parents/carers should have support from the oxygen supplier with regards to equipment.	10 To provide ongoing equipment and support.
11 The CYP may receive oxygen therapy while at school, if required.	11 To allow the CYP to access education.
12 The CYP should have open access to a local hospital (Balfour-Lynn et al. 2009).	12 To ensure swift intervention in an emergency.
13 Families and carers should be offered the option for learning basic life support. This can be from the hospital or from local service provision.	13 To empower families and carers in the care of their CYP in an acute emergency.

Chest drain management

Introduction

To enable efficient ventilation, expansion of the lungs and the parietal pleural spaces are necessary. A small amount of pleural fluid is normal and serves as lubrication for the surface of the pleural membranes during respiration. Small spontaneous air leaks do not cause symptoms, they reseal and air is absorbed back into the body. A moderate collection of fluid can be well tolerated, but large volumes of fluid compress normal lung tissue and limit space within the thoracic cavity, thereby interfering with gas exchange.

A chest drain may need to be inserted as an invasive procedure to:

- Remove the fluid or air from the pleural space or mediastinum.
- Re-expand the lungs and restore normal negative intrapleural pressure and respiratory function.

Conditions requiring a chest drain insertion include:

- **Pneumothorax:** A condition where a vacuum or an increase in negative pressure in the pleural spaces occurs, causing the lung to collapse and air to escape into the tissues. It is a clinical emergency. A pneumothorax can be spontaneous or the result of trauma (Figure 29.6).
- **Pleural effusion:** Often associated with pneumonia; there is a build-up of exudate fluid in the pleural space.
- **Haemothorax:** A condition where blood has built up in the chest cavity, compromising respiration.
- **Chylothorax:** The accumulation of lymph fluid in the pleural space; drainage of this fluid allows full expansion of the lungs.
- **Empyema:** The multiplication of bacteria in pleural effusion secondary to an infection or as a result of trauma (Jones et al. 2001).

This section includes the following guidelines:

- Preparation for insertion of a chest drain.
- Care of the CYP with a chest drain.
- Specific drain observations.
- Further care and prevention of complications.
- Changing the drainage chamber.
- Removal of a chest drain.

Insertion of a chest drain

The majority of chest drains are inserted in theatre following the guidelines drawn up by the British Thoracic Society (MacDuff et al. 2010) and the Association of Paediatric Anaesthetists of Great Britain and Ireland [APAGBI] (2012). A thoracotomy is performed to insert the chest drain. Placement of the catheter is dependent on the location of the collection of fluid or air. For a pneumothorax, the chest drain is usually inserted anteriorly, near the apex of the lung, in the vicinity of the third or fourth intercostal space. For a haemothorax or pleural effusion, the chest drain is inserted at the level of the seventh or eighth intercostal space. More than one chest drain may be required to drain the air or fluid. The catheter is secured with a purse string suture and the site is then covered with a sterile dressing. There are several different types of chest drain chambers; see Figure 29.7 (Sugarbaker et al. 2020; Haas and Nathans 2015).

Figure 29.6 Chest x-ray showing a pneumothorax.

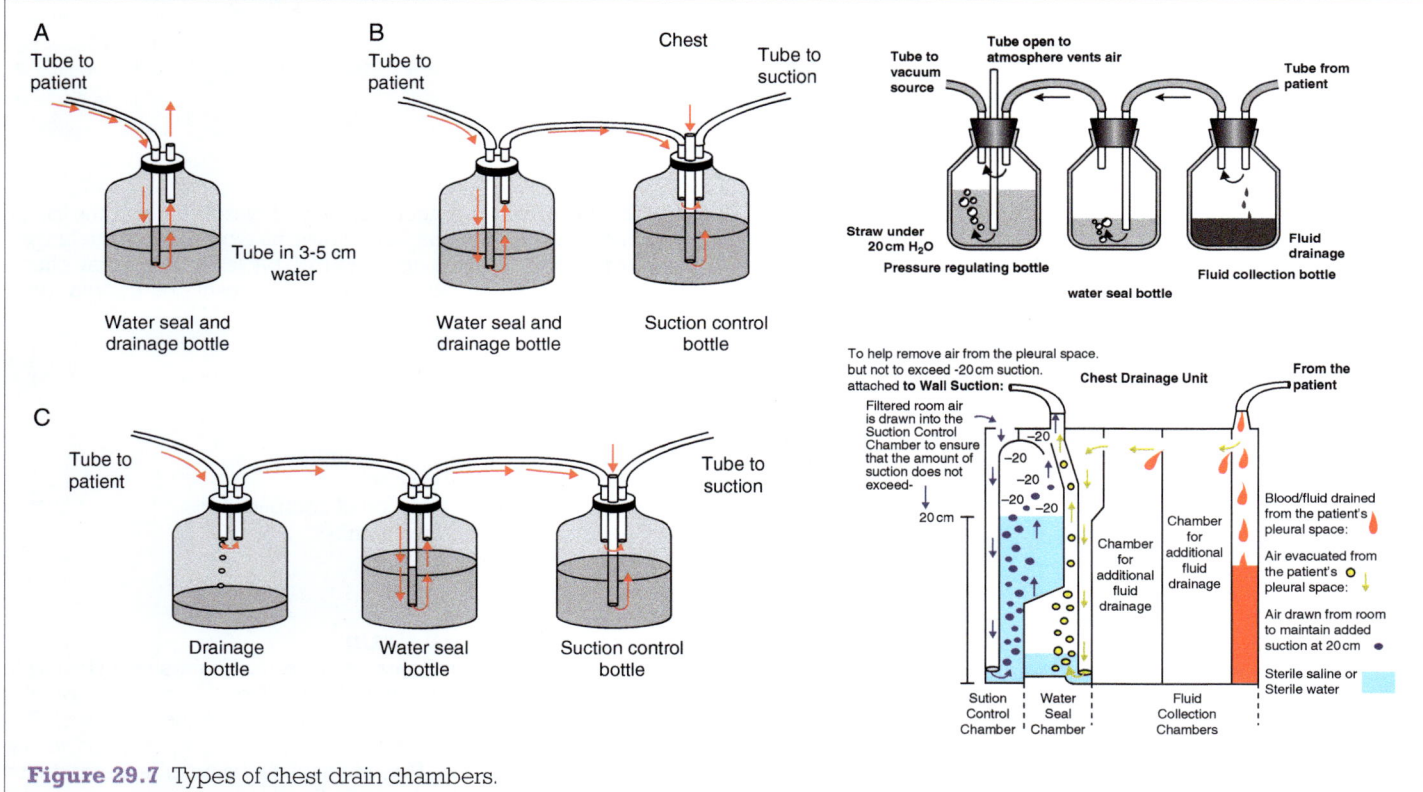

Figure 29.7 Types of chest drain chambers.

Chapter 29 Respiratory care

Procedure guideline 29.11 Preparation for insertion of a chest drain

Statement	Rationale
1 Ensure the CYP and family are informed of the following: • That a chest drain will need to be inserted. • What a chest drain is. • What the procedure and aftercare will entail. • The reasons for inserting a chest drain. • The likely duration of the procedure. • How long the chest drain will stay in situ. The family should be given written information about chest drains.	1 To provide information, reduce anxiety and facilitate informed consent (APAGBI 2012).
2 The CYP should be nil by mouth before the procedure as advised by the anaesthetist. The latest X-ray, bloods and ultrasound results must be available in addition to the normal pre-operative checklist.	2 To ensure all information is available for the team inserting the chest drain for the safety of the patient (Laws et al. 2003; Kirmani and Zacharias 2013).
3 If the procedure is being performed on the ward, gather and prepare the following equipment: • Obtain chest drainage system and chest drain insertion pack. • More than one chest drain may be required. • Sterile water for the underwater seal drain. • Sutures to secure chest drain in place. • Suction system.	3 To ensure immediate availability and a safe environment.
4 Give supplementary analgesia as prescribed, e.g. simple analgesics, opioids, local anaesthetic.	4, 5 To provide pain relief, minimise fear, and increase compliance (APAGBI 2012).
5 An anxiolytic may also be required for a younger or very fearful CYP.	

Procedure guideline 29.12 Postprocedure care of a chest drain

Statement	Rationale
1 Before the CYP returns from theatre, the bed space should be prepared and safety checks carried out.	1 To ensure that all equipment and monitoring is ready for the care of the CYP.
2 If the drain is to be on suction, a low suction unit must be available. **Two chest drain clamps should be with the CYP at all times** and these should come from theatre with the CYP.	2 To prevent air entering the chest in the case of accidental disconnection and fluid re-entering the chest when the drain is lifted above patient level.
3 On arrival to the ward, a full airway, breathing, and circulation assessment should be done and the PEW score calculated and recorded.	3 To provide a baseline set of observations. Any high PEWS should be reported to the medical team in line with the PEWS escalation policy (Pearson and Duncan 2011).
4 Using a stethoscope, the nurse should listen to the chest for bilateral breath sounds and the rate, regularity, depth, and ease of breathing noted.	4 A chest drain, if sited correctly, should not compromise breathing. If this happens the chest drain may need to be resited.
5 If suction is to be applied to the chest drain, the drain low-suction unit should be set at no greater than 20 mmHg. The water level on the suction compartment should be at the desired level (usually 5 or 10 cm of water). This will be determined by the surgical team and documented in the CYP's healthcare record.	5 To prevent trauma to the lungs.
6 The nurse attaching the suction must make sure that the suction switch is in the 'on' position and that the tube to the suction unit is not kinked or obstructed.	6 Suction needs to be continuous to ensure that the chest drain is patent and for the drain to be effective.
7 The chest drain should be placed securely on the floor below the CYP's chest.	7 To prevent fluid syphoning back into the chest and compromising the respiratory status.
8 A chest X-ray should be carried out within one hour of arrival on the ward.	8 To assess that the tube is in the correct position to enable the drain to function.
9 The initial drainage – amount, colour, and type – should be noted in the CYP's healthcare record.	9 To act as a baseline and initial assessment of the drainage.

(continued)

Procedure guideline 29.12 Postprocedure care of a chest drain *(continued)*

Statement	Rationale
10 The chest entry site should be checked and documented, checking the dressing is clean and dry, with no signs of redness and an accessible purse string, if sited.	10 To act as a baseline and initial assessment of the entry site.
11 The drain should be secured and the tubing will need an external omental tag tape.	11 To prevent accidental disconnection and trauma and pain to the CYP if the drain pulls.
12 For a newly sited drain, the drain should be assessed hourly for drainage, water seal, and the level of suction. These should be recorded on the fluid balance chart.	12 To provide an accurate record of the drain and the fluid loss.
13 Undertake pain assessment using an appropriate pain assessment tool and administer regular analgesia while the drain is in situ. It may be necessary to add dry gauze between the self-adhesive dressing and drain for comfort.	13 To assess and minimise pain. Insertion of a drain is a painful procedure and continues to be painful in the early postprocedure period (Bruce et al. 2006a,b; APABGI 2012). For more information, see Chapter 24: Pain Management.
14 The nurse should be able to answer any questions the patient or family may have on return to the ward.	14 To reassure the family about the procedure and the aftercare the CYP will be receiving.

Procedure guideline 29.13 Specific chest drain observations

Statement	Rationale
1 Check the water seal hourly to make sure there is enough water and that the water is moving to indicate it is working correctly. For a CYP breathing spontaneously, the water level in the water seal chamber should rise with inspiration and fall with expiration; this is called swinging.	1 The water seal acts as a one-way valve and prevents the air or fluid going back into the pleural space.
2 Observe for fluctuations (swinging) in the underwater seal drain chamber. If there are no fluctuations in the level of water in the water seal chamber, this may be due to one of the following factors: a) The tubing is kinked. b) The tubing is inadvertently clamped by the CYP lying on the tubing. c) There is a dependent fluid-filled loop in the tubing. d) Lung tissue or adhesions are blocking the drain during expiration. e) No more air is leaking into the pleural space as the lung is fully expanded. f) The medical team should be alerted if the water level does not start to fluctuate once kinking, clamping, and a fluid-filled loop have been eliminated as potential causes.	2 c) This will prevent the tube from draining effectively and will result in respiratory compromise. f) The drain may need to be replaced.
3 If the water in the water seal (blue dye) chamber evaporates, add water via the needleless access point on the back of the chamber using a luer-lock syringe. In the case of overfilling this chamber water can be removed in the same manner.	3 To maintain the correct level of water within the chamber (Figure 29.8). Refer to manufacturer's instructions.
4 In the case of a buildup of negative pressure within the chest drain unit, it may be necessary to release the pressure. Clamping is necessary during this manoeuver.	4 This is a rare but potentially dangerous procedure; the drain should be clamped to avoid excess pressure in the chest.
5 Not all drains will need to have suction applied. A plan of care should be documented for each individual CYP. Where fluid loss via the chest drain needs to be controlled or where the CYP will require intravenous volume replacement, high dependency level care should be provided (RCPCH 2014b).	5 Suction is not usually used, e.g. where fluid loss is excessive.

Procedure guideline 29.13 Specific chest drain observations *(continued)*

Statement	Rationale
6 If suction is required, attach to a low suction unit. The level of water in the suction chamber of the drain determines the level suction so wall suction should be turned to the minimum level to allow the water to bubble. It is necessary to check the suction hourly to ensure: • Bubbling is visible in the suction chamber. • The correct water level is in the suction chamber. • There are no loose connections between the drain and the suction unit, and that the suction unit is sealed.	6 It is vital to have the correct level of water in the suction chamber at all times so that the suction exerted on the drain is constant and correct. For the different types of chest drain chambers see Figure 29.7.
7 If the amount of water has dropped below the desired level: a) Disconnect suction. b) Open suction unit and top up with sterile water. Ensure unit is sealed after water is added (Figure 29.9).	7 To maintain the correct level of water in the chamber (Figure 29.9).
8 a) The need for suction should be reviewed by the medical team daily and the decision documented. b) If suction is no longer required, all suction tubing attached to the drain should be removed, not just turned off at the suction unit.	8 a) To ensure that suction is only used when required. b) Off suction means disconnecting the suction tube connection to the drain. Just turning off suction makes the drain system a closed one.
9 The amount, colour, and consistency of the drainage should be checked and recorded hourly. Any changes should be reported and investigated: a) Excessive drainage (>5ml/kg). There may need to be management of and a controlled loss of large fluid volumes. Excessive losses should be replaced with prescribed intravenous fluids. b) Any change in colour, e.g. milky or bloody drainage fluid: A sample should be taken; milky fluid suggests the presence of chyle and the CYP will require a dietetic review to determine if a low-fat diet is required. c) Sudden change in volume, either an increase or decrease. d) A change in the clinical observations and PEWS of the CYP.	9 To ensure prompt detection and treatment of any complications. a) Changes in the fluid loss could indicate a clinical change in the CYP. To prevent effects of excessive fluid loss on the circulation. b) To determine whether chyle or blood are present. These results may change the clinical care of the CYP and will confirm diagnosis. c) This may be caused by a blockage in the system or a change in the CYP's condition. d) A change in the PEWS will help predict clinical changes in the CYP.
10 Regularly manipulate tubing to empty any fluid filled loops into the collection chamber.	10 To allow for free drainage to the collection chamber.
11 Check drain insertion site and surrounding skin for signs of redness, swelling, pain, heat, and subcutaneous emphysema. These signs should be escalated.	11 To observe for signs of infection.

(continued)

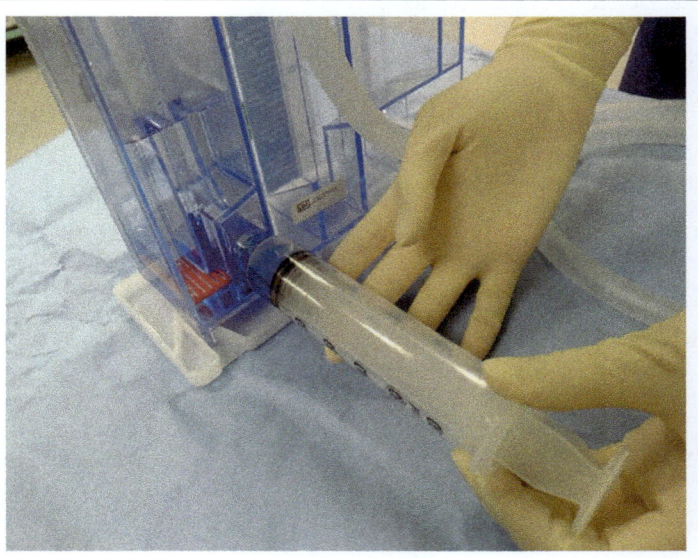

Figure 29.8 Adjusting the water level in the water seal chamber.

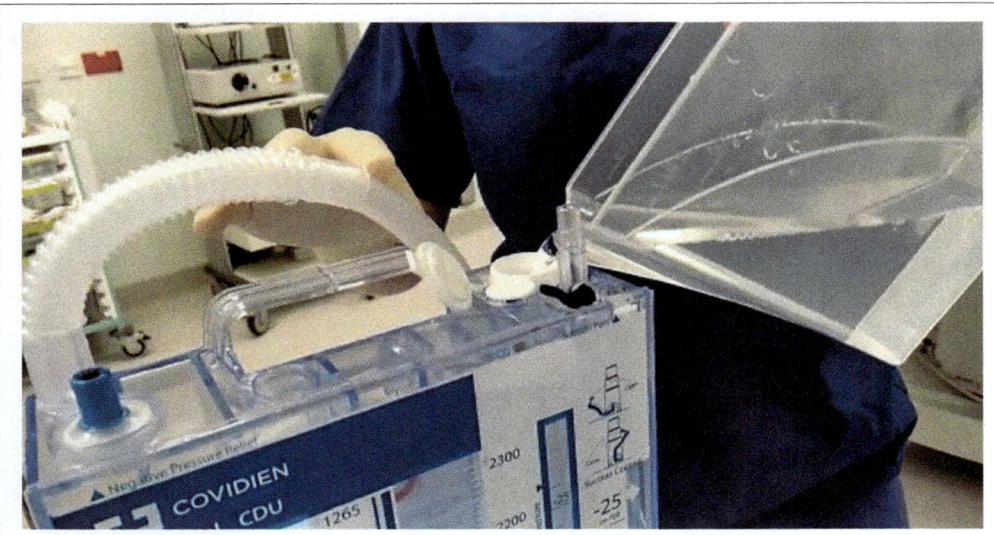

Figure 29.9 Topping up water in the suction chamber.

Procedure guideline 29.13 Specific chest drain observations *(continued)*

Statement	Rationale
12 Check for any drain-related complications not included above: **a) Tension pneumothorax:** Caused by interpleural pressure exceeding atmospheric, which could result from an incorrect water seal or if the suction tube from the suction limb of drain collection unit to the wall suction is in situ but the suction is not switched on. This will make this a closed circuit, and in the presence of air, can cause tension pneumothorax. **b) Bleeding:** Both around the site and excessive drain loss. This may be caused by blood vessel damage at time of insertion. The CYP will require a chest x-ray, ultrasound, pressure dressing, fluid resuscitation, and clotting screen to be sent. **c) Subcutaneous emphysema after initial period:** Can occur if drainage holes migrate to outside pleural space or if the drain is blocked or kinked. Contact the medical team as this will require a change in the position of drain or insertion of another drain. **d) Infection:** Can occur at any time while the drain is in situ. Monitor for clinical signs of infection such as pyrexia, redness, high PEWS, etc. Prophylactic antibiotics may be prescribed to be given before and after insertion in conjunction with local prescribing guidelines. **e) Displacement:** Can occur at any time. The drain should be clamped, tubing cleaned using an alcohol wipe and reconnected, and a chest X-ray performed. A full set of observations and PEW score should be calculated and recorded, taking particular note of the chest movement and work of breathing and oxygen saturations should be taken and documented.	12 a) This is a clinical emergency requiring another drain insertion immediately. b) To assess the amount of fluid loss and treat accordingly. c) This indicates incorrect positioning or a blocked drain (Jones et al. 2001). d) To ensure early detection and treatment of any infection. A drain site can be a focus for infection. e) Displacement can cause clinical complications including pain, internal damage and deterioration of the CYPs condition. Any displacement should be escalated rapidly to allow for a check of the drain site.
13 Ensure the drain is well secured.	13 To prevent it pulling on the skin and insertion site.

Procedure guideline 29.14 Ongoing chest drain care and prevention of complications

Statement	Rationale
Mobilisation	
1 If the drain is not on suction, the CYP can mobilise gently, taking care not to pull the tube.	1 Mobilisation reduces the risk of complications.
2 The drain should remain below chest height at all times and **two chest drain clamps should be carried at all times**.	2 To prevent backward flow of air or fluid into the thoracic cavity and to allow the drain to be clamped in case of accidental disconnection.
3 Parents and family should be taught safety care of the drain.	3 To ensure parents/carers know what to do in case the drain is accidentally removed or the tubing becomes disconnected.
4 If the CYP is immobilised, encourage a semi-upright position.	4 To facilitate drainage.
5 Early involvement of the physiotherapist is key to encourage deep breathing exercises in the immobile patient; e.g. encouragement to blow bubbles in a CYP old enough to do so.	5 Deep breathing will expand the lungs and encourage drainage.
6 When mobilising, always ensure the chest tube is supported so that it does not pull and that the collection unit is below the chest at all times.	6 To allow for drainage and prevent syphoning back into the chest.
7 To support the chest drain tube, create an omental tag allowing it to lie a little away from the chest wall.	7 To prevent pulls on the tube at connection and insertion sites.
8 Mobilisation often improves drainage. Viscous fluid (blood/pus) present in the tubing may be 'milked' to encourage drainage flow. However, this should NOT be carried out routinely unless the fluid is of a thick consistency.	8 To clear any thick viscous fluid from the tubing.
Dressing	
1 The entry site of the drain can be left with no dressing if dry. It should be covered with a dressing that is air permeable and with a self-adhesive woven fabric if the site is oozing.	1 To prevent infection around the site by keeping the entry site clean and dry.
2 The site should be reviewed for signs of redness, oozing and swelling.	2 To identify any infection early and initiate treatment.
3 If there is no dressing the site should be viewed six hourly.	
4 Check the suture is intact and secure daily.	4 To ensure the drain is secure.
Use of clamps	
1 The chest drainage tubing does not need to be clamped if the CYP is moved.	
2 The drain should only be clamped when it is necessary to: • Move the drain above chest height. • The collection unit requires changing. • If the drain tube becomes disconnected from the drain.	2 To prevent syphoning of drainage or air entry into the chest, as this would compromise the CYP's respiratory status.
3 Two clamps need to be available in the bed space at all times, or taken with the CYP if mobilising at all times, in case of accidental disconnection.	3 To clamp the drain immediately if disconnection occurs, to avoid pneumothorax.
Accidental disconnection or removal of the drain	
1 If accidental disconnection occurs: a) Clamp the drain. b) Clean with an alcohol wipe and reconnect the tubing. c) Unclamp the drain. d) Monitor the CYP's observations for any clinical changes.	1 To prevent further complications.
2 If accidental drain removal occurs: A small occlusive dressing such as paraffin gauze should be applied across the exit site.	2 To prevent entry of external air into the chest cavity.
3 Should either accidental disconnection or accidental removal of a drain occur: a) Alert the medical team to assess the CYP and plan further care. b) A chest X-ray should be done as soon as possible. c) A full set of observations and PEW score calculated, taking particular note of chest movement, work of breathing, and oxygen saturations. This must be documented in the CYP's healthcare record.	3 To escalate concerns for clinical review. a) To exclude pneumothorax. b) To note any early clinical changes in the CYP. c) To assess respiratory function and determine whether another drain is required to be inserted.

Procedure guideline 29.15 Changing a chest drain chamber

The chest drain chamber will need to be changed when it is full or when the chest drainage system sterility has been compromised such as in accidental disconnection of the drain.

Statement	Rationale
Gather equipment: • New chest drain drainage system chamber. • Dressing pack and cleaning solution. • Chest drain clamps. • Use standard precautions, and appropriate PPE, gloves, apron, and eye protection.	To ensure all equipment is prepared before starting the procedure.
Procedure: 1 Perform hand hygiene.	1 To minimise the risk of infection.
2 Use standard precautions and wear appropriate PPE.	2 To minimise the risk of infection. Protecting the person taking the sample from possible body fluid exposure, including eye protection in case of splashes.
3 Using an aseptic technique, remove the unit from packaging and place adjacent to old chamber.	3 To minimise the risk of infection.
4 Prepare the new underwater seal drainage chamber following the manufacturer's directions (supplied with chamber), paying particular attention to the amount of water needed to set the underwater seal and positive pressure in the drain. This will be advised by the surgeon.	4 To ensure the system is working as per the manufacturer's directions.
5 Ensure that the drain is double clamped before starting the procedure.	5 To prevent air being drawn into the chest cavity through the chest tube when the drainage system is removed for changing.
6 Clean the tube connection with the drain with chlorhexidine gluconate 0.5% in 70% alcohol wipe and allow to dry.	6 To prevent infection.
7 Disconnect the old chamber by gently pulling the chest drain tubing away from the chamber.	
8 Insert the new chamber tubing into the chest drain, then unclamp the drain.	
9 Recommence suction if required at the same pressure as per the individual care plan.	
10 Dispose of the old chamber in infectious waste bag and tie with cable clip.	
11 Perform hand hygiene and document the change and levels of fluid in the CYP's healthcare record.	

Procedure guideline 29.16 Removal of a chest drain

Statement	Rationale
1 **Pre-removal preparation:** a) Inform the CYP and family and prepare them for the removal. The indications for removing chest drains include: • Lung re-expansion on chest X-ray. • No evidence of air leak for 24 hours. • Fluctuations in water-seal chamber stops. • Drainage diminishes to little or nothing. • Comfortable respiratory effort. • Normal breath sounds over both lungs on auscultation (Martin et al. 2013). b) Negotiate the timing of the drain removal and whether parents wish to be present. Whenever possible the drain should be removed during the day so that the CYP can be monitored and observed and attend radiology department for a chest X-ray post removal. c) Members of the multidisciplinary team, such as the physiotherapist, may need to be informed. d) A play specialist may be involved for distraction therapy, adapting to the CYP and young person's level of understanding and psychological state.	a)–e) To prepare the CYP for the procedure and to minimise pain, anxiety, and risk (Akrofi et al. 2005; Bruce et al. 2006a,b; APAGBI 2012).

Procedure guideline 29.16 Removal of a chest drain *(continued)*

Statement	Rationale
e) Analgesia should be planned and administered in good time before the procedure (Akrofi et al. 2005). • Intravenous analgesia should be given at least 15 minutes before the procedure. • Oral analgesia should be given at least 40 minutes prior to the procedure. • If Entonox is to be used, the CYP must have enough time to practice their inhalation technique and feel confident in its use before the procedure starts. • Sublingual sedation is given five minutes before the procedure.	e) To allow time for the analgesia to work.
2 Preparation of equipment: a) Prepare a trolley by collecting the following: • Standard precautions and PPE: gloves, apron, and eye protection. • Skin-cleansing solution (such as chlorhexidine gluconate 0.5% in 70% alcohol or alcoholic betadine). • Sterile wound pack. • Sterile gauze. • Stitch cutter. • Appropriate dressing. • Paraffin gauze dressing. • Sterile skins closure strips, e.g. Steristrips™.	a) To ensure all equipment is prepared before commencing the procedure.
3 Preparing to remove the chest drain(s): a) Chest drain removal is a two-person procedure.	a) To allow removal of the drain with minimal risk of air entrainment; one person is required to remove the drain while the other is required to tie the purse string.
b) One of the healthcare workers removing the drain should be trained and experienced in the procedure.	b) To minimise risk.
c) Parental presence is encouraged, but this should be negotiated with them and the CYP.	c) Most CYPs find parental presence reassuring. However, the presence of an anxious parent may increase the anxiety in the CYP.
d) The aim is to remove the drain/s with the minimal risk of air entering the lung.	d) To minimise the risk of a pneumothorax.
e) If there are two drains to be removed, the lower drain should be removed first, followed by the higher drain.	e) So that apical drain will still function when the basal drain is removed.
4 To perform the procedure: a) Position the CYP so you have clear, easy access to the drain.	a) For ease of procedure.
b) Drains remain on suction unless specific instructions to the contrary are given. For example, in the case of a drain removed after a resolved pneumothorax, it is often requested that the drain is taken off suction for a few hours before removal.	b) To ensure standard of practice unless specific alternate instructions are given.
c) Wash hands as per trust policy and use standard precautions.	c) To protect the person undertaking the procedure as well as the patient.
d) Put on PPE.	d) To protect the person undertaking the procedure.
e) Using an aseptic non touch technique, expose and clean the drain site with saline.	e) To reduce the risk of infection.
f) Unwrap the purse string from around the drain if in situ.	f) To check purse string is in situ for skin closure when drain is removed.
g) Cut off the knot at the distal end of the purse string and give the ties to assistant to tie after removal.	g) Preparation and team work for safe practice.
h) If you assess that there may be a small gap on pulling the purse string, prepare a small paraffin gauze occlusive dressing. If you feel the purse string will not be adequate, contact the thoracic surgical registrar before removal.	h) To prepare for the procedure, check purse string and minimise risk of complications.
i) Clamp the second drain if there is more than one drainage system.	i) To prevent inadvertent air entry back into the thorax via an open check drain.
j) Cut the anchoring suture.	j) To allow the chest drain to be free.

(continued)

Procedure guideline 29.16 Removal of a chest drain *(continued)*

Statement	Rationale

5 **Timing of drain removal:**
  a) For CYPs who are spontaneously breathing and able to cooperate, ask them to practice taking a deep breath in and then remove the drain at the beginning of expiration. If the CYP is crying, intrathoracic pressure is elevated and it is therefore a good time to remove the drain (Cerfolio et al. 2013).
  b) For older CYPs the Vasalva manoeuvre (Laws et al. 2003) may be used: The CYP is instructed to take a deep breath, close their mouth and then blow their nose gently while at the same time, pinching it firmly shut.
	5
	  a) To reduce the risk of air entrainment, which is caused by the patient breathing in during drain removal.
	
	  b) To prevent air entering the thorax after chest drain removal.

6 Use one hand to withdraw the drain rapidly (within 1 second). It is sometimes easier to pull the drain vertically so that the drainage holes are pulled out almost together.	6 To prevent air entering the thorax after chest drain removal.

7 As soon as the drain is out, use the forefinger and thumb of the other hand to press the skin edges of the drain site together. Alternatively, if the skin cannot easily be pinched, a finger should press down from above the site directly over the hole.
  a) The second person should tie the purse string securely, taking care to avoid puckering the skin.
  b) If it has not been possible to tie the wound edges together, apply the prepared small occlusive dressing immediately.
  c) A large occlusive dressing should never be used on the site.
  d) Assess the drain site and leave it exposed if possible.
	7 To prevent air entering the thorax after chest drain removal if the usual safety measures to close the hole of the chest drain do not function.
	
	  a) To prevent air entering the thorax after chest drain removal.
	  b) To provide a seal for the puncture site.
	  c) A large occlusive dressing can prevent chest wall expansion (Laws et al. 2003).
	  d) For safety and visualisation.

8 Settle the CYP comfortably and conduct and document a full respiratory assessment.	8 To ensure there are no acute side effects from the chest drain removal.
9 Document the procedure in the CYP's healthcare record.	9 For communication with the clinical team.
10 Dispose equipment safely and wash hands.	10 For safety and infection control.
11 A chest X-ray may be performed routinely following drain removal, but unless there is a clinical sign of deterioration research has shown this to be unnecessary (Cunningham et al. 2014).	11 To check for ongoing lung issues post chest drain removal. To ensure that no lung collapse has occurred and that both lungs are fully expanded post removal.
12 Regular observations of vital signs and PEW score should continue every 30 minutes for four hours and then continued as appropriate for the CYP's condition and PEW score.	12 To do a full assessment as baseline post procedure and to act as an assessment scale for any problems.
13 Additional analgesia maybe required. Pain assessment should be undertaken.	13 To ensure patient comfort.
14 If the CYP is discharged within five days of the drain removal, the purse string suture must be removed by the community team and the family should be aware of possible signs of infection and who to report these to.	14 To maintain accurate communication and ensure any follow-up is provided for the CYP.
15 The local teams must be contacted before discharge and appropriate communication forwarded. This should be documented in the discharge plan.	15 To facilitate good communication and allow them to plan ahead. To ensure appropriate documentation and communication.

Noninvasive ventilation (NIV)

Introduction

Noninvasive ventilation (NIV) is the intervention of ventilatory support through the upper airway using a mask or other interface (Castro-Codesal et al. 2015). In most cases it relies on the patient being able to breathe spontaneously; when the CYP inhales, the NIV machine delivers positive pressure into the airway and supports that breath.

The use of NIV has markedly increased over the past two decades, and it has now become an integral tool in the management of both acute and chronic respiratory failure, in both the home setting and in the high dependency unit. NIV has been used as a replacement for invasive ventilation and its flexibility also allows it to be a valuable complement in patient management and very accessibly used in the home setting (Wallis et al. 2011).

NIV can be utilised for short- or long-term support. Short-term usage is usually for those CYPs with an acute episode of breathing difficulties. Long-term usage is primarily for CYPs with specific disease processes, and may be required on a permanent basis, or used until the CYP's airways have developed. If used long term, NIV is often only required during sleep (Castro-Codesal et al. 2015).

There are two main modes of NIV; continuous positive airway pressure (CPAP) and bi-level positive airway pressure (BIPAP).

CPAP provides a continuous positive pressure, prescribed by a clinician and aims to keep the airway open to maintain adequate gas exchange. It is used commonly in CYPs airway with upper airway obstruction.

BIPAP works by providing two pressures; an IPAP (inspiratory positive airway pressure) and an EPAP (expiratory positive airway pressure). It provides assistance during inspiration and prevents airway closure during expiration. BIPAP has multiple modes; three of the main modes are spontaneous, spontaneous timed, and timed. The mode used is dependent on the severity of the CYP's condition.

- Spontaneous mode: This triggers IPAP when the sensors in the machine detect inspiratory effort and then cycles back to EPAP. This would be used for CYPs with a good respiratory drive who are able to breathe spontaneously.
- Spontaneous timed mode: The device triggers to IPAP on inspiratory effort, but a 'backup' rate is also set to ensure that CYP still receives a minimum number of breaths per minute if they fail to breathe spontaneously.
- Timed mode: The IPAP/EPAP cycling is purely machine-triggered, at a set rate, typically expressed in breaths per minute.

Indications for NIV

There are many conditions that may be treated using NIV in CYPs; the main reasons for the use of CPAP or BIPAP are (Berry 2012):

- **Craniofacial disorders:** These include craniostenosis syndromes such as Aperts, Cruzons, and Pffifers syndromes and syndromes associated with micrognathia or midface abnormalities, such as Pierre Robin and Treacher Collins syndrome and Goldenhar syndrome. These anatomical defects can cause obstruction of the airways.
- **Neuromuscular disorders:** Conditions such as Duchenne muscular dystrophy (DMD) and spinal muscular atrophy cause muscular weakness, especially as the disease progresses, and this will cause hypoventilation (Marcus et al. 2012).
- **Obstructive sleep apnoea:** This can be due to enlarged tonsils and adenoids, macroglossia, or obesity, and is common in Down syndrome.
- **Malacia and stenosis:** Patients with tracheo/broncho/laryngeal malacia and/or stenosis may need CPAP to ensure their airways remain patent and are stented open.
- **Autonomic nervous system disorders:** The autonomic nervous system is responsible for all subconscious functions, including breathing. Central congenital hypoventilation syndrome (CCHS) causes hypoventilation due to impaired central respiratory drive.

Procedure guideline 29.17 Preparation for NIV

Statement	Rationale
1 Inform the CYP and family of the following: a) What NIV is and what the therapy will entail. b) The reasons for using a particular mask and ventilator. c) The likely duration of the therapy. d) Where to find NIV-related information	a) to ensure informed consent and understanding, and to meet expectations (Department of Health [DH] 2001). b) to explain that ventilators and masks are chosen depending on an individual's clinical need, reducing the risks associated with inappropriate mask and ventilator abilities (DH 2001). c) To prepare the family to plan for the future as the length and dependency of usage is based on clinical need (DH 2001). d) Patient information booklets on NIV are available on the internet for specific services or from the CYP's clinical nurse specialist.

Procedure guideline 29.18 NIV mask placement and care

Statement	Rationale
There are various products available for use with NIV, the most common ones used with CYPs being the nasal mask and the full-face mask. The masks are held in place by head straps. The decision of which device to use is made by the clinical team.	
1 **Nasal mask:** The nasal mask is generally used for CYPs who do not mouth breathe or who have a perceived/actual risk of aspiration. a) The bottom of the mask should sit below the septum, not obstructing the nostrils. b) The top of the mask should be positioned on the nasal bridge below the eye line. c) Head straps should be secure but with ability to fit a finger under straps either side of the mask. d) Apply mask before the ventilator turned on and pressure applied. e) Ensure exhalation valve is patent and not obstructed. f) Turn on the ventilator. g) Feel around mask to ensure no pressure leak, especially around the occipital region. h) Adjust mask or head strap accordingly until no leak felt. i) Ensure you can feel pressure leak from exhalation valve. j) Ensure patient comfort.	1 They are a less invasive option and reduce the feeling of claustrophobia. a) To ensure good nasal flow and comfort (British Thoracic Society Standards of Care Committee 2002). b) To reduce risk of pressure sores. c) To ensure a tight fit without causing too much pressure. d) To aid compliance and reduce anxiety. e) To reduce risk of carbon dioxide retention. g) To ensure comfort, good synchrony with the ventilator and to reduce the risk of pressure in the eyes. h) To ensure good synchrony, comfort and compliance. i) To reduce risk the of carbon dioxide retention. j) To improve tolerance and compliance.

(continued)

The Great Ormond Street Hospital Manual of Children and Young People's Nursing Practices

Procedure guideline 29.18 NIV mask placement and care *(continued)*

Statement	Rationale
2 **Full-face mask:** The full-face mask is generally used for CYPs who mouth-breathe, have a low aspiration risk, and who find ventilation synchrony more difficult with a nasal mask. a) Bottom of the mask needs to sit between bottom of chin and lower lip, which needs to be inside the mask. b) Top of mask to sit on the nasal bridge. c) Head straps should be secure but with ability to fit a finger under straps either side of the mask. d) Apply mask before the ventilator is turned on and pressure applied. e) Ensure exhalation valve is patent and not obscured. f) Turn on ventilator. g) Feel around mask to ensure no pressure leak, especially around the occipital region. h) Adjust mask or head strap accordingly until no leak felt. i) Ensure you can feel pressure leak from exhalation valve. j) Ensure patient comfort.	 a) To ensure comfort, good synchrony with the ventilator and to reduce the risk of pressure on the eyes. b) To reduce risk of pressure sores and good mask fit. c) To ensure a tight fit without causing too much pressure. d) To reduce anxiety and improve compliance. e) To reduce the risk of carbon dioxide retention g) To ensure comfort, good synchrony with the ventilator and to reduce the risk of pressure in the eyes. h) To ensure good synchrony, comfort and compliance. i) To ensure carbon dioxide can escape when mask applied j) Improve tolerance and compliance.
3 **Mask Care** a) Ensure the mask is clean before each use. b) Ensure the mask and headgear are intact and always have a spare available. c) Fully clean the mask and tubing once a week with warm soapy water and allow to dry. d) Leave to air-dry away from sinks and taps.	 a) To reduce the risk of pressure sore and skin damage. b) To enable a good fit and to ensure there is always a spare mask in case of an emergency. c) To reduce the risk of infection and maintain the integrity of the equipment. d) To reduce the risk of contamination.

Procedure guideline 29.19 NIV humidification and oxygen

Statement	Rationale
1 **Humidification** Humidification should be added if the CYP: a) Is prone to chest infections. b) Is using NIV for more than just overnight. c) Is reporting a dry nose or mouth that is affecting compliance. d) Has frequent nasal congestion which is exacerbated by NIV. e) A heat moisture exchanger (HME) should **never** be used for humidification.	 a) To reduce the viscosity and aid movement of secretions (Rodrigues et al. 2012). b) To minimise oral or nasal dryness and aid compliance and comfort. c) To reduce dryness of the oral and nasal cavity and improve compliance. d) To loosen secretions and maintain a patent nasal airway. e) HMEs can occlude the ventilator circuit when wet.
2 **Oxygen** a) Oxygen should only be added to NIV if there is a clinical need and this must be prescribed. b) Oxygen may be required if the patient has parenchymal changes or deterioration. c) In some patients, oxygen can be weaned with an increase in pressure via the NIV. This must lead by a clinician. d) To add oxygen to the ventilator, place an oxygen enrichment port or a filter with an oxygen port attachment between the ventilator and the tubing. e) There is no limit to the amount of oxygen you can add to the NIV circuit.	 a) NIV delivers pressurised air to overcome obstruction or to increase lung volumes. b) To maintain oxygen saturations. c) Increasing the pressures can improve gas exchange without the use of additional oxygen. NIV is a ventilation prescription and can only be changed on the advice of the medical team. d) Some ventilators have ventilator specific oxygen ports built into the back of them. Oxygen should be added using an oxygen enrichment port as they can be used on all ventilators. e) The percentage of oxygen being delivered by the flow metre is different from that which the CYP is receiving as you must allow for the dead space in the tubing.

Procedure guideline 29.20 NIV safety, tolerance, and compliance

1. **Troubleshooting Alarms**
   a) CPAP machines often do not have built-in alarms as they are used to deliver NIV for nondependent patients.
   b) There are two alarms that are a minimum requirement for patient using BIPAP.
      - High leak alarm; when the machine detects a leak over the set limit. Readjust mask and check the tubing for disconnections and cracks.
      - Nonvented mask alarm; will alarm within a set time if the vent detects use of therapy with a nonvented mask or blockage.
   c) Check the airway is patent, check the equipment is assembled correctly, check the exhalation port is not obstructed.

   a) To ensure that the patient or carer is alerted to a problem other than by an alarm to ensure patient safety.
   b) To ensure that the patient is receiving the correct pressure and that the patient or carer is alerted to a problem and can act swiftly to ensure patient safety.

   c) To ensure that the patient does not retain carbon dioxide due to a blocked exhalation port.

2. **Safety**
   a) A full set of observations and the PEW score must be undertaken and documented (RCN 2017). This should be repeated at four hourly intervals unless the patient's condition and PEW score indicates the CYP requires more frequent observation.
   b) Record the CYP's vital signs.
   c) Visually assess the CYP using an ABC approach.
   d) Check the ventilator and all equipment (including emergency equipment) and undertake all safety checks the beginning of every shift.
   e) Check that the pressures prescribed correspond with those being delivered by the ventilator.
   f) If the CYP is on BIPAP, check that the rise and fall of their chest is in synchrony with the ventilator.
   g) Check that the ventilator alarms are appropriate for the settings.
   h) Assess mask fit and appropriateness as previously explained.
   i) If humidification is used, check the temperature and alarms are set and that there is water in the humidifier chamber (no more than maximum line indicated).
   j) If the patient vomits, remove the NIV immediately and apply suction.
   k) If the CYP stops breathing, remove the mask and commence resuscitation.

   a) To ensure appropriate monitoring of the CYP and the early detection of any deterioration.

   b) To ensure that a full record of the CYP's care is maintained.

   d) To maintain safety.

   e) To ensure the CYP is receiving adequate ventilation as prescribed.
   f) To ensure comfort and to ensure that the CYP is not auto-cycling with the ventilator, as this may cause under- or overventilation.

   i) To ensure the correct level of humidification is delivered.

   j) To limit the risk of aspiration.
   k) The ventilator is a 'life-enhancing,' not a 'life-saving' device, and will not be effective in the event of a respiratory arrest.

3. **Tolerance and Compliance**
   a) If a CYP is finding it difficult to tolerate the mask and pressure, acclimatise using play and distraction (Koontz et al. 2003).
   b) Involve the parent/carer in all aspects of the NIV including the play and acclimatisation to reduce the fear the CYP may have.
   c) If the mask is uncomfortable for the CYP, consider changing to another shape or size more appropriate for the CYP.

   a) Desensitisation will reduce anxiety and age appropriate play can help the CYP have some understanding of why it is required.
   b) Parental involvement in key to compliance and tolerance. If the parent/carer is positive and aware of the benefits, it will reduce anxiety for the whole family.
   c) To improve comfort for the CYP and therefore compliance with NIV. Some ventilators have comfort settings built in to improve comfort and compliance.

Procedure guideline 29.21 Ongoing care of NIV

1.
   a) Pressure care management is vital to prevent the development of pressure damage from the mask.
   b) Assess the skin at least once a day and document in the CYP's record.
   c) If the skin becomes red or pressure damage occurs, adjust the position of the mask or change the type of mask and consider the use of barrier dressings.
   d) Should pressure damage occur, refer to the local tissue viability team as soon as possible.

1.
   a) The risk of pressure damage developing from the positioning of the mask is a significant risk for the CYP.
   b) To detect any problems early and ensure an accurate record.
   c) Changing the positioning of mask will alter the pressure points. Barrier dressings will help to cushion the pressure points.
   d) To enable effective and efficient treatment to be provided to manage the damage and prevent further damage.

2. Ensure parents are competent and confident in the care required and in managing any problems before discharge.

2. The CYP may need to use the NIV at home and this will be the responsibility of the parents.

3. It may be appropriate over time to change the ventilator or humidity settings. Contact the team that prescribed the ventilation to ensure this action is appropriate.

3. To ensure appropriate ongoing management of the CYP's NIV.

Long-term ventilation (LTV)

Introduction

Advances in paediatric respiratory technology and paediatric intensive care, accompanied by research and a greater understanding of disease processes, have revolutionised the provision of paediatric healthcare. Wallis et al. (2011) report a significant increase in the numbers of CYPs needing long-term ventilation (LTV) in order to survive. An increasing number of CYPs in need of acute medical and technical interventions during an acute illness are surviving but remain dependent on some form of technology for long-term survival (Jardine and Wallis 1998; RCPCH 2014b).

CYPs with complex long-term health needs may have been born with a congenital abnormality, survived deterioration within a chronic disease, or survived an acute and life-threatening illness such as trauma or major surgery. Stabilisation of the CYP's condition may often be achieved in a relatively short period. However, need for respiratory support may be long-term, and a decision about the long-term care of the CYP becomes a priority.

Once the decision to actively treat the chronically ill and long-term technology dependent CYP is made, then supporting that CYP within their home environment is preferable to a hospital environment. NHS England (2015) emphasise that patients who are supported by LTV can expect care to be provided at home, unless there is a clinical need for them to be within a hospital environment. Caring for CYPs who are dependent on noninvasive ventilation in their home environment has demonstrable psychological, social, and economic advantages, but it is important that early and careful planning takes place to ensure a smooth transition to home care (Jardine and Wallis 1998).

Long-term ventilatory support is defined as 'any child who, when medically stable, continued to need a mechanical aid for breathing, which may be acknowledged after a failure to wean, three months after the institution of ventilation' (Jardine and Wallis 1998).

CYPs with continuing LTV care needs, who are clinically well at home, will have differing and often complex care needs. The priority of care is to optimise quality of life through positive rehabilitation and ensuring as much normality and enjoyment as possible is maintained within the home and local care environment (NHS England 2015).

CYPs requiring LTV are usually divided in two groups:

- Invasive respiratory support through an artificial airway, such as a tracheostomy.
- Noninvasive respiratory support through externally fitted facial equipment.

Procedure guideline 29.22 Assessment for LTV and transitional care

Statement	Rationale
1 Accurate identification of those CYPs for whom LTV is appropriate is essential. CYPs must be medically stable, i.e. they must have: a) A stable airway. b) Stable ventilation on a portable respiratory support system/ventilator suitable for home use. c) Stable oxygen requirement (if required), usually less than 40%. d) All other medical conditions stable and well controlled (Jardine and Wallis 1998).	1 To identify CYPs requiring long-term respiratory support and ensure that the right preparation is undertaken. a-d) To differentiate from CYPs needing prolonged ventilation and the prospect of weaning in the intensive care/high dependency areas. To minimise risk.
2 Aim to transfer the CYP to a suitable hospital environment, e.g. a transitional care unit or paediatric ward (Murphy 2008).	2 The CYP needs the shift from the primary medical care to include the longer-term psychosocial aspects of care.
3 Care emphasis is placed on the CYP's long-term needs rather than short-term trouble shooting. The care is flexible and rigid hospital routines and rituals should be altered (Noyes 2001; NHS England 2015).	3 To limit the effects of hospitalisation that represent both an unsuitable environment for a growing CYP and an inappropriate use of resources (McDougal et al. 2013).

Procedure guideline 29.23 Management of a CYP on LTV

Statement	Rationale

1 **Select Ventilator/Respiratory Support Suitable for Home Use:**
a) Select equipment according the needs of the individual CYP.
 	
b) Home support machine should offer:
  i Single tubing system with exhalation valve.
  ii Flow auto-regulation.
  iii Independent of pressurised gas supply.
  iv Alarms.
  v Portability.
  vi Independent power supply (battery backup).
	a) To achieve optimal respiratory support for the CYP as simply as possible.
	b) For simplicity of handling.
	  i To compensate for small leaks.
	
	  iii No pressurised medical gases available in the CYP's home.
	  iv Safety feature.
	  v To allow the CYP mobility.
	  vi To allow mobility and independence for outings and as a safety feature in the event of a power outage.

Chapter 29 Respiratory care

Procedure guideline 29.23 Management of a CYP on LTV *(continued)*

Statement	Rationale
2 **Monitoring of the CYP:** a) Observe and record the normal pattern of breathing of the CYP. b) Carry out routine oxygen saturation monitoring while CYP is asleep. c) Oxygen saturation monitoring during daytime for clinical indication only. d) Sleep studies should be performed 6–12 monthly or as required.	a) To ensure safety and detect early indication of breathing abnormality. b) To provide early indication of respiratory deterioration. c) To assess effectiveness of respiratory support/ventilation. d) For long-term follow-up and consideration of changing ventilatory needs of growing CYP.
3 **Weaning Respiratory Support:** a) Respiratory support should be continually assessed as the CYP grows and develops regarding the continued need for ventilator support. This can be either in hospital or in the community. b) When weaning respiratory support allow only small changes (i.e. 1 cm H_2O per week). c) Increase time off respiratory support slowly. d) Develop an individualised weaning programme for the CYP and family. e) Wean BiPaP pressures first and aim for CPAP support prior to weaning further. f) Use clinical assessment and also how the CYP copes to prevent exhaustion. Capillary blood gases can support the weaning process as needed.	a) Any clinical improvement in respiratory ability/strength should be used to develop a weaning plan with the multiprofessional team and be assessed at regular intervals. b) To provide individualised care. c) To allow CYP to adjust and to continue with normal activities. d) To enable improvements or changes to be monitored and weaning progress documented. e) To avoid exhaustion. f) To assess readiness for self-ventilation.

Procedure guideline 29.24 Leaving the clinical area with LTV

Statement	Rationale
1 Clinically assess the CYP and ensure that he or she is fit to go on an outing from the ward: a) No restlessness, CYP is breathing comfortably. b) Normal O_2 saturations for that child. c) Minimum O_2 requirements. d) All equipment/batteries fully charged and checked.	1 To ensure the CYP is safe to leave the clinical area. a) The CYP needs to be comfortable and stable on the respiratory support before leaving the clinical area. b) These show the ventilation strategy is working well and supporting the individual. c) Oxygen can be taken when moving the individual but lower oxygen requirements mean increased respiratory stability.
2 Prepare an emergency bag with the following essential equipment, which should be kept with the CYP at all times: a) Tracheostomy tube same size and length. b) Tracheostomy tube half a size smaller, made of plastic. c) Scissors, tracheostomy tape, lubricant water based jelly. d) Suction catheters double the size of the tracheostomy tube. e) Self-inflating resuscitation bag. f) Disposable gloves. g) Yankeur suction. h) Nebuliser set. i) Normal saline, 5 ml syringes. j) Check suction unit working, ensure fully charged and all connections are secure. k) Manual foot pump. l) Check ventilator battery; ensure fully charged, take mains lead – may be able to plug ventilator in an emergency to electrical power source. m) Mobile phone.	2 To ensure safety of the individual outside the clinical environment. i) For suctioning j) Portable suction units last for one hour if used continuously. l) To plug ventilator in an emergency to electrical power source if possible. m) To summon emergency help if required.
3 Documents to check: • Parental consent. • If taking CYP home, provide information sheet with medical consultant, telephone number, diagnosis, and resuscitation status.	3 To ensure the safety of the CYP outside the clinical environment ensuring the availability of all key information in case of problems.

(continued)

The Great Ormond Street Hospital Manual of Children and Young People's Nursing Practices

Procedure guideline 29.24 Leaving the clinical area with LTV *(continued)*

Statement	Rationale
4 Oxygen requirements It is essential to calculate oxygen requirements for **any** travel (Box 29.2): a) C/D oxygen cylinders hold 460 litres when full. b) Always take out a full checked cylinder and ensure you have enough oxygen for the whole journey. c) Remember to observe the CYP all the time as you may not hear the alarms in a busy area.	4 To ensure sufficient oxygen is available for the CYP for the duration of the time away from the clinical area.

Box 29.2 Oxygen requirements for travel for safety.

> **Oxygen calculation:**
>
> How much oxygen required (Litres) per minute
>
> × 60 minutes (1 hour) = litres/hours needed
>
> **Examples:**
>
> If oxygen is required at 2 L per minute you need 120 L per hour:
>
> **2 × 60 minutes = 120** L oxygen per hour needed
>
> If oxygen is requires at 3 L per minute you need 180 L per hour:
>
> 3 × 60 = 180 L oxygen per hour needed
>
> **Always calculate the amount of oxygen you require for the outing. For safety, double this amount for the journey.**

Procedure guideline 29.25 Discharge planning for a CYP with LTV

Statement	Rationale
1 Multiprofessional planning is imperative for safe and effective complex care planning (NHS England 2015). A multidisciplinary approach is required to ensure effective rehabilitation. This will include input from: • Physiotherapy • Occupational therapist • Play specialist • Speech and language therapist • Teacher/education service • Healthcare workers • Family/carer competency based education • Specialist and generalist community paediatricians • Community children's services • Respite care services • Charity support • Dietician • Psychologist • Family support services • General practitioner	1 To ensure that long-term care is provided by the relevant teams. This could be either in the hospital environment or through working with local services in the community.
2 Needs assessment: a) Identify CYP's medical/nursing and psychosocial needs. b) Identify CYP's developmental needs (physical, cognitive). c) Consider psychosocial dynamics of family. d) Housing assessment. e) Identify availability of pre-existing local resources. f) Identify training needs of all involved in CYP's care.	2 a) Identify risks and needs to propose suitable care package (Hewitt-Taylor 2004). b) Review is based on an appraisal of the long-term needs of the family rather than on a short-term crisis intervention. c) Families with a CYP with long-term needs will have ongoing complex psychosocial needs. d) The CYP's home will need to be individually assessed and appropriate adaptions planned and implemented prior to discharge home. e) As part of the holistic assessment. f) To ensure safety and consistent training standards.

Procedure guideline 29.25 Discharge planning for a CYP with LTV *(continued)*

Statement	Rationale
3 Identify key workers: a) Community children's services b) Family/carers c) General practitioner d) Community paediatrician e) School /nursery f) Health visitor	3 To establish effective links and communication.
4 Develop and write a comprehensive discharge report detailing: a) Information regarding the CYP's medical and social history. b) Future care plan. c) A plan for discharge and follow-up care. d) Proposed skill mix for home care team. e) Identified training needs. f) A list detailing all equipment and equipment providers. g) Ongoing costs involved. h) Respite family services. i) Follow-up. j) Local hospital services. k) Local A&E. l) Planned future meetings.	4 This report is circulated to the family and all identified key workers prior to the first multidisciplinary planning meeting to establish effective communication.
5 Arrange multidisciplinary planning meetings.	5 To establish effective communication and individual action plan for discharge strategy.
6 Recruitment and selection home-care teams. a) This is a time-consuming process and should be initiated as early as possible, by the team responsible for delivering care to the CYP in the home setting. b) This should be undertaken in collaboration with the family.	6 a) To ensure safety of the CYP and adequate support for the families. b) As the care workers will be working in the family's home, it is of advantage for the families to be fully involved in the selection process.
7 Training: a) The team responsible for providing care to the CYP at home must organise a competency based training programme for staff and family depending on the technological needs of the CYP. b) The family and carers should be trained in • Basic life support. • Clinical deterioration signs. c) The family must know how to access emergency care if needed.	a) To reduce risks involved in CYP's care, and optimise safety in the community and home environment. To enable the family to meet all needs of the CYP. To ensure staff confidence and competence. To ensure consistent standards of care across professional and home care teams. b) To ensure clinical safety.
8 Moving to home: a) A phased discharge process, facilitating gradually lengthening trial periods at home when the family are fully responsible for care, will support the family in the establishment and development of the appropriate skills, knowledge and understanding of the care needs of their CYP and how working with their home care team will function.	a) To wean the CYP and family out of the hospital environment and to ensure confidence in home care provision.
9 Provision of equipment: a) Ensure the families have appropriate equipment required to support them at home. b) Equipment needed for home care includes: • Ventilator (×2). • Humidifier and leads. • Saturation monitor, portable saturation monitor. • Suction machine (×2). • Nebuliser. • Home oxygen concentrator or cylinders. • Back-up batteries. • Suctioning equipment disposables.	

Procedure guideline 29.26 The management of acute illness in a CYP with a tracheostomy at home

Statement	Rationale
1 Certain symptoms will require further assessment and treatment. These include: • Chesty cough. • Thick secretions or increased secretions. • Pyrexia (temperature over 37.6 C). • Altered sleep pattern. • Altered eating pattern or reduced appetite. • Diarrhoea or vomiting. • Altered or unusual behaviour/anxiety. (Warner and Norwood 1991)	1 CYPs on long-term ventilation can develop a range of illnesses which need to be assessed and treated. There may also be an increased anxiety and fear combined with clinical illness.
2 Action for symptoms noted. • Inform General Practitioner for advice, and the possible need for oral antibiotics. • Paracetamol to reduce pyrexia. • Encourage deep breathing/coughing. • Give extra 0.9% saline or hypertonic nebulisers if prescribed and tolerated. • Monitor O_2 saturations closely, on medical advice start or increase oxygen to ensure saturations are at an acceptable level. • May need increased ventilation with medical assessment/admission. • Inform Clinical Nurse Specialist or local team of change in condition. • Physio assessment and potential increase of physio regime.	2 Use the package of care set up to provide clear lines of care and local care services. The family/carers should use the package of care set-up and training. They should be able to access local hospital services if they are concerned.
3 Urgent medical assessment may be required if symptoms do not improve within 24 hours or CYP develops: • Difficulty in breathing. • Increased secretions or difficulty clearing secretions. • Altered breathing pattern. • Colour changes. • Low SO_2 saturation, usually 93% or less. • Headaches/lethargy/drowsiness. • Poor fluid intake.	3 To stabilise the CYP.
4 Ensure parents are fully involved in planning and decisions; take ventilator, humidifier, and emergency equipment with you (essential equipment must be with the CYP at all times).	4 For more information regarding the care of a CYP with a tracheostomy see Chapter 32: Tracheostomy Care and Management.

References

Ackerman, M.H. and Gugerty, B.P. (1990). The effects of normal saline bolus instillation on artificial airways. *The Journal of the Society of Otolaryngology Nursing Spring*: 14–17.

Akrofi, M., Miller, S., Colfar, S. et al. (2005). A randomized comparison of three methods of analgesia for chest drain removal in postcardiac surgical patients. *Anesthetic Analgesia* 100 (1): 205–209.

American Association for Respiratory Care (2010). Clinical practice guidelines: endotracheal suctioning of mechanically ventilated patients with artificial airways. *Respiratory Care* 55 (6): 758–764.

American Thoracic Society (2000). Care of the child with a chronic tracheostomy. *American Journal of Respiratory and Critical Care Medicine* 161 (1): 297–308.

Argent, A.C. (2009). Endotracheal suctioning is basic intensive care or is it? *Paediatric Research* 66 (4): 364–367.

Association of Paediatric Anaesthetists of Great Britain and Ireland (APAGBI) (2012). Good practice in postoperative and procedural pain management. *Pediatric Anesthesia* 22 (1): 1–79.

Association of Paediatric Chartered Physiotherapists (2020). Guidelines for nasopharyngeal suction of a child or young adult. https://apcp.csp.org.uk/publications/guidelines-nasopharyngeal-suction-child-or-young-adult (accessed 11 August 2022).

Balfour-Lynn, I. M., Shaw, N.J., Stevens, S., Sullivan C., Taylor, J.A., Wallis, C. (2009). BTS guidelines for home oxygen in children. https://thorax.bmj.com/content/thoraxjnl/64/Suppl_2/ii1.full.pdf (accessed 11 August 2022).

Berry, R. (2012). *Fundamentals of Sleep Medicine*. USA: Elsevier Saunders.

Blake, D.F., Shih, E.M., Mateos, P., and Brown, L.H. (2014). The efficacy of oxygen wafting using different delivery devices, flow rates and device positioning. *Australasian Emergency Nursing Journal* 17 (3): 119–125.

British National Formulary for Children (2022). Oxygen. https://bnfc.nice.org.uk/treatment-summaries/oxygen/ (accessed 11 August 2022).

British Thoracic Society Standards of Care Committee (2002). Non invasive ventilation in acute respiratory failure. *Thorax* 57 (3): 192–211.

Bruce, E., Franck, L., and Howard, R.F. (2006a). The efficacy of morphine and Entonox analgesia during chest drain removal in children. *Paediatric Anaesthetics* 16 (3): 302–308.

Bruce, E.A., Howard, R.F., and Franck, L.S. (2006b). Chest drain removal pain and its management: a literature review. *Journal of Clinical Nursing* 15 (2): 145–154.

Castro-Codesal, M.L., Featherstone, R., Carrosco, C.M. et al. (2015). Long-term non-invasive ventilation therapies in children: a scoping review protocol. *BMJ Open* 5 (8): e008697.

Cerfolio, R.J., Bryant, A.S., Skylizard, L., and Minnich, D.J. (2013). Optimal technique for the removal of chest tubes after pulmonary resection. *The Journal of Thoracic and Cardiovascular Surgery* 145 (6): 1535–1539.

Cunningham, J.P., Knott, E.M., Gasior, A.C. et al. (2014). Is routine chest radiograph necessary after chest tube removal? *Journal of Pediatric Surgery* 49 (10): 1493–1495.

Davies, P., Cheng, D., Fox, A., and Lee, L. (2002). The efficacy of noncontact oxygen delivery methods. *Pediatrics* 110 (5): 964–967.

Davies, K., Monterosso, L., Bulsara, M., and Ramelet, A.S. (2015). Clinical indicators for the initiation of endotracheal suction in children: An integrative review. *Australian Critical Care* 28 (1): 11–18.

Department of Health (2001). *Consent-What you Have a Right to Expect: A Guide for Parents*. London: DH.

Dinwiddie, R. (1997). *The Diagnosis and Management of Paediatric Respiratory Disease*, 2e, 81–85. New York: Churchill Livingstone.

Dougherty, L. and Lister, S. (2015). *The Royal Marsden NHS Trust Manual of Clinical Nursing Procedures*, 9e. London: Blackwell Science.

Edwards, E. (2018). Principles of suctioning in infants, children and young people. *Nursing Children and Young People* 30 (4): 46–54.

Evans, J., Syddall, S., Butt, W., and Kinney, S. (2014). Comparison of open and closed suction on safety, efficacy and nursing time in a paediatric intensive care unit. *Australian Critical Care* 27: 70–74.

Fisk, A. (2018). The effects of endotracheal suction in the paediatric population. An integrative review. *Dimensions of Critical Care Nursing* 37 (1): 44–56.

Gillies, D. and Spence, K. (2011). Deep versus shallow suction of endotracheal tubes in ventilated neonates and young infants. *Cochrane Database of Systematic Reviews* (7): CD003309. https://www.cochrane.org/CD003309/NEONATAL_deep-versus-shallow-suction-of-endotracheal-tubes-in-ventilated-neonates-and-young-infants (accessed 11 August 2022).

Haas, B., and Nathans, AB. (2015). Postoperative care including chest tube management. In McKee, MD., and Schemitsch EH. (eds) Injuries to the Chest Wall: Diagnosis and Management. pp143-54.

Hayward, R., Jones, B., Dunaway, D., and Evans, R. (eds.) (2004). *The Clinical Management of Craniosynostosis*. London: MacKeith Press.

Hellström, A., Smith, L.E., and Dammann, O. (2013). Retinopathy of prematurity. *The Lancet* 382 (9902): 1445–1457.

Hewitt-Taylor, J. (2004). Children who require long-term ventilation: staff education and training. *Intensive & Critical Care Nursing* 20 (2): 93–102.

Hoellering, A., Copnell, B., Dargaville, P. et al. (2008). Lung volume and cardiovascular stability changes during open and closed endotracheal suction in ventilated newborn infants. *Archive of Diseases in Childhood Fetal and Neonatal Edition* 93: F436–F441.

Jardine, E. and Wallis, C. (1998). Core guidelines for the discharge home of the child on long-term assisted ventilation in the United Kingdom. *Thorax* 53 (9): 762–767.

Jones, P.M., Hewer, R.D., Wolfenden, H.D., and Thomas, P.S. (2001). Subcutaneous emphysema associated with chest tube drainage. *Respirology* 6 (2): 87–89.

Kbar, F.A. and Campbell, I.A. (2006). Oxygen therapy in hospitalized patients: the impact of local guidelines. *Journal Evaluating Clinical Practice* 12 (1): 31–36.

Kirmani B, Zacharias J. (2013) Insertion of a chest drain for pneumothorax. *Anaesth Intensive Care Med.* 14 (4):163–165.

Koontz, K.L., Slifer, K.J., Cataldo, M.D., and Marcus, C.L. (2003). Improving pediatric compliance with positive airway pressure therapy: the impact of behavioural intervention. *Sleep* 26 (8): 1010–1015.

Laws, D., Neville, E., Duffy, J., and Pleural Diseases Group, Standards of Care Committee, British Thoracic Society (2003). BTS guidelines for the insertion of a chest drain. *Thorax* 58 (2): ii53–ii59.

Lee, J.H., Rehder, K.J., Williford, L. et al. (2013). Use of high flow nasal cannula in critically ill infants, children, and adults: a critical review of the literature. *Intensive Care Medicine* 39 (2): 247–257.

MacDuff, A., Arnold, A., and Harvey, J. (2010). Management of spontaneous pneumothorax: British Thoracic Society pleural disease guideline. *Thorax* 65 (2): ii18–ii31.

Marcus, C.L., Radcliffe, J., Konstantinopoulou, S. et al. (2012). Effects of positive airway pressure therapy on neurobehavioral outcomes in children with obstructive sleep apnea. *American Journal of Respiratory and Critical Care Medicine* 185 (9): 998–1003.

Martin, M., Schall, C.T., Anderson, C. et al. (2013). Results of a clinical practice algorithm for the management of thoracostomy tubes places for trauma mechanism. *Springerplus* 2 (642): 1–6.

Martin, S., Martin, J., and Seigler, T. (2015). Evidence-based protocols to guide pulse oximetry and oxygen weaning in inpatient children with asthma and bronchiolitis: a pilot project. *Journal of Pediatric Nursing* 30 (6): 888–895.

McDougal, C.M., Adderly, R.J., Wensley, D.F., and Seear, M.D. (2013). Long-term ventilation in children: longitudinal trends and outcomes. *Archives of Disease in Childhood* 98 (9): 660–665.

Morrow, B., Flutter, M., and Argent, A.C. (2006). Effects of endotracheal suction on lung dynamics in mechanically ventilated paediatric patients. *The Australian Journal of Physiotherapy* 52 (2): 121–126.

Murphy, J. (2008). Medically stable children in PICU: better at home. *Paediatric Nursing* 20 (1): 14–16.

Nakstad, E., Opdahl, H., Heyerdahl, F. et al. (2016). Manual ventilation and open suction procedure contribute to negative pressures in a mechanical lung model. *BMJ Open Respiratory Research* 4: e000176.

National Patient Safety Agency (2009). Oxygen safety in hospitals. Rapid response report NPSA/2009/RRR006. https://webarchive.nationalarchives.gov.uk/ukgwa/20180501163557/http://www.nrls.npsa.nhs.uk/resources/type/alerts/?entryid45=62811&p=2 (accessed 11 August 2022).

Neil, K. (2001). Normal saline instillation prior to endotracheal suction. *Nursing in Critical Care* 6 (1): 34–39.

NHS England (2015). Paediatric long-term ventilation. Service Specification. https://www.england.nhs.uk/wp-content/uploads/2018/08/Paediatric-long-term-ventilation.pdf (accessed 11 August 2022).

NHS Improvement (2016). Patient Safety Alert. Reducing the risk of oxygen tubing being connected to airflow meters. NHS/PSA/D/2016/009. https://www.england.nhs.uk/wp-content/uploads/2019/12/Patient_Safety_Alert_-_Reducing_the_risk_of_oxygen_tubing_being_connected_to_a_bDUb2KY.pdf (accessed 11 August 2022).

NHS (2020). Home oxygen therapy. https://www.nhs.uk/conditions/home-oxygen-treatment/ (accessed 11 August 2022).

Noyes, J. (2001). Ventilator-dependent' children who spend prolonged periods of time in intensive care units when they no longer have a medical need or want to be there. *Journal of Clinical Nursing* 9 (5): 774–783.

Ortega, R., Diaz Lobato, S., Galdiz Iturri, J.B. et al. (2014). Continuous home oxygen therapy. *Archives of Bronconeumology* 50 (5): 185–200.

Pandit, C. and Fitzgerald, D.A. (2012). Respiratory issues in downs syndrome. *Journal of Paediatrics and Child Health* 48 (3): E147–E152.

Pearson, G. and Duncan, H. (2011). Early warning systems for identifying sick children. *Paediatrics and Child Health* 21 (5): 232–233.

Resuscitation Council (2016). *Paediatric Immediate Life Support*, 3e. Resuscitation Council UK.

Ricard, J.D. and Boyer, A. (2009). Humidification during oxygen therapy and non-invasive ventilation: do we need some and how much? *Intensive Care Medicine* 35: 963–965.

Roberts, F.E. (2009). Consensus among physiotherapists in the United Kingdom on the use of normal saline instillation prior to endotracheal suction: a Delphi study. *Physiotherapy Canada* 61: 107–115.

Roberts, K., Whalley, H., and Bleetman, A. (2005). The nasopharyngeal airway: dispelling myths and establishing the facts. *Emergency Medical Journal* 22 (6): 394–396.

Robinson, P.D., Cooper, P., and Ranganathan, S.C. (2009). Evidence-based management of paediatric primary spontaneous pneumothorax. *Paediatric Respiratory Reviews* 10 (3): 110–117.

Rodrigues, A.M.E., Scala, R., Sorоksky, A. et al. (2012). Clinical review: humidification during noninvasive ventilation- key topics and practical implications. *Critical Care* 16 (1): 203.

Royal College of Nursing (2017). Standards for assessing, measuring and monitoring vital signs in infants, children and young people. https://www.rcn.org.uk/professional-development/publications/pub-005942 (accessed 11 August 2022).

Royal College of Paediatrics and Child Health (RCPCH) (2014a). Why children die: death in infants, children and young people in the UK. https://www.rcpch.ac.uk/resources/why-children-die-research-recommendations (accessed 11 August 2022).

Royal College of Paediatrics and Child Health (RCPCH) (2014b). High Dependency Care for Children – Times to Move On. https://www.rcpch.ac.uk/resources/high-dependency-care-children-time-move (accessed 11 August 2022).

Royal College of Paediatrics and Child Health (RCPCH) (2018). A Safe System Framework for Recognising and Responding to Children at Risk of Deterioration. London, RCPCH. https://www.rcpch.ac.uk/resources/safe-system-framework-children-risk-deterioration (accessed 11 August 2022).

Schoenwolf, G.C., Bleyl, S.B., Brauer, P.R. et al. (2014). *Larsen's Human Embryology*, 5e. New York/Edinburgh: Churchill Livingstone.

Simonds, A.K. (2007). *Non-invasive Respiratory Support- a Practical Handbook*. London: Hodder Arnold.

Sugarbaker, DJ. Bueno, R., Burt, BM., Groth, SS., Loor, G., Wolf, AS., Williams, M., Adams, A. (2020) Sugarbakers Adult Chest Surgery (3rd edition). New York: McGraw Hill.

Tume, L., Guerrero, R., Johnson, R. et al. (2017). Pilot study comparing closed versus open tracheal suction in postoperative neonates and infants with complex congenital heart disease. *Paediatric Critical Care Medicine* 18 (7): 647–654.

Tingay, D.G., Copnell, B., Grant, C.A. et al. (2010). The effect of endotracheal suction on regional tidal ventilation and end expiratory lung volume. *Intensive Care Medicine* 36 (5): 888–896.

Tweedie, D., Skilbeck, C.J., Lloyd-Thomas, A.R., and Albert, D.M. (2007). The nasopharyngeal prong airway: an effective postoperative adjunct after adenotonsillectomy for obstructive sleep apnoea in children. *International Journal of Paediatric Otolayngology* 71 (4): 563–569.

Wagstaff, T.A.J. and Soni, N. (2007). Performance of six types of oxygen delivery devices at varying respiratory rates. *Anaesthesia* 62 (5): 492–503.

Wallis, C., Paton, J.Y., Beaton, S., and Jardine, E. (2011). Children on long term ventilatory support: 10 years of progress. *Archives of Diseases in Children* 96 (11): 998–1002.

Walsh, B.K., Hood, K., and Merritt, G. (2011). Paediatric airway maintenance and clearance in the acute care setting: how to stay out of trouble. *Respiratory Care* 56 (9): 1424–1440.

Warner, J. and Norwood, S. (1991). Psychosocial concerns of the ventilator-dependent child in the pediatric intensive care unit. *AACN Clinical Issues in Critical Care Nursing* 2 (3): 432–445.

World Health Organisation (2016). Oxygen therapy for children. WHO Publications. Geneva. https://www.who.int/publications/i/item/9789241549554 (accessed 11 August 2022).

Chapter 30

Resuscitation

Denise Welsby

RN (Adult); EPALs Subcommittee faculty member, instructor and course director, Resuscitation Council UK; Head of Resuscitation Services, Great Ormond Street Hospital, London, UK

Chapter contents

Introduction	684
Early warning scoring (EWS)	684
Aetiology of cardiorespiratory arrest	684
Airway management	684
Recovery position	689
Circulation management	693
Basic life support	696
Choking	701
Cardiopulmonary arrest management	704
Defibrillation	707
Resuscitation team	710
Ethical considerations	710
References	711

Procedure guidelines

30.1	Head positioning (airway management)	687
30.2	Pharyngeal airways	688
30.3	Placing a child in a recovery position	690
30.4	Self-inflating bag mask valve ventilation	691
30.5	Preparation for insertion of an IO cannula	694
30.6	Procedure for a manually inserted cannula	695
30.7	Procedure for an EZ-IO inserted cannula	695
30.8	Using the IO cannula	696
30.9	Basic life support (BLS) provision	697
30.10	Management of the choking infant/child	702
30.11	Management of nonshockable rhythms (asystole and PEA)	704
30.12	Management of shockable rhythms (ventricular fibrillation and pulseless ventricular tachycardia)	705
30.13	Manual defibrillation with self-adhesive pads	707

The Great Ormond Street Hospital Manual of Children and Young People's Nursing Practices, Second Edition. Edited by Elizabeth Anne Bruce, Janet Williss, and Faith Gibson.
© 2023 John Wiley & Sons Ltd. Published 2023 by John Wiley & Sons Ltd.

Introduction

Cardiopulmonary resuscitation (CPR) is an all-encompassing intervention designed to improve and support the respiratory and/or circulatory systems. It is not merely a treatment aimed at the 'restoration' of a person's vital signs, but an intervention delivered in the hope of maintaining a quality of life acceptable for all patients, irrespective of age.

In recent years, scientific papers have confirmed that the early life-saving skills of CPR carried out by healthcare professionals and lay people serve as an important predictor of survival in both child and adult casualties. First responder interventions may almost double the chance of survival (Perman et al. 2021). However, response times remain poor, as there continues to be a great fear of doing harm. It follows then that first responders should be encouraged to 'do something rather than nothing', whether it be delivering mouth-to-mouth ventilations if safe to do so, or chest compressions, this may lead to better outcomes than doing nothing (Abella et al. 2007; Seethala et al. 2010).

There continues to be a paucity of evidence, specifically in relation to paediatric resuscitation practice, with some conclusions being drawn from experimental work or extrapolated from adult data. The International Liaison Councils on Resuscitation (ILCOR) of which the Resuscitation Council (UK) (hereafter RC UK) is affiliated, reviews current scientific-based evidence with the overall emphasis directed towards, knowledge retention, simplicity and a stronger focus on ensuring resuscitation quality (Skellett et al. 2021).

Age definitions
The age definitions used in paediatric resuscitation are:

- Newborn: Transition at birth (until the infant has made the transition to air breathing)
- Neonate: A baby from birth to 28 days old (irrespective of degree of prematurity)
- Infant: A baby from birth until the first birthday
- Child: From the first birthday until puberty

The question often asked is 'up to what age can the paediatric guidelines be used?' For simplicity the RC UK in 2021 suggested that the paediatric guidelines be used for patients from infancy to 18 years of age (Van de Voorde et al. 2021). This has the advantage of being easier to determine in contrast to an absolute age limit. In addition, training is standardised and avoids unnecessary confusion with healthcare staff. Similarly, from a practical perspective, adult guidelines can be used for anyone who appears to be an adult.

The primary difference in the approach to the resuscitation of a child lies in the knowledge that children are more likely to collapse due to respiratory causes related to an underlying illness or injury. A child deteriorates more gradually than an adult, as the body adjusts vital physiological parameters such as heart rate, respiratory rate, and blood pressure to maintain oxygenation and perfusion to end organs. Due to this inherent ability to compensate for the effects of the underlying cause, a cardiorespiratory arrest in paediatrics is rarely a sudden event. However, if undetected and untreated, this compensation phase leads to a decompensated state and hypoxia occurs as the body loses the ability to cope with the effects of the illness or injury.

Specific paediatric resuscitation algorithms exist for healthcare professionals with a duty of care for the paediatric patient (see Figures 30.1 and 30.2). Using these tools alongside enhanced training offers the best chance of a potential ROSC (Sutton et al. 2011).

Early warning scoring (EWS)

Early detection and intervention are the key elements in achieving a positive outcome for all acutely unwell patients, irrespective of age. Early warning scoring systems (EWS) exist in both paediatric and adult medicine to highlight predictive physiological markers, which identify the patient at risk and trigger the need for early intervention. There are a variety of systems utilised throughout the UK developed by individual hospitals. Here at GOSH our early warning score is called the Paediatric Early Warning Score (PEWS). These EWS, while improving the detection of patients at risk of clinical deterioration, still lack the sensitivity and specificity to allow accurate detection in all events (Austen et al. 2012). Healthcare professionals must appreciate that until they can be deemed 100% accurate and reliable, EWS should not replace high-quality clinical assessment, common sense judgments, and parental concern.

Aetiology of cardiorespiratory arrest

Unlike adults, the aetiology of paediatric cardiorespiratory arrest is rarely a primary cardiac event, but is usually secondary to hypoxia (Skellett et al. 2021). In the majority of children, this hypoxia is the result of respiratory failure. It is generally caused by underlying respiratory pathology (e.g. asthma, infection, foreign bodies), or may be due to a neurological problem (e.g. convulsions, raised intracranial pressure). Regardless of the primary cause, the resultant hypoxia and acidosis lead to the destruction and death of the cells in all body tissue, particularly the brain, kidneys, and liver. Once the myocardium is also affected, cardiac arrest will ensue. In some children, the primary problem may be circulatory in origin (e.g. loss or misdistribution of their circulating volume). The resultant inadequate delivery of oxygen and other nutrients to body tissue by the depleted circulating volume causes tissue hypoxia and acidosis, which again ultimately leads to cardiac arrest (van de Voorde et al. 2021).

The ABCDE approach to all deteriorating or critically ill patients is the same and follows a tried and tested approach based on an order of priority (Van de Voorde 2021):

- **A**irway (with cervical spine immobilisation if head/neck trauma is suspected)
- **B**reathing
- **C**irculation
- **D**isability
- **E**xposure

This approach is explained in Chapter 9: Early Recognition and Management of the Seriously Ill Child.

Airway management

Paediatric airway
There are a number of anatomical and physiological features that not only predispose infants and small children to hypoxia, but also necessitate specific management strategies (see Figure 30.3).

The anatomical features of the paediatric airway include:

- A relatively large tongue.
- 'U'-shaped epiglottis (which protrudes into the pharynx).
- Relatively high position of the larynx.
- Short and concave vocal cords.

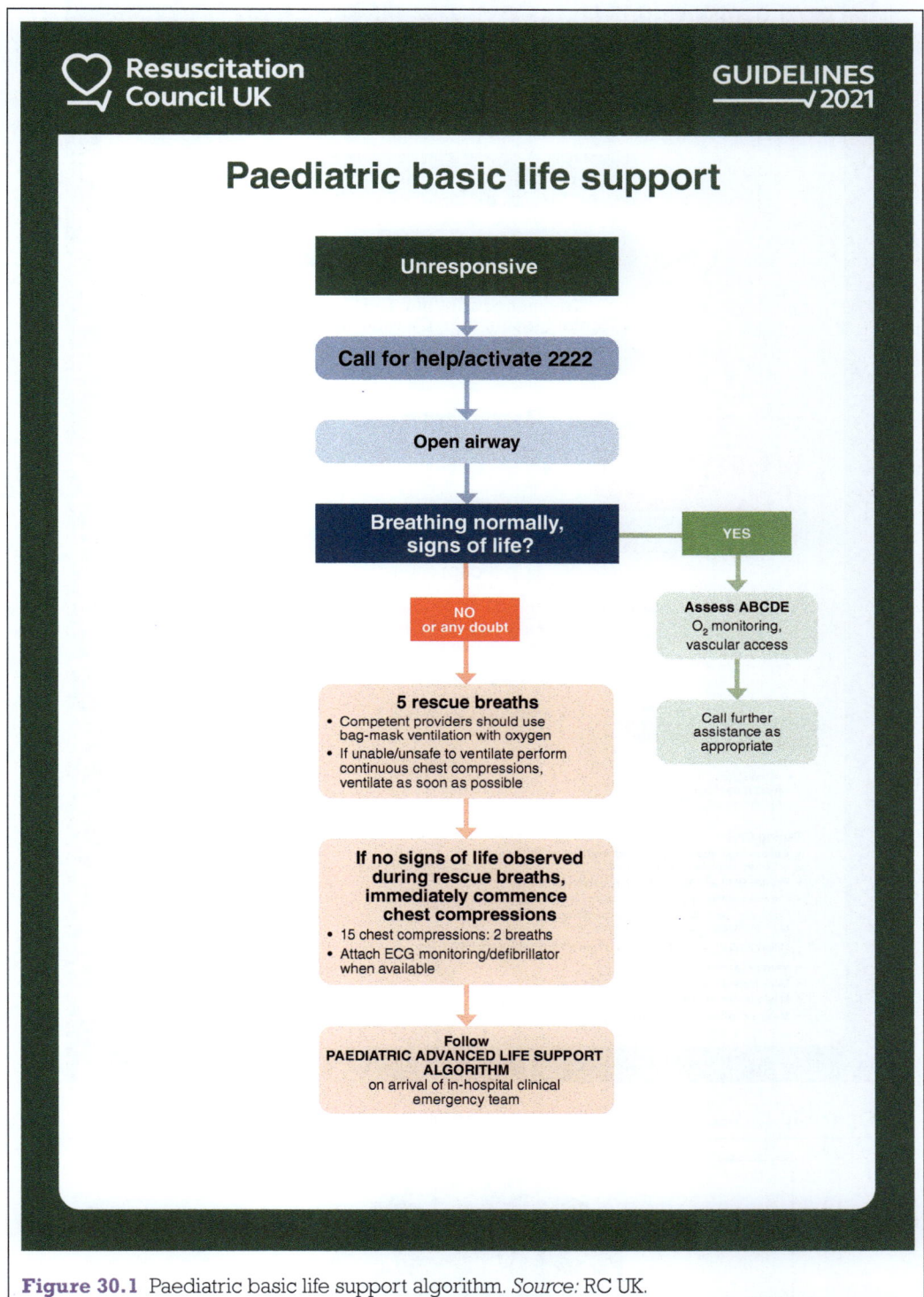

Figure 30.1 Paediatric basic life support algorithm. *Source:* RC UK.

- Narrow cricoid ring.
- Upper airway easily obstructed by flexion or hyperextension of head and neck.
- Preferential nasal breathers until approximately six months of age (patent nares [nostrils] and nasopharynx essential for adequate air flow).
- Small narrow airways (easily obstructed by swollen lymph tissue or secretions).
- Poorly developed lower airways (readily occluded by active constriction, e.g. oedema).
- Congenital abnormalities, e.g. vascular ring, tracheomalacia, or tumours (resulting in extrinsic obstruction).

Airway obstruction results in increased airway resistance. Even a minor reduction in the already small diameter of the paediatric airway can result in a large loss of the cross-sectional area; just 1 mm circumferential oedema at the level of the cricoid ring will produce a 50–75% reduction in the airway's diameter.

The degree of airway resistance is a primary factor in how infants and small children maintain adequate minute ventilation (i.e. The volume of any fluid or gas moved per minute.) With limited tidal volumes, sufficient minute ventilation is achieved by higher respiratory rates.

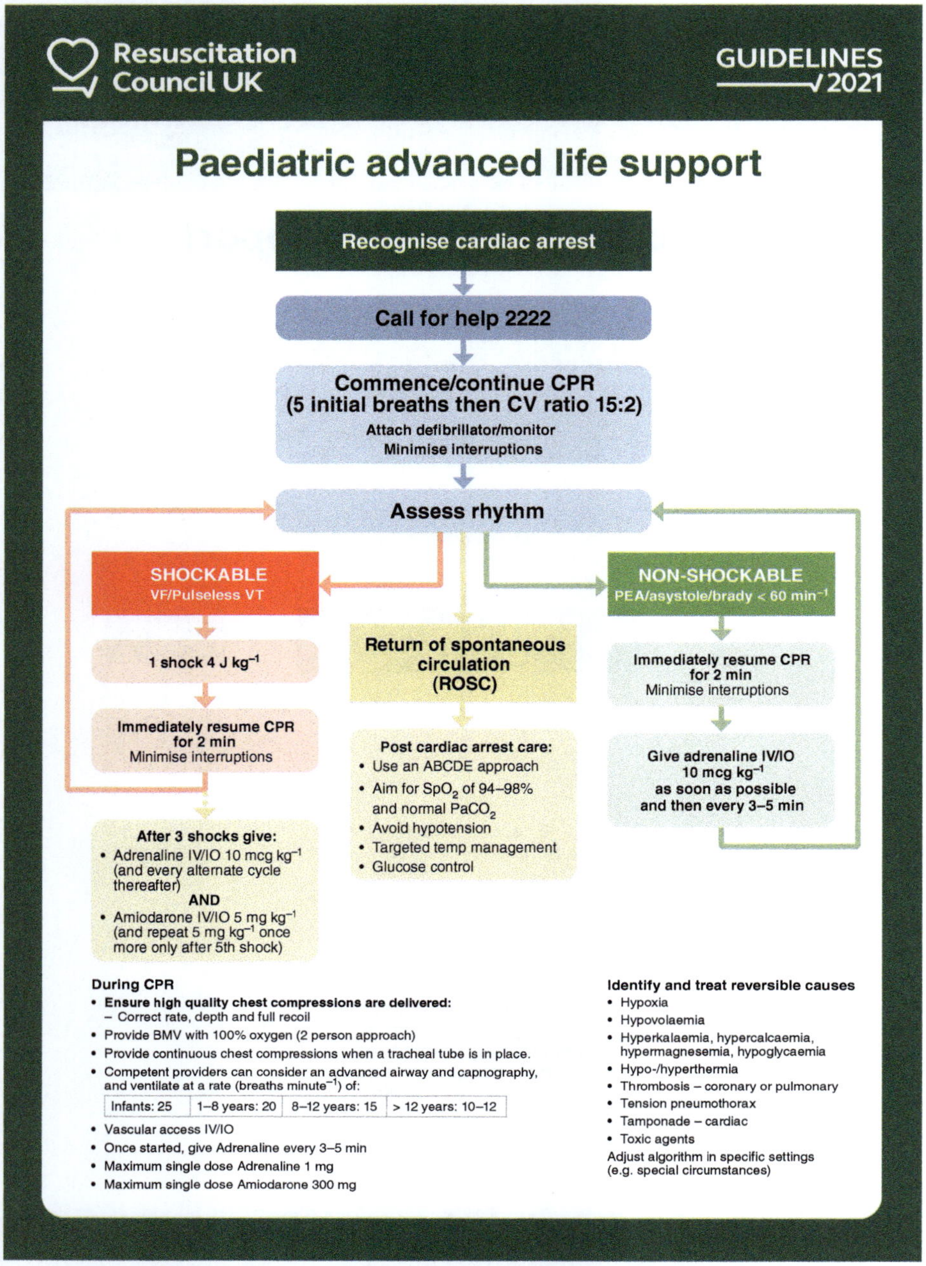

Paediatric advanced life support

Resuscitation Council UK — GUIDELINES 2021

- Recognise cardiac arrest
- Call for help 2222
- Commence/continue CPR (5 initial breaths then CV ratio 15:2)
  Attach defibrillator/monitor
  Minimise interruptions
- Assess rhythm

SHOCKABLE VF/Pulseless VT
- 1 shock 4 J kg^{-1}
- Immediately resume CPR for 2 min — Minimise interruptions
- After 3 shocks give:
  - Adrenaline IV/IO 10 mcg kg^{-1} (and every alternate cycle thereafter)
  - AND
  - Amiodarone IV/IO 5 mg kg^{-1} (and repeat 5 mg kg^{-1} once more only after 5th shock)

Return of spontaneous circulation (ROSC)
Post cardiac arrest care:
- Use an ABCDE approach
- Aim for SpO$_2$ of 94–98% and normal PaCO$_2$
- Avoid hypotension
- Targeted temp management
- Glucose control

NON-SHOCKABLE PEA/asystole/brady < 60 min^{-1}
- Immediately resume CPR for 2 min — Minimise interruptions
- Give adrenaline IV/IO 10 mcg kg^{-1} as soon as possible and then every 3–5 min

During CPR
- Ensure high quality chest compressions are delivered:
  – Correct rate, depth and full recoil
- Provide BMV with 100% oxygen (2 person approach)
- Provide continuous chest compressions when a tracheal tube is in place.
- Competent providers can consider an advanced airway and capnography, and ventilate at a rate (breaths minute^{-1}) of:

Infants: 25	1–8 years: 20	8–12 years: 15	> 12 years: 10–12

- Vascular access IV/IO
- Once started, give Adrenaline every 3–5 min
- Maximum single dose Adrenaline 1 mg
- Maximum single dose Amiodarone 300 mg

Identify and treat reversible causes
- Hypoxia
- Hypovolaemia
- Hyperkalaemia, hypercalcaemia, hypermagnesemia, hypoglycaemia
- Hypo-/hyperthermia
- Thrombosis – coronary or pulmonary
- Tension pneumothorax
- Tamponade – cardiac
- Toxic agents
Adjust algorithm in specific settings (e.g. special circumstances)

Figure 30.2 Paediatric advanced life support algorithm. *Source:* RC UK.

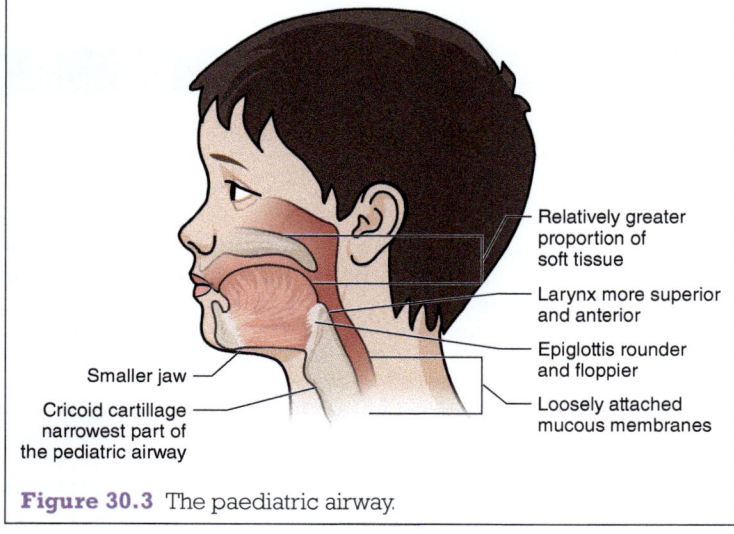

- Relatively greater proportion of soft tissue
- Larynx more superior and anterior
- Epiglottis rounder and floppier
- Loosely attached mucous membranes
- Smaller jaw
- Cricoid cartilage narrowest part of the pediatric airway

Figure 30.3 The paediatric airway.

Anatomical features in infants and small children that affect ventilation include:

- Horizontal placement of ribs means that elevation of them does not significantly increase intrathoracic volume.
- Diaphragm placement is also more horizontal and contraction tends to draw the lower ribs inwards.
- Immaturity of intercostal and accessory muscles and rib cartilage results in a very compliant thorax and contributes to the paradoxical movements (sternal and intercostal retractions) seen during active inspiration.

As tidal volume is very dependent on diaphragmatic functioning, any impedance from above (e.g. pulmonary hyperinflation in asthma) or below (e.g. gastric distension) seriously compromises respiration, as the chest wall cannot compensate. The main physiological features that predispose children to hypoxia are:

- High metabolic rate and oxygen consumption (6–8 ml/kg/min in children: 3–4 ml/kg/min in adults).
- Low resting lung volumes resulting in limited respiratory reserves.

Respiratory function may also be compromised by:

- CNS depression (coma/seizures, cranial trauma, metabolic disturbances, medications)
- Disease process (bronchospasm, atelectasis)
- Artificial airways (accumulated secretions)
- Inflammatory process (anaphylaxis, croup, post-surgery)
- Foreign bodies
- Dehydration (viscous secretions)

Regardless of the cause, any airway obstruction must be rapidly recognised and managed quickly.

Basic Airway Management
Suction

Suctioning is a basic airway management technique. Children with compromised airways frequently require suction to clear the upper airways of secretions and prevent aspiration. For further information and the clinical guideline for suctioning see Chapter 29: Respiratory Care. Standard suction devices in hospital are usually wall-mounted pipeline units. They consist of a wall terminal outlet, vacuum pressure regulator, a reservoir, tubing, and a connector for an appropriate suction catheter. All bed space suction units should be set up and ready for use with the appropriate suction tubing and Yankauer suction catheter while the space is occupied by a patient. Portable suction devices that run from both electrical outlet and battery should also be set up ready for use, especially if part of immediate resuscitation equipment on the emergency trolley.

Large-bore rigid suction catheters (Yankauer) are particularly useful for the clearance of thick or excessive secretions and vomit. Soft flexible catheters in a range of sizes should be available. They are particularly useful for nasal and endotracheal tube suctioning and may be less traumatic to use.

Whichever suction catheter type is used, it should have a side port that can be occluded by the rescuer's finger to allow greater control over the suction pressure generated.

Airway suction must be carried out cautiously if the child has an intact gag reflex as it may induce vomiting, which can lead to aspiration.

Basic airway management techniques

Procedure guideline 30.1 Head positioning (airway management)

Statement	Rationale
1 a) Children who have respiratory distress (increased effort of breathing) but are alert, will usually assume a position of optimal airway patency themselves.	1 a) The child will naturally maximise their own airway.
b) They should be supported in this position of choice, e.g. with pillows or in a carer's arms.	b) To provide comfort and keep the child calm, thus minimising oxygen consumption.
c) Placing the child in a supine position should be avoided.	c) This can potentiate airway obstruction (e.g. in epiglottitis).
d) The child should be monitored closely.	d) To rapidly initiate interventions if condition deteriorates.
e) If the child's conscious level is reduced, airway patency must be secured.	e) To prevent hypoxia.
2 a) There are two basic head positioning manoeuvres that can be used to achieve a patent airway: head tilt/chin lift or jaw thrust.	2 a) Head positioning can be safely and rapidly performed with minimal rescuer training.
b) The vast majority of children will require no airway adjuncts to secure a patent airway.	
Head tilt/chin lift	
3 a) With the child in a supine position, stand at one side of them. The rescuer's hand nearest the child's head should be placed on the forehead. Gentle downwards pressure is applied to tilt the head backwards.	3 a) To facilitate manoeuvre. To obtain functional alignment of the airway.

(continued)

Procedure guideline 30.1 Head positioning (airway management) (continued)

Statement	Rationale
b) The desired head position depends primarily on age, but abnormalities or injury may necessitate modifications.	b) Extension of the head and neck in infants results in airway occlusion due to kinking of their immature tracheal cartilage. As they grow, the cartilage rings mature and the airway lengthens, necessitating varying degrees of extension to achieve airway patency.
4 In general, *infants* should be placed in a neutral head position (the nares pointing at the ceiling) and the *child* should be in a slightly more extended head position. Sometimes referred to as 'sniffing'.	
5 The thumb and/or fingers of the other hand should be placed on the chin and if necessary, along the lower jaw. Pressing only on bony parts, the chin should be gently lifted upwards.	5 To lift the lower jaw forwards; this displaces the tongue and mandibular tissue away from the posterior pharyngeal wall.
6 Care must be taken to avoid pressing on the soft tissues under the chin.	6 To prevent airway occlusion from finger pressure on the tracheal rings.
Jaw thrust	
7 a) This is the manoeuvre of choice if there is any suspicion of cervical spine injury. It is also the recommended method when airway adjuncts or ventilatory devices are to be utilised.	7 a) Minimises risk of exacerbating injury. Facilitates easier use of airway and ventilatory equipment and allows for better access to the child by other rescuers.
b) With the child in a supine position, stand behind them and place a hand on each side of the child's face.	b) To facilitate manoeuvre.
c) Depending on the child's size, place one or two fingers from both hands under the angles of the lower jaw and gently lift it upwards.	c) To displace the mandibular block of tissue away from the posterior pharyngeal wall.
8 If this manoeuvre is being utilised where there is suspected spinal injury, the rescuer should position themselves with their elbows resting on the surface that the child is laid on.	8 To maximise control over immobilising the child's spine should they regain consciousness and attempt to move.
9 Whichever head positioning method is used to open the airway, ABC should be frequently reassessed.	9 To rapidly detect changes in condition and initiate appropriate interventions.

Procedure guideline 30.2 Pharyngeal airways

Statement	Rationale
1 If airway patency is difficult to maintain despite optimal head positioning, a pharyngeal airway may be inserted. These are available for oral or nasal insertion.	1 To minimise potential for airway obstruction related to the tongue and mandibular block of tissue.
Choice of pharyngeal airway	
2 a) Oropharyngeal (Guedel) airways should be used only in unconscious children except in very specific situations (e.g. initial management of neonates with bilateral choanal atresia).	2 a) Presence of a gag reflex means that an oral airway is unlikely to be tolerated and may induce vomiting with aspiration risk.
b) Nasopharyngeal airways are generally well tolerated even by conscious children.	b) They do not interfere with intact reflexes or activities such as suckling.
c) However, they are contraindicated where basal skull fracture is suspected and in some cases of nasal abnormality.	c) There is the potential to penetrate cerebral tissue or cause significant haemorrhage of the vascular nasal bed.
Sizing pharyngeal airways	
3 Select the appropriate size of: a) **Oral airway**, by measuring the total length of the oral airway against the side of the child's face. Place the flange at the centre of the child's incisors (or where they would be) to the angle of the mandible bone. b) **Nasal airway**, by measuring the distance from the tip of the child's nose to the tragus of their ear. An appropriate diameter is one that fits just inside the nostril without causing it sustained blanching (Papoff et al. 2021).	3 a), b) Too small an airway will be ineffective, while one that is too large may cause laryngospasm. Additionally, incorrect sizes can cause trauma and may result in worsened airway obstruction.

Procedure guideline 30.2 Pharyngeal airways *(continued)*

Statement	Rationale
Insertion of oropharyngeal airways	
5 a) Open the airway using jaw thrust manoeuvre and support the mouth in an open position.	5 a) To adequately visualise the mouth for placement of the airway.
b) If necessary, use a laryngoscope blade to depress the tongue gently and gently insert the airway as it will sit in situ (i.e. concave side down).	b) To prevent tongue being pushed back into pharynx. To prevent trauma to palate and ensure correct placement.
c) In older children, it is appropriate to use the standard 'adult' technique, i.e. the airway is inserted 'upside down' (concave side up) until it passes the soft palate. It is then rotated so that the natural curve follows that of the tongue and pharynx.	c) The risk of trauma while still present is much less than in infants and small children.
Insertion of nasopharyngeal airways	
6 a) Lubricate the airway with a water-soluble lubricant.	6 a) To facilitate insertion. To minimise discomfort for child.
b) If a commercially produced nasopharyngeal airway is to be used, insert the safety pin provided by the manufacturer through the side of the flange without obstructing the internal tube diameter.	b) The safety pin will ensure the airway is not inhaled or inserted too far. This also allows suction tubing to be inserted through the internal diameter to clear the airway if required.
c) If a shortened tracheal tube is to be used, an appropriate connector must be secured to the end of the tube.	c) To ensure the airway is not inhaled or inserted too far. This also helps secure it appropriately, and facilitates the application of continuous positive airway pressure (CPAP) if required.
7 a) Insert the tip of the airway into the nostril and gently direct it posteriorly (not upwards) along the nasal floor towards the tragus of the ear.	7 a) To minimise potential for trauma.
b) Gently progress the airway past the turbinates with a slight rotating movement until a 'give' is felt. Continue to gently insert the airway until the flange rests at the nostril.	b) To achieve correct placement. The loss of resistance indicates that the airway has entered the pharynx.
c) If difficulty is experienced inserting the airway, it should be removed and consideration given to using the other nostril or a smaller diameter of airway.	c) To minimise trauma.
8 Whichever pharyngeal airway route is used, observe the child for any signs of trauma to the oral or nasal cavity.	8 Difficulty in placement of the airway can lead to significant bleeding from mucous membranes or damage to teeth. Pressure ulceration can develop with improper placement or prolonged usage.
9 Reassess the child's ABC frequently.	9 Insertion of a pharyngeal airway should improve the child's condition. If it does not, its use should be reassessed.
10 Continue with clinical assessment and further interventions as appropriate.	10 To minimise the risk of morbidity and mortality.

Recovery position

The unresponsive child who is breathing spontaneously and has an adequate circulation should be placed in a safe, side-lying position unless contraindicated (e.g. suspected spinal injury). The purpose of this is to ensure that:

- The tongue does not fall back and obstruct the airway.
- The risk of aspiration of stomach contents is reduced.

There is no universally accepted recovery position, but the general principles are based on ensuring that the child:

- Is in as near a true lateral position as possible.
- Has a patent airway maintained.
- Can be easily observed and monitored.
- Is stable and cannot roll over.
- Can freely drain secretions/vomit from their mouth.
- Has no pressure on their chest that may impede breathing.
- Can be easily turned into a supine position for BLS if indicated.

Procedure Guideline 30.3 provides a description of one method of placing a child in a recovery position (Van de Voorde et al. 2021).

Procedure guideline 30.3 Placing a child in a recovery position

Statement	Rationale
1 a) The rescuer should kneel/stand at one side of the child. b) Straighten out the child's legs and arms. c) Remove any spectacles and sharp/bulky objects (e.g. large hair clips, items in their pockets, etc.).	1 a) To facilitate ease of positioning. b) To facilitate turning of child. c) To prevent trauma when they are turned on to their side.
2 Loosen any clothing around the child's neck.	2 To avoid airway constriction.
3 Extend the child's arm nearest to the rescuer to a 90% angle with the palm facing upward beside their head.	3 To minimise risk of trauma to child's limb during the manoeuvre.
4 Bring the child's opposite arm across their body towards the rescuer, and hold it against the cheek on the rescuer's side.	4 To facilitate turning of child.
5 a) With their other hand, the rescuer should bend up the child's farthest leg at the knee. b) Pressing against the child's knee, they should be gently rolled over towards the rescuer.	5 a) To facilitate turning the child safely. b) To minimise exertion required by the rescuer while placing child on their side.
6 The hand that was placed against the child's cheek previously (and is now underneath it) should be checked.	6 To ensure that it is not causing undue pressure on the face.
7 The child's head can then be positioned slightly backwards if necessary.	7 To ensure that the airway remains patent.
8 A rolled-up towel or blanket may need to be placed at the back of a small child or infant.	8 To prevent them from rolling onto their backs and potentially occluding their airway.
9 The child's breathing and circulation should be reassessed frequently while awaiting further assistance as indicated.	9 The child with a decreased conscious level is at increased risk of airway obstruction due to accumulated secretions or aspiration. To rapidly detect any deterioration, necessitating turning the child to a supine position for thorough ABC assessment.
10 If they are to be kept in a recovery position for any longer than 30 minutes, the infant/child should be turned onto their other side.	10 To minimise potential for pressure injuries or nerve damage.

Advanced airway and breathing management

Responders must always ensure initially that the patient has a patent airway, by performing an airway manoeuvre (see section on Airway Management). Bag valve mask (BVM) ventilation with high-concentration oxygen should be used as soon as this is available when an infant/child is unable to breathe adequately, or is in cardiorespiratory arrest (Stein et al. 2020). It is important to appreciate that hyperventilation with extreme force and speed is harmful and must be avoided. In a respiratory or cardiac arrest situation, oxygen should be administered at the highest concentration as soon as possible; concerns about the potential toxicity of oxygen should never prevent its use in initial resuscitation.

The equipment usually employed in paediatric resuscitation is a self-inflating bag device; with oxygen flow set at 10–15 l and a reservoir bag attached it is possible to achieve oxygenation of up to 98% concentration. Ideally this device should have a pressure-limiting (or 'pop off') valve incorporated in its design (Figure 30.4) to prevent inadvertent delivery of excessive inflation pressures (Nagler et al. 2021).

Ventilations should be delivered at the normal rate according to age (see Procedure Guideline 30.4).

In a cardiac arrest situation, as soon as experienced personnel arrive, advanced airway management can be performed, such as the insertion of an endotracheal (ET) tube, if this can be achieved with minimal interruptions to chest compressions. Once tracheal intubation has been achieved and the airway controlled, continual chest compressions can be delivered, which will improve circulation and coronary perfusion pressures. Once continuous chest compressions have been established, the respiratory rate will change from around 10 breaths per minute (bpm) (15:2 ratio) to age-related rates: infant = 25 bpm, 1–8 years = 20 bpm, 8–12 years = 15 bpm, and > 12 years = 10 bpm.

End tidal carbon dioxide (ETCO2) monitoring when attached to the Et tube will assist the resuscitation team to ensure that the tube is in the correct place and that good ventilations are being delivered (Nolan et al. 2014; Van de Voorde et al. 2021).

Laryngeal mask airways

Bag mask ventilation (BMV) remains the first line method for achieving airway control and ventilation (Van de Voorde et al. 2021). However the laryngeal mask airway (LMA) (Figure 30.5) has gained favour over recent years when BMV use is not possible due to supraglottic airway abnormalities, found in conditions such as Pierre Robin syndrome. Insertion of an LMA is simple, but requires specific training. They should be readily available as they can be lifesaving for a child with a difficult airway in whom adequate ventilation cannot be achieved by either BMV or tracheal intubation (Ostermayer and Gausche-Hill 2014; Stein et al. 2020).

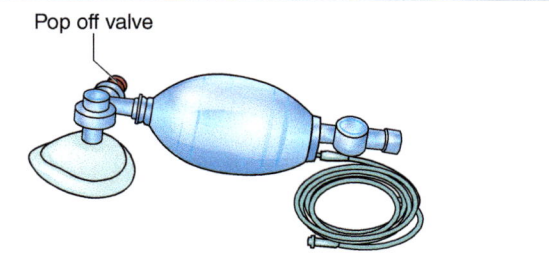

Figure 30.4 BMV with pressure relief valve. *Source:* https://uk.intersurgical.com/products/anaesthesia/bvms-and-resuscitation-mask © Intersurgical Ltd., 2021.

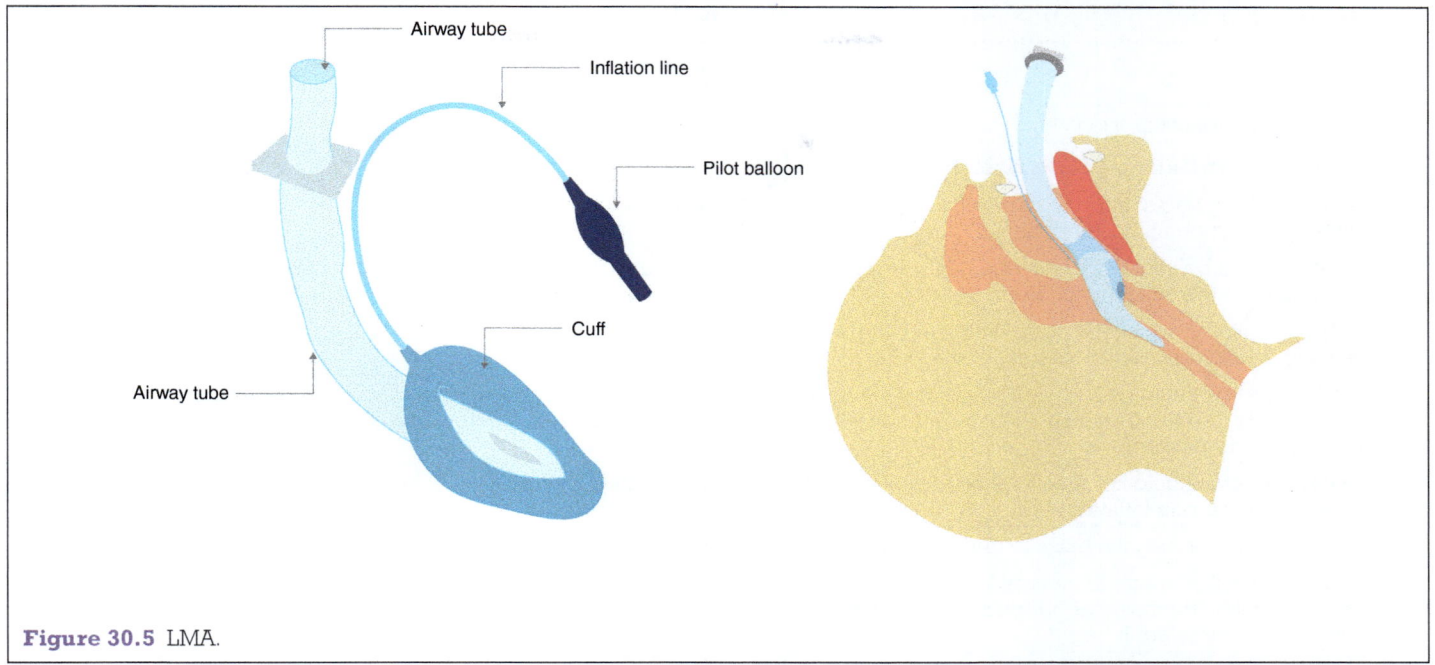

Figure 30.5 LMA.

Tracheal tubes

The placement of a tracheal tube is more usually undertaken as a planned procedure rather than an emergency one. This is because of the improvement in the early recognition of a seriously ill patient, which allows time for the responders to plan the tracheal tube insertion. However, when cardiorespiratory arrest occurs in a nonintubated child, the airway should be maintained and the patient oxygenated by noninvasive means before placement of a tracheal tube (see Procedure Guideline 30.4). Endotracheal intubation is a technically difficult procedure in children and not without complications (Lavonas et al. 2019; Nagler et al. 2021). It should therefore only be undertaken by someone competent in the procedure, and considered when:

- BMV fails to be effective.
- The airway is insecure.
- Ongoing ventilator support is anticipated.

Gastric tubes

When children have respiratory distress they tend to swallow large amounts of air, which distends the stomach and makes them prone to vomiting. The use of a BMV device compounds this, as some oxygen tends to be forced into the stomach. This can cause significant vagal stimulation, with potential risk of aspiration. Additionally, diaphragmatic splinting makes ventilation difficult. It is therefore important that a gastric tube is placed early to deflate the stomach. For procedure guidelines on insertion of a gastric tube, see Chapter 22: Nutrition and Feeding.

Procedure guideline 30.4 Self-inflating bag mask valve ventilation

Statement	Rationale
Selection of equipment	
1 A correctly sized facemask.	1
a) The required properties of the mask include: Transparency. Cover the mouth and nose. Avoid pressure on the eyes. Have a low dead space. b) If the mask has an inflatable rim, a check should be made to ensure this is adequately inflated.	a) To facilitate optimal ventilation: Observation of colour and detection of vomit. Create a good seal. Prevent trauma and vagal stimulation. Avoid CO_2 retention. b) To ensure an adequate seal.
2 Appropriate size of self-inflating bag.	2
a) These generally come in three sizes – 250 ml, 450–500 ml, and 1600–2000 ml. The smallest was designed for newborns but is generally considered ineffective as adequate tidal volumes may not be delivered. b) Either the middle or largest sizes can be used for children; however, not all manufacturers currently incorporate pressure-limiting devices into the large bags, which make them potentially less safe for use in infants and young children. The larger size is generally required in older children (above 20–30 kg) but individual responses need to be considered.	a) This is due to the inability to deliver prolonged inspiratory times required to inflate newborn lungs with it. b) This is designed to 'blow off' at a predetermined limit (approximately 30–40 cm H_2O pressure) thus minimising the risk of barotrauma to the lungs.

(continued)

Procedure guideline 30.4 Self-inflating bag mask valve ventilation *(continued)*

Statement	Rationale
3 Reservoir bag.	3, 4 To ensure the highest possible concentration of oxygen is administered.
4 Continuous supply of oxygen.	

Checking self-inflating bag-mask device

Statement	Rationale
1 The self-inflating bag should be checked for any visible defects (missing or faulty components).	1 To ensure safe functioning.
2 The bag should be squeezed with one hand, with the free hand held near the outlet (inspiratory) valve.	2 To ensure that air is felt on the free hand indicating that it has been expelled through the valve.
3 The bag should be squeezed again with one hand while the free hand is held against the inspiratory valve.	3 To check that the pressure limiting valve works (i.e. that excess air is vented through it).
4 While squeezing the bag again, the operator should use the thumb of their free hand to ensure that the pressure limiting valve can be depressed.	4 There is a metal spring in some of these valves which can rust and become ineffective (e.g. if the bag has been autoclaved).
5 The oxygen flow should be attached and turned on to check that the reservoir bag inflates.	5 To detect any leaks or defects in the system, which will reduce the oxygen concentration that can be delivered.
6 Attach the appropriate face mask to the bag device.	6 To ensure the device is ready for use.
7 Set the oxygen flow metre to an appropriate level (approximately 10 l/minute for 500 ml paediatric bag and 15 l/minute for large adult bag).	7 To maintain a high concentration of oxygen in the reservoir bag. If the flow metre is set too high the oxygen tubing can blow off.

Self-inflating bag-mask ventilation technique

Statement	Rationale
1 The child's airway should be opened by a jaw thrust manoeuvre (see Procedure Guideline 30.1).	1 To maintain airway patency. This places rescuer in optimal position for using airway adjuncts and ventilatory devices.
2 Place the correctly sized facemask on the child's face.	2 In preparation for ventilation.
3 Apply gentle downwards pressure to the mask, while gently lifting the child's mandible upwards into the mask by the continued application of jaw thrust.	3 To ensure a good seal and provide an adequate interface between child and ventilation device. To maintain airway patency.
4 In infants this is achieved by using the thumb and forefinger of one hand positioned in a C-shape to depress on the top of the mask. The remaining fingers of that hand perform the jaw thrust. The other hand is then used to gently squeeze the bag.	4 Ensures a good seal and prevents pressure on soft tissues under the chin.
5 In small children, the same technique is often possible. However, if there are two rescuers available, or it is an older child, one rescuer maintains the mask seal and jaw thrust with two hands, while the other squeezes the bag.	5 This technique is preferred for any child over 1 year of age as it can be difficult to maintain airway patency and perform ventilation single-handed.
6 The self-inflating bag should be gently squeezed until chest rise is observed.	6 To ensure oxygenation.
7 If no chest rise is seen, the airway position and facemask seal must be rechecked and corrected as necessary.	
8 If there is still no chest movement despite appropriate jaw thrust and a good facemask seal, the reason why must be sought. If necessary, BLS techniques should be attempted until the problem is rectified.	8 To minimise hypoxia.
9 The lack of chest movement may be related to faulty equipment, necessitating repair/replacement of the device.	9 An undetected defect or a disconnection of device.
10 The child's underlying clinical condition may also be the cause and this must be considered, e.g.: a) Airway obstruction due to a foreign body (FB) or intense swelling (e.g. in epiglottitis). b) 'Stiff' lungs due to underlying respiratory pathology (e.g. prematurity or asthma) – these children may require additional inflation pressure to be administered by over-riding of the pressure-limiting valve. c) NB: This should be performed with caution and for short periods only. d) In both of the scenarios above, depressing the pressure-limiting valve during delivery of the breath may also be effective.	10 A foreign body may completely obstruct the airway, which will require other airway and ventilation techniques to be employed. This may also be the same in epiglottitis c) To minimise the potential for trauma (e.g. pneumothorax). d) Higher airway pressures are generated, which may result in chest rise.
11 The rate of ventilation is generally 15–30 breaths/minute but is dependent on the age of the child.	11 Physiologically, younger children have higher respiratory rates.

Circulation management

When an infant/child is unable to maintain an adequate circulation, or is in cardiorespiratory arrest, it is essential that interventions are initiated rapidly. Performing good-quality chest compressions is vital, if ROSC is to be restored. Attention must be paid to all the essential components of compressions that are required for best quality; good depth, good rate, and a plan for pause times. Additionally, the use of CPR feedback devices, if available, to support quality compression delivery from all CPR providers. If no feedback device is available, it is recommended that an experienced member of the resuscitation team is designated as CPR coach, to ensure all aspects of quality compressions are achieved, during resuscitation attempts. Compression speed is the same for all age groups. CPR rate is *not* adjusted to the age of the patient as a speed of 100–120 compressions per minute (cpm) has been scientifically proven to achieve best end organ perfusion and chance of ROSC. During compressions CPR providers must be mindful not to lean on the patient's chest as full recoil or release of compression pressure is required between each compression to allow blood to refill the ventricles for the next compression (Niles et al. 2009). The depth of compressions in paediatric patients is still considered as one third of the anterior posterior diameter of the chest wall, which is approximately 4 cm in infants under the age of one year, 5 cm for children and 6 cm for young adults. Ideally, chest compressions should be delivered on a hard surface, otherwise the depth of compressions may be hard to achieve (Tisch and Abella 2020).

Once quality CPR is in progress the Team coordinator/clinical expert identifies which type of cardiopulmonary event the team are dealing with; shockable or non-shockable. This experienced member of the emergency team is able to guide all clinical emergency responders through the appropriate management for all paediatric resuscitation events and has the skills and ability identify and treat all potential reversal causes (4 H's 4T's). It is important that when compressions are being delivered CPR quality is not interrupted unless the patients shows signs of life, such as spontaneous moving, breathing, coughing, or gagging (Vaillancourt et al. 2020). Pauses in CPR are called the "NO Flow Time"; this means there is no blood flow and no perfusion to vital organs. Pauses can be planned for by the Team coordinator at the end of each 2 minute CPR cycle to deliver defibrillation therapy for cardiac arrhythmias, or pulse checks. In a clinical emergency situation, it is imperative to gain access to the circulation rapidly to enable swift delivery of medications and fluids. It is often extremely difficult to obtain IV access particularly if the child is already in a profoundly decompensated state (Bachmann 2005) and their circulation is poor, as the body diverts blood away from the peripheral circulation to the central core to protect vital organs. The ideal access route in a collapsed CYP is via a central vein to facilitate rapid onset of fluid support and administration of medications. However, this is a skilled procedure and should be attempted only by highly trained healthcare workers. A quicker option is intraosseous (IO) access (see the next section). However, this also requires the health worker to be skilled and trained in the insertion of the IO needle, as additional complications will arise if the needle is not sited properly (Dornhofer and Kellar 2022).

Intraosseous (IO) access

IO administration of medication is generally via the medullary cavity at the distal end of a long bone (i.e. tibia, distal femur, and humeral head). Access can be rapidly obtained, as the cancellous bone structure provides a rapid absorption of fluids and medication, which is as fast as the central venous route to the clinically compromised child. The tibial bone is the bone of choice in an obtund or arrested child who does not have existing IV access. In the long bones such as the tibia, femur, and humerus, the medullary cavity consists of a network of venous sinusoids. These sinusoids drain into large medullary venous channels, which in turn, drain into nutrient or emissary vessels. The emissary vessels exit the bone via the nutrient foramina and empty directly into the systemic venous circulation. This not only provides rapid systemic action of medications and fluids, but it is also more rapidly and easily achieved than other forms of central venous access. The need for rapid vascular access in collapsed children is essential to survival, the IO route is the route of choice in a clinical emergency situation where the child has no other venous or central venous access (Van de Voorde et al. 2021).

The IO route is often limited to young children because of the physiologic replacement of red bone marrow by the less vascular yellow marrow at around five to six years of age. However, it has been demonstrated that although less vascular, yellow marrow still facilitates absorption, and therefore the procedure can also be successfully used in older children and adults.

Benefits of the IO route

Unlike peripheral vessels, the medullary cavity does not collapse in the presence of hypovolaemia or circulatory failure. It acts like a rigid vein, making it an ideal site in a situation where vascular access is urgently required (e.g. clinical shock or cardiac arrest). The onset of action of medications administered via the IO route is as rapid as conventional central venous delivery and considerably quicker than those given via a peripheral vessel. Medications can be delivered as a bolus injection or continuous infusion. The IO route can be used to obtain bone marrow samples for emergency testing (e.g. cross-match in trauma).

Considerations for using the IO route

There are very few contraindications for the use of the IO route, but these include conditions that affect the integrity of the skin or bone (see Box 30.1). In general, any medication or fluid that can be delivered via a central venous route can be delivered via the IO route. Aseptic non-touch techniques should be adhered to due to the increased potential for infection in comparison with other routes used for administration of medications. Knowledge of potential complications and their early detection and management is essential to minimise risks (see Box 30.2).

Selection of insertion site

The preferred site is generally considered to be the anteriomedial aspect of the tibia, with the anteriolateral aspect of the femur being the next most commonly selected site. Both of these permit ease of access to the child's airway and thorax for other life-saving procedures. The anatomical landmarks for insertion of the IO cannula to these bones are:

- Tibia: 2–3 cm below the tibial tuberosity.
- Femur: 3 cm above the lateral condyle.
- Humeral head (preferred placement in older children and adults).

These sites specifically avoid the epiphyseal (growing) plates of the bone and the joint spaces, though many others may be chosen in particular circumstances. In general, infected skin or wounds should not be used as entry points to minimise infection risks.

Selection of Cannula or Needle

Commercially prepared, single use designated manual IO cannulae are available in a variety of sizes relative to age:

- 0–6 months = 18G
- 6–18 months = 16G
- >18 months = 14G

If a designated IO needle is not available, bone marrow or spinal needles can be used as an alternative in an emergency situation. There are also powered devices (e.g. EZ-IO drill), which are loaded with the cannula to allow very rapid insertion (Frascone et al. 2009). The cannulae for these devices come in several weight-based lengths:

- 3–39 kg = 15 mm
- >39 kg = 25 mm
- >39 kg, with excessive amounts of tissue over the chosen insertion site

Box 30.1 Contraindications to Using the IO Route

- Osteogenesis imperfecta
- Osteoporosis
- Osteopetrosis
- Fractures (select another site)
- Loss of skin integrity (select another site)

Box 30.2 Potential Complications

- Infection
- Extravasation
- Subperiosteal infusion
- Embolism
- Compartment syndrome
- Fracture
- Skin necrosis

Procedure guideline 30.5 Preparation for insertion of an IO cannula

Statement	Rationale
Equipment preparation:	
1 In preparation for insertion of an IO needle, the following equipment should be gathered:	1 To enable the procedure to be performed in a safe and timely manner.
a) Sterile gloves and apron.	a) To minimise infection potential.
b) Alcohol-based skin preparation fluid/wipes.	b) To cleanse skin in a rapid and effective manner.
c) Syringes.	
d) Needles.	
e) Sterile three-way tap with extension tubing.	e) To facilitate prompt administration of medication/fluids as per local and manufacturer's policies.
f) Draw up 10 ml of sodium chloride 0.9% for injection in an appropriately sized syringe and prime the three-way tap with extension tubing.	f) To facilitate checking of cannula patency and rapid delivery of medications.
Turn the three-way tap to the 'off' position.	To prevent introduction of air into the medullary cavity.
g) Sterile IO needle (appropriate gauge) – either manual insertion type or for powered device as appropriate.	g) To minimise infection potential.
h) Powered device (e.g. EZ-IO drill) if using.	h) To insert cannula appropriately.
i) Specimen bottles (as required).	i) To collect required specimens in a timely manner.
j) Local anaesthetic agent (if required) – this should be drawn up as prescribed, ready for use.	j) To minimise pain if the child is not deeply unconscious.
k) IV fluid administration set (if required).	k) To facilitate prompt administration of fluids.
l) Adhesive tape or dressing (if appropriate – see below).	l) To secure cannula and prevent accidental dislodgement.
m) If specific medication(s) and/or fluids are to be given, the following should also be prepared: Child's prescription chart Medication formulary Manufacturer's drug information Relevant medications and/or fluids	m) To facilitate prompt administration of medication/fluids.
Inform child and family:	
1 In a clinical emergency scenario, time for explanations may not be appropriate, but where possible, these should be given, in a manner appropriate to the child's age and condition.	1 To minimise fear, to gain cooperation and to provide reassurance and psychological support.
2 Family members must also receive appropriate explanations. • Information to the family should include: • Reason for IO cannulation • What it entails • Potential risks of IO cannulation • Duration of the procedure • Expected outcome of IO cannulation	2 To allay their anxieties and reassure them of the benefits of the procedure. To obtain informed consent. To minimise anxiety.
Preparation of child:	
1 a) Identify the site of insertion.	1 a) To ensure appropriate placement.
b) Using an appropriately briefed assistant, position the child in a safe position that provides ready access to the chosen insertion site.	b) To facilitate safe and prompt placement of the cannula and minimise trauma to the child.
2 If the insertion site is to be in a limb, it should be supported by placing a towel or nappy behind it.	2 To secure the limb and facilitate safe placement of cannula.

Chapter 30 Resuscitation

Procedure guideline 30.6 Procedure for a manually inserted cannula

Statement	Rationale
1 Check expiry date and open IO needle packaging.	1 To minimise risk of infection.
2 Remove device and check to ensure:	
a) Integrity – no cracks or bends in hub or cannula.	2 a) To ensure no damage to device that may hinder safe placement.
b) Internal trocar can be unscrewed and easily withdrawn from cannula.	b, c) To facilitate safe and easy placement of device.
c) When trocar is screwed into cannula it protrudes past the end of it, in readiness for insertion.	
3 Clean the skin around the selected insertion site with the alcohol-based solution/wipe and allow to dry.	3 To minimise risk of infection.
4 Infiltrate the skin through to the periosteum with local anaesthetic agent (if appropriate).	4 To minimise pain along the intended insertion track of the IO cannula.
5 Immobilise the relevant limb with the nondominant hand.	5 To secure the limb and facilitate safe placement of cannula.
a) Ensure the hand is not placed under the limb being cannulated.	a) To prevent injury to practitioner.
6 Holding the cannula in the dominant hand, it is positioned at an angle of 90° to the skin at the prepared site.	6 To avoid damaging epiphyseal plates.
7 Insertion is achieved by applying firm downwards pressure in a rotating action while maintaining the 90° angle until a loss of resistance ('give') is felt.	7 A 'give' indicates that the periosteum has been penetrated and the bone cortex accessed. The cannula should have penetrated the limb approximately 1–2 cm.
a) Care should be taken to avoid a 'rocking' motion during insertion.	a) To avoid 'splintering' of the bone.
8 Ensure cannula stands stable in an upright position without support.	8 To confirm correct placement.
9 Remove internal trocar; apply dressing.	9 To secure the IO for safe administration of fluids/drugs.

Procedure guideline 30.7 Procedure for an EZ-IO inserted cannula

Statement	Rationale
1 Check integrity of packaging and expiry date before opening appropriate size of IO cannula.	1 To minimise risk of infection.
2 Clean the skin around the selected insertion site with the alcohol-based solution/wipe and allow to dry.	2 To minimise risk of infection.
3 Infiltrate the skin through to the periosteum with local anaesthetic agent (if appropriate).	3 To minimise pain along the intended insertion track of the IO cannula.
4 Load the IO cannula on to the end of the drill (they fix together magnetically).	4 To prepare the device for use.
5 Hold the loaded drill in the dominant hand and place it on the skin at the selected insertion site at an angle of 90°.	5 To avoid damaging epiphyseal plates.
6 Immobilise the relevant limb with the nondominant hand.	6 To secure the limb and facilitate safe placement of cannula.
a) Ensure the hand is not placed under the limb being used.	a) To prevent injury to practitioner.
7 Without drilling, push the drill until the cannula penetrates through the child's skin and bone is felt.	7 To assist with correct placement of cannula and avoid injury.
8 Apply continuous pressure to the drill button until a loss of resistance ('give') is felt.	8 A 'give' indicates the periosteum has been penetrated and bone cortex accessed.
9 Ensure that the cannula stands stable in an upright position without support.	9 To confirm correct placement.
10 Detach the drill from the IO cannula and remove the trocar, the needle should stand proud.	10 To prepare the cannula for use.

Procedure guideline 30.8 Using the IO cannula

Statement	Rationale
1 a) If clinically appropriate, attach a 5 ml syringe and attempt aspiration of bone marrow. b) It is not always possible to obtain marrow easily.	1 a) To confirm correct placement. To obtain marrow for baseline testing. To rapidly identify a misplaced cannula. b) This is due to the narrow lumen of the cannula and the viscosity of marrow.
2 a) If no marrow is obtained, but the practitioner's clinical judgement is that the cannula is correctly placed (i.e. they felt loss of resistance on entering cortex and the cannula is standing in a stable unsupported position) they should assume it is sited correctly and use the cannula accordingly. b) Observations to detect possible extravasation or subperiosteal placement as described below should be made. c) NB: In cardiac arrest, the attempt at aspiration of bone marrow should be omitted.	2 The administration of first-line resuscitation medications must not be delayed. c) To ensure adrenaline administration is not delayed.
3 Attach the previously primed three-way tap and flush the cannula with 2–3 ml sodium chloride 0.9% for injection.	3 To confirm correct placement. To ensure patency of cannula.
4 Administer appropriate medications/fluids as prescribed.	4 To comply with treatment plan.
5 Observe site and relevant limb for any signs of extravasation, leakage, or development of compartment syndrome. If any of these complications are suspected, infusion or injection should be discontinued and advice sought immediately.	5 To minimise trauma and initiate appropriate treatments.
6 Ensure appropriate volume of sodium chloride 0.9% for injection is used to flush after and/or between each medication.	6 To ensure full dosage of medication is delivered. To ensure no drug interactions.
7 Ensure three-way tap is turned to 'off' position or fluid infusion is continued as prescribed following administration of medication.	7 To maintain patient safety. To minimise infection risks. To comply with prescribed treatment plan.
8 As the IO needle is generally only in situ for a short period (until more permanent vascular access can be secured), it is usually not necessary to secure it.	8 It is unlikely to become dislodged in the unconscious patient. To minimise potential for infection.
9 If the child's conscious level improves, or they need to be transported to another area, it may be necessary to secure the needle and/or extension tubing. **For the manually inserted cannula:** Place a gallipot over the top of the cannula. OR Place syringe barrels either side of the cannula under the hilt. Tape the gallipot or syringe barrels to the child's skin. **For the EZ-IO inserted cannula**: Use the designated fixation device as per manufacturer's instructions.	9 To minimise risk of accidental displacement. The site must be readily visible at all times.
10 Dispose of all equipment according to local policy.	10 To minimise potential for injury and infection.
11 Record medication(s) administered as per local policy and record procedure in child's clinical records.	11 To meet local and legal requirements.
12 Observe the site frequently (at least hourly) for any side effects such as extravasation, leakage, infection, or compartment syndrome.	12 Record and report to senior staff any potential problems so appropriate actions can be initiated.
13 Document in the child's clinical record.	13 To provide an accurate record of the procedure.

Basic life support

Basic life support (BLS) is a series of manoeuvres that can be performed to 'buy time' for the collapsed child (Figure 30.1). It is the basis of all advanced life support (ALS) techniques; without effective BLS, no amount of technological advances will improve patient outcome. Using no more than their hands and expired breath, the rescuer(s) can provide a level of oxygenation and perfusion that affords some protection from hypoxia until ALS measures are available.

It is recommended that when performing expired air ventilation, a protective barrier device (e.g. plastic face shield/pocket mask) should be used to minimise the potential risks of cross-infection. However, rescue breathing should not be delayed while the rescuer searches for a barrier device. Expired air ventilation alone will provide no more than 16–17% oxygen, so it is important to maximise oxygenation as equipment becomes available. Trained healthcare providers can utilise a BMV system attached to an oxygen supply (Figure 30.4) to support ventilation and deliver a high concentration of oxygen.

The sequence of events in paediatric BLS

To maximise the potential for a positive outcome, the steps to performing BLS follow a simple easily remembered algorithm (see Figure 30.1). All responders must remember that 'quality matters' if this potential is to be achieved. Unfortunately resuscitation quality is highly variable and often poorly preformed, even by trained healthcare providers. Recognition of a patient in cardiorespiratory arrest can be challenging for all rescuers. In 2021 the RC (UK) recommended that lay personnel should not be taught to feel for pulses as an assessment to commence CPR. Feeling for a palpable pulse is not a reliable way to determine if there is an effective or inadequate circulation and is not the sole determinant of the need for chest compressions. Responders, irrespective of experience, should be taught to look for 'signs of life' such as response to stimuli, normal breathing (rather than abnormal gasps), and spontaneous movement. Responders must not withhold BLS unless they are completely certain that the patient is showing signs of life. For the majority of children who suffer cardiorespiratory arrest this is usually a secondary event and not of cardiac origin. The most common cardiac arrhythmia encountered in arrests in children is severe bradycardia deteriorating to asystole; effective BLS is therefore more important than defibrillation.

If a child with a known cardiac condition, e.g. cardiomyopathy or congenital cardiac defect, suffers a sudden, witnessed collapse, it is likely that they may have suffered a primary cardiac event. In these patients, high-quality BLS and rapid defibrillation is essential. Defibrillation is more likely to stabilise the irritated myocardial muscle; in addition, good-quality chest compressions, as already discussed earlier in the chapter, will maintain the perfusion pressure required to drive the circulating blood to vital organs and achieve a ROSC. The lone rescuer should summon emergency assistance before commencing BLS in all patients known to have a cardiac condition as early access to a defibrillator will be necessary to terminate any potential shockable arrhythmia.

Paediatric BLS sequence

The sequence of actions in BLS is identical whether in or out of the hospital environment (see Figure 30.6). It can be easily remembered as:

- **S**afety
- **S**timulate
- **S**hout for Help
- **A**irway
- **B**reathing
- **C**irculation

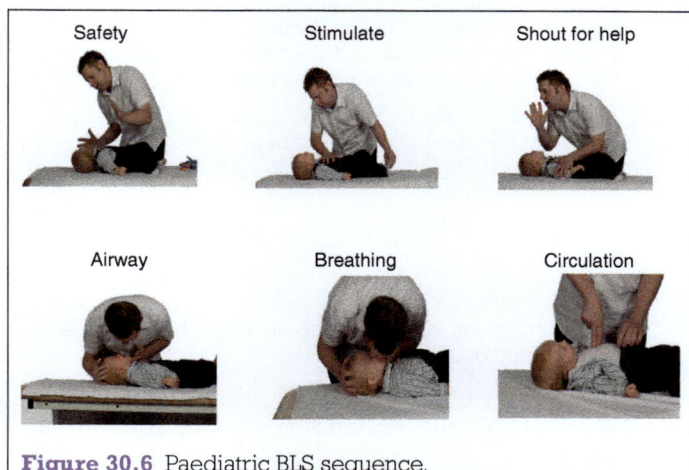

Figure 30.6 Paediatric BLS sequence.

Procedure guideline 30.9 Basic life support (BLS) provision

Statement	Rationale
Safety:	
1 The first priority is to ensure that rescuer(s) are not placed in danger. The second is to ensure that the child is in a 'safe' position.	1 Rescuer(s) are unable to assist child if they injure themselves. To prevent further injury.
2 Quickly check for potential environmental dangers in immediate vicinity. If necessary, move the child to a position of safety before initiating resuscitation. (This applies even if there is suspicion of trauma and movement should ideally be avoided.)	2 To avoid endangering the child and rescuers.
3 a) As all bodily fluids are potentially infectious, 'standard precautions' should be followed whenever practical. This includes gloves and barrier devices (e.g. face shields) if readily available. b) However, initiation of BLS to infants and children should not be delayed for the arrival of equipment.	3 a) To minimise risks of cross infection. b) Any delay in oxygenation will increase the likelihood of morbidity and mortality.
4 On approaching the child and before touching them, look for any clues as to what may have caused the emergency.	4 To modify initial management of the child (e.g. suspicion of head/neck trauma would necessitate consideration of immobilisation of the cervical spine).
Stimulate:	
1 a) Establish the responsiveness of the child through verbal and tactile stimulation. b) An appropriate way to do this is to stabilise child's head by placing one hand on their forehead and then use other hand to gently shake them.	1 a) To determine whether the child is actually in a critical condition requiring emergency help. b) To immobilise the cervical spine. To elicit a response through tactile stimulation.

(continued)

Procedure guideline 30.9 Basic life support (BLS) provision (continued)

Statement	Rationale
c) At the same time, loudly call the child's name or tell them to 'wake up.'	c) To elicit a response through verbal stimulation.
2 a) If the child responds (e.g. moving, crying or talking) their clinical status should be evaluated.	2 a) To determine whether their condition requires emergency medical service (EMS) activation.
b) To minimise delay in oxygenation and accessing EMS.	b) If there is no response to stimulation, proceed with the next step of BLS.

Shout:

Statement	Rationale
1 a) Shout out loudly for help/assistance. b) If there are 2 rescuers in attendance one should commence BLS whilst the other places a "2222" call if in hospital or "999" if in the community. c) If using a mobile phone put the call on speaker mode so the ambulance responder can support you.	1 To facilitate rapid access to EMS.
2 a) If there is only one rescuer they should carry out one minute of CPR before going for help. b) The exception to this is if the child is known to have a cardiac condition.	2 a) To avoid delay in ensuring child's airway patency and oxygenation. b) Early access to a defibrillator is crucial for these patients.
3 When calling for help you will need to provide the following information:	3
a) Precise location of the emergency.	a) To facilitate rapid arrival of EMS.
b) Telephone number from which the call is being made (community only).	
c) Number and age of victim(s) involved (community only).	c) To ensure appropriate personnel summoned.
d) Severity and urgency of situation – i.e. what has happened.	
4 a) The individual being sent to activate the EMS must be made aware that they should only hang up after the controller ends the call. b) They should also be instructed to return to the scene after they have alerted the EMS.	4 a) To ensure all necessary information has been relayed. b) To confirm that EMS has been summoned and to provide further assistance.

Airway

Statement	Rationale
1 To facilitate ventilation and oxygenation, airway patency must be achieved/maintained.	1 In the unconscious child, the combination of head flexion/hyper-extension and passive posterior displacement of the tongue is likely to at least partly occlude the airway.
2 If possible, place the child on their back in a supine/flat position on a firm, flat surface.	2 To facilitate BLS delivery.
3 Open the airway using either head tilt/chin lift or jaw thrust manoeuvres as described previously (Procedure Guideline 30.1).	3 To clear the tongue away from the posterior pharyngeal wall.
4 While opening the airway, look into the mouth. In infants, the nostrils should also be checked for patency.	4 To ensure no obvious foreign bodies. Blocked nostrils can cause apnoea in small infants who are preferential nasal breathers.
5 a) If there is a visible foreign body in the mouth that you are confident you can reach, consider attempting a single, gentle finger sweep. b) Blind finger sweeps must **not** be performed.	5 a) To clear the airway. b) To avoid further impacting a foreign body or risking soft tissue damage.
6 Once the airway has been opened, the rescuer must proceed with the next step of BLS.	6 To minimise delay in oxygenation.

Breathing

Statement	Rationale
1 While maintaining the airway open (as above), assess whether or not the child is making adequate spontaneous respiratory effort. To decide this, position your cheek a few centimetres above the child's face and look along the child's body towards their feet.	1 To determine the need for rescue breathing by **looking** (for chest/abdominal rise and fall), **listening** (for breath sounds), and **feeling** (for air movement).
2 No more than 10 seconds should be taken to determine if the CYP is breathing normally.	2 To minimise delay in oxygenation.

Procedure guideline 30.9 Basic life support (BLS) provision *(continued)*

Statement	Rationale
3 If there is adequate respiratory effort, the rescuer should continue to monitor the child and summon more assistance as appropriate.	3 To ensure no further deterioration in condition.
4 If there is no suspicion of head or spinal trauma, it would be appropriate to place the child in a safe, recovery position (Procedure Guideline 30.3).	4 To maintain airway patency and minimise potential risk of aspiration.
5 If the child is not making adequate respiratory effort and/or not breathing normally five rescue breaths should be delivered.	5 To deliver oxygen to the child's lungs.
6 While maintaining the airway position as described above, five initial rescue breaths should be delivered.	6 It is recognised that the first attempts at rescue breaths are often ineffective.
7 Each breath must be delivered (over approximately 1 to 1.5 seconds).	7 To minimise the potential for gastric distension.
8 Remove your mouth from the child's face between each breath.	8 To facilitate child's exhalation and avoid rebreathing of air.
9 You should take a breath between delivery of each rescue breath.	9 To maximise the amount of oxygen and minimise the amount of carbon dioxide in the expired air that they deliver to the child.
10 Delivery of rescue breaths can be performed either by mouth-to-mouth-and-nose (infants), or mouth-to-mouth (children and adults):	10 Choice is dependent on the size and/or anatomy of the child/adult's face.
11 a) **Mouth-to-mouth-and-nose:** Place your mouth over the infant's mouth and nose and create a seal. b) **Mouth-to-mouth:** Place your mouth directly over the child's, creating a seal. c) With the hand nearest the top of the child's head, the rescuer must occlude the child's nostrils.	11 a) Generally recommended for use in infants. This is more physiologically 'normal' as infants are preferential nasal breathers. b) Usually used in children or infants when a seal cannot be achieved in mouth-to-mouth-and-nose. c) To ensure that no air escapes from the nostrils during delivery of rescue breaths.
12 a) The effectiveness of rescue breaths must be determined by observing for chest rise and fall with each one. b) If chest movement is not observed, the child's head should be repositioned and the breaths repeated.	12 a) To ensure that air is being delivered to the child's lungs. b) The most common problem is inappropriate head positioning. An inadequate seal may be causing air to escape.
13 If, despite repositioning of the head, rescue breaths continue to fail to achieve chest rise, the likely cause must be sought and remedied.	13 The likelihood of a foreign body obstructing the airway should be considered and the rescuer should move straight to chest compression delivery.
14 Once initial rescue breaths have been delivered, the rescuer must proceed with the next step in BLS sequence.	14 To minimise delay in oxygenation and ensure circulation of oxygenised blood.

Circulation

Statement	Rationale
1 Continue to look for signs of life whilst delivering the 5 rescue breaths, e.g. spontaneous breathing, movement, gagging, or coughing.	1 To determine whether external chest compressions (ECC) are required to provide a circulation.
2 If there are signs of an effective circulation (i.e. pulse more than 60 beats per minute and/or spontaneous movement), the rescuer should reassess breathing.	2 ECC are not indicated. To determine the need for continuing appropriate rescue breathing (12–20 rescue breaths per minute and frequent reassessment of circulation).
3 If there are no signs of life, or if the rescuer is at all unsure, then ECC must be commenced.	3 All pulseless children and those with heart rates too low to adequately perfuse vital organs require ECC.
4 ECC are best delivered with the child in a supine position on a firm, flat surface.	4 To facilitate safe and effective delivery.
5 ECC are a series of rhythmic depressions of the anterior chest wall.	5 ECC deliver blood to the vital organs to keep them viable until the ROSC.
6 They should be delivered over the lower half of the sternum, in a smooth, rhythmic fashion. Rate of delivery is approximately 100 and no more than 120 times per minute.	6 To minimise trauma and optimise circulation.
7 The depth of compression should be approximately one-third of the anterior–posterior diameter of the thorax.	7 ECC have previously been noted to be too shallow. Compression depth should be: 4cm in Infants under 1 year 5cm in children over 1 year (Van de Voorde et al. 2021).

(continued)

Procedure guideline 30.9 Basic life support (BLS) provision (continued)

Statement	Rationale
8 Equal time should be spent in the depression and relaxation phases.	8 To optimise cardiac filling and emptying.
9 ECC are interspersed with rescue breaths.	9 To ensure blood being circulated is oxygenated.

Landmarking for ECC

Statement	Rationale
1 a) The area for delivery of ECC for both infants and children is the lower half of the sternum. This can be safely identified by locating the xiphisternum (the end of the breast bone where both rib margins meet), compressing approximately one finger's breadth above the xiphisternum.	1 a) To minimise risk of trauma.
b) However, it is essential to check that the rescuer's fingers are not over the xiphisternum.	b) To locate safe position for delivery (Clements and McGowan 2000).

ECC delivery

Statement	Rationale
1 The method of delivery of ECC is dependent on the: • Size of the child. • Number/expertise of rescuers.	
2 **Infant ECC** can be delivered by either the two-fingers of two-thumbs technique:	2
a) **Two-fingers technique**: Recommended for laypersons or the single rescuer. Two fingers from the hand nearest the infant's feet are placed in the correct position (as described above) on the centre of the lower sternum.	a) Considered the easiest method of ECC delivery for a single rescuer
b) **Two-thumbs technique**: One thumb is placed on top of the other in an infant, below the nipple line, and on the lower third of the sternum.	b) This is now the preferred approach in infants to achieve the best perfusion pressure to maintain end organ perfusion. Evidence suggests this method provides greater cardiac output.
3 **In children,** ECC is delivered by placing the heel of one hand along the long axis of the centre of their lower sternum.	3 To minimise risk of trauma.
4 The rescuer's shoulders should be directly over the child's chest, with their arm locked straight at the elbow.	4 The rescuer's body weight will help to reduce the physical effort required to achieve adequate compression depth.
5 a) If the rescuer finds it difficult to achieve a depth of at least one third of the anterior–posterior diameter of the thorax, they should use both hands; the second hand placed on top of the first with the fingers interlocked. When performing ECC only the heal of the lower hand is placed on the lower half of the sternum.	5 a) To allow the heart to refill with blood between compressions and optimise cardiac output.
b) During the relaxation phase of each individual compression, the rescuer must release/recoil the pressure completely. The heal of the compression hand can remain lightly in position until the next compression is delivered.	b) To minimise delay in recommencing ECC after ventilations.
6 If a single rescuer is providing both rescue breaths and ECC they must remove their fingers/hands to perform the chin lift at the end of each series of compressions.	6 To ensure airway patency and facilitate effective delivery of rescue breaths.
a) The recommended ratio in infants and children is a 15:2 ratio of compressions to breaths.	a) The hypoxic aetiology of children's cardiorespiratory arrests necessitates effective ventilation. Oxygenated blood is critical to minimise hypoxic tissue damage.
b) In newborn babies a ratio of 3:1 of compressions to breaths is recommended.	b) The physiological respiratory rates of a newborn is faster than in older children and adults; thus greater emphasis is placed on ventilation.

Reassessment

Statement	Rationale
1 In the community a lone rescuer should perform a full minute of BLS and then reassess, looking for signs of life. If there are no signs of life, ensure help is on the way and continue CPR until the EMS arrives.	1 To ensure access to ALS interventions is forthcoming as BLS alone is unlikely to achieve ROSC in cardiorespiratory arrest.

Procedure guideline 30.9 Basic life support (BLS) provision *(continued)*

Statement	Rationale
2 If a mobile telephone is available this should be placed on speaker when calling for help so that the EMS can offer guidance and support. Alternatively, if a mobile telephone is not available, and the victim is an infant or small child, the rescuer may be able to carry them safely to activate further assistance and then recommence BLS. If the means of summoning assistance is some distance away, the rescuer should stop on route every minute or so, place the child on the ground, and deliver a further minute of BLS before moving on again.	2 To contact the EMS for support while continuing to provide BLS to the child.
3 If the child is too large to carry safely, the rescuer would need to leave them to activate EMS and then return and recommence BLS as rapidly as possible.	3 To prevent injury to the child or themselves.
4 If EMS have already been alerted, the rescuer must immediately resume BLS as appropriate, unless there are obvious 'signs of life.'	4 To maximise oxygenation and minimise morbidity and mortality.
Continuing BLS	
1 The rescuer should only briefly stop to reassess the situation after the first minute of BLS. Thereafter, BLS should be continued until:	1 To maintain oxygenation.
a) The child exhibits any signs of response.	a) ABC should be reassessed and BLS continued as appropriate.
b) Another person competent in BLS takes over.	b–c) BLS is a physically demanding procedure.
c) The rescuer is too exhausted to continue.	
d) Resuscitation attempt is stopped by a medically qualified person.	d) It is deemed inappropriate to continue resuscitation attempt.

Choking

When a foreign body (FB) enters their airway, a person will immediately react by coughing in an attempt to expel it. Someone who is choking on a FB but is still able to cough effectively should be actively encouraged to do so (see Box 30.3). A spontaneous cough is not only safer, but is probably more effective than any manoeuvre that a rescuer might perform.

However, if coughing is absent or ineffective, the choking person is at extreme risk of complete airway obstruction with resultant rapid asphyxiation Chang et al. (2021). Anyone who is unable to effectively cough due to a FB in their airway requires immediate assistance.

Recognition of choking

Choking is characterised by the sudden onset of respiratory distress associated with coughing, gagging, and/or stridor. The majority of choking events in infants and children occur during feeding or playing, and are therefore usually witnessed by a caregiver. In an adolescent or adult, an FB is usually related to eating and again is frequently witnessed by another person. It is important to be aware that the signs and symptoms of choking can sometimes be confused with those of other causes of airway obstruction, such as laryngitis or epiglottitis, which require very different management (Nasir and Subha 2021).

General signs of choking in children

- Sudden onset
- Often a witnessed event
- Coughing, gagging, stridor
- History of playing with, or eating small objects immediately preceding the onset of symptoms

As with BLS, it is important to intervene quickly to prevent a manageable situation deteriorating into cardiorespiratory arrest. The steps for managing a choking infant/child who is conscious but unable to effectively cough are identical to the management of one who shows no 'signs of life.' Therefore, the procedure for BLS should be adhered to with the following additional considerations:

1. **Checking the mouth:** The mouth should be checked for the FB each time the airway is opened for rescue breaths. If it is visible, a single finger sweep should be used to try and remove the FB. However, blind or repeated finger sweeps must not be performed as these are likely to impact the FB further into the airway and/or cause trauma.

Box 30.3 Signs of Effective and Ineffective Coughing

Effective coughing	Ineffective coughing
• Crying or verbal response to questions • Able to cough forcefully • Able to inhale before coughing • Alert and responsive	• Inability to vocalise • Quiet or silent cough • Difficulty (or no) breathing • Cyanosis • Decreasing level of consciousness

2. **Initial rescue breaths:** If a rescue breath does not result in chest wall rise, the head should be repositioned before attempting the next breath. If all five initial breaths are ineffective (i.e. no visible chest rise), despite repositioning of the head, and the infant/child demonstrates no 'signs of life' the rescuer should proceed to external chest compressions (ECC).
3. **Continued BLS:** The cycle of BLS should be followed with a check for the FB in the child's mouth prior to delivery of each set of two breaths. If the first breath is ineffective, the head should be repositioned prior to the second. If the second is also ineffective, the rescuer should proceed again with ECCs.

Should rescue breaths be effective (i.e. there is visible chest rise), full BLS should continue until the child displays 'signs of life'. If 'signs of life' are displayed, the rescuer should rapidly assess the child's ABC and then continue as appropriate (Vilke et al. 2004).

Procedure guideline 30.10 Management of the choking infant/child

Statement	Rationale
1 Rapidly assess the situation (effectiveness of coughing; age of child) and ensure safety of both rescuer and child.	1 To identify the need for, and type of intervention required. To prevent injury to rescuer or child.
Stimulate	
2 The consciousness level of the child should be rapidly assessed.	2 To determine potential degree of hypoxia from airway obstruction.
Shout	
3 Shout for more assistance. Anyone answering this call for assistance should await further instructions from the rescuer depending on how the event progresses.	3 While many episodes of choking can be safely and quickly remedied, they also have the potential for rapidly deteriorating into a serious clinical emergency.
Back blows in infants (Figure 30.7a)	
4 Sit on a chair or kneel on the floor.	4 To minimise potential for injury if the infant should fall.
5 a) Place the thumb of one hand at the angle of the infant's lower jaw, and one or two fingers from this hand at the same point on the other side of the infant's face.	5 a) To support the infant's head and minimise risk of brain trauma. To maximise patency of the airway (modified jaw thrust).
b) Care must be taken not to compress the soft tissue under the chin.	b) To prevent airway occlusion.
6 Hold the infant in a head downwards, prone position along the length of your thigh or across your lap.	6 To provide some support. Gravity will assist with removal of the FB.
7 With the heel of your free hand, deliver up to five sharp blows to the middle of the infant's back, between the scapulae. Do not give all five unless necessary.	7 To loosen the object so that the infant can expel it and to relieve the obstruction with as few back blows as possible.
Back blows in children (Figure 30.7c)	
1 a) Depending on the size of both the rescuer and the child, try to support the child in a head downwards position.	1 a) Safety of both is the utmost priority.
b) If this is not possible, support them in a forward-leaning position, with the rescuer standing behind.	b) Gravity will help with removal of FB.
2 With the heel of your free hand, deliver up to five sharp blows to the middle of the child's back, between their scapulae. Do not give all five unless necessary.	2 To loosen the object so that the child can expel it and to relieve the obstruction with as few back blows as possible.
Thrusts	
Although guidelines for the delivery of thrusts state that abdominal thrusts can be used in children (i.e. over one year of age), it is important that the rescuer uses their clinical judgement to decide if it is safe to perform these. If the clinical judgement is that the child is too small, then they should deliver chest thrusts as for infants (Van de Voorde et al. 2021). **Abdominal thrusts should never be performed in infants due to the very high likelihood of trauma to their internal organs.**	
1 If back blows fail, and the infant or child is still conscious, the rescuer must administer thrusts; chest in the infant and abdominal in a child.	1 An alternative movement to relieve the airway obstruction.
Chest thrusts in an infant (see Figure 30.7b)	
2 Turn the infant from the head downwards, prone position they were in for back blows, to a head downwards, supine position.	2 To facilitate effective delivery of chest thrusts.
a) This can be achieved most easily by placing the free arm down the infant's back and cupping their occiput with the hand, and rolling the baby over into the supine head downwards position.	a) To support the infant's head throughout, to minimise risk of injury and to maximise safety.

Chapter 30 Resuscitation

Procedure guideline 30.10 Management of the choking infant/child *(continued)*

Statement	Rationale
b) If this is difficult, lay the baby flat on the ground, but avoid lifting their head higher than their trunk.	b) To prevent any loosened object falling back into the lower airway.
3 Hold the infant in a head downwards, supine position down the length of their thigh, or across their lap.	3 Gravity will assist with removal of the FB.
4 a) The landmark for ECC (i.e. a finger-breadth above the xiphisternum) should be identified and two fingers positioned on the sternum.	4 a) To minimise trauma.
b) Up to five sharp downward thrusts should be delivered. These thrusts are similar to ECC but are delivered at a slower rate and are sharper in nature. Do not give all five unless necessary.	b) The aim is to loosen the object in order that the infant can expel it and to relieve the obstruction with as few chest thrusts as possible.
Abdominal thrusts in a child (Figure 30.7d and e)	
5 a) Stand behind the child, place your arms underneath the chFVild's and encircle their torso.	5 a) To maximise safety.
b) You can then support them in a forward-leaning position.	b) To have a degree of control over the child if they lose consciousness andFV lower their body more safely to the floor.
6 Clench one of your fists and place this on the child's abdomen, midway between their umbilicus and the tip of their xiphisternum.	6 To minimise risk of trauma to internal organs.
7 Grasp the fist with your free hand and pull sharply upwards and inwards, to deliver up to five abdominal thrusts. Do not give all five unless necessary.	7 To cause a change in intrathoracic pressure, thus creating an artificial 'cough'. The aim is to loosen the object in order that the child can expel it and relieve the obstruction with as few abdominal thrusts as possible.
Reassessment	
1 Following delivery of the thrusts (chest or abdominal), briefly stop and reassess the situation.	1 To determine further management required.
2 If the FB has been successfully expelled, the child should be assessed and made comfortable until examined by a medical practitioner.	2 Any person who has required back blows and chest/abdominal thrusts needs to be assessed in case of internal trauma or retained FB.
3 If the FB has not been expelled, and the infant/child is still conscious, ensure that EMS is summoned (as in BLS support above) and the sequence of back blows and chest/abdominal thrusts is repeated as indicated.	3 To minimise delays in ALS availability and to try and relieve the FB while awaiting arrival of EMS.

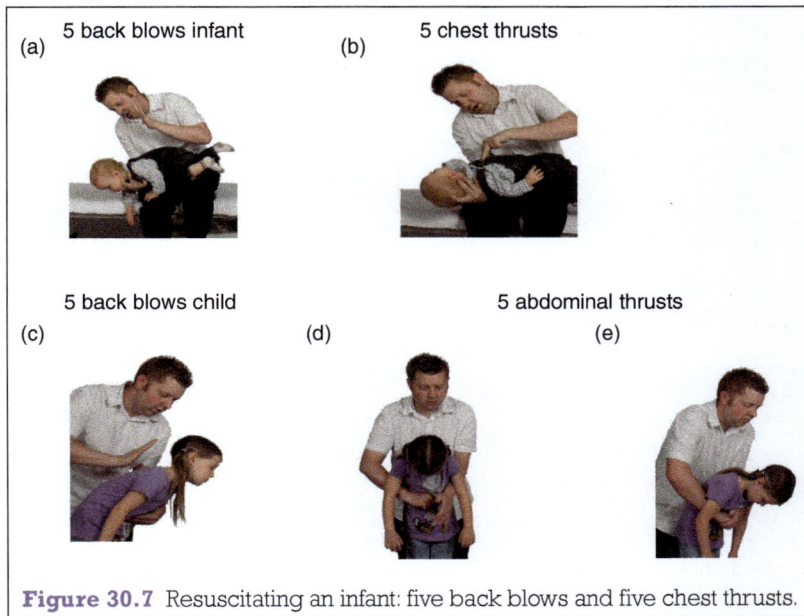

Figure 30.7 Resuscitating an infant: five back blows and five chest thrusts.

Cardiopulmonary arrest management

Cardiopulmonary arrest can be defined as the lack of palpable central pulses (Niles et al. 2018).

It is crucial that while quality and effective BLS is continued, specific ALS treatment strategies are incorporated in an attempt to re-establish circulation and achieve effective oxygenation. Cardiac arrest management will involve some or all of the following:

- ECG rhythm analysis
- Defibrillation/cardioversion
- Advanced airway management procedures with ET CO_2 (end-tidal carbon dioxide)
- Intravascular access/IO access
- Fluid and medication delivery
- Ongoing ABCDE assessment

Capnography: ET CO_2 Monitoring.

Monitoring the ET CO_2 with waveform capnography reliably confirms tracheal tube placement in a child weighing more than 2 kg with a perfusing rhythm and must be used after intubation and during transport of an intubated child (Dicembrino et al. 2021). The presence of a capnography waveform for more than four ventilated breaths indicates the tube is in the correct place in the trachea, both in the presence of a perfusing rhythm and during CPR. The absence of exhaled CO_2 during CPR does not guarantee tube misplacement because a low or absent CO_2 may reflect low or absent pulmonary blood flow. Capnography may therefore provide information of the efficiency of chest compressions, and a sudden rise in ET CO_2 can be an indication of a ROSC. The usual target for ET CO_2 in this setting is 4.4–5.0 kilo pascals (kPa) (Edelson et al. 2010).

ECG rhythm analysis

Early identification of the child's ECG rhythm is essential to influence appropriate management. There are essentially two categories of cardiac arrest arrhythmias: shockable and nonshockable (Skellett et al. 2021).

The *shockable* arrhythmias are ventricular fibrillation (VF) and pulseless ventricular tachycardia (pVT) (Figure 30.8).

The *nonshockable* rhythms are asystole and pulseless electrical activity (PEA) (Figure 30.9).

Profound bradycardia deteriorating to asystole is the most common ECG presentation of cardiac arrest in children. As with PEA, it should be treated with BLS and respiratory support following the ALS algorithm. For more information on performing an ECG see Chapter 15: Investigations.

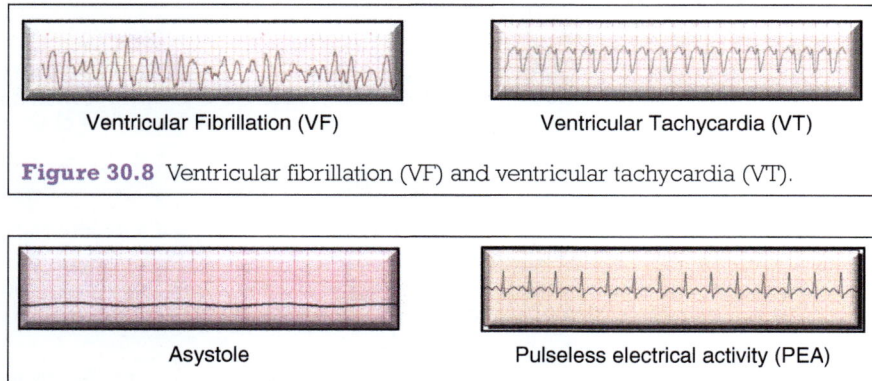

Figure 30.8 Ventricular fibrillation (VF) and ventricular tachycardia (VT).

Figure 30.9 Asystole pulseless electrical activity (PEA).

Procedure guideline 30.11 Management of nonshockable rhythms (asystole and PEA)

Statement	Rationale
1 a) Perform continuous CPR at 15 ECC:2 ventilations with high-concentration bag-mask ventilation as soon as available. b) Deliver ECC at a rate of 100–120/minute.	1 a, b) To maximise oxygenation to body tissues.
2 If the child's airway is secured with a tracheal tube, continuous ECC should be delivered.	2 Minimising interruptions to ECC results in increased coronary perfusion; the tracheal tube allows this as it protects the lower airways from potential aspiration of gastric contents.
3 Once the child is intubated, the ventilation rate should be: • Infant: 25 breaths per minute (bpm) • Child: 15 bpm • Young adult: 10–12 bpm	
4 End tidal CO_2 should be measured.	4 To monitor ventilation and ensure correct tracheal tube placement.
5 Adrenaline 10 µg/kg or 0.1 ml per kg must be given as soon as venous or IO access is achieved.	5 To increase contractility of heart muscle; any delay in administration reduces the likelihood of ROSC.
6 Continue CPR for 2 minutes, pausing briefly to check for rhythm change at the end. Pauses should be planned by the team coordinator.	6 To maximise oxygenation to body tissues. To ensure that all in the emergency team keep the pause time brief and minimise no flow time.
7 Administer adrenaline 10 µg/kg or 0.1 ml per kg every 4 minutes (i.e. every alternate cycle of CPR) while maintaining uninterrupted effective CPR.	7 Adrenaline induces vasoconstriction, increases coronary perfusion pressure, enhances the contractile state of the heart and stimulates spontaneous contractions.

Chapter 30 Resuscitation

Procedure guideline 30.11 Management of nonshockable rhythms (asystole and PEA) *(continued)*

Statement	Rationale
8 Examine the child and their records (e.g. drug chart and blood results) and consider any potentially reversible cause(s) of the arrest. These include: • Hypoxia • Hypovolaemia • Hypo/hyperkalaemia/-calcaemia/-magnesaemia and hypoglycaemia • Hypothermia • Tension pneumothorax • Toxic/therapeutic disturbances • Tamponade (cardiac) • Thromboembolism Correct all reversible causes and reassess intermittently.	8 It is particularly important to search for the underlying cause of the arrhythmia in children as it is unlikely to be due to coronary artery disease (the usual adult cause). The earlier these are identified and treated, the greater the likelihood of ROSC. Remember there may be more than one reversible cause and that new problems can occur during the resuscitation, necessitating frequent reassessment.
9 Consider other medications: Sodium bicarbonate is not a first-line medication, but may be useful in a prolonged event. b) Atropine may be useful in vagal induced bradycardia tone (e.g. after insertion of nasogastric tube). The dose is 20 µg/kg with a minimum dose of 100 µg.	9 a) In prolonged events, lactic acid accumulation may have occurred and require treating. NB: The best treatment for acidaemia in cardiac arrest is a combination of effective ECC and ventilation. b) A dose lower than 100 µg may cause a paradoxical bradycardic effect.

Procedure guideline 30.12 Management of shockable rhythms (ventricular fibrillation and pulseless ventricular tachycardia)

This is a much less common situation in paediatric practice, although the incidence is reported to be around 19% (Holmberg et al. 2019). A shockable rhythm may occur as a secondary event, and is likely when there has been a witnessed and sudden collapse. It is more commonly seen in paediatric intensive care units and cardiac wards.

Statement	Rationale
1 Continue with continuous CPR at 15 ECC to 2 ventilations with high-concentration bag-mask ventilation as soon as available, until defibrillator is ready to use.	1 To maximise oxygenation to body tissues.
2 Establish the energy level required: • 4 joules per kg if using manual defibrillator • A paediatric-attenuated dosage if using an Automated External Defibrillator (AED) for a child less than approximately 8 years of age. • If using an AED for a child over 8 years, use the standard adult dose.	2 A single 4 J/kg shock strategy improves first shock success rate and minimises interruption to ECC.
3 Charge the defibrillator while another rescuer continues chest compressions.	3 To minimise interruptions to ECC.
4 Once the defibrillator is charged, pause the chest compressions and quickly ensure that all rescuers are clear of the patient before promptly delivering the shock.	4 To adhere to best practice safe guidelines. To try and convert the rhythm to a perfusing one.
5 The shock may be delivered by the person doing compressions or by another trained rescuer. This decision should be planned before the ECC are stopped.	5 To minimise interruptions to ECC.
6 Immediately resume CPR without assessing the rhythm or checking for a pulse starting with ECC.	6 To minimise interruptions to ECC.
7 a) Examine the child, their records (e.g. drug chart and blood results) and consider any potentially reversible cause(s) of the arrest: • Hypoxia • Hypovolaemia • Hypo/hyperkalaemia (and other metabolic disturbances) • Hypothermia • Tension pneumothorax • Toxic/therapeutic disturbances • Tamponade (cardiac) • Thromboembolism b) Correct any reversible causes.	7 a) It is particularly important to search for the underlying cause of the arrhythmia in children as it is unlikely to be due to coronary artery disease (the usual adult cause). The earlier these are identified and treated, the greater the likelihood of ROSC. b) Remember there may be more than one reversible cause and that new problems can occur during the resuscitation, necessitating frequent reassessment.

(continued)

Procedure guideline 30.12 Management of shockable rhythms (ventricular fibrillation and pulseless ventricular tachycardia) *(continued)*

Statement	Rationale
8 Continue uninterrupted CPR for two minutes before briefly pausing to check the rhythm.	8 To maximise oxygenation to body tissues.
9 **If still VF/VT:** a) Give a second shock (identical to first). b) Immediately resume CPR without assessing the rhythm or checking for a pulse, starting with ECC. c) Continue uninterrupted CPR for two minutes before briefly pausing to check the rhythm.	9 a) To try and convert the rhythm to a perfusing one. b) To maximise oxygenation to body tissues. c) To maximise oxygenation to body tissues.
10 **If still VF/VT:** a) Give a third shock (identical to first and second). b) Immediately resume CPR without assessing the rhythm or checking for a pulse starting with ECC.	10 a) To try and convert the rhythm to a perfusing one. b) To maximise oxygenation to body tissues.
11 a) Administer adrenaline 10μg/kg (i.e. after the third shock and once CPR has resumed). b) Also administer amiodarone 5mg/kg. NB Amiodarone can cause thrombophlebitis when administered peripherally, and so should ideally be given via a central vein. If it has to be given peripherally in an emergency then it must be liberally flushed with sodium chloride 0.9% or 5% glucose.	11 a) Adrenaline induces vasoconstriction, increases coronary perfusion pressure, enhances the contractile state of the heart, stimulates spontaneous contractions and increases the intensity of VF, thereby increasing the likelihood of successful defibrillation. b) Amiodarone is a membrane-stabilising antiarrhythmic drug that increases the duration of the action potential and refractory period in atrial and ventricular myocardium. Atrioventricular conduction is slowed, and a similar effect is also seen in accessory pathways.
12 Administer adrenaline 10μg/kg every four minutes (i.e. every alternate cycle of CPR) while maintaining uninterrupted effective CPR.	12 Higher doses of intravascular adrenaline should not be used routinely in children as it may worsen outcome.
13 Repeat amiodarone 5mg/kg once more (after the fifth shock) if still in a shockable rhythm.	13 To try and convert the rhythm to a perfusing one.
14 Continue delivering shocks every two minutes, ensuring ECC are maintained during charging of defibrillator and minimising any interruptions to CPR as much as possible.	14 To try and convert the rhythm to a perfusing one.
15 After each two minutes of uninterrupted CPR pause briefly to assess the rhythm.	
16 **If still VF/VT:** Continue CPR with the shockable sequence.	16 To try and convert the rhythm to a perfusing one.
17 **If asystole:** Continue CPR but switch to nonshockable sequence as above.	17 To manage arrhythmia appropriately.
18 **If organised electrical activity is seen:** a) Check for 'signs of life' and central pulse. b) If there is ROSC commence post-resuscitation management. c) If there is **no** pulse or it is <60 beats per minute and there are no other 'signs of life,' continue CPR as for the nonshockable sequence described above.	18 b) To minimise/prevent hypoxic damage. c) To manage arrhythmia appropriately.
19 a) If defibrillation was successful but VF/VT recurs, resume the shockable CPR sequence with defibrillation. b) Give an amiodarone bolus (unless two doses have already been given) and start a continuous infusion.	19 a, b) To try and convert the rhythm back to a perfusing one.

N.B. Uninterrupted, good-quality CPR is vital; ECC and ventilation should only be paused for planned defibrillation. External ECC perfusion pressure requires at least 6–8 strikes of the chest to raise blood pressure and perfusion to the brain and the end vital organs, it is important that the CPR coach or team leader at any resuscitation event continuously assess the quality of the ECC, and change the provider delivering compressions approximately every 2 minutes to prevent fatigue (Abella et al. 2007; Gregson et al. 2017).

Defibrillation

Defibrillation is the delivery of an electrical current through the chest wall, to depolarise a maximum amount of myocardial tissue in order to allow the heart's natural pacemaker to resume control of cardiac conduction. The resultant depolarisation of the myocardium aims to restore the heart to an organised electrical ECG rhythm and create a life sustainable cardiac output.

Shockable arrhythmias (VF and pulseless VT) are uncommon in cardiac arrests in children. They are most commonly seen in children with underlying cardiac pathology, hypothermia, or tricyclic antidepressant poisoning. As with the adult in a shockable arrest rhythm, the paediatric patient should be defibrillated as soon as a defibrillator is available. ECC should continue uninterrupted for the duration of time that it takes for the defibrillators adhesive pad to be placed on the patient's chest and up to the point when the team leader needs to pause ECC to identify that the rhythm remains shockable.

Quick identification of the rhythm should be completed <10 seconds of pausing ECC as the patient becomes profoundly hypoxic during hands-off time. Therefore rhythm recognition should be carried out by an experienced healthcare professional. ECC should be recommenced immediately after this hand-off time and continued uninterrupted until the defibrillator is fully charged at the selected energy value and the shock is about to be delivered. This is classed as manual defibrillation.

Since 2005 it has been identified that patients who had no immediate access to a defibrillator, but received effective CPR first were more likely to have a successful outcome than those who received defibrillation first following collapse. This suggests that maintaining perfusion to the irritated myocardium helps to make it more responsive and amenable to the shock (Van de Voorde et al. 2021).

Automated external defibrillators

Automated external defibrillators (AEDs) are now widely available in both hospital and prehospital settings (see Figure 30.10). This has led to improvements in survival from VF for adults. Standard AED pads are suitable for use in children older than approximately eight years. Special paediatric pads that attenuate the current delivered during defibrillation should be used in children aged between one and eight years if they are available; if not, the AED should be used as it is. Shockable rhythms are uncommon in children of less than one year and the use of an AED is not generally recommended. However, if a shockable rhythm is present and an AED is the only defibrillator available, its use should be considered (Van de Voorde et al. 2021).

The current recommendation, therefore, is that variable energy defibrillators must still be available in areas where sick children are being cared for (Hoyme and Atkins 2021).

Defibrillation adhesive pads or paddles

Manual defibrillation can be performed using either self-adhesive pads (hands-free defibrillation), or the ridged paddles on the machine. Occasionally there may be times when the rigid paddles are required. While the ridged paddles are probably rarely used nowadays, they may still be necessary; e.g. for a very small infant in whom the paediatric pads (even in anterior–posterior placement) are too large (i.e. they touch one another) or certain skin conditions where the adhesive pads will not adhere. If paddles are to be used, then defibrillation gel pads must first be placed on the chest wall to ensure good contact, reduce transthoracic impedance, and prevent burning of the skin.

Self-adhesive pads are widely available in adult and paediatric sizes. They are safe, easy, and generally preferable to use (Figure 30.11).

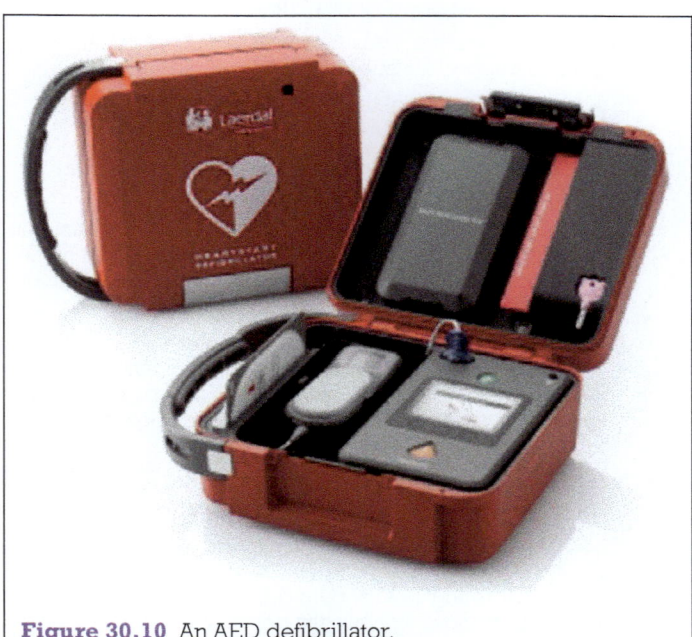

Figure 30.10 An AED defibrillator.

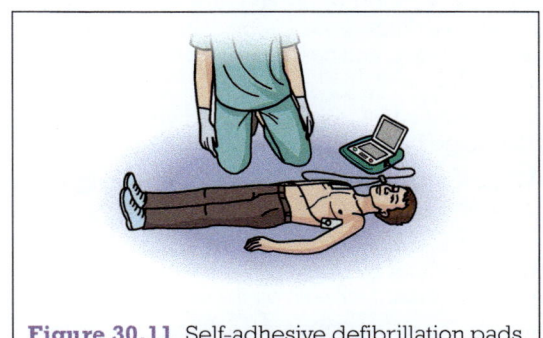

Figure 30.11 Self-adhesive defibrillation pads.

Procedure guideline 30.13 Manual defibrillation with self-adhesive pads

Statement	Rationale
1 Confirm the presence of shockable rhythm (VF/pulseless VT) via ECG and check for a central pulse during brief pause in ECC.	1 To ensure correct management.
2 Immediately resume ECC while the necessary equipment for defibrillation is prepared for use.	2 To maintain oxygenation.
3 Plan all actions before shock delivery and ensure all rescuers know what is expected of them.	3 To minimise interruption to CPR. To ensure shock delivery is safe and coordinated.

(continued)

Procedure guideline 30.13 Manual defibrillation with self-adhesive pads *(continued)*

Statement	Rationale
4 To facilitate prompt delivery, the child's weight must be determined.	4 To calculate the energy levels required.
5 Prompt, effective and safe defibrillation delivery is dependent on:	5
a) Pad size selection – choose largest available that still permits for space between them (infant pads are generally selected for babies <10 kg; manufacturer's guidelines should be followed).	a) To maximise contact with chest wall and to prevent arcing of current.
b) Placement of pads – bracket heart.	b) To allow for maximum current flow through the heart.
c) Skin-pad interface – ensure smoothed down on chest with no trapped air bubbles.	c) To decrease thoracic impedance to current flow.
d) Energy selection – determined by child's body weight.	d) To select lowest energy level likely to be effective, thus minimising potential for myocardial damage.
6 a) The self-adhesive pads should be positioned on the chest while ECC continues.	6 a) To minimise interruption to ECC and maintain coronary and cerebral artery perfusion.
b) The standard sites are one over the apex of the heart (left axilla region in small children) and one to the right of the sternum, just below the clavicle. In known dextrocardia, the pads should be applied in reverse position.	b) To bracket the heart appropriately for current delivery.
c) In a small infant where there are only large pads available, the baby is positioned on its side and essentially 'sandwiched' between one pad placed on the anterior chest and the other on their back between the scapulae.	c) To ensure the pads do not come into contact with one another and cause arcing of the delivered current.
7 The designated rescuer should select the energy for appropriate level of joules (4 J/kg) and presses the 'charge' button.	7 To charge the machine to the previously selected energy level. To inform other rescuers of stage in procedure.
8 While the defibrillator is charging, all rescuers other than the one performing ECC should be instructed to 'stand clear' and to remove any oxygen delivery devices as appropriate.	8 To facilitate prompt delivery of correct energy level. To minimise interruption to ECC and resultant fall in coronary and cerebral artery perfusion. There is a potential for combustion if the atmosphere is enriched with oxygen.
9 Once the machine is charged (change in audible tone), instruct the rescuer performing ECC to 'stand clear' while performing a quick visual check of the child and immediate surrounding area and confirming there is continued VF/pulseless VT.	9 To ensure that no one (including self) is in direct or indirect contact with the child or the surface on which they are lying. To confirm that the child is still in a shockable rhythm. To prevent delivery of an inappropriate shock if the child's rhythm has changed to a nonshockable one.
10 a) If the child is still in a shockable rhythm, press the discharge button on the machine.	10 a) To administer the shock effectively.
b) Without reassessing the rhythm or checking for a pulse, resume CPR starting with ECC.	b) To comply with current best practice treatment guidelines. Even if the defibrillation shock restores a rhythm, it is unlikely to be an effectively perfusing one initially.
11 Continue CPR for two minutes; consider reversible causes of arrest and prepare for next pause in ECC.	11 To rapidly identify and treat reversible causes. To minimise interruptions in CPR.
12 If after two minutes of CPR, VF/pulseless VT persists, proceed as before to deliver second shock.	12 To comply with current best practice treatment guidelines.
13 Following the resuscitation attempt, ensure that all defibrillation shocks are accurately documented in the child's healthcare records.	13 To record all interventions and maintain accurate records. To influence postresuscitation observations and management strategies.
14 The interventions should also be documented on clinical emergency audit forms as appropriate.	14 To help with data collection, which is vital to inform future practice guidelines.

Medications in cardiorespiratory arrest

Medications in a cardiac arrest can be delivered by intravenous, IO, or via a central vascular route. It is important that all medications are followed by a saline flush. There are few medications that are routinely used in cardiorespiratory arrest. There is no place for routine administration of alkalising agents e.g. sodium bicarbonate, unless indicated by the underlying condition or by biochemical results.

Body weight estimation

Medications and fluid management in children are weight dependent, therefore the child's weight should be determined as early as

Paediatric emergency drug chart — Resuscitation Council UK GUIDELINES 2021

| | | Adrenaline | Fluid bolus | Glucose | Sodium bicarbonate | | Tracheal tube | | Defibrillation |
							Uncuffed	Cuffed	
Strength		1:10 000	Balanced isotonic crystalloid OR, 0.9% Saline	10%	4.2%	8.4%			
Dose		10 mcg kg^{-1}	10 mL kg^{-1}	2 mL kg^{-1}	1 mmol kg^{-1}				4 joules kg^{-1}
Route		IV, IO	IV, IO	IV, IO	IV, IO, UVC	IV, IO			Transthoracic
Notes			Consider warmed fluids	For known hypoglycaemia				Monitor cuff pressure	Monophasic or biphasic
Age	Weight kg	mL	mL	mL (recheck glucose after dose and repeat as required)	mL	mL	ID mm	ID mm	Manual
< 1 month	3.5	0.35	35	7	7	–	3.0	–	20
1 month	4	0.4	40	8	8	–	3.0–3.5	3.0	20
3 months	5	0.5	50	10	10	–	3.5	3.0	20
6 months	7	0.7	70	14	–	7	3.5	3.0	30
1 year	10	1.0	100	20	–	10	4.0	3.5	40
2 years	12	1.2	120	24	–	12	4.5	4.0	50
3 years	14	1.4	140	28	–	14	4.5–5.0	4.0–4.5	60
4 years	16	1.6	160	32	–	16	5.0	4.5	60
5 years	18	1.8	180	36	–	18	5.0–5.5	4.5–5.0	70
6 years	20	2.0	200	40	–	20	5.5	5.0	80
7 years	23	2.3	230	46	–	23	5.5–6.0	5.0–5.5	100
8 years	26	2.6	260	50	–	26	–	6.0–6.5	100
10 years	30	3.0	300	50	–	30	–	7.0	120
12 years	38	3.8	380	50	–	38	–	7–7.5	120
14 years	50	5.0	500	50	–	50	–	7–8	120–150
Adolescent	50	5.0	500	50	–	50	–	7–8	120–150
Adult	70	10.0	500	50	–	50	–	7–8	120–150

Cardioversion	Synchronised Shock, 1.0 joules kg^{-1} escalating to 2.0 joules kg^{-1} if unsuccessful.
Amiodarone	5 mg kg^{-1} IV or IO bolus in arrest after 3rd and 5th shocks. Flush line with 0.9% saline or 5% glucose (max dose 300 mg).
Atropine	20 mcg kg^{-1}, maximum dose 600 mcg.
Calcium gluconate 10%	0.5 mL kg^{-1} for hypocalcaemia, hyperkalaemia (max dose 20 mL); IV over 2–5 min if unstable, over 15–20 min if stable.
Lorazepam	100 mcg kg^{-1} IV or IO for treatment of seizures. Can be repeated after 10 min. Maximum single dose 4 mg.
Adenosine	IV or IO for treatment of SVT: 150 mcg kg^{-1} (0–11 months of age); 100 mcg kg^{-1} (1–11 years of age) Increase dose in steps 50–100 mcg kg^{-1} every 1–2 min for repeat doses. 12–17 years: 3 mg, followed by 6 mg after 1–2 min if required, followed by 12 mg after 1–2 min if required. Requires large saline flush and ECG monitoring.
Anaphylaxis	Adrenaline 1:1000 IM: < 6 months 100–150 mcg (0.1–0.15 mL), 6 months–6 years 150 mcg (0.15 mL), 6–12 years 300 mcg (0.3 mL), > 12 years 500 mcg (0.5 mL); can be repeated after 5 min. After 2 IM injections treat as refractory anaphylaxis and start low dose adrenaline infusion IV.

Weights averaged on lean body mass from 50th centile weights for males and females.
Drug doses based on Resuscitation Council UK Guidelines 2021 recommendations.
Recommendations for tracheal tubes are based on full term neonates.
For newborns glucose at 2.5 mL kg^{-1} is recommended.

Figure 30.12 Paediatric emergency drug chart.

possible. If it is not already known, a recognised method of estimation, e.g. centile chart (Van de Voorde et al. 2021), or Paediatric Emergency chart (Figure 30.12) should be readily available. In many Accident and Emergency departments across the UK, systems such as the Broselow or Pawper tape systems are used to enhance the speed and accuracy of weight estimation of children requiring emergency treatments though the inclusion of body length/habitus. It is essential that whatever method is utilised, practitioners are familiar with it to minimise the potential for calculation errors in an emergency situation.

Adrenaline

Adrenaline is the first-line medication in cardiac arrest. It has an alpha-adrenergic effect that increases coronary artery perfusion and cardiac excitability. The dose is 0.1 ml/kg for IV or IO administration. It should be administered as a bolus injection and should be repeated every three to five minutes as necessary. Adrenaline is given immediately after access is obtained on the nonshockable side of the cardiac arrest algorithm, but not until after the third shock on the shockable side. The reason for withholding adrenaline in the early stages of a VF and pVT arrest lies in its ability to increase cardiac excitability and therefore has proarrhythmogenic properties, i.e. it causes arrhythmias. The endotracheal route for adrenaline administration is no longer recommended (Van de Voorde et al. 2021).

Amiodarone

Amiodarone is the antiarrhythmic medication of choice in shock-resistant VF and pulseless VT. The dosage is 5 mg/kg via rapid IV or IO bolus. It is given after the third defibrillation shock and may be repeated after the fifth shock.

If defibrillation has been successful but VF/pVT reoccurs, amiodarone can be repeated (unless two doses have already been given) and a continuous infusion started (Van de Voorde et al. 2021).

Glucose

Due to their high glucose requirements and low glycogen stores, sick infants and children can readily become hypoglycaemic. Low blood glucose levels (2.8–3.9 mmols/L) are known to be a common cause of seizures and also play a part in depressing myocardial contractility, so should be treated promptly. It is therefore important to ensure that glucose levels are monitored carefully. However, there is evidence to show a correlation between raised glucose levels and poor neurological outcome. Therefore, only proven hypoglycaemia merits the administration of glucose in resuscitation of children, with care being taken not to cause hyperglycaemia. The recommended dosage is 2 ml/kg of 10% glucose with reassessment of blood glucose every 10 minutes (Van de Voorde et al. 2021).

Intravascular fluids

Where circulatory failure has been the cause of the cardiorespiratory arrest (e.g. hypovolaemia or sepsis), the standard recommended volume of fluid is 10 ml/kg as a bolus via IV or IO routes. Isotonic fluid (balanced crystalloid solution) is preferable, but 0.9% sodium chloride is an acceptable alternative. If there is no improvement from 40–60 ml/kg, then ongoing losses must be suspected (e.g. bleeding, diarrhoea) and expert help must be sought (Van de Voorde et al. 2021).

In children with underlying structural cardiac disease the smaller volume of 5 ml/kg must be considered in the first instance in order to prevent cardiac failure, and expert help sought from a cardiac specialist.

Potentially reversible causes of cardiorespiratory arrest

It is essential to identify any potentially treatable causes of the cardiac arrest in order to treat them as rapidly as possible, and maximise the chances for ROSC. These causes are best remembered as the '4 Hs and 4 Ts' (Lott et al. 2021).

Hypoxia	**T**ension pneumothorax
Hypovolaemia	**T**amponade
Hypothermia	**T**oxicity
Hypo/hyperkalaemia	**T**hrombo-emboli

Rapid and appropriate treatment of these problems may result in ROSC and ultimate survival of the child. This is why ongoing reassessment of the ABCDE is so vital.

Post resuscitation care

Once ROSC is achieved, the child must be managed in an area capable of providing ongoing ALS measures. Immediate post resuscitation investigations should include:

- Arterial and central venous blood gases
- Chest X-ray
- 12-lead ECG
- Blood for:
- Glucose
  - Haemoglobin, haematocrit, and platelet count
  - Cross-match
  - Urea and electrolytes
  - Clotting screen

Ongoing management may necessitate transfer to a high dependency unit or intensive care. Any transfer (whether it is within the same institution or to another hospital) should be undertaken by staff skilled in intensive care.

Close monitoring of the child's vital signs postresuscitation is essential to rapidly detect any improvement or deterioration in the child's condition, and allow for modification of their treatment accordingly. This monitoring should include:

- Heart rate and rhythm
- BP
- O_2 saturation
- Core and peripheral skin temperature
- Urinary output
- Arterial blood gases
- CO_2 monitoring (capnography)

Consideration should be given to induced hypothermia and additional invasive monitoring such as central venous pressure (Hayashida et al. 2021).

Resuscitation team

Resuscitation teams may take many forms. A traditional cardiac arrest team is one that is called only when cardiac arrest is recognised. Alternatively, hospitals have developed additional teams who are called when patients show increased risk of deterioration and an immediate response is required to prevent them from cardiopulmonary arrest, e.g. medical emergency team, outreach team.

Together the team has a common goal or purpose, which is that by working together they contribute to the successful management of a critical life-saving situation. In resuscitation teams, members usually have complementary skills and through synergistically coordinate their effort, e.g. anaesthetist, medical/surgical physician, and nurse.

Characteristics of a good team member

- Competence: Has the skills required at a cardiopulmonary event and preforms them to the best of their ability.
- Commitment: Strives to achieve the best outcome for the patient.
- Communicates: Openly communicates with all other team members and listens to briefings and instructions from the team leader.
- Supportive: Allows others to achieve their best.
- Accountable: For their own and the team's actions.
- Prepared: Ready to admit when help is needed.
- Creative: Suggests different ways of interpreting the situation.
- Participates: Co-operates with team members in providing feedback.

Ethical considerations

Presence of family members during resuscitation attempts

It has become much more widespread practice to ask parents/carers (and sometimes other close family members) if they wish to be present during the resuscitation attempt. It is important that this is done in a supportive manner, allowing them to make a decision that feels most appropriate for them. While many will choose to be present, some will decline, and many will change their minds, perhaps choosing to be present for some time and leaving at another.

Whether the parents/carers are present or not, an experienced member of the healthcare team should be allocated to remain with them to ensure appropriate support and information is provided. Additionally, the team leader should at some point during the resuscitation attempt ensure that they take time out to speak directly with them. This is particularly important if the resuscitation attempt is prolonged, or if it seems likely to be unsuccessful (Dainty et al. 2021).

Ending resuscitation attempts

Resuscitation should be stopped only when all potential reversible causes have been robustly considered and the full team are in agreement that there are no signs of life. At this point, established biological death should be confirmed by the team leader, and a debrief of the event carried out with all staff involved as soon as possible. For more information about care after death, see Chapter 35: When a Child or Young Person Dies.

ReSPECT (recommendation on emergency summary plan and end of life care and treatment)

The ReSPECT (Recommendation on Emergency Summary Plan and End of Life Care and Treatment) process now replaces the older and more negative terms of DNAR or DNACPR used when recording whether patients are not for active resuscitation Hawkes et al. (2020). ReSPECT is a national document (see Figure 30.13) and may be used across a range of health and care settings, including the person's own home, an ambulance, a care home, a hospice, or a hospital. It was developed by the RC UK, Royal College of Nursing, and General Medical Council following a DNACPR review in 2014, which found:

- Variation in documentation
- Lack of communication between clinician and patient
- Negative public/patient/clinician/media perceptions of DNACPR decisions

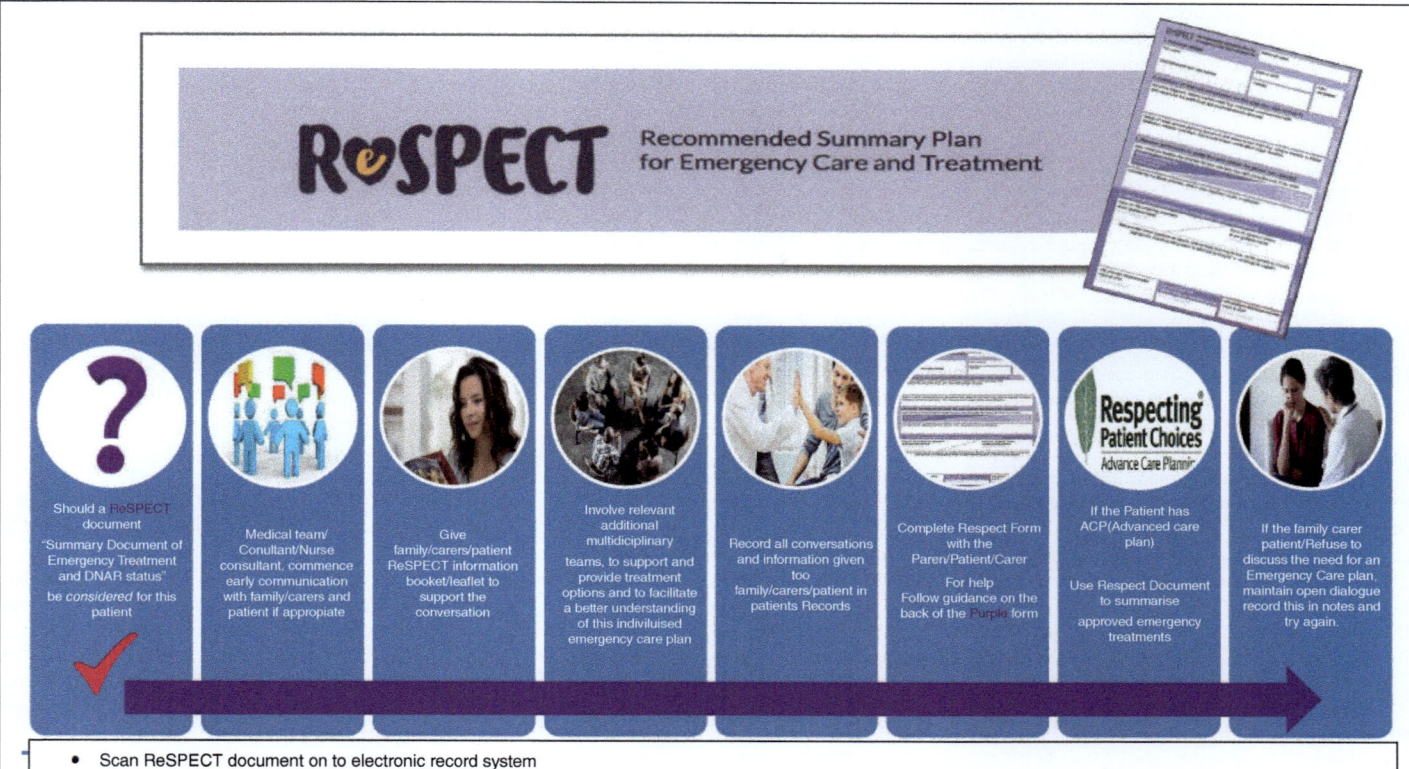

Figure 30.13 The ReSPECT process.

ReSPECT involves clear open communication and documentation of modified emergency care, agreed with the clinical staff, parents, and the child if Fraser competent. It is vitally important that all healthcare professionals understand what the parents and child hope for in the event of a clinical emergency or end of life event, should they be unable to make choices at the time of an emergency. Examples include the wish not to be in pain or to die at home. It is not limited to Do Not Attempt CPR recommendations.

Multiple meetings may be required in order for all involved to be fully informed in order to make these important decisions:

- Prognosis and expected quality of life and hope for the future
- Anticipated cardiorespiratory arrest
- Supportive modified treatments within resuscitation
- Specific palliative care measures to support end of life
- Effective open and honest communication

Once beneficial and/or support treatment options have been agreed, a ReSPECT form is completed to record these modified options and wishes and then stored placed in the patient's notes. On discharge from hospital the ReSPECT form should be rechecked by the clinical team and parent to ensure that all treatment options listed are still in the best interest of the child. This form is then given to the family so that it is immediately available to health and care professionals in the community faced with making decisions in an emergency to ensure that they are aware of agreed treatment options. This form is not a legally binding document and can be revoked at any time.

ReSPECT is a process for all ages and should be considered in particular for:

- Those patients with life-limiting conditions.
- All patients whose heath needs may involve sudden deterioration in health.
- Those with foreseeable risk of death.
- DNAR order can be revoked at any time.

A DNAR order relates only to active cardiorespiratory resuscitation interventions; all palliative care measures instituted to maintain dignity and comfort will be continued and increased as appropriate. For more information regarding palliative care, see Chapter 25: Palliative Care.

References

Abella, B.S., Edelson, D.P., Kim, S. et al. (2007). CPR quality improvement during in-hospital cardiac arrest using a real-time audiovisual feedback system. *Resuscitation* 73: 54–61.

Austen, C., Patterson, C., Poots, A., Green, S., Weldring, T., and Bell, D. (2012). Using a local early warning scoring system as a model for the introduction of a national system. *Acute Med* 11: 66–73.

Bachmann, D.C. (2005). Pediatric shock–pathophysiology, diagnosis and treatment. *Therapeutische Umschau* 62: 533–537.

Chang, D.T., Abdo, K., Bhatt, J.M. et al. (2021). Persistence of choking injuries in children. *International Journal of Pediatric Otorhinolaryngology* 144: 110685.

Clements, F. and McGowan, J. (2000). Finger position for chest compressions in cardiac arrest in infants. *Resuscitation* 44: 43–46.

Dainty, K.N., Atkins, D.L., Breckwoldt, J. et al. International Liaison Committee on Resuscitation's, P., Neonatal Life Support Task, F., Education, I. & Teams Task, F. (2021). Family presence during resuscitation in paediatric and neonatal cardiac arrest: A systematic review. *Resuscitation* 162: 20–34.

Dicembrino, M., Alejandra Barbieri, I., Pereyra, C., and Leske, V. (2021). End-tidal CO2 and transcutaneous CO2: Are we ready to replace arterial CO2 in awake children? *Pediatric Pulmonology* 56: 486–494.

Dornhofer, P. and Kellar, J.Z. (2022). Intraosseous Vascular Access. StatPearls [internet]. https://www.ncbi.nlm.nih.gov/books/NBK554373/ (accessed 08 November 2022).

Duval, S., Pepe, P.E., Aufderheide, T.P. et al. (2019). Optimal combination of compression rate and depth during cardiopulmonary resuscitation for functionally favorable survival. *JAMA Cardiology* 4: 900–908.

Edelson, D.P., Eilevstjonn, J., Weidman, E.K. et al. (2010). Capnography and chest-wall impedance algorithms for ventilation detection during cardiopulmonary resuscitation. *Resuscitation* 81: 317–322.

Fiser, D.H. (1990). Intraosseous infusion. *New England Journal of Medicine* 322 (220): 1579–1581.

Frascone, R.J., Salzman, J.G., Adams, A.B. et al. (2015). Evaluation of intraosseous pressure in a hypovolemic animal model. *The Journal of Surgical Research* 193: 383–390.

Gregson, R.K., Cole, T.J., Skellett, S. et al. (2017). Randomised crossover trial of rate feedback and force during chest compressions for paediatric cardiopulmonary resuscitation. *Archives of Disease in Childhood* 102: 403–409.

Hawkes, C., Fritz, Z., Deas, G. Development of the recommended summary plan for emergency care and treatment (ReSPECT) Resuscitation. 2020;148:98–107.

Hayashida, K., Takegawa, R., Nishikimi, M. et al. (2021). The interplay between bystander cardiopulmonary resuscitation and ambient temperature on neurological outcome after cardiac arrest: a nationwide observational cohort study. *Resuscitation* 164: 46–53.

Holmberg, M.J., Wiberg, S., Ross, C.E. et al. (2019). Trends in Survival After Pediatric In-Hospital Cardiac Arrest in the United States. *Circulation* 140: 1398–1408.

Hoyme, D.B. and Atkins, D.L. (2021). Reply to: "Improved survival to hospital discharge in paediatric in-hospital cardiac arrest using 2 Joules/kilogram as first defibrillation dose for initial pulseless ventricular arrhythmia" and "Optimal paediatric defibrillation dosage for children. We need a randomized clinical trial". *Resuscitation* 158: 293–294.

Lavonas, E.J., Ohshimo, S., Nation, K. et al. & International Liaison Committee on Resuscitation Pediatric Life Support Task, F. (2019). Advanced airway interventions for paediatric cardiac arrest: A systematic review and meta-analysis. *Resuscitation* 138: 114–128.

Lott, C., Truhlar, A., Alfonzo, A. et al. & Collaborators, E. R. C. S. C. W. G. (2021). European Resuscitation Council Guidelines 2021: Cardiac arrest in special circumstances. *Resuscitation* 161: 152–219.

McCrory, J.H. and Downs, C.E. (1984). Cardiopulmonary resuscitation in infants and children. In: *Nursing Care of the Critically ill Child* (ed. M.F. Hazinski), 39–54. St Louis: Mosby.

Nagler, J., Auerbach, M., Monuteaux, M.C. et al. (2021). Exposure and confidence across critical airway procedures in pediatric emergency medicine: An international survey study. *Am J Emerg Med* 42: 70–77.

Nasir, Z.M. and Subha, S.T. (2021). A Five-Year Review on Pediatric Foreign Body Aspiration. *Int Arch Otorhinolaryngol* 25: e193–e199.

Niles, D., Nysaether, J., Sutton, R. et al. (2009). Leaning is common during in-hospital pediatric CPR, and decreased with automated corrective feedback. *Resuscitation* 80: 553–557.

Niles, D.E., Duval-Arnould, J., Skellett, S. et al. (2018). Characterization of Pediatric In-Hospital Cardiopulmonary Resuscitation Quality Metrics Across an International Resuscitation Collaborative. *Pediatr Crit Care Med* 19: 421–432.

Ostermayer, D.G. and Gausche-Hill, M. (2014). Supraglottic airways: the history and current state of prehospital airway adjuncts. *Prehosp Emerg Care* 18: 106–115.

Perman, S.M., Wright, A. R., and Daugherty, S. L. (2021). Closing the Gap: How Telephone Assisted Cardiopulmonary Resuscitation (TA-CPR) Can Aid in Reducing the Sex Disparity in the Provision of Bystander CPR. Resuscitation.

Seethala, R.R., Esposito, E. C., and Abella, B.S. (2010). Approaches to improving cardiac arrest resuscitation performance. *Curr Opin Crit Care* 16: 196–202.

Skellett, S., Maconochie, I., Bingham, B. et al. (2021). Paediatric advanced life support guidelines. https://www.resus.org.uk/library/2021-resuscitation-guidelines/paediatric-advanced-life-support-guidelines (accessed 01 November 2022).

Stein, M.L., Park, R.S., and KovatsisS, P.G. (2020). Emerging trends, techniques, and equipment for airway management in pediatric patients. *Paediatr Anaesth* 30: 269–279.

Sutton, R.M., Niles, D., Meaney, P.A. et al. (2011). "Booster" training: evaluation of instructor-led bedside cardiopulmonary resuscitation skill training and automated corrective feedback to improve cardiopulmonary resuscitation compliance of Pediatric Basic Life Support providers during simulated cardiac arrest. *Pediatr Crit Care Med* 12: e116–e121.

Tisch, C.F. and Abella, B.S. (2020). What gaps in chest compressions tell us about gaps in CPR knowledge. *Resuscitation* 154: 119–120.

Vaillancourt, C., Petersen, A., Meier, E.N. et al. and Resuscitation Outcomes Consortium, I. (2020). The impact of increased chest compression fraction on survival for out-of-hospital cardiac arrest patients with a non-shockable initial rhythm. *Resuscitation* 154: 93–100.

Van De Voorde, P., Turner, N.M., Djakow, J. et al. (2021). European Resuscitation Council Guidelines 2021: Paediatric Life Support. *Resuscitation* 161: 327–387.

Vilke G.M., Smith, A.M., Ray, L.U., Steen, P.J., Murrin, P.A., and Chan, T.C. (2004). Airway obstruction in children aged less than 5 years: the prehospital experience. *Prehosp Emerg Care* 8: 196–199.

Chapter 31

Safeguarding children and young people

Janice Baker[1] and Danya Glaser[2]

[1] SCPHN-HV, RM, RN (Adult); formerly Head of Safeguarding, Great Ormond Street Hospital, London, UK

[2] MBBS, DCH, FRCPsych, Hon FRCPCH; Honorary Child and Adolescent Psychiatrist, GOSH

Chapter contents

Introduction	714
Safeguarding: An individual and corporate responsibility	714
Background	714
Defining child maltreatment	714
The effects of abuse and neglect	716
Intra-familial risk factors	716
Extra-familial risk factors	719
The legal framework	719
Improving child protection and safeguarding practice	719
Professional responsibilities	724
Procedures where there are concerns or suspicions about fabricated or induced illness (FII)	725
Pre-discharge planning procedure	725
Referral to children's social care	725
Looked after children (LAC)	726
Conclusion	726
References	726

The Great Ormond Street Hospital Manual of Children and Young People's Nursing Practices, Second Edition. Edited by Elizabeth Anne Bruce, Janet Williss, and Faith Gibson.
© 2023 John Wiley & Sons Ltd. Published 2023 by John Wiley & Sons Ltd.

Introduction

The United Nations Convention on the Rights of the Child (United Nations 1989) underpins our commitment to ensuring vulnerable children are cared for and protected from harm, stating that children should not have to live with any form of abuse or neglect. Safeguarding, the action we take to promote the welfare of children and protect them from harm, is everyone's responsibility. Everyone who comes into contact with children and families has a role to play, as outlined in the statutory guidance on inter-agency working to safeguard and promote the welfare of children 'Working Together to Safeguard Children' (HM Government 2018b, updated 2020). Child abuse and neglect are forms of maltreatment that occur across all social classes and within all cultures, and may be caused by an adult or adults, or another child. For professionals working with children and families there can be many challenges and uncertainties, where professionals will ask themselves if they have done the right thing, if they are over-reacting, or how they can possibly think the unthinkable. Public perceptions of professional roles are influenced in part through media reports of horrific child abuse and neglect and following cases where medical evidence appears to be in doubt and parents/carers are found innocent in the court. Personal sensitivity and awareness of the impact of the nurse's own personal experience of childhood, family life, and parenting can evoke strong emotions. Professionals should be supported by managers and safeguarding specialists in delivering their responsibilities to keep children safe. In managing and supporting children and families where there are concerns about abuse or neglect there are often no clear answers, and difficult decisions have to be made, together with partner professional agencies. Understanding the factors related to abuse and neglect and the actions required of professionals need to be considered from a holistic perspective, encompassing the child in the context of their family environment.

This chapter focuses on safeguarding children and young people (CYPs) in a hospital setting and the responsibilities of the nurses caring for them. For the most part, CYPs are described as children in this chapter; childhood is defined by the *Children Act 1989* as from birth until the 18th birthday). This covers England and Wales; there is separate legislation for Scotland and Northern Ireland. Young people with special needs up to 19 years old are regarded as children and subject to the same rights for protection from abuse and neglect. Safeguarding must be viewed as our core business, permeating throughout everything we do.

Safeguarding: An individual and corporate responsibility

There is national guidance to support professionals working with children to ensure that the correct processes and procedures are in place to keep them safe. This guidance is found in the document 'Working Together to Safeguard Children', first published in 2006. Safeguarding and promoting the welfare of children is defined in 'Working Together to Safeguard Children' (HM Government 2018b, updated 2020 p. 5) as:

- protecting children from maltreatment;
- preventing impairment of children's mental and physical health or development;
- ensuring that children grow up in circumstances consistent with the provision of safe and effective care; and
- taking action to enable all children to have the best outcomes.

'Working Together' clearly outlines how children are best protected when professionals are clear about what is required of them individually, and how they need to work together alongside professionals, having a clear understanding of the views and wishes of the children themselves, to ensure that a child-centred approach is taken. The document is updated regularly to reflect changes required to practices as a result of legal amendments, evidence-based research, and practice.

Background

The National Society for the Prevention of Cruelty to Children (NSPCC) estimates that on average in the past 5 years 62 children were killed each year. Children under one are more likely to suffer neglect and abuse than a child of any other age, and they are eight times more likely to be killed. Almost half, 154 (42%), of all Serious Case Reviews (SCRs) involve a child under one, and a large proportion of these 79 (51%) relate to the first three months of life (Brandon et al. 2020). Many more children will suffer harmful effects to their health and well-being for the rest of their lives. Child protection cannot be separated from policies to improve children's lives as a whole, and must be part of a spectrum of services to safeguard them.

The annual report 'Characteristics of Children in Need' (Department for Education (DfE) 2020) shows that the number of referrals in the year ending 31 March 2020 had decreased. The numbers of children in need at 31 March 2020 was 389,260 or 323.7 per 10,000 children – the lowest rate in the past 8 years.

Although unborn children currently have no legal rights under English law, concerns about unborn children may arise when thinking about safeguarding and protecting children, and a referral to children's social care should be considered as for any other child. Maternal health and welfare play a crucial part in the development of the unborn child, the mother and child relationship at birth, and the ability of the mother to safely care for her baby after birth.

Understanding what daily life is like for a child is crucial in order to identify and meet their needs (Horwath 2010). Nurses in their duty of care to CYPs need to be thoughtful, reflective, and ask themselves what it is it like for the child to live in this family, today, tomorrow, and at weekends. Nurses working with children have an absolute duty to safeguard and protect them from harm under the 'The Code: Professional Standards of Practice and Behaviour for Nurses, Midwives and Nursing Associates' (Nursing and Midwifery Council [NMC] 2018). This can mean breaking confidentiality by sharing information in order to protect, with a nurse's prime responsibility being to the child, to whom they have a crucial, assertive and professional role in upholding their welfare. All nurses should be familiar with their local safeguarding children policy and procedures, which set out the processes to be followed in safeguarding and promoting the welfare of children, including responding to concerns and taking action to protect a child who has been harmed.

Abused and neglected children can present in many ways, in any area within a hospital. The importance of listening to children and providing them with opportunities to feel safe enough to disclose distress and confusion about what may be happening in their lives cannot be over-emphasised. This may be the one opportunity they have to do so. Nurses need to develop working relationships with families, so that parents and carers feel confident about providing information about their children, themselves, and their circumstances. The challenge is to work in a trusting, supportive partnership with the child's parents or carers, and utilise their knowledge as one component of an assessment. Nurses working with children have an important role in communication, as well as other aspects that take place between professionals when abuse is suspected.

Defining child maltreatment

Four categories of child abuse and neglect are defined in 'Working Together'; physical abuse, neglect, sexual abuse, and emotional abuse (HM Government 2018b, updated 2020). While the purpose of this classification is to identify the predominant type of abuse to which a child is subject, there is often overlap between the different categories. The most common 'initial category of abuse' reported when a child becomes the subject of a plan in England is neglect (50.5%), followed by emotional abuse (35.7%). Both categories have increased in numbers over the past eight years, whereas physical (7.4%), sexual (3,8%), and multiple abuse (2.6%) have decreased. As of 31 March 2020 51,510 children were the subject of a child protection plan in England (DfE 2020). The National Institute for Health and Care Excellence (NICE) produces guidance to support professionals in managing safeguarding and child protection concerns (NICE 2009, updated 2017).

Physical abuse

Physical abuse is a form of abuse that may involve hitting, shaking, throwing, poisoning, burning or scalding, drowning, suffocating, or otherwise causing physical harm to a child. Physical harm may also be caused when a parent or carer fabricates the symptoms of, or deliberately induces, illness in a child.

Alerting factors may include:

- Unexplained bruising, marks, injuries, or burns.
- Multiple injuries of different ages/site.
- History incompatible with injury/illness, i.e. fractures in a nonmobile baby.

Research has shown that children who have been physically abused have higher rates of psychiatric problems, violence, and anti-social behaviour in later life (Kolko 2002; Springer et al. 2011).

Fabricated or induced illness

Fabricated or induced illness (FII) is a complex form of maltreatment that children's nurses may meet in the community and in paediatric and tertiary children's hospitals. Underlying FII is the caregiver's (usually the mother with or without the father) need for the child to be recognised and treated as more unwell (physically and/or psychologically) than the child actually is. The mother's words and sometimes actions are intended to convince health professionals (and others) about her beliefs and contentions.

There are three main ways of a parent or carer fabricating or inducing illness in a child. These are not mutually exclusive:

1. Erroneous reporting of signs and symptoms, history, and diagnoses, which may include significant exaggeration, fabrication, or deception.
2. Falsification of hospital charts and records, letters, and documents. This also includes interference with specimens of body fluids.
3. Induction of illness in the child by a variety of means, including, for example, interfering with IV lines, catheters, or feeding tubes; withholding medication or food; or administering harmful substances to a child (e.g. salt or medicines).

While erroneous reporting is far more common than the other ways and may or may not include an intention to deceive, the far rarer falsification or induction of illness (sometimes referred to as 'using hands') always involves deception on the part of the parent or carer.

The harm to the child comes about both directly as a result of the mother's behaviour and actions and also unintentionally, through health professionals' responses. The harmful effects to the child are significant, affecting them physically, emotionally, developmentally, and socially. Illness induction is additionally associated with occasional mortality, physical illness, and disability (Royal College of Paediatrics and Child Health [RCPCH] 2021). The child will often have undergone numerous investigations and treatments in primary care, hospital, or other settings before being referred to a tertiary or specialist hospital for further diagnostic tests. Many of these children also have a genuine health disorder.

The key to identifying possible FII is the finding of a number of alerting signs, which include discrepancies between parental reports and independent observations of the child. When alerting signs are accompanied by clear deception, illness induction, or clear indications of immediate serious risk to the child's health, referral should be made to children's social care. Otherwise, the alerting signs are termed 'perplexing presentations' and the key to the necessary response is to contact the named staff to determine the child's current actual state of health as well as to collate all medical information and diagnoses about the child from all sources.

Neglect

Neglect is defined as the persistent failure to meet a child's basic physical and/or psychological needs and is likely to result in the serious impairment of the child's health or development. Neglect may occur during pregnancy as a result of maternal substance abuse. Once a child is born, neglect may involve a parent or carer failing to:

- Provide adequate food, clothing and shelter (including exclusion from home or abandonment).
- Protect a child from physical and emotional harm or danger.
- Ensure adequate supervision (including the use of inadequate care-givers).
- Ensure access to appropriate medical care or treatment.

It may also include neglect of, or unresponsiveness to, a child's basic emotional needs as well as those CYPs who assume a young carer's role by taking responsibility for others.

An analysis of SCRs (Brandon et al. 2013) found that neglect had a much higher prevalence than previously thought, occurring in 60% of case reviews from 2009 to 2011, mostly evident as a secondary factor. It can also include the scapegoating of a single child within a family, as identified in the SCR following the death of Daniel Pelka in 2013 (Rogers 2013). Stevenson (2007) emphasises the serious effects of neglect and expresses major concern at the persistent high proportion of children registered under this category. The report by Brandon et al. (2014) on missed opportunities to identify neglect found that there are serious consequences of doing so for CYPs of all ages. Consideration will be given to criminalising the emotional neglect of children in England and Wales.

Alerting factors in health settings may include:

- Evidence of poor hygiene.
- Delays in seeking medical attention.
- A child who is underweight with no medical cause.
- Nonattendance at appointments or repeated cancellations of appointments.

Neglect occurs across all ages but predominates in infants and pre-school children. Neglect stems from a parental choice to prioritise something else above their child's basic needs. Identification of neglect is invariably made over a period of time, as opposed to abuse identified following isolated incidents of physical or sexual abuse. Neglectful behaviour would normally include all of the children in a care setting rather than a model of 'scapegoating' an individual child.

Sexual abuse

Sexual abuse involves forcing or enticing a CYP to take part in sexual activities, not necessarily involving a high level of violence, whether or not the child is aware of what is happening. The activities may involve physical contact, including assault by penetration (e.g., rape or oral sex) or non-penetrative acts such as masturbation, kissing, rubbing, and touching outside of clothing. It may also include non-contact activities, such as involving children in looking at or in the production of sexual images, watching sexual activities, encouraging children to behave in sexually inappropriate ways, or grooming a child in preparation for abuse, including via the internet.

Harmful sexual behaviour (HSB) is used to describe a continuum of sexual behaviours, ranging from inappropriate, to problematic, to abusive. There is a high proportion of contact sexual abuse (65.9%) reported of children under 17 years of age perpetrated by young people under 18 years old. This demonstrates the need for effective prevention, public education, and support for young people in negotiating respectful relationships (Radford et al. 2011).

Sexual abuse is not solely perpetrated by adult males; women also commit acts of sexual abuse, as do other children. On the basis of current evidence, two thirds of all child sexual abuse occurs in the family environment and victims are more likely to be female, with males likely to be under-represented in the data. Much of this type of abuse is hidden. Victims of child sexual abuse within families face differential access to support, with many failing to receive the help they need. It is reported that as few as one in eight victims of child sexual abuse come to the attention of authorities and that abuse within the family is a barrier to victims accessing help (Children's Commissioner for England 2015, 2017).

Police data shows that 73,620 sexual offences were recorded against children in England and Wales in the year ending March 2019; more than triple the figure of 24 085 recorded in 2013 (Office for National Statistics 2019). The sharp increase in numbers of recorded sexual offences against children is probably a result of increased disclosure, following a number of recent high-profile sexual abuse cases in the media (Jutte et al. 2015).

The *Sexual Offences Act 2003* introduced specific offences to deal with perpetrators who abuse or exploit CYPs through prostitution. Alerting factors related to child sexual abuse may include:

- Sexually transmitted disease.
- Pregnancy in a minor.
- Bruising or bleeding in the genital area.
- Children showing inappropriate sexualised behaviour, e.g. verbally or through play.

A sexual relationship can present a risk of significant harm to a child. A child under the age of 13 years is not legally capable of consenting to sexual activity, and such a case should always be discussed with a social worker. Any decision by professionals not to share information with children's social care regarding sexual activity involving children under 13 should be exceptional and made with the documented approval of a senior manager. Sexual activity with a child under 16 is also an offence, and in these cases the nurse must consult with the named nurse or children's social worker.

Child sexual exploitation is a form of child sexual abuse

Child sexual exploitation occurs where an individual or group takes advantage of an imbalance of power to coerce, manipulate, or deceive a CYP under the age of 18 into sexual activity, either in exchange for something the victim needs or wants, and/or for the financial advantage or increased status of the perpetrator or facilitator. The victim may have been sexually exploited even if the sexual activity appears consensual. Child sexual exploitation does not always involve physical contact; it can also occur through the use of technology (DfE 2017). The CYP may receive an item (e.g. food, accommodation, drugs, alcohol, cigarettes, affection, gifts, money) as a result of them performing, and/or another or others performing on them, sexual activities. Child sexual exploitation can occur through the use of technology without the child's immediate recognition; e.g. sexting; being persuaded to post sexual images (naked or semi-naked) on the internet, via a smartphone, tablet, laptop, or other device without immediate payment or gain. Children who are sexually exploited are a group with clearly identified risks to their physical, sexual, and mental health and well-being, and their familial and social relationships. They may run away from home, become dependent on drugs and alcohol, engage in gang activity, or be trafficked. The risk of significant harm to children and vulnerable young people cannot be underestimated, and a referral to children's social care is essential for their safety and protection.

Emotional abuse

Emotional abuse is the persistent emotional maltreatment of a child, such as to cause severe and persistent adverse effects on the child's emotional development. It may involve conveying to a child that they are worthless or unloved, inadequate, or valued only insofar as they meet the needs of another person. It may include not giving the child opportunities to express their views, deliberately silencing them, or 'making fun' of what they say, or how they communicate. It may feature age or developmentally inappropriate expectations being imposed on the child. Emotional abuse may include interactions that are beyond a child's developmental capability, overprotection and limitation of exploration and learning, or preventing them from participating in normal social interaction. It may involve seeing or hearing the ill-treatment of another, exploitation, corruption, or serious bullying (including cyber bullying), or causing children frequently to feel frightened or in danger. Some level of emotional abuse is involved in all types of maltreatment of a child, although it may also occur in isolation. Emotional abuse may be hard to identify, and the effects of this form of abuse may only become recognised over time through observation of a child and their interaction with their caregivers. Alerting factors may include:

- Excessive attention seeking.
- Low self-esteem, low self-confidence.
- Depression and/or withdrawal.
- Witnessing harm to another.

The effects of abuse and neglect

The sustained neglect or abuse of a child physically, emotionally, or sexually can have major long-term effects on all aspects of their health, development, and well-being. There is considerable literature on the traumatic impact of child abuse and neglect (Gerhardt 2004; Glaser 2003; Howe 2005; Reder and Duncan 1999). Glaser (2003) illustrates actual changes in the physically developing brain of maltreated infants, suggesting a wider and perhaps long-term damaging effect of neurological atrophy. Gerhardt (2004) interprets the findings in neuroscience, psychology, psychoanalysis and biochemistry, and explains why love is essential to brain development in the early years of life. Gerhardt describes how early interactions between babies and their parents/carers have lasting and serious consequences. Negative factors can occur in the context of how CYPs are cared for and nurtured by their parents and carers and how their developmental needs are responded to. Howe (2005) uses attachment theory to explain children's social and emotional development, and scientifically explores the formation of children's minds in the context of these early interactions or caregiving relationships, analysing the risks and consequences of child abuse, neglect, rejection, and trauma.

Some children are more vulnerable and others more resilient to negative impacts in their life. There will be strengths within some families and environments that help to offset negative effects, creating a protective resilience in the child. Examples of strengths are the presence of one nurturing and responsible parent/carer, positive friendships with peers, other supportive adult role models, and educational achievement and success (Cleaver et al. 1999).

Intra-familial risk factors

Research demonstrates that there are poor outcomes for children's health and welfare if they are affected by parental problems such as domestic abuse, drug and alcohol misuse, mental health problems, and learning difficulties (Advisory Council on the Misuse of Drugs [ACMD] 2011, Amiel and Heath 2003, Cleaver et al. 1999). It must be remembered that there is often overlap between these known key risk factors; one risk factor in a family can lead to another and the effects on the child are therefore compounded.

Domestic violence and abuse

Nurses and other health practitioners are in a key position to identify domestic abuse by recognising the indicators of abuse and offering support and referral for protection as needed (Department of Health and Social Care 2017). Domestic violence and abuse are the most prevalent of factors in SCRs, often coexisting with mental health and substance misuse. These three factors, termed 'the toxic trio' by Brandon et al. (2008), when coexisting, increase the risk exponentially to the child. Evidence of the toxic trio is highlighted in the Children Commissioner's report (Children's Commissioner for England 2020a). The currently soon to be replaced cross-government (non-statutory) definition of domestic violence and abuse, which was extended in March 2013 by the Home Office to include young people aged 16–to 17 and coercive or controlling behaviour. It is defined as:

> "Any incident or pattern of incidents of controlling, coercive, threatening behaviour, violence or abuse between those aged 16 or over who are or have been intimate partners or family members regardless of gender or sexuality. This can encompass but is not limited to the following types of abuse:
> - psychological
> - physical
> - sexual
> - financial
> - emotional"
>
> (Home Office 2013, p. 2).

Controlling and coercive behaviour is a form of domestic abuse and has been a criminal offence since December 2015 (Home Office 2018).

- *Controlling behaviour* is a range of acts designed to make a person subordinate and/or dependent by isolating them from sources of support, exploiting their resources and capacities for personal gain, depriving them of the means needed for independence, resistance and escape, and regulating their everyday behaviour.
- *Coercive behaviour* is an act or a pattern of acts of assault, threats, humiliation, and intimidation or other abuse that is used to harm, punish, or frighten their victim.

Coercion and control creates high levels of anxiety and fear with a significant impact on children both in their own right as a victim, but also from the impact of abuse on a non-abusing parent. This definition includes 'honour'-based violence, female genital mutilation (FGM), and forced marriage, and makes it clear that victims are not confined to one gender or ethnic group (Home Office 2015, 2018).

Approximately two million adults experienced domestic abuse in 2018. The Domestic Abuse Act 2021 creates, for the first time, a cross government statutory definition of domestic abuse to clarify understanding, what is acceptable behaviour, and to challenge across statutory agencies and public attitudes. It will introduce measures to:

- Address coercive control and economic abuse, and how domestic abuse affects children.
- Transform the response in the justice system.

The bill will also ban the distressing practice of domestic abuse victims being cross-examined by perpetrators in the family courts.

The Home Office (2018) published a report on the economic and social cost of domestic abuse, which reveals the crime cost England and Wales £66 billion in 2016–2017. The vast majority of this cost (£47 billion) was a result of the physical and emotional harm of domestic abuse, but it also includes other factors, such as cost to health services (£2.3 billion), police (£1.3 billion), and victim services (£724 million).

Partner abuse is the most prevalent form of domestic abuse. At least 26.6% of women and 15% of men aged 16–59 have, at some point, experienced some form of domestic abuse since the age of 16 (Strickland and Allen 2018). Several other criminal offences can apply to cases of domestic violence. These can range from murder, rape, and manslaughter, to assault and threatening behaviour. Civil measures include non-molestation orders, occupation orders and domestic violence protection orders (which can mean that suspected perpetrators have to leave their homes). Every year since 1995 approximately half of all women aged 16 or older murdered in England and Wales were killed by their partner or ex-partner (Smith et al. 2011).

Partner abuse among young people

Young people experience the highest rates of domestic abuse of any age group (SafeLives 2018a, b). Abuse can begin even earlier than age 16 for large numbers of young people. A survey of 13–17 year olds found that 25% of girls and 18% of boys reported having experienced some form of physical violence from an intimate partner. As stated previously, the Home Office (2013) definition of domestic violence and abuse now includes those aged 16–17 years. However partner violence is also prevalent in younger people's relationships. In the UK in 2009, 72% of girls and 51% of boys aged 13–16 reported experiencing emotional violence in an intimate partner relationship, 31% of girls and 16% of boys reported sexual violence, and 25% of girls and 18% of boys experienced physical violence (Meltzer et al. 2009).

Young people who harm a family member

Adolescent to parent violence is common and under-reported. For some young people, the experience of domestic abuse includes causing harm to those closest to them, including parents, siblings, and other family members. Nearly a quarter of 13- to 17-year-olds accessing specialist young people's domestic abuse services demonstrated harmful behaviour (SafeLives 2018a, b).

Domestic violence and abuse between parents

Domestic violence and abuse between parents is the most frequently reported form of trauma for children (Meltzer et al. 2009). In the UK, 24.8% of 18- to 24-year-olds reported that they experienced domestic violence and abuse during their childhood. Around 3% of those aged under 17 years reported exposure to it in the past 12 months (Radford et al. 2011). The prevalence of domestic violence starts or intensifies during and after pregnancy (Lewis and Drife 2001). There is a strong association between domestic violence and abuse and other forms of child maltreatment. It was a feature of family life in 64% of the SCRs carried out between 2014 and 2017 (Brandon et al. 2020). The *Adoption and Children Act 2002* identifies living with or witnessing domestic violence as a source of 'significant harm' for children, including domestic abuse in the definition of emotional abuse. Nurses must follow their safeguarding and child protection procedures if they suspect that a child is being exposed to domestic abuse and refer to the hospital social worker. The nurse must also know how to access services to support a mother to protect herself. It is often very hard for women, particularly in some cultures, to talk about domestic abuse. Nurses may be in situations where a mother feels safe to disclose such abuse. Comprehensive guidance that details the relevant legislation and inter-relationship between domestic violence and the abuse and neglect of children has been developed for health staff (Department of Health and Social Care 2017; National Institute for Health and Care Excellence (NICE) 2014). Evidence of the inter-relationship between the abuse of children, adults at risk, and animals is drawn mainly from studies in the USA that relate to cases of serious abuse, although there is also a growing evidence base in the United Kingdom (NSPCC 2012).

Female genital mutilation

Female genital mutilation (FGM) is illegal in the UK. For the purpose of the criminal law in England and Wales, FGM is defined by the World Health Organization (2022) as procedures that include the partial or total removal of the external female genital organs for non-medical reasons.

There are four main types of FGM:

- **Type 1 – clitoridectomy** – removing part or all of the clitoris.
- **Type 2 – excision** – removing part or all of the clitoris and the inner labia, with or without removal of the labia majora.

- **Type 3 – infibulation** – narrowing of the vaginal opening by creating a seal, formed by cutting and repositioning the labia.
- **Other harmful procedures** to the female genitals, which include pricking, piercing, cutting, scraping and burning the area.

It is illegal in the UK to subject a girl or woman to FGM, or to assist a non-UK person to carry out FGM overseas. A new mandatory reporting duty for FGM was introduced in the *Serious Crime Act 2015* and came into force on 31 October 2015. The duty requires all regulated health and social care professionals and teachers in England and Wales to report known cases of FGM in under 18-year-olds to the police by calling 101 (Home Office 2015). The duty is a personal duty, which requires the individual professional who becomes aware of the case to make a report; the responsibility cannot be transferred. Multiagency practice guidelines (HM Government 2018b, updated 2020) include general information about FGM and the best practice to follow in all cases was last updated in 2018. Where FGM is identified in NHS patients, it is now mandatory to record this in the patient's health record.

Mental health
There are important public health implications of not addressing the needs of families who experience mental health problems, as parental mental health can have an impact on parenting and on the child over time and across generations:

- Between one in four and one in five adults will experience a mental illness during their lifetime.
- At the time of their illness, at least 25-50% of these will be parents.
- Children of adults with mental health problems have an increased rate of developing mental health problems themselves, indicating a strong link between adult and child mental health.
- Parental mental illness has an adverse effect on child mental health and development, while child psychological and psychiatric disorders and the stress of parenting can impinge on adult mental health.
- The mental health of children is a strong predictor of their mental health in adulthood.
- The 2% of families who suffer the combined effect of parental illness, low income, educational attainment, and poor housing are among the most vulnerable in society (Social Care Institute for Excellence 2009).

Where a parent has mental health problems there should always be an assessment of parenting capacity and the implication for the child must be taken into consideration as part of this assessment. Many parents/carers with a mental illness care very well for their children, and are aware of and seek help for times when they are not. Some parents may need support to enable them to recognise their responsibilities as parents and some may be unable to provide for their child's physical needs, or are emotionally unavailable for the child. Without additional support, the parent's health condition will impact negatively on the child's developmental needs, leading to neglect and emotional harm.

Postnatal depression can also be linked to behavioural and physiological problems in the infants of affected mothers and it is important that healthcare professionals recognise this and support newly delivered mothers by ensuring they receive the appropriate support (Poobalan et al. 2007).

Substance misuse
Drug and alcohol misuse in a parent/carer has complex effects on children, and is related to the parents/carer's lifestyle and capacity to parent safely and responsibly. As with mental illness in a parent/carer, it is important not to generalise, and a thorough assessment is required. The effects on the child include harm caused by maternal transmission of substances during pregnancy and the reduced parenting capacity of those under the influence of drugs and/or alcohol. Children will also be physically affected and distressed by a parent/carer who may show bizarre, unpredictable, and dangerous behaviour when using some substances. Parental problem drug use can, and often does, compromise children's health and development at every stage from conception onwards. A report published in 2011 estimated that there were around 250 000 to 350 000 children of problem drug users in the UK; about one for every problem drug user (ACMD 2011). An analysis of longer-term effects of substance misuse during pregnancy are even more difficult to detect. Drugs can damage the foetus at any time during pregnancy, causing a wide range of abnormalities in growth and development. These can range from the immediate and catastrophic to much more subtle effects that may not emerge until many years later. There is considerable evidence that at least some drugs when used during pregnancy – notably tobacco, alcohol, and cocaine – have damaging effects on the foetus that are likely to affect the child's future health and well-being (ACMD 2011). The true extent of foetal damage due to maternal drug use remains unknown.

Parents with a learning disability
Parents/carers with a learning disability may experience stress and difficulty in bringing up their children. Again, it is important not to generalise, and a thorough assessment is required. A parent/carer may not have the capacity to respond safely or appropriately to a child's developmental needs, or anticipate what these may be. This is compounded when there are additional stressors such as social exclusion and other health and social issues. The nurse has an important role to assist the parent/carer to understand what is expected of them. This may involve the use of various learning media such as pictures to assist comprehension or arranging for an advocate to support the parent/carer. For more information see Chapter 16: Learning (Intellectual) Disabilities.

Social exclusion
Social exclusion may be caused by a range of factors, such as chronic poverty, poor housing, and social isolation as a result of racism and ethnic differences living in economically disadvantaged areas, homelessness, and living in temporary accommodation. Peruzzi (2013) suggests that all of these have a detrimental effect on the development and well-being of children. Children of young parents with little or no support may experience stresses if they are or they feel socially excluded.

Children with disabilities
Children with disabilities and additional needs are particularly vulnerable to abuse and neglect. There is a growing body of evidence that demonstrates that the presence of multiple disabilities increases the risk of both abuse and neglect. Specific guidance to support professionals in safeguarding disabled children is available (DCSF 2009). It is possible that additional health needs may cause added stresses on the parents and carers. There are greater demands practically, emotionally, and financially. There may be a lack of consideration given to the impact of the impairment or chronic illness on how the family functions. Signs of abuse or neglect may also be mistakenly attributed to a child's disability or health needs: '. . . physical injuries, challenging behaviours, developmental delays, poor growth, and unhygienic living conditions can all be left unchallenged or attributed to the child's disability rather than identified as symptomatic of abuse or chronic neglect. In some cases this may be compounded by parents actively deflecting attention from safeguarding concerns (Sidebotham et al. 2016, pp. 71–72).

Health practitioners working with disabled children need to remain alert to the possibility of maltreatment and consider this possibility when a child presents with signs and symptoms that might be considered indictors of abuse or neglect in a nondisabled child. Children with disabilities may have difficulty in communicating verbally, which can make it more difficult to disclose abuse and this may manifest in challenging or passive behaviours. In one study, disabled CYPs were found to be three times more likely to be abused or neglected than their nondisabled peers (Jones et al. 2012).

Difference and culture

All children have a right to grow up safe from harm and in England and Wales, children of all nationalities are entitled to protection under the *Children Act 1989*. Nurses must have awareness and knowledge of culture-specific child rearing practices within the context of child abuse and neglect; differences do not justify harm and all children have the right to be protected. Child abuse and neglect exists within all cultures, but the child's needs must come first. Certain practices, such as FGM, which is discussed in more detail earlier in the chapter, are illegal in the UK and many other countries.

Extra-familial risk factors

Assessment of Risk Outside the Home

As well as threats to the welfare of CYPs from within their families, they may also be vulnerable to abuse or exploitation external to their familial environment. Extra-familial threats might present from multiple sources; from within educational establishments, peer groups, the wider community or online. Exploitation can take a variety of different forms and children can be vulnerable to multiple threats, including exploitation by criminal gangs and organised crime groups such as county lines, trafficking, online abuse, teenage relationship abuse, sexual exploitation, and the influences of extremism which leads to radicalisation. Extremist groups make use of the internet to radicalise and recruit and to promote extremist materials. Any potential harmful effects to individuals identified as vulnerable to extremist ideologies or being drawn into terrorism should also be considered (HM Government 2018b, updated 2020).

The Children's Commissioner for England (2019) estimates 313,000 children aged 10–17 years know someone they would define as a gang member, and around 34 000 children in England are either in a gang or on the periphery of a gang and have experienced violence in the past 12 months. Just 6500 of these children are known to children's services or youth offending teams.

Preventing radicalisation and involvement in extremism

Vulnerable people, including CYPs, can be exploited by people who seek to involve them in terrorism or activity in support of terrorism. The Government Prevent Strategy (HM Government 2011, updated 2021) aims to stop people becoming terrorists or supporting terrorism. The focus of Prevent is on the significant threat posed by international terrorism and those in the UK who are inspired by it. But it is also concerned with reducing threats, risks, and vulnerabilities posed by domestic extremists such as those from the far right and far left, extreme animal rights activists and those involved in Northern Irish related terrorism. 'Raising awareness amongst healthcare workers of the health sector contribution to the Prevent strategy is crucial. Health are one of the best placed public sector to identify individuals who may be groomed in to terrorist activity, with 1.3 million people employed by the NHS and a further 700 000 private and charitable staff delivering services to NHS patients, we have 315 000 patient contacts per day in England alone. Staff must be able to recognise signs of radicalisation and be confident in referring individuals who can then receive support in the pre-criminal space' (NHS England 2015, p. 5). Training programmes have been implemented across all NHS Trusts throughout England to enable staff to recognise and report individuals who may have been or at risk of being radicalised.

The legal framework

The children act 1989

The *Children Act 1989* sets out the law and guidance for the care and protection of children, emphasising the need for shared responsibilities to safeguard children from abuse and neglect, and to promote their well-being.

The two key principles of the *Children Act 1989* are:

1 The child's welfare must always come first (this is paramount). This means that a child's needs and best interests must be put above all else. Due consideration must be given to the child's religious beliefs, racial origin and cultural and linguistic background.
2 Parental responsibility replaces the former concept of parental rights. Parental responsibility is defined as the duty of the parents/carers to care for their child physically, emotionally and morally.

Legislation does not clearly define abuse and neglect but the Act describes the concepts of risk; see Table 31.1.

Since the introduction of the *Children Act 1989* there has been significant development in policy and practice in children's services, with the aim of improving safeguards for CYPs.

The children act 2004

The *Children Act 2004* established the role of a Children's Commissioner, whose function was to promote the 'views and interests' of children in England. From 1st April 2014, the role was strengthened to 'promote and protect the rights of children'. LSCBs were implemented to perform a range of roles and statutory functions, including developing local policy and procedures, and overseeing local arrangements between partner agencies from public, voluntary, and private organisations with a responsibility to provide services for CYPs. Section 11 of the *Children Act 2004* reinforces the duty of all organisations (public, voluntary and private bodies) to safeguard and promote the welfare of CYPs and reinforces the need to ascertain the child's wishes and feelings regarding the provision of services. Statutory guidance from government on making arrangements under the *Children Act 2004* informs a strong and robust safeguarding culture within health organisations that are accountable to inspection by the Care Quality Commission (CQC). These inspections became part of multi-inspectorate programme in conjunction with the Office for Standards in Education (Ofsted). Internal governance arrangements within hospitals include a rigorous review of policies and procedures and audit activity to measure safeguarding capacity. Good nursing practice must reflect evidence-based practice in safeguarding including documentation, maintaining accurate records, and timely referral to appropriate named and designated professionals for advice and guidance.

Children and social work act 2017

The *Children and Social Work Act 2017* made amendments to sections of the *Children Act 2004* by establishing:

- A National Child Safeguarding Practice Review Panel to consider learning from serious incidents (formally Serious Case Reviews, SCRs) which will be of national interest for learning.
- Local child safeguarding practice reviews designed to identify serious child safeguarding cases which raise issues of importance in the area in relation to safeguard and promote the welfare of local.
- Safeguarding partners (representatives from the local authority, clinical commissioning groups and the police) to provide strategic leadership to local area safeguarding arrangements, following deregulation of Local Children Safeguarding Boards which have now become Local Safeguarding Children Partnerships.

Improving child protection and safeguarding practice

Child safeguarding practice reviews

A child safeguarding practice review is conducted when a child is seriously harmed, or dies, as a result of abuse or neglect. The review identifies how local professionals and organisations can improve the

Table 31.1 Key levels of risk to a child

Children Act 1989 Section	Definition of risk	Actions
Section 17 Child in need	A child who is unlikely to: achieve; or maintain a satisfactory level of health or development, or their health and development will be significantly impaired, without the provision of services; **or** a child who is disabled.	Assessments are carried out by a social worker in relation to a child's special educational needs, disabilities, or as a carer, or because they have committed a crime. The process for assessment should also be used for children whose parents are in prison and for asylum seeking children. Multiple assessments may be required and, where possible, should be coordinated so that the child and family experience a coherent process and a single plan of action.
Section 31 (9) Significant harm	'Harm' means ill-treatment or the impairment of health or development, including, for example impairment suffered from seeing or hearing the ill-treatment of another; 'Development' means physical or mental health; and 'Ill-treatment' includes sexual abuse and forms of ill-treatment which are not physical. There are no absolute criteria on which to rely when judging what constitutes 'significant harm' and different factors are taken into account, including the duration and frequency of the abuse and neglect and the degree of threat and coercion	Concerns about maltreatment may be the reason for a referral to local authority children's social care or concerns may arise during the course of providing services to the child and family. In these circumstances, local authority children's social care must initiate enquiries to find out what is happening to the child and whether protective action is required.
Section 47 Duty of local authority to intervene in a child's life.	Local authorities, with the help of other organisations as appropriate, have a duty to make enquiries if they have reasonable cause to suspect that a child is suffering, or is likely to suffer, significant harm.	Children's Social Care must decide whether they should take any action to safeguard and promote the child's welfare. There may be a need for immediate protection whilst the assessment is carried out.

way they work together. 'Working Together' (HM Government 2018b, updated 2020) set out the process for a new system of child safeguarding practice reviews at both local and national level, which replaces the various methodologies for SCRs. Responsibility for learning from serious child safeguarding incidents is the responsibility of the Child Safeguarding Practice Review Panel, and at local level, the safeguarding partners of Local Safeguarding Children Partnerships. The purpose of reviews of serious child safeguarding cases, at both local and national level, is to identify improvements to be made to safeguard and promote the welfare of children. Learning is relevant locally, but it has a wider importance for all practitioners working with children and families, and for the government and policy-makers. Understanding whether there are systemic issues, and whether and how policy and practice need to change, is critical to ensure that the system is dynamic and self-improving. For further information see 'Improving child protection and safeguarding practice' (HM Government 2018b, updated 2020 chapter 4). The purpose of reviews is to reduce the risk of repetition of similar events. They are not about blaming individuals, organisations, or agencies, for which there are other processes. Serious child safeguarding cases are those in which abuse or neglect of a child is known or suspected, and the child has either died or been seriously harmed. The definition of serious harm includes (but is not limited to) serious and/or long-term impairment of a child's mental health or intellectual, emotional, social, or behavioural development. It should also cover impairment of physical health. This is not an exhaustive list. When making decisions, judgement should be exercised in cases where impairment is likely to be long term, even if this is not immediately certain. Even if a child recovers, including from a one-off incident, serious harm may still have occurred.

National reviews

The Child Safeguarding Practice Review Panel will identify and oversee the review of serious child safeguarding cases that raise complex issues, or issues of national importance. The panel may review one or more cases that meet similar criteria, and may consider cases where previously identified improvements need reviewing, where legislative change to guidance is required, or where there are recurring themes. In addition, those cases where children have been educated other than at school, are in the care of the local authority, or are subject to (or recently removed from) a child protection plan, or involve a range of types of abuse, e.g. trafficking involving institutional settings.

Local reviews

Safeguarding partners within a local area must identify and review serious child safeguarding cases which are of importance to their local area. A rapid review is carried out to consider any urgent actions required to safeguard children and share any immediate learning. Once completed, the decision is notified to the national panel. The safeguarding partners may also consider cases where the Child Safeguarding Practice Review Panel have considered and concluded that a local review may be more appropriate, there have been concerns about the actions or a lack of by a single agency, involvement of the multi-agency network across several areas, or issues are related to actions within institutional settings. Other cases may be considered where important issues are raised pertaining to a local area, which can include good or poor practice and 'near miss events'. When professionals are involved in any type of review they should be offered support and reassurance that the process is about learning from serious incidents and not 'naming and blaming'.

Recurrent key themes of child safeguarding practice reviews

Formal reviews and enquiries following the death of, or very serious harm to, a child through abuse and neglect identify recurring themes. The series of biennial and triennial analyses of SCRs (Brandon et al. 2009, 2010, 2012, 2014, 2017) identified recurring findings that have significant implications for health professionals. The most recent triennial analysis (Brandon et al. 2020) considered 278 reports from SCRs that were available for the period 2014–2017 and focussed on the theme of complexity and challenge.

The subjects in the majority of SCRs were known to children's social care:

- 55% had current involvement.
- 22% had previous involvement.
- 15% were subject to a child protection plan and a similar number had been subject to plans previously.
- 42% were aged under one year.
- Domestic abuse was a factor in the majority of cases (64%).
- There were mental health issues in 56% of cases.

Other recurrent factors were substance misuse, poverty, crime, and adverse parental experiences as children.

Professionals faced complex challenges that were overwhelming in some cases. As already highlighted from the previous work of Brandon et al. (2013), neglect is a prevalent theme within SCRs, mostly evident as a secondary factor and one that has appeared within SCRs, stretching from Dennis O'Neill in 1945 (cited in Ferguson 2011) through to Daniel Pelka in 2013 (Rogers 2013).

Neglect may present in many ways including deprivation, co-morbidities with physical abuse, neglectful environments, suicide and self-harm in adolescents, and medical neglect, which is discussed in more detail below. It is important that nurses have an awareness of the impact of poverty and understand the interaction between socio-economic and other factors that can impact on parenting capacity and outcomes for children. Older children over 11 years of age featured in 31% of reviews, with risk taking, violent behaviour, and child sexual exploitation accounting for almost half of the cases (44%).

School-age children have predominantly been the focus of public inquiries, but account for only 10% of all SCRs (Ofsted 2011). While this group are more likely to spend time away from home in an educational setting where they can be independently observed, there are a significant number of children who are not educated in school due to physical or emotional factors, as well as parents choosing home education as an alternative, as in the case of Khyra Ishaq who had been withdrawn from school by her mother to be home educated (Birmingham LSCB 2010). While it is everyone's responsibility to safeguard and protect children, health agencies may be the only professionals involved with the family in the neonatal period. This emphasises the importance of effective universal services for babies and their families. Information sharing between the many agencies involved with children, including GPs, Health Visitors, A&E departments and minor injury units, 'urgent care' centres, nurseries, schools and social care is essential to effectively safeguard the child. In addition, a sound knowledge and understanding of child development is essential. In many of the case reviews involving toddlers and preschool aged children, a lack of understanding of child development amongst the professionals involved has meant that, potential concerns, such as an unusual pattern or site of bruising, which should have provoked curiosity regarding the cause of the bruising, was not challenged, and opportunities to safeguard children were lost. SCRs have consistently identified the invisibility of children who have remained hidden from authorities, partially due to the actions of their carers but also due to inaction by professionals who have not raised their concerns to the investigating agencies, as in the case of Daniel Pelka (Rogers 2013), who was noted by education staff to be scavenging for food and Victoria Climbie (Laming 2003), who despite coming into contact with the multiagency network, never had her educational status identified or challenged. Adolescents are a small (25%) but significant group who are often represented in SCRs as a result of their own risk-taking behaviours. Brandon et al. (2010 p. 53) identified that agencies struggle to engage this 'hard to help' cohort and 'neglect these challenging young people, because their needs have become too overwhelming'. The tendency for vulnerable 'hard to help' adolescents to be neglected by agencies, who give up on these challenging young people because their needs have become too overwhelming, was first identified in the 2003–2005 study (Brandon et al. 2008). This finding has also had resonance in later reviews (Brandon et al. 2009) and in other studies (Hicks and Stein 2010).

A number of SCRs have highlighted the issues of parental deceit and manipulation. Parents can present themselves to professionals as capable care givers; e.g., Daniel Pelka's mother presented herself as a capable caregiver by deceiving professionals through her assertive, but manipulative and deceitful behaviour. The SCR into Daniel's death concluded that emotional abuse or neglect were not considered as possible causes and that his mother's deceit and actions 'were not recognised for what they were, and her presenting image was too readily accepted' (Lock 2013 p. 70). Peter Connolly was 17 months old and subject to a child protection plan when he died of horrific inflicted injuries. His life and involvement with professionals reminds us of the need to focus on authoritative practice and intervention by all professionals and agencies involved with children. Authoritative practice challenges parents/carers with expectations of their responsibilities to parent and care for their child safely. It challenges other professionals in the expectations of their services, and assesses a child's experience thoroughly, with a low threshold of concern, and maintains the focus on the child at all times (Haringey 2009).

Bullying and cyberbullying (which takes place online), is a distinctive pattern of harming and humiliating others, and is a growing concern for many CYPs; it can be very damaging and causes considerable stress. Bullying affects over one million young people every year and may be carried out by one or more individuals. In the 2018 annual survey of bullying, which included more than 9000 respondents, 1 in 5 children disclosed that they had been bullied within the past 12 months (Ditch the label 2018). Both maintained and independent schools in England and Wales must have an anti-bullying policy or strategy in place (Education and Inspections Act 2006, Education (Independent School Standards) (England) (Amendment) Regulations 2012). Children may disclose to a nurse or other health care worker that they are being bullied by their peers, or sometimes a sibling. The nurse must listen and ensure that the child can discuss the issues with an appropriate person, such as the psychologist, social worker or child advocacy service, to ensure that they receive the right help. All hospitals should have anti-bullying policies and strategies in place, which should include education for staff, to protect the children in their care.

Nurses must be alert to the issue of children who are not brought to health appointments either in person or by virtual consultation. Repeated cancelling or rescheduling of health appointments by family members are important factors to consider in safeguarding children. It is the responsibility of the parent/carer to ensure that a child receives adequate health and dental care. Failure to do so, or to ignore medical advice, can lead to children suffering through their health needs not being met. Hospitals must have a clear published policy on the process for following up children who are not brought to health appointments or seen at virtual consultations. Nurses may be the best placed professionals to contact and inform the health visitor or school nurse, as well as through the normal process of notification of the family GP of a child's non-attendance. Where children are subject to a child protection plan, children's social care should be informed. Within his report, Lord Laming made recommendations for hospital Accident and Emergency departments (Laming 2009, p. 28). In many of the cases where a child had experienced significant harm or died as a result of abuse, they had at some point been taken to an Accident and Emergency department of a hospital. It is vital that nurses working in these departments are able to recognise abuse and are familiar with local procedures for making enquiries to find out whether a child is subject to a child protection plan. They also need information regarding whether a child has recently been seen in another Accident and Emergency department, ambulatory care unit, walk-in centre or minor injury unit. Where an injury is thought to be non-accidental, Children's Social Care Services and the child's GP must be notified as soon as possible.

Child death reviews

Child death reviews (CDRs) are mandatory for child death review partners in England. CDR partners must review the deaths of all children up to the age of 18 to understand why children die and put in place interventions to protect other children and reduce the risk of further deaths. (National Child Mortality Database [NCMD] 2020). The partners must collect information from all agencies that have had contact with the child during their life and after their death. In the year up to 31 March 2020, 2738 deaths were reviewed, with 862 identified as having modifiable factors. Deaths with a primary category of deliberately inflicted injury, abuse, or neglect had modifiable factors in 72% of cases. A large proportion of child deaths will be as a result of chronic illness, disability, and life-limiting conditions; others will be from accidents, and a minority as a consequence of abuse and neglect. In the former, nurses should be familiar with their Trust's policy for end-of-life plans. In the latter, any suspicious death will be managed as directed in the Trust's Safeguarding Children Policy. Further information can be found in 'Working Together' (HM Government 2018b, updated 2020). Of the CDRs completed in the year, a Child Safeguarding Practice Review was carried out for at least 48 child deaths and of these, 79% identified modifiable factors in the review (NCMD 2020).

A safeguarding culture

Skilled and competent staff, adequate managerial support and professional supervision are crucial elements in protecting children. Within every organisation there must be senior executive commitment to the importance of safeguarding and promoting welfare and a clear line of accountability, so that all staff know with whom they can discuss their concerns and to whom they can make a referral. There must be an environment that supports the sharing of appropriate information, values the expertise and skills of individual colleagues and professionals across disciplines, and works together in the best interests of the child. Hospitals must have safeguarding policies in place to ensure all staff are aware of the procedures for managing suspicions or actual concerns about a child's welfare or safety. These should be compatible with the principles and requirements of the London Safeguarding Children Partnership (LSCP), for example, London Child Protection Procedures and Practice Guidance (2020, updated October 2022). Arrangements for 'out of hours' concerns should be in place, with a key professional identified who has child protection expertise, to give advice and guidance, and to be available on a 24-hour basis. Children must also be protected from staff who would wish to harm them. Organisations must have safe recruitment and selection procedures in place. As well as obtaining recent references prior to employment, all staff are subject to a check with The Disclosure and Barring Service (DBS), which helps employers make safer recruitment decisions and (as far as possible) prevent unsuitable people from working with vulnerable groups, including children. It replaces the Criminal Records Bureau (CRB) and Independent Safeguarding Authority (ISA) under the Protection of Freedoms Act 2012.

The increased risk to vulnerable children due to the impact of the coronavirus pandemic

With all UK nations, having been under lockdown or high-level restrictions for long periods of time, many children and young people have had to stay at home. Even before the crisis, there were 2.2 million children in England living in households affected by the so-called 'toxic trio' of family issues: domestic abuse, parental drug and/or alcohol dependency, and severe parental mental health issues. After months of national anxiety, the stripping back of key support services and an emerging economic recession, the impact of lockdown on children is only just starting to become clear. Children can be both resilient and adaptable, but they can't do this on their own, and the crisis has shown how few resources some children – and their families – can rely upon when things go wrong. Some children have benefitted from aspects of lockdown, becoming less stressed due to respite of the routines of everyday life, enjoying quality time with families whose incomes remained stable or were furloughed. Covid-19 has exposed and exacerbated existing inequalities facing those children who have faced poorer life chances than others. The periods of lockdown reduced ways in which children were able to be identified as being at risk (Children's Commissioner Childhood in the Time of Covid 2020). Children have lost many sources of support that they may have previously had: education, health appointments, children's centres, health visitors, networks of family and friends, home visits from social workers – at the same time that their families have had to contend with changes in their day-to-day lives, from balancing working from home with looking after children and providing an educational environment, caring for relatives who may be shielding or unwell, and the potential for loss of employment and financial instability. Not having such regular face-to-face contact at scheduled health appointments reduces opportunities for professionals to recognise child protection concerns and provide appropriate support. Since the beginning of the Covid-19 pandemic, concerns have been raised over the potential increased risk of maltreatment for CYPs. The principles of safeguarding CYPs remain the same, with the child's welfare being paramount and at the centre of our work. The impact of the pandemic will continue to unfold in the coming years, but reports have highlighted particularly an increase in mental health and wellbeing issues, domestic abuse, and online sexual exploitation.

The Children's Commissioner for England publishes regular reports of child vulnerability, the most recent of which aids better identification of vulnerable children who need help during periods of lockdown and once the crisis has passed (Children's Commissioner for England 2020a). Subsequently the largest consultation with children has been launched to understand their priorities for improving childhood post-Covid. The Beveridge report 'The Big Ask', which will be published later this year, will provide the cornerstone of the 'Childhood Commission', the Children's Commissioner's blueprint for government (Children's Commissioner for England 2021).

Implications for practice
Education and training

Nurses having contact with children or their families need appropriate education and training to enable them to recognise abuse, to keep excellent records and clear documentation of concerns and communications with the child, the family, and professionals involved, and to know when to refer to Children's Social Care. Competencies for healthcare staff are underpinned by the knowledge and skills framework outlined in the Intercollegiate Document (Royal College of Nursing 2019), which clarifies training and education needs across the range of health practitioners, enabling individuals working in any healthcare environment to receive appropriate initial training and updates in relation to their specific roles and responsibilities. Children's nurses should receive core level 3 training as a minimum and progress to specialist level 3 training or level 4 depending on their level of responsibility and experience. Every hospital must have a dynamic training strategy that responds to the needs of its staff. Single agency training may be delivered through different mediums, which include e-learning, simulation, and face-to-face group training. Interagency training, available through the LSCP, helps to build trust and effective communication across professional boundaries by developing a shared understanding of each agency's roles and responsibilities, all of whom have a commitment to safeguarding and protecting children. This training is continually being refreshed and new areas covered in response to national issues and concerns, and should include raising awareness of current concerns, including FGM, radicalisation, and child sexual exploitation.

Safeguarding children supervision

Supervision can be defined as: 'an accountable process which supports, assures, and develops the knowledge, skills and values of an individual, group, or team. The purpose is to improve the quality of their work to achieve agreed outcomes' (Skills for Care and Children's Workforce Development Council 2007, p. 5). Working to safeguard children from abuse and neglect is demanding work that can be distressing and stressful. Effective professional supervision can play a critical role in ensuring a clear focus on a child's welfare, and all nurses involved in safeguarding children should have access to effective supervision (DH 2004; Morrison 2006). Supervision supports professionals to reflect critically on the impact of their decisions on the child and their family (HM Government 2018b, updated 2020).

A recurrent theme in many SCRs is the need for provision of supervision for staff involved in individual child protection cases. In the inquiry into the deaths of Victoria Climbie (Laming 2003) and progress report of actions taken following the death of Peter Connelly, Lord Laming expressed concern about the lack of supervision for health staff (Laming 2009). To be effective, supervision should take place at regularly defined intervals, either on an individual or group basis, and should also be available to any member of staff on an ad-hoc basis. In an acute setting a reflective model may be more appropriate, in order to meet the varying needs of the multidisciplinary professional workforce. Supervision may be provided by the named professionals or those with additional expertise in safeguarding.

Principles of collaborative working

Safeguarding and promoting the welfare of children, and in particular protecting them from significant harm, depends on effective joint working between agencies and professionals that have different roles and expertise. Ultimately, effective safeguarding can only be achieved by putting children at the centre of the system, and by every individual and agency playing their full part, and working together to meet the needs of our most vulnerable children (HM Government 2018b, updated 2020). Collaborative working involves effective information sharing and effective communication.

Information sharing

Effective information sharing by professionals makes an important contribution to safeguarding. If children's needs are identified at an early stage and information shared, then appropriate services and support can be provided for families, and more serious problems can be prevented. Nurses have a crucial responsibility to share information in their role as advocate for the child. Information that supports the safeguarding and protection of a child cannot remain confidential, and must be shared. The decision to share information is always based on professional judgement. 'Fears about sharing information cannot be allowed to stand in the way of the need to safeguard and promote the welfare of children at risk of abuse or neglect. No practitioner should assume that someone else will pass on information which may be critical to keeping a child safe' (HM Government 2018a, updated 2020, p. 6).

Information sharing is a key factor identified in many SCRs where poor information sharing has resulted in missed opportunities to take action to keep CYPs safe (Brandon et al. 2014). However the welfare of the child is paramount (HM Government 1989; United Nations 1989) and information that is relevant to safeguarding children must be shared with other professionals within health or other agencies as is necessary to safeguard a child's welfare. Patient data is kept confidential in line with current legislation and regulatory body guidance (NMC 2018). The General Data Protection Regulation (GDPR) (Information Commissions Office 2018) and the *Data Protection Act 2018* introduced new elements to the data protection regime, superseding the *Data Protection Act 1998*. Practitioners must have due regard to the relevant data protection principles that allow them to share personal information. The GDPR and *Data Protection Act 2018* place greater significance on organisations being transparent and accountable in relation to their use of data. They do not prevent, or limit, the sharing of information for the purposes of keeping CYPs safe. To effectively share information:

- All practitioners should be confident in the processing conditions which allow them to store and share the information that they need to carry out their safeguarding role. Information relevant to safeguarding will often be considered 'special category personal data', meaning it is sensitive and personal.
- Where practitioners need to share special category personal data, they should be aware that the *Data Protection Act 2018* includes 'safeguarding of children and individuals at risk' as a condition that allows practitioners to share information without consent.
- Information can be shared legally without consent if a practitioner is unable to, or cannot be reasonably expected to gain consent from the individual, or in instances where to gain consent could place a child at risk.
- Relevant personal information can be shared lawfully if it is to keep a child or individual at risk, safe from neglect or physical, emotional, or mental harm, or if it is protecting their physical, mental, or emotional well-being.

(HM Government 2018a)

The child protection information sharing system (CP-IS)

The CP-IS shares information about children subject to a Child Protection Plan, pregnant women with an Unborn Child Protection Plan, and children who are designated a Looked After Child (LAC), in particular those being cared for under the following sections of the *Children Act 1989*:

- Full Care Order (Section 31)
- Interim Care Order (Section 38)
- Voluntary Care Agreement (Section 20)

The CP-IS project ensures that health and care professionals in unscheduled health settings (see below) are alerted if a child or unborn baby is subject to a child protection plan or is looked after and provide contact details for the Children's Social Care team responsible for them. The system collects health audit data when healthcare professionals access the record. The information is sent back to the local authorities to inform them where a child has presented, and the health audit data details the previous unscheduled presentations of the child in healthcare settings (up to 25 presentations).

Currently, unscheduled healthcare settings are

- Emergency departments
- Minor injury units
- Walk-in centres
- GP out-of-hours services/111
- Unscheduled access to maternity units
- Unscheduled access to paediatric wards
- Ambulance services

Building on the success of the initial CP-IS programme through stakeholder engagement, this programme has now been extended in a second phase to include scheduled healthcare settings (NHS Digital 2020). GOSH was the first scheduled healthcare setting to be validated due to the unique environment of a specialist hospital setting without an A&E department whose patients reside across the UK.

Communication

Problems with communication are frequently identified between professionals in reviews of fatal child abuse. Reder and Duncan (2003) explore the psychology of communication and the complexities involved. They identify the responsibilities of both the message initiator and the message receiver to ensure that their communication is being understood, how meanings are attributed to messages both given and received, and how the contexts in which these communications occur can influence the understanding of the message. Ineffective communication can have a major impact on the safety of a child; e.g. Victoria Climbie was prematurely discharged from hospital, having been admitted with suspected non-accidental injuries. Sources of the confusion were multiple, but included a nurse's fax stating that Victoria was 'fit for discharge', which was interpreted by the social worker as meaning 'that the hospital no longer had any concerns about Victoria in the general sense'. By contrast, several hospital staff in their evidence to the inquiry said that 'fit for discharge' meant that Victoria was medically fit to leave and they assumed the social workers would make the necessary inquiries of her home and family before that actually happened' (Laming 2003, p. 148). Additionally, a paediatrician's entry in the medical notes, which stated '? Discharge', was understood by a nurse to indicate a definite discharge plan (Laming 2003, p. 274).

When discussing a child with another professional where there are suspected nonaccidental injuries, or concerns about the CYP's welfare, the language used should be clear and straightforward. It is important to clarify that the person receiving the message has understood what the giver has meant to relay. In addition, all communication must be recorded, dated, and signed as per the hospital policy and in accordance with the professional standards of practice (NMC 2018), and any written record about or involving the child should be unambiguous, and clearly understandable by anybody else who reads it.

Listening to the child's voice

Hearing the voice of the child is fundamental and may provide crucial clues to current or previous maltreatment that they may have experienced. In a busy and pressured work environment, the importance of asking curious questions about past experiences, culture, and beliefs should not be avoided for fear of being seen as overly intrusive, and may have a significant impact on the ability of professionals to make informed judgements and subsequent referrals to other services. If a CYP reveals they are at risk, the health professional must listen carefully and record the conversation, using the child's own words, reassuring them that they are right to tell. It is important not to promise to keep secrets, or jump to any conclusions. It is not the responsibility of the health professional to interrogate the child, but to follow the local safeguarding process immediately, ensuring that the safety of the child and any siblings or other children, and if appropriate to initiate a referral to children's social care. Care must be taken in the language we use when making such referrals, as this can be both supporting and a hindrance to effective safeguarding.

Professional responsibilities

Nurses must be familiar with their own local safeguarding and child protection procedures. They must know when it is appropriate to undertake an Early Help Assessment (EHA), and refer a child to children's social care for help as a 'child in need', and how to act on concerns that a child may be at risk of significant harm through abuse or neglect. Procedures in 'Working Together' (HM Government 2018b, updated 2020) and 'What to do if you are worried a child is being abused' (HM Government 2015) clearly summarise what action has to be taken. NICE has also issued clear guidance (NICE 2009, updated 2017). All anxieties and concerns about a CYP's safety and welfare must be discussed with the line manager, senior member of staff, consultant, named nurse, named doctor, or social worker from the hospital's social care department, or with children's social care as soon as possible on the same day, without delay. If there are disagreements between members of staff about making a referral, discussion with a named nurse or doctor must take place. All observations, discussions, and communications must be recorded in the child's healthcare record. Where a child presents with possible injuries, the named doctor will be called to undertake a detailed medical examination as part of the assessment.

Procedures for children attending A&E

Nurses have an important role in A&E departments, urgent care centres, etc., and are well placed to be able to recognise signs of abuse and neglect. They need to understand the local procedures and know who to contact both routinely and in emergency situations, internally and externally, on a 24-hour basis. Children suffering from abuse and neglect can be brought to any A&E department in the country for treatment and assessment, and staff must be aware of the risks and indicators of intentional injury. Children may also be transferred to one hospital directly from another A&E department, and it is important that the receiving nurse knows the processes that have taken place and when a referral to Children's Social Care has been made where a child is seriously injured, or abuse or neglect is a possibility.

The following questions must be considered and answered:

1. Has there been a delay in seeking medical help for which there is no satisfactory explanation?
2. Is the history consistent?
3. Are there unexplained injuries?
4. Is the child's behaviour and interaction with the adult appropriate?
5. Has the child attended another A&E department or health service provider recently?

If the answer to question 1 and 3 is 'Yes', and 2 and 4 is 'No', this must be treated as suspicious and further history taking, expert medical examination, and action must be taken to safeguard the child, according to the local procedures. This will involve close liaison with children's social care and may involve the police. If a Police Protection Order is required to keep the child in hospital while further plans for safety are made and investigations are carried out. The following indicators must raise concern:

1. Frequent attendee.
2. Any bruising or injury in a non-mobile infant.
3. Unexplained bruising, fracture, or head injury in a child under one year, or in a child who is not physically mobile.
4. Parents, especially young parent(s), presenting with crying or unsettled babies, or babies who are not feeding well.

Parent(s) who are very stressed and anxious with an unsettled baby may be actively seeking help because they cannot cope. Contacting the Health Visitor, General Practitioner, and other primary or secondary care professionals as appropriate is important to request early follow-up in the community. Admission to hospital should be considered for a period of observation.

Good recordkeeping is highlighted as an essential part of professional accountability where there is suspicion of abuse and neglect. If there is no record, there is no evidence for action to be taken. Recordkeeping, including detailed documentation of all communications with both the family and professionals should be very clear, including the rationale for actions taken.

Procedures for children admitted to hospital

When any child is seen for an investigation or examination in an outpatient setting, or is admitted to the ward as an in-patient, the following questions should be asked, or if already recorded, clarified with the parent/carer:

1. Does the child have a Health Visitor/School Nurse (or school)/Community Nurse?
2. Does the child have a Family Worker or a Social Worker? If so, is the child subject to a Child Protection Plan? Check whether there is an electronic alert.
3. Is the child's 'Parent-held record' book available?
4. Is the language spoken at home recorded? Translation and interpreting services will need to be considered to ensure questions are understood and information that is given to parents/carers verbally or in writing will be given in their preferred language where appropriate.

5 Who has parental responsibility?
6 Does the parent/carer have any physical or learning difficulties?

History-taking should be done on admission or attendance at an outpatient or a walk-in centre, or in an ambulatory care setting, and should include an accurate profile of the child's psychosocial background, as well as their health and developmental history. This facilitates seamless care and liaison with other professionals as required. It also supports a 'needs assessment' when appropriate, to aid the health and welfare of the child.

At GOSH, a dedicated section for sharing child protection information is included in a child's medical records once the threshold for a child protection referral has been met, – except where there are concerns regarding FII (see below) – and in all cases of head injuries to children under the age of two years, unless that injury has been sustained in a road traffic accident. The purpose of the separate section is to support effective information sharing, assisting staff to maintain an overview of the welfare of the child and refer as appropriate. It ensures that both a coherent account of the situation and the plans to protect the child are easily available to staff. It is imperative that all staff involved with the child record any aspect of their care that concerns the child protection issue; all relevant contacts from parents/carers and both internal and external agencies involved. If the child is under the care of more than one medical team, the consultant talking the lead for child protection concerns must be identified and documented in the child's healthcare record.

Procedures where there are concerns or suspicions about fabricated or induced illness (FII)

When CYPs present with complex or perplexing presentations, the key to identifying possible FII is the finding of a number of alerting signs, which include discrepancies between parental reports and independent observations of the child. When alerting signs are accompanied by clear deception, illness induction, or clear indications of immediate serious risk to the child's health, referral should be made to children's social care. Otherwise, the alerting signs are termed 'perplexing presentations' and the key to the necessary response is to contact the named professionals and to determine the child's current actual state of health, as well as to collate all medical information and diagnoses about the child from all sources. Refer to previous section, Fabricated and Induced Illness, for further information.

All records about a child's condition should clearly state who reported the concerns, what was observed, and by whom. Records of key discussions and safeguarding supervision notes about the child's care should be kept within every organisation's main health record pertaining to the child to ensure that they do not come to further harm, as per recommendations from the Victoria Climbié Inquiry (Laming 2003). The child protection section should not be inserted into the records until all possible diagnoses/medical causes have been excluded. If illness induction or interference with specimens and apparatus is suspected, all specimens and apparatus need to be retained and stored safely for forensic purposes (RCPCH 2021) and the organisational Safeguarding Policy must be followed.

Pre-discharge planning procedure

When child protection concerns have been raised, plans for discharge must be documented in the child's healthcare record by the lead consultant. The plan should be summarised in the Child Protection section of the child's records, indicating that there is full cooperation and agreement with the social worker, medical, nursing, and allied health professionals involved. This will include details of the outcomes of any strategy meetings held. In keeping with the Laming Report (2003), p. 379), no child about whom there are child protection concerns may be discharged from hospital, either to another hospital or to home, without a documented plan for their future, including follow-up arrangements.

To ensure that a child for whom there are safeguarding or child protection concerns is discharged safely there must be:

1 A clear plan for discharge in the child's medical record that includes a summary of the issues and future plan for protecting the child, including out-patient follow-up.
2 A clear plan for discharge with respect to child protection concerns, documented in the Child Protection section in the child's medical record, signed by the lead consultant and the CYP's social care worker.
3 A record in the nursing record that child protection concerns have been passed verbally prior to transfer of the child, between the nurse in charge of the ward and the receiving hospital or community nursing team as appropriate.
4 A record in the medical notes that the lead consultant or the registrar has verbally notified the receiving consultant or the GP as appropriate (if discharging to home).
5 Discharge plan (medical summary) to include names of professionals to whom this information has been conveyed, both internally and externally, e.g. child's social worker, consultant at the receiving hospital, GP, and health visitor/community nurse/school nurse as appropriate. A written copy should be faxed to the GP and/or receiving hospital, as per hospital policy.
6 If child protection concerns have been raised and on investigation not substantiated this should be indicated in the discharge plan as 'child protection concerns not founded, case closed with respect to this issue.'
7 All record entries signed, with date and times recorded.

The early help assessment tool

Effective early help relies upon local agencies working together to identify children and families who would benefit from this approach. Multi-agency working is supported through a variety of tools to aide professional judgements, but not replace them. In recent years, the Common Assessment Framework (CAF) has been replaced by an Early Help Assessment Tool (EHAT), which is based on the same principles as the CAF but it is more user-friendly and simpler to use. The EHAT is an initial assessment and planning tool that facilitates and coordinates multi-agency support. It standardises the assessment to identify the needs of both the children and the adults in the family to promote early intervention, with the aim of preventing any escalation of needs. It is a multi-agency tool, which can be used to develop a coordinated response, thereby improving involvement between agencies and ensuring that the child and their family are offered the support they need from wherever they need it.

Referral to children's social care

Where abuse or neglect are considered likely or have already occurred the health professional must make a referral to Children's Social Care. The welfare of the child must remain the focus. The process will be clearly defined within the Trust's Safeguarding Children Policy and Procedures, including what must be done if immediate action is required to ensure the safety of the child. Where the nurse is uncertain about what to do advice can be sought from a number of professionals, including a line manager or senior member of the team, named professionals, Children's Social Care, or those taking responsibility for safeguarding children 'Out of Hours'. 2021This might take the form of a multi-agency meeting or phone calls, and more than one discussion may be necessary. A strategy discussion can take place following a referral or at any other time, including during the assessment process. The nurse's role is to participate in the discussions and considerations about the child and a plan of safety, and know what services their organisation can offer. The nurse should be supported by the named professional for safeguarding and child protection or a senior colleague with appropriate experience. A decision will be made about what and how information will be shared with the parents/carers and the child.

Child protection conference

An initial child protection conference will be convened within 15 working days if child protection concerns are identified. This will bring the family members, and the CYP where appropriate, together with any advocates or supporters and the key professionals involved, including the consultant and the nurse, to make decisions about the future safety, health, and development of the CYP and to identify the key professionals involved with them and their family. Nurses may be asked to contribute to the assessment and the analysis of the findings as required by children's social care.

Where the threshold for the likelihood or actual significant harm has been met, CYPs will become subject to an individual child protection plan.

- A copy of the child protection plan should be available to the child's lead consultant, named professionals, and hospital social worker.
- A core group of key professionals involved with the CYP will meet in between conferences to develop and monitor progress of the plan.
- A further review conference will be held within three months of the initial conference and thereafter at least six monthly, to consider the effectiveness and impact of actions taken so far. A decision will be made to either discontinue the plan for the child, or consider other options, such as legal planning.
- Hospitals make internal arrangements for appropriate senior nursing staff to access the local Children's Social Care Emergency Duty Team (EDT) 'out of hours' or the local social work team when hospital social workers are not available.

When a nurse is alerted to the fact that a CYP attending hospital is already subject to a child protection plan the hospital social worker should be notified immediately, and the child's consultant and other professionals directly involved with the child's care should also be informed. For more information, see the section *Child Protection Information Sharing System*. The nurse or hospital social worker must inform the child's key worker in the local Children's Social Care team of the reason for admission (or attendance at an A&E or out-patient department). The nurse will be informed of the relevant details of the Child Protection Plan for the child, including who and what services are involved and who the key worker co-ordinating the plan is. Information is shared on a 'need to know' basis.

Family Group Conference

A family group conference (FGC) is a voluntary decision-making process led by family members supported by an independent FGC coordinator to assist the family to identify their own solutions to problems. The meeting empowers the wider family network to consider their strengths and abilities to make a safe plan for the child.

Looked after children (LAC)

Under the *Children Act 1989*, a child is looked after by a local authority if he or she is:

- Provided with accommodation for a continuous period of more than 24 hours (*Children Act 1989*, Section 20 [by voluntary agreement] and 21).
- Subject to a care order [Children Act 1989, Part IV] (forming the largest group).
- Subject to a placement order (for adoption).

At the end of March 2020, there were 80,080 looked after children (LAC) in England, an increase of 2% on the previous year. Children aged 10–15 years old comprise the largest group (39%), with under one-year-olds the smallest at 5%. The majority of children (65%), become LAC due to abuse or neglect, which has seen a gradual increase in recent years. The remainder are due to absent or dysfunctional parenting, families in acute distress, or other reasons (HM Government 2010; DfE 2020). Children who are looked after may have worse outcomes than those who are not in terms of physical and mental health, and educational attainment. Nurses should be familiar with the potential additional needs of this cohort and refer to the competency framework in the intercollegiate document "Looked after Children: roles and competencies of healthcare staff" (RCN RCPCH 2020). Children stop being looked after if they return to the family home or are adopted. If they remain in care when they reach their 18th birthday, children's services have a duty to continue to support them until 21 years of age or beyond.

Conclusion

All nurses involved in the care of CYPs must have sufficient knowledge and understanding of risks to children, how to recognise them, and how to seek help and report these concerns, and must also have an understanding of the roles of other professionals in the provision of services. All healthcare professionals need to be aware of risks posed by adult behaviours that affect parenting and other family and environmental factors, and must share concerns with appropriate professionals at an early stage.

No one professional has the full picture of a child's needs and circumstances. Professionals must work collaboratively to ensure a coordinated and child-centred approach to safeguarding and promoting the welfare of the child: We all have a responsibility for keeping children and young people safe.

References

Adoption and Children Act 2002. https://www.legislation.gov.uk/ukpga/2002/38/contents (accessed 23 August 2022).

Amiel, S. and Heath, I. (eds.) (2003). *Family Violence in Primary Care*. Oxford: Oxford University Press.

Birmingham LSCB (2010). *Serious Case Review for Khyra Ishaq*. Birmingham: LSCB.

Brandon, M., Belderson, P., Warren, C., et al. (2008). Research report DCFS-RR023. Analysing child deaths and serious injury through abuse and neglect: what can we learn? A biennial analysis of serious case reviews 2003–2005. London, DCSF. https://dera.ioe.ac.uk/7190/1/dcsf-rr023.pdf (accessed 23 August 2022).

Brandon, M., Bailey, S., Belderson, P. et al. (2009). *Understanding Serious Case Reviews and Their Impact. A Biennial Analysis of Serious Case Reviews 2005–2007*. London: DFES Research Report DCSF-RR129.

Brandon, M., Bailey, S., and Belderson, P. (2010). *Building on the Learning from Serious Case Reviews: A Two-Year Analysis of Child Protection Database Notifications 2007–2009*. London: Department for Education.

Brandon, M., Sidebotham, P., Bailey, S. et al. (2012). *New Learning from Serious Case Reviews: A Two Year Report for 2009–2011*. London: Department for Education.

Brandon, M., Bailey, S., Belderson, P., & Larsson, B. (2013). Neglect and Serious Case Reviews. A report from the University of East Anglia commissioned by the NSPCC. University of East Anglia/NSPCC. https://learning.nspcc.org.uk/research-resources/2013/neglect-serious-case-reviews (accessed 23 August 2022).

Brandon, M., Glaser, D., Maguire, S., McCrory, E., Lushey, C. & Ward, H. (2014). Missed opportunities: indicators of neglect – what is ignored, why, and what can be done? Research report. Childhood Wellbeing Research Centre. Loughborough University Institutional Repository. https://www.gov.uk/government/publications/indicators-of-neglect-missed-opportunities (accessed 23 August 2022).

Brandon, M., Sidebotham, P., Belderson, P. et al. (2020). *Complexity and challenge: a triennial analysis of SCRs 2014-2017: final report*. London:

Department for Education (DfE). https://assets.publishing.service.gov.uk/government/uploads/system/uploads/attachment_data/file/869586/TRIENNIAL_SCR_REPORT_2014_to_2017.pdf (accessed 23 August 2022).

Care Quality Commission (CQC) (2009). *Safeguarding Children: a review of arrangements in the NHS for safeguarding children.* London.

Chamberlain, T; George, N; Golden, S; Walker, F and Benton, T (2010). Tellus4 National Report DCSF Research Report DFE-RR218 DCSF.

Children Act. (1989). www.legislation.gov.uk/ukpga/1989/41/contents (accessed 23 August 2022).

Children Act 2004. Chapter 31. www.legislation.gov.uk/ukpga/2004/31/pdfs/ukpga_20040031_en.pdf (accessed 23 August 2022).

Children and Social Work Act (2017). https://www.legislation.gov.uk/ukpga/2017/16/contents (accessed 23 August 2022).

Children's Commissioner for England (2021). Launching the biggest ever consultation with children in England as part of Beveridge-style report into post-Covid childhood. https://www.childrenscommissioner.gov.uk/2021/04/19/launching-the-biggest-ever-consultation-with-children-in-england-as-part-of-beveridge-style-report-into-post-covid-childhood/ (accessed 23 August 2022).

Children's Commissioner for England (2015). Protecting children from harm. https://www.childrenscommissioner.gov.uk/report/protecting-children-from-harm/ (accessed 23 August 2022).

Children's Commissioner for England (2017). Barnahus: improving the response to child sexual abuse in England. https://www.childrenscommissioner.gov.uk/report/barnahus-improving-the-response-to-child-sexual-abuse-in-england/ (accessed 10 November 2022).

Children's Commissioner for England (2019). Keeping kids safe: Improving safeguarding responses to gang violence and criminal exploitation. https://www.childrenscommissioner.gov.uk/report/keeping-kids-safe/ (accessed 09 November 2022).

Children's Commissioner for England (2020a). Annual study of childhood vulnerability in England. https://www.childrenscommissioner.gov.uk/about-us/corporate-governance/annual-report-2019-20/ (accessed 10 November 2022).

Children's Commissioner for England (2020b). Childhood in the time of Covid (September). https://www.childrenscommissioner.gov.uk/report/childhood-in-the-time-of-covid/ (accessed 09 November 2022).

Cleaver, H., Unell, I., and Aldgate, J. (1999). *Children's Needs – Parenting Capacity: The Impact of Parental Mental Illness, Problem Alcohol and Drug Use, and Domestic Violence on children's Development.* London: HMSO.

Department for Children, Schools and Families (DCSF) (2009). Safeguarding disabled children: Practice guidance. https://www.gov.uk/government/publications/safeguarding-disabled-children-practice-guidance (accessed 10 November 2022).

Department for Education (DfE) (2017). Child sexual exploitation: definition and a guide for practitioners, local leaders and decision makers working to protect children from child sexual exploitation. https://www.gov.uk/government/publications/child-sexual-exploitation-definition-and-guide-for-practitioners (accessed 10 November 2022).

Department for Education (DfE) (2020). Reporting Year 2020: Characteristics of children in need. https://explore-education-statistics.service.gov.uk/find-statistics/characteristics-of-children-in-need/2020 (accessed 10 November 2022).

Department of Health (DH) (2004). *The National Service Framework for Children, Young People and Maternity Services.* London: HMSO.

Department of Health and Social Care (2017). Responding to domestic abuse: a resource for health professionals. https://www.basw.co.uk/resources/responding-domestic-abuse-resource-health-professionals (accessed 10 November 2022).

Ditch the label (2018). The annual bullying survey 2018. https://www.ditchthelabel.org/research-papers/the-annual-bullying-survey-2018/ (accessed 10 November 2022).

Education (Independent School Standards) (England) (Amendment) Regulations 2012. https://www.legislation.gov.uk/uksi/2012/2962/made (accessed 09 Novemmber 2022).

Education and Inspections Act 2006. https://www.legislation.gov.uk/ukpga/2006/40/contents (accessed 10 November 2022).

Ferguson, H. (2011). *Child Protection Practice.* Hampshire: Palgrave-MacMillan.

Gerhardt, S. (2004). *Why Love Matters: How Affection Shapes a baby's Brain.* Sussex, Hove: Routledge.

Glaser, D. (2003). Early experience, attachment and the brain. In: *Revolutionary Connections: Psychotherapy & Neuroscience* (eds. J. Corrigall and H. Wilkinson), 117–134. London: Karnac.

Haringey (2009). *Serious Case Review for Peter Connolly.* Haringey: LSCB.

Hicks, L. and Stein, M. (2010). *Neglect Matters a Multi-Agency Guide for Professionals Working Together on Behalf of Teenagers.* London: Department for Children, Schools and Families.

HM Government (2011, updated 2021). Revised Prevent Duty Guidance for England and Wales. https://www.gov.uk/government/publications/prevent-duty-guidance/revised-prevent-duty-guidance-for-england-and-wales (accessed 23 August 2022).

HM Government (2015). What to do if you're worried a child is being abused. https://assets.publishing.service.gov.uk/government/uploads/system/uploads/attachment_data/file/419604/What_to_do_if_you_re_worried_a_child_is_being_abused.pdf (accessed 23 August 2022).

HM Government (2018a). Information sharing: advice for practitioners providing safeguarding services to children, young people, parents and carers. https://assets.publishing.service.gov.uk/government/uploads/system/uploads/attachment_data/file/721581/Information_sharing_advice_practitioners_safeguarding_services.pdf (accessed 10 November 2022).

HM Government (2018b, updated 2020). Working Together to Safeguard Children: A guide to inter-agency working to safeguard and promote the welfare of children. https://www.basw.co.uk/resources/working-together-safeguard-children-guide-inter-agency-working-safeguard-and-promote (accessed 10 November 2022).

HM Government (2021). Children looked after in England including adoption: 2020 to 2021. https://www.gov.uk/government/statistics/children-looked-after-in-england-including-adoption-2020-to-2021 (accessed 10 November 2022).

Home Office (2013). Information for Local Areas on the change to the Definition of Domestic Violence and Abuse. https://www.gov.uk/government/publications/definition-of-domestic-violence-and-abuse-guide-for-local-areas (accessed 10 November 2022).

Home Office (2015). Mandatory reporting of female genital mutilation: procedural information. https://www.gov.uk/government/publications/mandatory-reporting-of-female-genital-mutilation-procedural-information (accessed 10 November 2022).

Home Office (2018). *Domestic Abuse: How to Get Help.* London: Home Office.

Home Office (2019, updated 2021). Domestic Abuse Bill. Policy paper. https://www.gov.uk/government/collections/domestic-abuse-bill (accessed 10 November 2022).

Horwath, J. (2010). Assessing children in need: background and context. In: *The Child's World. The Comprehensive Guide to Assessing Children in Need*, 2e (ed. J. Horwath). London: Jessica Kingsley, pp. 18–33.

Howe, D. (2005). *Child Abuse and Neglect: Attachment, Development and Intervention.* Basingstoke: Palgrave Macmillan.

Information Commissions Office (2018) Guide to the General Data Protection Regulation (GDPR). https://ico.org.uk/for-organisations/guide-to-data-protection/ (accessed 10 November 2022).

Jones, L., Bellis, M.A., Wood, S., et al. (2012). Prevalence and risk of violence against children with disabilities: a systematic review and meta-analysis of observational studies. The Lancet https://www.thelancet.com/pdfs/journals/lancet/PIIS0140-6736(12)60692-8.pdf (accessed 09 November 2022).

Jutte, S., Bentley, H., Tallis, D. et al. (2015). *How Safe Are Our Children? The Most Comprehensive Overview of Child Protection in the UK.* London: NSPCC.

Kolko, D.J. (2002). Child physical abuse. In: *APSAC Handbook of Child Maltreatment*, 2e (eds. J.E.B. Myers, L. Berliner, J. Briere, et al.). Thousand Oaks: Sage, pp. 21–54.

Laming, L. (2003a). *The Victoria Climbie Inquiry: Report of an Inquiry by Lord Laming.* London: The Stationery Office.

Lord Laming (2003b). The Victoria Climbié Inquiry. Crown Copyright 2003. https://www.gov.uk/government/publications/the-victoria-climbie-inquiry-report-of-an-inquiry-by-lord-laming (accessed 09 November 2022).

Laming, L. (2009). *The Protection of Children in England: A Progress Report.* London: The Stationery Office.

Lewis, G. and Drife, J. (2001). *Why Mothers Die: Report from the Confidential Enquiries into Maternal Deaths in the UK 1997–9; Commissioned by Department of Health from RCOG and NICE*. London: RCOG Press.

Lock R (2013). Serious case review re: Daniel Pelka: born 15th July 2007 died 3rd March 2012: overview report. Coventry Safeguarding Board.

London Safeguarding Children Partnership (2020, updated 2022). London Child Protection Procedures and Practice Guidance 7th edition. https://www.londoncp.co.uk (accessed 10 November 2022).

Meltzer, H., Doos, L., Vostanis, P. et al. (2009). The mental health of children who witness domestic violence. *Child & Family Social Work* 14 (4): 491–501.

Morrison, T. (2006). *Staff Supervision in Social Care: Making a Real Difference for Staff and Service Users*. Southampton: Pavilion Publishing.

National Child Mortality Database (2020). CDR Data: 2019/20. https://www.ncmd.info/publications/cdr-data-2019-20/ (accessed 10 November 2022).

National Institute for Health and Care Excellence (NICE) (2014). *Domestic Violence and Abuse: multi-agency working (PH50)*. https://www.nice.org.uk/guidance/ph50 (accessed 10 November 2022).

National Institute of Health and Clinical Excellence (NICE) (2009, updated 2017). Child maltreatment: when to suspect maltreatment in under 18s. When to Suspect Child maltreatment Guidance No 89. National Institute for Health and Care Excellence. www.nice.org.uk/guidance/cg89 (accessed 10 November 2022).

National Society for the Prevention of Cruelty to Children (NSPCC) (2012). Understanding the links: child abuse, animal abuse and domestic violence. Information for professionals. https://lx.iriss.org.uk/content/understanding-links-child-abuse-animal-abuse-and-domestic-violence (accessed 10 November 2022).

National Society for the Prevention of Cruelty to Children (NSPCC) (2020). How safe are our children? https://learning.nspcc.org.uk/research-resources/how-safe-are-our-children (accessed 10 November 2022).

NHS Digital (2020) Child protection information sharing service. https://digital.nhs.uk/services/child-protection-information-sharing-service (accessed 10 November 2022).

NHS England (2015). *Prevent Training and Competencies Framework*. London: NHS England.

Nursing and Midwifery Council (NMC) (2018). *The Code: Professional Standards of Practice and Behaviour for Nurses, Midwives and Nursing Associates*. London.

Office for National Statistics (2019). Child Sexual Abuse in England and Wales: a year ending March 2019. https://www.ons.gov.uk/peoplepopulationandcommunity/crimeandjustice/articles/childsexualabuseinenglandandwales/yearendingmarch2019 (accessed 10 November 2022).

Ofsted (2011). *Ages of Concern: Learning Lessons from Serious Case Reviews. A Thematic Report of Ofsted's Evaluation of Serious Case Reviews from 1 April 2007 to 31 March 2011*. London: Office for Standards in Education, Children's Services and Skills.

Peruzzi, A. (2013). From Childhood Deprivation to Adult Social Exclusion: Evidence from the 1970 British Cohort Study, Working paper 2013/5. Centre for Longitudinal Studies (University of London).

Poobalan, S., Aucott, L.S., and Ross, W.C.S. (2007). Effects of treating postnatal depression on mother–infant interaction and child development; systematic review. *The British Journal of Psychiatry* 191: 378–386.

Protection of Freedoms Act 2012. https://www.legislation.gov.uk/ukpga/2012/9/contents/enacted (accessed 10 November 2022).

Radford, L., Corral, S., Bradley, C. et al. (2011). *Child Abuse and Neglect in the UK Today*. London: NSPCC.

Reder, P. and Duncan, S. (1999). *Lost Innocents. A Follow-Up Study of Fatal Child Abuse*. London: Routledge.

Reder, P. and Duncan, S. (2003). Understanding communication in child protection networks. *Child Abuse Review* 12 (2): 82–100.

Rogers, M. (2013). *Daniel Pelka Serious Case Review*. Coventry: LSCB.

Royal College of Nursing (2019). Safeguarding Children and Young People: Roles and Competencies for Healthcare staff. 4th edition. www.rcn.org.uk/professional-development/publications/007-366 (accessed 10 November 2022).

Royal College of Nursing and Royal College of Paediatrics and Child Health (2020) Looked after Children: roles and competencies of healthcare staff. https://www.rcn.org.uk/professional-development/publications/rcn-looked-after-children-roles-and-competencies-of-healthcare-staff-uk-pub-009486 (accessed 10 November 2022).

Royal College of Paediatrics and Child Health (RCPCH) (2021). *Perplexing Presentations (PP)/Fabricated or Induced Illness (FII) in Children Guidance*. https://www.rcpch.ac.uk/news-events/news/new-guidance-perplexing-presentations-fabricated-or-induced-illness-children (accessed 10 November 2022).

SafeLives (2018a). Safe Young Lives; Young People and Domestic Abuse. http://safelives.org.uk/sites/default/files/resources/Safe%20Young%20Lives%20web.pdf (accessed 10 November 2022).

SafeLives (2018b). SafeLives Impact Report 2017–18. Getting it right the first time. https://safelives.org.uk/node/1395 (accessed 10 November 2022).

Serious Crime Act (2015). www.legislation.gov.uk/ukpga/2015/9/contents/enacted (accessed 10 November 2022).

Sexual Offences Act (2003). https://www.legislation.gov.uk/ukpga/2003/42/contents (accessed 10 November 2022).

Sidebotham, P., Brandon, M., Bailey, S., et al. (2016). Pathways to harm, pathways to protection: a triennial analysis of serious case reviews 2011 to 2014. Final report. Department for Education. https://www.gov.uk/government/publications/analysis-of-serious-case-reviews-2011-to-2014 (accessed 10 November 2022).

Skills for Care and Children's Workforce Development Council (2007). Providing effective supervision: a workforce development tool, including a unit of competence and supporting guidance. https://www.scie-socialcareonline.org.uk/providing-effective-supervision-a-workforce-development-tool-including-a-unit-of-competence-and-supporting-guidance/r/a11G00000017sifIAA (accessed 10 November 2022).

Smith, K., Chaplin, K., Elder, S., et al. (2011). Homicides, firearm offences and intimate violence 2009/10 (Supplementary volume 2 to Crime in England and Wales 2009/10 (2nd Edition]. Home Office Statistical Bulletin 01/11). https://www.gov.uk/government/uploads/system/uploads/attachment_data/file/116512/hosb0111.pdf (accessed 10 November 2022).

Social Care Institute for Excellence (2009). Think child, think parent, think family: a guide to parental mental health and child welfare. SCIE accredited Guide 30. www.scie.org.uk/publications/guides/guide30 (accessed 10 November 2022).

Springer, K.W., Sheridan, J., Kuo, D., and Carnes, M. (2011). Long-term physical and mental health consequences of childhood physical abuse: results from a large population-based sample of men and women. *Child Abuse & Neglect* 31 (5): 517–530.

Stevenson, O. (2007). *Neglected Children and their Families*, 2e. Oxford: Blackwell.

Strickland P. Allen G (2018). Domestic Violence in England and Wales. Briefing Paper number 6337. https://researchbriefings.parliament.uk/ResearchBriefing/Summary/SN06337 (accessed 10 November 2022).

United Nations (1989). The United Nations Convention on the Rights of the Child. https://www.unicef.org.uk/what-we-do/un-convention-child-rights/ (accessed 10 November 2022).

World Health Organisation (2022). Female genital mutilation. Key facts. https://www.who.int/news-room/fact-sheets/detail/female-genital-mutilation (accessed 10 November 2022).

Chapter 32

Tracheostomy care and management

Joanne Cooke

TD, MSc, BSc (hons), RN (adult), RN (child), NT: Advanced Nurse Practitioner, ENT/Tracheostomies, Great Ormond Street Hospital NHS Foundation Trust, London, UK

Chapter contents

Introduction	730
Care of the CYP with a tracheostomy	730
Ongoing care and management: TRACHE care bundle	735
Tracheostomy tube changes (planned)	745
Tracheostomy tubes for CYPs	746
Discharge planning	749
Decannulation	749
References	750
Further reading	751

Procedure guidelines

32.1 Preparation of the bed space for a new tracheostomy	731
32.2 Care and assessment of potential complications of a new tracheostomy	733
32.3 Other tracheostomy care needs	735
32.4 Tape changes (cotton)	737
32.5 Tracheostomy resuscitation	742
32.6 Suctioning a tracheostomy tube	743
32.7 Tube changes	746
32.8 Preparation for discharge	749

Principles table

32.1 Introducing feeding to a CYP with a new tracheostomy	734

The Great Ormond Street Hospital Manual of Children and Young People's Nursing Practices, Second Edition. Edited by Elizabeth Anne Bruce, Janet Williss, and Faith Gibson.
© 2023 John Wiley & Sons Ltd. Published 2023 by John Wiley & Sons Ltd.

Introduction

A tracheostomy is an artificial opening in the trachea, into which a tube is inserted to facilitate breathing. It is usually inserted between the second and fourth tracheal rings, depending on the size/anatomy of the child or young person (CYP) (see Figure 32.1). The formation of a tracheostomy can be a lifesaving procedure but can also be life threatening if it is not cared for appropriately and kept clear from secretions and blockages 24 hours a day.

Surgical tracheostomy in the paediatric population is indicated when a safe and protected airway is required in the long term. However, as with all surgical procedures, it is associated with certain risks and complications. More CYPs with chronic medical conditions are surviving, largely due to advances in tracheostomy care and technology support. The vast majority are now being cared for in their own homes and at school.

Morbidity and mortality rates in CYPs with a tracheostomy are reportedly two to three times higher than those seen in adults (Alladi et al. 2004). The overall mortality rate for a complication directly related to a paediatric tracheostomy is 0.7% (Carr et al. 2001). The majority of reported adverse incidents do not occur in the immediate postoperative period; late complications occurring a week or more after tracheostomy formation are four times more common (Corbett et al. 2007). Consistent high-quality tracheostomy care is essential and must be delivered by all those caring for these CYPs in both the hospital and community environments. Training in the management of paediatric tracheostomy care, based on formalised standards, would improve the consistency and quality of care.

Currently, there are no formally accepted national standards in the United Kingdom (UK) for paediatric tracheostomy management. Tracheostomy management has been the focus of a number of reviews in the UK over the last decade; however, paediatric patients have thus far been excluded from the analysis (Thomas and McGrath 2009; National Confidential Enquiry into Patient Outcome and Death [NCEPOD] 2014). The author of this guideline is a member of the National Tracheostomy Safety Project and has collaborated widely with the key stakeholders in tracheostomy care and developed guidance by consensus. The guidelines in this chapter are intended to support practitioners caring for CYPs with a tracheostomy. They do not negate the need to have appropriate clinical experience to care safely for this group of patients.

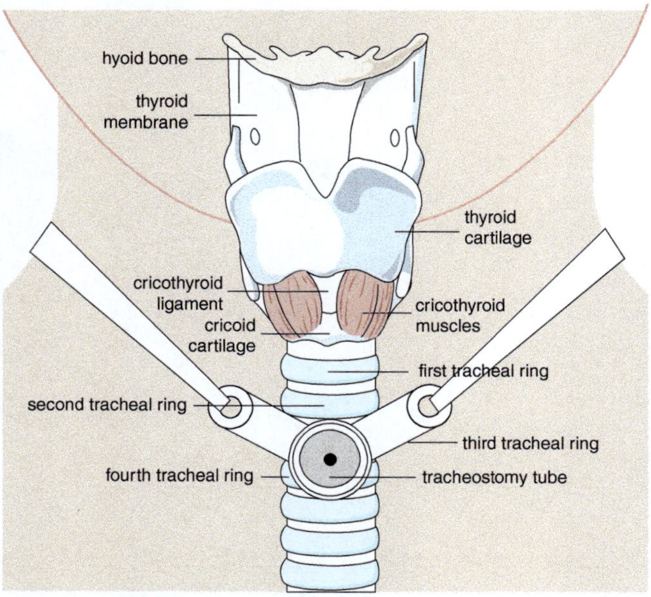

These resources are supported by local algorithms especially in resuscitation. Other useful resources include *Living with a Tracheostomy* and the UK National Tracheostomy Safety Project (www.tracheostomy.org.uk). For further information, see McGrath (2014).

Care of the CYP with a tracheostomy

CYPs with tracheostomies require constant supervision from those fully trained in its care.

Initial care: care of the new tracheostomy (less than seven days)
Caring for a newly formed tracheostomy

The initial care of a tracheostomy is very different from that for an established stoma. While there is no consensus about the timing of the first tube change, at GOSH, the first tube change occurs after one week. This is to ensure that the tube has been in situ long enough for the tract to form. The first tube change should be performed by someone experienced in the procedure, e.g. a Tracheostomy Nurse Practitioner (TNP) or the ears, nose, and throat (ENT) surgeon. Displacement of the tracheostomy tube is a potentially fatal complication. To ensure the safety of the airway, the trachea is sometimes sutured onto the skin at the time of surgery with tiny interrupted disposable sutures called maturation sutures. These provide an extra safety measure, which facilitates tube replacement (Craig et al. 2005). In addition, two long looped 'stay' sutures extend from inside the stoma and are taped to the chest (Figure 32.2). These sutures are attached to the tracheal wall on either side of the stoma. They assist with the opening of the stoma during the first week by raising the trachea to the surface of the skin and pulling the stoma apart so that a tube can be inserted. Tape on the CYP's chest will be labelled 'DO NOT REMOVE.' Stay sutures are removed after the first tube change when the stoma is more stable.

The CYP will have a portable chest X-ray immediately postoperatively to confirm tube position and to rule out a pneumothorax and surgical emphysema (Tarnoff, et al. 1998). The X-ray must be reviewed by the ENT team.

Early postinsertion complications

All equipment must be checked whenever a practitioner takes over the care of a CYP with a tracheostomy, including breaks and transfers. They must never be left alone and the accompanying carer (including parents where applicable) must, at a minimum, be able to recognise the signs of tracheostomy obstruction and initiate suctioning of the tracheostomy tube.

Figure 32.1 Placement of the paediatric tracheostomy.

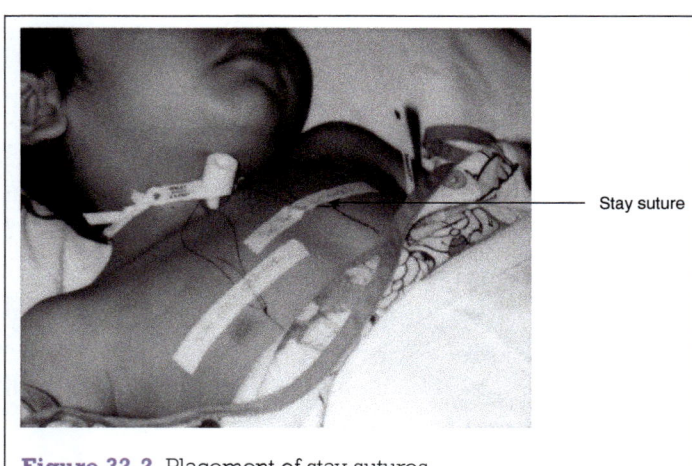

Figure 32.2 Placement of stay sutures.

Chapter 32 Tracheostomy care and management

Procedure guideline 32.1 Preparation of the bed space for a new tracheostomy

Principle	Rationale
1 The bed area must be easily accessible from both sides without obstruction for emergency and rapid access. The area should be free from luggage, chairs, etc.	1 To facilitate swift access to the CYP if required. The airway is potentially at risk and they may need immediate attention.
2 Appropriate resuscitation and suction equipment with correct tracheostomy fittings (15 mm Smiths Medical (Portex®) swivel connector and a male Smiths Medical (Portex®) adaptor for GOSH, Silver, and Montgomery tubes), checked and in full working order.	2 To facilitate emergency care quickly.
3 The CYP should have a dedicated tracheostomy trolley by the bedside containing: a) Oxygen saturation monitoring – if oxygen therapy is required. b) Suction catheters – of the correct size – see Suctioning a tracheostomy tube, procedure guideline 32.6 for more details. c) Gloves and appropriate personal protective equipment (PPE). d) Clean gauze. e) Bowl of clean water. f) 2 ml syringe. g) Ampoule 0.9% sodium chloride. h) Clinical waste bag 'for incineration'.	3 Specific emergency equipment must be rapidly accessible. a) To enable continual assessment of any supplementary oxygen requirements. b) To safely suction the tracheostomy tube. Refer to individual tube chart (Figure 32.3). c) To minimise the risk of cross-contamination. d) To clean stoma/secretions. e) To flush through suction tubing after use. f) To draw up saline for instillation. g) For irrigation. h) To meet local waste disposal guidelines.

Bivona Tracheostomy Tube

Tube Contains Metal

Great Ormond Street Hospital for Children NHS Foundation Trust

Made from opaque white silicone PVC. The silicone is reinforced with wire, producing a flexible tube that conforms to the shape of the trachea, and has a fixed flange which is kink resistant.

SPECIAL INSTRUCTIONS

Ferromagnetic coil precludes use during MRI, please change to a Shiley tube for scans

Ideal for children requiring long-term ventilation

Disconnection wedge must be used to facilitate separation from the tube

Changed – Monthly or PRN

The latex free-hydrophobic tube hinders protein adhesion thereby limiting secretion build up and bacterial colonisation

Tube can be sterilised in HSDU and re-used (5 times)

Ensure introducer kept with tube

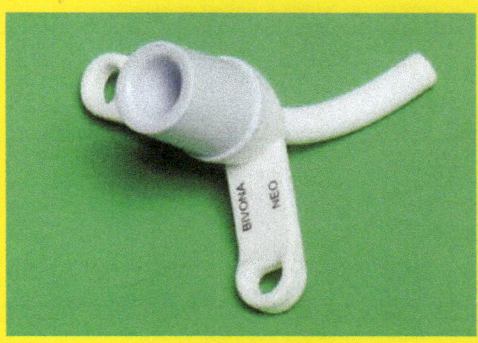

Tube size ……… fg NEO/PAED (delete as appropriate)

Suction Length ……… cm   Catheter Size ………… fg

Last Tube Change …/…/…

Contact ANP or ENT on call bleep if you have any concerns

STOMA CARE

Daily/PRN tape changes must be carried out.

Use of cotton tapes and Trachi-Dress

Correction tension – one finger space between tapes and child's neck

Emergency Box
Tube of the same size (Paed/Neo)
Tube ½ size smaller (Shiley)
Suction Catheter (same size as suctioning)
KY Jelly
Tracheostomy Tapes
Round Ended Scissors

© Great Ormond Street Hospital for Children NHS Foundation Trust November 2016 (Jo Cooke ANP)

Figure 32.3 Specific tube details.

(continued)

Procedure guideline 32.1 Preparation of the bed space for a new tracheostomy (*continued*)

Principle	Rationale
4 An emergency tracheostomy box containing: Two spare tracheostomy tubes: a) One the same size and type. b) One a half size smaller; must be a Shiley. c) A water-based lubricant such as Aqua lube® or K-Y jelly®. d) Round-ended scissors. e) Spare tracheostomy tapes. f) A suction catheter (same internal diameter ID) as the suction catheter used to suction the CYP).	4 To replace a blocked tube. a) To replace tube with like for like. b) For use if the stomal opening closes. c) For smoother insertion of the tracheostomy tube. d) To prevent trauma to the neck/tube when cutting the ties. e) To secure the tube. f) To 'railroad' the tube into the stoma (Seldinger technique; refer to Tracheostomy Resuscitation, Procedure Guideline 32.5).
5 PPE including apron, goggles or protective eye wear.	5 To minimise the risk of infection and ensure safety of staff caring for the CYP.
6 A resuscitator (ambu bag or t-piece) must be available at the bedside.	6 To enable effective emergency attention if required. This allows a more flexible approach to ventilating the CYP, if required.
7 A non-15 mm termination tube (flat-ended) requires an appropriately sized tracheal tube adapter that will 'fit into' the tube as required to create a 15 mm termination that will be compatible with resuscitation equipment.	7 To enable effective emergency attention if required. The size must be checked for a 'tight fit'.
8 Following an audit on dilators, practitioners are now taught the Seldinger technique, which has proven to be effective at replacing tracheostomy tubes (Lyons et al. 2007).	8 This is a noninvasive method of reinserting the tube using a suction catheter.

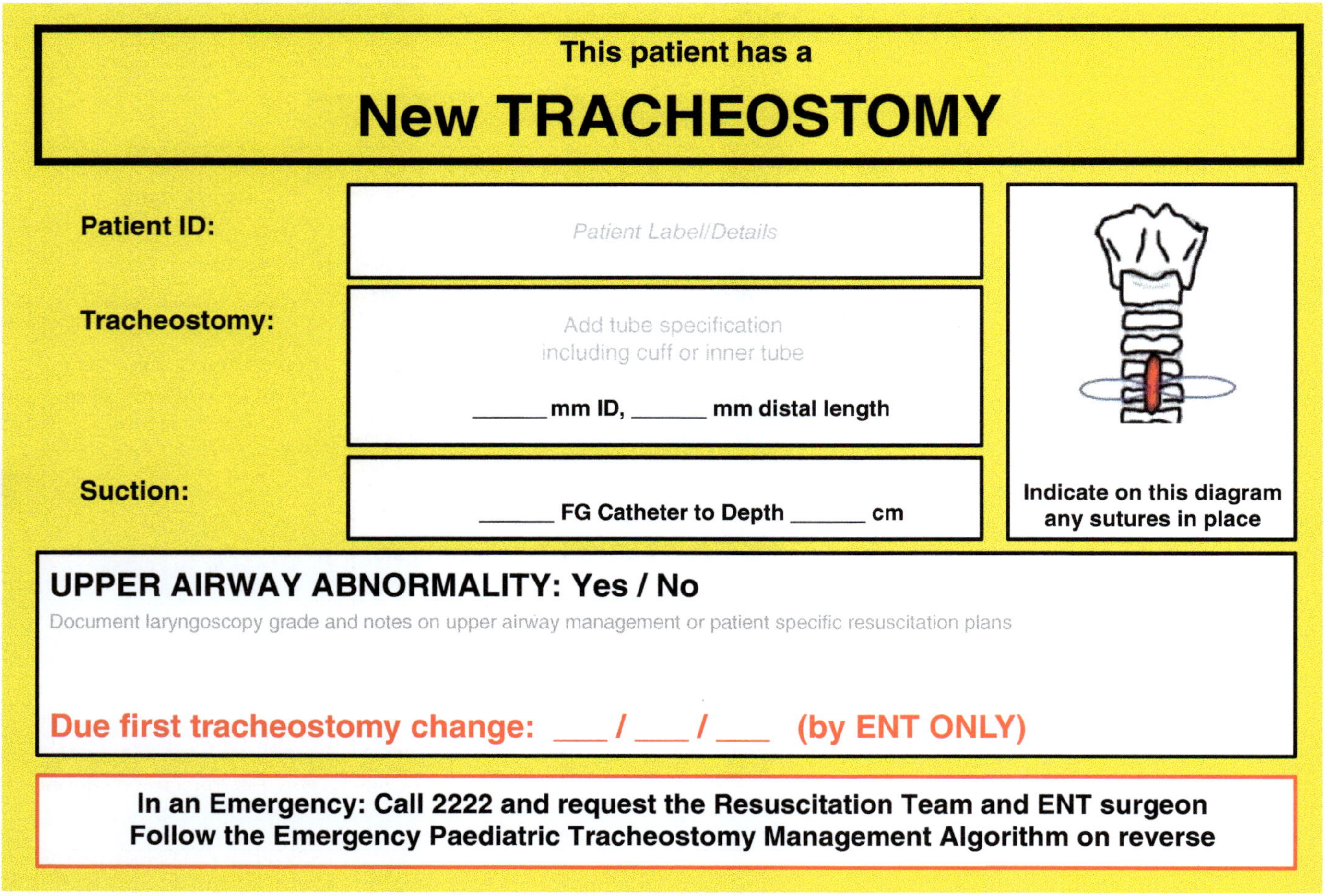

This patient has a

New TRACHEOSTOMY

Patient ID: *Patient Label/Details*

Tracheostomy: Add tube specification including cuff or inner tube

_____ mm ID, _____ mm distal length

Suction: _____ FG Catheter to Depth _____ cm

Indicate on this diagram any sutures in place

UPPER AIRWAY ABNORMALITY: Yes / No

Document laryngoscopy grade and notes on upper airway management or patient specific resuscitation plans

Due first tracheostomy change: ___ / ___ / ___ (by ENT ONLY)

In an Emergency: Call 2222 and request the Resuscitation Team and ENT surgeon
Follow the Emergency Paediatric Tracheostomy Management Algorithm on reverse

Figure 32.4 New tracheostomy bed head.

Chapter 32 Tracheostomy care and management

Initial complications following formation of a tracheostomy include haemorrhage, tube blockage, accidental decannulation, infection, and surgical emphysema. These are largely avoidable if the tracheostomy is carefully performed together with diligent and effective postoperative management. The stomal opening is made as safe as possible with the use of stay and maturation sutures. However, decannulation of the tube within the first few days may occur. This will compromise the airway and can make reinsertion of a tube difficult. Nursing care must be concentrated on maintaining patency with good humidity, securing the tube, regular suctioning, observing for potential complications, and training the carers.

A 'New tracheostomy' sign (Figure 32.4) should be placed at the head of the CYP's cot/bed for easy recognition and to alert all practitioners. This was developed as part of the National Tracheostomy Safety project (www.tracheostomy.org.uk) and highlights the basic first response to secure an airway. It is important that practitioners caring for the CYP know if the upper airway adjuncts are options should it become impossible to replace the tracheostomy in an emergency.

Procedure guideline 32.2 Care and assessment of potential complications of a new tracheostomy

Statement	Rationale
Initial observations and complications:	
1 The CYP's vital signs should be recorded in accordance with local policy, with the frequency reducing as their condition dictates. Refer to paediatric early warning scores.	1 To ensure the safe recovery from effects of anaesthesia. For more information regarding early warning scores, see Chapter 9: Early Recognition and Management of the Seriously Ill Child.
2 Practitioners should also carry out routine noninvasive observations: a) Check that the tape tension is correct and able to support the tracheostomy tube. b) Observe any neck swelling (surgical emphysema). c) Check for air entry through tube; place a finger above the tube opening and feel for a passage of air. d) Inspect the chest for bilateral chest movement. e) Auscultate the chest for equal air entry.	2 Early detection of potential complications. a) To prevent accidental decannulation and check for presence of surgical emphysema. b) To ensure early detection of complications. More information on surgical emphysema is provided later in this section. c–e) To confirm the position of the tracheostomy tube and rule out complications such as pneumothorax and surgical emphysema. d–e) These should be performed by an advanced practitioner or doctor.
Postprocedural tube check	
1 a) For the majority of cases a chest X-ray is performed in recovery. If this has not been done a portable chest X-ray must be performed as soon as possible after the CYP has returned to the ward, ideally within 1 hour. b) If the CYP is distressed or coughing a flexible endoscopy may be performed post operatively.	1 a) To confirm tube tip position, presence of a pneumothorax or in some cases surgical emphysema (Tarnoff et al. 1998). b) An endoscopy will also confirm the tube tip position.
2 Where possible, the CYP should not leave the ward during the first week unless medically indicated.	2 Their airway is at risk and they must remain in an environment that can effectively manage any complications. For any transfer between units, the CYP must be escorted by an ENT surgeon or the TNP.
Haemorrhage	
1 Observe the CYP and document any bleeding from the tracheostomy.	1 This may be primary, reactionary, or secondary. A large haemorrhage may be fatal. Secretions may initially be bloodstained, but should settle within a few hours.
2 If bleeding continues, contact the TNP or ENT team.	2 This may be suction trauma beyond the tube tip and the CYP may require a flexible endoscopy.
3 If any large haemorrhages occur, immediately call the ENT and/or clinical emergency teams as required.	3 The CYP may need to return to theatre.
Tube blockage	
1 a) Suction should be performed a minimum of: • ½-hourly suction for the first 24 hours. • Then 'as required' until first tube change (Park et al. 1999; Seay et al. 2002; Friedman et al. 2003; Onakoya et al. 2003; Yaremchuck 2003). Document in the CYP's healthcare record.	1 a) To prevent tube occlusion. Although research has shown that CYPs should be suctioned only when required, it is imperative that the tracheostomy tube is kept clear at all times during the first week, so practitioners must be mindful and carry out frequent checks on the tube.

(continued)

Procedure guideline 32.2 Care and assessment of potential complications of a new tracheostomy *(continued)*

Statement	Rationale
2 The CYP must be nursed in continuous humidity for the first week. The humidity may be discontinued for short periods, for bathing or playing.	2 To keep secretions loose and thus easily retrieved from the tube.
Accidental decannulation or tube displacement	
1 Care must be taken to ensure that the tube is correctly secured and does not become displaced/dislodged.	1 Early recognition of decannulation or tube displacement is essential as this could be life-threatening. Contact the ENT team/TNP or clinical emergency team for immediate assistance.
2 Check correct tension of the tapes, ensuring that only one finger width can be inserted between the neck and tapes.	2 To check that the tension of the tapes support the tube, reducing the risk of tube displacement (tapes too loose) or skin injury (tapes too tight).
3 Ensure close observation and recording of respiratory rate, effort, chest movements, and air entry on return to the ward.	3 To ensure prompt detection of decannulation or tube displacement.
Infection (chest/stoma site)	
1 • The stoma site must be cleaned daily. • The wound must be inspected for signs of inflammation, granulation, breakdown, and/or infection. • Observe and record in the CYP's healthcare record, the colour and nature of secretions. • Report to TNP or medical teams and document all signs of infection.	1 To ensure that any infection or skin breakdown is detected and treated appropriately and as quickly as possible.
Surgical emphysema	
1 a) Air may leak around the tube into the surrounding tissue. Contact the ENT team. b) Observe the CYP for neck/face swelling or any complaints of discomfort, pain, or difficulty with breathing. c) Regularly check tape tension for increased tightness.	1 a) The child may need to return to theatre for review. b) To detect emphysema. c) This not only confirms that the tube is secured correctly but may also indicate swelling.

Principles table 32.1 Introducing feeding to a CYP with a new tracheostomy

Principle	Rationale
1 If there have been no previous feeding concerns, the CYP may recommence their normal feeds after a specified time of being 'nil orally'. This is normally 3 hours postoperation, but practitioners must confirm this with the anaesthetic chart instructions.	1 The vocal cords are sprayed during procedure, making them less responsive and effective in protecting the airway from aspiration. The effect of the local anaesthetic can continue for up to 3 hours.
2 Water should be offered initially. If the CYP shows signs of aspiration (e.g. coughing after/during drinking, or visible drink coming out of the tracheostomy), keep them nil orally and contact the ENT team and speech and language therapist (SALT).	2 To ensure they are not put at risk of aspiration and that individual feeding issues are addressed.
3 For a CYP who has had feeding difficulties or has never fed orally, consultation with a SALT should be sought before commencing oral feeds.	3 To ensure they are not put at risk of aspiration and that individual feeding issues are addressed.
4 It is important that the CYP with a tracheostomy remains systemically hydrated and an increase their fluid intake should be considered during illnesses such as vomiting, diarrhoea, pyrexia, etc.	4 Good systemic hydration will help keep secretions loose and allow for easy retrieval on suctioning.

Procedure guideline 32.3 Other tracheostomy care needs

Statement	Rationale
1 Change the tapes at least daily. Observe stoma condition. Record in CYP's health care record.	1 To minimise bacterial colonisation of the skin/stoma area and monitor stoma healing.
2 a) A suitable dressing, such as Trachi-dress®, should be inserted behind the flanges (shiny side to skin). b) Avoid using bulky substitutes.	2 a) To protect the skin. Use of the correct dressing will enhance skin protection and reduce the risk of complications. b) These may pull the tube away from the neck precipitating accidental decannulation.
3 Never use cotton wool or cut keyhole gauze dressings.	3 Flecks of displaced cotton may enter the respiratory tract.
4 The tracheostomy tube should be changed for the first time 7 days after surgery. The tracheostomy tube should normally be changed for the first time by someone experienced and competent to do so, e.g. ENT surgeon or TNP. The stay sutures will be removed at this time. Document in the CYP's healthcare record.	4 The stoma is still new and not fully formed.
5 Once the stability of the tracheostomy stoma and tract has been verified the CYP may be allowed off the ward with a person appropriately trained in routine and emergency tracheostomy skills.	5 Continuous risk assessment of the tracheostomy stoma will ensure the appropriate staff care for the CYP in each environment.

Ongoing care and management: TRACHE care bundle

Following a multidisciplinary review of morbidity associated with paediatric tracheostomy a TRACHE care bundle (Figure 32.5) was developed. It highlighted the six main areas of concern relating to tracheostomy care.

T = Tapes: Keep tube secure

A tracheostomy tube is held in place with cotton tapes around the neck. Security of the tracheostomy tube is a key principle in maintaining airway safety. Paediatric patients provide a variety of challenges in achieving this with accidental decannulation occurring in around 5% of paediatric tracheostomies (Thomas and McGrath 2009). It had been noted that Velcro® neck tapes were more easily undone by the patient or became attached to clothing and that, as a method of fixation, were associated with a higher rate of accidental decannulation. Accordingly, the departmental policy now is for the exclusive use of hand-tied cotton tapes to secure tracheostomy tubes. To address issues related to these ties, a new product was developed with Marpac® from Platon Medical to offer increased comfort and safety. These were implemented across the hospital in 2013. If families arrive in the trust with Velcro tapes, they are changed to cotton for the duration of their stay. If Velcro ties are used then a risk assessment must be completed in accordance with Trust policy and documented in the local and trust risk registers.

A rolled-up towel or blanket should be placed under the shoulders to extend the neck and give a better visibility of the tube and stoma (Figure 32.6). Tape tension should allow one finger between the neck and the tracheostomy tapes (Figure 32.7).

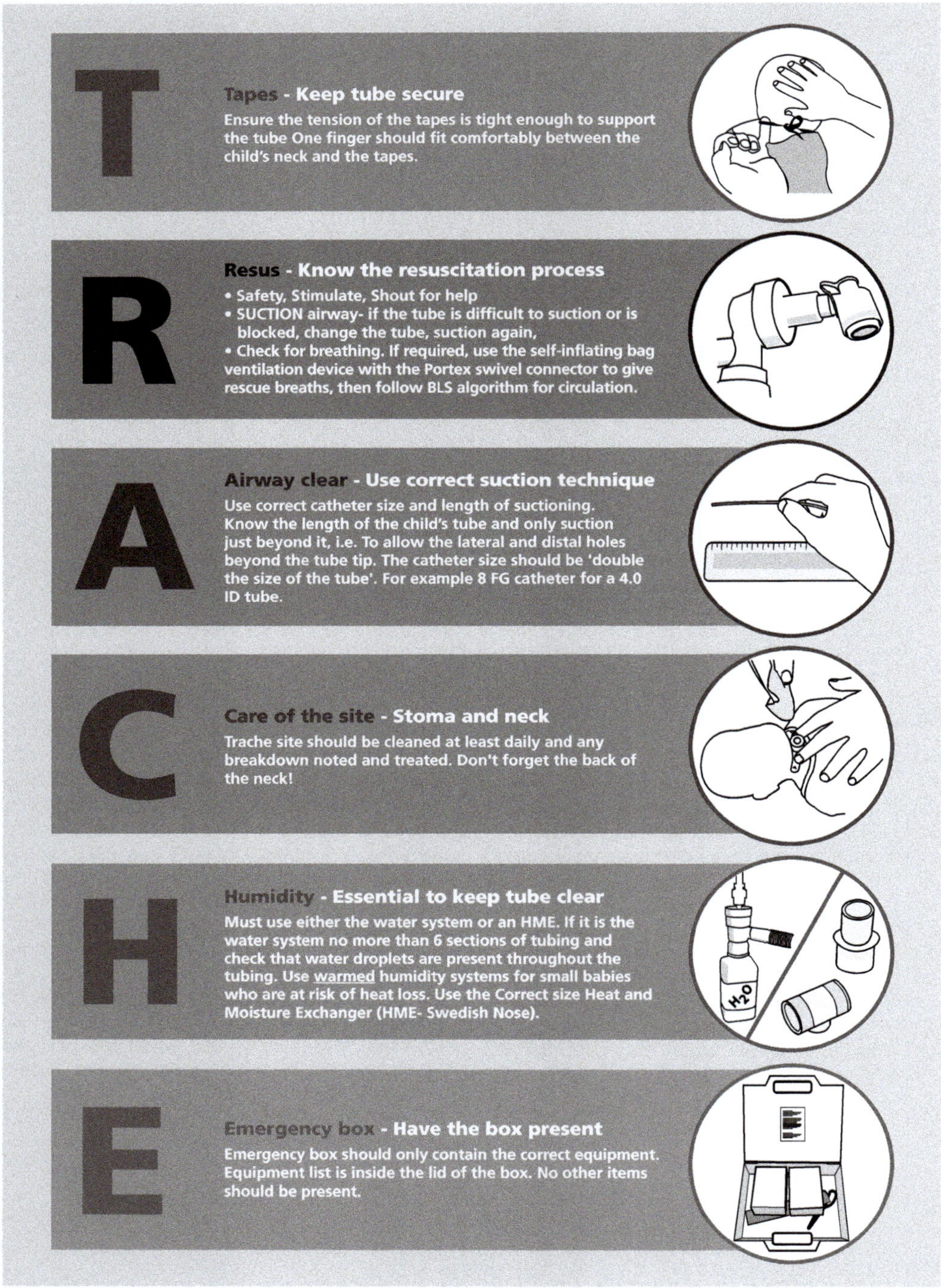

Tapes - Keep tube secure
Ensure the tension of the tapes is tight enough to support the tube One finger should fit comfortably between the child's neck and the tapes.

Resus - Know the resuscitation process
- Safety, Stimulate, Shout for help
- SUCTION airway- if the tube is difficult to suction or is blocked, change the tube, suction again,
- Check for breathing. If required, use the self-inflating bag ventilation device with the Portex swivel connector to give rescue breaths, then follow BLS algorithm for circulation.

Airway clear - Use correct suction technique
Use correct catheter size and length of suctioning. Know the length of the child's tube and only suction just beyond it, i.e. To allow the lateral and distal holes beyond the tube tip. The catheter size should be 'double the size of the tube'. For example 8 FG catheter for a 4.0 ID tube.

Care of the site - Stoma and neck
Trache site should be cleaned at least daily and any breakdown noted and treated. Don't forget the back of the neck!

Humidity - Essential to keep tube clear
Must use either the water system or an HME. If it is the water system no more than 6 sections of tubing and check that water droplets are present throughout the tubing. Use warmed humidity systems for small babies who are at risk of heat loss. Use the Correct size Heat and Moisture Exchanger (HME- Swedish Nose).

Emergency box - Have the box present
Emergency box should only contain the correct equipment. Equipment list is inside the lid of the box. No other items should be present.

Figure 32.5 TRACHE care bundle.

Chapter 32 Tracheostomy care and management

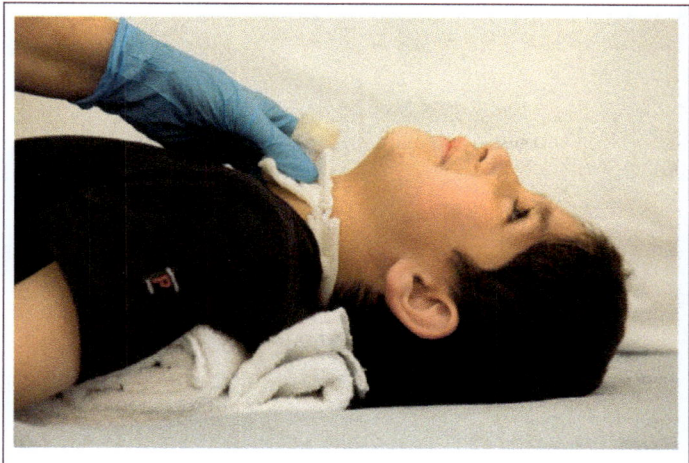

Figure 32.6 Demonstrating tube/tape change position.

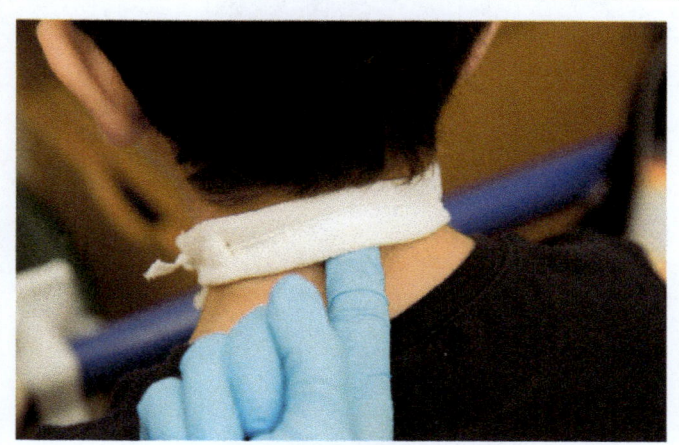

Figure 32.7 Confirming correct tape tension.

Procedure guideline 32.4 Tape changes (cotton)

A tracheostomy tube is held in place with cotton tapes around the neck. It is essential that the ties are secure and the tension is correct. The tapes are secured with knots tied either side of the tracheostomy tube. Velcro ties are not routinely used at GOSH as they can be easily undone by young children (Hall et al. 2017). Velcro tapes should not be used with silcone tracheostomy tubes as they can damage the silicone.

Statement	Rationale
1 All staff/parents/carers should be taught to tie the tapes in the same way.	1 To ensure continuity of training. Ensure they watch the tape changing webcast (https://youtu.be/6vrYRKlhZSg)
2 Tracheostomy tape changes are normally performed daily.	2 To ensure comfort and cleanliness and to assess the stoma site.
3 Only personnel competent in the technique should change tracheostomy tapes. Two people are required for the procedure.	3 To ensure the CYP's safety during the procedure.
4 The following equipment should be prepared and readily available: a) Appropriate emergency equipment. b) Gauze swabs and 0.9% saline/alternative cleaning solution. c) GOSH uses Marpac® tracheostomy ties d) Round-ended scissors. e) A towel or pillow to place under the shoulders. f) A blanket to swaddle a baby or toddler g) Suction equipment available (see Procedure Guideline 32.6). h) Appropriate PPE. i) CYP's own comforter, e.g. dummy, as appropriate.	4 a) For management of accidental decannulation. c) Marpac tapes are padded for comfort and have cotton ties for security. e) To hyperextend the neck, making observation and cleaning of the stoma easier. f) To minimise the risk of accidental decannulation.

(continued)

Procedure guideline 32.4 Tape changes (cotton) *(continued)*

Statement	Rationale
5 Options for keeping the young child still must be discussed, as swaddling may cause increased distress. Involve the play specialist where possible. Most children will settle once they get used to the procedure, especially when parents/carers begin to do it. An older CYP may not require holding. Some children assist with the procedure by holding the tracheostomy tube in place and some may even prefer to sit during a change.	5 To ensure the CYP is as comfortable as possible during the procedure and has a say in the procedure as their age and mental capability allows.
6 **To change the tracheostomy tapes:**	
a) Perform hand hygiene, put on gloves, apron, and protective eye wear (parents/carers do not need to wear the protective clothing).	a) To reduce the risk of infection/cross contamination.
b) The warmed saline should be poured onto the gauze swabs.	
c) Assistant to swaddle baby, exposing the shoulders and above.	c, d) To provide easy access to the tracheostomy.
d) Place baby/child in supine position, with a rolled up towel under shoulders. As mentioned above, some older CYPs may wish to sit. The rest of this procedure is described for babies and younger children in mind and can be adapted for the older/more co-operative child. **NB. Do not compromise safety for child's position preference.**	
e) Assistant should hold tube in position using either their thumb and index finger or index and middle finger (see Figure 32.6). Minimal pressure should be applied.	e) To support the tracheostomy tube and prevent an accidental decannulation.
f) Tape changer should cut the tapes between the knot and the flange and remove ties.	f) For comfort and to prevent any risk to the CYP.
g) The stoma site (above, below, and under each flange and back of the neck should be cleaned and thoroughly dried with the saline and gauze using a clean technique.	g) For patient comfort and to prevent infection and loss of skin integrity.
h) Place the tapes behind the child's neck (ensure they have already been cut to size). Thread the new tape through the flange on the side *furthest* away from the tape changer.	
i) Tie the tapes using three knots, ensuring the tape is flat to the skin.	
j) Thread tape through *near* side flange, tie once, and make a bow.	
k) Check tape tension by raising baby/child to a sitting position while the assistant continues to hold the tube in position. With their head bent forward it should be possible to slip one finger comfortably between the ties and the neck (Figure 32.7).	k) To ensure the tapes are firm enough to hold the tube safely in position.
l) If the ties are too tight or loose, lay the baby/child back down, undo the bow, and readjust.	
m) If the tension is correct, lay the baby/child down and change the bow into three knots by pulling the loops of the bow through to create a second knot.	m) So that the tension is not lost.
n) Tie one further knot to secure the ties.	
o) Cut off excess tape to leave 1 cm remaining.	
p) Assistant may release the tube ONLY when instructed to do so.	
q) Ensure baby/child is made comfortable.	
r) Clear away equipment according to local waste disposal policy. Wash hands.	r) To reduce risk of cross-infection and contamination.
s) Record the tape change in the CYP's healthcare records.	s) To ensure good communication between colleagues.
t) Check all equipment is replaced and restocked as necessary.	

This patient has a
TRACHEOSTOMY

Patient ID : _Patient Details_

Tracheostomy: Add tube specification including cuff or inner tube
_____ mm ID, _____ mm distal length

Suction: _____ FG Catheter to Depth _____ cm

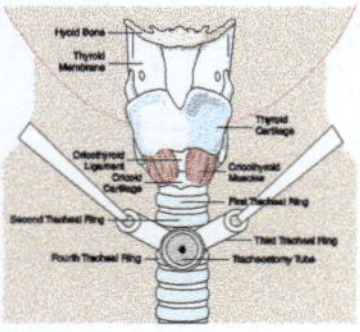

UPPER AIRWAY ABNORMALITY: Yes / No please give details of any expected difficulty

Emergency Paediatric Tracheostomy Management

Basic Response

SAFETY - STIMULATE - SHOUT FOR HELP - OXYGEN

- **SAFE:** Check Safe area, Stimulate, and Shout for help, CALL 2222 (hospital) or 999 (home)
- **AIRWAY:** Open child's airway: head tilt / chin lift / pillow or towel under shoulders may help
- **OXYGEN:** Ensure high flow oxygen to the tracheostomy AND the face as soon as oxygen available
- **Capnograph:** Exhaled carbon dioxide waveform may indicate a patent airway (secondary responders)

SUCTION TO ASSESS TRACHEOSTOMY PATENCY

Remove any attachments: humidifier (HME), speaking valve and change inner tube (if present)
Inner tubes need re-inserting to connect to bagging circuits

Can you pass a SUCTION catheter? — Yes →

The tracheostomy tube is patent
- Perform tracheal suction
- Consider partial obstruction
- Consider tracheostomy tube change

CONTINUE ASSESSMENT (ABCDE)

No ↓

EMERGENCY TRACHEOSTOMY TUBE CHANGE

Deflate cuff (if present). Reassess patency after any tube change
1st – same size tube, 2nd – smaller size tube
* 3rd – smaller size tube sited over suction catheter to guide
IF UNSUCCESSFUL – REMOVE THE TUBE

IS THE PATIENT BREATHING? - Look, listen and feel at the mouth and tracheostomy/stoma

No ↓   Yes →

5 RESCUE BREATHS – USE TRACHEOSTOMY IF PATENT

Patent Upper Airway – deliver breath to the mouth
Obstructed Upper Airway – deliver breath to tracheostomy/stoma

CHECK FOR SIGNS OF LIFE ? – START CPR

15 compressions : 2 rescue breaths
Ensure help or resuscitation team called

RESPONDS: continue oxygen, reassessment and stabilisation

Plan for definitive airway if tube change failure

*3-smaller size tube sited over suction catheter to guide: to be used if out of hospital

Figure 32.8 Tracheostomy emergency algorithm with tube requirements.

R = Resuscitation: Know the resuscitation process

The basics of cardiopulmonary resuscitation (CPR) and basic life support (BLS) are universal to all protocols for emergency care: airway management; rescue breathing; circulatory support.

The airway element of BLS will require modification in CYPs with tracheostomies. It is therefore essential that practitioners have received training in both routine and tracheostomy BLS. BLS is similar in the sequence of skills to be performed for those with a tracheostomy: Safety, Stimulate, Shout, Suction/Site (tube is in situ), Airway, Breathing, Circulation. When applied to a patient with a tracheostomy, CPR may be more difficult to teach and to learn because additional processes are required to determine and correct the cause of the collapse. Practitioners caring for a CYP with a tracheostomy must familiarise themselves with the tracheostomy resuscitation algorithm (Figure 32.8). Patients with a tracheostomy must always have their specific emergency equipment correctly assembled and easily accessible as previously discussed.

Paediatric Intermediate Life Support courses (PILS) for clinical staff include teaching about resuscitation in CYPs with tracheostomies. This information can be further reinforced by attendance at dedicated tracheostomy simulation training and study days.

The resuscitation algorithms used at GOSH (Figures 32.8 to 32.10) incorporate the bed head with the hospital algorithm for the emergency response to a tracheostomy concern.

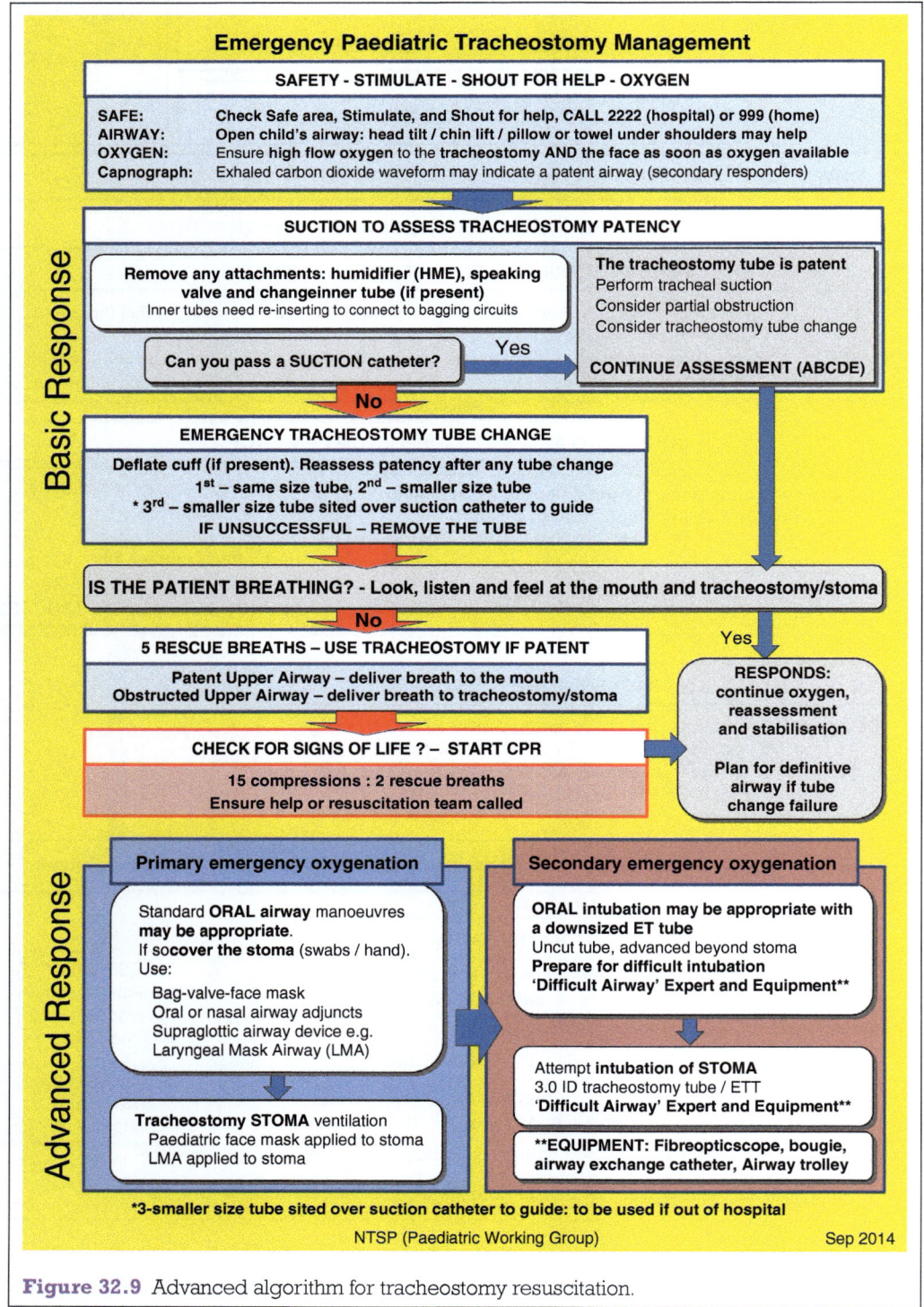

Figure 32.9 Advanced algorithm for tracheostomy resuscitation.

Chapter 32 Tracheostomy care and management

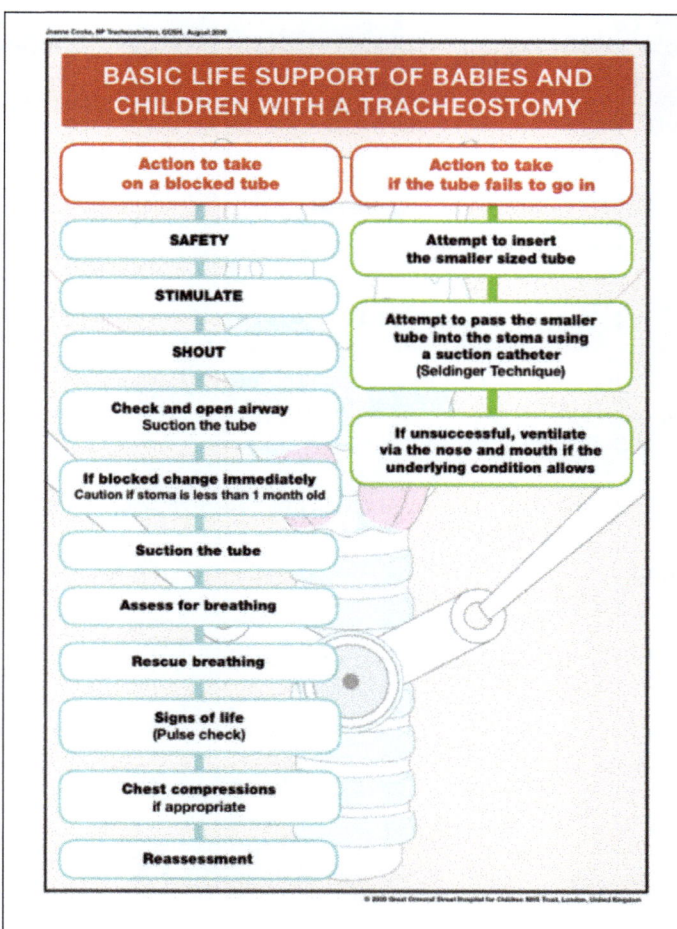

Figure 32.10 Basic tracheostomy emergency algorithm (parents and carers).

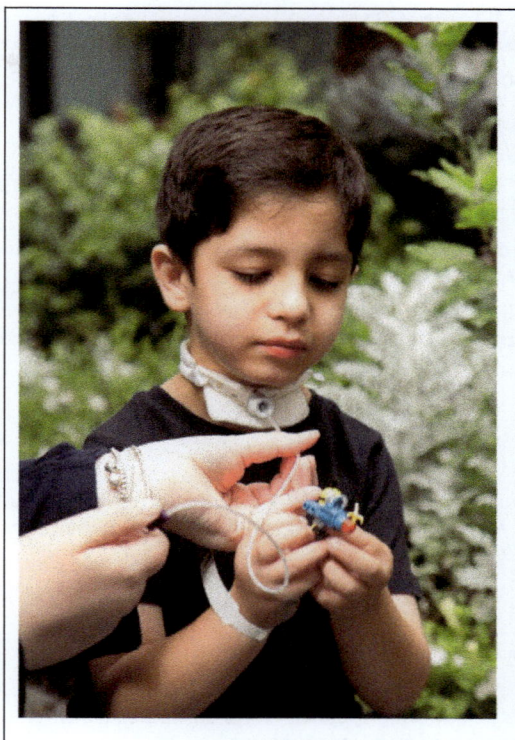

Figure 32.11 Suctioning a tracheostomy tube.

The aim of airway suction is to clear secretions to maintain a patent airway. Suction is used to clear retained or excessive respiratory tract secretions in those CYPs who are unable to do so effectively for themselves. This could be due to the presence of an artificial airway, such as an endotracheal or tracheostomy tube, or a poor cough, e.g. due to excessive sedation or a neurological condition. Having an artificial airway in situ impairs the cough reflex and may increase mucus production (Walsh et al. 2011). Therefore, in neonatal and paediatric intensive care units, suctioning of an artificial airway is likely to be a common procedure.

Suction is a procedure that is regularly carried out by healthcare workers (HCWs) and in some cases by parents or carers. The aim is to clear the airway and in doing so to reduce work of breathing and the risk of atelectasis, thereby maintaining or improving gas exchange. Those performing suction should be aware of the potentially harmful side effects and have the skills and competence to assess the need for suction and to perform it safely and effectively while minimising the potential side effects. The effects that need to be minimised during suction are:

- Tracheobronchial trauma
- Atelectasis
- Hypoxia
- Cardiovascular changes
- Alterations in intracranial pressure
- Pneumothorax
- Infection
- Formation of distal granulation tissue or ulceration.

(Davies et al. 2015; Edwards 2018).

Although care should be taken to minimise the occurrence of the above side effects it is of paramount importance that the objective, the maintenance of a patent airway, is achieved. When suctioning is indicated, the decision to withhold suction to avoid potential adverse events may result in, for example, a blocked endotracheal tube (ETT) and the risks associated with an emergency reintubation (Davies et al. 2015).

The CYP and equipment should be prepared and the procedure should be carried out as quickly as possible to prevent loss of lung volume. This may be caused by taking too long to perform suction (Tingay et al. 2010).

A = Airway: Use Correct Suction Equipment

The importance of precise suctioning cannot be underestimated in paediatric tracheostomy care (see Figure 32.11). If the suction length is too short, the patient is at risk of tube blockage, yet if the suction length is too long it may lead to tracheal trauma and can result in distal soft tissue trauma and overgrowth.

Procedure guideline 32.5 Tracheostomy resuscitation

Statement	Rationale
1 Starting BLS quickly is extremely important.	1 To prevent/minimise hypoxia and subsequent tissue death. Early intervention may prevent progression into full cardiorespiratory arrest.
2 Ensure safety of yourself and the CYP including appropriate PPE.	
3 Stimulate the CYP and call their name, taking care to support their head and body.	3 This may be sufficient to rouse them.
4 Call for assistance from colleagues. If non responsive, **summon the clinical emergency team immediately.**	4 Always summon more help, to assist in tube changes, bringing other equipment, etc.
5 If you are by yourself, **do not** leave the CYP at this stage.	5 Commencing airway breathing, respiratory support is of primary importance as per basic life support policy.
6 Open and check the CYP's airway by placing them supine on a flat firm surface.	6 To tilt the head and expose the airway.
7 It may be helpful to put a folded towel under the shoulders, but only if this is immediately available. Do not waste time by collecting this equipment.	7 To extend the neck and visualise the airway stoma. To start BLS as quickly as possible.
8 Gently tilt the tip of the chin upward, taking care not to press on soft tissue underneath.	8 To visualise the tube.
9 Inspect tube for obvious problems, i.e. signs of blockage: crusts, kinks, or dislodgement.	9 Initial assessment of the airway is important for effective future support.
10 If in any doubt about the CYP's condition, summon the clinical emergency team immediately.	
11 Suction the tracheostomy tube.	11 In most circumstances suctioning will clear the obstruction.
12 Change the tracheostomy tube immediately if the tube appears blocked or any resistance is felt and the CYP is in distress. **Exercise caution if the stoma is less than 1 week old; if there is time, contact the TNP/ENT team/Emergency team first.** However, if the CYP's condition is unstable, summon the Clinical Emergency Team immediately.	12 If there is a physical airway obstruction changing the tracheotomy tube will improve their condition.
13 The same size tube should be inserted. If unable to insert the same size tube try to insert the smaller, stiffer one.	13 On occasions the stomal opening can close, so attempts to replace a narrower airway must be attempted.
14 If the stoma closes and the smaller tube cannot be replaced, remove the obturator from the smaller tube and pass a suction catheter through the tube. Then attempt to insert the end of the catheter through the stoma opening and guide the tracheostomy tube along the catheter and through the stoma - Seldinger technique (Lyons et al 2007).	
15 If this is also unsuccessful, consider conventional rescue breaths (e.g. mouth-to-mouth or BVM to nose and mouth and/or LMA over the stoma). These options may not be appropriate for some CYPs due to their underlying airway problem; practitioners must therefore always be aware of the underlying disease/anatomy.	15 Practitioners must be aware of the airway aetiology so that they can decide the most appropriate way to manage the airway.
16 **Assess breathing:** Supporting the new tube, place the side of your face over the tracheostomy tube to listen and feel for any breathing. At the same time look at the CYP's chest to observe any breathing movement. Take up to a maximum of 10 seconds to do this.	16–19 To adhere to national life support assessment criteria (Resuscitation Council [UK] [RCUK] 2021).
17 If the CYP is breathing adequately, give oxygen and keep their airway open by regular suction and wait for the clinical emergency team or other support e.g. ENT/TNP. Secure the tube.	

Chapter 32 Tracheostomy care and management

Procedure guideline 32.5 Tracheostomy resuscitation (continued)

Statement	Rationale
18 If the CYP is not breathing (or only making agonal gasps), commence artificial respiration with a bag-valve system directly connected to the tracheostomy tube and administer five rescue breaths.	18 Refer to Resuscitation Guidelines (RCUK 2021) regarding the use of a Bag Valve Mask (BVM).
19 Ensure that the breaths are effective by observing chest movement. If the chest doesn't move, consider suctioning / changing the tube/repositioning the CYP.	19 The tube may be displaced or occluded beyond the tube tip.
20 Oxygen should be set at a minimum of 15 litres.	20 To ensure adequate oxygen delivery.
21 Parents/carers will be taught mouth to tracheostomy resuscitation by a suitably qualified BLS instructor before discharge. They are given a Laerdal Valve Pocket Mask to facilitate this.	21 To enable parents to secure the airway and perform BLS in an emergency situation at home.
22 Although community teams will supply the equipment for discharge, the parents/carers should be given two pairs of Velcro tapes, two disconnection wedges, and a laerdal valve. Practitioners should seek advice from the TNP; these items should be added to their emergency boxes when they get home. A rebreathing circuit will be provided for a ventilator dependent or high risk CYP.	22 To ensure that the family are fully equipped to deal with any emergency situations.
23 Parents/carers require both theoretical and practical teaching, practice of both emergency algorithms, management of a blocked tube, and action to take if the tracheostomy tube cannot be replaced (Seldinger technique). Practitioners teaching parents/carers must have appropriate knowledge and experience in both areas. A modified 'Resus baby' and 'Little Junior' can be used for BLS and a Smiths Medical (Portex®) percutaneous tracheostomy manikin for parents/carers to practice the Seldinger technique.	23 Education to assess carer's knowledge and competence is vital to ensure the CYP's safety. Practitioners / carer must watch the emergency management podcast (https://youtu.be/5wd7KLo32fU).

BLS instructions can be found on the RCUK Guidelines (2021) and in Chapter 30: Resuscitation.

Procedure guideline 32.6 Suctioning a tracheostomy tube

Statement	Rationale
1 Gather the following equipment: • Suction catheters of the correct size. • Suction unit with variable vacuum control. • Appropriate PPE. • Bottled water (to flush tubing). • 2 ml syringe with 0.9% sodium chloride for irrigation (**not for routine suctioning**). • Waste bag 'for incineration'.	
2 Perform hand hygiene.	2, 3 To minimise the risk of infection.
3 Sanitise hands using an alcohol based gel	
4 Turn the suction unit on, check the vacuum pressure and set to the appropriate level, for the CYP's age.	4 To use the correct suction pressure that maximises suction, and minimises complications.
5 a) The carer MUST know the length and type of the tracheostomy tube. b) If the tube is fenestrated then an un-fenestrated inner tube should be inserted prior to suctioning.	5 a) To prevent distal trauma from deep suctioning. b) To prevent the catheter going through the fenestration and causing trauma to the posterior tracheal wall.
6 a) Insert the catheter gently into the tracheostomy tube, far enough to ensure that the lateral and distal holes just pass through the tip of the tube. Use the graduations on the catheter as a guide. b) Do not apply suction on insertion.	6 To prevent distal tracheal damage. Adult literature suggests longer distances (Luce et al. 1998); the distance between the tube tip and the carina may be only a few millimetres.

(continued)

Procedure guideline 32.6 Suctioning a tracheostomy tube (continued)

Statement	Rationale
7 Handle only the proximal end of the catheter. Catheters should be discarded if the end has been touched before insertion.	7 To minimise the risk of infection.
8 a) Once the catheter has been inserted, apply suction by placing thumb over the valve, found either on catheter or suction tubing. Do not kink the catheter (Czarnik et al. 1991). b) Do not employ an intermittent suction technique.	8 a) To prevent a vacuum build-up, which on release may cause high suction pressures, resulting in biopsies of fragile tracheal mucosa.
9 Slowly withdraw the catheter straight out of the tube, maintaining the vacuum. There is no need to rotate the suction catheter on withdrawal.	9 Both the distal and lateral holes on the new style of catheter allow for circumferential suctioning.
10 The maximum duration of each suction attempt should be determined by the clinical response, but should not exceed 5–10 seconds (Young 1984; Sumner 1990).	10 Limiting the suctioning time minimises hypoxia, which is significantly related to duration of suction attempts. Most of the evidence is based on the adult population.
11 Where possible, secretions should be cleared on the first attempt.	11 To limit potential side effects and maximise the recovery period (Luce et al. 1998; Day et al. 2002).
12 The catheter may be re-used if immediate suction is required, as long as secretions have not occluded the suction ports and the distal end of the catheter has not been contaminated prior to the suctioning episode.	12 There is no evidence to suggest that using the same catheter up to three times at the same suctioning episode increases the risk of infection. In fact with effective re-training on technique, some institutions have repeatedly used the same catheter on the same patient for a 24-hour period and have reported no increase in infection (Scoble et al. 2001).
13 Wrap the catheter around the gloved hand; remove the glove by inserting it over the used catheter, and discard in clinical waste bag according to local waste policy.	13 To prevent infection risks and contamination of staff and other patients.
14 Flush suction tubing with tap water and connect a new catheter to the tubing.	14 To clear the tubing of secretions.
15 Observe and record secretions that are bloody, purulent, foul-smelling or unusually thick in the CYP's healthcare records. Take samples as required and inform medical team of changes.	15 Accurate and early documentation will ensure early alert of infection risks.
16 Deep suctioning may be required in certain circumstances, but this should not be routine practice (Bailey et al. 1988).	16 To provide the most appropriate care for the CYP's needs.
17 Instillation of saline should not be done routinely (Hudak and Bond-Domb 1996; Ackerman and Mick 1998; Blackwood 1999; Pritchard et al. 2001; Scoble et al. 2001).	17 Other methods, such as continuous humidity, nebulisers, and good systemic hydration are far better ways of keeping secretions loose enough to ensure the tracheostomy tube does not become occluded.

Practitioners must be competent in respiratory assessment and the indications for suctioning and suction technique; this will minimise complications and maximise the effect of treatment.

C = Care of the site: Stoma and neck

During a morbidity audit at GOSH, cases of trauma and excoriation to the skin around the neck and stoma were carefully documented. The results showed that neck injuries and skin damage were reduced from 20% in 2008 to 8% in 2014. Neonates and those with increased susceptibility to skin trauma, e.g. vascular and lymphatic malformations or Epidermolysis Bullosa, are most at risk.

The sternum and chin are areas of potential skin breakdown, as a result of abrasion from the tracheostomy tube or ventilation tubing over long periods of time. CYPs requiring ventilation and those with challenging anatomy were particularly at risk. The use of the Bivona Flextend® tube is preferential for those with lymphatic malformations due to the increased length of the tube outside the airway. The recommended practice is to review the stoma, assess the skin of the neck, and clean the local area around a tracheostomy each day. This should be documented in the patient healthcare record. The Monolyke® range of thin and flexible hydrocolloid dressings are preferred due to their excellent skin protection and their limited impact on the positioning of the tracheostomy tube. Bulkier dressings have the potential to alter the angle of the tracheostomy affecting the stoma as well as abrading the tracheal wall.

GOSH now uses the silicone range of tracheostomy tubes from Bivona® in the vast majority of cases. Stomal granulation tissue has almost been completely eradicated, a dramatic reduction from the report of our own data from 2007 (refer to the tape changing section within the guidelines).

H = Humidity: Essential to keep the tube clear

In the first week after a new tracheostomy is formed, warm humidification should be used as much as possible to counter thick secretions that can occlude the tracheostomy tube. This is a potential cause of an emergency first tracheostomy tube change before the stoma has matured.

Humidification

Maintenance of the humidity and warmth of inspired air is an essential part of tracheostomy management, as the normal functions of the upper respiratory tract have been bypassed. The nose and nasopharynx normally ensure that inspired air reaches the optimum temperature and humidity. Bypassing these with a tracheostomy dedicates such functions to the lower airways, which are poorly suited to the task. Inspiration of cool and dry air may create many problems for the CYP with a tracheostomy. Impairment and destruction of cilia reduces the proximal transportation of mucus (Jackson 1996). Secretions become increasingly thick and tenacious, making their expulsion difficult. This may lead to blockage of the tube. Additionally, cold inspired air increases heat loss from the respiratory tract, a particular danger for the small infant (American Thoracic Society 2000).

Heat and moisture exchangers (HME)

After the first tube change, it is recommended that an appropriately sized Heat Moisture Exchange (HME) device is used. The size is calculated from the CYP's estimated tidal volume. HME's consist of multiple layers of water repellent paper or foam membranes, which trap heat and moisture during exhalation. Cold inhaled air is then warmed and moisturised, thus maintaining the optimum respiratory tract environment.

Several varieties of HME may be used. The internal volume of the HME will add to respiratory dead space, increasing the work of breathing. This may be further increased by the accumulation of secretions within the device; manufacturers therefore recommend changing the HME daily or whenever contaminated.

There are several types available and care should be taken to ensure that the correct HME is used based on the CYP's weight:

- Gibeck Mini Vent® is used for infants under one year (usually under 10kgs); they have smaller tidal volumes and cause minimal resistance to breathing.
- Thermovent T™ from Smiths Medical is for those over 10kg.
- Trachphone™ from Platon Medical is for infants and children requiring supplementary oxygen; it has an integrated suction port and can support phonation (Figure 32.12).

An alternative to the HME are Buchanan bibs which contain a foam layer that absorbs moisture from the CYP's expired gases and can easily be tucked into clothing.

Alternatives to the HME

The ill/hospitalised CYP with a tracheostomy may require extra humidity and this can be delivered via a nebuliser or by a continuous humidity system. Nebulisers provide aerosol droplets in a saturated vapour. The advantage of using water droplets in the respiratory tract is not well documented or understood and some argue that excessive saturation of the lower airways may cause atelectasis and impair the function of distal cilia (Conway et al. 1992). For this reason nebulisers should be used as an addition to and not replace a primary method of humidification.

Water humidifiers are particularly useful when there is a higher requirement for humidification, e.g. when the CYP requires a high minute volume during an acute respiratory illness or post anaesthesia (Klein and Graves 1974). Care must be taken when assessing the effectiveness of water humidifiers; water droplets must be visible along the whole of the elephant tubing. Warmed humidity must be used for small and vulnerable infants and those receiving oxygen therapies.

E = Emergency box: Have the box present

The contents of the emergency tracheostomy box are designed to include the absolute essential equipment required in case of an accidental decannulation or for an emergency tube change. The emergency box accompanies the CYP at all times, reducing the time and potential consequences of unavailable equipment. The 'Kapitex Trachi Box'® is easily recognisable and is used for all our patients.

Items for each tube will vary.

A 'tube box content' chart should be used to ensure the consents are correct (Figure 32.13).

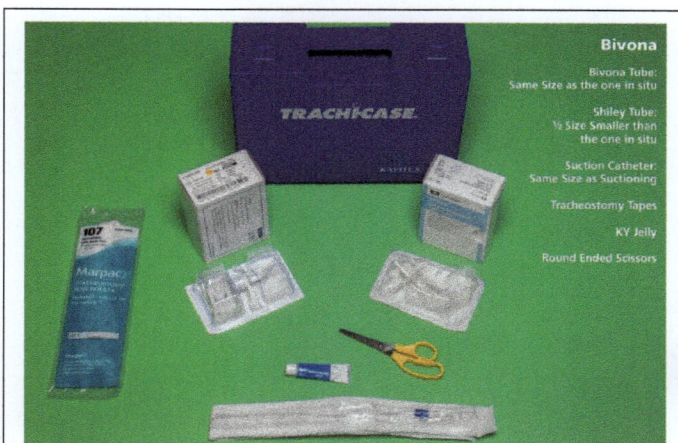

Figure 32.13 Tube box and contents.

Tracheostomy tube changes (planned)

Tracheostomy tubes can be changed weekly or monthly. Only personnel trained and competent in the techniques involved must perform a tracheostomy tube change. See below for further tube information. Alternative advice can be sought from the manufacturers.

Some children may need to be swaddled to maintain their safety during the tube change; older CYPs may prefer to sit. Some CYPs assist with the procedure by, e.g. holding the tracheostomy tube. Practitioners must assess each CYP individually.

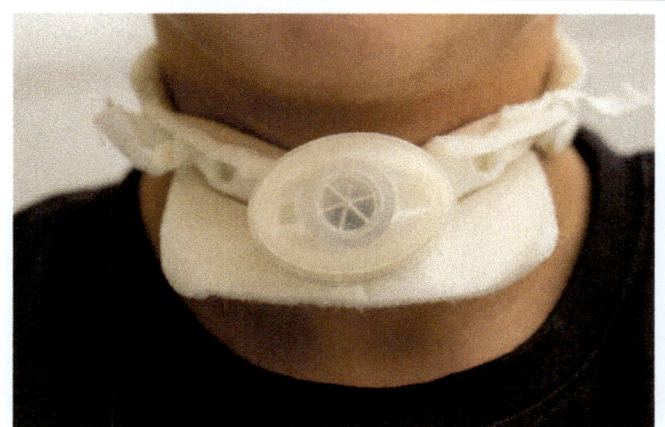

Figure 32.12 Trachphone HME.

Tracheostomy tubes for CYPs

The first types of tracheostomy tubes were made of sterling silver. As other synthetic materials have developed they have improved the flexibility and comfort of paediatric tracheostomy tubes (Hall et al. 2017). See Figure 32.14 for a chart showing the range of tracheostomy tubes.

Tube Parts

All tracheostomy tubes have similar parts. In particular, paediatric tubes are designed to accommodate the paediatric neck shape; they provide stability and a means of securing the tube in place.

Ports: A universal 15mm termination providing the means of connecting additional equipment, such as speaking valves and HMEs, or ventilator/ resuscitation equipment. A port also provides an extension to prevent occlusion from the CYP's chin (not present on the GOS Rusch®, Silver tubes).

Cannula: Paediatric tubes generally have a single cannula to allow for maximum internal diameter (ID). However, tubes are available with both an inner and outer cannula for older CYPs; the cannula may be fenestrated to allow air to pass upwards through the vocal cords to aid phonation.

Procedure guideline 32.7 Tube changes

Statement	Rationale
1 Ensure that all staff involved in the procedure have watched the training podcast (https://youtu.be/6vrYRKlhZSg).	1 To ensure staff and carers are adequately trained.
2 Prepare equipment: • Emergency equipment, oxygen and suction. • A tracheostomy tube of the same size. • A tracheostomy tube that is a size smaller. • A water based lubricant such as Aqualube® or K-Y jelly. • Gauze swabs. • Saline sachets. • Marpac trache tapes cut to size. • Round-ended scissors. • A pillow / towel. • Appropriate PPE. Equipment may vary due to different tube styles; always refer to tube charts for reference..	2 To support any emergency event and ensure all equipment is at hand during the procedure.
To change a tracheostomy tube:	
2 Perform hand hygiene. 3 Don appropriate PPE.	2, 3 To minimise the risk of infection.
4 Assistant to swaddle baby, exposing shoulders and above (baby in supine position if appropriate).	4 For patient comfort and safety.
5 Lubricate new tube with a 'dot' of water-based lubricant on the outside bend of the tube.	5 For patient safety and to reduce risk of trauma to the stoma.
6 a) Measure the length of the tracheostomy tube before inserting the obturator. b) Insert obturator (introducer) into the tube.	6 a) To confirm suction length b) To stiffen the tube.
7 Position the rolled up towel under the shoulders, as per tape changes.	7 To hyper-extend the neck and expose the stoma, facilitating an easier change.
8 Assistant should hold the tube in position using either their thumb and index finger, or index and middle finger.	8 To maximise comfort by not pushing down on the tube.
9 Tube changer should cut the ties between knot and flange.	
10 Remove the ties.	
11 a) Prepare the CYP as appropriate and ensure that the assistant is ready. b) Remove the tube from the stoma with a curved action and dispose.	
12 Insert new tube with a curved action.	
13 Remove obturator.	13 This occludes the tube, so the CYP will not be able to breathe with it in.
14 The assistant should take over and hold the tube in position.	
15 The stomal area and back of the neck should be cleaned and dried with saline and gauze using a clean technique.	
16 The ties are then tied using the method previously described.	
17 Ensure that the CYP is comfortable, clear away all equipment and perform hand hygiene.	17 To maintain comfort and minimise the risk of infection.

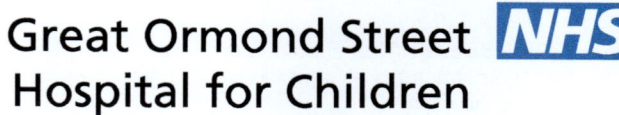

Figure 32.14 Paediatric airways. *Source:* Tweedie et al. (2018).

Obturator (introducer): This should always be used when inserting the tracheostomy tube, as it provides rigidity to the tube, allowing a smoother insertion.

Tube types

Extensive selections of paediatric tubes are currently available, driven by a variety of specific clinical requirements. Choosing an appropriate tube is just one of the preliminary steps in the management of a tracheostomy. The Consultant and/or TNP will decide the design and size of tube to suit the CYP. They should be consulted if it is necessary to change the size or style of the tube in the future.

Sizes of tubes are generally measured by the ID. For the majority of CYPs this is the only measurement required. However, some require specifically shorter or longer tubes. The list below briefly summarises the tubes that are most commonly used at GOSH. Seek advice from the TNP, ENT team, and manufacturer if more information is required.

Bivona®

The Bivona range is the most commonly used tube at GOSH, largely replacing other varieties on grounds of comfort and versatility. The range is based around a standard shaft, manufactured from opaque, white siliconised PVC. It is latex free and hydrophobic, hindering protein adhesion and thereby limiting secretion build-up and bacterial colonisation. For this reason, these tubes can remain in place for up to 28 days. The silicone is reinforced with wire, producing a tube that is flexible, conforming to the shape of the trachea, but resists kinking. An integrating 15 mm swivelling adapter reduces torque on the shaft and is universally compatible with ventilation appliances. There are two versions: Paediatric (of standard length) and Neonatal (shorter length). The tubes come in a variety of styles, some with independent flexing proximal and distal shafts, which are beneficial for those requiring ventilation (Flextend®); some tubes also have adjustable flanges so that the shaft length can be altered (Hyperflex®). The tubes can be uncuffed or cuffed. The Fome cuff® is a self-inflating tube, providing a high level of protection from aspiration while providing optimal comfort. Practitioners must ensure that they are familiar with the specifics of this tube when removing and inserting it as it is very different from other tubes. The Tight To Shaft (TTS) is a high-pressure low-volume cuff. The cuff is filled with sterile water, not air. Care must be taken not to overfill the cuff, and practitioners should inflate the cuff only enough to support artificial ventilation. The cuff can be deflated completely to assume the profile of an uncuffed tube, which makes it very useful when weaning from the ventilator. Bivona tubes can be sterilised and reused (maximum of five times or when the integrity of the tube is broken). 'In hospital and at home' cleaning solutions are now available from the TNP or the company direct. These tubes contain metal so require caution with MRI scanning.

The Great Ormond Street hospital tube

This series is still produced, but no longer commonly used. There are two versions: flat and extended (external fenestrated extension). The extended version is suitable when the chin may obstruct the standard flat tube. Both types of tube are made of polyvinyl chloride (PVC) and are clear/brown in colour, with a bevelled tip to facilitate introduction into the stoma and soft, atraumatic flanges. They are available in sizes from 3.0 to 7.0 mm ID, designed for single use only. More importantly, these tubes are not compatible with ventilator tubing or resuscitation equipment. A Smiths Portex® male/female adapter of appropriate size will be required in such situations but this method is only temporary. If long-term ventilation is required then practitioners should change the tube to one with a 15 mm termination.

Shiley®

The Shiley range is not commonly used at GOSH. This product range is manufactured from opaque, thermosensitive, latex-free PVC, with a thin-walled shaft, tapered tip, and universal 15 mm connector. Tubes are available in neonatal, standard paediatric, and long paediatric varieties, with optional cuffs for the paediatric series. The sizing system used for the Shiley range was updated several years ago: the ID (mm) is now quoted for reference, in line with other manufacturers' products. From our experiences a weekly tube change is recommended. The Shiley tube has been superseded by the Bivona as the product of first choice at GOSH. However, a long paediatric tube (size 5.0–6.5) is not made by other manufacturers, such that the Shiley remains a unique option for a few CYPs who require a tube that is midway between typical paediatric and adult lengths.

Smiths portex™

This tube is not commonly used at GOSH. There are two versions available, one without a termination and the other with a 15 mm standard termination. This enables them to be used with anaesthetic and ventilatory equipment. They are made of a clear PVC material with a blue radio-opaque line. Paediatric sizes range from 3.0 to 7.0 mm ID. Cuffed and fenestrated (to facilitate vocalisation) versions are available.

Silver tubes

A number of silver tubes have been developed. Their designs and general principles remain unchanged for a number of years now. While seldom used at GOSH, silver tubes have some important qualities that confer advantages over plastic varieties in certain circumstances. Most significantly, the tubes can be manufactured with very thin walls, permitting the use of an inner tube without compromising airflow. This can be removed and cleaned without taking out the whole tube. Silver tubes may remain in situ for up to one month, a particular advantage for those requiring long-term tracheostomy. However, silver tubes have certain disadvantages. For example, they are rigid and do not conform to the trachea, which some CYPs find uncomfortable. Additionally, each tube is unique; the unit cost is high (although far fewer tubes are required in the long term) and the components are not interchangeable, creating compatibility problems. Sizes are measured in the French gauge (Fr) and are not comparable to the metric measurements of the plastic tubes. For resuscitation and ventilator purposes, a Smiths Portex male/female adapter of appropriate size will be required. The Sheffield® tube is the only silver product commonly used at Great Ormond Street Hospital. Note that silver tubes are not compatible with MRI scanning and they may distort CT scan pictures of the head, neck, and chest. After discussion with the TNP or consultant a suitable alternative must be inserted for the duration of the scan.

One way valves

A tracheostomy alters a CYP's ability to communicate (speak) by affecting the passage of air through the voice box (larynx) and mouth for speech. Air from the lungs passes out of the tracheostomy tube, instead of passing up through the larynx and out of the mouth. A one-way valve sits on the end of the tracheostomy tube and opens as the CYP breathes in and closes as they breathe out, directing air up through the larynx and out of their mouth. Not all CYPs will tolerate a one way valve, as a good air leak around and above the tube is essential. The valve is NOT be used while the CYP is asleep or when using a cuffed tracheostomy tube. Some variations include the facility for oxygen delivery. Several manufacturers, e.g. Smiths Portex, Shiley, and Rusch make these. A joint decision is made between the ENT Consultant, TNP, and the SALT to use a speaking valve, as changes often need to be made to the existing tracheostomy tube to accommodate it. They must not be fitted or used without a full assessment by the SALT or TNP. The Rusch valve is commonly used for initial assessments and then the Passy Muir® is used for long-term use.

Discharge planning

Procedure guideline 32.8 Preparation for discharge

Statement	Rationale
1 The formation of a tracheostomy must be communicated to local teams.	
2 Most CYPs will be discharged back via their local hospital, which will allow local services and support to be activated.	2 To ensure safe and timely discharge.
3 The CYP's parents, or two main carers, must be taught and be deemed as competent in the following: • Tracheostomy tube changes (minimum of two) • Tracheostomy tape changes • Stoma care • Suctioning • Resuscitation skills/emergency care The carer must stay with their CYP and carry out all care overnight. It is important that the carer feels confident in their ability to take the CYP out of the hospital. This can be an extremely difficult time for parents; there is a difference between completing the practical skills and feeling confident to carry these out independently at home.	3 To enable them to safely care for their child.
4 Tracheostomy and resuscitation booklets and podcasts are available to support training. All training provided must be recorded on the discharge planner and kept in their health record for future reference.	4 To ensure that parents/carers receive competency based training.
5 Follow up times vary. An ENT outpatient appointment will be arranged.	

Decannulation

Decannulation can occur within the ward setting over a period of five days, or can be undertaken as a surgical procedure.

Surgical decannulation

Surgical decannulation is carried out under a general anaesthetic and usually involves reconstruction of the upper airway or stomal area. The tracheostomy is removed at the time of surgery and the stomal opening surgically closed. The CYP will be routinely intubated and cared for on the intensive care unit for up to seven days and have an elective microlaryngoscopy and bronchoscopy (MLB), downsize (MLB), and elective extubation.

Ward decannulation

Ward decannulation is the most common method to remove the tracheostomy tube. It is noninvasive and does not require intubation and/or admission to a paediatric intensive care unit.

Endoscopic evaluation of the airway is required to confirm the patency at all levels and to exclude (and treat) peristomal complications such as granulation or collapse. The decannulation trial itself must take place within six weeks of the assessment.

If the decannulation is carried out straight after the MLB (this would be unusual), then the patient must have a 'rest day' to allow any potential oedema to settle, before the trial period begins.

The CYP remains in hospital during the most critical stage of the programme, to allow appropriate airway monitoring as well as intervention, including halting the procedure and replacing the tracheostomy tube if indicated.

Ward decannulation usually requires a five-day admission but this will vary according to the age of the CYP and the type of tracheostomy tube they have in situ.

Principles of decannulation

For the CYP with a tracheostomy tube with an ID greater than 3.0mm, smaller tracheostomy tubes should be inserted until a tube size of 3.0mm is reached. The tube size should only be downsized to allow the stoma to shrink and the CYP to adjust to breathing through the nose and mouth. For small infants/children weighing less than 12kg, where a tracheostomy tube with a 3.0mm ID will occupy much of their airway, the decannulation process will be different. This will include downsizing the tracheostomy tube to a 2.5 ID rather than the 3.0 ID or removing the tracheostomy tube without going through the process of downsizing or capping (Kubba et al. 2004).

The child must have a tracheostomy tube with a 15mm standard termination in place to allow fitting of the decannulation cap.

During the decannulation process, observe and record for any signs of increased respiratory effort.

- Skin colour change (cyanosis, pale)
- Irritability/anxious (associated with breathing)
- Restlessness, particularly when asleep
- Loss of appetite
- Tracheal tug/nasal flaring
- Lethargy when normally active/ breathlessness on exertion
- Sternal/intercostal/subcostal recession
- Stridor/stertor
- Change in general observations (increased heart/respiratory rate)
- Increased respiratory effort

Should complications arise, indicative of deterioration, effective urgent response is required, DO NOT delay following the appropriate escalation processes.

Record half-hourly observations of pulse and respiratory rate, while asleep. Routine observations in line with the CYP's general condition should be undertaken while awake and recorded in the healthcare record throughout the decannulation period.

On the second day, the CYP's progress will be assessed and reviewed and, if stable during the previous 24 hours, the tracheostomy tube will be covered with a red 'occlusion cap.' This cap can be easily seen and easily removed in case of any difficulty. The CYP should be able to cough around the tube. Removing the cap during coughing or suctioning the tube is classed as a failed attempt, so this should not be done. The CYP must learn to clear secretions on their own. If they become overly distressed, remove the cap immediately and inform the ENT team TNP.

The tracheostomy tube is removed on day three following a reassessment by the ENT team TNP. The stoma should be covered with clean gauze secured with a waterproof, airtight dressing such as Duoderm or P3 Tracheseal®. Both will provide an airtight occlusion around the opening, preventing the CYP from breathing through it. Practitioners should ensure that the dressing remains airtight. Record the decannulation in the healthcare record. The CYP must not leave the ward for the next 24 hours.

Change the tracheostomy swivel connection to a face mask on rebreathe circuit – but keep the swivel connector in the emergency box. Keep the tracheostomy box by the bedside, containing a size 3.0 mm ID tube.

If the 24 hours after tube removal has been uneventful, the airtight dressing can be removed to review stoma site. Renew dressing as before, using an aseptic nontouch technique. The CYP can then leave the ward accompanied by someone competent in the mouth-to-mouth resuscitation technique. The nurse should discuss the CYP's ongoing care needs with the family, in particular the general care of the stoma, equipment needed, emergency procedures, schooling, and care of the stomal opening, to ensure they are confident to manage these aspects of care once discharged. This must be documented in the healthcare record. If the decannulation process has been without complication the CYP will be discharged home.

If the stoma remains large or there is excessive exudate, the dressing will need to be replaced as necessary. The stoma may/may not close by itself; if it hasn't closed after six to nine months, then it will be surgically closed.

Contact Community team and GP to inform them of the outcome of the decannulation process and to arrange for replacement dressings to be ordered.

If at any stage the trial fails, the ENT/Tracheostomy NP will reinsert the tracheostomy tube. If the stoma has closed it may need to be dilated with smaller tubes until the original size is reached or the CYP may need to return to theatre for the stoma to be dilated. They are then discharged with a follow-up plan.

References

Ackerman, M.H. and Mick, D.J. (1998). Instillation of normal saline before suctioning in patients with pulmonary infections: a prospective randomized controlled trial. *American Journal of Critical Care* 7 (4): 261–266.

Alladi, A., Rao, S., Das, K. et al. (2004). Pediatric tracheostomy: a 13-year experience. *Pediatric Surgery International* 20 (9): 695–698.

American Thoracic Society (2000). Care of the child with a chronic tracheostomy. *American Journal of Respiratory and Critical Care Medicine* 161: 297–308.

Bailey, C., Kattwinkel, J., Teja, K., and Buckley, T. (1988). Shallow versus deep endotracheal suctioning in young rabbits: pathologic effects on the tracheobronchial wall. *Pediatric* 82 (5): 746–751.

Blackwood, B. (1999). Normal saline instillation with endotracheal suctioning: primum non nocere (first do no harm). *Journal of Advanced Nursing* 29 (4): 928–934.

Carr, M.M., Poje, C.P., Kingston, L. et al. (2001). Complications in pediatric tracheostomies. *The Laryngoscope* 111: 1995–1998.

Conway, J.H., Fleming, J.S., Perring, S., and Holgate, S.T. (1992). Humidification as an adjunct to chest physiotherapy in aiding trachobronchial clearance in patients with bronchiectasis. *Respiratory Medicine* 86 (2): 109–114.

Corbett, H.J., Mann, K.S., Mitra, I. et al. (2007). Tracheostomy – a 10-year experience from a UK pediatric surgical center. *Journal of Pediatric Surgery* 42 (7): 1251–1254.

Craig, M.F., Bajaj, Y., and Hartley, B.E. (2005). Maturation sutures for the paediatric tracheostomy – an extra safety measure. *Journal of Laryngology and Otology* 119 (12): 985–987.

Czarnik, R.E., Stone, K.S., Everhart, C.C. Jr., and Preusser, B.A. (1991). Differential effects of continuous versus intermittent suction on tracheal tissue. *Heart & Lung* 20 (2): 144–151.

Davies, K., Monterosso, L., Bulsara, M., and Ramelet, A.S. (2015). Clinical indicators for the initiation of endotracheal suction in children: An integrative review. *Australian Critical Care* 28 (1): 11–18.

Day, T., Farnell, S., and Wilson-Barnett, J. (2002). Suctioning: a review of current research recommendations. *Intensive and Critical Care Nursing* 18 (2): 79–89.

Edwards, E. (2018). Principles of suctioning in infants, children and young people. *Nursing Children and Young People* 30 (4): 46–54.

Evans, J., Syddall, S., Butt, W., and Kinney, S. (2014). Comparison of open and closed suction on safety, efficacy and nursing time in a paediatric intensive care unit. *Australian Critical Care* 27: 70–74.

Friedman, E., Kennedy, A., and Neitzschman, H.R. (2003). Innominate artery compression of the trachea: an unusual cause of apnea in a 12-year-old boy. *Southern Medical Journal* 96 (11): 1161–1164.

Hall, A., Bates, J., Ifeacho, S. et al. (2017). Implementation of the TRACHE care bundle: improving safety in paediatric tracheostomy management. *Archives of Disease in Childhood* 102: 563–565.

Hudak, M. and Bond-Domb, A. (1996). Postoperative head and neck cancer patients with artificial airways: the effect of saline lavage on tracheal mucus evacuation and oxygen saturation. *ORL-Head and Neck Nursing* 14 (1): 17–21.

Jackson, C. (1996). Humidification in the upper respiratory tract: a physiological overview. *Intensive and Critical Care Nursing* 12 (1): 27–32.

Klein, E.F.J. and Graves, S.A. (1974). 'Hot pot' tracheitis. *Chest* 65 (2): 225–226.

Kubba, H., Cooke, J., and Hartley, B. (2004). Can we develop a protocol for the safe decannulation of tracheostomies in children less than 18 months old? *International Journal of Pediatric Otorhinolaryngology* 68 (7): 935–937.

Luce, J.M., Pierson, D.J., and Tyler, M.L. (1998). Intensive Respiratory Therapy, 2e. Philadelphia, W.B.: Saunders Co.

Lyons, M.J., Cooke, J., Cochrane, L.A., and Albert, D.M. (2007). Safe reliable atraumatic replacement of misplaced paediatric tracheostomy tubes. *International Journal of Pediatric Otorhinolaryngology* 71 (11): 1743–1746.

McGrath, B. (ed.) (2014). Comprehensive Tracheostomy Care: The National Tracheostomy Safety Project Manual. Wiley Blackwell Publications.

National Confidential Enquiry into Patient Outcome and Death (NCEPOD) (2014) Tracheostomy Care: On the Right Trach? National Confidential Enquiry into Patient Outcome and Death. London.

Onakoya, P.A., Nwaorgu, O.G., and Adebusoye, L.A. (2003). Complications of classical tracheostomy and management. *Tropical Doctor* 33 (3): 148–150.

Park, J.Y., Suskind, D.L., Prater, D. et al. (1999). Maturation of the pediatric tracheostomy stoma: effect on complications. *Annals of Otology, Rhinology and Laryngology* 108 (12): 1115–1119.

Pritchard, M., Flenady, V., and Woodgate, P. (2001). Preoxygenation for tracheal suctioning in intubated, ventilated newborn infants. *The Cochrane Database of Systematic Reviews* 3: CD000427.

Resuscitation Council (UK) (RC UK) (2021) Resuscitation Guidelines. www.resus.org.uk/resuscitation-guidelines (accessed 1 June 2019).

Scoble, M.K., Copnell, B., Taylor, A. et al. (2001). Effect of reusing suction catheters on the occurrence of pneumonia in children. *Heart & Lung* 30 (3): 225–233.

Seay, S.J., Gay, S.L., and Strauss, M. (2002). Tracheostomy emergencies. *American Journal of Nursing* 102 (3): 59, 61, 63.

Sumner, E. (1990). Artificial ventilation of children. In: The Diagnosis and Management of Paediatric Respiratory Care (ed. R. Dinwiddie), 267–287. London: Churchill Livingstone.

Tarnoff, M., Moncure, M., Jones, F. et al. (1998). The value of routine posttracheostomy chest radiography. *Chest* 113 (6): 1647–1649.

Thomas, A.N. and McGrath, B.A. (2009). Patient safety incidents associated with airway devices in critical care: a review of reports to the UK National Patient Safety Agency. *Anaesthesia* 64 (4): 358–365.

Tingay, D.G., Copnell, B., Grant, C.A. et al. (2010). The effect of endotracheal suction on regional tidal ventilation and end expiratory lung volume. *Intensive Care Medicine* 36 (5): 888–896.

Tweedie, D.J., Cooke, J., Stephenson, K.A. et al. (2018). Paediatric tracheostomy tubes: recent developments and our current practice. *Journal of Laryngology & Otology* 132 (11): 961–968.

Yaremchuck, K. (2003). Regular tube changes to prevent formation of granulation tissue. *The Laryngoscope* 113 (1): 1–10.

Young, C.S. (1984). Recommendation for suction. *Physiotherapy* 70 (3): 104–106.

Further reading

National Tracheostomy Safety Project Paediatric emergency algorithms. www.tracheostomy.org.uk/storage/files/Paeds%20Bedhead%20Algorithm%20Combo.pdf (accessed 6 January 2019).

Chapter 33

Urinary catheter care

Donna Wyan

DipHE (Child), BSc (Hons), Independent Prescriber, Urology Nurse Practitioner, Great Ormond Street Hospital, London, UK

The author would like to thank Mr Alexander Cho, Consultant Urologist, for his review of this chapter.

Chapter contents

Introduction	754	Risk factors	754
Types of catheters	754	References	767

Procedure guidelines

33.1 Catheter insertion: preparation	756	33.6 Maintaining catheter drainage	763
33.2 Urethral catheter insertion	757	33.7 Flushing suprapubic, urethral or mitrofanoff catheters	763
33.3 Catheter care: general	759	33.8 Removal of suprapubic and urethral catheters	765
33.4 Catheter care: entry site	761	33.9 Discharge planning	766
33.5 Emptying a catheter drainage bag	762		

Principles table

33.1 Inform child or young person and family	755

The Great Ormond Street Hospital Manual of Children and Young People's Nursing Practices, Second Edition. Edited by Elizabeth Anne Bruce, Janet Williss, and Faith Gibson.
© 2023 John Wiley & Sons Ltd. Published 2023 by John Wiley & Sons Ltd.

Introduction

This chapter covers the fundamental principles of urinary catheter care, including insertion, caring for an indwelling urinary catheter, and its safe removal. For information regarding obtaining a urine specimen from a catheter, see Chapter 15: Investigations.

The main purpose of a urinary catheter is to drain and collect urine. Less commonly, it can also be used to instil fluid (Bray and Sanders 2006). The risks of catheterisation need to be fully evaluated to ensure the decision to catheterise best suits the clinical needs of the child or young person (CYP), and takes into consideration the impact of having a catheter on their physical and emotional wellbeing (Bray and Sanders 2006; Gokula et al. 2012; National Institute for Health and Care Excellence [NICE] 2012).

Indications for a urinary catheter include:

- To promote healing and prevent impact on the renal system by allowing for optimal drainage following urological surgery (Nasir et al. 2011).
- To drain the bladder if urinary retention occurs (Steggall et al. 2013). This can be due to a variety of reasons, the commonest being medication-related side effects, surgical complications, and trauma (Wright 2012).
- To drain urine if there is an obstruction in the urinary tract, for example in males born with posterior urethral valves (PUV) (Krishnan et al. 2006).
- To calculate accurate urinary output (McLafferty et al. 2014).
- Bladder irrigation (Cutts 2005).
- To obtain a urine specimen (not a routine procedure in CYPs) (NICE 2007).
- Long-term continence management (Gurung et al. 2007).
- For invasive urodynamic testing (Shaban et al. 2010).
- Reduced mobility (Farringdon et al. 2013).

There are different types of urinary catheters and the decision regarding preference requires detailed consideration by the health care professionals (HCPs) involved to ensure it meets the clinical needs of the CYP, with the potential risks thoroughly evaluated.

Urethral catheterisation is the commonest form of artificial urinary drainage; a catheter is passed through the urethra into the bladder using an aseptic technique. In the hospital setting this can be performed as an intermittent procedure for treatment of urinary retention or specimen collection, or for more long-term management of urinary drainage an indwelling catheter will be passed. This intervention should only be undertaken by a HCP who has undergone training and gained clinical competence (RCN 2021; NICE 2012, 2015).

Suprapubic catheterisation (SPC) is a procedure whereby a catheter is inserted through an incision made in the abdominal wall into the bladder using an aseptic technique (Sanders 2001). If this is a new insertion it is usually performed under general anaesthetic by a suitably trained doctor. A change of an SPC with an established tract does not routinely require an anaesthetic and can be performed by a suitably trained HCP on the ward or in the community.

Clean intermittent catheterisation (CIC) is taught to parents and CYPs and can be undertaken urethrally or via a mitrofanoff (a surgically made channel for intermittent catheterisation) (McMonnies 2002; Minkin and Baskin 2003). This can be required for many conditions, including myelomeningocele, bladder exstrophy, and PUV. The aim of this procedure is to provide optimal urinary drainage which minimises the risk of infection, maintains the safety of the urinary tract and renal system and/or for urinary continence to be gained (Bray and Sanders 2006; Woodward et al. 2013). This skill is taught to the parents or the CYP so they can perform this at home and school. It is a significant undertaking for the family, so it is essential that they are monitored regularly by appropriately skilled professionals to ensure that they remain clinically well and supported from a psychosocial point of view (Bray and Sanders 2006). Information for families is available at www.gosh.nhs.uk/medical-information-0/procedures-and-treatments/clean-intermittent-catheterisation.

Types of catheters

There are a variety of urinary catheters available, making it essential to ensure that the correct one is chosen to suit its purpose. Silicone catheters, such as Foley™, are indicated for long term indwelling catheterisation and can remain in situ for up to 12 weeks.

A Foley catheter is a balloon device which enables the catheter to remain in place within the bladder. If used for a SPC and when inserted under GA, especially for new tracts, it can be sutured to secure in position. Silicone catheters are robust and are less likely to be troubled with encrustations (Nazarko 2007). Hydrogel coated catheters can remain in situ for up to 14 days and have been found to cause less inflammation, discomfort, and infection, as they are less prone to bacterial adherence (Gould et al. 2010). The circumference of the catheter is the French (Fr). The size used is dependent on the age and weight of the CYP (Bowden and Greenbers 2011). It is recommended that the smallest size that will allow optimal drainage is used to minimise the risk of trauma on insertion and further long-term damage (Smith 2003). For guidance on choosing the correct size, see Table 33.1.

Risk factors

The most common risk factor associated with a urinary catheter is a urinary tract infection (UTI) (Parry et al. 2013). UTIs account for 40% of all hospital acquired infections in adults, 80% of which are related to urinary catheters (Boybeyi et al. 2013). The risk of developing a UTI is directly related to the length of time the catheter remains in situ (Parry et al. 2013). HCPs should evaluate the need for the urinary catheter to remain in situ and these should be removed at the earliest opportunity or changed within the time frame recommended by the manufacturer (Cedeno 2008; NICE 2012, 2015). Other risk factors associated with UTIs include trauma during insertion and poor catheter care (Pomfret 2010).

Urinary catheters can block, which prevents them from draining effectively. This needs to be dealt with immediately so as not to compromise the urology and/or renal systems. Reasons for reduced drainage or blocking of urinary catheters include:

- Kinking of the tube or catheter displacement (Spinks 2013)
- Constipation (Pomfret 2010)
- Blood clots or debris following surgery (Cutts 2005).
- Encrustation on the tip of the catheter from the formation of crystals and potential stones (Yates 2004).
- Mucous build up; often seen in CYPs who have undergone an ileocystoplasty (Cutts 2005).

See flushing guidelines for advice on management of a blocked catheter.

An indwelling urinary catheter can irritate the bladder wall or sphincter and cause spasms, which can be very painful and increase anxiety and stress for the CYP and family (Bray and Sanders 2006; Nazarko 2007). To minimise the risk of bladder spasms, the catheter should be taped securely, preferably to the suprapubic area of the abdomen, as this limits movement of the catheter tube when mobilising (Spinks 2013). This will also minimise the risk of accidental removal or displacement of the catheter. Medications such as oxybutynin and tolterodine can be helpful for the management of bladder spasms as they inhibit the parasympathetic nerve impulses that can cause involuntary muscle

Chapter 33 Urinary catheter care

Table 33.1 Catheter size chart

M/F	Age/Gestation	Weight	Size and length of catheter	Type
M or F	Premature	<3 kg	5 Fr 30 cm paediatric length	Nelation/PVC non-balloon urinary catheter
M or F	Term	3–4 kg	6 Fr 30 cm paediatric length	Nelation/PVC non-balloon urinary catheter If balloon required (e.g. being discharged): Balloon urinary catheter Foley™
M or F	Term to 3 months (of LGA – Large for gestational age)	4–6 kg	6 or 8 Fr 30 cm Paediatric Length	Nelation/PVC non-balloon urinary catheter If Balloon required (e.g. being discharged): Balloon urinary catheter Foley™
M	1 year	<12 kg	6 or 8 Fr	Balloon urinary catheter Foley™
F	1 year	<12 kg	8 Fr	Balloon urinary catheter Foley™
M	1–5 years	<25 kg	8 Fr	Balloon urinary catheter Foley™
F	1–5 years	<25 kg	10 Fr	Balloon urinary catheter Foley™
Version 2: October 2019				
M	5–10 years	<25 kg	10 Fr	Balloon urinary catheter Foley™
F	5–10 years	<25 kg	12 Fr	Balloon urinary catheter Foley™
M	10–16 years		12–14 Fr	Balloon urinary catheter Foley™
F	10–16 years		10–12 Fr	Balloon urinary catheter Foley™

Source: © Great Ormond Street Hospital for Children NHS Foundation Trust.
Length of insertion: insert the catheter until urine drains freely into the receiver. If using a Foley catheter insert to the hub **BEFORE** inflating the balloon, to prevent trauma from incorrect balloon position.
Top tip: Where a size range occurs if you cannot retract the foreskin and see the meatus then use the smaller size catheter.

contractions in the bladder (Abrams et al. 2006; Bray and Sanders 2006). For more information regarding the management of bladder spasm see Figure 33.3.

As with all potentially painful and frightening procedures, adequate preparation, explanation, analgesia, and sedation (if necessary) must be planned well in advance to manage both the fear and pain associated with the procedure (Association of Paediatric Anaesthetists of Great Britain and Ireland 2012; Twycross et al. 2014). For more information on procedural pain management, see Chapter 24: Pain Management and Chapter 27: Play as a Therapeutic Tool.

Thorough documentation is essential, to provide accurate information; this also allows for care to be audited and evaluated, facilitating future improvements in care. Care bundles and pathways used locally should encompass all aspects of catheter care, from insertion to its removal and after care (Nursing & Midwifery Council [NMC] 2015 (updated 2018); RCN 2021).

The guidelines below provide information for all HCPs involved in the care of urinary catheters; they should have received training and be competent to perform these procedures and should not undertake care that is beyond their expertise.

Principles table 33.1 Inform child or young person and family

Principle	Rationale
1 a) Discuss with the CYP and family: • Why a catheter is necessary. • How the catheter will be inserted. • The likely duration of the procedure. • How long the catheter is likely to remain in situ. b) Answer any questions as they arise	1 To provide information and enable informed consent to be given.
2 Preparation • Consider gender, culture, and religious beliefs. • Privacy and dignity. • Discuss techniques to reduce upset, where needed.	2 To encourage co-operation and ensure that the procedure causes the minimum possible psychological distress.
3 If restraint, or 'clinical holding', is required, the parents need to be informed and staff should refer to local and national guidelines.	3 To ensure the safety of the CYP (RCN 2019). For more information on clinical holding see the Introduction.
4 Any discussion must be recorded in the CYP's healthcare record.	4 To provide an accurate record.
5 Written information should be available for all CYPs being discharged with a catheter in situ.	5 To reinforce verbal explanations (GOSH 2012).

Procedure guideline 33.1 Catheter insertion: preparation

Statement	Rationale
1 Catheterisation must be performed only by or under the supervision of staff who are competent in the procedure: a) Ensure that the CYP and their family are fully prepared and that the procedure is discussed, including the use of sedation, distraction, and restraining techniques, if required. b) The procedure normally involves at least two members of staff. Ensure all those involved including carers are aware of their role during the procedure.	1 To minimise trauma, discomfort, and the potential for catheter-associated infections (Loveday et al. 2014; NICE 2012, 2015). a) To minimise distress. b) To facilitate the procedure and maintain the CYP's safety.
2 When choosing a catheter this should be: a) Latex free. b) The correct diameter; the smallest diameter catheter that will effectively empty the bladder should be used (Smith 2003). c) The correct length; insert catheters to the hub of the catheter. d) Choosing the correct length is particularly important in neonates.	2 a) To minimise the risk of latex allergy (Wilson 2012). b) Smaller gauge catheters minimise trauma and mucosal irritation, which can lead to catheter-associated infection (Loveday et al. 2014; NICE 2012, 2015). c) To prevent intravesical knotting of the catheter (Turner 2004). d) For catheter sizes, lengths, and models see Table 33.1.
3 a) Gather the following equipment: • Catheterisation pack. • Catheter of appropriate size and design for intended purpose. • Appropriate catheter drainage system. • Latex-free sterile gloves. • Plastic apron. • Sachet 0.9% sodium chloride. • Sterile lubrication agent. • Water-based anaesthetic gel (males), e.g. lidocaine 2%. • Water-based gel (females), e.g. Optilube (TM). b) If Foley catheter: • Luer lock syringe and sterile water for injection. • Hypoallergenic and latex free adhesive strapping, e.g. Mefix™.	a) To ensure that everything is prepared for the procedure. b) Sterile water is preferred for filling the catheter ballon as saline solutions can cause crystallisation and subsequent difficulty in catheter removal.
4 Lay the CYP in a comfortable position with their head on a pillow: • **Females** should be supine, with their knees bent and flexed outwards. • **Males** should be semi-supine if possible.	4 To provide ease of access for catheterisation.
5 Place an absorbent pad under their buttocks.	5 To protect the mattress and bedding.
6 The abdomen and lower legs may be covered with a sheet.	6 To maintain dignity and privacy.
7 A parent or carer should remain by the CYP's head.	7 To provide comfort and restrain hands if necessary.
8 Place a sachet of 0.9% sodium chloride in a bowl of warm water.	8 A cold solution can cause discomfort.
9 Put on an apron. Perform hand hygiene and dry hands thoroughly.	9 To minimise the risk of infection (Loveday et al. 2014; NICE 2012, 2015).
10 Open catheter pack and prepare sterile field, adding lubricating agent and catheter.	10–13 To avoid delays and ensure that the necessary equipment is ready for use.
11 Add contents of 0.9% sodium chloride sachet to sterile field.	
12 Apply alcohol gel to hands and put on gloves.	
13 If using a Foley catheter, place syringe and water for injection on sterile field.	
14 Tear a circular hole in the centre of the sterile sheet and place over the groin area.	14 To give access to groin area.

Chapter 33 Urinary catheter care

Procedure guideline 33.2 Urethral catheter insertion

Statement	Rationale
To insert a catheter into a female (Figure 33.1):	
1 Using non dominant hand, hold labia open with sterile gauze.	
2 Using gauze soaked in 0.9% sodium chloride, clean the vulva using a downward motion.	2, 3 To minimise the risk of infection.
3 Clean the outer labia, then the inner labia and then the vulval groove using new gauze for each area.	
4 Position receiver close by.	4 To collect urine.
5 Lubricate tip of catheter with sterile gel.	5 To reduce friction and discomfort from a dry catheter.
6 Ensure that the CYP is ready for catheter insertion.	6 To psychologically prepare the CYP.
7 Gently insert catheter tip into urethral meatus. Ensure that only the inner wrapper is touched and not the catheter itself.	7 To ensure that the catheter remains sterile.
8 Insert the catheter using a smooth steady horizontal motion.	
To insert a catheter into a male (Figure 33.2):	
1 Gently hold penis with non-dominant hand using sterile gauze and place through the hole in the sterile sheet.	1 To give access to penis.
2 Hold the penis vertically and prepare to clean it.	2 To enable effective cleaning.
3 Using gauze soaked in 0.9% sodium chloride, clean prepuce with a singular circular motion. Where possible continue to retract the prepuce.	3 The prepuce is non retractable in boys under five years and excessive force will cause trauma (Thomas et al. 2008). However, this varies in individuals and some males can never fully retract their foreskin, therefore never force a foreskin to retract.
4 Clean each area of the prepuce/glans with new gauze until prepuce will retract no further or until urethral meatus is visible.	
5 Whilst holding the penis at a 90° angle, insert nozzle of lidocaine gel into the urethral meatus/prepuce.	5 Gravity will aid administration of gel.
6 Administer the gel, massaging it downwards into urethra by digital stroking and wait for four minutes.	6 Facilitates action of the gel (Addison 2000).
7 Position the receiver close by.	7 To collect urine.
8 Ensure the CYP is ready for catheter insertion.	8 To ensure that they are psychologically prepared for the procedure.
9 a) Remove the stylet if present. b) Lubricate the tip of the catheter with lidocaine gel.	9 a) To reduce the risk of urethral trauma. b) To reduce friction from a dry catheter (Loveday et al. 2014; NICE 2012, 2015).
10 Gently insert the catheter tip into the urethral meatus.	
11 Insert the catheter using a smooth steady motion. When the posterior urethra is approached, where resistance is felt, direct the penis towards the foot of the bed.	11 To enable the catheter to pass around the posterior urethra into the bladder without resistance.
For both sexes:	
1 Resistance will be felt on reaching the bladder neck.	
2 Encourage the CYP to take deep breaths.	2 To act as a distraction and to relax them.
3 Continue to insert the catheter until urine drains freely into the receiver.	
4 If using a Foley catheter: a) Insert the catheter to the hilt. b) Insert a syringe of sterile water into the one-way valve on the side of the catheter; the volume used will be dependent on the size of the catheter. c) Remove the syringe. d) Pull back the catheter. e) In males, ensure the foreskin is reduced to the normal position at the end of the procedure.	4 a) To prevent trauma from incorrect balloon position. b) To inflate the balloon at the bladder neck and prevent the catheter from falling out. d) To ensure it is sitting comfortably. e) To prevent paraphimosis (Garg et al. 2016).

(continued)

Procedure guideline 33.2 Urethral catheter insertion *(continued)*

Statement	Rationale
5 a) Secure the catheter to the abdomen or groin using adhesive hypoallergenic and latex free strapping. b) Do not tape the catheter to the CYP's leg.	5 a) To prevent accidental catheter removal (Spinks 2013). b) To minimise trauma to the urethral meatus and bladder neck. This is a greater risk when mobilising with a Foley catheter (Hanchett 2002).
6 Attach a sterile drainage bag.	6 To create a closed system (Loveday et al. 2014; NICE 2012, 2015).
7 Place the bag below the level of bladder using a drainage bag hanger/stand. Do not put it on floor.	7 To promote urine drainage via gravity and minimise the risk of infection (Loveday et al. 2014; NICE 2012, 2015).
8 Dispose of equipment according to local waste policy. Perform a social hand-wash and dry hands thoroughly.	8 To minimise the risk of cross infection.
9 Following catheterisation the following must be recorded in the CYP's healthcare records: • Reasons for catheterisation • Date and time of catheterisation • Type of catheter, including length and size • Volume of sterile water injected into the balloon • Batch number • Manufacturer • Any problems encountered during the procedure • Review date/date to change catheter (RCN 2021)	9 To provide an accurate record.

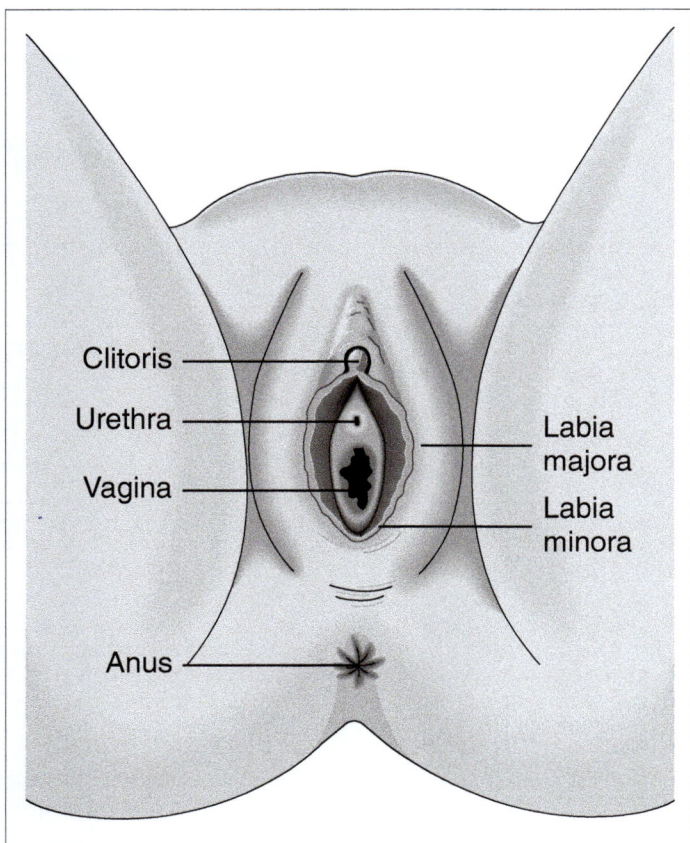

Figure 33.1 Anatomy of the female genitourinary system. *Source:* © Great Ormond Street Hospital for Children NHS Foundation Trust.

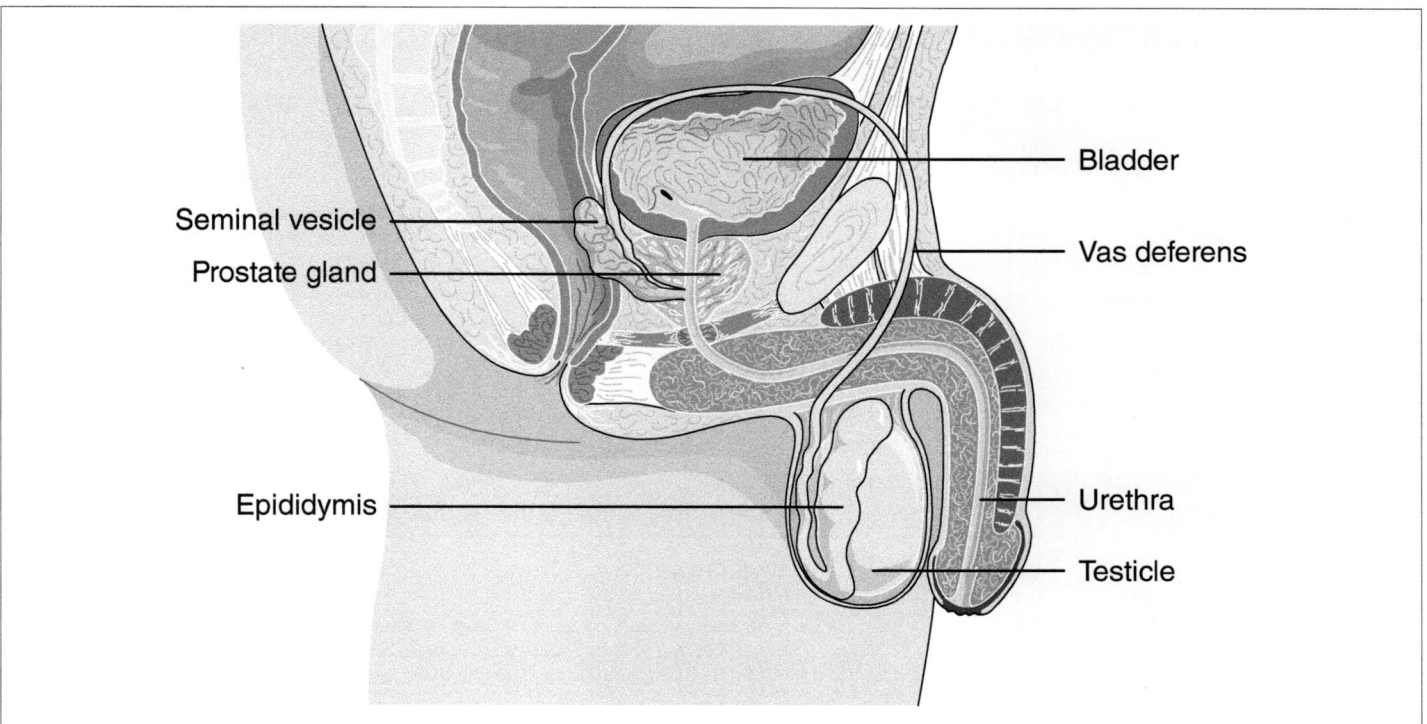

Figure 33.2 Anatomy of the male genitourinary system. *Source:* © Great Ormond Street Hospital for Children NHS Foundation Trust.

Procedure guideline 33.3 Catheter care: general

Statement	Rationale
1 Ensure catheter is securely taped.	1 To provide comfort and prevent accidental removal of the catheter.
2 Encourage adequate fluid intake.	2 To encourage drainage and reduce the risk of complications such as infection and bladder spasms.
3 Analgesia should be given as prescribed on an 'as required' basis.	3 To reduce pain – the level of discomfort from an indwelling catheter can vary considerably, even if it is the correct size and correctly positioned.
4 Administer anticholinergics as prescribed.	4 To reduce the likelihood of bladder spasms (Bray and Sanders 2006). See bladder spasm protocol (Figure 33.3).

Management of Acute Bladder Spasm (e.g. post-operative Kelly procedure, bladder augmentation, hypospadias)

Bladder spasm symptoms:

Pain:
- Lower abdominal
- Perineal
- Intermittent/spasmodic

Patient may also have:
- Urgency to void
- Leaking around catheter
- Peri-anal itch

Exclude other potential problems:

Constipation Management
- Assessment using validated tool: e.g. Bristol Stool Chart
- Optimise fluid intake (e.g. ice-lollies, jelly, smoothies)
- Increase dietary fibre (fruit, vegetables, whole grains)
- Consider glycerine suppository or stool softeners

Blocked catheter? Monitor catheter tubing for:
- kinks
- blood clots
- mucous

Postoperative pain management:

Treatment of wound pain:
Paediatric Analgesia & Antiemetic guideline (poster)

Consider increasing rate of epidural analgesia if in use. Assess risk/benefit of prolonged use of epidural if oral route not available.

Spasm management — If patient is allowed oral intake

OXYBUTININ	Dose by mouth	REGULAR
> 1 month and < 10 kg	0.1 mg/kg	twice a day
> 10 kg and < 2 years	0.1 mg/kg	3 times a day, increase to 0.2 mg/kg 3 times a day (max. per dose 1.25 mg)
2–4 years	1.25 mg	3 times a day, increase if necessary up to 2.5 mg 3 times a day
5–11 years	2.5 mg	3 times a day, increase if necessary up to 5 mg 3 times a day
12–17 years	5 mg	3 times a day, increase if necessary up to 5 mg 4 times a day

- Oral oxybutynin is available in 2.5 mg and 5 mg tablets. Tablets can be halved, crushed and dispersed in a small amount of water
- Oxybutynin 5 mg in 5 mL oral solution is available for doses less than 1.25 mg
- The frequency can be reduced to twice a day if patient is affected by side-effects

Avoid administering alongside antimuscarinics (anticholinergics) with similar properties (e.g. hyoscine butylbromide, hyoscine hydrobromide)

Add in as needed

DIAZEPAM	Dose by mouth	PRN
> 1 month	0.1–0.2 mg/kg	2–4 times a day (max. per dose 2 mg)
5–11 years	2.5 mg	2–4 times a day
12–17 years	2.5 mg–5 mg	2–4 times a day

- Oral diazepam is available in 2 mg in 5 ml oral solution, 2 mg and 5 mg tablets
- Use with care due to combined sedative effect with opioids
- **Discuss the use of diazepam with consultant before prescribing.**

Spasm management — If patient is nil by mouth (NBM)

Please note: Switch to oral treatment once patient is tolerating oral intake and absorption can be assured

HYOSCINE BUTYLBROMIDE	Dose by intravenous injection	REGULAR
> 1 month	300–500 micrograms/kg	3–4 times a day (max. per dose 5 mg)
5–11 years	5–10 mg	3–4 times a day (max. 30 mg per day)
12–17 years	10–20 mg	3–4 times a day (max. 80 mg per day)

Avoid administering alongside antimuscarinics (anticholinergics) with similar properties (e.g. oxybutynin, hyoscine hydrobromide)

Add in as needed

DIAZEPAM	Dose by rectum	PRN
≥ 12.5 kg	2.5 mg	2–4 times a day
12–17 years	2.5–5 mg	2–4 times a day

- Rectal diazepam is available in 2.5 mg and 5 mg rectal tubes
- Use with care due to combined sedative effect with opioids
- Avoid rectal medications if patient is neutropenic
- **Discuss the use of diazepam with consultant before prescribing.**

If spasm persists, contact the Pain Control Service for advice (bleep 0577)

- **Co-prescribing antimuscarinics:** When transitioning from intravenous to oral antimuscarinics, the co-prescription of a single dose of intravenous hyoscine butylbromide may be considered, along with the 1st dose of oral oxybutynin.
- **Stopping antimuscarinics:** Stop oxybutynin the night before catheter removal to prevent urine retention.
- **Patients with ureteric JJ-stent:** Oxybutynin contraindicated unless urethral catheter in situ
- **Interactions:** The antimuscarinic effect of oxybutynin and hyoscine butylbromide may be intensified by the following medications: antihistamines, atropine and related compounds, tri- and tetracyclic antidepressants and any other antimuscarinics.

Figure 33.3 GOSH protocol for the management of acute bladder spasm. Source: Saul et al. (2021).

Procedure guideline 33.4 Catheter care: entry site

Statement	Rationale
1 The catheter must be secured to the abdomen using hypoallergenic adhesive strapping at all times.	1 To prevent accidental removal and trauma to the entry site/urethral meatus.
2 The strapping, and retention suture for suprapubic catheters and stents, should be checked for security whenever the catheter bag is emptied.	2 To maintain the security of the catheter.
3 Usual hygiene appropriate for age should be maintained while the catheter is in situ (Loveday et al. 2014; NICE 2012, 2015).	3
a) For suprapubic catheters, a shallow bath should be used to avoid soaking the entry site.	a) To minimise the risk of infection.
b) Observe the entry site/urethral meatus for trauma and infection.	b) To ensure prevention or early detection and treatment of complications.
c) The doctor should be informed of any bleeding, discharge or inflammation.	c) To ensure effective treatment of complications.
d) If present this must be recorded in the CYP's health care records.	d) To maintain an accurate record.
4 If an infection is suspected a swab should be taken for microbiological examination.	4 To enable identification of micro-organisms (Higgins 2013).
5 Entry site or meatal cleaning should be performed daily.	
6 Gather the following equipment:	6
a) Nonsterile latex free gloves and a plastic apron.	a) To minimise the risk of cross infection (NICE 2012; Sanders 2001).
b) Dressing pack and additional sterile gauze.	
c) Clean non linting gauze.	c) Cotton wool should not be used as it can deposit fibres around the entry site, which can cause irritation and increase the risk of infection.
d) Foil bowl containing soap and water (urethral catheters). OR Sachet sterile 0.9% sodium chloride (suprapubic catheters and stents).	d) Soap and water provides effective cleansing for urethral catheters. There is no advantage in using antiseptic preparations for cleansing (Sanders 2001).
e) Hypoallergenic, latex free adhesive strapping, e.g. Mefix.	e) To replace the strapping if necessary.
f) Adhesive remover if necessary.	f) To remove any old tape.
7 To clean a bleeding or infected entry site:	7
a) Explain the procedure.	a) To promote co-operation and involvement and relieve anxiety.
b) Fill a clean foil bowl with warm soap and water. For suprapubic catheters and stents, warm a sachet of 0.9% sodium chloride.	b) Warm solution causes less discomfort.
c) Put on plastic apron and perform hand hygiene.	c) To minimise the risk of infection (Loveday et al. 2014; NICE 2012, 2015).
d) Remove any strapping. Remove dressings on suprapubic catheters using adhesive remover.	d) To enable entry site/meatus to be accessed and to minimise discomfort.
e) Perform hand hygiene.	e) To minimise the risk of infection.
f) Apply alcohol-based gel to hands and put on gloves.	f) To prevent contamination of gloves.
g) With non-dominant hand, hold catheter using sterile gauze.	g) To minimise the risk of infection.
For urethral catheters (males):	
h) Using gauze soaked in warm soapy water, clean the prepuce/meatus with a circular motion.	
i) Ensure all soap is rinsed off.	
For urethral catheters (females):	
j) Using gauze soaked in warm soapy water, clean the outer/inner labia and vulval groove using a vertical downward motion.	j) To minimise the risk of spreading infection.
k) Ensure all soap is rinsed off.	

(continued)

The Great Ormond Street Hospital Manual of Children and Young People's Nursing Practices

Procedure guideline 33.4 Catheter care: entry site *(continued)*

Statement	Rationale
For suprapubic catheters and stents:	
l) Using gauze soaked in 0.9% saline wipe around the entry site once.	
For all catheters:	
m) A new piece of non linting gauze must be used each time until the entry site/meatus is cleaned.	
n) Ensure the area is dry once the procedure is complete.	
o) Re-secure the catheter.	o) To prevent trauma and accidental removal of the catheter.
p) Dispose of equipment according to the trust's waste policy.	p) To minimise the risk of cross infection.
q) Remove gloves and apron (dispose of in clinical waste bag). Perform a social hand-wash and dry hands thoroughly.	
r) Record procedure in CYP's healthcare records.	r) To provide an accurate record.

Procedure guideline 33.5 Emptying a catheter drainage bag

Statement	Rationale
1 To empty a catheter drainage bag:	1
a) Inform the CYP and family.	a) To promote cooperation and involvement.
b) Put on an apron, perform a social hand-wash, dry hands thoroughly, and put on clean nonsterile gloves.	b) To minimise risk of cross infection and colonisation of the exit port (Loveday et al. 2014; NICE 2012, 2015).
c) Clean the exit port of the drainage bag using a 2% chlorhexidine/ 70% alcohol wipe.	c) To minimise risk of cross infection.
d) Empty the urine into a pulp or foil bowl, taking care not to allow the container to touch the exit port.	d) To ensure accurate fluid balance recording and minimise risk of catheter associated infections (Loveday et al. 2014; NICE 2012, 2015).
e) Wipe the exit port again with 2% chlorhexidine/70% alcohol wipe.	
f) Use a new receptacle for each catheter.	f) To avoid risk of cross infection (Loveday et al. 2014; NICE 2012, 2015).
g) Measure urine by weighing in bowl (i.e. 1 g = 1 ml). Ensure dry bowl weight is removed from total.	g) To ensure accuracy of measurement.
h) Discard urine in the sluice.	h) To avoid cross infection.
i) Discard pulp bottle/ bowl in macerator.	i) As per local infection control hospital policy
j) Remove gloves and apron and dispose of as per local waste policy; perform hand hygiene and dry hands thoroughly.	j) To safely dispose of waste and minimise risk of cross infection (Loveday et al. 2014; NICE 2012, 2015).
k) Record urinary output on the fluid balance chart in millilitres.	k) To ensure accurate fluid balance recording.
l) Also record in the CYP's nursing notes: • The colour of their urine. • Any signs of infection. • Any debris observed.	l) To monitor for signs of infection.

Chapter 33 Urinary catheter care

Procedure guideline 33.5 Emptying a catheter drainage bag *(continued)*

Statement	Rationale
Open drainage system with suprapubic/urethral catheters (double nappies)	
1 The double nappy method involves using two nappies, instead of a catheter bag, with the catheter placed in the outer nappy to avoid contamination of stool. This method can be used for a child under the age of three or those CYPs still wearing nappies at home. This must be discussed and agreed with the medical team.	1 Double nappies may be safer for the CYP who is at risk of pulling at or falling over the tubing of a catheter bag. It is practical for CYPs discharged with a catheter on a short-term basis and provides reassurance for carers who can change their nappies as they would at home, providing they have received information upon how to care for the catheter.
2 Place the first nappy on the child, then gently bring the catheter out of the leg or over the top of the inner nappy and place it into the outer nappy. Be careful to ensure that there are no kinks or twists in the catheter.	2 To allow drainage of urine into the second nappy.
3 It is important to note that a hole must <u>not</u> be made in the first nappy.	3 Studies have identified that granules in the nappy can block the catheter, which causes obstruction (Bertozzi et al. 2010).
4 This method is unsuitable for an immunocompromised child.	4 To avoid an increased risk of infection.

Procedure guideline 33.6 Maintaining catheter drainage

Statement	Rationale
1 If urinary drainage decreases or the CYP is experiencing increased discomfort:	
a) Check the catheter and tubing for kinking or obstruction.	a) Kinking will prevent drainage and cause discomfort.
b) Position the catheter drainage bag below the level of the bladder, but ensure that is not in contact with the floor.	b) To prevent reflux, promote drainage and minimise the risk of infection (Loveday et al. 2014; NICE 2012, 2015).
c) Calculate fluid balance.	c) To assess whether decreased output is related to reduced intake (Methany 2010).
d) Look for blockages in the drainage bag tubing caused by debris, blood clots, or mucus. If these are present, gently squeeze the catheter above the location of the blockage.	d) To break up the blockage and create a vacuum in the tubing, which can mobilise the blockage.
2 Calculate the urine output; this should be above 1 ml/kg/hr. in CYPs. If this is not achieved:	2 This is considered the least amount for the kidneys to produce in order to ensure adequate fluid and electrolyte balance (Methany 2010).
a) Encourage an increase in oral intake if appropriate.	
b) Consult the medical team; an intravenous infusion may need to be commenced or the rate of an existing infusion increased.	b) To ensure adequate hydration and increase urine output.
c) It is recommended that all CYPs with an indwelling catheter increase fluids from their normal intake.	c) To avoid the colonisation of bacteria in the urine and flush out any micro-organisms or debris in long-term catheterisation.

Procedure guideline 33.7 Flushing suprapubic, urethral or mitrofanoff catheters

Statement	Rationale
1 Suprapubic, urethral, and Mitrofanoff catheters may be flushed if the catheter has stopped draining or as part of postoperative/long-term care of an indwelling catheter.	1 To dislodge blockages, such as blood and mucus, which can cause a build-up of urine, bladder spasms, and urine to bypass the catheter (Fillingham and Douglas 2004). An unresolved blockage can also lead to bladder distension, which can compromise the bladder's blood supply and leave the bladder vulnerable to infection (McLeod et al. 2013).
To flush a urethral, suprapubic or Mitrofanoff catheter	
2 Gather the following equipment:	
a) Plastic apron.	
b) Latex free non-sterile gloves.	
c) Sachet of 0.9% sodium chloride.	

(continued)

Procedure guideline 33.7 Flushing suprapubic, urethral or mitrofanoff catheters *(continued)*

Statement	Rationale
d) Two 2% chlorhexidine/70% alcohol wipes.	
e) New catheter drainage bag if required.	
f) A 50ml bladder syringe.	f) To reduce the pressure imposed on the bladder mucosa while flushing and minimise the risk of trauma (Fillingham and Douglas 2004).
3 a) Explain the procedure.	3 a) To relieve anxiety and promote cooperation and involvement.
b) Place a sachet of saline in a clean foil bowl, containing warm water.	b) Warm solution reduces discomfort.
c) Put on a plastic apron.	c) To minimise the risk of cross infection (Loveday et al. 2014; NICE 2012, 2015).
d) Perform hand hygiene and dry hands thoroughly.	
e) Dry the sachet of 0.9% saline.	
f) Open 2% chlorhexidine/70% alcohol wipes.	
g) Apply alcohol gel to hands and put on non sterile gloves.	
h) Using an aseptic non touch technique, draw up the prescribed volume of saline into the syringe and place back into packaging of syringe.	h) To minimise the risk of infection. The volume used is dependent on the underlying condition or nature of the surgery.
i) In one circular motion, clean around the join of the catheter and the drainage bag using one 2% chlorhexidine/70% alcohol wipe.	
j) Allow to dry.	
k) Kink the catheter and remove the drainage bag.	k) To prevent leakage of urine from the catheter.
l) Wipe the end of the catheter with a second 2% Chlorhexidine/70% alcohol wipe.	l) To minimise the risk of infection.
m) Allow to dry.	
n) Insert the syringe into the end of the catheter and unkink the tubing.	
o) If there is **no** resistance push the fluid into the catheter with a smooth and steady motion.	
p) If there is resistance push the catheter a little more firmly.	
q) Do not continue pushing if resistance increases.	q) To prevent damage to the bladder mucosa (Fillingham and Douglas 2004).
r) If necessary, draw back on the syringe. This should be done gently.	r) To prevent trauma to the urothelium, blockage of the catheter, pain and an increased risk of infection (Fillingham and Douglas 2004).
s) Kink tubing again.	s) To prevent leakage of urine.
t) Remove the syringe.	
u) Unkink the catheter and ensure drainage occurs.	
v) Connect a new drainage bag.	
w) Secure the catheter to the CYP's abdomen with hypo-allergenic, latex free adhesive strapping.	w) To prevent trauma (Spinks 2013).
x) Dispose of equipment as per local waste disposal policy.	x, y) To prevent cross infection (Loveday et al. 2014; NICE 2012, 2015).
y) Remove gloves and apron and dispose of as per local policy. Perform hand hygiene and dry hands thoroughly.	
4 Record procedure and amount drained in CYP's healthcare records.	4 To ensure accurate record keeping and good communication.
5 Inform the medical team if there was resistance to flushing and/or no drainage occurred following the flush.	5 Further investigations may be needed to assess reasons for poor drainage.

Procedure guideline 33.8 Removal of suprapubic and urethral catheters

Once the decision to remove an indwelling catheter has be made this may be done by, or under the supervision of a nurse or doctor experienced in the technique (Loveday et al. 2014; NICE 2012, 2015, RCN 2021).

Statement	Rationale
1 Gather the following equipment: 　a) An appropriate sized syringe for a Foley catheter. 　b) Nonsterile latex-free gloves. 　c) Stitch cutter if required. 　d) Plastic apron. 　e) Adhesive remover wipe.	1 To enable the procedure to be performed safely and efficiently.
2 Standard precautions and an aseptic non touch technique must be used.	2 To minimise the risk of infection.
3 Give analgesia well in advance of the procedure.	3 To relieve any discomfort from catheter removal and first micturition.
4 If the CYP is prescribed oxybutynin they should not have a dose within 8 hours of a planned catheter removal.	4 This reduces bladder tone, which could delay micturition after catheter removal (Abrams et al. 2006).

To remove the catheter:

Statement	Rationale
1 Prepare the CYP and family.	1 To promote cooperation and involvement and reduce anxiety.
2 Put on an apron.	2–4 To minimise the risk of cross infection.
3 Perform hand hygiene and dry hands thoroughly.	
4 Put on gloves.	
5 Using adhesive remover, remove adhesive strapping from abdomen, while supporting the weight of the catheter.	5, 6 To reduce trauma to the skin.
6 Cut retaining suture if in situ.	
7 Deflate balloon (Foley catheters): 　a) Insert syringe into the one-way valve. 　b) Withdraw the documented volume of sterile water. 　c) If the sterile water cannot be withdrawn consult the CYP's doctor.	7 To avoid trauma to urethra 　a) To enable balloon on catheter to be deflated. 　d) Occasionally the one-way valve fails to release the sterile water.
8 Hold catheter at the entry site.	8 To enable catheter to be gently pulled.
9 Encourage deep breaths.	9 To relax abdominal wall and bladder neck.
10 While the CYP exhales, gently pull on the catheter in one steady motion until it is completely removed.	10 To minimise risk of the catheter catching on the bladder neck or urethra, as this can cause pain, mucosal damage, and bladder spasms.

For suprapubic catheters:

Statement	Rationale
1 Do not use excessive force.	1 To prevent the catheter from breaking.
2 Contact the CYP's doctor if the catheter cannot be removed.	2 The internal suture may still be intact or it may be caught in oedematous tissue.
3 Following removal, apply pressure to the entry site for one minute with sterile gauze.	3, 4 To promote closure of the bladder and abdominal wall and prevent bleeding and leakage of urine.
4 Leave gauze in situ and apply strapping to secure.	
5 If site is bleeding/leaking urine, inform the CYP's doctor.	5 The entry site may not have sealed following the application of initial pressure.

For all catheters

Statement	Rationale
1 Dispose of urine and equipment according to the Trust's Waste Policy.	1, 2 To minimise the risk of cross infection.
2 Remove gloves and apron, perform a social hand-wash and dry hands thoroughly.	
3 Record volume of urine in drainage bag on fluid balance chart.	3, 4 To maintain an accurate record.
4 Record procedure in the CYP's healthcare records.	

(continued)

Procedure guideline 33.8 Removal of suprapubic and urethral catheters *(continued)*

Statement	Rationale
Care after catheter removal	
1 Observe the CYP to ensure that they are able to pass urine normally.	1 To ensure they are not retaining urine.
2 The time limit to first micturition should be determined by the CYP's doctor.	2 There is a risk of urine leakage due to excess pressure following bladder or urethral surgery.
3 The CYP and family must be informed that the first micturition may be painful.	3 To provide information.
4 Document the first micturition on the fluid balance chart and in the CYP's healthcare record.	4 To maintain an accurate record.
5 The CYP's doctor must be informed if they: a) Are unable to pass urine. b) Have dysuria.	5 a) The bladder neck or urethra may be oedematous, which can cause pain and/or obstruction. b) To identify any possible complications.
In addition, for suprapubic catheters	
1 The doctor should be informed if the entry site leaks on first micturition.	1 Increased bladder pressure may cause a leak.
2 a) The entry site must be observed for haemorrhage and urine leakage. b) If either occurs, pressure must be applied and the CYP's doctor informed.	2 a) If the bladder bleeds or leaks urine, a haematoma or urinoma may form, creating a risk of infection (Fillingham and Douglas 2004). b) To ensure that the complication is treated swiftly.
3 The dressing should be removed after 24 hours.	3 To promote healing. Once the site is healed a dressing will no longer be required.

Procedure guideline 33.9 Discharge planning

Statement	Rationale
1 If the CYP is being discharged with a catheter in situ it is essential that teaching takes place and local support is organised (Samwell 2012). a) Parents/carers must have been taught and be competent in the following: • Catheter drainage. • Care of catheter site. Securing the catheter. • Signs and symptoms of a UTI. • What to do if the catheter stops draining. • What to do if the catheter is accidentally removed b) Written information should also be given on discharge, including emergency contact information. c) Ensure that the family have enough supplies to last until they return for removal of the catheter or until supplies are organised locally. This includes catheter bags, catheter syringes and securement devices.	1 a) To ensure the safety of the CYP and minimise risks with the urinary catheter (RCN 2021) b) Available online at www.gosh.nhs.uk/medical-information-0/procedures-and-treatments/looking-after-your-childs-urethral-catheter. c) To enable them to effectively care for the catheter at home.
2 Liaise with the community children's nursing team, providing information on the CYP's medical history and needs.	2 To provide support for the parents and carers at home following discharge from hospital (Samwell 2012). Communication between teams is essential for the safe transition of care from the hospital to the home setting.
3 Medication teaching, including dosage, frequency, and side effects.	3 To ensure that the CYP receives the correct medication at home.
4 Ensure appropriate follow-up is organised and communicated to the family or carer.	4 To ensure the CYP's safety through regular reviews with the care titrated to their needs including dates for catheter removal/or change, teaching, radiology investigations.

References

Abrams, P., Cardozo, L., Chapple, C. et al. (2006). Comparison of the efficacy, safety, and tolerability of the propiverine and oxybutynin for the treatment of overactive bladder syndrome. *International Journal of Urology* 13 (6): 692–698.

Addison, R. (2000). Catheterisation using lignocaine gel. *Nursing Times* 96 (41): 43–44.

Association of Paediatric Anaesthetists of Great Britain and Ireland (APAGBI) (2012). Good practice in postoperative and procedural pain management. 2nd edition. Pediatric Anesthesia, 22 (1): 1–79.

Bertozzi, M., Prestipino, M., Nardi, N., and Appignani, A. (2010). Care on double diaper technique after hypospadias repair. *Journal of Pediatric Surgical Specialities* 4: 44–45.

Bowden, V.R. and Greenbers, C.S. (2011). *Paediatric Nursing Procedures*, 3e. London: Lippincott Williams and Wilkins.

Boybeyi, O., Karnak, I., Tanyel, F.C., and Senocak, M.E. (2013). Risk factors of catheter associated urinary tract infections in paediatric surgical patients. *Surgical Practice* 17: 7–12.

Bray, L. and Sanders, C. (2006). Nursing management of paediatric urethral catheterisation. *Nursing Standard* 20 (24): 51–60.

Cedeno, D.P. (2008). Preventing Unnecessary Urinary Catheter Use. The 19th International Nursing Research Congress: Focusing on Evidence Practice.

Cutts, B. (2005). Developing and implementing a new bladder irrigation chart. *Nursing Standard* 20 (8): 48–52.

Farringdon, N., Fader, M., and Richardson, A. (2013). Managing urinary incontinence at the end of life: an examination of the evidence that informs practice. *International Journal of Palliative Care* 19 (9): 449–456.

Fillingham, S. and Douglas, J. (2004). *Urological Nursing*, 3e. London: Bailliere Tindall.

Gokula, M., Smolen, D., Gaspar, P.M. et al. (2012). Designing a protocol to reduce catheter-associated urinary tract infections among hospitalised patients. *American Journal of Infection Control* 40: 1000–1002.

GOSH (2012). Looking after your child's urethral catheter. https://www.gosh.nhs.uk/conditions-and-treatments/procedures-and-treatments/looking-after-your-childs-urethral-catheter/ (accessed 28 June 2022).

Gould, C.V., Umscheid, C.A., Agarwal, R.K. et al. (2010). Guideline for prevention of catheter-associated urinary tract infections 2009. *Infection Control and Hospital Epidemiology* 31: 319–326.

Gurung, P. Banks, F. Fell, S. (2007). Reconstruction options in adolescent urology. *Continence UK*, 1 (4): 9–14.

Hanchett, M. (2002). Techniques for stabilising urinary catheters. Tape maybe the oldest method but it's the only one. *American Journal of Nursing* 102 (3): 44–48.

Higgins, C. (2013). *Understanding Laboratory Investigations. A Text for Healthcare Professionals*, vol. 3. Oxford: Blackwell Science.

Krishnan, A., de Souza, A., Konijeti, R., and Baskin, L.S. (2006). The anatomy and embryology of posterior urethral valves. *Journal of Urology* 175 (4): 1214–1220.

Loveday, H.P., Wilson, J.A., Pratt, R.J. et al. (2014). epic3: National evidence-based guidelines for preventing healthcare-associated infections in NHS hospitals in England. *Journal of Hospital Infection* 86S1: S1–S70.

McLafferty, E., Johnstone, C., Hendry, C., and Farley, A. (2014). The urinary system. *Nursing Standard* 28 (27): 42–49.

McLeod, L., Southerland, K., and Bond, J. (2013). A clinical audit of postoperative urinary retention in the postanesthesia care unit. *Journal of PeriAnesthesia Nursing* 28 (4): 210–216.

McMonnies, G. (2002). Paediatric continence in children with neurogenic bladders. *British Journal of Nursing* 11 (11): 765–772.

Methany, N.M. (2010). *Fluid and Electrolyte Balance: Nursing Considerations*, 5e. Philadelphia: Lippincott.

Minkin, G.C. and Baskin, L.S. (2003). Surgical management of the neurogenic bladder and bowel. *International Brazilian Journal of Urology* 29 (1): 53–61.

Nasir, A., Emmanuel, A., Lukman, A.R. et al. (2011). Posterior urethral valve. *World Journal of Pediatrics* 7 (3): 205–216.

National Institute for Health and Care Excellence (NICE) (2007). Urinary tract infection in under 16s: diagnosis and management [CG54]. https://www.nice.org.uk/Guidance/CG54 (accessed 28 June 2022).

National Institute for Health and Care Excellence (NICE) (2012) Healthcare-associated infections: prevention and control in primary and community care. Clinical guideline [CG139]. https://www.nice.org.uk/Guidance/CG139 (accessed 1 April 2021).

Nazarko, L. (2007). Avoiding the pitfalls and perils of catheter care. *British Journal of Nursing* 16 (8): 468–472.

Nursing & Midwifery Council. (2015, updated 2018). The Code: Professional standards of practice and behaviour for nurses, midwives and nursing associates. https://www.nmc.org.uk/standards/code/ (accessed 24 June 2022).

Parry, M.F., Grant, B., and Sestovic, M. (2013). Successful reduction in catheter-associated urinary tract infections: focus on nurse-directed catheter removal. *American Journal of Infection Control* 41: 1178–1181.

Pomfret, I. (2010). Catheter care: is it really improving. *Journal of Community Nursing* 24 (5): 26–28.

Royal College of Nursing (RCN) (2021). Catheter Care: Guidance for Health Care Professionals. London: RCN. https://www.rcn.org.uk/professional-development/publications/catheter-care-guidance-for-health-care-professionals-uk-pub-009-915 (accessed 28 June 2022).

Royal College of Nursing (RCN) (2019) Restrictive physical interventions and the clinical holding of children and young people. Guidance for nursing staff. London: RCN. https://www.rcn.org.uk/Professional-Development/publications/pub-007746 (accessed 24 June 2022).

Samwell, B. (2012). From hospital to home: journey of a child with special care needs. *Nursing Children and Young People* (14): 16–19.

Sanders, C. (2001). Suprapubic catheterisation: risk management. *Paediatric Nursing* 13 (10): 14–18.

Saul, B., McElligott, I., Cleary, K., Sawyer, N., Ooi, K., Urology Team (2021). Management of acute bladder spasm. GOSH Protocol.

Shaban, A., Drake, M.J., and Hashim, H. (2010). The medical management of urinary incontinence. *Autonomic Neuroscience: Basic and Clinical* 152 (1–2): 4–9.

Smith, L. (2003). Which catheter? Criteria for selection of urinary catheters for children. *Paediatric Nursing* 15 (3): 14–18.

Spinks, J. (2013). Urinary incontinence and the importance of catheter fixation. *Journal of Community Nursing* 27 (5): 24–29.

Steggall, M., Treacy, C., and Jones, M. (2013). Post-operative urinary retention. *Nursing Standard* 28 (5): 43–48.

Thomas, D.F.M., Rickwood, A.M.K., and Duffy, P.G. (eds.) (2008). *Essentials of Paediatric Urology*, 2e. London: Martin Dunitz.

Turner, T.W. (2004). Intravesical catheter knotting: an uncommon complication of urinary catheterisation. *Paediatric Emergency Care* 2 (2): 115–117.

Twycross, A., Dowden, S.J., and Stinson, J. (eds.) (2014). *Managing Pain in Children: A Clinical Guide for Nurses and Healthcare Professionals*, 2e. Oxford: Wiley.

Wilson, M. (2012). Addressing the problems of long-term urethral catheterisation: part 2. *British Journal of Nursing* 21 (1): 16–25.

Woodward, S., Steggal, M., and Juliana, T. (2013). Clean intermittent self-catheterisation: improving quality of life. *British Journal of Nursing* suppl. Urology supplement 22 (9): S20–S22–S25.

Wright, E. (2012). Reviewing urinary complications of epidural analgesia in children with orthopaedic conditions. *Nursing Children and Young People* 24 (2): 32–36.

Yates, A. (2004). Crisis management in catheter care. *Journal of Community Nursing* 18 (5): 28.

Chapter 34

Drug withdrawal: prevention and management

Rebecca Saul

RN (Child), RN (Adult), MSc, Clinical Nurse Specialist, Pain Control Service, GOSH

Chapter contents

Introduction	770	Prevention of withdrawal symptoms	771
Definitions	770	Assessment of the symptoms of withdrawal	771
Incidence of withdrawal	770	Management of withdrawal of opioid and benzodiazepine therapy	771
Mechanisms of tolerance	770	Pharmacological weaning management	772
Overall aims of withdrawal management	770	References	777

Procedure guidelines

34.1 Prevention of opioid or benzodiazepine withdrawal symptoms	772	34.5 Conversion from intravenous to oral medication	775
34.2 Assessment of opioid and benzodiazepine withdrawal	773	34.6 Clonidine	776
34.3 Taking a patient history	773	34.7 Non-pharmacological management	776
34.4 Creating a weaning plan	774		

The Great Ormond Street Hospital Manual of Children and Young People's Nursing Practices, Second Edition. Edited by Elizabeth Anne Bruce, Janet Williss, and Faith Gibson.
© 2023 John Wiley & Sons Ltd. Published 2023 by John Wiley & Sons Ltd.

Introduction

Clinically significant iatrogenic withdrawal has been linked to the continuous infusion of opioids and/or benzodiazepines, the duration of exposure to such agents, and the rate at which drug reductions are made (Grant et al. 2013). The prolonged use of opioids (e.g. morphine, fentanyl) and benzodiazepines (e.g. midazolam) for pain management and sedation in children and young people (CYPs) are well-established practices that reduce the emotional, physiological, and metabolic response to critical illness (Cho et al. 2007; Birchley 2009). However, the use of any opioid or benzodiazepine has inherent consequences, which may include drug tolerance, physical dependence, cross-tolerance with similar pharmacological agents, and drug withdrawal (Anand et al. 2010).

Definitions

Misconceptions related to the nature of withdrawal from opioids and benzodiazepines are common; therefore it is vital that the healthcare professional is familiar with some standard definitions (see Box 34.1).

Incidence of withdrawal

Clinical studies have identified a 13% incidence of withdrawal symptoms in critically ill CYPs, for whom morphine and midazolam were the most commonly used analgesic and sedative agents (Jenkins et al. 2007). This ranges from 17 to 30% in CYPs receiving midazolam (Playfor et al. 2006), to as high as 57% in those receiving potent opioids such as fentanyl (Katz et al. 1994). Tolerance to opioids is more frequent following prolonged administration of short-acting opioids; it may develop earlier in younger children, and is more commonly seen in the critical care setting (Anand et al. 2010). Strategies and treatment regimens are required to manage these patients effectively (Galinkin and Koh 2014), and the use of nurse-driven protocols in paediatric intensive care settings can reduce the occurrence of withdrawal symptoms in CYPs (Neunhoeffer et al. 2015).

Mechanisms of tolerance

The mechanisms of tolerance and dependence are not clearly understood (Franck et al. 2012). It has been hypothesised that when opioids and benzodiazepines are administered continuously to a CYP, adaptation occurs in the central nervous system in response to prolonged receptor site occupancy (Yaster et al. 1996). Kosten & George (2002) outline the physiology of withdrawal as follows:

Within the locus coeruleus of the brain, naturally occurring opioids attach to mu receptors on nerves (neurones), activating an enzyme that converts adenosine triphosphate (ATP) into cyclic adenosine monophosphate (cAMP), and the release of noradrenaline (NA), a neurotransmitter that plays a role in arousal, respiration, and muscle tone. Opioid drugs attaching to mu opioid receptors inhibit the converting enzyme and thus levels of cAMP, and the release of noradrenaline declines respectively, which results in a corresponding reduction in respiration, alertness and muscle tone. In response to constant mu receptor occupancy over time the neurones build-up greater amounts of ATP and converting enzyme, such that increased levels of cAMP are produced in the neurones' efforts to maintain near-normal levels of noradrenaline. In response, the patient appears to become tolerant to the opioid drug. Sudden withdrawal of the opioid without a tapered reduction leaves the neurones functioning on abnormally elevated levels of ATP and converting enzyme, resulting in higher than normal levels cAMP and an excessive release of noradrenaline, causing the patient to experience increased levels of arousal, insomnia, and muscle tone (jittering). The introduction of N-methyl-D-aspartic acid (NMDA) receptor antagonists (such as ketamine) has been shown to reduce opioid tolerance, as NMDA receptor sensitivity may also be a factor in the desensitisation of mu-opioid receptors to opioids (Stein 2013).

Overall aims of withdrawal management

The health professional's role in the treatment of CYPs receiving long-term opioids or benzodiazepines includes the slow reduction of these drugs to prevent the onset of withdrawal symptoms (Ista et al. 2009), close monitoring for symptoms (Franck et al. 2012), and the complimentary use of nonpharmacological therapies (Playfor et al. 2006). In addition, good practice in opioid and benzodiazepine management should include avoidance of excessive sedation and maintenance of a normal sleep–wake pattern where possible (Puntillo et al. 1997). Clinically significant iatrogenic withdrawal (i.e. resulting from medical treatment) should be recognised as an adverse event in the intensive care setting (Grant et al. 2013). The aim of care should be to ensure that the CYP's medical condition is not compromised by the physical effects of drug withdrawal, as this may prolong their hospitalisation (Osborn et al. 2003).

Healthcare workers may be concerned that slow reduction of opioids or benzodiazepines as part of the weaning process may prolong the duration of mechanical ventilation (Ducharme et al. 2005). However, research suggests that tolerance to the respiratory depressive effects of opioids occurs rapidly (Franck et al. 2004), whereas a rapid reduction in sedatives may be associated with increased episodes of agitation, distress, and other physical

Box 34.1 Definitions

Tolerance	Reduction in a drug's efficacy over a period of time of repeated exposure, requiring the increase of the drug dose to produce the same initial response (Jage 2005).
Physical dependence	Adaptation of neurones, whereby abrupt cessation of the analgesic or sedative agent results in characteristic withdrawal symptoms (Anand et al. 2010).
Cross-tolerance	A CYP who is tolerant to one drug may also exhibit some tolerance to other similar drugs, e.g. a CYP who has developed tolerance to morphine may also show signs of tolerance to other opioids (Jage 2005).
Withdrawal syndrome	A response to sudden discontinuation of long-term sedative or analgesic drug treatment, characterised by a wide range of symptoms. This condition may affect the CYP's physical well-being and ultimately delay their recovery (Anand et al. 2010).
Addiction	Describes a multifaceted pattern of behaviours, which includes psychological, as well as a physiological dependence, due to habitual administration of a drug for its nonmedicinal qualities. It may be influenced by genetic, psychosocial, or environmental factors, and is a chronic neurological disease (Galinkin and Koh 2014). The use of this term can be confusing and is not appropriate in describing iatrogenic withdrawal (i.e. withdrawal induced by medical treatment).
Pseudo-addiction	Seemingly inappropriate analgesia seeking behaviours that result from under-treatment of pain, and which usually resolve when pain relief is adequate (Schug et al. 2015).

symptoms, which can obstruct the process of weaning mechanical ventilation (Alexander et al. 2002). Extubation or early discharge from the intensive care unit should not necessitate an excessively rapid reduction of opioids or benzodiazepines, as it is unlikely that appropriate weaning will disrupt the CYP's ongoing treatment (Tobias 2003). Many CYPs can be effectively weaned from the ventilator before opioid or benzodiazepine drugs are discontinued, often while still receiving relatively high-dose therapy (Tobias 2003).

Prevention of withdrawal symptoms

Interpreting the Symptoms of Withdrawal

The use of an appropriate withdrawal assessment tool is fundamental to the management of sedation and analgesic requirements of ventilated CYPs. Symptoms may vary from one individual to another (Ista et al. 2009), and while the characteristics of withdrawal from opioids or benzodiazepines are often similar, they may also be indicative of the specific analgesic or sedative agent being weaned (Ista et al. 2007, 2009). The signs and symptoms of withdrawal may be grouped under the following headings: dysregulation of the autonomic nervous system (evident as physiological changes), central nervous system dysregulation; abnormal motor movements (which are more pronounced with benzodiazepine withdrawal), and gastrointestinal disturbances which are not seen in benzodiazepine withdrawal (see Box 34.2) (Ista et al. 2009). It is important that symptoms of a worsening clinical condition are not mistaken for withdrawal symptoms and therefore other potential causes, such as metabolic, neurological problems are excluded before a diagnosis of withdrawal is made (see Box 34.3).

Assessment of the symptoms of withdrawal

Withdrawal Assessment Tools

The 'Sedation Withdrawal Score' (SWS) (Cunliffe et al. 2004) is a simple, 12-item scale. Each parameter is scored from 0 to 2 dependant on severity of symptoms, every 6 hours to achieve a maximum score of 24. Scores of greater than 6 indicate drug withdrawal of differing intensity. The SWS has been found to be clinically sensitive in detecting withdrawal symptoms in CYPs discharged from intensive care to the ward (see Box 34.4).

The *Withdrawal Assessment Tool-1* (WAT-1) (Franck et al. 2008, 2012) is an 11-item (12-point) multifactorial assessment tool, designed to be carried out every 12 hours. It has been tested in the intensive care setting in CYPs aged 2 weeks to 18 years, with a WAT-1 score *greater than* 3 indicating clinically significant symptoms of withdrawal. This is available online at http://www.marthaaqcurley.com/wat-1.html.

The *Sophia Observation Withdrawal Symptoms Scale* (SOS) (Ista et al. 2013) is a 15-item behavioural scale validated for use in critically ill children from 0 to 42 months. The score is based on the nurse's observations of the CYP over a previous four hour period and a score of *less than* 3 indicates 'no withdrawal syndrome' and *greater than* 4 'withdrawal syndrome'. This is available online at: https://www.comfortassessment.nl/web/index.php/instruments/sophia-observation-withdrawal-symptoms-scale-sos/scoring-form-sos/.

Management of withdrawal of opioid and benzodiazepine therapy

Withdrawal Protocols in CYPs

There is no standardised withdrawal protocol used in UK paediatric intensive care settings (Birchley 2009; Hudak and Tan 2012). Nevertheless, the duration of opioid and benzodiazepine therapy has been identified as a key indicator in predicting the risk of withdrawal symptoms (Ista et al. 2007). Continuous therapy over a number of days increases the risk of withdrawal symptoms developing. Fisher et al. (2013) identified a relationship between duration of opioid exposure and the risk of symptoms of physical dependence; however they found no relationship between the cumulative or peak opioid doses given to CYPs and the incidence of withdrawal symptoms. For more information see Table 34.1.

Box 34.2 Clinical symptoms of withdrawal of opioid and benzodiazepine medication

	Central nervous system dysregulation	**Gastrointestinal disturbances**	**Dysregulation of the autonomic nervous system**
Opioids	Increased muscle tone Uncoordinated movements Pupil dilation (>4 mm) High-pitched crying Myoclonus (sudden muscle contraction)	Nausea Vomiting Diarrhoea Poor feeding Uncoordinated/constant sucking	Tachypnoea Yawning Sneezing Hypertension Mottling
Benzodiazepines	Muscle twitching Inconsolable crying Jittering Visual/auditory hallucinations Disorientation Seizures, particularly in some infants Movement disorder		Increased secretions (frequent suctioning)
Opioids & Benzodiazepines	Tremors Anxiety Agitation Insomnia/sleep disturbance Involuntary movements (upper extremities)		Pyrexia Sweating Tachycardia

Adapted from Ista et al. 2007, 2009; additional references: Katz et al. 1994, Fisher et al. 2013.

Box 34.3 Other potential causes of withdrawal-like symptoms

- Inadequate sedation
- Inadequate analgesia
- Ventilator distress
- Infection
- Noisy surroundings
- Delirium
- Hypoxia
- Hypercarbia
- Cerebral hypoperfusion (due to alterations in cardiac output or cerebral vascular disease)
- Bladder distension
- Surgical lesions

(Tobias 2003, Ista et al. 2007)

Box 34.4 Sedation withdrawal score (Cunliffe et al. 2004)

Tremor	Sneezing
Irritability	Respiratory distress
Hypertonicity	Fever
Hyperactivity	Diarrhoea
Vomiting	Sweating
High-pitched cry	Convulsions

For each parameter score 0 = absent, 1 = mild, 2 = severe.
Maximum possible score = 24.
Instructions
Score (six hourly)
<6 Current regimen to remain
6–12 Do not reduce regimen further
12–18 Revert to former regimen
>18 Seek advice

Table 34.1 Categorising the risk of developing withdrawal symptoms

Risk category	Duration of opioid/benzodiazepine
Category 1 (low risk)	Less than 5 days
Category 2 (medium risk)	5–14 days
Category 3 (high risk)	More than 14 days

(Cunliffe et al. 2004; Saul et al. 2018)

Pharmacological weaning management

Procedure guideline 34.1 Prevention of opioid or benzodiazepine withdrawal symptoms

Principle	Rationale
1 a) All CYPs should have regular pain and sedation assessment using a validated tool such as the COMFORT tool, which is validated for the assessment of pain and sedation in both ventilated and nonventilated CYPs (Wolf and Jenkins 2005).	1 a) To monitor the effect of the drug(s) being administered, avoid inappropriate dose administration, and inform decisions regarding weaning (Wolf and Jenkins 2005).
b) Analgesic or sedative drug administration should be kept to the minimum required for efficacy.	b) To minimise the risk of tolerance and the development of physical dependence.
2 Nonsteroidal anti-inflammatory agents or paracetamol may be considered for use as adjunct therapy.	2 Nonsteroidal anti-inflammatory agents or paracetamol have been found to have an opioid-sparing effect in the perioperative (Wong et al. 2013) and postoperative setting (Hong et al. 2010) and may reduce overall opioid requirements in the critically ill patient, although further research to confirm this is required (Playfor et al. 2006).
3 Drug strategies that may limit the impact of prolonged sedative and analgesic therapy may be considered. These include: a) NMDA receptor antagonists (such as ketamine) b) Opioid rotation	3 To minimise withdrawal symptoms a) Combined use of ketamine and opioids may limit opioid tolerance, although the efficacy of this in critically ill CYPs requires further investigation (Anand et al. 2010). b) Opioid rotation is theoretically believed to delay the onset of tolerance but studies are needed to establish the efficacy of this strategy (Tobias 2000).

Chapter 34 Drug withdrawal: prevention and management

Procedure guideline 34.2 Assessment of opioid and benzodiazepine withdrawal

Principle	Rationale
1 A validated withdrawal assessment tool should be chosen by the unit based on its clinical utility. When choosing a withdrawal assessment tool, the following should be considered: • Ease of application. • Willingness of all members of the MDT to use the tool. • A strategy for staff education in the use and interpretation of the tool. • Availability of a flexible weaning protocol. (Easley and Nichols 2008)	1 No 'gold standard' assessment of withdrawal currently exists (Franck et al. 2008) and there are a limited number of tools that may be used for assessing withdrawal in CYPs who have been exposed to opioids or benzodiazepines (Ista et al. 2009).
2 Assessment scores should be used to: • Identify existing symptoms. • Establish a baseline score for any weaning plan implemented.	2 Withdrawal assessment tools should be used to objectively observe for signs and symptoms of withdrawal (Fisher et al. 2013).
3 The CYP should be assessed for level of risk, depending on the length of time they have received an opioid or benzodiazepine infusion (see Table 34.1).	3 To identify the likelihood of withdrawal symptoms and assist in planning the speed of the drug reduction (Ducharme et al. 2005).
4 The interval between assessments should be based on the specific withdrawal assessment tool chosen:	4 To use the validated tool as recommended. • The *Withdrawal Assessment Tool-1* (WAT-1) is designed to be carried out every 12 hours (Franck et al. 2012). • The *Sedation Withdrawal Score* suggests 6 hourly scores (Cunliffe et al. 2004) (Box 34.4). • The *Sophia Observation Withdrawal Symptoms Scale* (SOS) is performed 4 hourly (Ista et al. 2013).
5 Nurses' judgment should be taken into account when evaluating the score using a withdrawal assessment tool.	5 There is a strong correlation between nurses' clinical judgement and the occurrence of withdrawal (Frank et al. (2012).
6 Scoring tools may be modified on an individual basis to exclude symptoms of underlying conditions that may influence the withdrawal score and result in unnecessary treatment. For example, the occurrence of loose stools in a CYP with an ileostomy should be discounted as a symptom of withdrawal, as this is a normal event for this child (Franck et al. 1998).	6 To ensure that any underlying condition does not skew the withdrawal score and delay the weaning process unnecessarily (Franck and Vilardi 1995).

Procedure guideline 34.3 Taking a patient history

Principle	Rationale
1 Prior to weaning, a history of drug usage should be taken, including:	1 Withdrawal syndrome is thought to be related to the total drug doses received (Playfor et al. 2006) and the length of time a drug has been continuously infused (Ducharme et al. 2005).
a) Analgesic and sedative drug dosages, including the highest (peak) dose administered during treatment.	a) While the peak opioid dose does not affect the degree of opioid withdrawal symptoms experienced (Fisher et al. 2013), the percentage of the drug weaned per day is calculated from the highest dose administered, unless this was only maintained for a few hours.
b) Duration of opioid or benzodiazepine therapy.	b) Physical dependence to opioids generally occurs after 2 weeks of morphine administration, but may occur after as little as 2–3 days of therapy (Fisher et al. 2013). In a prospective observational study of critically ill children in 20 UK paediatric intensive care units, most episodes of withdrawal occurred within the first 7 days of admission, with symptoms emerging at around day 5 (Jenkins et al. 2007). The UK consensus guidelines on sedation and analgesia in critically ill children recommend that opioid and benzodiazepine withdrawal symptoms may occur after 7 days of continuous therapy (Playfor et al. 2006). Neonates and infants who received fentanyl infusions for more than 9 days had a 100% incidence of withdrawal symptoms (Katz et al. 1994). Withdrawal symptoms have also been observed after administration of continuous midazolam for more than 7 days (Sury et al. 1989), and for as few as 5 days (Ista et al. 2008).

(continued)

Procedure guideline 34.3 Taking a patient history *(continued)*

Principle	Rationale
c) Any weaning already undertaken (as a percentage of the peak dose).	c) To determine the effect of the weaning already undertaken and inform decisions regarding the appropriate rate for future weaning.
d) The use of any muscle relaxants.	d) Neuro-muscular blocking agents may increase the risk of withdrawal symptoms by masking the signs normally displayed that would otherwise prompt weaning of sedation. CYPs receiving neuromuscular blocking agents tend to receive higher doses of opioids and benzodiazepines (Tobias 2000; Birchley 2009).
e) Any previous history of opioid or benzodiazepine use or withdrawal problems.	e) This information assists the healthcare worker to identify those at risk of developing withdrawal symptoms and to provide individualised care (Tobias 2003).
4 A diagnosis of withdrawal syndrome should only be made if there has been a recent reduction or abrupt discontinuation of opioids or benzodiazepines and all other possible causes have been excluded (see Box 34.3).	4 To correctly identify and treat the underlying cause. Ongoing or associated conditions may have similar symptoms and these should be considered and discounted before a diagnosis of withdrawal syndrome is made (Ista et al. 2007, 2009; Playfor et al. 2006).
5 The onset of withdrawal symptoms may occur within hours or days of stopping analgesic or sedation therapy.	5 Opioid or benzodiazepine withdrawal typically occurs 8–48 hours after discontinuing the drug (Ista et al. 2007). Delayed manifestation of withdrawal symptoms may occur as a result of delayed metabolism or excretion of opioids or benzodiazepines due to changes in hepatic or renal blood flow.

Procedure guideline 34.4 Creating a weaning plan

Principle	Rationale
1 A weaning plan should be considered as soon as opioids or benzodiazepines are commenced and reassessed daily by the multidisciplinary team (MDT), who should be aware of the adverse effects of prolonged analgesia and sedation therapy. Whatever the weaning protocol adopted, it should be based on the premise of the regular delivery of decreasing amounts of the drug responsible for the actual or potential cause of withdrawal symptoms.	1 A therapeutic plan of analgesia should be formulated and reviewed to ensure that inadequate or excessive sedation is avoided (Playfor et al. 2006).
2 Depending on the duration of exposure to continuous opioid or benzodiazepine infusions, a CYP's risk of withdrawal should be categorised as 'low', 'moderate' or 'high' (Table 34.1).	2 The rate of weaning is based on the level of risk (see Table 34.1); the percentage reduction from the peak dose can then be agreed and its effect monitored.
3 The following protocols may form the basis of a weaning strategy for patients:	3 No one standardised withdrawal protocol is observed in UK paediatric intensive care settings (Birchley 2009; Hudak and Tan 2012).
4 **Category 1 patients (minimal risk)** CYPs on continuous opioids or benzodiazepine therapy for **fewer than 5 days** a) Taper sedation and analgesic drugs a as clinically indicated, e.g. prior to extubation. b) Assess the CYP using a validated withdrawal assessment tool. c) If withdrawal symptoms are observed, cease weaning and initiate treatment indicated by scores.	4 The literature suggests that those on short-term therapy (less than 3–5 days) may be weaned as rapidly as 50% per day (Jin et al. 2007), or in incremental dose reductions of 10–15% every 6–8 hours (Tobias 2000); although some authors suggest a daily wean of 20% following 1–3 days of therapy and 13–20% following continuous therapy for 4–7 days (Ducharme et al. 2005).
5 **Category 2 patients (moderate risk)** CYPs on continuous opioid or benzodiazepine therapy for **5 to 14 days** a) Reduce opioid and/or benzodiazepine infusion rate by **20% of the baseline dose** every 24 hours. b) Assess the CYP using a validated withdrawal assessment c) Initially, only one medication should be weaned at a time. d) If withdrawal symptoms persist/develop consider the following options: • Reduce weaning rate to **10% per day**. • Consider suspending weaning for a 24 hour period. • Revert to the last opioid/benzodiazepine dose at which acceptable withdrawal scores were maintained. • Re-commence previously discontinued benzodiazepine/opioid therapy if symptoms indicate withdrawal (see Box 34.2). • When symptoms resolve, consider weaning more slowly to prevent symptom recurrence. • Consider consultation from MDT at any point.	5 a) Weaning of longer term therapy (more than 5 days) may begin with daily dose reductions of 20% (Franck et al. 2004) or 10–25% every 12–24 hours (Jin et al. 2007), but may be as little as 8–13% following 8–14 days of continuous therapy (Ducharme et al. 2005). Weaning is usually accomplished by decreasing the dose every 24 to 48 hours (Galinkin and Koh 2014). b) To determine whether there are already any signs of withdrawal. c) Further studies are required to identify weaning criteria for tapering both opioid and benzodiazepine infusions at the same time (Ducharme et al. 2005). Reduction of one medication at a time may be beneficial so that any signs of withdrawal may be more clearly attributed to a single medication (Galinkin and Koh 2014). d) Movement disorders, grimacing, inconsolable crying, and hallucinations result from withdrawal of benzodiazepines (Ista et al. 2013). Gastrointestinal symptoms associated with opioid withdrawal include vomiting, diarrhoea and poor appetite (Anand et al. 2010).

Procedure guideline 34.4 Creating a weaning plan *(continued)*

Principle	Rationale
6 **Category 3 patients (highest risk)** CYPs on continuous opioid or benzodiazepine therapy for **more than 14 days** a) Reduce opioid and benzodiazepine infusions more slowly, e.g. by **10% of the baseline dose**, (Rationale 27) every 24 hours (Rationale 22) b) Assess the CYP using a validated withdrawal assessment c) Initially, only one medication should be weaned at a time. d) If withdrawal symptoms persist/develop consider the following options: • Reduce weaning rate to **5% per day**. • Consider suspending weaning for a 24 hour period. • Revert to the last opioid/benzodiazepine does at which acceptable withdrawal scores were maintained. • Recommence previously discontinued benzodiazepine/opioid therapy if symptoms indicate (see Box 34.2). • When symptoms resolve, consider weaning more slowly to prevent symptoms reoccurring. • Consider consultation from MDT at any point.	6a) Patients receiving continuous therapy for more than 14 days may require a daily dose reduction of 10% (Franck et al. 2004) or 8% for those weaning after 15–21 days; and 2–4% for CYPs who have received continuous therapy for more than 21 days (Ducharme et al. 2005). d) To minimise withdrawal symptoms. Throughout this process, dose reduction is slowed or suspended if withdrawal symptoms are observed and reinstated as symptoms subside (Franck et al. 2004).

Procedure guideline 34.5 Conversion from intravenous to oral medication

Statement	Rationale
1 Intravenous opioids and benzodiazepines should be converted to an oral equivalent as soon as possible (Birchley 2009). Criteria for conversion include:	1 While intravenous routes are essential during the CYP's stay in critical care, enteral medications should be introduced as soon as possible (Wolf and Jenkins 2005). Converting from an intravenous to an oral drug simplifies the weaning process and may allow for earlier discharge from ITU and subsequently from hospital (Tobias 2003).
a) The CYP must be tolerating enteral feeds.	a) Inability to tolerate or absorb the oral drug may lead to increase in withdrawal symptoms.
b) Withdrawal scores should be consistently low.	b) The efficacy of the oral dose cannot be accurately ascertained if the CYP is already showing signs of withdrawal.
c) The intravenous dose, when converted to the oral equivalent, should not exceed the dose recommended in the Trust's paediatric formulary. **NB:** If these criteria are not met, weaning management should continue on intravenous therapy.	c) To minimise the risk of errors.
2 Particular caution is required when converting to a different drug in the same group (e.g. from intravenous midazolam to oral diazepam).	2 Changing from one drug to another may require a reduction in the total dose administered, as cross-tolerance may vary (Indelicato and Portnoy 2002; Tobias 2003).

Suggested Conversion Factors

Route / drug		Conversion factor
From	**to**	
IV Morphine	Oral Morphine	× 3
IV Midazolam	Oral Diazepam	÷ 3

3 When a drug has been converted from intravenous to oral the following observations should be documented regularly: • Withdrawal assessment scoring • Respiratory rate (for signs of respiratory depression) • Sedation score (for signs of excessive sedation) • Blood pressure (hypotension)	3 To detect for early signs of respiratory depression, hypotension and withdrawal. The risk of over or underdosing is significant during the conversion phase and careful monitoring is essential (Tobias 2000).

Procedure guideline 34.6 Clonidine

Principle	Rationale
1 Clonidine is sometimes introduced as an adjunct to opioid or benzodiazepine weaning in patients with persistently raised withdrawal scores; however, it should be used with caution and only after discussion with the MDT. The health professional should be aware of its potential adverse effects, which include hypotension and bradycardia (Playfor et al 2006).	1 Clonidine is a sedative agent. There is limited information to support its use as an adjunct to the tapering process in the paediatric population (Osborn et al. 2003).
2 If clonidine has been administered for more than 2 weeks it should be weaned over 1 to 2 week period.	2 Stopping clonidine abruptly may cause severe symptoms such as rebound hypertension (D'Apolito 2009).
3 Regular vital signs monitoring, including heart-rate and blood pressure, should be undertaken throughout the use of clonidine.	3 Abrupt discontinuation of clonidine after extended administration may result in hypertension and/or seizures (Playfor et al. 2006).

Procedure guideline 34.7 Non-pharmacological management

Statement	Rationale
1 Ensure that all CYPs receive appropriate nonpharmacological interventions to prevent or minimise the symptoms of withdrawal, even if they are also receiving drug therapy.	1 Supportive nursing interventions should be used when managing the child with opioid withdrawal (Osborn et al. 2003; Anand et al. 2010) as they may reduce observed irritability and distress (Wolf and Jenkins 2005).
2 To reduce environmental stimulation: • Nurse the CYP in a quiet area of the ward, if possible and appropriate. • Liaise with family or carer to limit unnecessary visitors. • Sequence nursing procedures to promote minimal disturbance. • Remove balloons and noisy toys. Keep a few familiar and comforting toys nearby. • Turn off televisions and ensure that music is kept at a low level. • Dim lights if possible. • Keep bed sheets plain. Brightly coloured or patterned curtains should be avoided.	2 Clustering procedures, such as venipuncture, turning, physiotherapy, etc., allows analgesia and sedation to be administered at targeted intervals. Noise reduction, distraction with music and toys, and dimming lights at the child's usual bedtime may be helpful in minimising distress and restlessness (Wolf and Jenkins 2005).
3 For small children, comfort measures can be helpful. These include: a) Swaddling b) Holding or rocking c) Bathing and massage d) Nonnutritive sucking, e.g. dummies	3 a) b) Hyperirritability and agitation may be managed by swaddling, containment, and rocking (Wong et al. 2003), c) Massage and relaxation baths may be used as supportive treatments to ameliorate the symptoms of opioid withdrawal (Osborn et al. 2003). d) Dummies may be useful in reducing behavioural stress (Osborn et al. 2003; Wolf and Jenkins 2005).
4 Nutritional concerns: Monitor nutritional intake and feeding tolerance. Advice should be sought from the dietician when necessary, in consultation with the MDT.	Withdrawal from opioids and benzodiazepines (e.g., tremors) increases the CYP's calorie requirements. Gastrointestinal disturbances may also lead to nutritional concerns (Tobias 2000).
5 Maintenance of skin integrity: Close attention should be paid to pressure area care, particularly the skin integrity of the heels, toes, and nappy area. Assess and document the skin integrity using a recognised risk assessment tool. Introduce appropriate pressure relieving measures, and reassess regularly. Consider the use of pressure-relieving equipment.	Repetitive movements in an irritable child may cause redness or skin abrasions. Diarrhoea may also result in skin breakdown (Franck and Vilardi 1995). For more information regarding pressure area care, see Chapter 11: Personal Hygiene and Pressure Ulcer Prevention.
6 Education: a) Families should be given clear information, including explanations relating to: • The reversible neurological adaptation that takes place during the development of tolerance, and physical dependence. • The symptoms of withdrawal. • Misconceptions related to addiction. b) All members of the MDT should be educated in the practical aspects of the weaning process (Easley and Nichols 2008). A clear policy for analgesia and sedation management should be adopted by all members of the MDT (Wolf and Jenkins 2005).	a) In some cases families may mistakenly believe that the symptoms they are witnessing are the result of a neurological assault, psychological damage, or worsening of their child's disease process or clinical condition. Families may be reassured that it is unusual for a CYP with physical dependence or tolerance to opioids to develop an addictive disorder (Galinkin & Koh 2014). b) The management of analgesic and sedative reduction should be based on shared goals and effective communication between members of the MDT (Cho et al. 2007).

References

Alexander E, Carnevale F, Razack S. (2002) Evaluation of a sedation protocol for intubated critically ill children. *Intensive & Critical Care Nursing*, 18, 292–301.

Anand, KJS., Willson DF, Berger J, Harrison R, Meert KL, Zimmerman J, Carcillo J, Newth CJL, Prodhan P, Dean JM, Nicholson C, for the Eunice Kennedy Shriver National Institute of Child Health and Human Development Collaborative Pediatric Critical Care Research Network (2010) Tolerance and withdrawal from prolonged opioid use in critically ill children. *Pediatrics*, 125, 1208–1225.

Birchley, G. (2009). Opioid and benzodiazepine withdrawal syndromes in the paediatric intensive care unit: a review of recent literature. *Nursing in Critical Care* 14 (1): 26–37.

Cho, H.H., O'Connell, J.P., Cooney, M.F., and Inchiosa, M.A. (2007). Minimising tolerance and withdrawal to prolonged pediatric sedation: case report and review of the literature. *Journal of Intensive Care Medicine* 22 (3): 173–179.

Cunliffe, M., McArthur, L., and Dooley, F. (2004). Managing sedation withdrawal in children who undergo prolonged PICU admission after discharge to the ward. *Pediatric Anesthesia* 14: 293–298.

D'Apolito, K. (2009). Neonatal opiate withdrawal: pharmacologic management. *Newborn and Infant Nursing Reviews* 9 (1): 62–69.

Ducharme, C., Carnevale, F.A., Clermont, M., and Shea, S. (2005). A prospective study of adverse reactions to the weaning of opioids and benzodiazepines among critically ill children. *Intensive & Critical Care Nursing* 21: 179–186.

Easley, R.B. and Nichols, D.G. (2008). Withdrawal assessment in the pediatric intensive care unit: quantifying a morbidity of pain and sedation management in the critically ill child. *Critical Care Medicine* 36 (8): 2479–2480.

Fisher D. Grap, M.J. Younger, J.B. Ameringer, S. Elswick, R.K. (2013) Opioid withdrawal signs and symptoms in children: frequency and determinants. *Heart & Lung* 42 407–413 Franck L, Vilardi J. (1995). Assessment and management of opioid withdrawal in ill neonates. *Neonatal Network*, 14(2), 39–49.

Franck, L., Vilardi, J., Durand, D., and Powers, R. (1998). Opioid withdrawal in neonates after continuous infusions of morphine or fentanyl during extracopporeal membrane oxygenation. *American Journal of Critical Care* 7 (5): 364–369.

Franck, L., Naughton, I., and Winter, I. (2004). Opioid and benzodiazepine withdrawal symptoms in paediatric intensive care patients. *Intensive & Critical Care Nursing* 20: 344–351.

Franck, L., Harris, S., Soetenga, D. et al. (2008). The withdrawal assessment tool–1 (WAT–1): an assessment instrument for monitoring opioid and benzodiazepine withdrawal symptoms in pediatric patients. *Pediatric Critical Care Medicine* 9 (6): 573–580.

Franck, L., Scoppettuolo, L.A., Wypij, D., and Curley, M.A.Q. (2012). Validity and generalizability of the withdrawal assessment tool–1 (WAT–1) for monitoring iatrogenic withdrawal syndrome in pediatric patients. *Pain* 153: 142–148.

Galinkin, J. and Koh, J.L. (2014). Recognition and management of iatrogenically Induced opioid dependance and withdrawal in children. *American Academy of Pediatrics* 133: 152–155.

Grant, M.J.C., Balas, M.C., Curley, M.A., and for the RESTORE Investigative Team (2013). Defining sedation-related adverse events in the pediatric intensive care unit. *Heart & Lung* 42: 171–176.

Hong, J.Y., Kim, W.O., Koo, B.N. et al. (2010). Fentanyl-sparing effect of acetaminophen as a mixture of fentanyl in intravenous parent-/nurse-controlled analgesia after pediatric Ureteroneocystostomy. *Anesthesiology* 113: 672–677.

Hudak, M.L. and Tan, R.C. (2012). The committee on drugs and the committee on fetus and newborn. *Paediatrics* 129 (2): e540.

Indelicato, R. and Portnoy, R.K. (2002). Opioid rotation in the management of refractory cancer pain. *Journal of Clinical Oncology* 20 (1): 348–352.

Ista, E., van Dijk, M., Gamel, C. et al. (2007). Withdrawal symptoms in children after long term administration of sedatives and/or analgesics: a literature review. 'Assessment remains troublesome'. *Intensive Care Medicine* 33: 1396–1406.

Ista, E., van Dijk, M., Gamel, C. et al. (2008). Withdrawal symptoms in critically ill children after long-term administration of sedatives and/or analgesics: a first evaluation. *Critical Care Medicine* 36 (8): 2427–2432.

Ista, E., van Dijk, M., de Hoog, M. et al. (2009). Construction of the Sophia observation withdrawal symptom scale (SOS) for critically ill children. *Intensive Care Medicine* 35: 1075–1081.

Ista, E., de Hoog, M., Tibboel, D. et al. (2013). Psychometric evaluation of the Sophia observation withdrawal symptoms scale in critically ill children. *Pediatric Critical Care Medicine* 14 (8): 761–769.

Jage, J. (2005). Opioid tolerance and dependence – do they matter? *European Journal of Pain* 9: 157–162.

Jenkins, I.A., Playfor, D.M., Bevan, C. et al. (2007). Current United Kingdom sedation practice in pediatric intensive care. *Pediatric Anesthesia* 17: 675–683.

Jin, H.S., Yum, M.S., Kim, S.L. et al. (2007). The efficacy of the COMFORT scale in assessing optimal sedation in critically ill children requiring mechanical ventilation. *Journal of Korean Medical Science* 22: 693–697;

Katz, R., Kelly, H.W., and His, A. (1994). Prospective study on the occurrence of withdrawal in critically ill children who receive fentanyl by continuous infusion. *Critical Care Medicine* 22 (5): 763–767.

Kosten, T.R. and George, T.P. (2002). The neurobiology of opioid dependence: implications for treatment. *Science & Practice Perspectives* 1 (1): 13–20.

Neunhoeffer, F., Kumpf, M., Renk, H. et al. (2015). Nurse-driven pediatric analgesia and sedation protocol reduces withdrawal symptoms in critically ill medical pediatric patients. *Pediatric Anaesthesia* 25 (8): 786–794.

Osborn DA, Jeffery HE, Cole MJ. (2003) Sedatives for opiate withdrawal in newborn infants The Cochrane Library, 2003 4

Playfor, S., Jenkins, I., Boyles, C. et al. (2006). Consensus guidelines on sedation and analgesia in critically ill children. *Intensive Care Medicine* 32: 1125–1136.

Puntillo, K., Casella, V., and Reid, M. (1997). Opioid and benzodiazepine tolerance and dependence: application of theory to critical care practice. *Heart and Lung* 26 (4): 310–344.

Saul R, Robinson L, Ooi K (2018) Clinical Guidelines: Drug (Opioid or Benzodiazepine) Withdrawal Syndrome – Prevention and Management. Great Ormond Street Hospital for Children NHS Foundation Trust.

Schug SA, Palmer GM, Scott DA, Halliwell R, Trinca J; APM:SE (2015) *Australian and New Zealand College of Anaesthetists and Faculty of Pain Medicine, Acute Pain Management: Scientific Evidence* (4). Melbourne, ANZCA & FPM.

Stein, C. (2013). Opioids, sensory systems and chronic pain. *European Journal of Pharmacology* 716: 179–187.

Sury, M., Russell, G., Hopkins, C. et al. (1989). Acute benzodiazepine withdrawal syndrome after midazolam infusions in children. *Critical Care Medicine* 17: 301–302.

Tobias, J.D. (2000). Tolerance withdrawal and physical dependency after long term sedation and analgesia of children in the pediatric intensive care unit. *Critical Care Medicine* 3 (6): 2122–2132.

Tobias, D.J. (2003). Pain management for the critically ill child in the pediatric intensive care unit. In: *Pain in Infants and Children*, 2nde (eds. N. Schecter, C. Berde and M. Yaster). Philadelphia: Lippincott Williams and Wilkins, pp. 807–840.

Williams, J.T., Ingram, S.L., Henderson, G. et al. (2013). Regulation of m-Opioid Receptors: Desensitization, Phosphorylation, Internalization, and Tolerance. *Pharmacological Reviews* 65: 223–254.

Wolf, A.R. and Jenkins, I.A. (2005). Sedation of the critically ill child. *Current Paediatrics* 15: 316–323.

Wong, M.C., McIntosh, N., Menon, G., and Frank, L.S. (2003). Pain (and stress) in infants in a neonatal intensive care unit. In: *Pain in Infants and Children*, 2e (eds. N. Schecter, C. Berde and M. Yaster). Philadelphia: Lippincott Williams and Wilkins, chapter 37.

Wong, I., St John-Green, C., and Walker, S.M. (2013). Opioid-sparing effects of perioperative paracetamol and nonsteroidal anti-inflammatory drugs (NSAIDs) in children. *Pediatric Anesthesia* 23: 475–495.

Yaster, M., Kost-Byerly, S., Berde, C., and Billet, C. (1996). The management of opioid and benzodiazepine dependence in infants, children and adolescents. *Pediatrics* 98 (1): 135–140.

Chapter 35

When a child or young person dies

Rachel Cooke
RN (Child), Bereavement Services Manager, Great Ormond Street Hospital, London, UK

The author would like to acknowledge the contribution of Lydia Judge-Kronis, formerly Mortuary Manager, Senior APT, GOSH to this chapter. Thank you also, to Angela Scales, Practice Development Specialist, NHS Blood and Transplant, for the advice on organ donation.

Chapter contents

Introduction	780	Moving the CYP to the mortuary and aftercare	788
Communication and responsibilities following a death of a CYP	780	Post-mortem	792
		Bereavement	792
Legal aspects: Certification, notification, and registration	780	Self-care and debrief	792
Personal care of the CYP (previously known as last offices)	787	References	794
		Further reading	794

Procedure guidelines

35.1 Communication and responsibilities	783	35.3 Personal care of a CYP (previously known as last offices)	788
35.2 Legal aspects: certification, registration, post-mortem, and organ and tissue donation	785	35.4 Moving a CYP to the mortuary and aftercare	790

The Great Ormond Street Hospital Manual of Children and Young People's Nursing Practices, Second Edition. Edited by Elizabeth Anne Bruce, Janet Williss, and Faith Gibson.
© 2023 John Wiley & Sons Ltd. Published 2023 by John Wiley & Sons Ltd.

Introduction

It is essential to ensure that a high standard of care is maintained after a child or young person (CYP) dies. The following guidelines relate predominantly to the death of a CYP in the hospital setting. However, much of this guidance, particularly the legal requirements, are also relevant to the death of a CYP at home or in the community setting. National recommendations are provided by Together for Short Lives (Bennett 2012). Family involvement at this stage is paramount and the nurse should ascertain by sensitive enquiry how much the parents/carers wish to be involved in the preparation of their child's body and with the legal requirements concerning the death. In response to the recent coronavirus pandemic the process for registration of death has changed and these changes may well remain in the long term. It is essential that health care professionals are aware of local process and policies. For more information, see procedure guideline 35.2.

The family will be emotional, distressed, and possibly in shock at this time, even if the death was expected. Sensitivity is required when assisting them. The desire to be of assistance and support to the family can at times lead the nurse to take over actions the parents/carers might prefer to do for themselves. Sensitivity and allowing the parents/carers time to make decisions with the support of the healthcare team should avoid this situation. Knowledge of the legal requirements following the death will ensure that families are able to make the necessary arrangements with the minimum of difficulty and distress.

We live in a multicultural society and rituals and practices around death may be influenced by families' culture, religion and beliefs. There are numerous texts available describing practices associated with different faiths (West Midlands Paediatric Palliative Care Network 2018). These should be used as guidelines only; it is essential to remember that although a family might profess a recognised faith, their beliefs may be individual, and so it is important to avoid making assumptions. When in doubt, asking the family about their wishes rarely causes offence if done sensitively. The behaviour they exhibit will also be influenced by their culture, previous experiences, and coping mechanisms. Cultural expressions of grief vary and should be supported by the nurse, even if the nurse perceives them to be inappropriate.

Communication and responsibilities following a death of a CYP

Many hospitals, hospices, and community settings will have local guidance for communication and responsibilities following the death of a CYP. Figures 35.1 and 35.2 provide a summary of the guidance provided for nurses and doctors at GOSH which can be adapted for local use.

Legal aspects: Certification, notification, and registration

There are legal requirements following a death of a CYP; these are certification, notification, and registration. The death must be documented in the medical and nursing healthcare records. Organ donation procedure is outlined in Procedure Guideline 35.2.

Certification

The family should be given their child's Medical Certificate of Cause of Death (MCCD). Guidance for doctors completing medical certification of cause of death in England and Wales is available (Office for National Statistics and HM Passport Office 2018). There are two MCCD books: one for babies dying within the first 28 days of life (form 65) and one for those who die after 28 days (form 66). The MCCD should be given to the family with an explanation of what is written on it before they go to register their child's death. This will not be possible if the death is to be investigated by the coroner.

The details on the MCCD should be checked for legibility; abbreviations should not be used. The signature should be accompanied by a printed name and by the Doctor's GMC registration number. The CYP's details, particularly their names, should be clarified with the family. Neonates may have a change of surname, so it is vital to check first with family. On the reverse of the MCCD is a box that may be ticked to indicate that further information may be available later. The registrar may then contact the doctor for the underlying cause of death. This should always be ticked. Any healthcare-associated infection must be noted on the MCCD. It is also important to discuss information with regards to cremation with the family. For cremation, legal documentation needs to be completed by two medical doctors, as explained in the cremation regulations (Ministry of Justice 2012).

Notification of a death
Sudden unexpected death

A sudden unexpected death is defined as one which:
- Was not anticipated as a significant possibility 24 hours before the death; or
- Involved a similarly unexpected collapse or incident leading to or precipitating the events which led to the death. This definition is especially relevant when there is a significant time delay between the collapse of the CYP and their eventual death.

Unexpected deaths include those of CYPs with existing medical conditions or disabilities, including those that are life limiting or threatening but where, at the time that it occurred, death was not expected as a natural cause. When the death is sudden and unexpected national guidance must be followed (The Royal College of Pathologists 2016). When a CYP dies the following should be notified within 24 hours (or the next working day):

- Child Death Overview Panel administrator where the child is resident: This is the completion of Form A (this is completed by Bereavement service at GOSH).
- General Practitioner: Inform them of the facts and circumstances of the death, so that the GP is able to support the family.
- Other professionals as appropriate: Health visitor, school nurse, hospital/community medical team.

Registration

The death is registered at the registry office local to where the CYP dies. It is possible to register the CYP's death in their home area but paperwork may take more than a week to process and the family should be informed of this. Please refer to local information; for example 'When a child dies. Information for families' (Great Ormond Street Hospital 2015).

Registration of death must take place within five days in England, Wales and Northern Ireland and eight days in Scotland. This is normally done by the parents and can be a helpful beginning to their grief journey. Therefore offering to register the death on their behalf is not always in their best interests. However, after discussion with the registrar (of deaths), it is sometimes possible for a relative, friend, or member of hospital staff to do it on the parents behalf, as long as they are able to identify the CYP's body.

Chapter 35 When a child or young person dies

Child Dies

↓

Practicalities

Perform final personal care–as per guidance
- Ask parents if they would like keepsakes, e.g. photograph, foot-or handprints, lock of hair
- Memory work, i.e. hand-and footprints, lock of hair
- Ensure two name bands are attached to child
- Wrap child in sheet
- Please use the cotton bag for child's belongings; do not use plastic property bag (When A Child Dies (WACD) box)
- Favourite toy or item to be labeled if staying with the child
- Expected death: the family may wish to take the child home as an alternative to the mortuary.
- Moving the child-home, hospice or funeral directors via mortuary. Children's hospice may offer use of a cool room (if available)
- Arrange transport as per guidance – hand them 'transfer of care' form to give to their funeral director
- Provide parents with the booklet, 'When a Child Dies' and Child Death Helpline details, all included in the parent's information pack from WACD Box
- Family accommodation informed and key returned
- Support parents to make funeral arrangements. If advice is required, please contact the Bereavement Service Manager or Chaplains

↓

Communication immediately after the death

The following are also to be contacted as soon as possible, but this must be within 24 hours of the child's death
- Appropriate clinical staff/teams
- Mortuary
- Clinical Site Practitioner
- Bereavement Service
- Book appointment at local registry office on line for parents to take Medical Certificate of Cause of Death (MCCD)

↓

Communication – when practical

- Embassy (if applicable)
- Interpreters, if required or previously involved
- Social Care Team (if applicable)
- Religious representative, if requested by the family
- Clinical Nurse Specialists (if applicable)
- Health visitor or school nurse
- Community children's nurse (if applicable)
- Midwife, if the child was a newborn or infant under 28 days old
- Decide how to inform other families on the ward of the child's death

Figure 35.1 Guidance for nurses when a child or young person dies.

The Great Ormond Street Hospital Manual of Children and Young People's Nursing Practices

Child Dies

Practicalities

- Verify and certify the death and record in the child's healthcare record.
- Initiate response to sudden unexpected death, if this was not noted as having been anticipated within the last 24 hours
- Notify the Infection Prevention and Control Team and Public Health England of any Health Care Acquired Infection (HCAI) or notifiable disease complete DATIX incident report if the HCAI is thought to be/have contributed to the cause of death
- Seek advice from Coroner, if necessary, using the form and guidance on the intranet
- Request the post–mortem, if appropriate, and discuss with pathologist. Obtain consent form from histopathology team.
- Discuss organ donation (see section on organ donation).
- Complete and sign Medical Certificate of Cause of Death
- Enter details from the (MCCD) onto the self-adhesive checklist on the front of the medical notes or on ICU's fill the bereavement form in on Carevue
- Complete a Cremation form 4, in case a cremation is requested (WACD box)

Communication within 24 hrs

- Discuss postmortem, postdeath biopsies and organ or tissue retention with the family. Give parent's a copy of the postmortem information leaflet in WACD box.

To contact

- The child's GP
- Referring hospital Consultant (if applicable)
- Explain need for Coroners post mortem (if necessary)

Communication – when practical

- Arrange for a discussion of the postmortem results with the parents on the earliest possible date
- Ensure the Lead consultant is aware so that a letter of condolence is written and sent, along with a bereavement followup appointment giving opportunity for the family to discuss any issues for six to eight weeks after the child's death

Figure 35.2 Guidance for doctors when a child or young person dies.

Procedure guideline 35.1 Communication and responsibilities

Statement	Rationale
1 If the parents or carers are not present they must be informed of their child's death immediately.	1 To facilitate good communication.
2 If the CYP has died in hospital the following need to be advised as soon as possible: • Appropriate clinical staff • Site managers (GOSH: Clinical site practitioner) • Bereavement Service (24-hour voicemail) • The CYP's general practitioner (GP) • Referring hospital Consultant (if applicable) • Mortuary staff	2 To initiate practical help and support. To facilitate good communication.
3 The following also need to be advised, as appropriate, that the CYP has died if this has occurred in hospital: • Clinical Nurse Specialists involved in their care • Health visitor • School nurse • Community nurse • Referring hospital • Hospice (if involved) • Bed manager • Embassy/sponsoring body • Interpreters • Religious/spiritual representative • Midwife if infant is under 28 days old • Social care team	3 To ensure the hospital and local services are informed and ready to support the family before and on their return home.
4 a) When a CYP dies expectedly at home there is no urgency for nursing staff to contact anybody. b) The following need to be informed at an appropriate time: • GP, including the out-of-hours service, ensuring that the authorities are aware that the death was expected • Religious/spiritual representative • Local Child Death Overview Panel (CDOP) using Form A (Notification form) • Health visitor • School nurse • Community nurse • Local hospital • Tertiary centre (if appropriate) • Hospice (if involved) • Other professionals involved in the care of the CYP	4 a) To empower the family and give them control over the situation. b) To prevent unnecessary processes requiring investigation into the death by the Child Death Review Panel: • To certify the death • To support the family and facilitate funeral arrangements • To facilitate good communication
5 Ensure that the death is recorded in all the appropriate documentation and any electronic records.	5 To ensure subsequent communications with the family are accurate.
6 If the CYP has died in hospital, ensure they have two legible name bands; one on the wrist and one on the ankle.	6 To ensure continued identification and care of the CYP after they leave the ward.
7 a) If the CYP has died during surgery, the relevant ward must be informed and arrangements made for transfer of the CYP to an appropriate area. b) Inform mortuary staff if the CYP is to go directly there.	7 a) To enhance communication between appropriate personnel and allow parents time to say goodbye in more appropriate surroundings. b) To ensure they are prepared for the arrival of the CYP.
8 Local procedure should be followed for the CYP who has an infectious disease such as hepatitis or meningitis.	8 To minimise the risk of cross infection.
9 **In hospital the medical staff should:** a) Discuss organ donation (if not previously discussed). b) If appropriate, discuss: • Post-mortem, • Post-death biopsies • Organ or tissue retention c) Request these and obtain consent.	9 a) To obtain consent and to maximise viability of organs for donation. b) To provide information, facilitate informed consent and ensure that the parents' wishes are met. c) To ensure good communication. There is a legal obligation to obtain informed consent. Local requirement is that this must be in writing for any of the post-mortem procedures.

(continued)

Procedure guideline 35.1 Communication and responsibilities *(continued)*

Statement	Rationale
d) Confirm death and enter into the healthcare records.	d) To meet legal requirements.
e) Inform the mortuary if there is to be a post-mortem and what type of post-mortem the family have agreed to.	e) To ensure a timely examination can be arranged. To enhance communication.
f) Ensure completed consent form and notes are taken to the mortuary as soon as possible during working hours.	f) To enable the mortuary team to make the necessary requirements to facilitate the post-mortem examination as soon as practical. This will not proceed until the 'cooling off' period had reached its end.
g) Explain the need for coroner's post-mortem if required.	
h) A medical doctor must complete the Medical Certificate of Cause of Death (MCCD), ensuring that they sign and record their GMC number legibly.	h) So the registrar is able to register the death without further delay to the family.
i) Give the death certificate to the family before they go to register their CYP's death.	
If the family have chosen cremation for their child:	
i) The doctor should complete the medical certificate for cremation, forms 4 (cremation 4) and 5 (cremation 5). Ensure contact numbers are included on the form to enable the next doctor to contact the relevant people.	i) This document is necessary for the cremation to be held. It should be completed for every CYP, as parents often change their mind.
j) Inform the mortuary of any implant or device present, such as pacemakers, defibrillators, or fixion nails.	j) These have to be deactivated and/or removed prior to a cremation being held. Early identification of such things can prevent any delay.
k) Arrange for the cremation form and notes to be taken to the mortuary as soon as possible during working hours to enable the second part of the form, crematorium 5 to be completed. The doctor completing the crematorium 5 form will need to contact the person who signed the crematorium 4 form and a member of the nursing team to discuss the patient.	k) This is a legal requirement.
l) Arrange family follow-up and discussion of post-mortem results.	l) To initiate later support for family.
m) Notify GP and referring hospital of death.	
10 **In hospital the nursing staff should:** • Arrange for keepsakes. • Perform personal care and transfer the CYP to the mortuary. • Provide parents/carers with relevant leaflets. • Arrange for parents/carers to view their child at a later date. • Advise parents/carers about funeral arrangements (support the family if they require assistance in making plans for CYP's funeral). • Ensure suitable travel arrangements are in place for the family to go home. • Ensure that other staff members are informed of the death. • Consider informing other families on the ward.	10 To ensure good communication, to provide psychological support for the family, and to provide practical advice.
11 **If the child or young person dies at home:**	
a) It may still be appropriate to discuss donation of tissue if this has not been done previously.	a) To obtain consent and to maximise viability of tissue for donation.
b) It may be appropriate to discuss post-mortem.	b) To ensure good communication and parent's/carer's knowledge of legal and practical requirements.

Chapter 35 When a child or young person dies

Procedure guideline 35.2 Legal aspects: certification, registration, post-mortem, and organ and tissue donation

Statement	Rationale
Certification and registration of death	
1 A doctor must examine the CYP after death.	1 To verify and certify death.
2 The death must be entered into the medical and nursing notes and recorded on the patient information system (PIMs).	2 To document that they have died.
3 The doctor should explain what they have written on the CYP's medical certification of the cause of death (MCCD) then:	3 The MCCD is required to register a death.
a) The MCCD is scanned into the CYP's healthcare records and sent via email to the local registry office. The original copy is sent to the local registry office by post via the hospital bereavement office.	
b) An appointment must be booked for the parents at the registry office local to the place of death. This can be done either by phone or online.	b) To avoid the family returning at a later date and having to wait with families registering the birth of their child, as this can be distressing.
c) This will not be possible if the death is to be investigated by the Coroner or if a post-mortem is to be performed.	c) The cause of death will not yet be established.
4 a) The details on the MCCD should be checked for legibility. It should also be clarified with the family.	4 a) To avoid difficulties when the death is registered.
b) An additional 'Certificate of Examination' is required for cremation. Part 4 of this form is completed by the doctor writing the MCCD and this is then taken to the mortuary to enable part 5 to be completed.	b) This is a legal requirement.
c) The doctor signing part 5 will need to speak to the doctor who signed part 4 and a nurse who cared for the CYP.	c) Part 5 must be completed by a doctor who was not involved in the patient's care.
5 When the medical staff complete the MCCD of a CYP with HIV, the cause of death should be written as: a) Final illness, e.g. pneumonia, septicaemia. b) Immune deficiency may be added but not HIV or AIDS. c) On the reverse of the MCCD is a box that may be ticked indicating that further information may be available later. This should be ticked. The Registrar may then contact the doctor for the underlying cause of death.	5 To provide information while maintaining confidentiality.
6 Registration of death in England and Wales **must** take place within 5 days (or 8 days in Scotland).	6 To meet legal requirements.
a) This is normally done by the CYP's parents/carers; however, after discussion with the family and the Registrar (of deaths), it is sometimes possible for a relative, friend, or member of hospital staff to do it on the parents'/carers' behalf as long as they are able to identify the body.	a) If a family feels unable to do it themselves.
7 The following is required to register a death: • An MCCD stating the cause of death. • Date and place of death. • The CYP's full name, home address, place, and date of birth. • The parents'/carers' full names, home addresses and occupations.	7 To meet legal requirements.
8 An appointment for the local registry office to register the death is made online, by staff or parents.	8 To avoid unnecessary distress and time wasting for family members.
9 It is possible to register the CYP's death in their home area, but paper work may take more than a week to process.	
10 The Registrar will provide:	10
a) A certificate for burial or cremation for the undertakers (known as the green certificate). b) Form BD8 (revised) notification of death. c) They will be asked to fill out 'Tell me once' documentation as well, which will in time replace form BD8 (revised).	a) To enable the funeral to proceed. b) To inform government organisation that the CYP has died. c) This is needed to arrange a funeral abroad or if the CYP had a savings account.

(continued)

Procedure guideline 35.2 Legal aspects: certification, registration, post-mortem, and organ and tissue donation *(continued)*

Statement	Rationale
11 The registration and issue of certificates has a nominal fee. Ensure that the family have monies to purchase the death certificates.	11 To avoid unnecessary distress and time wasting for family members.
12 If a post-mortem is required by the coroner, the coroner's office, will advise when and where the family may collect the death certificate and how they may then proceed.	12 To enable the funeral to be planned.
13 If a new-born baby dies, and their birth has not been registered, a declaration of birth can be made at the same time as registration of death. The birth certificate will be sent at a later date. • Parents can still register the birth locally within the normal 6 weeks if they wish to do so. • If the parents are not married, the mother **must** be present. If they wish for the baby to be registered with the father's surname, both parents **must** be present.	13 To meet legal requirements.
14 It is the responsibility of the parents/carers to contact Social Services to cancel any benefits that they received for their child.	14 To meet legal requirements.

Post-Mortem Examination

Statement	Rationale
1 Post-mortems may be: • Ordered by the Coroner • Requested by medical staff • Requested by the family • A full post-mortem is not always required.	1 To establish cause of death.
2 The post-mortem may be limited to specific areas of the body and include imaging.	2 To further medical knowledge.
3 Consent is not a legal requirement for a coroner's post-mortem but good practice requires discussion and information to be given. Consent regarding blocks and slides (tissue samples) will be discussed with the family. a) If the medical team or family request a post-mortem written consent MUST be given. This may be faxed or emailed. Verbal assent is unacceptable. b) Consent forms are available on the wards or from Histopathology. c) Completed forms should be kept with the CYP's medical notes.	3 To comply with good practice. a) To comply with good practice. c) To ensure the CYPs records are complete and for future reference.
4 If a post-mortem is to be performed, the appropriately trained practitioner should explain the procedure and obtain consent.	4 To obtain informed consent, to provide any additional information related to their child's death, and to comply with recommended good practice. Human Tissue Authority (HTA) (2020a) outline the need for the family to give informed consent.
5 If a post-mortem is to be performed, an appointment with the family and lead doctor for about 6–8 weeks later must be made to discuss the findings/results with the family.	5 To ensure the family are informed of the results and have the opportunity to ask any questions.
6 When obtaining consent it is important to: a) Have a thorough discussion to ensure there are no objections. b) Include all appropriate family members. c) Be accurate about what needs to be done. d) Ensure consent is clear on how to proceed with tissue samples and/or organs to be retained or used in the future. e) Advise when and where it is likely to occur.	6 a)–e) To ensure there are no objections, and to comply with recommended good practice and the newly operational consent forms (National Institute for Health and Care Excellence 2011). c)–e) To adhere to HTA guidance (HTA 2020a).
7 All the same issues of consent apply when a sample of body tissue is to be taken from the body of a deceased CYP. a) Consent may occasionally be obtained in advance of death.	7 To ensure there are no objections. a) To enable samples to be taken immediately on death.

Procedure guideline 35.2 Legal aspects: certification, registration, post-mortem, and organ and tissue donation (*continued*)

Statement	Rationale
8 Once consent has been given the mortuary team should be informed and arrangements made for them to receive the case notes and consent form.	8 To provide background information for investigation. It may enable the post-mortem to be limited. They will be able to provide advice on the time frame for the examination.
9 If a post-mortem is to be done, the CYP should be taken to the mortuary as soon as possible.	9 To prevent serious degeneration of the tissues, which would render the investigation less useful.

Organ donation

1 The medical team must contact the specialist donation services team to discuss the potential for donation if the following criteria are met. • There is a plan to withdraw life-sustaining treatment and death is thought to be imminent. • Brain Stem Death is suspected. Donation of solid organ occurs under these circumstances. Tissue donation can potentially occur following any death. And advice can be sought from the specialist organ donation nurse. **UK Organ donor referral line: 0300 123 23 23**	
2 The Specialist Nurse - Organ Donation (SNOD) will be able to: a) Advise on the suitability for organ donation. It may be appropriate for the assessment to be made following arrival of the specialist at the hospital. Sufficient time should be allowed for a full assessment to be made. b) Approach the family regarding donation once an agreed plan is in place.	2 a) Donation should only be offered to families only if it is a real possibility. Expert advice on this should be sought. b) To ensure that the families are given the full information they require to make an informed choice and are fully supported in their decision.
3 Should the family wish to consider a donation, the specialist team in conjunction with the medical team will seek appropriate consent from the coroner and family. Normal procedures for final cares will still apply.	3 The specialist team are best placed to provide advice on the legal requirements for the processes.
4 Donation of tissues, e.g. cornea, heart valves, and skin, should also be considered following the death of any CYP. Advice on this can be gained from the specialist teams and the PICU family Liaison Team. Or follow your local advice on tissue donation policy.	4 Donation should be considered in all cases where it is a possibility.
5 CYPs who die at home can still potentially donate tissues. Advice should be sought from the palliative care team or from the organ donation referral line number above.	

The following is required to register a death:
A certificate stating:

- The cause of death.
- Date and place of death.
- The CYP's full name, home address, place and date of birth. Names should be confirmed with parent/s, as these do sometimes change, particularly for neonates.
- The parent/s' full names, home addresses, and occupations.

The registrar will provide:

- A certificate for burial or cremation for the undertakers, required for release of the body (green form).
- Form BD8 (revised) notification of death.
- Form for social security purposes.

The registration and issue of certificates and any extra certified copies of the death certificate are available for a small fee. If a post-mortem is required by the coroner, normally the coroner's officer will advise about collecting the death certificate and how the family may then proceed.

If a new-born baby dies and their birth has not been registered, a declaration of birth can be made at the same time as registration of death. The birth certificate will be sent at a later date. Parents can still register the birth locally within the normal six weeks if they wish. If the parents are not married, the mother must be present. If they wish for the baby to be registered with the father's surname both parents must be present. It is the responsibility of the parents to contact their benefits office to cancel any benefits that they received for their child. Families may need to be reminded and supported in this task.

Personal care of the CYP (previously known as last offices)

Whether a CYP dies at home or in hospital, washing and dressing the body may be performed by the family, nurse or religious leader. It is important to discuss this with the family in order to support them and adhere to their wishes. The following guidelines relate to the preparation of the body in hospital. If this is performed at home they should be adapted as appropriate.

When a CYP dies, allow the family to spend time with them. Families may need to be supported and helped to be with or touch/cuddle their child if that is their wish. If a CYP dies at home there is no rush to move the body to the funeral director. If families wish for the body to remain at home support should be provided on cooling measures to prevent the body from deteriorating too quickly. Unless the CYP is referred to the coroner, it is considerate to seek the family's wishes in performing 'final personal care'. It is appropriate to involve them fully and support them in carrying out as much or as little of the practical aspects as they wish to.

Moving the CYP to the mortuary and aftercare

Once the family have left or are ready, arrange for the CYP to be taken to the mortuary. There are a number of ways to transfer the CYP to the mortuary department. Smaller babies may be carried, a Moses basket, or the child's bed from the ward may be used, and alternatively a concealment trolley will be available. How an infant, child, or young person is transferred to the mortuary is an individual decision, although staff should be mindful of issues such as moving and handling, infection control, and protecting other children and families in the hospital. Hospital policies should be strictly followed to ensure that the CYP's body is appropriately identified with two Identification bracelets in place.

Procedure guideline 35.3 Personal care of a CYP (previously known as last offices)

Statement	Rationale
1 Prepare equipment for washing and dressing the CYP.	1 To ensure availability of equipment.
a) Standard Infection Prevention and Control Precautions must be taken.	a) To prevent cross infection. For more information see Chapter 13: Infection Prevention and Control.
2 Tidy bed space, switch off all monitoring equipment, and wherever possible remove it from the bed area.	2 To normalise the environment.
3 a) If possible, lay the CYP flat with their limbs straight.	3 a) To help them look more natural after rigor mortis occurs.
b) Their eyes should be gently closed. If their eyes do not close, do not force them. Attaching things to the lids damages the sensitive skin area around the eye.	
c) Aspirate any secretions. • If secretions are copious the orifices **must** be packed. • The mouth should be gently closed. • No packing should be visible if used. It may be better to place the CYP on pads in the region of secretions. • Express the bladder into a foil bowl or nappy, gently pressing on the abdomen below the belly button. • Leave a clean nappy on if this is usual for the CYP.	c) To prevent oozing of secretions. To minimise leakage during transportation.
4 a) All drains, tubes, cannula etc. should be left in situ until the CYP is released from the hospital. This is particularly necessary if a coroner's post-mortem examination is to be held.	4 a) To prevent leaking onto clothes and surfaces. It may be necessary to trace their insertion sites during post-mortem examination.
b) Occasionally the parents may request that they are removed. If this is permitted, the parents should be advised that this may cause some leakage, but they may be removed and disposed of in waste disposal bags for incineration.	
c) Medical devices such as intravenous equipment should be removed or disconnected.	
d) If a post-mortem is to be performed they must not be removed. Airways can be cut down to teeth level. All other lines are to be left and covered and if they have been removed, they must be placed in bags and accompany the CYP.	d) To comply with legal requirements. To facilitate investigation of cause of death.
5 Renew dressings and secure them using waterproof adhesive tape.	5 To prevent oozing of secretions.
6 If the CYP has a high intestinal stoma, a new stoma appliance or a larger than usual nappy may be applied rather than a gauze dressing.	6 To avoid later leakage onto clothing.
7 Wash the CYP as appropriate.	7 a) To leave them in a 'natural' state.
b) Brush their hair into their usual style.	
c) Dress the CYP in the chosen clothes. Inform the family that due to some changes in temperature the clothes may become soiled.	c) To comply with the wishes of the family. Clothes often become damp and bloodstained.
8 Clean the bed and remake using clean bed linen.	8 To ensure the bed is aesthetically clean.

Procedure guideline 35.3 Personal care of a CYP (previously known as last offices) *(continued)*

Statement	Rationale
9 a) Check that the CYP's identity band clearly displays the following: • Full name • Hospital number • Date of birth • NHS umber	9 a) To ensure full accurate information is recorded.
b) A second identity band with the same information must be applied to another limb.	b) To facilitate ease of identification.
10 Leave the CYP as if 'asleep' with any special toys, etc. Their head should be straight and not tilted to the side.	10 To leave them in a 'natural' state. To prevent fluid collection in soft tissue.

Keepsakes

Statement	Rationale
1 a) Parents/carers may ask to take photographs or a video during the CYP's last days or after death. b) If families do not have their own camera, medical illustration (if available) may be contacted during office hours and at other times the intensive care areas may be able to help.	1 To provide a source of comfort.
c) Mementoes of the CYP should be offered to the family before they leave the hospital, e.g. photographs, lock of hair, hand- and/or footprints. This can be done on behalf of the family but only with their consent. The family should be advised that the funeral directors can assist with this if they choose this option a later time.	c) To aid grieving and be a source of comfort.
2 If the parents/carers do not wish to take the mementos apart from hair at this time, staff may offer to retain the items in the CYP's notes until a later time.	2 To provide comfort at a later date.

Special considerations: infectious precautions

Statement	Rationale
1 If the CYP has died from a potentially highly infectious disease, e.g. HIV, viral hepatitis, open pulmonary tuberculosis, they should be placed in a body bag. They can still be dressed and visited in hospital.	1–4 To prevent cross infection and meet government recommendations (Public Health England 2010).
2 The mortuary team must be informed of the Infectious status of the CYP.	
3 Body bags are kept in the mortuary. • The CYP should only be placed in a body bag once they are in the mortuary if there is an infection risk or significant leakage. • The CYP may be removed from the body bag for viewing but must be put back into the bag afterwards. • If the CYP is removed from the body bag for viewing or examination, infectious precautions **must** be maintained as when they were alive, i.e. the wearing of protective clothing, handwashing, etc.	
4 Used linen should be disposed of and other items in the child's room should be cleaned and/or disposed of in line with local linen, infection control, and waste management guidelines and policies.	

Special considerations: family support

Statement	Rationale
1 a) After the family have spent time with their child, if they do not want to assist with personal care, they should be provided with a quiet room away from the bedside.	1 a) To ensure privacy.
b) The family should be given the opportunity to telephone a friend or relative to join them.	b) To obtain support.
2 a) If the CYP has died in hospital, the family should be informed of the following before leaving: • What will happen to their child. • That they may return to see their child but need to call first and set up an agreed time. • To contact the ward in advance of this. • The phone number for the ward. • A name of a specific staff member to ask for (wherever possible). • That they will receive an appointment to return to the hospital to meet their child's consultant and other staff to talk over anything they wish to discuss.	2 a) To ensure they are kept informed and to enable the visit to be organised.

(continued)

Procedure guideline 35.3 Personal care of a CYP (previously known as last offices) *(continued)*

Statement	Rationale
b) They should be given any relevant booklets produced by the local government, NHS Trust, or other relevant agencies.	b) These contain a summary of the actions that need to be taken after a CYP has died.
3 The following advice may be offered to lactating mothers: • To wear a firm, well-supporting bra. • To take regular analgesia. • Hormone therapy is no longer considered appropriate. • To seek advice from their own midwife or health visitor.	3 To offer guidance and support.
4 a) The nurse should establish how the family are returning home. Transport, e.g. a taxi, may have to be arranged and possibly paid for by the Trust. b) If a CYP dies at home the nurse should ascertain from the family the level and type of contact and support that they would find appropriate in the time immediately following their child's death.	4 a) To ensure their safety. b) To provide support.

Procedure guideline 35.4 Moving a CYP to the mortuary and aftercare

Statement	Rationale
To the mortuary 1 The CYP may be transferred to the mortuary: a) On their bed. b) In a Moses basket. c) In the arms of a nurse or carer, wrapped in a blanket, which is replaced with a sheet on arrival to the mortuary. d) In the mortuary concealment trolley if of appropriate size. NB: Fully covering the CYP's face may draw unnecessary attention. On occasion other methods can be used; a discussion with the mortuary staff will help.	1 To facilitate the transfer in the most acceptable way and reduce the distress of all involved.
2 A nurse should accompany the CYP.	2 To complete the caring process.
3 The portering team may collect a trolley from the mortuary and deliver it to the ward. The Security staff will allow access out of working hours but the nursing team will take the CYP to the mortuary.	3 To facilitate the safe and smooth transfer of the CYP.
4 When bringing a CYP to the mortuary it is important to: a) Prepare a mortuary tray for the CYP. b) Place a sheet on the mortuary tray and then place the CYP onto the sheet. If they are already wrapped in a sheet this can be used instead of a clean one; however it is best to have one ready in case of any leaks. c) Lay the CYP on their back, using a low pillow to keep their head straight. d) Put their arms by their side and legs as straight as possible. If their eyes will not close, do not force them nor use any other method to seal them. e) Check there is a legible wristband on both a wrist and an ankle that has the full name, date of birth, and hospital number so there are three identifiers. f) Label any toys and leave these and any property with the CYP. If any of the property is fragile leave this uncovered so it is easy to recognise. g) Fold the sheet over the CYP so they are completely covered. This does not need to be wrapped around them, simply folded over to maintain privacy and dignity. h) Push the tray back into the correct space in the fridge/cold area and ensure the door is closed properly. i) Write the name on the relevant section of the white board and complete an admission form and remember to add on any special instructions. j) Leave the admission form along with any other paperwork on the table NOT with the CYP. k) Ensure you dispose of any gloves/aprons used and leave the area as you found it.	4 To maintain the CYP in as optimal condition as possible until they are collected by the funeral directors. c)–d) To position them properly and to ensure continuation of care. e) To comply with legal requirements and facilitate identification. f) These familiar items can provide comfort to the family.

Chapter 35 When a child or young person dies

Procedure guideline 35.4 Moving a CYP to the mortuary and aftercare *(continued)*

Statement	Rationale
5 a) It is not recommended that valuable jewellery is left with the CYP. If parents/carers wish to leave jewellery with their child, it is advisable to keep the quantities to a minimum. Rings and bracelets should be secured with tape. b) If jewellery or religious artefacts are left, these must be indicated in the 'comments' section of the Admission form along with a full description of the items.	5 a) Large quantities of valuables are a security risk. b) To ensure there is a record of items remaining with the CYP.
6 Ensure all details are written on the white board by the refrigerators as appropriate.	
7 If a CYP has a notifiable infectious disease, this need to be written on the admission form for the mortuary.	
Collection of the body	
1 Some families may wish to take their child home from the hospital themselves.	1 Unless a post-mortem is required and as long as there is suitable transport there is no legal reason why they cannot do so.
2 The family must have the death certificate before taking their child home.	
3 a) The CYP may be taken home using undertakers or the parent's/carer's own transport. b) It is not advisable for the parent/carer to be the driver of the transport. c) A Transfer of Care Form must be completed and sent to the mortuary. This will include the name of whoever has taken the CYP and where they have gone.	
4 If the parents/carers wish to take their child home using their own transport they should also receive a proforma letter detailing the circumstances of their journey.	4 To provide additional information as required. To avoid distressing enquires, e.g. from the police.
5 Families should be reminded that they should register their child's death within five days in England or eight days in Scotland.	5 To meet legal requirements.

The mortuary is staffed by anatomical pathology technologists (APTs); a team of staff each specially trained to work with CYPs who have died. They aim to provide high standards of care and a suitable environment. The APTs are able to help with all aspects of mortuary related information and will often help with speaking to the family if they would find that beneficial.

The mortuary is similar to a ward in a hospital. It is a secure area with limited access to prevent unauthorised visitors gaining access. The area is specifically designed to look after CYPs after death. There is a specific bedroom area where families come to visit their child and are welcome to bring siblings along. If siblings are going to be visiting their brother or sister in the mortuary they should be prepared for what will happen and be accompanied by a family member where possible.

Parents can visit their child with the APTs during working hours and with the clinical site practitioners/senior nurse or ward staff out of hours. All visits are by appointment only and are usually for one hour (refer to local policy), although this can be discussed at the time of booking. It is usual for a nurse from the ward/department to accompany the family during their entire visit to provide practical and emotional support. The APTs may assist if requested; they will usually welcome everyone and give some information about the CYP to prepare the nurse and the family. If the nurse is not available to support the family during the visit then others such as a member of the chaplaincy and bereavement service maybe available to assist.

Collection

Collecting a CYP from the hospital mortuary can be done by anyone who has permission from the parents and the relevant paperwork; there may be occasions when it is appropriate for the family to collect their child themselves. All arrangements should be made with the mortuary during working hours and the site managers/senior nurse out of hours.

There are a number of documents needed before a CYP can leave the hospital. These always include a transfer of care form signed by the family stating who will be collecting their child and where they are going. The documents **may** also include a copy of the green form, a death certificate, an out of England order (repatriation only), cremation forms and freedom of infection form (Ministry of Justice 2012).

A suitable time and location may be agreed with the mortuary. The CYP will be checked for identification and then placed into/onto a Moses basket, baby carrier, or stretcher. Any property will be checked and placed with them. They will be secured to ensure their safety on the journey and will be covered for dignity. All documentation will be checked and occasionally copies will be made. The person collecting and the person transferring care will sign the necessary books/papers and then the CYP will be escorted to the vehicle by a member of the mortuary staff.

In the period between death and the funeral the CYP's body may be cared for at home, in a mortuary, hospice cool room, which is often referred to as the tranquil suite, or a funeral director's premises. These options should be discussed with the family if not already decided or stated in the CYP's care plan. A hospital mortuary can also be used when a CYP dies at home, if such arrangements have been discussed before the CYP's death.

Post-mortem

A post-mortem may be performed for a variety of reasons including (but not exclusive to) confirmation of cause of death, to provide more detailed information about the illness, to enable further testing in the future by gathering tissues (e.g. for genetic testing). A post-mortem may be performed at either the coroner's or the family's request. Police can also request a forensic post-mortem to establish third-party involvement or suspicious circumstances. A consented post-mortem examination is a detailed procedure that is tailored to each individual family's wishes. This can be a very important part of a CYP's care after death and is provided by specialist trained professionals.

There are four types of post-mortem examination available:

1. A full post-mortem, in which everything is examined carefully and in detail and samples are taken.
2. A limited post-mortem, in which only specific areas are targeted and samples are taken.
3. A minimally invasive or less invasive post-mortem, in which imaging is used to look at everything, and then samples are taken from all areas possible but using a smaller incision, giving maximum access.
4. Imaging/external examination.

Asking a family about a post-mortem may seem difficult but it is an option that many families are happy to discuss. There is no obligation for them to consider this but it is a procedure that may help the family and others if they decide it is right for their child. There are professionals specifically trained in taking post-mortem consent who can support the professionals caring for the family. A post-mortem required by the coroner is a legal requirement. If the Coroner is involved, the family do not have any choice about the procedure, only about what happens to any samples afterwards.

The consent process for a post-mortem needs to be handled sensitively for each individual family. It can be a detailed process for staff involved in providing families with appropriate information and allowing time for questions and reflection. The storage of samples, how and when the post-mortem report will be available, and the aftercare for the family will need to be carefully explained (Human Tissue Authority [HTA] 2020a). There are decisions for the family to make about what to do with the samples after the post-mortem examination. Most families agree to keep these as part of their child's medical records. This means the samples are stored and can be re-examined or used for other scheduled purposes at the family's request in the future. If the samples are kept then many families also agree for them to be used for other scheduled purposes such as teaching and education, research, quality control, and audit. There is no expectation for the family to choose any of the extra options and they should be provided with adequate information to help them make an informed choice. Other options are to have the samples sensitively disposed of, or returned at a later time for burial or cremation (HTA 2020b). All the options will be explained very sensitively to the family as part of the consenting process.

Bereavement

The key to supporting bereaved families is good communication skills in difficult circumstances. It is important to be aware of the families' own networks, which include the extended family, community, and faith groups. Local resources available to families can be quite variable; it is good practice to research what is available to the family locally. Bereavement support varies, with a number of different models used in practice. No one support model will suit all families. It is important to offer a bereaved family choice at this difficult time. Options such as telephone helplines, face-to-face support, and support groups are just some of the services that can be made available. Bereavement support can be provided locally or via national helplines, depending on individual needs. It is important to remember the whole family, including siblings, grandparents, and other significant people. Bereavement services within the hospital are a resource; they can help signpost and may continue to follow up once the family has left the hospital.

Immediately following the death, families will often experience a range of emotions and try to make sense of all the confusion. Some families like to focus on what to do next and the practicalities. As a clinician it is important to be there to answer questions and 'just be' with them.

It is important to ask families what they would like as a keepsake, which may include a lock of their child's hair, a photograph, or hand- and footprints. This is discussed in more detail in Procedure Guideline 35.3. Further information is available at the Bereavement Advice Centre: https://www.bereavementadvice.org.

A bereavement care pathway is provided below (see Figure 35.3). This highlights the role of the bereavement key worker, a role that can be carried out by any health care professional who takes the lead to support the family.

Definition of Terms

Bereavement contact: Named nurse contacting the family within 24 hours of CYP's death, to answer practical questions, ask about further support.

Bereavement information pack: Information leaflets given to the family when a CYP dies. This includes:
- When a Child Dies Information for Families.
- Child Death Helpline.
- Other information leaflets can be added as appropriate.

Bereavement support sessions: Face to face or telephone support offered by a bereavement service, which includes:
- Memory work, understanding the grief process, coping strategies.
- Parents, siblings, wider family who have no local bereavement support.
- Referral discussed and agreed with family
- Referrals for high-risk families (suicidal, self-harm, other mental health diagnosis) are not appropriate.

Medical bereavement follow-up: Doctors and medical team review the CYP's clinical case with the family.

Memory work: Work with the CYP and family at the time of death (e.g. photos, handprints, lock of hair), visits to mortuary, chaplaincy.

Named professional: A member of the Multi-Disciplinary Team (MDT) who knew the family prior to the CYP dying, e.g. consultant, Clinical Nurse Specialist, Family Liaison Nurse. Named professional should be identified in the MDT/Psychosocial meeting.

Self-care and debrief

It is important that all staff caring for a CYP who has died and their family after the death are offered the opportunity to "debrief", or discuss events in an appropriate setting such as clinical supervision sessions. Supporting families after the death of a CYP can be distressing, and it is important that health care professionals recognise their own feelings of loss, reflect, and consider what their own coping strategies will be (Bennett 2012). The purpose of a debrief is to review what happened, to evaluate the care provided, to explore the impact of the death on the staff, and to identify the needs of the family. On the day of the death, it is important to check with all members of staff involved to ensure they feel suitably supported before they leave the shift. A more reflective debrief, including all members of the team around the CYP, should be offered at a time that is suitable for most of the staff involved and could be repeated if necessary. This is best held while any issues are fresh; within two weeks is considered best practice. Debriefings can be facilitated by palliative care staff, the bereavement service manager, chaplain, or psychosocial staff (Keene et al. 2010).

Great Ormond Street Hospital Bereavement Care Pathway

GOSH patients (For children expected to die)

Information gathered

Information gathered pre bereavement
- Identify bereavement **key worker** (e.g. palliative care team, CNS, family liaison nurse)
- Discussed practical issues in appropriate MDT (e.g. Palliative care team meeting, psychosocial, ward round) e.g. funeral
- Identify if further local support or GOSH psychology, social work, family support, chaplaincy is needed, make appropriate referrals. (transfer to Hospice)

CHILD DIES

Within 48 hrs (or 2 working days)

All GOSH patients:
- Tranquil suite at a local hospice to be offered
- **Named bereavement key worker** carries out (minimum) one **bereavement contact** telephone call.
  - Check if family have been given **bereavement information pack** or would like this sent
  - Identify who else is involved to support
  - Notify MDT of death, inform bereavement services and EPIC
- Inpatients only:
  - **Memory Work** (i.e. hand and footprints, visits to mortuary etc.) Liaise with bereavement service, mortuary service, play, chaplaincy
  - Viewings of deceased child to be arranged with the mortuary team
- **Bereavement information pack** to be given to family by ward staff with the name and contact details of the bereavement key worker

2 weeks

- **Named bereavement key worker.** Identify appropriate service to carry out bereavement follow up (e.g. community, hospice, GOSH) – record this in the notes, inform appropriate teams and family
- If appropriate on going bereavement support offered to family by psychology, social work, chaplaincy, bereavement services
- Palliative Care Team: one **bereavement contact** appointment (at home/hospital) offered to the family
- Bereavement service send letter 2 weeks post bereavement to all bereaved families (including opt in for further support)

6–8 weeks

- **Medical bereavement follow up** appointment with consultant and bereavement key worker
  - Referral to bereavement services for support if necessary <u>and with families' consent</u>
- Chaplaincy: Invite family to have child's name in book of remembrance

Up to 2 years

- Bereavement Services: Anniversary contacts/card on dates of birth and death for 2 years
- Ongoing **bereavement key worker support** (Coronial process)
- Chaplaincy: Invites to memorial service, memory days
- Bereavement survey

Figure 35.3 Great Ormond Street Hospital bereavement care pathway.

References

Bennett H (2012). *A Guide to End of Life Care: Care of children and young people before death, at the time of death and after death.* Together for Short Lives. https://www.togetherforshortlives.org.uk/app/uploads/2018/01/ProRes-A-Guide-To-End-Of-Life-Care.pdf (accessed 17 August 2022).

Great Ormond Street Hospital (2015). When a child dies. Information for families. https://media.gosh.nhs.uk/documents/When_a_child_dies_F0587_FINAL_Jun15.pdf (accessed 22 November 2022).

Human Tissue Authority (HTA) (2020a). Code A: Guiding principles and the fundamental principle of consent. https://content.hta.gov.uk/sites/default/files/2021-07/Public%20guide%20to%20principles%20and%20consent.pdf (accessed 22 November 2022).

Human Tissue Authority HTA (2020b). Code B. Post-mortem examination. Standards and guidance. https://content.hta.gov.uk/sites/default/files/2020-11/Code%20B%20standards.pdf (accessed 17 August 2022).

Keene, E.A., Hutton, N., Hal, B., and Rushton, C. (2010). Bereavement debriefing sessions: an intervention to support health care professionals in managing their grief after the death of a patient. *Paediatric Nursing* 36 (4): 185–189.

Ministry of Justice (2012). Crematorium managers: guidance on cremation regulations and forms. https://www.gov.uk/government/publications/crematorium-managers-guidance-on-cremation-regulations-and-forms (accessed 22 November 2022).

National Institute for Health and Care Excellence (2011). Organ donation for transplantation: improving donor identification and consent rates for deceased organ donation. https://www.nice.org.uk/guidance/cg135 (accessed 17 August 2022).

Office for National Statistics and HM Passport Office (2018). *Guidance for Doctors Completing Medical Certificates of Cause of Death in England and Wales.* (Updated March 2022) https://assets.publishing.service.gov.uk/government/uploads/system/uploads/attachment_data/file/1062236/Guidance_for_Doctors_completing_medical_certificates_Mar_22.pdf (accessed 17 August 2022).

Public Health England (2010). Guidance on notifiable diseases and causative organisms: how to report. (Updated 2022). https://www.gov.uk/guidance/notifiable-diseases-and-causative-organisms-how-to-report (accessed 17 August 2022).

The Royal College of Pathologists working group (2016). Sudden unexpected death in infancy and childhood Multi-agency guidelines for care and investigation (2nd edition). https://www.rcpath.org/uploads/assets/874ae50e-c754-4933-995a804e0ef728a4/Sudden-unexpected-death-in-infancy-and-childhood-2e.pdf (accessed 17 August 2022).

West Midlands Paediatric Palliative Care Network (2018). West Midlands Children and Young People's Palliative Care Toolkit. https://www.togetherforshortlives.org.uk/resource/west-midlands-toolkit/ (accessed 17 August 2022).

Further reading

Chambers L. (2019). Caring for a child at end of life. A guide for professionals on the care of children and young people before death, at the time of death and after death. Bristol: Together for Short Lives. https://www.togetherforshortlives.org.uk/app/uploads/2019/11/TfSL-Caring-for-a-child-at-end-of-life-Professionals.pdf (accessed 17 August 2022).

Child Death Review Statutory and Operational Guidance (England) 2018. https://www.gov.uk/government/publications/child-death-review-statutory-and-operational-guidance-england (accessed 17 August 2022).

Crown Office and Procurator Fiscal Service (2015). Reporting Deaths to the Procurator Fiscal. Information and Guidance for Medical Practitioners. https://www.copfs.gov.uk/for-professionals/reporting-deaths/reporting-deaths/ (accessed 22 November 2022).

Department for Education (2018). Working together to safeguard children: July 2018. Chapter 5: Child Death Reviews. https://www.workingtogetheronline.co.uk/chapters/chapter_five.html (accessed 17 August 2022).

Hospice UK (2022). Care after death. Advice for staff responsible for care after death. Fourth edition. https://www.hospiceuk.org/what-we-offer/clinicaland-care-support/clinical-resources (accessed 17 August 2022).

Index

Page locators in **bold** indicate tables. Page locators in *italics* indicate figures. This index uses letter-by-letter alphabetization.

A&E *see* accident and emergency
ABCDE assessment tool, 125–130, *125*, *129*
abdominal pain, 74
abdominal thrusts, 702–703, *703*
abdominal X-ray, 75
abduction traction, 527, *528*
absence, 469
accident and emergency (A&E), 724
ACE *see* antegrade colonic enema
acetylcysteine, 638, *638–639*
acquired immunodeficiency syndrome (AIDS)
    blood components and products, 62
    infection prevention and control, 240–242
    nutrition and feeding, 483
ACS *see* acute compartment syndrome
activated charcoal, 640
active immunity, 203–204
acupuncture, 100, *101*
acute bladder spasm, *760*
acute compartment syndrome (ACS), 520, 526, **532**
acute kidney injury (AKI), 134, 137, **137**, 151–153
addiction, 770
adenotonsillectomy, 650
adenovirus, **222**
ADHD *see* attention deficit and hyperactivity disorder
administration of medicines, 367–404
    buccal route, 372–373, *373*, 386
    checking the prescription, 370
    child development considerations, 370
    concepts and definitions, 368
    documentation and record keeping, 369
    drug calculations, 370–371
    enteral via tube or device, 372, 384–386
    epidural route, 381
    general guidelines, **382–383**
    independent check of medicines, 369
    inhalation route, 374–375, 388–390
    intradermal route, 376–377, 393
    intramuscular route, 376, 378–380, *379*, 396–397, *396*
    intranasal route, 374, 387–388
    intraosseous route, 380, 398
    intrathecal route, 380–381, 398–401
    intravenous route, 380
    oral route, 371–372, 384
    pain management, 544, 552–565
    patient group/specific directions, 368–369
    patient self-administration, 369
    procedure guidelines, 384–402, *395–396*
    rectal route, 375–376, 390–391
    subcutaneous route, 376–377, *377–378*, 394–395, *395*
    sublingual route, 373–374, 386, *395*
    timeliness of administration, 369
    transdermal (skin) patches, 381–382, 402
adrenaline
    allergy and anaphylaxis, 32–34, **33**
    cardiopulmonary resuscitation, 704, 710
advanced life support (ALS), 686, 704
adverse events following immunisations (AEFI), 40, 205–206, 214
AED *see* automated external defibrillator
AEFI *see* adverse events following immunisations
aerosolisers, 374–375
agitation, 582, 589–590
air enema, 350
airway
    cardiopulmonary resuscitation, 684–689, *686*, 698
    investigations, 352
    perioperative care, 611
    poisoning and overdose, 639
    respiratory care, 646–657
    seriously ill child, 127–128
    tracheostomy care and management, 741–744, *741*
AKI *see* acute kidney injury
albumin, 67
alcohol poisoning, 638–639
allergic rhinitis, 37–39, *37–38*
allergy and anaphylaxis, 29–42
    allergens in healthcare settings, 39–41, **40**
    assessment, 5
    classification and immune response, 30, *30*, **30**
    concepts and definitions, 30
    diagnosis and management of allergy, 30–32, *31*, **32**
    food allergy, 34–36, **35**
    management of anaphylaxis, 32–34, **32–33**, *33*
    nutrition and feeding, 486
    perioperative care, 597
    personal hygiene, 162, 165
    respiratory allergy, 37, *37–38*
ALS *see* advanced life support
alteplase, 281, **282**, 284–286, *284–285*
amiodarone, 709
anaesthesia
    pain management, 543, 550–555, *552*, 561–562
    perioperative care, 596–597, *596*, *598*, 601–602
anaesthetic T-piece, 659
analgesia *see* pain management
anal irrigation, 78, 80–81
anaphylaxis *see* allergy and anaphylaxis
anatomical pathology technologists (APT), 791
ano-rectal manometry, 75
anorexia nervosa, 409
antegrade colonic enema (ACE), 78, 81–82
antibiotics
    antibiotic resistance and antimicrobial stewardship, 219, **226**
    intravenous and intra-arterial access, 269, 280
    investigations, 315
    personal hygiene, 170
anticoagulation, 136
antifungals, 164, 190
antihistamines, 37
antiseptic detergents, 232
ANTT *see* aseptic nontouch technique
anxiety disorders, 407
anxiety/distress, 360–361, 623–624, 630
apheresis central venous catheters, **254**
aprons/gowns, 115, 237, **237**
APT *see* anatomical pathology technologists
aromatherapy, 101–102
arrhythmias, 639
arterial compression, 532
arterio-venous (AV) fistulas, 136
arts in health, 633
ASC *see* autistic spectrum condition
aseptic nontouch technique (ANTT), **119**, 288, 290, 295, 315, 491
    administration of medicines, 392
    intravenous and intra-arterial access, 250–253, **250**, 295
    investigations, 314–315, 339, 342
aspergillosis, **222**
aspiration, 353
assessment, 1–27
    body systems review, 1, 19–25
    burns and scalds, 90, *91*

The Great Ormond Street Hospital Manual of Children and Young People's Nursing Practices, Second Edition. Edited by Elizabeth Anne Bruce, Janet Williss, and Faith Gibson.
© 2023 John Wiley & Sons Ltd. Published 2023 by John Wiley & Sons Ltd.

Index

assessment (cont'd)
  cardiac, **19**, 126
  drug withdrawal, 771, 773
  family history, 1, 5
  fluid balance, 134, **135**, **140–141**
  general principles, 1–3
  mental health, 410
  moving and handling, **423**
  neurological care, 454–457, 473
  orthopaedic care, 520, **521**, *522–523*, 524–525, *525–526*, 532
  pain management, 545–551, 556
  palliative care, 579–580, *579*, **580**, 584–585
  past history, 1, 4–5
  perioperative care, 611–614, **613**
  personal hygiene, 160–162, **162**, 166–167, **167–168**, 173, 185, 187–188
  poisoning and overdose, **641**
  present illness, 1, 4
  respiratory care, 647, 661–662, 676
  safeguarding, 719
  vital signs and baseline measurements, 1, 6–18
  see also risk assessment
associative play, 623
asthma, 37
asystole, 704–705, *704*
atonic seizures, 470
atopy, 30
atropine, 705
attention deficit and hyperactivity disorder (ADHD), 407
atypical absence, 469
auscultation, 7, 128
autistic spectrum condition (ASC), 628
automated external defibrillator (AED), 705, 707–710, *707*
autonomic nervous system disorders, 673, 771
AV *see* arterio-venous fistulas
AVPU consciousness scale, 127, *127*, 130
axillary temperature, 6

Babytherms, **429**
baby wipes, 162
bacillus Calmette-Guerin (BCG), 203, 215
back blows, 702–703, *703*
bag mask valve (BMV), 658, 659, 690–692, *690*, 696
barium enema, 75
barium follow-through, 349
basic life support (BLS), 696–701
  choking, 701
  paediatric algorithm, *685*
  procedure guidelines, 697–701
  sequence of events, 697, *697*
  tracheostomy care and management, 740
bassinettes, **430**
bathing, 158–159, *160*, 178–182
BCG *see* bacillus Calmette-Guerin
bed bathing, 181
bedwetting, 160–161
behavioural assessment tools, **549**, 550
benzodiazepines, 771–776, **772**
best motor response, 455–456
bilevel positive airway pressure (BiPAP), 659, 672–675
biofeedback, 76
biopsy, 43–60
  bone marrow aspirate/trephine, 57–59
  investigations, 320, 353
  liver biopsy, 44–49, *44*

  punch skin biopsy, 49–54
  renal biopsy, 54–56
biopsychosocial model, 579, *579*
BiPAP *see* bilevel positive airway pressure
birth history, 4
Bivona tracheostomy tubes, 748
bladder cuffs, 8–10, *11*
bladder spasm, *760*
bleeding/haemorrhage
  biopsy, 45, 49, 57
  intravenous and intra-arterial access, 293, 305
  neonatal care, 435, **435–436**
  palliative care, 582, 590
  perioperative care, 604–605
  respiratory care, 668
  tracheostomy care and management, 733
  urinary catheter care, 761
blood components and products, 61–71
  administration of blood components, 66–70
  coagulation factors, 70–71
  concepts and definitions, 62
  intravenous and intra-arterial access, 295
  overview of blood transfusion, 62–66
blood glucose monitoring, 331–333, **331**
blood pressure (BP)
  assessment, 8–10, *11–13*
  intravenous and intra-arterial access, 298
  perioperative care, **48**, **55**, **66**
  seriously ill child, *129*
blood sampling
  blood culture, 315–316
  intravenous and intra-arterial access, 265–267, 303–304
  investigations, 315–319, **316**, *318–319*, **318**
  neonatal care, 438–442, **438–439**, *442*, **443**
bloodstream infections, 218, 280
blood volume, **613**
BLS *see* basic life support
BMF *see* breast milk fortifiers
BMI *see* body mass index
BMV *see* bag mask valve
body mass index (BMI), 17
body surface area (BSA), *138*
body systems review
  assessment, 1, 19–25
  development, 25
  elimination and sexual development, 22–23
  mobility, 24
  neurological system, 20, **21–22**
  nutrition, 22
  respiratory and cardiovascular systems, 19–20
  skin and hygiene, 23–24
body weight estimation, 708–709
bolus feeds, 507
bolus medications, 262–263, 273–274, 295
bone marrow aspirate/trephine, 57–59
  complications, 57
  procedure guidelines, 57–59
Books Beyond Words, 364
Bordetella pertussis
  immunisation, 211, 215
  infection prevention and control, **226**, **230**
  investigations, 325, 326
bottle-feeding, 22, 487, 491
bowel care, 73–85
  concepts and definitions, 74
  constipation, 74–76
  diarrhoea, 74

  factors to note, 84–85
  faecal soiling/incontinence, 76–78, *77*
  laxatives, 75–76
  personal hygiene, 163
  preparation for investigations or surgery, 76
  procedure guidelines, 78–84
  stoma care, 78, 82–85, **82–84**
BP *see* blood pressure
brain tumour, 110
breastfeeding
  assessment, 22
  investigations, 340
  nutrition and feeding, 483–486, **485**, 488–489, 491, **495**
breast milk fortifiers (BMF), 485, **485**, **495**, 496
breast pumps, **492**
breath activated inhalers, 375, 390
breathing
  cardiopulmonary resuscitation, 690–692, *690–691*, 698–699
  pain management, 544
  perioperative care, 612, **613**
  poisoning and overdose, 639
  seriously ill child, 128
  tracheostomy care and management, 742–743
Bromage score, *559–560*
bronchiolitis, **222**
brucellosis, **222**
bruises, 24
BSA *see* body surface area
buccal route, 372–373, *373*, 386
bulimia nervosa, 409
bullying, 721
burns and scalds, 87–97
  anatomy and physiology, 88
  assessment, 90, *91*
  classification of burns, 89
  common causes in children, 88
  concepts and definitions, 88
  first aid, 89–90
  fluid resuscitation, 90–91, **91**
  nutrition, 94
  procedure guidelines, 89–90, 92–96
  wound healing/wound care, 91–94, **92**

CAHN *see* clinician-assisted hydration and nutrition
calcium, **449**
CAM *see* complementary and alternative medicine
CAMHS *see* Child and Adolescent Mental Health Services
Campylobacter spp., **222**
Candida spp., 163–164, 190, 193
capacity, 346, 361–362
capillary blood sampling, 316–319, **316**, *318–319*, **318**
capnography, 690, 704
carbapenemase-producing *Enterobacteriaceae* (CPE), 219
cardiac monitoring, 130
cardiopulmonary resuscitation (CPR), 683–711
  advanced life support, *686*, 704
  aetiology of cardiorespiratory arrest, 684
  age definitions, 684, *685–686*
  airway management, 684–689, *686*, 698
  basic life support, *685*, 696–701, *697*, 703
  breathing management, 690–692, *690–691*, 698–699

Index

choking, 701–704, *703*
circulation management, 693–696, 699
concepts and definitions, 684
defibrillation, 705, 707–710, *707*
electrocardiography, 704–706, *704*
ending resuscitation attempts, 710
ethical considerations, 710–711
paediatric early warning score, 684
post resuscitation care, 70
procedure guidelines, 687–692, 694–706
recovery position, 689–690
ReSPECT process, 710–711, *710*
resuscitation teams, 710
tracheostomy care and management, 740–744, *740–741*
cardiorespiratory/cardiopulmonary arrest, 684, 690–691, 693, 697, 700–701, 704–705, 707–710
cardiovascular status, 19–20, 305
care planning, 173–175
Care Quality Commission (CQC) criteria, 218
catheter hubs, 252
catheter-related bloodstream infections (CRBSI), 280
CBT *see* cognitive behavioural therapy
CCN *see* community children's nursing
CD *see* controlled drugs
CDR *see* child death reviews
central nervous system disorders, 771
Central venous access devices (CVAD), 116, 250, 268, 491
central venous catheters, **253**
cerebrospinal fluid (CSF)
assessment, 18, 20
investigations, 320
neurological care, 470–479, *472*, *479*
certification of death, 780, 785–787, 791
CEWS *see* Children's Early Warning Score
CF *see* cystic fibrosis
chain of infection, 219–220
chain of prevention, 124, *124*
challenging behaviour
learning (intellectual) disability, 359–361, **360**
mental health, 407
play as a therapeutic tool, 627
charcoal, 640
chemical burns, 88
chemotherapy *see* systemic anti-cancer treatment
chest drains, 663–672
changing a chamber, 670
indications, 663, *664*
insertion, 663–665, *664*
investigations, 320
observations, 666–668, *667–668*
ongoing care and preventing complications, 669
postprocedure care, 665–666
procedure guidelines, 665–672
removal, 670–672
chest thrusts, 702–703, *703*
chest X-ray, *664*
chickenpox
immunisation, 215
infection prevention and control, **222**, **229**
investigations, 328
Child and Adolescent Mental Health Services (CAMHS), 406–408, 410, 636
child death reviews (CDR), 722
child protection *see* safeguarding
child protection conference, 726

Child Protection Information Sharing System (CP-IS), 723, 726
Children Act (1989), 714, 719, **720**, 726
Children Act (2004), 719
Children and Social Work Act (2017), 719
Children's Early Warning Score (CEWS), 46, 127
Children's Social Care, 725–726
child sexual exploitation, 716
chin lift, 687–688
chiropractic, 100
chlorhexidine
intravenous and intra-arterial access, 269
personal hygiene, 190
urinary catheter care, 764
choking, 701–704, *702*
chronic illness
assessment, 4
complementary and alternative medicine, 109
immunisation, 203, **203**
CHT *see* congenital hypothyroidism
chylothorax, 663
CIC *see* clean intermittent catheterisation
CIPOLD *see* Confidential Inquiry into the Premature Deaths of People with Learning Disabilities
circulation
cardiopulmonary resuscitation, 693–696, 699
circulation compromise, 305
perioperative care, 612, **613**
poisoning and overdose, 639
seriously ill child, 128–129
clamps, 669
cleaning, 243–244
cleaning trays, 250
clean intermittent catheterisation (CIC), 754
cleft lip and palate, 650
clinician-assisted hydration and nutrition (CAHN), 583
clitoridectomy, 717
clonic seizures, 468
clonidine, 776
Clostridium spp., 213, 218, **222**
clove hitch knots, *536*
CMV *see* cytomegalovirus
coagulation factors, 70–71
coanalgesics, 544
codeine, 544
coercive behaviour, 717
cognitive behavioural therapy (CBT), 407, 544
cold stress, **431–432**, *432*
collaborative working, 723
colonic transit studies, 75
colonoscopy, 75
colonostomy, 391
colostomy irrigation, 85
colour, 524
communication
assessment, 3, 25–26
deaths, 780, *781–782*, *783–784*
documentation, 173
learning (intellectual) disability, 358, 362, 364
neurological care, **458**, 472
play as a therapeutic tool, 623, 624
safeguarding, 723–724
SBARD, 124, *126*, 646
community children's nursing (CCN) team, 94
community practitioner nurse prescribers, 368
compensated shocked state, 129, *129*

complementary and alternative medicine (CAM), 99–111
case studies, 109–110
categorisation, 100
concepts and definitions, 99
disclosure to healthcare practitioners, 102
five most commonly used CAMs, 101–102
history and legislation, 100–101
massage therapy, 102–110, **103**, *104–109*
complementary foods, 486–487, **486–487**
component vaccines, 204
computer tomography (CT), 351
conductive heat loss, *430*
Confidential Inquiry into the Premature Deaths of People with Learning Disabilities (CIPOLD), 359
congenital hypothyroidism (CHT), 438
conjugate vaccines, 204
consciousness
neurological observations, 454–457, **457–458**, *459–464*, *462–463*
seizures, 465, 468
seriously ill child, 127, *127*, 130
consent
investigations, 352
learning (intellectual) disability, 361–362
mental health, 412
perioperative care, **599**
poisoning and overdose, 642
systemic anti-cancer treatment, 114
constipation
bowel care, 74–76
palliative care, 580–581, 587
personal hygiene, 161
contact burns, 88
contact lenses, 170, 196
contamination/decontamination, 115, 243–245, **244–245**
continence/incontinence
bowel care, 76–78, *77*
personal hygiene, 159–165, **162**, *163–164*, 182–186
continuing care, 488
continuous feeds, 507–508, 512
continuous positive airway pressure (CPAP), 659, 672–675
continuous renal replacement therapy (CRRT), 136, 139, 142–147, *148*
contrast enema, 350
controlled drugs (CD), 368
controlling behaviour, 717
convective heat loss, *430*
co-operative play, 623
core temperature, 6
corticosteroids
allergy and anaphylaxis, 37, *38*
personal hygiene, 163–164, 170
Corynebacterium spp., 206–207
cots, **430**
cough, 20
cough swabs, 321, 323
Covid-19/SARS-CoV-2, **222**, **228**, 722
CPAP *see* continuous positive airway pressure
CPE *see* carbapenemase-producing *Enterobacteriaceae*
CP-IS *see* Child Protection Information Sharing System
CPR *see* cardiopulmonary resuscitation
CQC *see* Care Quality Commission
cranial nerves, **21–22**

Index

craniofacial disorders, 650, 673
CRBSI *see* catheter-related bloodstream infections
Creutzfeldt-Jakob disease, **222**
croup, **222**
CRRT *see* continuous renal replacement therapy
crutches, 521, 533, **534–535**
cryoprecipitate, 67
Cryptosporidium spp., **222**
CSF *see* cerebrospinal fluid
CT *see* computer tomography
culture/religion, 62, 719
cyanosis, 19
cyberbullying, 721
cyclical feeds, 513
cystic fibrosis (CF), 438
cytomegalovirus (CMV), 62, **223**
cytotoxic chemotherapy *see* systemic anti-cancer treatment

dampened trace, 304
Data Protection Act (2018), 723
deaths, 779–794
    bereavement, 792, *793*
    cardiopulmonary resuscitation, 710–711
    collection of body, 791
    communication and responsibilities, 780, *781–782*, 783–784
    concepts and definitions, 780
    learning (intellectual) disability, 359
    legal requirements, 780, 785–787
    moving CYP to mortuary and aftercare, 788, 790–791
    organ donation, 787
    palliative care, 584, 590
    personal care of CYP (last offices), 787–790
    post-mortem examination, 786–787, 792
    procedure guidelines, 783–791
    safeguarding, 714, 721–722
    self-care and debrief, 792
debrief, 792
decompensated shocked state, 129
defibrillation, 705, 707–710, *707*
dehydration *see* hydration/dehydration
delayed haemorrhage, 49
delusions, 408
dental caries, 486
dental floss, 190
dental hygiene, 486–487
dentition, 166
depression, 408
desensitisation, 632–633
detachable chamber spacers, 375
development
    administration of medicines, 370
    assessment, 25
    neonatal care, 433, **433–435**, *434*
    play as a therapeutic tool, 622–623
diagnostic overshadowing, 359, 360–361
diarrhoea
    bowel care, 74
    nutrition and feeding, 509
    palliative care, 580–581, 587
diet *see* nutrition and feeding
difference, 719
digital rectal examination (DRE), 75
dignity, 604
diphtheria, 206–207
disability
    personal hygiene, 160, 184
    safeguarding, 718
    seriously ill child, 130
    see also learning (intellectual) disability
disability distress assessment tool (DisDAT), 360–361
discharge planning
    biopsy, 46, 49
    perioperative care, 617
    respiratory care, 656–657, 662–663, 678–679
    safeguarding, 725
    tracheostomy care and management, 749
    urinary catheter care, 766
DisDAT *see* disability distress assessment tool
disimpaction, 75
disinfection, 244, 252
distraction techniques, 544, 628–630
DNAR/DNACPR orders *see* ReSPECT process
documentation and record keeping
    administration of medicines, 369
    assessment, 2–3, 18
    deaths, 780, 785–787, 791
    immunisation, 214
    infection prevention and control, 242–243
    investigations, 314
    moving and handling, 421
    neurological care, **465–466**
    pain management, 547, 549, 551, 558
    personal hygiene, *177*
    safeguarding, 723, 724–726
domestic violence/abuse, 716–717
do not resuscitate (DNAR/DNACPR) orders *see* ReSPECT process
Doppler ultrasound, 9
dosage charts, *638*
double nappies, 763
DPI *see* dry powder inhalers
drain insertion, 353
DRE *see* digital rectal examination
dressings and wound care
    assessment, 24
    biopsy, 49, 57
    burns and scalds, 91–94, **92**
    entry/exit site care, **478**
    intravenous and intra-arterial access, 259, 269–271, *270*, 296–297
    investigations, 327, 328
    neurological care, 478
    orthopaedic care, 524
    pain management, 562–563
    respiratory care, 669
    tracheostomy care and management, 735
    urinary catheter care, 761–762
drug allergy, 39–40
drug calculations, 370–371
drug withdrawal, 769–777
    assessment of symptoms, 771, 773
    clonidine, 776
    concepts and definitions, 770
    conversion from intravenous to oral medication, 775
    creating a weaning plan, 774–775
    incidence, 770
    mechanisms of tolerance, 770
    nonpharmacological management, 776
    opioids and benzodiazepines, 771–776, **772**
    overall aims of withdrawal management, 770–771
    pharmacological weaning management, 772–776
    prevention of withdrawal symptoms, 771, 772
    taking a patient history, 773–774
dry powder inhalers (DPI), 375
dysphagia swallow, 349
dyspnoea, 581, 587–588

Early Help Assessment (EHA), 724, 725
early warning score (EWS), 126–127, *126–127*, **127**
ear, nose, and throat (ENT), 20
ears
    investigations, 324
    personal hygiene, 170, 197
eating disorders, 408–413
    assessment, 410
    treatment, 410–413
EBM *see* expressed breast milk
Ebola virus, **230**
EBV *see* Epstein–Barr virus
ECC *see* external chest compressions
ECG *see* electrocardiography
ECV *see* extracorporeal volume
education and training
    moving and handling, 418–421, *420*
    neurological care, **458**
    pain management, 551
    personal hygiene, 176
    play as a therapeutic tool, 624–625
    poisoning and overdose, **641**
    respiratory care, 679
    safeguarding, 722
    seriously ill child, 124, 127
    systemic anti-cancer treatment, 116
    tracheostomy care and management, 740
    see also health promotion/education
egg allergy, 40, **40**
EHA *see* Early Help Assessment
electrical burns, 88, 96
electrocardiography (ECG)
    cardiopulmonary resuscitation, 704–706, *704*
    investigations, 333–338, *334–337*
    seriously ill child, 130
electrolytes *see* fluid balance
electrosurgical diathermy, 605–607
elimination
    assessment, 22–23
    bowel care, 72–73
    personal hygiene, 159–161, 182–184
    seriously ill child, 130
emergency care *see* medical emergencies
emergency medical services (EMS), 700–701
emotional abuse, 714, 716
empyema, 663
EMS *see* emergency medical services
endotracheal tube (ET), 690–691, 741
end-stage renal failure (ESRF), 134
end-tidal carbon dioxide monitoring, 690, 704
enemas
    administration of medicines, 375–376, 390–391
    bowel care, 76–79, 81–82
ENT *see* ear, nose, and throat
enteral route
    administration of medicines, 372, 384–386
    nutrition and feeding, 488, **488**, 489–490, **497–498**, 498–509
Entonox, 550–555, *552*
entry/exit site care *see* dressings and wound care
EPC *see* epilepsia partialis continua

Index

epidermolysis bullosa, 193, 325
epidural route
  administration of medicines, 381
  pain management, 555–565, **556–557**, *558–559*, 571
epilepsia partialis continua (EPC), 468
epilepsy, 470
epileptic spasm, 470
Epstein–Barr virus (EBV), **223**
ESBL *see* extended spectrum beta-lactamase
Escherichia coli, **223**
ESRF *see* end-stage renal failure
essential oils, 101–102
ET *see* endotracheal tube
ethanol, 638–639
evaporative heat loss, *431*
EVD *see* external ventricular drainage
EWS *see* early warning score
excision, 717
exposure, 130
expressed breast milk (EBM), 483–485, 489, **492–495**, 496
extended spectrum beta-lactamase (ESBL), 219
external chest compressions (ECC), 699–700, 702–706
external ventricular drainage (EVD), 470–479
  administration of medicines, 399
  drainage system, *472*
  procedure guidelines, 471–479
  zero reference point, *474*
extracorporeal volume (ECV), 136, **137**
extravasation, 116–117, 121
extremism, 719
eyelid myoclonia, 469
eye opening, 454–455
eye protection, 115
eyes
  investigations, 324
  personal hygiene, 169–170, 194–196

fabricated or induced illness (FII), 715, 725
face masks, 659, 673–674
facial protection, 238, **238–239**
faecal samples, 321, 323
faecal soiling, 76–78, *77*
family
  cardiopulmonary resuscitation, 710
  deaths, 784, 789, 792
  mental health, 411
  neonatal care, **435**
  neurological care, **458**, 472
  play as a therapeutic tool, 624
  poisoning and overdose, 640
  respiratory care, 647
  safeguarding, 714–719
family group conference (FGC), 726
family history, 1, 5, 20, 24, 26
fasting, **599–600**
FB *see* foreign bodies
female genital mutilation (FGM), 717–718
FFP *see* fresh frozen plasma
FGC *see* family group conference
FGM *see* female genital mutilation
FII *see* fabricated or induced illness
finger prick sampling, 316, **316**
first aid, 89–90
FLACC (revised) Scale, **549**
fluid balance, 133–155
  bowel care, 84–85
  burns and scalds, 90–91, **91**
  cardiopulmonary resuscitation, 710
  concepts and definitions, 133
  electrolytes, 134
  haemodialysis, 136–139, **136–138**, *138*, 142–143, 149–150
  haemofiltration, 136, 139, 142–147, *148*
  intravenous and intra-arterial access, 136, 142–143
  maintenance of fluid requirements, 133, **133**
  neonatal care, 444, **448–449**
  neurological care, 477
  nutrition and feeding, 490
  observations in ill CYP, 134, **135**, **140–141**
  palliative care, 582, *583*, 588
  perioperative care, 616
  peritoneal dialysis, 136, 139–140, **140**, 150–154
  procedure guidelines, 141–154
  renal replacement therapy, 134–136
  seriously ill child, 129
fluoride toothpaste, 189
fluoroscopy, 349
foam cleaning sponges, 189–190
focal seizures, 468, *469*
food allergy, 34–36, **35**, 486
food refusal, 412–413
foot movement, 524, *525–526*
foot protection, 239
foreign bodies (FB), 701–704, *703*
formula feeds, 485–486, **485**
fortifiers, 485, **485**, **495**, 496
Frankfurt plane, 15, *16*
fresh frozen plasma (FFP), 67

GA1 *see* glutaric acidemia type 1
gallows traction, 521
gastral washings, 320
gastric lavage, 640–643, **641**
gastric tubes, 691
gastroenteritis, **222**
gastrointestinal tract
  drug withdrawal, 771
  investigations, 352
  perioperative care, 616
gastrostomy tubes, 385, 489–490, **503–507**, 579
GCS *see* Glasgow Coma Scale
GDPR *see* General Data Protection Regulation
Gell-Coombs classification, **30**
General Data Protection Regulation (GDPR), 723
generalised anxiety disorder, 407
genetically engineered vaccines, 204
genetic disorders, 470
German measles *see* rubella
GFR *see* glomerular filtration rate
Giardia lamblia, **223**
glandular fever *see* infectious mononucleosis
Glasgow Coma Scale (GCS), 454
glaucoma, 170
glomerular filtration rate (GFR), 338–344
gloves, 235, **236–237**, 250
glucose
  cardiopulmonary resuscitation, 710
  neonatal care, **449**
  seriously ill child, 130
glutaric acidemia type 1 (GA1), 439
goggles, 238, **238–239**
GOSH tracheostomy tubes, 748
growth, 14–18
grunting, 20
guided imagery, 631

haematoma, 55
haemodialysis (HD)
  fluid balance, 136–139, **136–138**, *138*, 142–143, 149–150
  intravenous and intra-arterial access, 254, 269
haemofiltration (HF), 136, 139, 142–147, *148*
Haemophilus influenzae, 207, **223**, 225
haemorrhage *see* bleeding/haemorrhage
haemothorax, 663
hair, 320, 321
half-hitch knots, *536*
hallucinations, 408
halo traction, *538*
hand, foot, and mouth disease, **223**
hand hygiene
  infection prevention and control, 221, **231–232**, 232–234, *234–235*
  investigations, 314
hand movement, 525, *525–526*
handover, 617
hand protection, 115
hazardous waste, 245, **245**
HCA *see* homocystinuria
HCAI *see* infection prevention and control
HD *see* haemodialysis
head circumference, 18, 20
head lice, **223**, **226**
head tilt, 687–688
health and safety measures
  intravenous and intra-arterial access, 287
  investigations, 314–315
  moving and handling, 415–426
  systemic anti-cancer treatment, 114
Health and Social Care Act (2008), 218
healthcare associated infections (HCAI) *see* infection prevention and control
health play specialists (HPS), 624–625, 631–633
health promotion/education
  burns and scalds, 95–96
  drug withdrawal, 776
  neurological care, **458**, 472
  nutrition and feeding, 487
  orthopaedic care, 533
  personal hygiene, 167, 173, 192
  poisoning and overdose, 637
  respiratory care, 660
  urinary catheters, **755**
heart rate, 7, **613**
heat and moisture exchangers (HME), 745, *745*
heat stress, **433**
heel prick sampling, 316, **316**, *318–319*, **318**
height, 15–16, *16*
heparinisation, 252, **252–254**, 298, 302
hepatitis viruses
  blood components and products, 62
  immunisation, 203, 207, 215
  infection prevention and control, **223**, 240–242
herbal medicines, 100, 102
herd immunity, 206, 213–214
herpes simplex virus (HSV), **223**, 328
herpes zoster virus, 215
HF *see* haemofiltration
high concentration oxygen therapy, 658
high-flow nasal cannula, 659
histamine, 30
HLA *see* human leukocyte antigen
HME *see* heat and moisture exchangers
hMPV *see* human metapneumovirus
hoists, 421–422, **425**

Index

home care, 676–680
home parenteral nutrition (HPN), 491
homocystinuria (HCA), 439
homoeopathy, 100, 101
hoop traction, 527
hospital passports, 362, *363–364*
HPN *see* home parenteral nutrition
HPS *see* health play specialists
HPV *see* human papillomavirus
HSV *see* herpes simplex virus
HTLV *see* human T-cell leukaemia viruses
human immunodeficiency virus (HIV)
    blood components and products, 62
    infection prevention and control, 240–242
    nutrition and feeding, 483
human leukocyte antigen (HLA), 66
human metapneumovirus (hMPV), **224**
human papillomavirus (HPV), 207–208
human T-cell leukaemia viruses (HTLV), 62
humidification, 659, 674
humidity, 744–745, *745*
hydration/dehydration
    bowel care, 85
    fluid balance, 134, **134–135**, **137**
    palliative care, 582, *583*, 588
hydrocolloids, 163
hydrocortisone, 163–164
hyperglycaemia, **331**
hypoglycaemia, **331**
hypovolaemia, **136**
hypoxia, 684, 696, 700

IAD *see* incontinence associated dermatitis
ICP *see* intracranial pressure
ID *see* intradermal route
idiopathic constipation, 74
IDT *see* intradermal testing
Ig *see* immunoglobulins
ileostomy, 391
IM *see* intramuscular route
immune disorders, 470
immune response, 30
immunisation, 201–216
    adverse reactions and vaccine safety, 205–206, 214
    allergy and anaphylaxis, 39–40, **40**
    assessment, 5
    concepts and definitions, 202
    contraindications, 204–205
    efficacy of vaccines, 206
    ensuring high vaccine uptake, 213–214
    healthcare workers, 203, 214–215
    herd immunity, 206
    passive versus active immunity, 203–204
    procedure guidelines, 205
    routine immunisation schedules in UK, 202, **202**
    special risk groups, 203, **203**
    specific diseases/vaccines, 206–213
    storage and administration of vaccines, 213
    types of vaccine, 204, **204**
    vaccines not in general use in UK, 213
immunocompromised patients, 193
immunoglobulins (Ig), 30–32, 35–36, **35**, 67–70
impetigo, **224**
incontinence associated dermatitis (IAD), 161–165, **162**, *163–164*, 184–186
incontinence/continence *see* continence/incontinence
incubators, **429**
induced emesis, 640

infection prevention and control, 217–247
    antibiotic resistance and antimicrobial stewardship, 219
    Care Quality Commission criteria, 218
    chain of infection, 219–220
    colonisation and infection, 221
    deaths, 789
    decontamination of equipment/environment, 243–245, **244–245**
    exposure to blood and body fluids, 240–242
    financial burden of healthcare associated infections, 218
    hand hygiene, 221, **231–232**, 232–234, *234–235*
    Health and Social Care Act (2008), 218
    Health care acquired Infection (HCAI), 239
    intravenous and intra-arterial access, 280
    investigations, 314–315
    isolation precautions, 221, **222–230**, 239–240
    neurological care, 470
    nutrition and feeding, 506
    pain management, 563
    personal protective equipment, 235–239, **236–239**
    reporting and dangerous occurrences regulations, 242–243
    respiratory care, 668
    standard precautions, 221–239
    tracheostomy care and management, 734
    urinary catheter care, 754, 761
infectious mononucleosis, **224**
inferior vena cava (IVC), 294–295
infibulation, 718
influenza viruses, 208–209, 215, **224**
information sharing, 723
infused medications, 263–265, 274–277, 295, 301
infusion feeds, 511–513
inhalation route, 374–375, 388–390
interventional radiology (IR), 351–352, **352–353**
intracerebroventricular access, 399–400
intracranial pressure (ICP), **458**, 615
intradermal route (ID), 376–377, 393
intradermal testing (IDT), 39
intramuscular route (IM), 376, 378–380, *379*, 396–397, *396*
intranasal route, 374, 387–388
intraosseous (IO) route, 380, 398, 693–696
intraperitoneal haemorrhage, 45
intrathecal route
    administration of medicines, 380–381, 398–401
    neurological care, 478
    systemic anti-cancer treatment, 117
intravenous and intra-arterial access, 249–311
    accessing/de-accessing an implanted port, 277–279
    administration of bolus/infused medications, 262–265, 273–277, 295, 301
    administration of medicines, 380
    arterial lines, 298–306
    aseptic nontouch technique, 250–253, **250**, 295, **564**
    blood sampling, 265–267, 303–304
    common CVAD complications, 280–286, **280–282**, *284–285*, 293
    concepts and definitions, 249
    CVAD dressings, 269–271, *270*
    CVAD repair, 288–292
    dressings, 259, 269–271, *270*, 296–297
    drug withdrawal, 775

    fluid balance, 136, 142–143
    flushing techniques, 254, 261, 272–273, 280
    flush volumes and heparinisation, 252, **252–254**, 298, 302
    investigations, 342–344, 352
    maintenance of arterial lines, 301–303
    needle-free access devices, 252, 272
    neonatal care, 444
    neonatal longlines: nursing management, 294–298, *297*
    nutrition and feeding, 491, 510
    pain management, 571
    palliative care, 579
    procedure guidelines, 251, 255–259, **258–259**, 261–267, 271–279, 283–294, 296–306
    removal of arterial cannula, 306
    removal of CVADs, 293–294
    removal of peripheral cannula, 267
    safety aspects for staff and families, 287
    seriously ill child, 129
    syringe pumps, 274–275
    syringe size, 254–255
    systemic anti-cancer treatment, 116, **118–121**
    troubleshooting, 304–305
    types of central venous access devices, **253–254**, 254, 268
    visual infusion phlebitis, 260–261, **260**
    volumetric pumps, 275–277
intraventricular access, 401
investigations, 313–355
    analysis of antibiotic levels, 315
    biopsy material, 320
    blood culture, 315–316
    blood glucose monitoring, 331–333, **331**
    blood sampling, 315–319, **316**, *318–319*, **318**
    cerebrospinal fluid, 320
    chest drain fluid, 320
    collection of microbiological specimens, 314–330
    concepts and definitions, 314
    cough swabs, 321, 323
    ear swabs, 324
    electrocardiograph monitoring, 333–338, *334–337*
    equipment, 315
    eye swabs, 324
    fungal samples, 320, 321
    gastral washings, 320, 321
    glomerular filtration rate, 338–344
    nasopharyngeal aspirate, 320–321, 322
    nose swabs, 325
    pregnancy testing, 345–346
    preparation, 314–315
    procedure guidelines, 315–330, 332–333, 335–344, 347–348
    radiological investigations, 346–352, **350–353**
    rationale for specimen collection, 314
    sputum samples, 321, 322
    stool samples, 321, 323
    transport to the laboratory, 315
    urine samples, 327–330, 345–346
    vesicular fluid samples, 328, 330
    ward-based investigations, 331–346
    see also biopsy
IO *see* intraosseous route
ipecacuanha, 640
IR *see* interventional radiology
isolation precautions, 221, **222–230**, 239–240
isopropyl alcohol, 269

isovaleria acidemia, 439
IVC *see* inferior vena cava

jaundice, neonatal care, 443–444, *445*, **445–448**, *447*
jaw thrust, 688
jejunostomy tubes, 385, 489–490
just in case/just in time training, 127

keepsakes, 789
keratoconjunctivitis, **222**
knots, *536*
Korotkoff sounds, 9–10

LAC *see* looked after children
laryngeal mask airway (LMA), 690, *691*
laser therapy, 352
Lassa virus, **230**
last offices, 787–790
latex allergy, 41, 597
laundry
    infection prevention and control, 244, **244**
    moving and handling, 422
laxatives, 75–76
learning (intellectual) disability, 357–365
    becoming an adult, 361–362
    Books Beyond Words, 364
    challenges faced by health professionals, 359
    communication, 358, 362, 364
    concepts and definitions, 358–359
    consent and decision-making, 361–362
    diagnostic overshadowing, 359, 360–361
    families as allies, 358
    getting care right in practice, 362
    health needs, 362
    hospital passports, 362, *363–364*
    need for change in services and practice, 359
    pictures and images, 364
    play as a therapeutic tool, 627–628
    positive behaviour support, 361
    preparation for theatre and recovery, 364
    principles underpinning practice, 358
    protocols to improve care outcomes, 362–364
    reasonable care adjustments, 362
    safeguarding, 718
    seeing the person and understanding behaviour, 359–360, **360**
lice, **223**, **224**, **226**
life-limiting conditions (LLC), 578, *581*
light management, **434**
limb movement, **21**, 457, 524
linogram, 350
liver biopsy, 44–49
    anatomy and physiology, 44, *44*
    complications, 45–46
    contraindications, 45
    discharge planning, 46, 49
    equipment, 45
    indications, 44
    procedure guidelines, 46–49
live vaccines, 204
LLC *see* life-limiting conditions
LMA *see* laryngeal mask airway
local anaesthesia, 543, 561–562
long-term oxygen therapy (LTOT), 658
long-term ventilation (LTV), 676–680
looked after children (LAC), 726
low concentration oxygen therapy, 658
LTOT *see* long-term oxygen therapy

LTV *see* long-term ventilation
lumbar puncture, 400–401

magnetic resonance imaging (MRI), 351, 628
malacia, 673
malaria, **224**
malignancy
    biopsy, 45, 353
    complementary and alternative medicine, 110
    systemic anti-cancer treatment, 113–122
manual defibrillation, 707–708, *707*
Manual Handling Operations Regulations (MHOR), 416–418, 420
maple syrup urine disease (MSUD), 439
Marburg virus, **230**
masks, 238, **238–239**
massage therapy, 102–110
    basic techniques, 103, *104–109*
    case studies, 109–110
    principles, **103**
MCADD *see* medium-chain acyl-CoA dehydrogenase deficiency
MCCD *see* Medical Certificate of Cause of Death
meal management, 411, 412
measles, 209, **224**
measles, mumps, rubella (MMR) vaccine, 39, 205–206, 209, 211, 213, 214
mechanical occlusions, 280
Medical Certificate of Cause of Death (MCCD), 780, 785–786
medical emergencies
    cardiopulmonary resuscitation, 683–711
    nasopharyngeal airway, 650
    oxygen therapy, 657, 659
    status epilepticus, **467–468**
    tracheostomy care and management, *739*, *741*, 745, *745*
medically unexplained symptoms, 407
medication history, 5, 130
medium-chain acyl-CoA dehydrogenase deficiency (MCADD), 438
memory work, 792
meningitis, **224–225**
meningococcal disease, **225**
meningococcal vaccines, 210
menstruation, 23
mental health, 405–413
    adjustment to illness, 406–407
    anxiety disorders, 407
    available help, 406
    concepts and definitions, 406
    depression, 408
    eating disorders, 408–413
    incidence and prevalence, 406
    poisoning and overdose, 636, *637*
    psychosis, 407, 408
    safeguarding, 718
    self-harm, 408
    somatoform disorders and medically unexplained symptoms, 407
MERS *see* Middle East respiratory syndrome
metabolic disorders, 470
metastatic rhabdomyosarcoma, 110
meticillin-resistant *Staphylococcus aureus* (MRSA), 218, **226**
MHOR *see* Manual Handling Operations Regulations
micturating cystourethrogram, 350
Middle East respiratory syndrome (MERS), **225**
Mitrofanoff catheters, 763–764

MMR *see* measles, mumps, rubella
mobilisation, **531**
mobility, 24
modified gallows traction, 527
molluscum contagiosum, **225**
mortuaries, 788, 790–791
mottling, 19
mouthwashes, 190
moving and handling, 415–426
    concepts and definitions, 416
    documentation and record keeping, 421
    education and training, 418–421, *420*
    equipment, 421–422, **421**, **424**
    general guidelines, **422**
    hoists and slings, 421–422, **425**
    legislation, 416
    musculoskeletal health and wellbeing, 417–418, *419*
    patient assessment, **423**
    patient positioning, **424**
    perioperative care, 603
    risk assessment, 416–417, **424–425**
MRI *see* magnetic resonance imaging
MRSA *see* meticillin-resistant *Staphylococcus aureus*
MSD *see* musculoskeletal disorders
MSUD *see* maple syrup urine disease
multidrug resistance, 219, **226**
mumps, 210–211, **226**
muscle relaxation, 631
musculoskeletal disorders (MSD), 416
musculoskeletal health and wellbeing, 417–418, *419*
Mycobacterium spp.
    immunisation, 213
    infection prevention and control, **226**
    investigations, 320
mydriatic drugs, 170
myoclonic absence, 469
myoclonic seizures, 470

nails
    investigations, 320, 321
    personal hygiene, 165, *165*, 187–188
naloxone, 570
named professional, 792
nappy rash, 161–165, **162**, *163–164*, 184–186
nasal masks, 673
nasal sprays, 37, *38*
nasoduodenal tube, 385
nasogastric tubes, 385, 413, 489–490, 498–501, 581
nasojejunal tubes, 385, 489–490, 501–503, **501**
nasopharyngeal airway (NPA), 649–657
    cardiopulmonary resuscitation, 689
    indications, 650
    insertion, 654, *655*
    observations, 656, *656*
    ongoing care and discharge planning, 656–657
    preparation, 651–652, *652–653*
    size and length, 649, *650*
nasopharyngeal aspirate (NPA), 320–321, *322*
National Society for the Prevention of Cruelty to Children (NSPCC), 714
nausea and vomiting
    pain management, 570–571
    palliative care, 580, *581*, 585
    perioperative care, 615

Index

NCA see nurse-controlled analgesia
nebulisers, 374–375, 388
necrotising enterocolitis, **226**
needle-free access devices, 252, 272
negative myoclonus, 470
neglect, 714–715, 716
Neisseria spp., 210, **225**
neonatal care, 427–451
    Babytherms, **429**
    bassinettes/cots, **430**
    cold stress, **431–432**, *432*
    concepts and definitions, 428
    developmental care, 433, **433–435**, *434*
    family involvement, **435**
    fluid management, 444, **448–449**
    heat stress, **433**
    incubators, **429**
    light/noise management, **434–435**
    monitoring temperature, **428**
    newborn blood spot screening, 438–442, **438–439**, *442*, **443**
    phototherapy for neonatal jaundice, 443–444, *445*, **445–448**, *447*
    positioning, **433**, *434*
    prevention of heat loss, **430–431**, **430**
    procedure guidelines, 437–442
    thermoregulation, 428, **428–433**, *430–432*
    umbilical cord care, 436–438
    vitamin K administration/management, 435, **435–436**
neonatal history, 4
neonatal longlines, 294–298, *297*
nephrology interventions, 353
nerve compression, 532
nerve compromise, 526
neurological care, 453–480
    assessment, 20, **21–22**
    education and training, **458**
    external ventricular drainage, 470–479, *472*, *479*
    Glasgow Coma Scale, 454
    GOSH coma chart, *459–461*
    informing CYP and family, **458**, 472
    intracranial pressure, **458**
    neurological observations, 454–457, **457–458**, *459–461*, 473
    painful stimuli, 454–455, 462–463, *462–464*, 471–479
    pain management, 563
    perioperative care, 614
    procedure guidelines, 454–457, 466–467
    seizures, 463–470, **465–468**, *469*
    seriously ill child, 127, *127*, 130
neuromuscular disorders, 673
neurovascular observations, 520, **521**, *522–523*, 524–525, *525–526*
newborn blood spot screening, 438–442, **438–439**, *442*, **443**
nitrous oxide, 550–555, *552*
NIV see noninvasive ventilation
noise management, **435**
noninvasive ventilation (NIV), 672–675
    indications, 673
    procedure guidelines, 673–675
nonograms, *639*
nonsteroidal anti-inflammatory drugs (NSAID), 544
normalisation, 623
norovirus, **226**
nose swabs, 325

notification of death, 780
NPA see nasopharyngeal airway; nasopharyngeal aspirate
NSAID see nonsteroidal anti-inflammatory drugs
NSPCC see National Society for the Prevention of Cruelty to Children
NST see Nutrition Support Team
nuclear medicine, 350
nurse-controlled analgesia (NCA), 565–569, 580, 585–586
nurse independent prescribers, 368
nutrition and feeding, 481–517
    assessment, 22
    bowel care, 76, 84–85
    breastfeeding, 483–486, **485**, 488–489, 491, **495**
    breast milk fortifiers, 485, **485**, **495**, 496
    breast pumps and expressed breast milk, **492–495**, 496
    burns and scalds, 94
    continuing care, 488
    diet through childhood and adolescence, 487, **487**
    drug withdrawal, 776
    enteral feeding, 488, **488**, 489–490, **497–498**, 498–509
    feeding the preterm infant, 483–485, **485**, **495**
    feeding the term infant, 485, **485**
    feed preparation and administration, 485–486
    health promotion, 487
    introduction of complementary foods, 486–487, **486–487**
    mental health, 411–413
    nutritional requirements, 482–483, **483–484**
    palliative care, 582, *583*, 588
    parenteral nutrition, 490–491, 510–511
    preterm to adolescence, 483–488, **485–488**
    procedure guidelines, 496, 498–503, 507–515
    screening tools, 482
    sham feeding, 491, 513–515
    supplementary feeding, 488, **488**
    tracheostomy care and management, **734**
Nutrition Support Team (NST), 490

obdurators, 748
obsessive–compulsive disorder (OCD), 407
obstructive sleep apnoea (OSA), 673
occlusions
    intravenous and intra-arterial access, 280–286, **280–282**, *284–285*
    pain management, 563–564
    tracheostomy care and management, 733–734
occupational therapy, 490
OCD see obsessive–compulsive disorder
oedema, 19
oesophagostomy, 491
OFC see oral food challenge
Ommaya reservoirs, 401
one way valves, 748
ooze, 524
open drainage systems, 763
opioids
    drug withdrawal, 771–776, **772**
    pain management, 543–544, 566, 569–571
oppositional defiant disorder, 407
OPQRSTU mnemonic, **580**
oral fluid swabs, 325–326
oral food challenge (OFC), 36, **35**, 40

oral hygiene, 165–169, *166*, **167–169**, 188–193
oral phobia, 193
oral route, 371–372, 384
    drug withdrawal, 775
    systemic anti-cancer treatment, 116, **121**
oral stimulation programmes, 490, 509
oral temperature, 7
organ donation, 787
organisational culture, 722
orogastric tubes, 385, 489–490
oropharyngeal airway, 689
orthopaedic care, 519–540
    acute compartment syndrome, 520, 526, **532**
    concepts and definitions, 520
    crutches, 521, 533, **534–535**
    neurovascular observations, 520, **521**, *522–523*, 524–525, *525–526*
    plaster casts, 520–521, 526–527, *527*, 529–531, **530–532**
    procedure guidelines, 524–527, *525–527*, 529–533, 536–539
    skeletal pin site care, 520
    traction, 520, 521, 527–528, *528*, **535–536**, 536–539, *536–538*
    walking aids, 532, **532–533**
OSA see obstructive sleep apnoea
osteopathy, 100, 101
OTC see over-the-counter
otitis externa, 170
otitis media, 170
overdose see poisoning and overdose
overgranulation, 507
over-the-counter (OTC) medicines, 368
oxygen saturation, 14
oxygen therapy, 657–663
    cardiopulmonary resuscitation, 696
    indications, 658
    methods and equipment, 659, *659*
    prescribing oxygen, 658
    procedure guidelines, 660–663
    pulse oximetry, 658
    types, 658
    ventilation and humidification, 659, 674, 676–677

PACS see paediatric acute compartment syndrome
paediatric acute compartment syndrome (PACS), 520, 526, **532**
paediatric early warning score (PEWS)
    cardiopulmonary resuscitation, 684
    respiratory care, 646, 658, 668–669, 675
    seriously ill child, 126–127, *126–127*, **127**
    see also Children's Early Warning Score (CEWS); early warning score (EWS)
paediatric intensive care units (PICU), 136, 193, 578
painful stimuli, 454–455, 462–463, *462–464*, 471–479
pain management, 541–575
    administration of Entonox, 550–555, *552*
    analgesic ladder, *545*
    assessment, 545–551, 556
    complementary and alternative medicine, 110
    concepts and definitions, 542
    documentation and record keeping, *548*, *550*, *552*
    education and training, 551
    epidural analgesia, 555–565, **556–557**, *559–560*, 571

general principles, **542–544**
learning (intellectual) disability, 360–361
palliative care, 581, *582*, 585–586
patient- and nurse-controlled analgesia, 565–569
perioperative care, 615
play as a therapeutic tool, 628
prevention and management of opioid complications, 566, 569–571
procedure guidelines, 548–549, 551–555, 557–572
sucrose, 571
United Kingdom guidelines and recommendations, 542
pain score, 524
palliative care, 577–593
agitation, 582, 590–591
assessment of symptoms, 579–580, *579*, **580**, 584–585
concepts and definitions, 578–579
constipation and diarrhoea, 581, 586–587
dyspnoea, 581, 587–588
haemorrhage, 582, 589
hydration and nutrition, 582, *583*, 588
nausea and vomiting, 580–581, *581*, 586
pain management, 580, 585–586
procedure guidelines, 584–590
seizures, 582–583, 591
signs of impending death, 586, 592
pallor, 19
palpation, 7
panic disorder, 407
paracetamol
pain management, 544
poisoning and overdose, 636, 637–638, *638–639*
parainfluenza virus, **226**
parallel play, 623
parental responsibility (PR), 3
parenteral nutrition (PN), 490–491, 510–511
Parkland formula, 91
partner abuse, 717
parvovirus B19, **226**
passive immunity, 203
past history
assessment, 1, 4–5
drug withdrawal, 773–774
seriously ill child, 130
patient-controlled analgesia (PCA), 110, 565–569, 580, 585–586
patient group directions (PGD), 368–369
patient self-administration, 369
patient specific directions (PSD), 368–369
PBS *see* positive behaviour support
PCA *see* patient-controlled analgesia
PCHR *see* Personal Child Health Record
PCR *see* polymerase chain reaction
PD *see* peritoneal dialysis
PEA *see* pulseless electrical activity
peer support, 411
perioperative care, 595–619
admission to hospital, 598–599
care in anaesthetic room, 601–602
care in operating theatre, 602–609
care in recovery, 609–617, *610*, **613**
concepts and definitions, 596
consent, **599**
fasting, **599–600**
immediately prior to theatre, 600–601
intra operative care, 597

pre-admission, 598
premedication, **600**
preparation, 596, *596*
procedure guidelines, 598–617
recovery, 597, *598*, 609–617, *610*, **613**
peripherally inserted central catheters (PICC), **252**, 254, 268–269, *270*, 287–289, 293–298, *297*
peripheral temperature, 6
peripheral venous catheters **252**, 255–267, **258–259**, 342–343
peritoneal dialysis (PD), 136, 139–140, **140**, 150–154
pernasal swabs, 325, 326
peroneal nerve, *525–526*
Personal Child Health Record (PCHR), 214
personal hygiene, 157–200
anatomy and physiology, 158–159, *158*
assessment, 23–24
bathing and washing, 158–159, *160*, 178–182
concepts and definitions, 158
ear care, 170, 197
eye care, 169–170, 194–196
nail care, 165, *165*, 187–188
nappy and incontinence pad care, 161–165, **162**, *163–164*, 184–186
oral hygiene, 165–169, *166*, **167–169**, 188–193
orthopaedic care, 531
pressure ulcer prevention and management, 171–177, *171–172*, *174–175*, *177*
procedure guidelines, 178–197
toileting, 159–161, 182–184
personal protective equipment (PPE)
infection prevention and control, 235–239, **236–239**
investigations, 314–315
systemic anti-cancer treatment, 115
pertussis
infection prevention and control, 211, 215, **226**, 230
investigations, 325, 326
pest control, 245
PEWS *see* paediatric early warning score
PGD *see* patient group directions
pharmacological weaning management, 772–776
pharmacy-only medicines, 368
pharyngeal airway, 688–689
phenylketonuria (PKU), 438
phlebitis, 260–261, **260**
phobias, 407
phototherapy, 443–444, *445*, **445–448**, *447*
physical abuse, 714–715
physical dependence, 770
PICC *see* peripherally inserted central catheters
PICU *see* paediatric intensive care units
Pierre Robin Sequence (PRS), 650
pinch up technique, 397
pinworm, **226**
PKU *see* phenylketonuria
plaster casts, 520–521, 526–527, *527*, **530–532**
platelets, 66
play as a therapeutic tool, 621–634
additional needs or learning disability, 627–628
adolescents, 627
aims of play preparation, 625–626
arts in health, 633

case studies, 628, 631–633
concepts and definitions, 622
desensitisation, 632–633
development of play, 623
development of play in hospital, 622
distraction techniques, 628–630
education and training, 624–625
following the procedure, 627
functions of play, 623
functions of play in hospital, 623–624
guided imagery, 631
health play specialists, 624–625, 631–633
importance of play in hospital, 623
normal play for development, 622–623
outcomes, 627
play workers, 625
postprocedural play, 627
preadmission programmes, 626
preparation for surgery and procedures, 625
preparation session/resources, 626
procedure guidelines, 629–630
process/action, 626–627
relaxation techniques, 630–631
reluctant CYPs, 627
siblings, 624
therapeutic play, 631–632
types of play, 623
pleural effusion, 663
pMDI *see* pressurised metered dose inhalers
PN *see* parenteral nutrition
pneumococcal disease, 211–212
pneumonia, **227**
pneumothorax, 663, *664*, 668
poisoning and overdose, 635–644
accidental ingestion, 636
care of the parent/carer, 640
common ingestions, 636, 637–639, *638–639*
concepts and definitions, 636
gastric lavage, 640–643, **641**
health promotion strategies, 637
initial management, 639
nonaccidental ingestion and self-harm, 636, *637*
procedure guidelines, 642–643
treatment of ingested poisons, 640
poliomyelitis, 212, **227**
polymerase chain reaction (PCR), 328, 330
POM *see* prescription-only medicines
positioning
cardiopulmonary resuscitation, 687, 689–690
moving and handling, **424**
neonatal care, **433**, *434*
orthopaedic care, **530**
perioperative care, 603
personal hygiene, 175–176, *175*
positive behaviour support (PBS), 361
positive pressure flushing, 254
postcraniofacial mid-facial advancement, 650
posterior fossa syndrome, 109
post-mortem examination, 786–787, 792
post-traumatic stress disorder (PTSD), 407
posture, 19
potassium, **449**
PPCA *see* proxy patient-controlled analgesia
PPE *see* personal protective equipment
PR *see* parental responsibility
preadmission programmes, 626
pregnancy, 340, 349
pregnancy testing, 345–346
premedication, **600**
prenatal history, 4

Index

prescription-only medicines (POM), 368
present illness, 1, 4
pressure care, 604, 776
pressure points, *537*
pressure ulcers
  care planning, 173–175
  extrinsic/intrinsic risk factors, 171, *171*
  management, 176–177, *177*
  parent and carer education, 173
  personal hygiene, 171–177
  repositioning, 175–176, *175*
  risk assessment, 171–173, *174*
  skin assessment, 173
  SSKIN care bundle, 171, *172*
  staff education, 176
  support surfaces, mattresses, and cushions, 176
pressurised metered dose inhalers (pMDI), 375, 390
prevention
  ABCDE assessment tool, 125–130, *125*, *129*
  AVPU consciousness scale, 127, *127*, 130
  chain of prevention, 124, *124*
  concepts and definitions, 124
  drug withdrawal, 771, 772
  early recognition, 124
  early warning score, 126–127, *126–127*, **127**
  just in case/just in time training, 127
  opioid complications, 566, 569–571
  SBARD communication tool, 124, *126*
  seriously ill child, 123–131
  situational awareness, 127
  see also infection prevention and control
prion disease, **227**
privacy
  bowel care, 85
  investigations, 345
  perioperative care, 604
protein (dietary), 94
proxy patient-controlled analgesia (PPCA), 580, 585–586
PRS *see* Pierre Robin Sequence
pruritus, 571
PSD *see* patient specific directions
pseudo-addiction, 770
psychological care, 616
psychosis, 407, 408
psychotropic medications, 410
PTSD *see* post-traumatic stress disorder
puberty, 23
Pugh's traction, 527, *528*
pulsatile flush technique, 254
pulse, 7, 524
pulseless electrical activity (PEA), 704–705, *704*
pulse oximetry, 14, 658
punch skin biopsy, 49–54
pupil reaction, 456–457

quality control (QC), 332–333

radiative heat loss, *431*
radicalisation, 719
radiological investigations, 346–352, **350–353**
  concepts and definitions, 346–347
  environment and physical safety, 349
  interventional radiology, 351–352, **352–353**
  pregnancy status, 349
  preparation and patient care, 347–349
  types, 349–351, **350–351**
RAS *see* reticular activating system

rashes
  assessment, 23–24
  personal hygiene, 161–165, **162**, *163–164*
ready to feed (RTF) formulas, 485–486
reasonable care adjustments, 362
recession, 19
record keeping *see* documentation
recovery and rehabilitation
  perioperative care, 597, *598*, 609–617, *610*, **613**
  play as a therapeutic tool, 623, 624
recovery position, 689–690
rectal route, 375–376, 390–391
rectal temperature, 7
rectal washout, 80
red cells, 66
registration of death, 780, 785–786
relaxation techniques, 407, 630–631
renal biopsy, 54–56
  complications, 54–55
  contraindications, 54
  indications, 54
  investigations, 353
  procedure guidelines, 55–56
renal replacement therapy (RRT), 134–136
rescue breaths, 702
reservoir devices, 399–400, 401
ReSPECT process, 710–711, *710*
respirators, 238, **238–239**
respiratory allergy, 36–37, *37*
respiratory care, 645–682
  airway suction, 646–649
  assessment, 19–20
  chest drain management, 663–672, *664*, *667–668*
  concepts and definitions, 646
  long-term ventilation, 676–680
  nasopharyngeal airway, 649–657, *650*, *652–653*, *655–656*
  noninvasive ventilation, 672–675
  oxygen therapy, 657–663, *659*, *674*, 676–677
respiratory depression, 570
respiratory rate, 8, **613**
respiratory syncytial virus (RSV), 213, **227**
respiratory tract disease, **222**
resuscitation *see* cardiopulmonary resuscitation
reticular activating system (RAS), 454
rhinovirus, **227**
RIDDOR reporting, 242
ringworm, **227**, **229**
risk assessment
  drug withdrawal, **772**, 774–775
  immunisation, 203
  mental health, 411
  moving and handling, 416–417, **424–425**
  pressure ulcers, 171–173, *174*
rotaviruses, 212, **227**
RRT *see* renal replacement therapy
RSV *see* respiratory syncytial virus
RTF *see* ready to feed
rubella, 212–213, **223**, **227**

SACT *see* systemic anti-cancer treatment
safeguarding, 713–728
  background, 714
  child death reviews, 722
  collaborative working, 723
  communication, 723–724
  Covid-19/SARS-CoV-2, 722
  defining child maltreatment, 714–715

education and training, 722
  effects of abuse and neglect, 716
  extrafamilial risk factors, 719
  fabricated or induced illness, 715, 725
  improving child protection and safeguarding practice, 719–724
  individual and corporate responsibility, 714
  information sharing, 723
  intra-familial risk factors, 716–719
  legislation and guidance, 714, 719, **720**
  listening to the child's voice, 724
  looked after children, 726
  organisational culture, 722
  practice reviews, 719–722
  pre-discharge planning procedure, 725
  professional responsibilities, 724–725
  referral to Children's Social Care, 725–726
  supervision, 723
saliva, 325–326
Salmonella spp., **228**
SALT *see* speech and language therapy
SARS *see* severe acute respiratory syndrome
SBARD communication tool, 124, *126*
SC *see* subcutaneous route
scabies, **228**
scalds *see* burns and scalds
scarlet fever, **228**
scars, 19, 95
SCD *see* sickle cell disease
school attendance, 5
sclerotherapy, 352
sedation
  drug withdrawal, 771–772, **772**
  pain management, 544, 550, 571
seizures, 463–470
  care of CYP with seizures, 465–467, **466**
  classification, 468–470, *469*
  concepts and definitions, 463–464
  documentation on admission, 465–466
  palliative care, 583–584, 591
  physiology of seizures, 464–465, **465**
  status epilepticus, **467–468**
self-adhesive defibrillation pads/paddles, 707–708, *707*
self-care, 792
self-harm, 408, 636, *637*
self-inflating bag mask valve, 691–692
self-report measures, 580
semantic pragmatic communication disorder (SPCD), 628
sensation, 524–525, *525–526*
sepsis, 129, 130, 134, 280, 315
Serious Crime Act (2015), 718
Serious Hazards of Transfusion (SHOT), 62
seriously ill child, 123–131
  ABCDE assessment tool, 125–130, *125*, *129*
  AVPU consciousness scale, 127, *127*, 130
  chain of prevention, 124, *124*
  concepts and definitions, 124
  early recognition, 124
  early warning score, 126–127, *126–127*, **127**
  just in case/just in time training, 127
  SBARD communication tool, 124, *126*
  sepsis, 130
  situational awareness, 127
SES *see* socioeconomic status
severe acute respiratory syndrome (SARS), **228**
sexual abuse, 327, 714–716
sexual development, 22–23
sham feeding, 491, 513–515

Index

sharps bins, 241, 251–252
Shigella spp., **228**
Shiley tracheostomy tubes, 748
shingles, **228–229**, 328
shock
  poisoning and overdose, 639
  seriously ill child, 128–129, *129*
  toxic shock syndrome, **229**
shoe covers, 239
short-term nontunnelled central venous catheters, **254**
SHOT *see* Serious Hazards of Transfusion
siblings, 624
sickle cell disease (SCD), 438
sigmoidoscopy, 75
silver tubes, 748
simple nasal cannula, 659
sip feeds, 488, **488**
situational awareness, 127
skeletal pin site care, 520
skin
  administration of medicines, 381–382, 402
  assessment, 23–24
  drug withdrawal, 776
  investigations, 320, 321, 325, 326
  nutrition and feeding, 506
  see also personal hygiene
skin cleansers, 161–162, 269
skin prick testing (SPT), 31, *31*, **32**, 35, 39
skin stretch technique, 397
skin traction, 527, *528*, 537, *537*
skin tunnelled central venous catheters, **253**, 268, 287–292
slings, 421–422, **425**
slings and springs suspension, 528, *528*
small-volume extended mouthpiece spacers, 375, 389
Smiths portex tracheostomy tubes, 748
social anxiety disorder, 407
social exclusion, 718
socioeconomic status (SES), 5
SOCRATES mnemonic, **580**
sodium, **449**
solitary play, 623
somatoform disorders, 407
spacers, 375, 389
spastic flexion, **21**
SPC *see* suprapubic catheterisation
SPCD *see* semantic pragmatic communication disorder
special/additional needs
  personal hygiene, 160, 182, 184
  play as a therapeutic tool, 627–628
specific IgE testing (SpIgE), 32, 35
speech and language therapy (SALT), 490, 582
SpIgE *see* specific IgE testing
spillages, 115, 242–243
spinal traction, 528, 539
SPT *see* skin prick testing
sputum samples, 321, 322
squint repair, 170
SSKIN care bundle, 171, *172*
Staphylococcus spp., **228**
status epilepticus, **467–468**
stay sutures, *730*
stenosis, 673
sterilisation, 244
sternal rub, 463
stethoscopes, 9–10
stoma care
  bowel care, 78, 82–85, **82–84**
  nutrition and feeding, 506
  tracheostomy care and management, 734–735, 744
stomatitis, 193
stool samples, 321, 323
Streptococcus spp., 211–212, **228**
stridor, 20
stroke volume, 129
structural disorders, 470
subcutaneous emphysema, 668
subcutaneous implanted ports, **253–254**, 268, 277–279
subcutaneous route (SC), 376–377, *377–378*, 394–395, *395*
sublingual route, 373–374, 386, *395*
substance misuse, 718
sucrose, 571–572
suction
  respiratory care, 646–649
  tracheostomy care and management, 741, *741*, 743–744
sudden unexpected deaths, 780
sunburn, 88
superior vena cava (SVC), 294–295
supervision, 723
supplementary feeding, 488, **488**
support surfaces, mattresses, and cushions, 176
suppositories
  administration of medicines, 375–376, 390–391
  bowel care, 76–77, 78–79
supraorbital pressure, 463
suprapubic catheterisation (SPC), 754, 762–766
surgery
  bowel care, 76, 85
  learning (intellectual) disability, 364
  perioperative care, 595–619
  personal hygiene, 170
  play as a therapeutic tool, 625
surgical count, 608
surgical decannulation, 749
surgical emphysema, 734
SVC *see* superior vena cava
swabs, 321, 323–327
swelling, 524
syringe pumps, 274–275
systemic anti-cancer treatment (SACT), 113–122
  administration of medicines, 400–401
  chemo, 114–115, **117–118**
  concepts and definitions, 114
  consent, 114
  legislation and recommendations, 114
  personal protective equipment, 115
  prescribing cytotoxic therapy, **117–118**
  procedure guidelines, 121
  reconstitution and preparation of chemotherapeutic agents, 114–115
  routes of administration, 116–117, **118–121**
  safe administration, 115–116
  safe handling, 114
  work practices, 115

tapeworm, **229**
TB *see* tuberculosis
temperature
  assessment, 6–7
  neonatal care, 428, **428–433**, *430–432*
  orthopaedic care, 524
  perioperative care, 603, 614
tension pneumothorax, 668
tetanus, 213, **229**
therapeutic play, 631–632
therapeutic relationship, 411
throat packs, 602
throat swabs, 326–327
thrombosis, 293
thrombotic occlusions, 280–281
tibial nerve, *525–526*
toddler diarrhoea, 74
toileting
  bowel care, 76
  personal hygiene, 159–161, 182–184
tolerance, 770
tonic–clonic seizures, 468
tonic seizures, 469
toothbrushes, 189
topping and tailing, 180
tourniquets, 607
toxic shock syndrome, **229**
toxoids, 204
toxoplasmosis, **229**
tracheal tubes, 691
TRACHE care bundle, 735–745, *736*
tracheostomy, 729–751
  care of stoma/neck site, 744
  concepts and definitions, 730
  decannulation, 749–750
  discharge planning, 749
  early postinsertion complications, 730, 733–734
  emergency algorithms, *739*, *741*
  emergency box, 745, *745*
  humidity, 744–745, *745*
  introducing feeding, **734**
  long-term ventilation, 680
  newly formed tracheostomy, 730, *730*
  oxygen therapy, 659
  placement of paediatric tracheostomy, *730*
  preparation of bed space, 731–732, *731–732*
  procedure guidelines, 731–735, *731–732*, 737–738, 742–744, 746, 749
  resuscitation, 740–744, *740–741*
  suction, 741, *741*, 743–744
  tapes, 735, 737–738, *737*
  TRACHE care bundle, 735–745, *736*
  tube changes (planned), 745–748, *746*
traction, 520, 521, 527–528, *528*, **535–536**, 536–539, *536–538*
training *see* education and training
tramadol, 544
transanal colonic irrigation, 78
transdermal route, 381–382, 402
trapezium squeeze, 462
treatment protocols, 116
tube oesophagram, 350
tuberculosis (TB), 213, **229**
tumour biopsy, 45, 353
tumour seeding, 45
turbulent flush technique, 254
two-fingers technique, 700
two-thumbs technique, 700
tympanic temperature, 7
typhoid fever, **229**
typical absence, 469

ultrasound, 9, 350, 353
umbilical cord care, 436–438
uniforms, 244–245
upper gastrointestinal series, 349

Index

urethral catheterisation, 754, 761, 763–766
urinary catheters, 753–767
   concepts and definitions, 754–755
   discharge planning, 766
   emptying a drainage bag, 762
   entry site care, 761–762
   flushing catheters, 763–764
   general care, 759
   informing CYP and family, **755**
   maintaining drainage, 763
   management of acute bladder spasm, *760*
   open drainage systems, 763
   preparation and insertion, 756–758, *758–759*
   procedure guidelines, 756–766
   removing catheters, 765–766
   sizing chart, **755**
urinary retention, 561
urinary tract infections (UTI), 754
urine output, 130, **613**
urine samples, 327–330, 345–346
urology interventions, 353
UTI *see* urinary tract infections

vaccination *see* immunisation
vagal reactions, 293
vaginal discharge, 327
variant Creutzfeldt-Jakob disease (vCJD), 62
varicella zoster virus (VZV)
   immunisation, 213
   infection prevention and control, **222, 228–229**
   investigations, 328
vascular access *see* intravenous and intra-arterial access

vaseline, 190
vCJD *see* variant Creutzfeldt-Jakob disease
venous compression, 532
venous spasm, 293
ventilation
   cardiopulmonary resuscitation, 690–692, *690–691*, 696
   long-term ventilation, 676–680
   noninvasive ventilation, 672–675
   oxygen therapy, 659, 674, 676–677
ventricular fibrillation (VF), 704, *704*, 705–706
ventricular tachycardia (VT), 704, *704*, 705–706
verbal response, 455
vesicular fluid samples, 328, 330
VF *see* ventricular fibrillation
videofluoroscopy, 349
VIP *see* visual infusion phlebitis
visible pulsations, 19
visors, 238, **238–239**
visual infusion phlebitis (VIP) score, 260–261, **260**
vital signs and baseline measurements
   assessment, 1, 6–18
   blood pressure, 8–10, *11–13*
   growth assessment, 14–18, *16*
   heart rate, 7
   oxygen saturation, 14
   perioperative care, 613
   respiratory rate, 8
   temperature, 6–7
vitamin C, 94
vitamin K deficiency bleeding (VKDB), 435, **435–436**
volumetric pumps, 275–277
VT *see* ventricular tachycardia

vulval swabs, 327
VZV *see* varicella zoster virus

wafting, 659
walking aids, 532, **532–533**
ward-based investigations, 331–346
   blood glucose monitoring, 331–333, **331**
   electrocardiograph monitoring, 333–338, *334–337*
   glomerular filtration rate, 338–344
   pregnancy testing, 345–346
ward decannulation, 749
washing, 158–159, *160*, 178–182
waste management and disposal
   infection prevention and control, 245, **245**
   systemic anti-cancer treatment, 115
weight
   assessment, 16–17
   mental health, 411
wheezing, 20
whole cell vaccines, 204
whooping cough *see* pertussis
WHO Surgical Safety Checklist Sign Out, 608
WHO Surgical Safety Checklist Time Out, 604
withdrawal *see* drug withdrawal
work-related back injuries, 417–418
wound care *see* dressings and wound care

X-ray
   investigations, 349, 353
   respiratory care, *664*

zero reference point, *474*
zinc, 94
Z-track technique, 397